SECOND EDITION

GENERAL PRACTICE

SECOND EDITION

GENERAL PRACTICE

John Murtagh

AM, MBBS, MD, BSc, BEd, FRACGP, DipObstRCOG
Professor of General Practice Monash University

The McGraw-Hill Companies, Inc
Sydney   New York   San Francisco   Auckland
Bangkok   Bogotá   Caracas   Hong Kong
Kuala Lumpur   Lisbon   London   Madrid
Mexico City   Milan   New Delhi   San Juan
Seoul   Singapore   Taipei   Toronto

First published 1994
Hardcover edition 1994
Reprinted 1994, 1995
Paperback edition 1996, 1997
Second edition 1998
Hardcover edition 1998
Reprinted 1999 (twice)
Paperback edition, 1999
Reprinted 2000, 2001

National Library of Australia Cataloguing-in-Publication data:

Murtagh, John, 1936–.
  General practice.

  2nd ed.
  Includes index.
  ISBN 0 07 470719 1.

  1. Family medicine. 2. Physicians (General practice). 3. Family practice. 4. Physicians, Family. I. Title.

610

Published in Australia by
McGraw-Hill Book Company Australia Pty Limited
4 Barcoo Street, Roseville NSW 2069, Australia
Typeset in Australia by Midland Typesetters, Victoria
Printed in Hong Kong by Best Tri Colour Printing Co. Ltd

Acquisitions Editor: Kristen Baragwanath
Production Editor: Geraldine Chan
Cover Designer: Steve Miller, Miller Hare
Illustrators: Chris Sorrell, John Murtagh and Trade Wind Creations

THE AUTHOR

John Murtagh

AM, MBBS, MD, BSc, BEd, FRACGP, DipObstRCOG
Professor of General Practice,
Department of Community Medicine and General Practice,
Monash University.
General Practitioner, East Bentleigh Medical Group.

John Murtagh was a science master teaching chemistry, biology and physics in Victorian secondary schools when he was admitted to the first intake of the newly established Medical School at Monash University, graduating in 1966. Following a comprehensive postgraduate training program, which included surgical registrarship, he practised in partnership with his medical wife, Dr Jill Rosenblatt, for ten years in the rural community of Neerim South, Victoria.

He was appointed Senior Lecturer (part-time) in the Department of Community Medicine at Monash University and eventually returned to Melbourne as a full-time Senior Lecturer. He was appointed to a professorial chair in Community Medicine at Box Hill Hospital in 1988 and subsequently as chairman of the extended department and Professor of General Practice in 1993. He combines this position with part-time general practice, including a special interest in musculoskeletal medicine.

He was appointed Associate Medical Editor of *Australian Family Physician* in 1980 and Medical Editor in 1986, a position held until 1995. He achieved the Doctor of Medicine degree in 1988 for his thesis 'The management of back pain in general practice'. In 1995 he was awarded the Member of the Order of Australia for services to medicine, particularly in the areas of medical education, research and publishing.

*To my wife, Jill, and our children, Paul, Julie,
Caroline, Luke and Clare, for their understanding,
patience and support
and
To all my medical colleagues, past and present,
who have provided the vast reservoir of
knowledge from which the content of this book
was made possible*

Foreword

In 1960 a young schoolmaster, then teaching biology and chemistry in a secondary school in rural Victoria, decided to become a country doctor. He was admitted to the first intake of students into the Medical School of the newly established Monash University and at the end of the six-year undergraduate medical course and subsequent intern and resident appointments his resolve to practise community medicine remained firm.

During his years of undergraduate and early postgraduate study Dr Murtagh continued to gather and record data relating to the diagnostic and therapeutic procedures and clinical skills he would require in solo country practice. These records, subsequently greatly expanded, were to provide at least the foundation of this book. Happily, after graduation, he married Dr Jill Rosenblatt, a young graduate from Melbourne University, who shared his vocational interests. Subsequently they also shared the fulfilment of family life and the intellectual and emotional satisfaction of serving as doctors in a rural setting.

In the meantime the Royal Australian College of General Practitioners had established postgraduate training programs that had a significant influence on standards of professional practice. At the same time Monash University established a Department of Community Medicine at one of its suburban teaching hospitals, under the Chairmanship of Professor Neil Carson and staffed by practitioners in the local community.

While in practice Dr Murtagh gained a Fellowship of the College through examination. The College recognised his unique clinical, educational and communication skills and immediately commissioned him to prepare educational programs, especially the CHECK programs. His outstanding expertise as a primary care physician led to his appointment as a senior lecturer in the University Department of Community Medicine.

The success of the initial academic development in Community Medicine at Monash University, and its influence on the clinical skills of its graduates as they relate to primary care, led to a University decision to establish a further Department of Community Medicine at another suburban teaching hospital in Melbourne. It was considered by the University to be entirely appropriate that Dr Murtagh be invited to accept appointment as Professor and Head of that Department. Four years later Professor Murtagh was appointed Head of the extended Department and the first Professor of General Practice at Monash University.

John Murtagh has now become a national and international authority on the content and teaching of primary care medicine. As Medical Editor of *Australian Family Physician* from 1986 to 1995 he took that journal to the stage where it was the most widely read medical journal in Australia.

This textbook provides a distillate of the vast experience gained by a once-upon-a-time rural doctor whose career has embraced teaching from first to last, whose interest is ensuring that disease, whether minor or life-threatening, is recognised quickly, and whose concern is that strategies to match each contingency are well understood.

General Practice is the outcome of the vision of a young schoolteacher of great talent who made a firm decision to become a country doctor; through this book his dream has become a reality for all who are privileged to practise medicine in a community setting.

The first edition of this book, published in 1994, has achieved remarkable success on both the national and international scene. This second edition has been updated and expanded, and has retained the successful format of the first edition.

John Murtagh's works have already been translated into Italian by McGraw-Hill Libri Italia s.r.l., Portuguese by McGraw-Hill Nova Iorque and Spanish by McGraw-Hill Interamericana Mexico. In the second edition of this work, translations are under way in Italian by McGraw-Hill Libri Italia s.r.l., and Russian and Bulgarian, and the People's Medical Publishing House in Beijing, China, is planning to translate the work into Mandarin.

G.C. SCHOFIELD
OBE, MD, ChB(NZ), DPhil(Oxon), FRACP, FRACMA, FAMA
Professor of Anatomy, Monash
University 1961–77
Dean of Medicine, Monash University 1977–88

Contents

———

Foreword vii
Preface xiii
Acknowledgments xv
Laboratory reference values xvii
Abbreviations used in this text xix

Part 1   The basis of general practice

1. The nature and content of
   general practice 3
2. The family 9
3. Consulting skills 17
4. Communication skills 25
5. Counselling skills 34
6. Difficult, demanding and angry
   patients 43
7. Palliative care 47
8. The elderly patient 55
9. Prevention in general
   practice 65
10. Health promotion and patient
    education 76
11. Whole person approach to
    management 85
12. Travel and tropical
    medicine 91
13. Research in general
    practice 110

Part 2   Diagnostic perspective in general practice

14. Inspection as a clinical
    skill 121
15. A safe diagnostic strategy 125

Masquerades in general practice

16. Depression 130
17. Diabetes mellitus 137

18. Drug problems 147
19. Anaemia 156
20. Thyroid and other endocrine
    disorders 163
21. Spinal dysfunction 172
22. Urinary tract infection 174
23. Malignant disease 181
24. Human immunodeficiency
    virus infection—could it be
    HIV? 187
25. Baffling viral and protozoal
    infections 198
26. Baffling bacterial infections   206
27. Chronic renal failure 218
28. Connective tissue disorders
    and the vasculitides 223
29. Neurological dilemmas 231

Part 3   Problem solving in general practice

30. Abdominal pain 247
31. Arthritis 267
32. Anorectal disorders 287
33. Low back pain 294
34. Thoracic back pain 318
35. Bruising and bleeding 331
36. Chest pain 337
37. Constipation 360
38. Cough 371
39. Deafness and hearing loss ... 385
40. Diarrhoea 393
41. The disturbed patient 409
42. Dizziness 426
43. Dyspepsia (indigestion) 435
44. Dysphagia 445
45. Dyspnoea 448
46. The painful ear 463
47. The red and tender eye 475
48. Pain in the face 487

49. Fever and chills 496
50. Faints, fits and funny turns .. 505
51. Haematemesis and
    melaena 512
52. Headache 515
53. Jaundice 532
54. Nausea and vomiting 547
55. Neck lumps 551
56. Neck pain 555
57. Shoulder pain 568
58. Pain in the arm and hand ... 580
59. Hip and buttock pain 596
60. Pain in the leg 608
61. The painful knee 626
62. Pain in the foot and ankle .. 644
63. Walking difficulty 659
64. Palpitations 666
65. Sore throat 679
66. Tiredness 687
67. The unconscious patient 696
68. Urinary disorders 703
69. Visual failure 712
70. Weight gain 724
71. Weight loss 732

86. The menopause and
    osteoporosis 857
87. Vaginal discharge 866
88. Domestic violence and
    sexual assault 874
89. Basic antenatal care 878
90. High-risk pregnancy 886
91. Postnatal care 891

Part 6 Men's health

92. Scrotal pain 899
93. Inguinoscrotal lumps 903
94. Disorders of the penis 912
95. Disorders of the prostate 917

Part 7 Sexually related problems

96. The infertile couple 925
97. Sexual dysfunction 932
98. Sexually transmitted
    diseases 942

Part 4 Child and adolescent health

72. An approach to the child ... 741
73. Specific problems of
    children 747
74. Common childhood infectious
    diseases (including skin
    eruptions) 758
75. Behaviour disorders in
    children 769
76. Child abuse 776
77. Emergencies in children 782
78. Adolescent health 795

Part 8 Problems of the skin

 99. A diagnostic and
     management approach to
     skin problems 955
100. Pruritus 965
101. Common skin problems 972
102. Acute skin eruptions 989
103. Skin ulcers 999
104. Common lumps and
     bumps 1006
105. Pigmented skin lesions 1019

Part 5 Women's health

79. Cervical cancer and Pap
    smears 803
80. Family planning 810
81. Breast pain (mastalgia) 818
82. Lumps in the breast 824
83. Abnormal uterine bleeding ... 834
84. Lower abdominal and pelvic
    pain in women 840
85. Premenstrual syndrome 853

Part 9 Common continuing management problems

106. Alcohol problems 1029
107. Allergic disorders including
     hay fever 1036
108. Anxiety 1043
109. Asthma 1051
110. Epilepsy 1063
111. Hypertension 1071
112. Dyslipidaemia 1090
113. Rational prescribing 1094

Part 10 Accident and emergency medicine

114. Emergency care 1111
115. Stroke and transient ischaemic attacks 1127
116. Common skin wounds and foreign bodies 1132
117. Common fractures and dislocations 1145
118. Major trauma 1166
119. The doctor's bag and other emergency equipment 1174
120. The treatment room and equipment 1179
121. Common sporting injuries 1183

Part 11 Aboriginal health

122. The health of Aboriginal and Torres Strait Islander peoples 1199

Part 12 Everyday practice tips

123. Nitty-gritty problems A–Z (a summary) 1209

Appendices

I   Percentile charts: infant girls 1240
II Percentile charts: infant boys 1241
III Percentile charts: girls 1242
IV Percentile charts: boys 1243
V Predicted values for peak expiratory flow rate 1244
VI The Australian Nutrition Foundation: weight for height chart 1245

Index 1247

CHAPTER 12

Preface

The discipline of general practice has become complex, diffuse and challenging. With the ever-burgeoning phenomenon of specialisation in medicine, with its associated complex technology and hospital basis, the need for competent, caring generalists is more important than ever before.

This textbook attempts to address the issue of the broad knowledge and skills required in modern general practice. Some of the basics of primary health care remain the same. In fact, there is an everlasting quality about many of the medical problems that affect the human being, be it a splinter under a nail, a stye of the eyelid, a terminal illness or simply stress-related anxiety. Many of the treatments and approaches to caring management are universal and timeless. Unfortunately, the modern general practitioner has lost a considerable amount of counselling and therapeutic skills compared with his or her counterpart of 50 years ago and this book encourages GPs to develop these basic skills.

General practice remains the most cost-effective health service and there is evidence that the consumer and government agencies are focusing more on general practitioners as a solution to the high-cost, high-technology, depersonalised services in the health care system. They are searching for value, satisfaction, early diagnosis and holistic management without inappropriate invasive investigations and potent medication.

This textbook of general practice attempts to take these issues into account and adopts an approach typical of Western medicine: strategies for solving common problems, continuing care, basic medical skills and 'tricks of the trade'.

The discipline of general practice can at times be overwhelming in its breadth and depth, especially with patients presenting with undifferentiated problems with an overlap of organic and psychosocial aspects. There is the constant challenge to make an appropriate early diagnosis and detect the ever-lurking life-threatening illness. The approach in this book is to promote relatively fail-safe strategies to reduce the margin of error. This diagnostic model, which pervades all the chapters on problem solving, is based on my own experience, but readers can draw on their own experience to make the model work effectively for themselves.

Guidelines for early referral are included.

Another feature is the prominence given to 'masquerades' in general practice so that an increased awareness of these baffling problems will lead to improved diagnostic skills and more interesting practice.

A particular challenge in the preparation of this book was to identify as much evidence-based material as possible. At present there is a limited amount of accessible information. Consequently, I have relied on considerable collective wisdom from experts, especially from the Therapeutic Guidelines series. For the everyday nitty-gritty problems of general practice, recommended treatments include those that have worked effectively for myself and my colleagues.

Such a book cannot possibly present all the medical problems likely to be encountered, but an attempt has been made to select those problems that are common, significant, preventable and treatable. I am confident that my general practice colleagues will identify with the book's content and methodology.

General Practice is written with the recent graduate and the medical student in mind. It is a comprehensive textbook that focuses on the very basics of medical principles and management. However, it is hoped that all practitioners will gain useful information from the book's content.

Acknowledgments

—

The author would like to thank the Publication Division of the Royal Australian College of General Practitioners for supporting my role as Medical Editor of *Australian Family Physician*, which has provided an excellent opportunity to gather material for this book. Acknowledgment is also due to those medical organisations that have given permission to use selected information from their publications. They include the Preventive and Community Medicine committee of the RACGP (Guidelines for Preventive Activities in General Practice), the Victorian Medical Postgraduate Foundation (Therapeutic Guidelines series), the Hypertension Guideline Committee: Research Unit RACGP (South Australian Faculty), and the *Medical Observer*, publishers of *A Manual for Primary Health Care*, for permitting reproduction of Appendices I–IV.

I am indebted to the many consultants for their help and advice after reviewing various parts of the manuscript that covered material in their particular area of expertise. They are:

Dr Roy Beran	epilepsy; fits and funny turns; neurological dilemmas
Dr Peter Berger	a diagnostic and management approach to skin problems
Professor Geoff Bishop	basic antenatal care
Dr John Boxall	palpitations
Professor Bob Burrows	high-risk pregnancy
Dr Paul Coughlin and Professor Hatem Salem	bruising and bleeding
Mr Rod Dalziel	shoulder pain
Dr David Dunn	the health of Aboriginal and Torres Strait Islander peoples
Dr Robert Dunne	common skin wounds and foreign bodies
Dr Lindsay Grayson	medical advice for travellers
Dr Michael Gribble	anaemia
Mr John Griffiths	pain in the hip and buttock
Professor Michael Grigg	pain in the leg
Dr Gary Grossbard	the painful knee
Dr Peter Hardy-Smith	the red and tender eye; visual failure
Dr David Healy	abnormal uterine bleeding
Dr Peter Holmes	cough; dyspnoea; asthma
Professor Gab Kovacs	abnormal uterine bleeding; the infertile couple
Professor Even Laerum	research in general practice
Dr Barry Lauritz	common skin problems; pigmented skin lesions
Mr Peter Lawson	disorders of the penis; prostatic disorders
Dr Peter Lowthian	arthritis
Mr Frank Lyons	common fractures and dislocations
Dr Ron McCoy and Dr Alex Welborn	human immunodeficiency virus infection
Professor Barry McGrath	hypertension
Dr Joe McKendrick	malignant disease
Professor Robyn O'Hehir	allergic disorders including hay fever
Dr Michael Oldmeadow	tiredness
Dr Frank Panetta	chest pain
Dr Geoff Quail	pain in the face
Mr Ronald Quirk	pain in the foot and ankle

Dr Ian Rogers	emergency care; major trauma
Dr Jill Rosenblatt	the menopause
Professor Avni Sali	abdominal pain; lumps in the breast; jaundice; constipation; dyspepsia; prevention in general practice
Dr Hugo Standish	urinary tract infection; chronic renal failure; urinary disorders
Dr Paul Tallman	stroke and transient ischaemic attacks
Dr Alan Yung	fever and chills; sore throat
Dr Ronnie Yuen	diabetes mellitus; thyroid and other endocrine disorders
Dr Arthur Zulman	'nitty-gritty problems'

Special thanks to Chris Sorrell, graphic designer, for his art illustration, and to Nicki Cooper, Jenny Green and Caroline Menara for their skill and patience in typing the manuscript.

Figures 60.6, 104.7c, 104.7d were provided by Dr Levent Efe.

Many of the quotations at the beginning of chapters appear in either Robert Wilkins (ed), *The Doctor's Quotation Book*, Robert Hale Ltd, London, 1991 or Maurice B. Strauss (ed), *Familiar Medical Quotations*, Little, Brown & Co., New York, 1958.

Thanks are also due to Lesley Rowe, Deputy Director of Pharmacy, Nepean Hospital, Penrith, NSW, for reviewing the manuscript, and to John Rowe and his team for their patience and assistance in so many ways.

Laboratory reference values

The reference values and ranges for these blood tests are given in the system of international units (SI) and may vary from laboratory to laboratory. An asterisk (*) indicates that paediatric reference ranges differ from the adult range given.

Electrolytes/renal
Sodium	(135–145 mmol/L)
*Potassium	(3.5–5.0 mmol/L)
Chloride	(95–107 mmol/L)
Bicarbonate	(23–32 mmol/L)
Urea	(2.5–8.0 mmol/L)
Creatinine	(M 0.04–0.13, F 0.04–0.1 mmol/L)
*Calcium	(2.10–2.60 mmol/L)
Phosphate	(0.90–1.35 mmol/L)
*Magnesium	(0.65–1.30 mmol/L)
*Uric acid	(M 0.17–0.45, F 0.12–0.40 mmol/L)

Liver function/pancreas
*Bilirubin (total)	($<$ 19 µmol/L)
(direct)	($<$ 3 µmol/L)
*AST	($<$ 40 U/L)
*GGT	(F $<$ 45; M $<$ 65 U/L)
*Alkaline phos	($<$ 120 U/L)
Total protein	(60–80 g/L)
Albumin	(38–50 g/L)
Amylase	(30–110 U/L)

Therapeutic drugs
*Digoxin	(Ther. 1.3–2.6 nmol/L)
*Phenytoin	(Ther. 40–80 µmol/L)
*Valproate	(Ther. 300–700 µmol/L)
*Carbamazepine	(Ther. 10–50 µmol/L)
Gentamicin (pre)	($<$ 2.0 µg/mL)
(post)	($<$ 12.0 µg/mL)
Lithium	(Ther. 0.5–1.0 mmol/L)

Cardiac/lipids
*AST	($<$ 40 U/L)
CK (total)	(F $<$ 200; M $<$ 300 U/L)
CK-MB	($<$ 25 U/L)
*Cholesterol	($<$ 5.5 mmol/L)
*Triglycerides	($<$ 2.0 mmol/L)
HDL cholesterol	($>$ 1.00 mmol/L)
LDL cholesterol	($<$ 3.5 mmol/L)

Thyroid tests
Free T-4	(10.0–20.0 pmol/L)
*Ultra sens TSH	(0.3–5.0 mU/L)
Free T-3	(3.3–8.2 pmol/L)

Other endocrine tests
s Cortisol 8 am	(130–700 nmol/L)
4 pm	(80–350 nmol/L)

FSH adult	(1.9 IU/L)
ovulation	(10–30 IU/L)
post menopausal	(4–200 IU/L)
Oestradiol menopausal	($<$ 200 pmol/L)
Testosterone	(M 10–35 F $<$ 3.5 nmol/L)

Tumour markers
PSA	(0–4.0 µg/L)
CEA	($<$ 7.5 µg/L)
AFP	($<$ 10 µg/mL)
CA 125	($<$ 35 U/mL)

Iron studies
Ferritin	(20–200 µg/L)
Iron	(14–30 µmol/L)
Iron binding capacity	(45–80 µmol/L)

Blood gases/arterial
*pH	(7.38–7.43)
*pO$_2$	(85–105 mmHg)
*pCO$_2$	(36–44 mmHg)
*Bicarbonate	(20–28 mmol/L)
*Base excess	(-3 to $+3$ mmol/L)

Glucose
Glucose (fasting)	(3.5–5.9 mmol/L)
Glucose (random)	(3.5–7.9 mmol/L)
Hb A1c	(4.7–6.1%)

Haematology
*Hb	(F 115–165 M 130–180 g/L)
*PCV	(F 37–47 M 40–54%)
*MCV	(81–98 fl)
Reticulocytes	(0.5–2.0%)
*Leucocytes	(4.0–11.0 $\times$ 10^9/L)
Platelets	(150–400 $\times$ 10^9/L)
ESR	($<$ 20 mm)

Paul Bunnell (IM test)	%	Abs. values	Ranges
*Brand neutro			0.0–5 $\times$ 10^9/L
*Mature neutro			2.0–7.5 $\times$ 10^9/L
*Lymphocytes			1.0–4.0 $\times$ 10^9/L
*Monocytes			0.2–0.8 $\times$ 10^9/L
*Eosinophils			0.0–0.4 $\times$ 10^9/L

Coagulation
Bleeding time	(2.0–8.5 min.)
Fibrinogen	(2.0–4.0 g/L)
Prothrombin time	sec.
Prothrombin ratio (INR)	
APTT	sec.

Others
s Creatine (phospho) kinase	($<$ 90 U/L)
s Lead	(2 µmol/L)
s C-reactive protein	($<$ 10 mg/L)

Abbreviations used in this text

AAA   aortic abdominal aneurysm
AAFP   American Academy of Family Physicians
ABC   airway, breathing, circulation
ABCD   airway, breathing, circulation, dextrose
ABFP   American Board of Family Practice
AC   air conduction
ACE   angiotensin-converting enzyme
ACL   anterior cruciate ligament
ACTH   adrenocorticotrophic hormone
ADHD   attention deficit hyperactivity disorder
ADT   adult diphtheria vaccine
AFP   alpha fetoprotein
AI   aortic incompetence
AICD   automatic implantable cardiac defibrillator
AIDS   acquired immunodeficiency syndrome
ALL   acute lymphocytic leukaemia
ALTE   apparent life-threatening episode
AMI   acute myocardial infarction
AML   acute myeloid leukaemia
AP   anterior–posterior
APF   Australian pharmaceutical formulary
APTT   activated partial thromboplastin time
ARC   AIDS-related complex
ASD   atrial septal defect
ASIS   anterior superior iliac spine
ASOT   antistreptolysin 0 titre
AST   aspartate aminotransferase
AV   atrioventricular
AZT   azidothymidine

BC   bone conduction
BCC   basal cell carcinoma
BCG   bacille Calmette-Guérin
BMI   body mass index
BP   blood pressure
BPH   benign prostatic hyperplasia
BPPV   benign paroxysmal positional vertigo
BSE   breast self-examination

Ca   carcinoma
CABG   coronary artery bypass grafting
CAD   coronary artery disease
CBE   clinical breast examination
CCF   congestive cardiac failure
CCU   coronary care unit
CD_4 T helper cell
CD_8 T suppressor cell
CDT   combined diphtheria/tetanus vaccine
CEA   carcinoembryonic antigen
CFS   chronic fatigue syndrome
CHD   coronary heart disease
CIN   cervical intraepithelial neoplasia
CK   creatinine kinase
CK–MB   creatinine kinase–myocardial bound fraction
CMC   carpometacarpal
CMV   cytomegalovirus
CNS   central nervous system
co   compound
COAD   chronic obstructive airways disease
COC   combined oral contraceptive
COPD   chronic obstructive pulmonary disease
CPA   cardiopulmonary arrest
CPPD   calcium pyrophosphate dihydrate
CPR   cardiopulmonary resuscitation
CPS   complex partial seizures
CRD   computerised reference database system

CREST	calcinosis cutis; Raynaud's phenomenon; oesophageal involvement; sclerodactyly; telangiectasia	ERCP	endoscopic retrograde cholangiopancreatography
CRF	chronic renal failure	ESR	erythrocyte sedimentation rate
CRFM	chloroquine-resistant falciparum malaria	ET	embryo transfer
CRP	C-reactive protein	FBE	full blood count
CSF	cerebrospinal fluid	FDL	flexor digitorum longus
CSFM	chloroquine-sensitive falciparum malaria	FEV_1	forced expiratory volume in 1 second
CT	computerised tomography	fL	femto-litre (10^{-15})
CTS	carpal tunnel syndrome	FSH	follicle stimulating hormone
CVA	cerebrovascular accident	FTA–ABS	fluorescent treponemal antibody absorption test
CVS	cardiovascular system	FTT	failure to thrive
CXR	chest X-ray	FUO	fever of undetermined origin
		FXS	fragile X syndrome
DA	dissecting aneurysm	g	gram
DBP	diastolic blood pressure	GA	general anaesthetic
DC	direct current	GABHS	group A beta-haemolytic streptococcus
DDH	developmental dysplasia of the hip	GBS	Guillain-Barré syndrome
DIC	disseminated intravascular coagulation	GGT	gamma glutamyl transferase
		GI	gastrointestinal
DIP	distal interphalangeal	GIFT	gamete intrafallopian transfer
dL	decilitre	GIT	gastrointestinal tract
DNA	deoxyribose-nucleic acid	GnRH	gonadotrophin-releasing hormone
DOM	direction of movement	GO	gastro-oesophageal
drug dosage bd	—twice daily	GP	general practitioner
tid, tds	—three times daily	G_6PD	glucose-6-phosphate dehydrogenase
qid, qds	—four times daily	GSI	genuine stress incontinence
ds	double strand	GU	gastric ulcer
DS	double strength	HAV	hepatitis A virus
DSM	diagnostic and statistical manual (of mental disorders)	anti-HAV	hepatitis A antibody
		Hb	haemoglobin
DU	duodenal ulcer	anti-HBc	hepatitis B core antibody
DUB	dysfunctional uterine bleeding	HBeAg	hepatitis Be antigen
DVT	deep venous thrombosis	anti-HBs	hepatitis B surface antibody
		HBsAg	hepatitis B surface antigen
EAR	expired air resuscitation	HBV	hepatitis B virus
EBM	Epstein-Barr mononucleosis (glandular fever)	HCG	human chorionic gonadotrophin
		HCV	hepatitis C virus
EBV	Epstein-Barr virus	anti-HCV	hepatitis C virus antibody
ECG	electrocardiogram	HDL	high-density lipoprotein
ECT	electroconvulsive therapy	HDV	hepatitis D (Delta) virus
EDD	expected due date	HEV	hepatitis E virus
EEG	electroencephalogram	HFV	hepatitis F virus
ELISA	enzyme linked immunosorbent assay	HGV	hepatitis G virus
		HIDA	hepatobiliary iminodiacetic acid
EMG	electromyogram	HIV	human immunodeficiency virus
EPL	extensor pollicis longus	$HLA(B_{27})$	human leucocyte antigen
EPS	expressed prostatic secretions	HMGCoA	hydroxymethylglutaryl CoA
ER	external rotation	HPV	human papilloma virus

HRT	hormone replacement therapy	MAIS	*Mycobacterium avium intracellulare* or *M. sacrofulaceum*
HSV	herpes simplex viral infection		
HT	hypertension	mane	in morning
		MAOI	monoamine oxidase inhibitor
IBS	irritable bowel syndrome	MAST	medical anti-shock trousers
ICE	ice, compression, elevation	MB	myocardial base
ICS	intercondyler separation	MCL	medial collateral ligament
IDDM	insulin dependent diabetes mellitus	MCP	metacarpal phalangeal
		MCU	microscopy and culture of urine
IDU	injecting drug user	MCV	mean corpuscular volume
IgE	immunoglobulin E	MDI	metered dose inhaler
IgG	immunoglobulin G	MG	myaesthenia gravis
IgM	immunoglobulin M	MI	mitral incompetence
IM / IMI	intramuscular injection	MID	minor intervertebral derangement
		MRI	magnetic resonance imaging
IMS	intermalleolar separation	MS	multiple sclerosis
INR	international normalised ratio	MSU	midstream urine
IOFB	intraocular foreign body	MTP	metatarsophalangeal
IP	interphalangeal	MVA	motor vehicle accident
IR	internal rotation		
ITP	idiopathic (or immune) thrombocytopenia purpura	N saline	normal saline
		NAD	no abnormality detected
IUCD	intrauterine contraceptive device	NGU	non-gonococcal urethritis
IV	intravenous	NHL	non-Hodgkin's lymphoma
IVF	in vitro fertilisation	NH&MRC	National Health and Medical Research Council
IVI	intravenous injection		
IVP	intravenous pyelogram	NIDDM	non-insulin dependent diabetes mellitus
IVU	intravenous urogram		
		nocte	at night
JCA	juvenile chronic arthritis	NR	normal range
JVP	jugular venous pulse	NSAIDs	non-steroidal anti-inflammatory drugs
		NSU	non-specific urethritis
KA	keratoacanthoma		
kg	kilogram	(o)	taken orally
KOH	potassium hydroxide	OA	oestoarthritis
		OCP	oral contraceptive pill
LA	local anaesthetic	OSA	obstructive sleep apnoea
LBBB	left branch bundle block	OSD	Osgood-Schlatter disorder
LBP	low back pain	OTC	over the counter
LDH/LH	lactic dehydrogenase		
LDL	low-density lipoprotein	PA	posterior–anterior
LFTs	liver function tests	Pap	Papanicolaou
LH	luteinising hormone	PCL	posterior cruciate ligament
LHRH	luteinising hormone releasing hormone	PCP	pneumocystitis pneumonia
		PCR	polymerase chain reaction
LIF	left iliac fossa	PCV	packed cell volume
LMN	lower motor neurone	PD	Parkinson's disease
LRTI	lower respiratory tract infection	PDA	patent ductus arteriosus
LSD	lysergic acid	PEF	peak expiratory flow
LUQ	left upper quadrant	PEFR	peak expiratory flow rate
LUTS	lower urinary tract symptoms	PET	pre-eclamptic toxaemia
LVH	left ventricular hypertrophy	PET	positron emission tomography

PGL	persistent generalised lymphadenopathy		SL	sublingual
PH	past history		SLD	specific learning disability
PHR	personal health record		SLE	systemic lupus erythematosus
PID	pelvic inflammatory disease		SLR	straight leg raising
PIP	proximal interphalangeal		SND	sensorineural deafness
PKU	phenylketonuria		SNHL	sensorineural hearing loss
PLISSIT	permission: limited information: specific suggestion: intensive therapy		SNRI	serotonin noradrenaline reuptake inhibitor
PMS	premenstrual syndrome		SOB	shortness of breath
PR	per rectum		sp	species
prn	as and when needed		SPECT	single photon emission computerised tomography
PSA	prostate specific antigen		SPF	sun penetration factor
PSIS	posterior superior iliac spine		SR	sustained release
PSVT	paroxysmal supraventricular tachycardia		SSRI	selective serotonin reuptake inhibitor
PT	prothrombin time		SSS	sick sinus syndrome
PU	peptic ulcer		statim	at once
PUO	pyrexia of undetermined origin		STD	sexually transmitted disease
PUVA	psoralen + UVA		STD	sodium tetradecyl sulfate
PVC	polyvinyl chloride		SVC	superior vena cava
PVD	peripheral vascular disease		SVT	supraventricular tachycardia
qds, qid	four times daily		T_3	tri-iodothyronine
			T_4	thyroxine
			TA	temporal arteritis
RA	rheumatoid arthritis		TB	tuberculosis
RACGP	Royal Australian College of General Practitioners		tds, tid	three times daily
			TENS	transcutaneous electrical nerve stimulation
RAP	recurrent abdominal pain			
RF	rheumatic fever		TFTs	thyroid function tests
RFT	respiratory function test		TIA	transient ischaemic attack
Rh	rhesus		TM	tympanic membrane
RIB	rest in bed		TMJ	temporomandibular joint
RICE	rest, ice, compression, elevation		TOF	tracheo-oesophageal fistula
RIF	right iliac fossa		TORCH	toxoplasmosis, rubella, cytomegalovirus, herpes virus
RPR	rapid plasma reagin			
RSD	reflex sympathetic dystrophy		TPHA	Treponema pallidum haemoglutination test
RSI	repetition strain injury			
RT	reverse transcriptase		TSE	testicular self-examination
rt-PA	recombinant tissue plasminogen activator		TSH	thyroid-stimulating hormone
			TUIP	transurethral incision of prostate
RUQ	right upper quadrant		TURP	transurethral resection of prostate
SAH	subarachnoid haemorrhage		U	units
SBE	subacute bacterial endocarditis		UC	ulcerative colitis
SBO	small bowel obstruction		U&E	urea and electrolytes
SBP	systolic blood pressure		μg	microgram
SC/SCI	subcutaneous/subcutaneous injection		UMN	upper motor neurone
			URTI	upper respiratory tract infection
SCC	squamous cell carcinoma		US	ultrasound
SCFE	slipped capital femoral epiphysis		UTI	urinary tract infection
SIDS	sudden infant death syndrome		UV	ultraviolet
SIJ	sacroiliac joint			

VBI	vertebrobasilar insufficiency		VT	ventricular tachycardia
VC	vital capacity			
VDRL	Venereal Disease Reference		WBC	white blood cells
	Laboratory		WBR	white→blue→red
VF	ventricular fibrillation		WCC	white cell count
VMA	vanillylmandelic acid		WHO	World Health Organisation
VSD	ventricular septal defect		WPW	Wolff-Parkinson-White

PART 1

THE BASIS OF
GENERAL PRACTICE

—

1
The nature and content of general practice

—

Medical practice is not knitting and weaving and the labour of the hands, but it must be inspired with soul and be filled with understanding and equipped with the gift of keen observation; these together with accurate scientific knowledge are the indispensable requisites for proficient medical practice.

Moses ben Maimon (1135–1204)

General practice is a traditional method of bringing primary health care to the community. It is a medical discipline in its own right, linking the vast amount of accumulated medical knowledge with the art of communication.

Definitions

General practice can be defined as that medical discipline which provides 'community-based, continuing, comprehensive, preventive primary care', sometimes referred to as the CCCP model.

The Royal Australian College of General Practitioners (RACGP) uses the following definitions of general practice and primary care:

General practice is that component of the health care system which provides initial, continuing, comprehensive and co-ordinated medical care for all individuals, families and communities and which integrates current biomedical, psychological and social understandings of health.

General practitioner is a medical practitioner with recognised generalist training, experience and skills, who provides and co-ordinates comprehensive medical care for individuals, families and communities.

Primary care involves the ability to take responsible action on any problem the patient presents, whether or not it forms part of an ongoing doctor–patient

relationship. In managing the patient, the general/ family practitioner may make appropriate referral to other doctors, health care professionals and community services. General/family practice is the point of first contact for the majority of people seeking health care. In the provision of primary care, much ill-defined illness is seen; the general/family practitioner often deals with problem complexes rather than with established diseases.

The practitioner must be able to make a total assessment of the person's condition without subjecting the person to unnecessary investigations, procedure and treatment.

The American Academy of Family Physicians (AAFP)[1] and the American Board of Family Practice (ABFP) have defined family practice as:

. . . the medical specialty that provides continuing and comprehensive health care for the individual and the family. It is the specialty in breadth that integrates the biological, clinical and behavioural sciences. The scope of family practice encompasses all ages, both sexes, each organ system and disease entity.

The AAFP has emphasised that the primary objective of the specialty of family practice is to deliver primary health care, described as:

. . . a form of medical care delivery that emphasises first contact care and assumes ongoing responsibility for the patient in both health maintenance and therapy of illness. It is personal care involving a unique interaction and communication between the patient and the physician. It is comprehensive in scope and includes the overall co-ordination of care of the patient's health problems, be they biological, behavioural or social. The appropriate use of consultants and community resources is an important part of effective primary care.

The AAFP has expanded on the function of delivery of primary health care.[1,2]

Primary care is a form of delivery of medical care that encompasses the following functions:

1. *It is 'first-contact' care, serving as a point-of-entry for patients into the health care system.*
2. *It includes continuity by virtue of caring for patients over a period of time, both in sickness and in health.*
3. *It is comprehensive care, drawing from all the traditional major disciplines for its functional content.*
4. *It serves a co-ordinative function for all the health care needs of the patient.*
5. *It assumes continuing responsibility for individual patient follow-up and community health problems; and*
6. *It is a highly personalised type of care.*

Pereira Gray[3] identifies six principles—primary care, family care, domiciliary care and continuing care—all designed to achieve preventive and personal care. 'We see the patient as a whole person and this involves breadth of knowledge about each person, not just depth of disease.'

General practice is not the summation of specialties practised at a superficial level and we must avoid the temptation to become 'specialoids'. In the current climate where medicine is often fragmented there is a greater than ever need for the generalist. The patient requires a trusted focal point in the often bewildering health service jungle. Who is to do this better than the caring family doctor taking full responsibility for the welfare of the patient and intervening on his or her behalf? Specialists also need highly competent generalists to whom they can entrust ongoing care.

Unique features of general practice

Anderson, Bridges-Webb and Chancellor[4] emphasise that 'the unique and important work of the general practitioner is to provide availability and continuity of care, competence in the realm of diagnosis, care of acute and chronic illness, prompt treatment of emergencies and a preventive approach to health care'.

The features that make general practice different from hospital- or specialist-based medical practices include:

- first contact
- diagnostic methodology
- early diagnosis of life-threatening and serious disease

- continuity and availability of care
- personalised care
- care of acute and chronic illness
- domiciliary care
- emergency care (prompt treatment at home or in the community)
- family care
- palliative care (at home)
- preventive care
- scope for health promotion
- holistic approach
- health care co-ordination

Apart from these processes the general practitioner has to manage very common problems including a whole variety of problems not normally taught in medical school or in postgraduate programs. Many of these problems are unusual yet common and can be regarded as the 'nitty gritty' or 'bread and butter' problems of primary health care.

Continuing care

The essence of general practice is continuity of care. The doctor–patient relationship is unique in general practice in the sense that it covers a span of time which is not restricted to a specific major illness. The continuing relationship involving many separate episodes of illness provides an opportunity for the doctor to develop considerable knowledge and understanding of the patient, the family and its stresses, and the patient's work and recreational environment.

Strategies to enhance continuing care

A philosophical commitment

Underlying appropriate patient care is the attitude of the provider. A caring, responsible practitioner who is competent, available and a trusted friend is 'like gold' to his or her patients.

Medical records

An efficient medical record system is fundamental. Ideally it should include a patient profile, a database, problem lists, special investigation lists, medication lists, adverse drug reactions and 'at risk' details.

Checklists

The use of checklists or questionnaires to assemble information on presenting problems may enhance knowledge as well as assist earlier diagnosis.

Home visits

Home visits are a goldmine of information about intrafamily dynamics. They should cement the doctor–patient relationship if used appropriately and discreetly. We are the only doctors who practise domiciliary care. We must treasure it. Sitting in the office chair practising 'conveyor belt' medicine is contrary to the ideals of general practice.

Anticipatory guidance

Unfortunately patients do not usually perceive the family doctor as a counsellor, but opportunities should be taken to offer advice about anticipated problems in situations such as pre-marital visits, antenatal care and preadolescent contact.

Patient education

Whenever possible, patients should be given insight into the nature of their illness, and reasons for the treatment and prognosis. Patient education leaflets, such as those published in journals, can be used as a starting point although there is no substitute for careful personal explanation. This should lead to better compliance and an improved relationship between doctor and patient.

Personal health records

These excellent wallets, which are handed to parents of newborn babies, have a very important place in the ongoing care of children. Their purpose is to supply an outline of preventive health care, beginning from birth. They provide an inbuilt recall list directed at a most compliant source—mothers. In fact they provide a complete record of health care throughout a person's lifetime.

Patient register

An age-and-sex register of all patients in the practice is a very useful acquisition. The main strategy is to find out who are the patients, what are their basic characteristics and who suffers from chronic diseases such as cancer, diabetes and emphysema.

Recall lists

Use of recall lists based on the patient register should significantly improve health care delivery. Dentists have been using this technique successfully for some time. In the United States of America and Canada doctors use recall lists regularly to remind patients that preventive items such as immunisation schedules and cancer smear tests are due.

Computers

Computers have simplified and streamlined the design and use of practice registers and patient-recall systems in addition to their use for accounting purposes. Their potential for patient education and doctor education is considerable.

Common presenting symptoms

Common presenting symptoms in Australian practices are presented in Table 1.1,[5] where they are compared with the United States of America.[6] The similarity is noticed but the different classification system does not permit an accurate comparison. In the third national survey of morbidity in general practice in Australia[5] the most common symptoms described by patients were cough (7.5 per 100 encounters), throat complaints (4.7 per 100), back complaints (3.8 per 100) and skin symptoms (3.6 per 100). In addition very common presentations included a check-up (13.6 per 100) and a request for prescription (8.8 per 100). McWhinney lists the ten most common presenting symptoms from representative Canadian and British practices but they are divided between males and females.[7]

For males in the Canadian study these symptoms are (in order, starting from the most common) cough, sore throat, colds, abdominal/pelvic pain, rash, fever/chills, earache, back problems, skin inflammation and chest pain.

For females the five other symptoms that are included are menstrual disorders, depression, vaginal discharge, anxiety and headache.

In the British study the most common symptoms are virtually identical between males and females and include cough, rash, sore throat, abdominal pain, bowel symptoms, chest pain, back pain, spots, sores and ulcers, and headache.

Most frequent presenting symptoms in the author's practice

The most common presenting symptoms in the author's practice[8] were identified, with the emphasis being on pain syndromes:

- cough
- disturbance of bowel function

Table 1.1 *Most frequent presenting problems/symptoms (excluding pregnancy, hypertension, immunisation and routine check-up)*

	Australia	United States
Cough	1	1
Throat complaints	2	2
Back pain	3	4
Rash	4	5
Abdominal pain	5	6
Headache	6	10
Weakness/tiredness	7	
Swelling	8	
Ear pain	9	3
Fever	10	7
URTI	11	
Nasal congestion/sneeze	12	12
Diarrhoea	13	
Chest pain	14	13
Foot, toe complaints	15	
Vertigo/dizziness	16	
Visual dysfunction		8
Knee symptoms		9
Head cold		11

Source: Australian figures: Bridges-Webb et al.[5];
United States figures (all specialties): De Lozier & Gagnon[6]

- pain in abdomen
- pain in back
- pain in chest
- pain in head
- pain in neck
- pain in ear
- pain in throat
- pain in joints/limbs
- rashes
- sleep problems
- tiredness/fatigue
- vaginal discomfort

These symptoms should accurately reflect Australian general practice since the rural practice would represent an appropriate cross-section of the community's morbidity, and the recording and classification of data from the one practitioner would be consistent.

Common managed disorders

Excluding a general medical examination, hypertension and upper respiratory tract infection (URTI) were the two most common problems encountered in both the Australian and USA[9] studies. The 23 most frequent individual disorders are listed in Table 1.2 and accounted for over 40% of all problems managed.[10]

Most commonly diagnosed disease classes

Although there is a similar general trend in the distribution of problems managed across body systems in these two Australian studies, a notable difference occurs in the diagnosis of psychological problems (Table 1.3).

The content of this textbook reflects what is fundamental to the nature and content of general practice—that which is common but is significant, relevant, preventable and treatable.

Table 1.2 *Most frequently managed disorders/diagnoses (rank order)*

	Australia	United States
General medical examination	1	1
Hypertension	2	3
URTI	3	2
Asthma	4	29
Osteoarthritis	5	10
Acute bronchitis	6	13
Immunisation	7	*
Anxiety	8	6†
Sprain/strain	9	5
Arthritis (excluding osteoarthritis)	10	27
Depression	11	6†
Contact dermatitis	12	9
Acute otitis media	13	18
Diabetes mellitus	14	8
Lipid metabolism disorder	15	*
Tonsillitis	16	—
Sinusitis	17	25
Urinary tract infection	18	11
Heart failure	19	—
Sleep disorders/insomnia	20	—
Female genital check-up, Pap smear	21	(under 1)
Viral diseases (other)	22	—
Solar/hyper keratosis	23	—
Soft tissue injuries		4
Ischaemic heart disease		7

* not listed   † combined
Source: Australian figures: reference 5;
United States figures: reference 9

Table 1.3 *Most frequently diagnosed disease classes*

	Author's country practice (1974–78)[8]	Australian morbidity study (1990–91)[5]
	%	%
Respiratory	24.3	16.7
Psychological	12.8	6.6
Musculoskeletal	12.2	12.0
Cardiovascular	7.5	12.5
Skin	7.0	12.4
Preventive medicine	5.4	5.6
Digestive	4.4	7.1
Genitourinary	4.4	6.7
Reproductive	3.8	3.4

References

1. American Academy of Family Physicians. Official definition of Family Practice and Family Physician (AAFP Publication No. 303). Kansas City, Mo, AAFP, 1986.

2. Rakel RE. *Essentials of family practice*. Philadelphia: WB Saunders Company, 1993, 2–3.

3. Pereira Gray DJ. Just a GP. JR Coll Gen Pract, 1980; 30:231–239.

4. Anderson NA, Bridges-Webb C, Chancellor AHB. *General practice in Australia*. Sydney: Sydney University Press, 1986, 3–4.

5. Bridges-Webb C, Britt H, Miles D et al. Morbidity and treatment in general practice in Australia 1990–1991. Med J Aust (supplement), 19 October 1992.

6. De Lozier JE, Gagnon RO. 1989 Summary: National Ambulatory Medical Care Survey. Hyattsville, Md, National Centre for Health Statistics, 1991.

7. McWhinney IR. *A textbook of family medicine* (2nd edn). New York: Oxford University Press, 1997, 40–44.

8. Murtagh JE. *The anatomy of a rural practice*. Melbourne: Monash University, Department of Community Practice Publication, 1980, 8–13.

9. Rosenblatt RA, Cherkin DC, Schneeweiss R et al. The structure and content of family practice: Current status and future trends. J Fam Pract, 1982; 15(4):681–722.

10. Bridges-Webb C, Britt H, Miles D et al. Morbidity and treatment in general practice in Australia. Aust Fam Physician, 1993; 22:336–346.

2
The family

—

*The family only represents one aspect, however
important an aspect, of a human being's functions and
activities—A life is beautiful and ideal, or the reverse,
only when we have taken into our consideration the
social as well as the family relationship.*

Havelock Ellis 1922
Little Essays of Love and Virtue

Working with families is the basis of family practice. Families living in relative harmony provide the basis for the good mental health of their members and also for social stability.

However, the traditional concept of the nuclear family where the wife stays at home to care for the children occurs in only about 15% of Australian families, and approximately 40% of Australian marriages end in separation. This results in many psychosocial problems that family doctors will have to address.

Family therapy is ideally undertaken by general practitioners, who are in a unique position as providers of continuing care and family care. It is important for them to work together with families in the counselling process and to avoid the common pitfalls of working in isolation and assuming personal responsibility for changing the family.

Bader[1] summarises working with families succinctly:

*From the perspective of family therapy, working with
families means avoiding the trap of being too
directive, too responsible for the family's welfare, with
the result that the family becomes overly dependent on
the general practitioner for its health and
development. From the perspective of family
education, working with families means developing
the skills of anticipating guidance, helping families to
prepare, not only for the normal changes occurring as
the family develops, but also for the impact of illness
on the family system.*

Characteristics of healthy families

Successful families have certain characteristics, an understanding of which can give the family doctor a basis for assessing the health of the family and a goal to help set targets for change in disrupted families. Such characteristics are:

- *Healthy communication*. In this situation family members have freedom of expression for their feelings and emotions.
- *Personal autonomy*. This includes appropriate use of power sharing between spouses.
- *Flexibility*. This leads to appropriate 'give and take' with adaptation to individual needs and changing circumstances.
- *Appreciation*. This involves encouragement and praise so that members develop a healthy sense of self-esteem.
- *Support networks*. Adequate support from within and without the family engenders security, resistance to stress and a healthy environment in general. The family doctor is part of this network.
- *Family time and involvement*. Studies have shown that the most satisfying hallmark of a happy family is 'doing things together'.
- *Spouse bonding*. The importance of a sound marital relationship becomes obvious when family therapy is undertaken.
- *Growth*. There needs to be appropriate opportunities for growth of individual family members in an encouraging atmosphere.
- *Spiritual and religious values*. An attachment to spiritual beliefs and values is known to be associated with positive family health, supporting the saying 'The family that prays together stays together'.

Families in crisis

Doctors are closely involved with families who experience unexpected crises, which include illnesses, accidents, divorce, separation, unemployment, death of a family member and financial disasters.

The effect of illness

Serious illness often precipitates crises in individual members of the family, crises which have not previously surfaced in the apparently balanced family system. It is recognised, for example, that bereavement over the unexpected loss of a child may lead to marital breakdown, separation or divorce.

In the long term, other family members may be affected more than the patient. This may apply particularly to children and manifest as school underachievement and behaviour disturbances.

During the crisis the obvious priority of the doctor is to the patient but the less obvious needs of the family should not be ignored.

Guidelines for the doctor

- Include the family as much as possible, starting early in the acute phase of the illness. It may necessitate family conferences.
- Include the family on a continuing basis, especially if a long-term illness is anticipated. It is helpful to be alert for changes in attitudes, such as anger and resentment towards the sick member.
- Include the family in hospital discharge planning.
- If a serious change in family dynamics is observed the use of experts may be needed.

Significant presentations of family dysfunction

The following presentations may be indicators that all is not well in the family, and so the doctor needs to 'think family':

- marital or sexual difficulties
- multiple presentations of a family member—'the thick file syndrome'
- multiple presentations by multiple family members
- abnormal behaviour in a child
- the 'difficult patient'

- inappropriate behaviour in the antenatal and/or postpartum period
- drug or alcohol abuse in a family member
- evidence of physical or sexual abuse in wife or child
- psychiatric disorders
- susceptibility to illness
- increased stress/anxiety
- complaints of chronic fatigue or insomnia

It is important that the family doctor remains alert to the diversity of presentations and takes the responsibility for identifying an underlying family-based problem.

The patient and family dynamics

Family doctors see many patients who present with physical symptoms that have primarily an emotional or psychosocial basis with either little or no organic pathology. As many as 50–75% of patients utilising primary care clinics have a psychosocial precipitant as opposed to biomedical problems as the main cause of their visit.[2]

In order to understand the clinical manifestations of the sick role of patients, family doctors should first understand the individual's response to stress stimuli, which may come from external (family, work or sexual behaviour) or internal (personality trait or psychosocial) sources (Fig. 2.1 and Table 2.1).

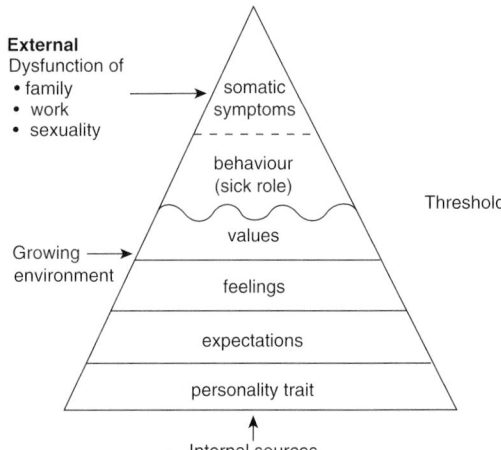

Fig. 2.1 *Family dynamics and psychosomatic illness iceberg*

Table 2.1 *Areas of possible biopsychosocial dysfunction*

Work	Family	Sex
• Type of work	• Present family (change of structure and function)	• Sexual dysfunction
• Workload		• Disharmony
• Work environment	• Extended family (parents and relatives)	• Deprivation
• Goals		• Guilt
• Work satisfaction	• Growing environment (family tree)	

How to evaluate the family dynamics

- Carefully observe family members interacting.
- Invite the whole family to a counselling session (if possible).
- Visit the home: an impromptu home visit (with some pretext such as a concern about a blood test result) on the way home from work may be very revealing.
- Prepare a genogram (Fig. 2.2): family dynamics and behaviour can be understood by drawing a family map—genogram (a diagrammatic representation of family structure and relationships).[3,4]

The genogram

The genogram is a very valuable pedigree chart that usually covers three generations of a family tree.[3] It is a simple and disciplined way of gathering data about an individual, couple or family, especially for inheritance patterns. The data has to be gathered with tact and care. Genograms are also a useful strategy for involving family members who may have been reluctant to be involved in discussions on family matters.[4] An example including the use of symbols is shown in Figure 2.2.

The family life cycle

Helpful in understanding the dynamics of the family is the concept of the family life cycle,[5] which identifies several clearly defined stages of development (Table 2.2). Such an understanding can help the doctor form appropriate hypotheses about the problems patients are experiencing at a particular stage. Each stage brings its own tasks, happiness, crises and difficulties.

Family assessment

The assessment of families with problems can be formalised through a questionnaire which allows the collection of information in a systematic way in order to give an understanding of the functioning of the family in question.

The questionnaire[1]

1. *Family of origin*

- Could each of you tell us something about the families you grew up in?
- Where do you come in the family?
- Were you particularly close to anyone else in the family?
- Were there any severe conflicts between family members?
- Did anyone abuse you in any way?
- Do you have much contact with any of your family now?
- Have you tried to model (or avoid) any features for your own family?

2. *History of the couple's relationship*

- How did you two meet?
- What attracted you to each other?
- Why did you marry this person rather than someone else?
- How did your families react to your choice?
- How did the birth of your children affect your relationship?
- When was your relationship at its best? Why?

3. *Experience in counselling and enrichment*

- Have any of you been to 'marriage encounter' or similar programs?

- 'What is your mood like? Do you feel sad or happy?'

Trouble

Enquire about how the patient's problems are troubling the patient.

- 'What about the situation troubles you most?'
- 'What troubles or worries you most in your life?'
- 'What worries you most at home?'
- 'How stressed and upset are you about this problem?'
- 'How do you think this problem affects you?'

Handling

- 'How are you handling this problem?'
- 'Do you think that you have mishandled anything?'
- 'Do you get support at home to help handle the problem?'
- 'What does your support come from?'
- 'How do you feel that you are coping?'

Empathy

Indicate an understanding of the patient's distress and legitimise his or her feelings.

- 'That must be very difficult for you.'
- 'That sounds really tough on you.'

Steps to bring about behaviour change

Fabb and Fleming have introduced the model of change which is fundamental to initiating therapy. The five steps are:

| 1. *Dissatisfaction* |

There must be dissatisfaction with the present pattern of behaviour.

| 2. *Alternative* |

There must be an acceptable alternative behaviour pattern available.

| 3. *Emotional commitment* |

There must be an emotional commitment to the new pattern of behaviour over the old.

| 4. *Practice with feedback* |

There must be practice of the new behaviour, with feedback, to establish the new pattern as an available behaviour.

| 5. *Habituation with support* |

There must be installation of the new behaviour in the normal work/living situation *with support*.

All of these must be present for change to occur. Steps 4 and 5 are often neglected with the result that change does not occur or is less successful.

Marital disharmony

Family doctors often have to provide marital counselling for one or both partners. The problems may be resolved quite simply or be so complex that marital breakdown is inevitable despite optimal opportunities for counselling.

Opportunities for prevention, including anticipatory guidance about marital problems, do exist and the wise practitioner will offer appropriate advice and counselling. Examples include an accident to a child attributable to neglect by a parent, or similar situation in which that parent may be the focus of blame leading to resentment and tension. The practitioner could intervene from the outset to alleviate possible feelings of guilt and anger in that marriage.

Some common causes of marital disharmony are:

- selfishness
- unrealistic expectations
- financial problems/meanness
- not listening to each other
- sickness (e.g. depression)
- drug or alcohol excess
- jealousy, especially in men
- fault finding
- 'playing games' with each other
- driving ambition
- immaturity
- poor communication

Basic counselling of couples

The following text on basic counselling of couples,[7] which should be regarded as a patient education sheet, includes useful advice for couples:

'The two big secrets of marital success are *caring* and *responsibility*.

Some important facts

- Research has shown that we tend to choose partners who are similar to our parents and that we may take our childish and selfish attitudes into our marriage.
- The trouble spots listed above reflect this childishness; we often expect our partners to change and meet our needs.
- If we take proper care and responsibility, we can keep these problems to a minimum.
- Physical passion is not enough to hold a marriage together—'when it burns out, only ashes will be left'.
- While a good sexual relationship is great, most experts agree that what goes on *out* of bed counts for more.
- When we do something wrong, it is most important that we feel forgiven by our partner.

Positive guidelines for success

1. *Know yourself.* The better you know yourself, the better you will know your mate. Learn about sex and reproduction.
2. *Share interests and goals.* Do not become too independent of each other. Develop mutual friends, interests and hobbies. Tell your partner 'I love you' regularly at the right moments.
3. *Continue courtship after marriage.* Spouses should continue to court and desire each other. Going out regularly for romantic evenings and giving unexpected gifts (such as flowers) are ways to help this love relationship. Engage in some high-energy fun activities such as massaging and dancing.
4. *Make love, not war.* A good sexual relationship can take years to develop; so work at making it better. Explore the techniques of lovemaking without feeling shy or inhibited. This can be helped by books such as *The Joy of Sex* and videos on lovemaking. Good grooming and a clean body are important.
5. *Cherish your mate.* Be proud of each other, not competitive or ambitious at the other's expense. Talk kindly about your spouse to others—do not put him or her down.
6. *Prepare yourself for parenthood.* Plan your family wisely and learn about child bearing and rearing. Learn about family-planning methods and avoid the anxieties of an unplanned pregnancy. The best environment for a child is a happy marriage.

7. *Seek proper help when necessary.* If difficulties arise and are causing problems, seek help. Your general practitioner will be able to help. Stress-related problems and depression in particular can be lethal in a marriage—they must be 'nipped in the bud'.
8. *Do unto your mate as you would have your mate do unto you.* This gets back to the unconscious childhood needs. Be aware of each other's feelings and be sensitive to each other's needs. Any marriage based on this rule has an excellent chance of success.

The **B**e **A**ttitudes (virtues to help achieve success)

BE honest	**BE** loyal
BE loving	**BE** desiring
BE patient	**BE** fun to live with
BE forgiving	**BE** one
BE generous	**BE** caring

Making lists—a practical task

Make lists for each other to compare and discuss.

- List qualities (desirable and undesirable) of your parents.
- List qualities of each other.
- List examples of behaviour each would like the other to change.
- List things you would like the other to do for you.

Put aside special quiet times each week to share these things.'

Pitfalls[1]

The general practitioner who is too closely attached to one or more members of the family can easily become trapped in the role of the 'rescuer' or 'saviour' of those members. The best defence against this trap is to respect the family's autonomy and work with the family to achieve the goals the family sets for itself, thus avoiding three major pitfalls for the general practitioner in treating families:

1. assuming personal responsibility for changing the family
2. working alone, neglecting the assistance of the family
3. becoming a 'rescuer' or 'saviour'

Other pitfalls

- conducting therapy in the absence of a significant member
- breaching confidentiality of individuals within the family
- failing to recognise the 'ganging-up effect'
- taking sides
- failing to use available resources
- overrelating to your own experiences

Possible solutions to avoid pitfalls[1]

- Let the patients do the work.
- Share the burden with a colleague or other resources.
- Ensure that the goals for therapy are realistic.
- Point out that all family members have to work together and that therapy works best when there is openness on all sides.
- Identify any tendency to look for scapegoats within the family.
- Avoid trying to achieve quick solutions.
- Obtain clear-cut agreements on confidential matters and record this in the history.
- Keep an open mind and avoid forcing your own values on to the family.

References

1. Bader E. Working with families. Aust Fam Physician, 1990; 19:522–528.
2. Fabb W. *Handbook for medical students.* Hong Kong: Chinese University of Hong Kong, 1995, 31.
3. McGoldrick M, Gerson R. *Genograms in family assessment.* New York: WW Norton, 1985, chs 1–4.
4. Jackson L, Tisher M. Family therapy skills for general practitioners. Aust Fam Physician, 1996; 25:1265–1269.
5. Van Doorn H. *Common problems checklist for general practice.* Melbourne: Royal Australian College of General Practitioners, 1989, 19.
6. Stuart MR, Leiberman JA III. *The 15-minute hour: Applied psychotherapy for the primary care physician.* New York: Praeger, 1986.
7. Murtagh JE. *Patient education* (2nd edn), Sydney: McGraw-Hill, 1996, 3.

3
Consulting skills

—

The essential unit of medical practice is the occasion when in the intimacy of the consulting room the person who is ill or believes himself (or herself) to be ill, seeks the advice of a doctor whom he (she) trusts. This is the consultation and all else in the practice of medicine derives from it.

Sir James Spence 1960

The consultation is a formalised interaction between doctor and patient in settings that may vary from a clearly defined task such as suturing a simple wound to the complexities of vague undifferentiated illness with profound psychological issues.

The *objectives of the consultation* are to:

- determine the exact reason for the presentation
- achieve a good therapeutic outcome for the patient
- develop a strong doctor–patient relationship

The skills of general practice

A successful outcome to the medical consultation depends on a whole array of skills required by the general practitioner. Although interrelated, these skills, which can be collectively termed 'consulting skills', include clinical skills, diagnostic skills, management skills, communication skills, educative skills, therapeutic skills, manual skills and counselling skills.

Communication skills, which are fundamental to consulting skills, are the key to the effectiveness of the doctor as a professional, and expertise with these skills is fundamental to the doctor–patient relationship. Communication skill is essential in obtaining a good history and constitutes one of the cornerstones of therapy.

A skilled interviewer will succeed in transmitting his or her findings to the patient so that they are clearly understood, are not unduly disturbing, and inspire trust and confidence in the physician.

Models of the consultation

Several models that formalise the general practice consultation can be very useful for developing an understanding of the process of the consultation. Two classic models are those by Pendleton and his colleagues, and by Stott and Davis. Pendleton and colleagues in their landmark book *The consultation: An approach to learning and teaching*[1] defined seven key tasks to the consultation, which serve as helpful guidelines:

1. To define the reason for the patient's attendance, including:
   - the nature and history of problems
   - their aetiology
   - the patient's ideas, concerns and expectations
   - the effect of the problems
2. To consider other issues:
   - continuing problems
   - risk factors
3. To choose, with the patient, an appropriate action for each problem
4. To achieve a shared understanding of the problems with the patient
5. To involve the patient in the management and encourage him or her to accept appropriate responsibility
6. To use time and resources efficiently and appropriately:
   - in the consultation
   - in the long term
7. To establish or maintain a relationship with the patient that helps to achieve the other tasks.

The exceptional potential in each primary care consultation described by Stott and Davis,[2] which is presented in Table 3.1, also acts as an excellent *aide-mémoire* to achieve maximal benefit from the consultation.

Table 3.1 *The potential in each primary care consultation*

A	B
Management of presenting problems	Modification of health-seeking behaviour
C	D
Management of continuing problems	Opportunistic health promotion

Source: Stott & Davis[2]

Phases of the consultation

The consultation can be considered in three phases, as follows:

1. Establishment of rapport
2. Diagnostic phase
   • the history
   • the physical and mental examination
   • investigations
3. Management phase
   • explanation and education
   • prescribing medication
   • procedural—therapeutic or extended diagnostic
   • referral
   • follow-up

Establishing rapport

Although rapport building occurs throughout all phases of the consultation the initial encounter with the patient sets the foundation for the relationship during the consultation. It is good policy to walk into the waiting room and call the patient by the most appropriate name. Valuable clinical information can be gleaned by observing the patient's affect, movements and walking. It is also most appropriate to quickly familiarise oneself with the patient's notes from well-kept records, preferably before seeing the patient. Rapport-establishing techniques include:

• Greet the patient with a friendly interested manner.
• Treat the patient with respect and courtesy.
• Greet the patient by his or her preferred name.
• Shake hands if appropriate.
• Make the patient feel comfortable.
• Be 'unhurried' and relaxed.
• Be well briefed about prior consultations.

• Focus firmly on the patient.
• Listen carefully and appropriately.
• Make appropriate reassuring gestures.
• Start with: 'What would you like to tell me?' or 'How can I help you?'

The history

The doctor has four basic tasks to perform during the history-taking phase of the consultation. These are to determine:

• the patient's stated reason for attending
• why the patient is attending today, or at this particular time in the course of this illness
• a list of problems or supplementary symptoms
• any other initially unspoken or hidden reason for attending, e.g. the fear of cancer

The old medical cliché that 'a good history is the basis of the clinical examination' is as relevant as always. The art of history taking, which is based on good communication, is the most fundamental skill in general practice and requires a disciplined approach.

Guidelines include:[3]

• Commence by eliciting the presenting complaint.
• Permit an uninterrupted history.
• Use appropriate language—keep the questions simple.
• Use specific questions to clarify the presenting complaint.
• Write notes or use the keyboard to record information but maintain as much eye contact as possible.
• Enquire about general symptoms such as fatigue, weight changes, fever, headache, sleep and coping ability.
• Undertake a relevant systems review.
• A historical checklist includes past medical history, complete medication history, drug habits and sensitivities, family history, psychosocial history and preventive care history.
• Give feedback to the patient about your understanding of the problems and agenda, and correct any misconceptions.

Good questions

In order to determine any underlying agenda or significant psychosocial problems it is very helpful to use analytical questions. Such questions and inviting statements could include:

• 'Do you have any particular concern about your health?'

- 'That really interests me—tell me more—it seems important.'
- 'Where would you put your real feelings between 0 and 100%?'
- 'What is it that's really upsetting or bothering you?'
- 'What do you really think deep down is the cause of your problem?'
- 'Are you basically satisfied with your life?'
- 'Is there anything that I haven't asked you and that you should tell me about?'
- 'Tell me about things at home.'
- 'Tell me about things at work.'
- 'Are you afraid that something bad is going to happen to you?'
- 'Is your relationship with any particular loved one/person causing you stress?' (This may lead to information about sensitive issues such as domestic violence or sexual problems.)
- 'Is there anything in your life that you would like changed?'
- 'I'm concerned about what you are not telling me.'

Basic interviewing techniques

There are a number of basic interviewing techniques[1] that encourage communication. It is important to use the least controlling interview techniques, before embarking on direct questioning.

The open-ended question

The open-ended question is essential in initiating the interview. A question such as 'What kind of troubles have you been having?' says to the patient 'I'm interested in anything you may feel is important enough for you to tell me'.

The open-ended question gives the patient an opportunity to take temporary control of the consultation and to outline problems and concerns.

Listening and silence

Silence is a means of encouraging communication. While the patient is communicating freely, the doctor's behaviour of choice is an interested, attentive and relaxed silence. An attentive facial expression and posture tells the patient non-verbally that he or she has an interested listener. Silence can also encourage communication but one has to be careful that the person does not feel uncomfortable with the process. There is one time when it is mandatory for the doctor to use silence—this is when the patient has stopped speaking from being overwhelmed with emotion.

Facilitation

Facilitation encourages communication by using manner, gesture or words that do not specify the kind of information that is being sought. It suggests that the doctor is interested and encourages the patient to continue. Silence and facilitation go hand in hand.

A common mode of facilitation is the nod of the head, conveying 'I'm listening', 'I understand what you are saying' or 'Go on'. A similar message is conveyed to the patient with an occasional 'mmm-mmm' or by postural shifts towards the patient or into a position of greater alertness. The doctor may also interject short words or phrases, such as 'Yes' or 'I see', without interrupting the flow of the patient's narrative or following a pause saying: 'Yes, I understand—please continue'.

Confrontation

When one senses that the patient is not speaking freely or clearly, the technique of confrontation may be used whereby the interviewer describes to the patient something striking about his or her verbal or non-verbal behaviour. Examples are: 'You look sad', 'You seem frightened', 'You sound angry' or 'I notice that you have been rubbing the back of your neck'. Confrontation has to be used with tact and skill, and should reflect sympathetic interest in the patient. It is appropriate too to confront a patient when his or her voice, posture, facial expression or bodily movements betray emotions, for example 'You seem tense' or 'You're trembling'.

Questions

When the patient is asked a question the doctor tends to take control of the interview, and so directs it along the lines of his or her own thinking or hypothesis generation. The problem is that if questions are used too early in the interview, the amount of desirable information is restricted and may disrupt the true priorities of the patient's concerns.

Open-ended questions and direct questions are very useful at appropriate times, while other questions are very restrictive. Examples, using pain as the 'problem', are:
- Open-ended question: 'Tell me about the pain.'
- Direct question: 'Where is the pain?'
- Closed question: 'Is the pain severe?'
- Leading question: 'The pain is severe?'

• Reflected question: 'You want to know the cause of the pain?'

Support and reassurance

The doctor's ability to be appropriately supportive and reassuring helps to create an atmosphere in which the patient is encouraged to communicate. Examples of supportive statements are: 'I understand' or 'That must be very upsetting'. Reassurance includes words or actions which tend to restore the patient's sense of well-being, worthiness or confidence.

Summarising

Summarising what the patient has said can keep the patient on track and check the accuracy of the information by providing the patient with the opportunity to revise any misunderstandings, e.g. 'If I've understood you correctly you have told me . . .'

Information from other sources

Sometimes it is important to obtain information from other sources, especially friends or relatives. Off-handed comments from others may be loaded with 'cues' and one should be listening intently.

Problem definition

Part of the diagnostic process is defining the patient's problem or problems. The more complex the presentation, the more necessary it is to have an orderly approach. It is clearly important to list the problems in a priority order. These problems may have been 'offered' by the patient, 'observed' by the doctor, 'derived' during the interview or 'known' from the past history. Problems can be conveniently considered as organic or physiological, and intrapersonal or social.[5]

Touching the patient

Sometimes a natural response is to touch the distressed patient as a reassuring gesture. It is best to adopt a caring-and-support gesture such as offering a box of tissues to the weeping patient, but it may be quite acceptable in most patients to give a reassuring momentary touch somewhere between the shoulder and wrist on the arm nearest to you. Touching should be a natural gesture that is comfortable for both the doctor and patient. Touch elsewhere should generally be avoided.

The physical and mental examination

If a diagnostic hypothesis based on the history is being tested, the examination may be confined to one system or to one anatomical region. However, other regions, systems or a general examination may be undertaken for medicolegal or preventive reasons. Patients tend to feel vulnerable during the physical examination; so their sensitivity and modesty have to be respected. Generally the examination is conducted in relative silence, with the doctor instructing the patient what to do.

Patients need to be warned of possible discomfort or pain that may accompany certain examinations, of the reason for the examination, and of its immediate results particularly if normal. Continued silence on the doctor's part is often interpreted by patients as being indicative of something serious or unusual being found. For the same reason the doctor's non-verbal behaviour is important.

Investigations

It is often necessary to arrange for special tests to assist in the diagnostic process or to monitor the progress of certain illnesses or response to treatment. The informed consent of patients must be obtained. A collaborative decision for or against certain tests may be negotiated.

General practitioners have a responsibility (clinical and economic) to be very discerning and selective in the investigations that they choose. The questions that should be asked in decision making include:

• 'Is this investigation necessary?'
• 'Will it change my management?'

Richard Asher (1954) listed the questions a clinician should ask before requesting an investigation:[6]

• 'Why am I ordering this test?'
• 'What am I going to look for in the result?'
• 'If I find it, will it affect my diagnosis?'
• 'How will this affect my management of the case?'
• 'Will this ultimately benefit the patient?'

In general, investigations should be performed only when the following criteria are satisfied.[1]

• The consequence of the result of the investigation could not be obtained by a cheaper, less intrusive method, e.g. taking a better history or using time.

- The risks of the investigation should relate to the value of the information likely to be gained.
- The result will directly assist in the diagnosis or have an effect on subsequent management.

Management phase of the consultation

The management phase of the consultation may immediately follow the information-gathering interview, or it may take place on review, after diagnostic tests or referral. It should be remembered that there are at least two people concerned in management: the doctor *and* the patient. Poor patient compliance with any proposed therapy can be a result of a poorly conducted management phase. It is necessary not only for the doctor to make statements concerning therapy and the reasons for the chosen therapy, but also for the information to be conveyed in a language appropriate to each patient's understanding.

Management includes immediate care, prevention and long-term care. Doctors generally tend to be authoritarian in their management proposals. Whole-person management, however, implies that the patient's views are listened to, explanations are offered where necessary by the doctor, and an educative approach is adopted to encourage the patient to actively participate in management and preventive behaviour, where possible.

No longer can the patient be expected to act as the passive receiver of advice or to submit without question to procedures as in the past. There is evidence that the patient's compliance with management plans is improved if the patient has been involved in the decision making.

The objectives of the management phase of the consultation are summarised in Table 3.2.

The sequence of the management interview

The following is a suggested *10-point plan* or sequence for conducting a management interview. These guidelines will not always need to be applied in their entirety, and may need to be staged over a number of consultations. The use of this sequence should ensure identification of all the patient's problems by the doctor (including fears, feelings and expectations); adequate patient understanding of their problems; an acceptable and appropriate treatment plan being defined for each problem; preventive opportunities being addressed; and the patient being satisfied with the consultation and being clear about follow-up arrangements.

The sequence is as follows.

1. *Tell the patient the diagnosis*

If a diagnosis is not possible describe the problem as it relates to the presenting symptoms.

2. *Establish the patient's knowledge of the diagnosis*

This information provides a clear-cut baseline of information from which to launch the management phase of the consultation.

3. *Establish the patient's attitude to the diagnosis and management*

Unless this is done the doctor may already have begun to enter a conflicting relationship with the patient without knowing why and be unaware of underlying fears.

4. *Educate the patient about diagnosis*

- Correct any incorrect health beliefs recognised in point 2.
- Supplement the patient's existing knowledge to a level appropriate to the needs of the patient and the doctor.

Table 3.2 *Objectives of the management phase of the consultation*

- To make use of the doctor–patient relationship in therapy
- To involve the patient as far as possible in the management of his or her own problem
- To educate the patient about the illness
- To promote rational prescribing
- To achieve compliance in therapy
- To emphasise preventive opportunities
- To provide appropriate reassurance
- To encourage continuity of ongoing care

Such illness education will be facilitated by the use of appropriate language, special charts and diagrams, models, investigation reports and other relevant aids, e.g. X-rays and ECGs.

5. *Develop a management plan for the presenting problem*

With precise instructions using three headings:
- Immediate: always included, even if no action is proposed
- Long term: for chronic, long-term or recurrent illnesses
- Preventive: sometimes specific measures apply—often patient education is the method required

The patient should be encouraged at this stage to participate in decision making regarding management and to make a commitment to the plans.

6. *Explore other preventive opportunities*

Common examples of preventive opportunities include immunisation, screening status (e.g. Pap smear), and advice about smoking and alcohol problems, and safe sex.

7. *Reinforce the information*

Emphasise information already given about the diagnosis and management by the use of other techniques, for example:
- Use the patient's own results, e.g. X-rays and ECGs.
- Encourage the patient to participate in the decision making and in accepting some degree of responsibility for his or her own management.

This process may be facilitated by having patients learn drug names and dosages, record body weight and urine tests, and monitor temperatures and blood pressure—when relevant.

8. *Provide takeaway information*

Examples of this important strategy include patient instruction leaflets and resource contacts.

9. *Evaluate the consultation*

When time permits the doctor should encourage feedback regarding the patient's reaction to the way the consultation has been conducted, and establish whether the objectives of both have been met and the patient is happy with the outcome.

10. *Arrange follow-up*

Clear instructions for review need to be made, preferably by providing appointments or stating that no further review is needed. Follow-up not only shows patient response to management, but also enables the reinforcement and clarification of preventive measures and information given. It also allows involvement of others, particularly family members where appropriate.

Discussion

The first three points should be attended to clearly right at the start of the management phase, to avoid any conflict or misunderstanding between doctor and patient. The doctor can then commence education about the diagnosis, correcting any incorrect health beliefs recognised in point 2, and supplement the patient's existing knowledge to a level appropriate to the needs of the patient and doctor.

The management plan for the presenting problem must be clear and specific—if complicated, the steps involved should be written down for the patient to take home. Immediate management should always be included even if no action is proposed. Long-term management strategies are useful for chronic or recurrent illness to help the patient envisage what the future holds. Preventive measures may be a specific part of the long-term management or just require patient education. The patient encouraged to participate in decision making should indicate commitment to the plans, which reinforces the essential information and encourages the patient to accept some degree of responsibility for the management of his or her own illness.

The final, yet essential, step in the management consultation is precise follow-up. Follow-up strengthens an ongoing doctor–patient relationship where the doctor indicates genuine concern and interest in that patient's long-term health needs.

A patient management strategy

Brian McAvoy, writing in Fraser's excellent book *Clinical method: A general practice approach*, presents a helpful *aide-mémoire* in the approach to patient management:[6]

1. reassurance and/or explanation
2. advice

3. prescription
4. referral
5. investigation
6. observation (follow-up)
7. prevention

Prescriptions

It is worth emphasising that prescribing medicine is a relatively complex skill that requires considerable knowledge of the disease, patient's expectations, the drugs prescribed, their interactions and their adverse reactions. Part of this skill is making a decision not to prescribe medication when it is not absolutely necessary and then explaining the reasons and including non-pharmacological measures. This decision may be made in the context of a patient expecting a biochemical solution for his or her problem. As McAvoy points out, 'If in doubt whether or not to give a drug—don't'.[1]

Referral

The decision to refer a patient is also another important skill. It is often difficult to find the right balance. Some practitioners refer excessively—others cling to the patients inappropriately. It is a mistake not to refer a patient with a serious chronic or life-threatening disease. Apart from consultants and hospitals, referral should be considered to GP colleagues or partners with special interests or expertise, support groups and other members of the primary health care team such as physiotherapists, dietitians, chiropodists and social workers. At all times the GP should act as the focal reference point and maintain control of patient management.

The 'gatekeeper' role of the general practitioner

The patient's general practitioner is the obvious and ideal lynchpin in the health care system to take responsibility for the patient's health concerns and management. The patient may become confused with the system, especially if his or her problems are many and complex. The patient's GP has a vital role in acting as a 'gatekeeper' between primary and secondary care, and between paramedical services. He or she should always act in the patient's best interests and intervene, if necessary, to ensure that the patient is getting the best possible care.

The healing art of the doctor

The counselling process in general practice is based on the therapeutic effect of the doctor. This well-recorded feature is reinforced if the doctor has a certain professional charisma, and is caring and competent. We cannot underestimate the dependency of our patients on this healing factor, especially where significant psychic factors are involved.

Making the patient feel good about the consultation

Many patients do not particularly enjoy visiting the general practitioner and some, for a variety of reasons, visit as a last resort. It is important to make patients feel good about their visit. They should feel accepted, believed and important in the sense that they have reached out to a friend in whom they can trust and be confident with. This is where appropriate explanation, reassurance and basic counselling are so important in patient management. Even seemingly trivial complaints should be managed with understanding and explanation. Patient education handouts are appreciated. Attention to even simple problems with simple therapies such as the palpation of a tender trigger spot on the back followed by the application of an 'analgesic' spray or rub with gentle massage is much more powerful than a disinterested, albeit reassuring, dismissal that the problem is 'nothing much to worry about'.

Key points on patient management

- It is difficult, perhaps impossible, to reassure patients in the absence of an appropriate physical examination and certain investigations.
- Reassurance must always be appropriate and therefore based on a substantial foundation: inappropriate reassurance damages the credibility of both the doctor and his or her profession.
- The two key characteristics of the doctor in establishing the basis of a successful outcome for the doctor–patient relationship are caring and responsibility.
- Vital factors included in this relationship are good communication, genuine interest and trust.

References

1. Pendleton D et al. *The consultation: An approach to learning and teaching.* Oxford: Oxford University Press, 1984.

2. Stott N, Davis R. The exceptional potential in each primary care consultation. JR Coll Gen Pract, 1979; 29: 201–205.

3. Nyman KC. *Successful consulting.* Melbourne: Royal Australian College of General Practitioners, 1996, 11–32.

4. Rose AT. Basic interview techniques. In Kidd M, Rose A. *An introduction to consulting skills*, Community Medicine Student Handbook. Melbourne: Monash University, 1991, 32–40.

5. Barrard J. The consultation in general practice: Patients, problems and resources. Med J Aust, 1991; 154:671–676.

6. Fraser RC. Clinical method, a general practice approach (2nd edn). Oxford: Butterworth–Heinemann, 1992, 59–76.

4

Communication skills

Most people have a furious itch to talk about themselves and are restrained only by the disinclination of others to listen. Reserve is an artificial quality that is developed in most of us as a result of innumerable rebuffs. The doctor is discreet. It is his business to listen and no details are too intimate for his ears.

W. Somerset Maugham (1874–1965)
Summing up

Hippocrates wrote:

In the art of medicine there are three factors—the disease, the patient and the doctor . . . It is not easy for the ordinary people to understand why they are ill or why they get better or worse, but if it is explained by someone else, it can seem quite a simple matter— if the doctor fails to make himself understood he may miss the truth of the illness.[1]

Francis Macnab, Doctor of Divinity and patient, wrote: 'The style of the doctor, the communication of the doctor and the person of the doctor at the level of primary contact and primary care can be crucial in a person's life'.[2]

Much of the art of general practice lies in the ability to communicate.

Communication

Communication can be defined as 'the successful passing of a message from one person to another'.

There are five basic elements in the communication process:

- the communicator
- the message
- the method of communicating
- the recipient
- the response

Important principles facilitating the communication process are:

- the rapport between the people involved
- the time factor, facilitated by devoting more time
- the message, which needs to be clear, correct, concise, unambiguous and in context
- the attitudes of both the communicator and the recipient

Communication in the consultation

The doctor requires appropriate communication skills for complete diagnosis (physical, emotional and social) and competent management. The majority of interaction between doctor and patient occurs in the traditional consultation. Table 4.1 shows where the communication pattern swings between being 'patient focused' and 'doctor focused'.[3]

Important positive doctor behaviour

At first contact:

- Address the patient by his or her preferred name.
- Make the patient feel comfortable.
- Be 'unhurried' and relaxed.
- Focus firmly on the patient.
- Use open-ended questions where possible.
- Make appropriate reassuring gestures.

Active listening

Listening is the single most important skill.[3] Listening is an active process, described by Egan as follows:

One does not listen with just his ears: he listens with his eyes and with his sense of touch. He listens by becoming aware of the feelings and emotions that arise within himself because of his contact with others (that is, his own emotional resonance is another

Table 4.1 *Phases of doctor–patient communication*[3]

Phase 1 Patient focus	Phase 2 Doctor focus	Phase 3 Mutual focus
Introduction Present complaint Other medical history Family history Social history	Examination Investigation	Management discussion Follow-up Sign-off

'ear'), he listens with his mind, his heart, and his imagination. He listens to the words of others, but he also listens to the messages that are buried in the words or encoded in all the cues that surround the words. He listens to the voice, the demeanour, the vocabulary, and the gestures of the other. He listens to the context, verbal messages and linguistic pattern, and the bodily movements of others. He listens to the sounds, and to the silences.[4]

Listening includes four essential elements:
• checking facts
• checking feelings
• encouragement
• reflection

Listen with understanding, in a relaxed, attentive silence. Use reflective questions, such as:
• 'You seem very sad today.'
• 'You seem upset about your husband.'
• 'It seems you're having trouble coping.'
• 'You seem to be telling me that . . .'
• 'Your main concern seems to me to . . .'

Attitudes
• caring
• empathy
• respect
• interest
• concern
• confidence
• competence
• responsibility
• trust
• sensitivity
• perceptiveness
• diligence

Communicating strategies
• Modify language.
• Avoid jargon.
• Provide clear explanations.
• Give clear treatment instructions.
• Evaluate the patient's understanding.
• Summarise and repeat.

• Avoid uncertainty.
• Avoid inappropriate reassurance.
• Arrange appropriate referral (if necessary).
• Ensure patient is satisfied.
• Obtain informed consent.

Follow-up
• Be available for phone calls.
• Ensure patients obtain results of investigations ordered, including Pap smears.
• Ensure any promised follow-up is carried out.
• Phone the patient if you have any lingering concerns (this could be handled by the receptionist).
• Arrange referral if inadequate response to treatment.
• Act as an advocate if necessary, e.g. pressing for hospital admission.

Difficulties in communication

The Victorian Medical Board lists poor communication as the most important factor causing complaints from patients and relatives against doctors.[5]

Effective communication depends on four interrelated factors concerning the message—the doctor (the sender), the patient (the recipient), the message itself and the environment in which the message is sent (Fig. 4.1).[6]

Environment

The physical environment is important (Table 4.2). The appearance, size and layout of consulting rooms, waiting rooms and patients' rooms will affect communication, sometimes adversely, especially if privacy is threatened by, say, leaving the consulting room door open. The doctor can create an obstacle simply by a physical 'barrier', for example a large desk distancing the doctor from the patient (Figure 4.2).

The hospital environment will encourage the 'sick' role and generally is not conducive to

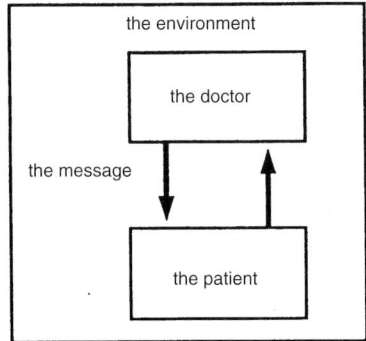

Fig. 4.1 *The four key factors affecting communication*

good communication because of a low level of privacy.

A busy practice affected by time constraints on doctor or patient will influence communications seriously. A doctor in Wales has a notice in his waiting room: 'If the doctor is a long time with a patient don't get mad: it might be you'.

The message

The nature and content of the message may be uncomfortable for the doctor or the patient or both (Table 4.3). This applies to emotionally charged, complex or subtle content such as sexual problems, malignant disease, drug abuse, bereavement, malingering and psychiatric disorders.

The patient may find the message difficult to comprehend because of inappropriate delivery or explanation by the doctor. Failure to use good follow-up strategies, including appointment times and appropriate patient education material, will aggravate communication breakdown. Language difficulties can distort the

Fig. 4.2 *The physical barrier*

message and generate frustration in both parties. Good interpreters often help.

The doctor may also fail to appreciate that certain symptoms such as chronic pain or the presence of a lump mean 'cancer' to the patient. Failure to reassure the patient (where appropriate) distracts the patient.

Doctor–patient interaction

There are several general characteristics that affect communication between doctor and patient. These include:

- poor past relationships and experiences leading to unresolved interpersonal conflict, e.g. an incorrect diagnosis or poor treatment outcome and indifferent compliance in following treatment or paying accounts

Table 4.2 *Summary of environmental factors that can adversely influence communication*

Waiting room	Poor physical layout
	Length of waiting time
Time pressure	'Traffic' level
	? busy
	? noisy
	? sense of urgency
Physical factors	Desk—barriers
	Layout inappropriate
	Poor record system
	Substandard examination couch
Privacy	Dressing/undressing
	Sound
	Interruptions—phone

Table 4.3 *Negative communication related to the message*

Language difficulties

Complex problems

Emotional problems

Uncertainty and doubt

Examples:
- sexuality, such as incest, STDs
- malignancy
- multiple complaints: 'the shopping list'
- infertility
- unwanted pregnancy
- abortion

Table 4.4 *The doctor's personal factors that influence communication*

Age	Elderly, young
Sex	Opposite
Senses	Deafness, speech idiosyncrasy
Handicap	
Competence	Health understanding
	Professional training
	Social awareness
	Empathy
Attitudes	Bias—patient attending other doctors or alternative practitioners
Communication style differences	Religion, sexual practices
	Social class
	Ethnic group
	Political group
	Dress
	Eccentricities
	Familiarity

- personal differences, openly expressed, which may create subtle barriers, including differences in age, sex, religion, culture, social status and doctor/patient roles (occasionally influenced by political factors)
- the communication skills of doctor and patient, both as the sender and receiver of messages
- the personal honesty and integrity of both parties in dealing with difficult messages
- psychosocial problems that will establish barriers, e.g. psychiatric illness or speech impediments
- familiarity between patient and doctor, e.g. friends or relatives

The doctor

Although we believe that most doctors satisfactorily meet professional standards, there are times when the communication factor is adversely affected by inbuilt negative forces, including chronic tiredness, stress, domestic problems and poor health (Table 4.4).

Furthermore, there are many strategies, roles, 'games' or 'hobby-horses' that some of us appear to rely on, especially when confronted with difficult or threatening circumstances, such as the management of the terminally ill.

Dare we recognise in ourselves some of the following unkind caricatures of doctors, i.e. personality types who may generate unfavourable communication?[7,8]

Dr Al Oof (Fig. 4.3). The prima donna doctor (not necessarily a surgeon); aloof; omnipotent; dark suit with matching Mercedes; club tie or bow-tie; feared by medical students; partial to Scotch; pronounces certain cures; powerfully dispels doubts; no faith in the healing process before surgery but unshakeable faith after surgery; unavailable in the patient's decline.

Dr N. Zyme (Fig. 4.4). The scientific doctor; machine-like; cool; assured; obsessive; drives an Italian car; orders a new test and drug at every visit; conversant with the cellular biochemistry of the disease process but ignorant of its host.

Dr G. Rumble. The gruff doctor; grunts in monosyllables; brilliant but appears tough and unapproachable; actually quite shy, soft and kind behind the facade; drives a Ford.

Fig. 4.3 *Dr Al Oof*

Fig. 4.4 *Dr N. Zyme*

Dr No Komento. The secretive doctor; strong and silent, or is he weak and silent, threatened? In another world! Drives a BMW; a computer buff.

Dr I. Knowall (Fig. 4.5). Glib; assured; garrulous; drives latest red sports car; drapes stethoscope around neck; accepts invitations to lecture on all subjects; rarely available on the phone; keeps patients waiting for hours.

Dr S. Winger. Modern, swinging and trendy; superficial; on first name terms with patients; drives beaten-up Renault held together by political stickers; works only 35 hours a week; cavalier; undiplomatically blunt.

Dr X. Cytabull. Fanatic; madly enthusiastic about rarities; overreacts to physical abnormalities; compulsive writer to medical editors; refers patients ad nauseam; drives yellow Porsche.

Dr Genghis M. Pyre. Longs for a mega-practice, assistants (not partners) and a pathology service; addicted to conferences and cocktail parties; also yearns for a Daimler, a halo and New Year's honours.

Dr Buzz Bee. Ever busy; flits from one consulting room to another; frequent phone user during consultation; creates a sense of urgency everywhere; charming to patients but intimidates them; overservices; holds pilot's licence; drives Landcruiser when licence not suspended.

Dr Go Along Cassidy. Feels comfortable when he is giving patients what they ask for; has a 'conveyor belt' type practice; rarely leaves his chair and doesn't examine his patients; drives a Colt.

Dr I. Kling. Protective and possessive; hangs on to patients; refers only under pressure; overconfident; likes to be liked; indifferent medical record system; compulsive drug prescriber; still drives 1969 Volvo.

Dr Nat Ure. Strong on 'alternatives'; pleasant chap; keen on Blackmore's publications and remedies; health shop (run by spouse) next door for fibre, sprouts and vitamin pills; attracts an attractive clientele; mutters audibly while writing the rare script; into massage, yoga and transcendental meditation; wears a knitted tie; rides a bicycle.

Fig. 4.5 *Dr I. Knowall*

Dr Fi Mayle. The invisible doctor; juggles patients, children and the PC with one hand while cooking dinner with the other; earns less, pays more; shuns cocktail parties in preference to continuing medical education (CME) meetings with child care; prefers to be really achieving something through her division rather than waiting for the power boys to do it for her; finds continuing care and collegiate relationships difficult; drives whatever will take her reliably from A to B many times a day.[9] (reprinted with permission)

Dr Amy Preschool. Ever late to start surgery; smartly dressed in three-year-old fashions (bought before the baby was born) bearing telltale infant food stains; babysitting problems; caring of mums and kids; constant attender of paediatric continuing education programs to find the cause of her child's continual diarrhoea; drives a late model Japanese-built station-wagon with a recommended car seat in the back.[10]

Dr Family Practice. The conservative doctor; married to a university sweetheart; practising from home for many years with her husband; prescribes mist magnesium trisilicate for peptic ulceration, Relaxa-Tabs for panic states and the 'Red tonic' for depression; children grown up and at university; both left at home with the ageing parents, two dogs and two cars; she drives the Austin A30.[10]

Dr Susie Nirvana. Pap smear queen; always working, never in the same place twice; takes her entourage of similar searching patients with her. Drives someone else's car.[10]

Dr Magoo. Always in court; popular with solicitors; never examines patients; great conversationalist; rarely looks; misses obvious signs; can't afford a car.

Dr Ann Osmia. Socialite doctor with 'special' clientele; senseless to sensory signs such as abnormal smells, sights and sounds; has difficulty with diagnosing alcohol abuse, gastrointestinal disorders and diabetes; harbours secret bad experiences with neurology tutor; drives a Saab cabriolet with matching poodle.

Dr Otto Sclerosis. The clinic's unpopular doctor; doesn't listen; doesn't hear; preoccupied; has gambling and drinking problem; drives Range Rover when driver's licence not suspended.

These caricatures mirror something of ourselves, so that, it is to be hoped, we can understand our own attitudes and behaviour. The stereotypes portrayed may well adversely affect our relationship with our patients and colleagues.

The patient

Do we recognise, with significant emotion, these patients in our practice?
- 'Smith speaking—I insist on speaking to you directly and not to the "iron curtain" out front.'
- 'Doctor, I've lost my script again—be a good fellow and . . .'
- 'Those pills you prescribed yesterday are doing nothing for me.'
- 'Doctor, you're the only one who can help me.'

Yes, doctors are human and can harbour hostility towards the difficult patient, including the demanding patient, the seductive patient, the 'compo' patient, the difficult 'ethnic' patient, the hypochondriac, the bad debtor or the manipulative patient.

Some patients appear to have the irrepressible ability to create conflict, so often heralded by an upset receptionist, thus setting the scene for a potentially difficult consultation (Table 4.5).

However, doctors have a professional responsibility to transcend interpersonal conflict and facilitate productive communication by establishing a caring and responsible relationship even with 'difficult' patients. Not surprisingly, such patients can also be found to be warm and

pleasantly human beneath their 'shoulder-chip' facade and so be helped immeasurably by an empathetic doctor.

It is important to bear in mind that medical communication often occurs in an emotional environment, because 'disease' has important emotional connotations for patients and their relatives and friends. Inappropriate communication and management can generate hostility.

The doctor-become-patient in the hands of his colleagues learns fast, but possibly too late. Illness plus defective communication can bring confusion, anxiety and pain; suspicion and confinement add new dimensions to suffering.

Sooner or later we come to see ourselves as persons, both as doctor and as patient ('wearing his moccasins'). The patient in us longs for the ideal doctor who is truly professional with sound knowledge and sane judgment, who is available, unhurried, caring and responsible.

Table 4.5 *Patient characteristics that can influence communication*

Age	Adolescent, elderly
Sex	Opposite
Senses	Deaf, blind, speech impairment
Handicapped	Speech disorders, visual impairment
Illness	Acutely ill/injured
Psychological	
Attitudes	Aggressive, hostile
	Demanding
	Aggrieved, e.g. fees, mistakes
	Perception of doctor's authority

Anxiety/depression
Dementia
Fears and phobias, e.g. AIDS
Health understanding
Hysteria
Hypochondriasis
Personality disorders
Sensitive issues, e.g. sexuality, bereavement, malignancy

Social
Social class
Ethnic group
Education
Dress
Political group
Familarity

Non-verbal communication

Non-verbal communication or body language is a most important feature of the communication process. Birdwhistle[11] has shown that more human communication takes place by the use of gestures, postures, position and distances (non-verbal communication or *body language*) than by any other method. Albert Mehrabian showed that non-verbal cues comprise the majority of the impact of any communicated message (Table 4.6).[12]

Recognition of non-verbal cues in our communication is important especially in a doctor–patient relationship. The ability to recognise non-verbal cues improves communication, rapport and understanding of the patient's fears and concerns. Recognising body language can allow doctors to modify their behaviour, thus promoting optimum communication.[13]

Interpreting body language[11,13]

The interpretation of body language, which differs between cultures, is a special study in its own right but there are certain cues and gestures that can be readily interpreted. Examples illustrated include the depressed patient (Fig. 4.6), barrier-type signals often used as a defensive mechanism to provide comfort or indicate a negative attitude (Figs 4.7 a,b,c) and a readiness gesture indicating a desire to terminate the communication (Fig. 4.8).

Having noted the non-verbal communication the doctor must then deal with it. This may require confrontation, that is, diplomatically bringing these cues to the patient's attention and exploring the associated feeling further.

It is not difficult to appreciate the importance of body language in the doctor–patient relationship. A hunch or gut feeling can be better understood, reinforced or corrected by skilled observation and interpretation of body language. A doctor can recognise a patient's non-verbal cues and explore the issues raised. By improving

one's skills, and modifying one's behaviour (and consulting room configuration) the doctor can encourage communication and a better understanding of the patient.

The skill to interpret non-verbal cues can be achieved by conscious observation of people's interaction, including our own. A technique suggested by Pease[11] is to watch television without sound for 15 minutes each day and check your interpretation each five minutes. By the end of three weeks, he suggests, you will have become a more skilled body language observer.

Rapport-building techniques

A person can develop rapport with another by mimicking their body language, speech, posture, pace and other characteristics. This method is a type of neuro-linguistic programming based on the work of Bandler and Grinder.[14] Such techniques can be used to help the doctor communicate better with the patient and also to improve a patient's attitude by changing the patient's body language position. It will be difficult for the patient to maintain a negative attitude if the body language position is not congruent.[13]

Mirroring

Mirroring is a useful technique whereby the limb positions and body angles of the person you are talking to can be copied. A mirror image is formed of their position so that when they look at you they see themselves as in a mirror. It is not necessary to copy uncomfortable gestures or unusual limb positions such as hands behind the head. A partial mirror is often sufficient.

Fig. 4.6 *Posture of a depressed person—head down, slumped, inanimate; postion of desk and people correct*

Table 4.6 *Impact of the message*

	%
Words alone	7
Tone of voice	38
Non-verbal communication	55

Fig. 4.7 *Body language—barrier signals:* **(a)** *arms folded;* **(b)** *legs crossed;* **(c)** *'ankle lock' pose*

Fig. 4.8 *Body language—'readiness to go' gestures*

Pacing

People exhibit a certain rhythm or pace that can be revealed through their breathing, talking, and movements of the head, hands or feet. If you can copy the pace of another person, it will establish a sense of oneness or rapport with them. Once this pace is established you can change their pace by changing yours. This is called *leading*.

Vocal copying

Vocal copying is a rapid and effective way to develop rapport with people. It involves copying intonation, pitch, volume, pace, rhythm, breathing and length of the sentence before pausing.

Engaging in these strategies will bring you into such close rapport that you can intuitively pick up all kinds of things about people that were not obvious beforehand. It may also have the unfortunate effect of making you feel that you are 'drowning' in their problems. If you feel overwhelmed, then break the rapport and diplomatically go into a leading phase.[15]

Practice tips

- A fundamental prerequisite for effective communication is listening; this includes not only hearing the words but also understanding their meaning in addition to being sensitive to the feelings accompanying the words.[16]
- Undertake the strategies of paraphrasing and summarising during the consultation to emphasise that listening is occurring and to provide a basis for defining the problems.
- Associated with listening is the observation of the non-verbal language, which may in many instances be the most significant part of the communication process.
- Good communication between doctors and patients decreases the chance of dissatisfaction with professional services, even with failed therapy, and the likelihood of litigation.

References

1. Elliott-Binns E. *Medicine: The forgotten art.* Tunbridge Wells, Kent: Pitman Books, 1978, 35.

2. Macnab F. Changing levels of susceptibility in sickness and in health. Aust Fam Physician, 1986; 15:1370.

3. Mansfield F. Basic communicating skills. Aust Fam Physician, 1987; 16:216–222.

4. Kidd M, Rose A. *An introduction to consulting skills.* Community Medicine Student Handbook. Melbourne: Monash University, 1991, 15.

5. Medical Board of Victoria. Third Annual Report, 1982/3. Melbourne: FD Atkinson, Government Printers, 1983, 12.

6. Carson N, Findlay D. *Communication skills.* Student Handbook. Melbourne: Monash University, Department of Community Medicine, 1986, 31.

7. Elliott CE. 'How am I doing?' Med J Aust, 1979; 2:644–645.

8. Murtagh JE, Elliott CE. Barriers to communication. Aust Fam Physician, 1987; 16:223–226.

9. Ivory K. The invisible doctor. Medical Observer, 12 April 1996, 19.

10. Saltman D. Rectifying a sexual bias (Letter to the editor). Aus Fam Physician, 1987; 16:545.

11. Pease A. *Body language.* London: Camel Publishing, 1985, 1–63.

12. Mehrabian A. *Silent messages.* Belmont, Calif: Wadsworth, 1971.

13. Findlay D. Body language. Aust Fam Physician, 1987; 16:229.

14. Bandler R, Grinder J. *Re-framing: Neuro-linguistic programming and the transformation of meaning.* Moab, Utah: Real People Press, 1982, 1–203.

15. Oldham J. Neuro-linguistic programming. Aust Fam Physician, 1987; 16:237–240.

16. Lloyd M, Bor R. *Communication skills for medicine.* London: Churchill Livingstone, 1996, 17–25.

5
Counselling skills

—

The doctor should have a kind disposition, great patience, self-possession, meticulous freedom from prejudice, an understanding of human nature resulting from an abundant knowledge of the world, adroitness in conversation and a special love of his calling.

G. Griesinger 1840

The Macquarie Dictionary says that counselling is 'giving advice': that it is 'opinion or instruction given in directing the judgment or conduct of another'. In the clinical context counselling can be defined as 'the therapeutic process of helping a patient to explore the nature of his or her problem in such a way that he or she determines his or her decisions about what to do, without direct advice or reassurance from the counsellor'.

The counselling process in general practice is based on the therapeutic effect of the doctor. There is an enormous and ever-increasing need for people in the community to have many of their emotional and social problems addressed by the health profession. Modern medicine has acquired a much more scientific face over recent years at the expense of its once respected humanistic one. Medicine is primarily a humanitarian pursuit, not an economic or scientific one, and uses science as a tool. Many feel that medicine is losing sight of this, at the considerable expense of its standing in the community.[1]

The public perceives that general practitioners can and do counsel people, because more people go to their GP for counselling than to any other group of health workers, including psychologists, psychiatrists, social workers, marriage guidance counsellors and clergy.[1] People do not generally tell the doctor or even realise that counselling is exactly what led them to come to

the doctor in the first place. The GP is therefore ideally placed in the community to make the most significant contribution to fill the community's needs in this area.

The GP as an effective counsellor

General practitioners can be effective counsellors for the following reasons:[2]

- They have the opportunity to observe and understand the patients and their environment.
- General practitioners are ideally placed to treat the whole patient.
- Their generalist skills and holistic approach permit them to have a broad grasp of the patient's problems and a multifaceted approach to treatment.
- They can provide treatment in comfortable and familiar surroundings including the GP's rooms and the patient's home.
- They are skilled at working as a member of a professional team and directing patients to more expert members of the team as necessary.
- They can readily organise 'contracts' with the patient.
- They have an intimate knowledge of the family and the family dynamics.
- They fit comfortably into continuing patient care with appropriate follow-up treatment programs.

To be an effective counsellor the general practitioner must first prepare for this role. Following a commitment to its importance the general practitioner can acquire the knowledge and skills for basic counselling by reading, by attending workshops and by discussing cases with colleagues who are skilled in counselling.[2] Well-developed interviewing skills are essential, as is self-discipline to appreciate one's strengths and limitations.

Features of counselling

Doctors can respond to patients' problems and distress by a spectrum of behaviours from doctor-centred directive behaviour or advice at one end, to patient-centred non-directive behaviour at the other. In handling psychosocial problems, advice giving is at one end of the spectrum and psychotherapy at the other.

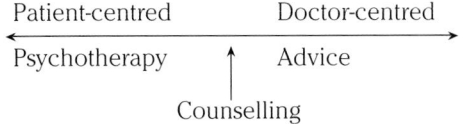

Counselling, as an activity in general practice, can be represented by a moving point between these two extremes.[1]

Counselling can be seen as having the following features:[1]

- It is a clear-cut treatment option like a course of antibiotics.
- It is a co-operative problem-solving process.
- It is an educational venture where patients learn new information and new activities.
- It is a developmental process for patients.
- It is a change process—often moving a patient from a 'stuck state'.
- It is a goal-directed activity.
- It is a process of energising patients and lifting their morale.
- It is a sensitive response to problems within a caring relationship.

A problem-solving approach

Defining the problem (what the matter really is) is the most important step in the process of patient care. The following outline is one approach to counselling that is applicable to a general practice context.[1]

1. Listen to the problem of first presentation: this involves listening not only to issues, events and experiences, but also to the patient's feelings and distress. The emphasis here is more on the communication skills of facilitation, silence, clarification, reflection, paraphrasing, confrontation and summary, than on questioning. In many cases this phase of the counselling constitutes the major part of the therapy; e.g. in grief or bereavement counselling, where the doctor supports the patient through a natural but distressing process.

2. Define a problem, if possible in behavioural terms:

   Beneath the feeling is the experience, beneath the experience is the event, the event is related to a problem.[3]

3. Establish a contract for counselling, with an agreed number of visits initially, e.g. weekly half hour or hour appointments for 4 to 6 weeks.

4. Define short-term and long-term goals for action.

5. Decide on one option—'experimental action'.

6. Build an action program with the patient—negotiate 'homework' for the patient between visits.

7. Evaluate progress.

8. Continue action or select another option.

9. Evaluate progress.

10. Terminate or refer.

Counselling models

The PLISSIT model

The PLISSIT model, developed by Annon (1974)[4] as an aid in therapy for sexual problems, is a very useful model for problems presented as feelings where there is limited scope for intervention by the therapist.

The mnemonic PLISSIT stands for the following:

- P is for permission giving.
- LI is for limited information.
- SS is for specific suggestion.
- IT is for intensive therapy.

Annon emphasises that every primary care practitioner should be competent to offer 'permission giving' and 'limited information'.

The Colagiuri and Craig model

The medical counselling model was developed by Colagiuri and Craig (Fig. 5.1)[5] as a useful tool for teaching contraceptive, abortion and sterilisation counselling. It can be applied in most situations as it empowers the patients to make their own decisions through facilitation as opposed to the directive and advisory learning model.

Fig. 5.1 *Medical counselling model*   AFTER COLAGIURI AND CRAIG, REPRINTED WITH PERMISSION

The value of patient-centred counselling

There is evidence that the use of non-directive counselling techniques leads to more accurate diagnosis and therefore to more appropriate management and an improved outcome.[6]

Jerome Frank wrote in 1967: 'The field of counselling and psychotherapy has for years presented the puzzling spectacle of unabating enthusiasm for forms of treatment where effectiveness could not be objectively demonstrated'.[7] Traux and Carkhuff[8] measured important aspects of the psychotherapeutic relationship and demonstrated what had long been recognised: the outcome was enhanced if practitioners had such qualities as accurate and sensitive awareness of the patient's feelings, deep concern for the patient's welfare (without attempting to dominate) and openness about their own reactions.

The essential feature of the patient-centred approach is that the counsellor is more like a facilitator; that is, by the asking of well-directed questions it is hoped that patients can realise their own solutions for their problems.[1] This encourages patients to attain understanding and personal growth themselves rather than just put their personal affairs in the hands of someone else. This does not mean to say that the facilitator is passive in the process of assessing the relative merit of various solutions produced by the patient. The doctor-centred approach is most applicable for patients who are so confused or distraught that their ability to reflect usefully is temporarily or permanently inaccessible. Here, taking a more active and authoritarian role may be just what is required. It is therefore important to be flexible and move between the two ends of the spectrum as needed.

Basics of counselling or psychotherapy

- Listening and empathy are the beginning of counselling.
- Good communication is the basis of counselling.
- The therapist must really care about the patient.
- Always be aware of the family context.
- It is important for therapists to handle and monitor their own feelings and emotions.
- Maintain eye contact.
- The therapist must tolerate and be comfortable with what the patient says.
- Confidentiality is essential.
- Counselling is easier if there is a good rapport with the patient, especially if a long-standing relationship exists.
- Counselling is difficult if a social relationship is present.
- Don't say to the patient, 'I'm counselling you' or 'I'm giving you psychotherapy'—make it a natural communication process.
- The therapist must be versatile and adapt a counselling style to the clinical occasion.
- Characteristics of the effective counsellor have

been demonstrated to be genuineness, non-possessive warmth for the patient, and accurate and empathic understanding.

Some useful interviewing skills used in counselling are summarised in Table 5.1.

Table 5.1 *Interview skills used in counselling*

- Use reflected statements.
- Use silence.
- Allow expressions of emotion.
- Offer supportive comments.
- Paraphrase and summarise.
- Allow patients to correct your interpretations of their feelings.
- Observe lack of congruence.
- Try to understand what the patient is feeling:
  — anger
  — hostility
  — fear
  — manipulation
  — seduction
  — insecurity
- Make intelligent guesses to prompt patient to continue.
- Don't reassure too soon.

Counselling strategies[3,6]
- The therapy should be patient-centred.
- Use gentle, clever, probing questions.
- Facilitate the discussion to draw out relevant areas.
- It is important to be non-judgmental.
- Counsel through intuition and base it on common sense.
- Do not tell the patient what to do.
- Do not try to rush patients into achieving a happy ending.
- Provide guidance to allow the patient to gain insight.
- Wherever possible, make therapy non-authoritarian and non-directional.
- Use appropriate 'gentle' confrontation to allow self-examination.
- Help patients to explore their own situation and express emotions such as anxiety, guilt, fear, anger, hope, sadness, self-hate, hostility to others and hurt feelings.
- Explore possible feelings of insecurity and allow free expression of such feelings.
- Explore patients' belief systems and consider and respect their spiritual aspirations and conflicts.

- Ask key searching questions such as:
  — 'What would be different in your life if you were well?'
  — 'Who are you mad at?'
  — 'If I understand you correctly you are telling me that . . .'
  — 'You seem to be telling me that . . .'
  — 'Correct me if I'm on the wrong track, but you are saying that . . .'
  — 'What do you think deep down is the cause of your problem?'
  — 'What does your illness do to you?'
  — 'Do you really worry about any things in particular?'
  — 'How do you think your problem should be treated?'
  — 'If you could change anything in your life what would it be?'

Avoid:
- telling patients what they must do/offering solutions
- giving advice based on your own personal experiences and beliefs
- bringing up problems that the patient does not produce voluntarily

What counselling is not:
- giving information
- giving advice
- being judgmental
- imposing one's own values, behaviour and practices
- the same as interviewing
- handing out patient education material

Cautions[1]
- Individual doctors cannot be useful to all patients; so be selective.
- We cannot solve patients' problems for them.
- Patients' problems belong to them and not to their counsellors.
- Patients often have to change by only an inch in order to move a mile.
- If a counselling relationship is no longer productive, then terminate and refer.
- Most patients in primary care need information, support and a lift in morale, not long-term psychotherapy.

Patients unlikely to benefit

The following groups of patients are not likely to benefit from counselling therapy[1] (i.e. relative contraindications):

- psychotic patients
- patients who have had an unrewarding experience with psychiatrists and other psychotherapists
- people who are antagonistic to the notion of a psychosocial diagnosis, subsequently found to be organic
- patients with little awareness or language to express emotional difficulty
- patients who do not believe doctors can treat psychosocial problems
- patients who are dependent on contact with the doctor and are willing to do almost anything to maintain the relationship
- patients with a vested interest in remaining unwell who are therefore resistant to change, e.g. patients with work-related disabilities awaiting legal settlement
- patients with chronic psychosomatic tendencies who are willing to do almost anything to maintain the relationship
- those in an intractable life situation who are unable or unwilling to change
- patients who are unwilling to examine and work on painful or uncomfortable areas of their life

Specific areas of counselling

Opportunities for basic counselling by the general practitioner are ubiquitous in medical practice. Complex problems require referral but, irrespective of that situation, the general practitioner still has an important role in continuing management.

Areas demanding counselling include:

- any crisis situation
- bereavement or grief
- terminal illness/palliative care (Chapter 7)
- marital problems (Chapter 2)
- family problems (Chapter 2)
- sexual dysfunction (Chapter 97)
- chronic pain
- anxiety and stress (Chapter 108)
- depression (Chapter 16)
- intellectual handicap in a child
- infertility (Chapter 96)
- any disease or illness, especially severe illness
- sexual abuse/child abuse (Chapter 76)
- domestic violence (Chapter 88)

Crisis management

Crisis situations are not uncommon in general practice and people in crisis are usually highly aroused and demanding. Examples include tragic deaths such as children drowning or sudden infant death syndrome (SIDS), unexpected marital break-up and breaking bad news.

Aims of crisis intervention

- Resolve the crisis and restore psychological equilibrium as quickly and constructively as possible.
- Encourage the person in crisis to regain control and take appropriate action.

Principles of management

- Intervene early—actively and directly.
- Establish an empathic alliance.
- Be accessible.
- Attend to family and social supports.
- Be prepared for the difficult phase of 24–48 hours.
- Do not carry the burden of crisis.
- Aim for brief time-limited intervention (no more than six interviews over six weeks).
- When necessary, be prepared to provide short-term use of psychotropic drugs, e.g. a hypnotic, for two or three nights of good sleep.

Ten rules to help those in distress

The following rules are given to those in crisis (personal explanation followed by a take-home handout):

1. *Give expression to your emotions.*
   You simply must accept your reactions as normal and not be afraid to cry or call out. Do not bottle up feelings.
2. *Talk things over with your friends.*
   Do not overburden them but seek their advice and listen to them. Do not avoid talking about what has happened.
3. *Focus on things as they are now—at this moment.*
   Do not brood on the past and your misfortune. Concentrate on the future in a positive way.
4. *Consider your problems one at a time.*
   Do not allow your mind to race wildly over a wide range of problems. You can cope with one problem at a time.
5. *Act firmly and promptly to solve a problem.*
   Once you have worked out a way to tackle a problem, go for it. Taking positive action is a step in allowing you to get on with life.
6. *Occupy yourself and your mind as much as possible.*
   Any social activity—sports, theatre, cards,

discussion groups, club activity—is better than sitting around alone. Many people find benefit from a holiday visit to an understanding friend or relative. Religious people usually find their faith and prayer life a great source of strength at this time.

7. *Do not nurse grudges or blame other people.* This is not easy but you must avoid getting hostile. In particular, do not get angry with yourself and your family, especially your spouse.

8. *Set aside some time every day for physical relaxation.*
   Make a point of doing something physical such as going for a walk, swimming or enjoying an easy exercise routine.

9. *Stick to your daily routine as much as possible.*
   At times of crisis a familiar pattern of regular meals and chores can bring a sense of order and security. Avoid taking your problems to bed and thus ensuring sleepless nights. Try to 'switch off' after 8 p.m. Taking sleeping tablets for those few bad nights will help.

10. *Consult your family doctor when you need help.*
    Your doctor will clearly understand your problem because stress and crisis problems are probably the commonest he or she handles. Consult your doctor sooner rather than later.

- Remember that there are many community resources to help you cope, e.g. ministers, social workers, community nurses, crisis centres and church organisers.
- Take care: do drive carefully and avoid accidents, which are more common at this time.

Bereavement

Bereavement or grief may be defined as deep or intense sorrow or distress following loss.[9] Raphael uses the term to connote 'the emotional response to loss: the complex amalgam of painful affects including sadness, anger, helplessness, guilt, despair'.[10]

The general practitioner will see grief in all its forms over a wide variety of losses. Although the nature of loss and patient reaction to it varies enormously the principles of management are similar.

Stages of normal bereavement

1. *Shock or disbelief.* Feelings include numbness and emptiness, searching, anxiety, fear and suicidal ideation, 'I don't believe it'. Concentration is difficult and spontaneous emotions such as crying, screaming or laughing tend to occur. There may be a sense of the deceased's presence, and hallucinations (visual and auditory) may occur.

2. *Grief and despair.* Feelings include anger, 'Why me?', guilt and self-blame, and yearning. Social withdrawal and memory impairment may occur. The feeling of intense grief usually lasts about 6 weeks and the overall stage of grief and despair for about 6 months, but it can resurface occasionally for a few years. The last few months involve feelings of sadness and helplessness.

3. *Adaptation and acceptance.* Features of the third stage include significant feelings of apathy and depression. This phase takes a year or more. Physical illness is common and includes problems such as insomnia, asthma, bowel dysfunction, headache and appetite disturbances.

Pathological bereavement

Pathological bereavement can occur and may manifest as intense emotion, particularly anger, and multiple visits with somatic complaints; the patient often gets around to long dissertations about the deceased and the circumstances surrounding death. Extreme anger is likely when the sense of rejection is great as with divorce or sudden death. Guilt can also be intense.[9]

Raphael's classification of the patterns of pathological grief and its various resolutions are presented in Table 5.2.[10]

The GP as counsellor[1]

Important rules to bear in mind:

- The bereaved may be feeling very guilty.
- They may be angry towards their doctor or the medical profession in general.
- They need a clear explanation as to the exact cause and manner of death. Autopsy reports should be obtained and discussed.
- The bereaved tend to view an apparent lack of concern and support as disinterest or guilt.[9]
- Early intervention averts pathological grief.

The general practitioner probably had a close relationship with the deceased and the family. The GP will have a special awareness of those at

Table 5.2 *Patterns and resolution of pathological grief*[10]

Morbid or pathological patterns
- Absence, inhibition or delay of bereavement
- Distorted bereavement
- Chronic grief (intense anguish continues unabated)

Outcome
- Normal resolution, satisfactory adjustment; reintegration in life, satisfying attachments
- General symptomatology (leading to increased care eliciting behaviour)
- Depression, suicidal behaviour
- Other psychiatric disorders (anxiety state, phobia, mania, alcoholism, criminal activity such as shoplifting)
- Altered relationship patterns
- Vulnerability to loss
- Anniversary phenomenon
- Death (more likely in the first 12 months)

risk and the nature of the relationships within the family. The family is likely to maintain the relationship with the GP, expressing the physical and psychological effects of grief and consulting about intercurrent problems.[9]

Working through the stages of grief with patients will allow general practitioners to reach some acceptance of their own emotions, as well as ensure that patients feel supported and cared for, rather than distanced by embarrassment.

Help from religious sources is highly valued as it can meet both spiritual and personal needs. Other resources include funeral directors, hospice (and other) counsellors and support groups such as those for sudden infant death syndrome.[9]

At least 30 minutes should be allowed for consultations.

Long-term counselling

Normal bereavement can persist for years. Ongoing counselling is indicated if it continues unabated or psychiatric referral sought if grief is extreme. Regular enquiries during routine consultations or meetings are important if the patient appears to be coping.

Breaking bad news

Good communication skills are fundamental to giving bad news appropriately. When bad news is broken insensitively or inadequately the impact can be distressing for both giver and recipient, leaving lasting scars for the latter.

Doctors should have a plan for this difficult process and learn how to cope with the recipient's reaction. Most of the circumstances described apply to unexpected death.

Optimal approach

Some basic initial rules:[11]
- If relatives have to be contacted it is preferable for the doctor (if at all possible) or a sympathetic police officer to make the contact personally, rather than a relatively matter-of-fact telephone call from the hospital or elsewhere.
- If a telephone message is necessary it should be given by an experienced person.
- The relatives or close friends should not drive to the clinic alone.

The setting for the interview:
- Use a suitable quiet private room if possible.
- See the recipients of the news alone in the room.
- Advise that the meeting should be undisturbed.

Guidelines for the doctor

- Always ask those involved if they have heard any news or know the reasons for the consultation.
- Always assess their understanding.
- Give information in an unhurried, honest, balanced, empathic manner.[12]
- Look directly at the person you are talking to, be honest and direct, and keep information simple (avoid technical language).
- The sad news must be accompanied by positive support, understanding and encouragement.
- Give recipients time to react (offer time and moments of silence to allow the facts to sink in) and opportunities to ask questions.
- Avoid false reassurance.
- Remember that relatives appreciate the truth and genuine empathy.
- In the event of death, relatives should be given a clear explanation of the cause of death.

A list of guidelines for the interview is summarised in Table 5.3.[11]

Coping with patient responses

- The responses cover a wide range—stunned silence, disbelief, acute distress, anger, extreme guilt.
- Be prepared for any of these responses.
- Appropriate training using simulated patients,

Table 5.3 *Breaking bad news: Recommended actions during the interview*

Allow
- time
- opportunities to react
- silence
- touching
- free expression of emotions
- questions
- viewing of a dead or injured body

Avoid
- rushing
- bluntness
- withholding the truth
- platitudes
- protecting own inadequacies
- euphemisms
- the notion 'nothing more can be done'

Source: After McLauchlan[11]

video replays and skilled feedback improves communication skills.
- Give permission and encouragement for reactions such as crying and screaming.
- Have a box of facial tissues available.
- A comforting hand on the shoulder or arm or holding a hand is an acceptable comfort zone.
- Offer a cup of tea or a cool drink if available.
- Ask the patients or relatives how they feel, what they would like to do and if they want you to contact anyone.
- Arrange follow-up.
- Give appropriate patient education material.
- Provide information about support services.

The depressed patient
Studies have emphasised the importance and therapeutic efficacy of counselling in the management of the depressed patient.[13] The most practical approach by the general practitioner to the depressed patient is empathy, support and a logical explanation of their malaise. The author gives the following explanation to the patient.

Depression is a very real illness that affects the entire mind and body. It seriously dampens the five basic activities of humans, namely their energy for activity, sex drive, sleep, appetite and ability to cope with life. They cannot seem to lift themselves out of their misery or fight it themselves. Superficial advice to 'snap out

of it' is unhelpful because the person has no control over it.

The cause is somewhat mysterious but it has been found that an important chemical is present in smaller amounts than usual in the nervous system. It is rather like a person low in iron becoming anaemic.

Depression can follow a severe loss such as the death of a loved one, a marital separation or financial loss. On the other hand it can develop for no apparent reason although it may follow an illness such as glandular fever or influenza, an operation or childbirth.

Emphasising the 'missing chemical' theory really helps patients and family come to terms with an illness that tends to have socially embarrassing connotations. It also helps compliance with therapy when antidepressant medication is prescribed.

Ongoing contact, support and availability are an important component of counselling with appropriate referral to someone with more expertise, should that be required.

Chronic pain
Patients suffering from long-term pain are a special problem, especially those with back pain who seem to be on a merry-go-round of failed multiple treatments and complex psychosocial problems. These patients are frequently treated in pain clinics. As family doctors we often observe an apparently normal, pleasant person transformed into a person who seems neurotic, pain-driven and doctor-dependent. The problem is very frustrating to the practitioner, often provoking feelings of suspicion, uncertainty and discomfort.

De Vaul et al.[14] list five subgroups of patients where perplexing pain presents as the major symptom.[3]

1. Pain as a symptom of depression
2. Pain as a delusional symptom of psychosis
3. Pain as a conversion symptom of hysterical neurosis
4. Pain as a symptom of an unresolved bereavement reaction
5. Pain as a symptom of a 'need to suffer'

Patients who somatise their symptoms present one of the most difficult challenges to our skills and usually require a multidisciplinary team approach.

Management involves:

- thorough medical assessment
- psychological assessment

- detailed explanations to the patient and family about treatment
- rational explanations about the cause of the pain
- management of associated problems, e.g. depression, sexual dysfunction
- behavioural modification to encourage increased activity and a gradual return to normality

A useful explanation

The author finds the following account a most useful method of explaining perplexing continuing back pain or neuralgia to patients (where there is no evidence of a persisting organic lesion).

Part of the problem is that psychological factors continue to aggravate and maintain the problem even though the reason for the pain in the first place may have disappeared. It is a similar problem to a person who has had a painful leg amputated. Even though it has been removed, the patient can still feel the leg and maybe even the pain. The patient has a 'phantom limb'. The nervous system, especially the brain, can play funny tricks on us in this way.

This means that even though the original disc injury has settled after several weeks, the body can still register the pain. This is more likely to occur in people who have become anxious and depressed about their problem. The pain continues. Someone once described it as a 'tension headache that has slipped down to the back'.

References

1. Hassed C. Counselling. In: Final Year Handbook. Melbourne: Monash University, Department of Community Medicine, 1992, 97–104.

2. Ramsay AT. The general practitioner as an effective counsellor. Aust Fam Physician, 1990; 19:473–479.

3. Harris RD, Ramsay AT. *Health care counselling*. Sydney: Williams and Wilkins, 1988, 68–95.

4. Annon JS. *The behavioural treatment of sexual problems*. Vols 1 and 2. Honolulu: Enabling Systems Inc, 1974.

5. Craig S. A medical model for infertility counselling. Aust Fam Physician, 1990; 19:491–500.

6. Cook H. Counselling in general practice: Principles and strategies. Aust Fam Physician, 1986, 15:979–981.

7. Frank JF. Foreword. In: Traux CB, Carkhuff RR, *Towards effective counselling and psychotherapy: Training in practice*. New York: Aldine, 1967:ix.

8. Traux CB, Carkhuff RR. *Towards effective counselling and psychotherapy*. New York: Aldine, 1967.

9. Williams AS. Grief counselling. Aust Fam Physician, 1986; 15:995–1002.

10. Raphael B. *The anatomy of bereavement: A handbook for the caring professions*. London: Hutchinson, 1984, 33–62.

11. McLauchlan CAJ. Handling distressed relatives and breaking bad news. In: Skinner D, *ABC of major trauma*. London: British Medical Association, 1991, 102–106.

12. Cunningham C, Morgan P, McGucken R. Down syndrome: Is dissatisfaction with disclosure of diagnosis inevitable? Devel Med Child Neurol, 1984; 26:33–39.

13. Jackson HJ, Moss JD, Solinski S. Social skills training: An effective treatment for unipolar non-psychotic depression? Aust & NZ J Psychiatry, 1985; 19:342–353.

14. De Vaul RA, Zisook S, Stuart HJ. Patients with psychogenic pain. J Fam Prac, 1977; 4(1):53–55.

6

Difficult, demanding and angry patients

—

There are patients in every practice who give the doctor and staff a feeling of 'heartsink' every time they consult.

Thomas O'Dowd 1988

Weston defines a 'difficult patient' as one with whom the physician has trouble forming an effective working relationship.[1] However it is more appropriate to refer to difficult problems rather than difficult patients—it is the patients who have the problems while doctors have the difficulties.

Some characteristics of problematic patients, from the doctor's perspective, include:

• frequent attenders with trivial illness
• multiple symptomatology
• undifferentiated illness
• chronic tiredness
• negative investigations
• dissatisfaction with treatment, especially procedures
• non-compliant
• hostile or angry
• attending multiple therapists
• demanding on staff
• inconsiderate of the doctor's time
• taking multiple drugs
• seductive, then demanding
• garrulous
• manipulative
• taciturn and uncommunicative
• all knowing

Such patients are often referred to as the 'heartsink' patients,[2] referring to that certain sinking feeling on seeing them in the waiting room or their name on the booking list. They can provoke negative feelings in us and we have to discipline ourselves to be patient, responsible and professional.

An inevitably poor consultation will follow if we allow feelings of hostility to affect our communication with the difficult patient, especially the demanding, angry or 'compo' patient.

However it is important not to misdiagnose organic disease and also to consider the possibilities of the following disorders, which may be masked:

• anxiety
• depression
• obsessive compulsive disorder
• bipolar disorder (manic depression)
• drug dependency
• alcohol abuse
• schizophrenia

It is therefore appropriate to maintain traditional standards by continually updating the data-base, integrating psychosocial aspects, carefully evaluating new symptoms, conducting an appropriate physical examination and being discriminating with investigations.

Management strategies

Our professional responsibility is to rise above interpersonal conflict and facilitate productive communication by establishing a caring and responsible relationship with such patients. An appropriate strategy is to follow Professor Aldrich's precepts[3] for the 'difficult' patients who do not have an organic disorder or a psychiatric illness.

1. Give up trying to cure them—they are using their symptoms to maintain their relationship with you: accept them as they are.
2. Accept their symptoms as expressions of their neurosis. Make a primary positive diagnosis—only test if you have to.
3. Structure a program for them, e.g. 'Mrs Jones, I have decided that we should meet for 15 minutes every second Wednesday at 10 a.m.'
4. During the consultation, demonstrate your genuine interest in the person's life, garden, work and so on; show less interest, even boredom, for the litany of complaints.

Other management guidelines include:

- Use reassurance with caution—it is insufficient by itself and should be soundly based.
- Be honest and maintain trust.
- Allow the patient a fair share of your time—this is your part of the contract. At the same time indicate that there are limits to your time (set rules).
- Be polite yet assertive.
- Avoid using labels of convenience and placebo therapy.
- Be honest about your understanding (or lack of understanding) of the problems.
- Remember that the consultation is often the therapy, without a prescription.
- Do not undermine other doctors. Avoid collusion.
- Have limited objectives—zealous attempts to cure may be inappropriate.
- Do not abandon the patient, however frustrating the relationship. Accept this as a legitimate role.
- Remain available if alternative therapies are sought by the patient.
- Take extra care with the 'familiar' patient and sometimes the patient who brings gifts. Maintain your professional role.
- If you are uncomfortable with counselling, consider early referral to a counsellor while maintaining contact in the future.
- You may have to accept that there are some people no one can help.

A 'heartsink' survival kit

A pilot workshop of managing 'heartsink' patients described by Mathers and Gask[4] led to the formulation of a 'heartsink survival' model for the management of patients with somatic symptoms of emotional distress.

The first part of the three-part model, which is called 'feeling understood', includes a full history of symptoms, exploration of psychosocial cues and health beliefs, and a brief focused physical examination. In the second stage, termed 'broadening the agenda', the basic aim is to involve discussion of both emotional and physical aspects during the consultation. It includes reframing the patient's symptoms and complaints to provide insight into the link between physical, psychological and life events.

In the third stage, 'making the link', simple patient education methods are used to explain the causation of somatic symptoms such as the way in which stress, anxiety or depression can exaggerate symptoms. It also includes projection or identification techniques using other sufferers as examples.

The angry patient

Anger in patients and their relatives is a common reaction in the emotive area of sickness and healing. The anger, which may be concealed or overt, might be a communication of fear and insecurity. It is important to bear in mind that many apparently calm patients may be harbouring controlled anger. The practice of our healing art is highly emotive and can provoke feelings of frustration and anger in our patients, their friends and their relatives.

Anger is a normal and powerful emotion, common to every human being, yet with an enormous variety of expression. The many circumstances in medicine that provoke feelings of anger include:[5]

- disappointment at unmet expectations
- crisis situations, including grief
- any illness, especially an unexpected one
- the development of a fatal illness
- iatrogenic illness
- chronic illness, such as asthma
- financial transactions, such as high cost for services
- referral to colleagues, which is often perceived as failure
- poor service, such as long waits for an appointment
- problems with medical certificates
- poor response to treatment

- inappropriate doctor behaviour, e.g. brusqueness, sarcasm, moralistic comments, aloofness, superiority

The patient's anger may manifest as a direct confrontation with the doctor or perhaps with the receptionist, with litigation or with public condemnation.

In an extreme example, a Melbourne doctor was shot and killed by an angry patient who had been denied a worker's compensation certificate for a claim considered unjustified.

When a patient expresses anger about the medical profession or our colleagues it may be directed at us personally and, conversely, if directed to us it may be displaced from someone else such as a spouse, employer or other figure of authority.

What is anger?

Anger is a person's emotional response to provocation or to a threat to his or her equilibrium. If inappropriate, it is almost always the manifestation of a deeper fear and of hidden insecurity. Angry abusive behaviour may be a veiled expression of frustration, fear, self-rejection or even guilt.

On the other hand, its expression may be a defence against the threat of feeling too close to the doctor, who could have an overfamiliar, patronising or overly friendly attitude towards the patient. Some patients cannot handle this threatening feeling.

Basically anger may be a communication of fear and insecurity. The patient could be saying, 'I am afraid there is something seriously wrong with me. Are you doing everything to help me?'

Consulting strategies[6]

When one feels attacked unfairly, to react with anger is a natural human response. This response, however, must be avoided since it will damage the doctor–patient relationship and possibly aggravate the problem.

- The initial response should be to remain calm, keep still and establish eye contact.
- 'Step back' from the emotionally charged situation and try to analyse what is happening.
- Ask the patient to sit down and try to adopt a similar position (the mirroring strategy) without any aggressive pose.
- Address the patient (or relative) with appropriate name, be it Mr or Mrs Jones or a first name.

- Appear comfortable and controlled.
- Be interested and concerned about the patient and the problem.
- Use clear, firm, non-emotive language.
- Listen intently.
- Allow patients to ventilate their feelings and help to relieve their burdens.
- Allow patients to 'be themselves'.
- Give appropriate reassurance (do not go overboard to appease the patient).
- Allow time (at least 20 minutes).

Analysing the responses

- Search for any 'hidden agenda'.
- Recognise the relationship between anger and fear.

Recognising distress signals

It is important to recognise signs of deteriorating emotional distress:[7]

- body language (demonstrative agitated movements or closing in)
- speech (either becoming quiet or more rapid and louder)
- colour (either becoming flushed or pale)
- facial expression (as above, tense, tightening of muscles of eye and mouth, loss of eye contact)
- manner (impatient, threatening)

Skilful consulting strategies should then be employed. It is worthwhile having a contingency plan such as memorising a telephone number to summon security help.

Questions to uncover the true source of anger

The following represent some typical questions or responses that could be used during the interview.

Rapport building
'I can appreciate how you feel.'
'It concerns me that you feel so strongly about this.'
'Tell me how I can make it easier for you.'

Confrontation
'You seem very angry.'
'It's unlike you to be like this.'
'I get the feeling that you are upset with . . .'
'What is it that's upsetting you?'
'What really makes you feel this way?'

Facilitation, clarification

'I find it puzzling that you are angry with me.'

'So you feel that . . .'

'You seem to be telling me . . .'

'If I understand you correctly . . .'

'Tell me more about this . . .'

'I would like you to enlarge on this point—it seems important.'

Searching

'Do you have any special concerns about your health?'

'Tell me about things at home.'

'How are things at work?'

'How are you sleeping?'

'Do you have any special dreams?'

'Do you relate to anyone who has a problem like yours?'

'If there's any one thing in your life that you would like to change, what would it be?'

Some important guidelines are summarised in Table 6.1.

Table 6.1 *Guidelines for handling the angry patient*

Do	Don't
Listen	Touch the patient
Be calm	Meet anger with anger
Be comfortable	Reject the patient
Show interest and concern	Be a 'wimp'
Be conciliatory	Evade the situation
Be genuine	Be overfamiliar
Allay any guilt	Talk too much
Be sincere	Be judgmental
Give time	Be patronising
Arrange follow-up	
Act as a catalyst and guide	

Management

When confronted with an angry patient the practitioner should be prepared to remain calm, interested and concerned. It is important to listen intently and allow time for the patient to ventilate his or her feelings.

A skilful consultation should provide both doctor and patient with insight into the cause of the anger and result in a contract in which both parties agree to work in a therapeutic relationship. The objective should be to come to amicable terms which, of course, may not be possible, depending on the nature of the patient's grievance.

If the problem cannot be resolved in the time available a further appointment should be made to continue the interview.

Sometimes it may be appropriate to advise the patient to seek another opinion. If the angry patient does have problems with relationships and seeks help, it would be appropriate to arrange counselling so that the patient acquires a more realistic self-image, thus leading to improved self-esteem and effectiveness in dealing with people. In addition it should lead to the ability to withstand frustration and cope with the many vicissitudes of life—a most rewarding outcome for a consultation that began with confrontation.

References

1. McWhinney I. *A textbook of family medicine*. New York: Oxford, 1989, 96–98.

2. O'Dowd TC. Five years of 'heartsink' patients in general practice. BMJ, 1988; 297:528–530.

3. Elliott CE. 'How am I doing?' Med J Aust, 1979; 2:644–645.

4. Mathers NJ, Gask L. Surviving the 'heartsink' experience. Fam Practice, 1995; 12:176–183.

5. Murtagh JE. The angry patient. Aus Fam Physician, 1991; 20:388–389.

6. Mongtomery B, Morris L. *Surviving: Coping with a crisis*. Melbourne: Lothian, 1989, 179–186.

7. Lloyd M, Bor R. *Communication skills for medicine*. London: Churchill Livingstone, 1996, 135–137.

7

Palliative care

—

When the cancer that later took his life was first diagnosed, Senator Richard L. Neuberger remarked upon his 'new appreciation of things I once took for granted—eating lunch with a friend, scratching my cat Muffet's ears and listening to his purrs, the company of my wife, reading a book or magazine in the quiet of my bed lamp at night, raiding the refrigerator for a glass of orange juice or a slice of toast. For the first time, I think I actually am savouring life'.

Better Homes and Gardens magazine

Palliative care is an approach to the management of a person with a terminal illness. It implies that at some point in the management process there is a change from the objective of curing the disease to that of controlling and alleviating symptoms.[1]

To enable a person to live in dignity, peace and comfort throughout their illnesses means responding to physical, psychological, emotional, social and spiritual needs.[1]

Palliative care is comprehensive, continuing, multidisciplinary patient care that involves the patients and their carers, consultants, domiciliary nurses, social workers, clergy and other health professionals who are able to contribute to optimal team care.

The fundamental principles of palliative care are:[2]

- good communication
- management planning
- symptom control
- emotional, social and spiritual support
- medical counselling and education
- patient involvement in decision making
- support for carers

The diseases

Palliative care applies not only to incurable malignant disease and HIV/AIDS but also to several other diseases such as end-stage organ failure (heart failure, renal failure, respiratory failure and hepatic failure) and degenerative neuromuscular diseases.

The special role of the family doctor

The general practitioner is the ideal person to manage palliative care for a variety of reasons—availability, knowledge of the patient and family, and the relevant psychosocial influences. A key feature is the ability to provide the patient with independence and dignity by managing palliative care at home. Someone has to take the responsibility for leadership of the team and the most appropriate professional is a trusted family doctor.

Most patients and their families require answers to six questions:[3]

- What is wrong?
- What can medical science offer?
- Will I suffer?
- Will you look after me?
- How long will I live?
- Can I be looked after at home?

Caring honesty is the best policy when discussing the answers to these questions with the patient and family. Never lie to a patient and avoid thoughtless candour.

Support for patients and carers

Studies have indicated that the most common complaints of patients are boredom and fear of the unknown. This highlights the importance for the attending doctor of the following points:

- Give emotional support.
- Listen and be receptive to unexpressed 'messages'.
- Treat the sufferer normally, openly, enthusiastically and confidently.
- Show empathy and compassion.
- Employ good communication skills.
- Give honest answers without labouring the point or giving false hope.
- Provide opportunities for questions and clarification.
- Show an understanding of the patient's needs and culture.
- Adopt a whole person approach: attend to physical, psychosocial and spiritual needs.
- Anticipate and be prepared for likely problems.

Special points worth emphasising are:

- The patient needs a feeling of security.
- Provide reassurance that the patient will not suffer unnecessarily.
- Be prepared to take the initiative and call in others who could help, e.g. clergy, cancer support group, massage therapists.
- Patients must not be made to feel isolated or be victims of the so-called 'conspiracy of silence' in which families collude with doctors to withhold information from the patient.
- The worst feeling a dying patient can sense is one of rejection and discomfort on the part of the doctor.
- Always be prepared to refer to an oncologist or appropriate therapist for another opinion about further management. The family and patient appreciate the feeling that every possible avenue is being explored.

Note: Always establish what the patient knows and wants to know.

Symptom control
Common symptoms
- boredom (the commonest symptom)
- loneliness/isolation
- fear
- pain
  — physical
  — emotional
  — spiritual
  — social
- anorexia
- nausea and vomiting
- constipation

The grief reaction

This follows five stages, as identified by Kübler-Ross:[4]

1. denial and isolation
2. anger
3. bargaining
4. depression
5. acceptance

This model provides a useful guideline in understanding the stages a patient and family will be experiencing.

The principles of symptom management are summarised in Table 7.1, and the goals of treatment according to the different stages of cancer are presented in Figure 7.1.

Table 7.1 *Principles of symptom management*[2]

Determine the cause.

Treat simply.

Provide appropriate explanation of symptoms and treatment.

Provide regular review.

Give medication regularly around the clock, not ad hoc.

Plan 'breakthrough' pain-relieving doses.

Provide physical treatment as necessary
   e.g. paracentesis, pleural tap, nerve block.

Provide complementary conservative therapy
   e.g. massage, physiotherapy, occupational therapy, dietary advice, relaxation therapy.

Provide close supervision.

Pain control in cancer

Achieving pain relief is one of the most important functions of palliative care and patients need reassurance that they can expect such relief. The principles of relief of cancer pain are:[1]

1. Treat the cancer.
2. Raise the pain threshold:
   - Provide appropriate explanation.
   - Allow the patient to ventilate feelings and concepts.
   - Give good psychosocial support.
   - Use antidepressants or hypnotics.
3. Add analgesics according to level of pain, e.g. opioids (if necessary).
4. Use specific drugs for specific pain—not all pain responds to analgesics (refer Table 7.2).
5. Set realistic goals.
6. Organise supervision of pain control.

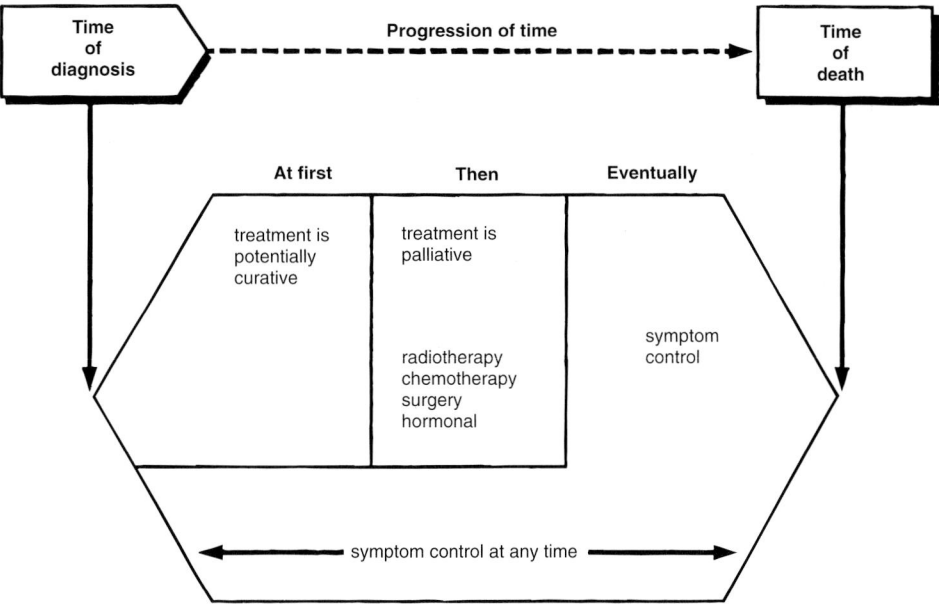

Fig. 7.1 *Stages of cancer management: the goals of treatment differ according to the different stages*
AFTER J. BUCHANAN ET AL.[6]

Table 7.2   *Treatment options for cancer pain[5] (based on aetiology)*

Aetiology	1st line treatment	2nd line treatment	Other treatment modalities to consider
Nociceptive pain (stimulation sensory nerves)	aspirin	opioids corticosteroids antidepressants NSAIDs	radiotherapy neurosurgery
Neuropathic pain (direct nerve involvement) e.g. brachialgia, sciatica	opioids antidepressants antiepileptics e.g. carbamazepine		spinal morphine local anaesthetic
Dysaesthesia: superficial burning pain	antidepressants	opioids	local anaesthetic TENS
Pressure pain • Tumour-associated oedema, e.g. raised intracranial pressure	corticosteroids aspirin	opioids	radiotherapy neurosurgery
Bony metastases and other tissue destruction •	NSAIDs aspirin	opioids	radiotherapy (the most effective) hormones orthopaedic surgery
Muscle spasm pain	diazepam clonazepam baclofen	opioids	
Viscus (hollow organ) obstruction, e.g. colic, tenesmus	antispasmodics	opioids chlorpromazine corticosteroids	palliative surgery radiotherapy
Metabolic effects • Hypercalcaemia	biphosphonates (APD)		
Skin infiltration/ulceration	aspirin opioids	corticosteroids	treat infection dressings palliative surgery radiotherapy

Note: The right drug, in the right dose, given at the right time relieves 80–90% of the pain.[1]

Use of analgesics[5]

These should be given by the clock and administered according to the three-step method:

> Step 1: Mild pain

Start with basic non-opioid analgesics:
    aspirin 600–900 mg (o) 4 hourly (preferred)
                        or
    paracetamol 1 g (o) 4 hourly

> Step 2: Moderate pain

Use low dose or weak opioids or in combination with non-opioid analgesics (consider NSAIDs):
    add morphine 5 to 10 mg (o) 4 hourly
                        or
    oxycodone up to 10 mg (o) 4 hourly
                        or
    30 mg, rectally, 8 hourly

> Step 3: Severe pain

Maintain non-opioid analgesics. Larger doses of opioids should be used and morphine is the drug of choice:
    morphine 10 mg (o) 4 hourly
                        or
    morphine SR tabs or caps (o) 12 hourly

- Give dosage according to individual needs (morphine SR comes in 10, 20, 30, 50, 60, 100, 200 mg tablets or capsules).
- The proper dosage is that which is sufficient to alleviate pain.
- The usual starting dose is 20–30 mg bd.
- Give usual morphine 10 mg with first dose of morphine SR and then as necessary for 'rescue dosing'.
- Gauge the probable dose of the long-acting morphine from the standard dosage.
- To convert to morphine SR calculate the daily oral dose of regular morphine and divide by 2 to get the 12 hourly dose.
- Do not crush or chew the tablets or capsules.

Guidelines

- Ensure that pain is likely to be opioid-sensitive.
- Give morphine orally (if possible) either by mixture or tablets.
- Starting doses are usually in the range of 5–20 mg (average 10 mg).
- If analgesia is inadequate, the next dose should be increased by 50% until pain control is achieved.
- Give it regularly, usually 4 hourly, before the return of the pain (see Fig. 7.2).
- Many patients find a mixture easier to swallow than tablets, e.g. 10 mg/10 mL solution.

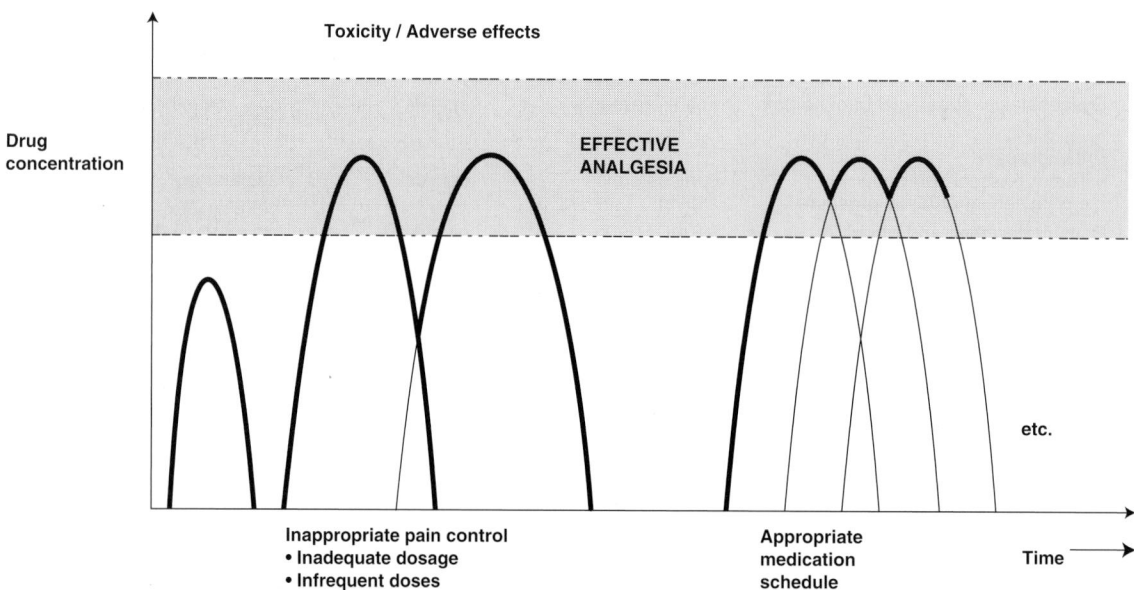

Fig. 7.2 *Appropriate scheduling of analgesia to achieve optimal pain control*

- Constipation is a problem, so treat prophylactically with regular laxatives and carefully monitor bowel function.
- Order a 'rescue dose' (usually 5 mg) for breakthrough pain or anticipated pain (e.g. going to toilet).
- Order antiemetics, e.g. haloperidol prn at first (usually can discontinue in 1 to 2 weeks as tolerance develops).
- Reassure the patient and family about the safety and efficacy of morphine (see Table 7.3). (Beware of opiophobia.)
- Using morphine as a mixture with other substances, e.g. Brompton's cocktail, has no particular advantage.
- Pethidine is not recommended (short half-life, toxic metabolites) and codeine and IM morphine should be avoided.
- Other opioids are sometimes used instead of morphine (Table 7.4).
- Fentanyl is a potent synthetic opioid which is available as a transdermal system.

Parenteral morphine
This is generally given subcutaneously (not IV or IM). Indications are:[6]

1. Unable to swallow, e.g. severe oral mucositis; dysphagia; oesophageal obstruction
2. Bowel obstruction
3. Severe nausea and vomiting
4. At high oral dose, i.e. above 100–200 mg dose, there appears to be no additional benefit from further dose increments.

Adjuvant therapy
Refer to Table 7.2.

In all three steps of pain control consider the use of adjuvant 'analgesics'; while not strictly speaking analgesics, they contribute to pain

Table 7.3 *Common myths about morphine* [5]

- Morphine is a last resort.
  This is not so, and there is no maximum dose.
- The patient will become addicted.
  This is rare and probably irrelevant in the context of palliative care.
- The patient will need ever-increasing amounts.
  The drug does not lose its effect but is usually increased according to disease progression.
- Morphine will cause respiratory depression.
  This is rarely a problem and may even help those with dyspnoea. An overdose can be reversed with an injection of naloxone.
- Morphine will shorten life.
  The reverse may in fact apply. It is not being used for euthanasia but to control pain.

relief. Examples are corticosteroids, antidepressants, psychotropic agents and anticonvulsants.

Pain control
Bone pain
- aspirin, paracetamol, NSAIDs are helpful co-analgesics

Neuropathic pain (direct involvement of nerves)
- antidepressants, e.g. amitriptyline
- anticonvulsants, e.g. carbamazepine

Neurological pressure
- corticosteroids for spinal cord compression and raised intracranial pressure
  e.g. dexamethasone 4–16 mg (o) daily
  or
  prednisolone 25–100 mg (o) daily

Continuous subcutaneous infusion of morphine
When the oral and/or rectal routes are not possible or ineffective a subcutaneous infusion with a syringe pump can be used.

Table 7.4 *Non-morphine opioids used in pain control* [1]

Opioid	Duration of action (hours)	Dose equivalent to oral morphine 10 mg
Codeine	3–5	60 mg
Oxycodone		
Endone (oral)	3–5	10 mg
Proladone (rectal)	6–12	10 mg
Methadone	variable 8–24	15 mg
Dextromoramide (Palfium)	2	20 mg
Fentanyl (transdermal)	72	100 mg

It is also useful for symptom control when there is a need for a combination of drugs, e.g. for pain, nausea and agitation. It may avoid bolus peak effects (sedation, nausea or vomiting) or trough effects (breakthrough pain) with intermittent parenteral morphine injections.

Practical aspects

- Access to the subcutaneous space is via a 21 g butterfly needle, which is replaced regularly (1, 2, 3 or 4 days).
- Most regions are suitable. The more convenient are the abdomen, the anterior thigh, and the anterior upper arm (usually the anterior abdominal wall is used).
- The infusion can be managed at home.
- About one-half to two-thirds of the 24 hour oral morphine requirement is placed in the syringe.
- The syringe is placed into the pump driver, which is set for 24 hour delivery.
- Areas of oedema are not suitable.

Spinal morphine

Epidural or intrathecal morphine is sometimes indicated for pain below the head and neck, where oral or parenteral opioids have been ineffective. It is necessary to insert an epidural or intrathecal catheter (anaesthetist or neurosurgeon).[5]

Common symptom control

Common symptoms can be controlled as follows:[1]

Anorexia

metoclopramide 10 mg tds
    or
corticosteroids, e.g. dexamethasone 2–8 mg tds
high-energy drink supplements

Constipation

If opioids need to be maintained, the laxatives need to be peristaltic stimulants, not bulk-forming agents. Aim for firm faeces with bowels open about every third day.

e.g. senna (Senokot) 2 daily or bd
    bisacodyl (Durolax) 5–10 mg bd

Rectal suppositories, microenemas or enemas may be required, e.g. Microlax.

Shaw's cocktail is useful for severe constipation. With a small quantity of water melt one tablespoon of Senokot granules in a microwave oven. Add 20 mL Agarol and constitute to 100 mL with cold milk or ice-cream.

Death rattles

Hyoscine 0.4–0.8 mg, 4–8 hourly, can be used to dry secretions and stop the 'death rattle'.

Dyspnoea

Identify the cause, such as a pleural effusion, and treat as appropriate. Pleural taps can be performed readily in the home. Corticosteroids can be given for lung metastases. Oxygen may be necessary to help respiratory distress in the terminal stages and bedside oxygen can be readily obtained. Morphine can be used for intractable dyspnoea, together with haloperidol or a phenothiazine for nausea.

Terminal distress/restlessness[7,8]

(exclude reversal causes, e.g. drugs, fear, faecal impaction, urinary retention)

1st choice: clonazepam 0.3–0.5 mg SC bolus
                 12 hourly[7] or (o)
                 drops
          or   2–4 mg over 12 hours
                 in SC syringe driver
          midazolam very effective but
          expensive

If very severe: add phenobarbitone as SC
                 infusion
                 or (with care because of
                 fitting) haloperidol

Nausea and vomiting

If due to morphine:
    haloperidol 1.5–5 mg daily[1]
        can be reduced after 10 days
            or
    prochlorperazine (Stemetil)
        5–10 mg (o) qid
            or
        25 mg rectally bd

Consider ondansetron (Zofran) for nausea and vomiting induced by cytotoxic chemotherapy and radiotherapy.

Cerebral metastases

Common symptoms are headache and nausea. Consider corticosteroid therapy e.g. dexamethasone 4–16 mg daily. Analgesics and antiemetics such as haloperidol are effective.

Paraplegia

Paraplegia is especially prone to occur with carcinoma of the prostate, even when treated with LHRH analogues. The warning signs are the development of new back pain, paraesthesia in limbs or the recent development of urinary retention.[1] The objective is to prevent paraplegia developing. High-dose corticosteroids are given while arranging urgent hospital admission.

Hiccoughs

Try a starting dose of
chlorpromazine 25 mg tds or 25 mg IM as bolus
              or
haloperidol 2.5 mg bd
Swallowing granulated sugar with or without vinegar does not appear to be effective.

Weakness and weight loss

This problem may be assisted by a high-calorie and high-protein diet. A list of high-energy drink supplements is provided in *Palliative care: The nitty gritty handbook.*[1]

Examples
Banana Sustagen milk

• milk	2 cups
• banana	one
• egg	one
• Sustagen powder	3 dessertspoons
• skim milk powder	1 dessertspoon
• Glucodin	1 dessertspoon
• ice	crushed

(Vitamise all together.)

Egg flip

• egg	one
• milk	one cup
• vanilla syrup or essence	to taste (1–3 drops)
• sugar	1 teaspoon
• brandy	(optional)

(Vitamise all together, strain, sprinkle with nutmeg.)
High-energy cordial

• cordial	1 tablespoon
• Glucodin	1 teaspoon
• water	1 cup
• ice	crushed

(Blend cordial and Glucodin till smooth, stir in water.)

High-energy juice

• juice	1 cup
• Glucodin	1 dessertspoon

(Blend Glucodin with a little juice till smooth. Stir in remaining juice.)

The AIDS patient

The same principles of management apply to the person suffering from the many manifestations of terminal AIDS. Many of these patients wish to die at home and there are excellent caring support groups to help. It is important to become acquainted with the service network. Because of opportunistic infections there are many challenges facing the palliative care of such patients and some management guidelines are included in Chapter 24.

Dying and grieving

The stages of the grieving process as described by Kübler-Ross may be experienced by both the patient and family, albeit not exactly according to the five stages. The grieving process following the death of a loved one can vary enormously but many people are devastated.

The principles of care and counselling include:[1]

- Be available and be patient.
- Allow them to talk while you listen.
- Reassure them that their feelings are normal.
- Accept any show of anger passively.
- Avoid inappropriate reassurance.
- Encourage as much companionship as possible, if desired.

(See guidelines for crisis counselling given in Chapter 5.)

Communicating with the dying patient

Good communication is essential between the doctor and patient in order to inform, explain, encourage and show empathy. However, it can be very difficult, especially with the cancer patient.

Good communication is dependent on honesty and integrity in the relationship. Telling the truth can be painful and requires sensitivity, but it builds trust that enables optimal sharing of other difficult concerns and decisions such as abandoning curative treatment, explaining the dying process and perhaps addressing thoughts on euthanasia.

Improved communication will lead not only to better 'spiritual' care but also to better symptom control.[1] Give patients every opportunity to talk about their illness and future expectations, and be available and patient in offering help and support.

Spiritual issues

Spirituality is an important issue for all people, especially when faced with inevitable death. Many people are innately spiritual or religious and those with deep faith and a belief in 'paradise' appear to cope better with the dying process. Others begin to reflect seriously about spirituality and search for a meaning for life in this situation; carers, including the attending doctor, should be sensitive to their needs and turmoil and reach out a helping hand, which may simply involve contacting a minister of religion.

Spiritual care builds on patients' existing resources to enable them to rise above the physical, emotional and social effects of their terminal illness.[1]

The question of euthanasia

It should be a rare experience to be confronted with a request for the use of euthanasia,[3] especially as the media clichés of '*extreme* suffering' and 'agonising death' are rarely encountered in the context of attentive whole-person continuing care. The non-use of life support systems, the use of 'round the clock' morphine, cessation of cytotoxic drugs, the use of ancillary drugs such as antidepressants and antiemetics, various nerve blocks and loving attention almost always help the patient cope without undue pain and suffering.

Practice tips

- Consider prescribing antidepressants routinely for patients in pain.
- Remember the 'sit down rule' whereby the home visit is treated as a social visit—sitting down with the patient and family, having a 'cuppa' and sharing medical and social talk.[3]
- Early referral of terminal patients with difficult-to-control problems, especially pain, to a hospice or multidisciplinary team can enhance the quality of care. However the patient's family doctor must still be the focus of the team.

References

1. Fairbank E, Banks T. *Palliative care: The nitty gritty handbook*. Melbourne: RACGP Services Division, 1993, 1–18.
2. McGuckin R, Currow D, Redelman P. Palliative care: Your role. Medical Observer, 27 November 1992, 41–42.
3. Carson NE, Miller C. *Care of the terminally ill*. Melbourne: Monash University Department of Community Medicine Handbook, 1993, 107–115.
4. Kübler-Ross E. *On death and dying*. London: Tavistock, 1970.
5. Moulds RFW et al. *Analgesic guidelines*. Melbourne: Victorian Medical Postgraduate Foundation, 1992–93, 39–48.
6. Buchanan J et al. *Management of pain in cancer*. Melbourne: Sigma Clinical Review, 1991; 18:8–10.
7. Burke AL. Palliative care: An update on 'terminal restlessness'. Med J Aust, 1997; 166:39–42.
8. Twycross R. *Introducing palliative care*. Oxford: Radcliffe Medical Press, 1996, 147.

8
The elderly patient

—

Last scene of all,
That ends this strange eventful history,
Is second childishness, and mere oblivion,
Sans teeth, sans eyes, sans taste, sans everything
(sans = without)

William Shakespeare (1564–1616)
As You Like It

The ageing (over 65 years) are the fastest growing section of the Australian population. The number of 'old-old' (over 85 years) is increasing at an even faster rate.[1]

The over 65s in 1988 made up 10.8% of the Australian population (12% in the United States). It is expected that this group will make up 13.4% in 2011 and 20% in the year 2031. A similar trend is expected in the United States with 13% by the year 2000 and 18% in 2040.[2]

The over 65s use twice the number of health services per head of population. They account for 25% of all hospital costs and 75% of all nursing home costs. They represent 25% of all general practice consultations.[1] Many are affected by multisystem disease. All are affected to a greater or lesser extent by the normal physiological changes of organ ageing.

Ageing is characterised by the following:[1]

- decrease in metabolic mass
- reduction in the functional capacity of organs
- reduced capacity to adapt to stress
- increased vulnerability to disease
- increased probability of death

Age-associated deterioration occurs with hearing, vision, glucose tolerance, systolic blood pressure, renal function, pulmonary function, immune function, bone density, cognitive function, mastication and bladder function.

One of the main contributing factors is the problem of disuse. Encourage exercise, especially walking and water aerobics.

Ageing and disease

Degenerative cardiovascular disease emerges with ageing according to the following approximate guidelines:

aged 40	—	obesity
50	—	diabetes
55	—	ischaemic heart disease
65	—	myocardial infarction
70	—	cardiac arrhythmias
75	—	heart failure
80	—	cerebrovascular accidents

Deterioration in health and the 'masquerades'

Unexpected illness including mental confusion (one of the major hallmarks of disease in the elderly) can be caused commonly by any of the so-called masquerades outlined in Chapter 15:

- depression
- drugs, including alcohol
- diabetes mellitus
- anaemia
- thyroid disease
- urinary tract infection
- neurological dilemmas
  - Parkinson's disease
  - cerebrovascular accident
- infections, e.g. bronchopneumonia
- neoplasia
- giant cell arteritis/polymyalgia rheumatica

Common significant management disorders encountered in the elderly include:

- hypertension
- ischaemic heart disease and heart failure
- depression
- diabetes (NIDDM)
- dementia
- social and physical isolation

- osteoarthritis
- disorders of the prostate
- urinary incontinence
- locomotive (lower limb) disorders
  - neurological
    - peripheral neuropathy
    - ataxia
  - claudication due to vascular insufficiency
  - other peripheral vascular disease
  - claudication due to spinal canal stenosis
  - sciatica/nerve root paresis
  - osteoarthritis: hips, knees, feet
  - foot disorders, e.g. ingrown toenails
  - leg ulceration

Important problems affecting the elderly are presented in Figure 8.1.

The 'classic' triad[3]

Be mindful of the classic triad:

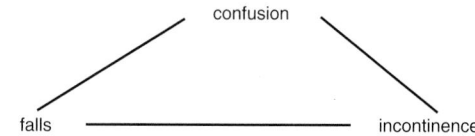

This can represent non-specific signs of acute illness, particularly infection. Aggressive antibiotic treatment is worth considering while awaiting the results of culture or clinical developments.

Changes in sensory thresholds and homeostasis

A clinically significant feature in some elderly patients is the raising of the pain threshold and changes in homeostatic mechanisms such as temperature control. Consequently these patients may have an abnormal response to diseases such as appendicitis, pyelonephritis, internal abscess, pneumonia and septicaemia. There may be no complaints of pain and no significant fever but simply general malaise and abnormal behaviour such as . delirium, agitation and restlessness.

Establishing rapport with the elderly patient

The elderly patient especially requires considerable support, understanding, caring and attention from a general practitioner who can instil confidence and security in a patient who is likely

to be lonely, insecure and fragile. This means taking time, showing a genuine interest and a modicum of humour, and always leaving detailed instructions.

One of the best ways to generate a good relationship is through home visitation. The value of home visits can be considered under the concepts of the Royal Australian College of General Practitioners.[4]

1. Assessment, both initial and continuing: 'You don't know your patient until you've visited their home'.
2. Continuing care:
   - security to the patient
   - support for 'caring' family
   - effective monitoring/intervention role
   - effective liaison with patient/family
   - checking medication

Home visits can be considered in three categories:

1. an 'unexpected' visit (especially to a new patient)
2. a patient-initiated but routine request for a 'check-up and tablets'
3. the regular call—usually 2 to 4 weeks

These home visits are a 'security gesture' to the patient—evidence that they are supported in their desire to remain independent for as long as possible in their own home. They strengthen the patient–doctor relationship as a position of trust, which is of special importance to frail, elderly people feeling increasingly insecure and threatened.

If the patient is being supported by a spouse or relative the doctor can provide continuous reassurance and support to all concerned as well as continual assessment, both physical and mental. Finally, the home visit may become part of the terminal care of a dying patient, something that is very important to the elderly patient. Home visits can enhance the quality of life, both physical and mental, of an ageing person.

Doctor behaviour that can irritate and confuse elderly patients

Ellard[5] has written a most interesting paper, based on a compendium of complaints by the elderly about their doctors, on behaviour that upsets the elderly.

- Having a consulting room with slippery steps, poor lighting and inadequate handrails

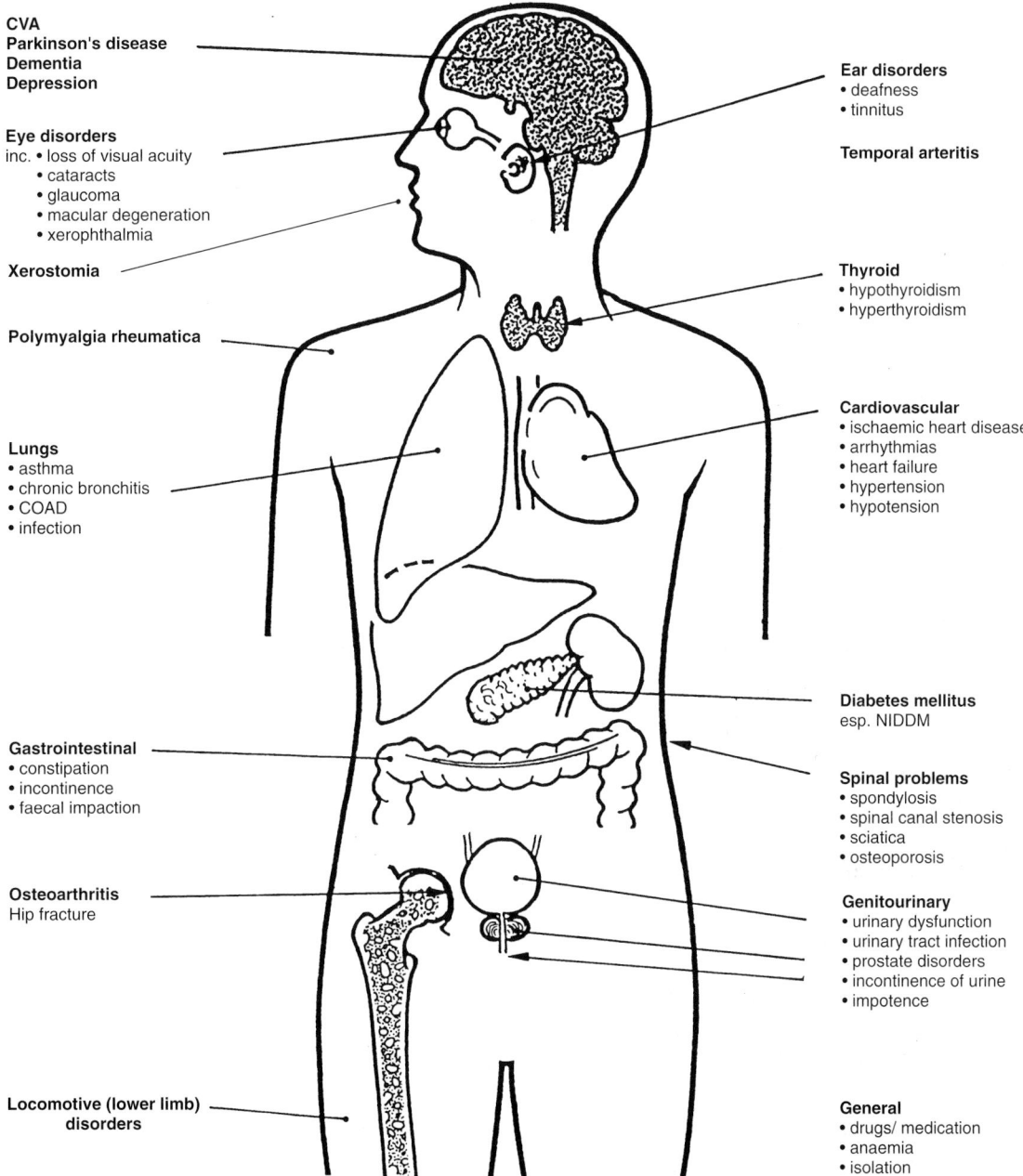

Fig. 8.1 *Significant problems affecting the elderly*

CVA
Parkinson's disease
Dementia
Depression

Eye disorders
inc. • loss of visual acuity
    • cataracts
    • glaucoma
    • macular degeneration
    • xerophthalmia

Xerostomia

Polymyalgia rheumatica

Lungs
• asthma
• chronic bronchitis
• COAD
• infection

Gastrointestinal
• constipation
• incontinence
• faecal impaction

Osteoarthritis
Hip fracture

Locomotive (lower limb)
    disorders

Ear disorders
• deafness
• tinnitus

Temporal arteritis

Thyroid
• hypothyroidism
• hyperthyroidism

Cardiovascular
• ischaemic heart disease
• arrhythmias
• heart failure
• hypertension
• hypotension

Diabetes mellitus
esp. NIDDM

Spinal problems
• spondylosis
• spinal canal stenosis
• sciatica
• osteoporosis

Genitourinary
• urinary dysfunction
• urinary tract infection
• prostate disorders
• incontinence of urine
• impotence

General
• drugs/ medication
• anaemia
• isolation

- Non-attention to simple courtesies by receptionist staff
- Keeping them waiting
- Having low soft chairs in the waiting room and surgery
- Being overfamiliar, with addresses such as 'Pop' or first names for elderly females
- Shouting at them on the assumption that they are deaf
- Appearing rushed and keen to get the consultation over quickly
- Forgetting their psychosocial problems and concentrating only on their physical problems, i.e. not treating the whole person

- Forgetting that they have several things wrong with them and using a different priority list from theirs
- Being unaware that they may have seen other practitioners or may be taking additional medication
- Failing to ask patients to give their understanding of what is wrong
- Omitting to give printed patient education handouts about their problems and medications
- Omitting to explain how the medication will work
- Treating them as though they would have little comprehension of their health and treatment
- Failing to respect their privacy such as not knocking before entering the examination room
- Failing to provide appropriate advice on various social services such as meals on wheels and other support groups
- Failing to re-evaluate carefully their health and medication
- Failing to take steps to reverse any deterioration in their health including reluctance to refer

Assessment of the elderly patient

The initial consultation should include a thorough clinical examination on the traditional lines of history, physical examination and selective laboratory investigation. At regular intervals during continuing care this careful assessment may need to be repeated.

History

The medical history may be difficult to obtain and the help of a family member is recommended. The use of questionnaires, which can be completed at leisure at home with the help of family members, is most helpful as complementary to the medical interview.

Important specific areas to focus on are:

- previous medical history and hospitalisation
- immunisation status
- medications and OTC drugs
- alcohol intake, smoking
- problem list of complaints
- dependence on others
- members of household
- household problems

- comforts: heating, cooling, bedding, etc.
- ambulation/mobility
- meals: diet
- hygiene: bathing
- toileting: continence
- teeth: condition, ? dentures
- vision
- hearing (always ask about this)
- systems review, especially:
  — genitourinary function
  — gastrointestinal
  — cardiorespiratory
- locomotion including feet
- nervous system, ? falls, giddiness, faints
- emotional and mental health
- evidence of depression
- history of bereavement
- history of abuse by carers, family members
- financial/insurance status

A thorough family history and psychosocial history is of prime importance. At all times concentrate on a general assessment of the patients' ability to communicate by evaluating mental status, comprehension, hearing, vision, mood and speech.

Physical examination

The routine for the physical examination is similar to that of the younger adult but certain areas require more attention. The elderly patient expects to be examined adequately (especially having the blood pressure measured) but requires appropriate dignity. It is recommended that the practice nurse supervise dressing and undressing and prepares the patient for examination.

The following areas should be examined.

Practice nurse

- prepares for examination
- helps with questionnaire
- records weight and height
- takes temperature, pulse and respiration
- checks audiometry (if hearing problem)
- checks ocular tension (if appropriate)
- prepares cervical smear tray for female patient (if relevant)

Doctor

- general appearance including skin, hair and face (evaluate nutritional status)
- mental status examination (Fig. 8.2)[6]
- eyes: visual acuity

Introduction

'I'd like to ask you some questions about your health.'
'What's your sleep been like?'_____ 'Your appetite?'_____
'Your interest?'_____ 'Your energy?'_____ 'Your concentration?'_____
'What's your memory like these days? Do you mind if I test it?'

Memory registration

'What I want to do is give you three things I want you to try to remember for me. First I want you to repeat them, then in a few minutes I'll ask you how many you can recall. Here are the three things I want you to remember for me.'
'MELBOURNE, CRICKET, BLUE.'

—/3 'Can you repeat them for me?' (Score number of attempts required —/3, for example, CORRECT FIRST TRY = 3; SECOND TRY = 2; THIRD TRY = 1)
'Good, now can you try to remember those three things for me, because I'm going to ask you to recall them shortly. But first I'd like to get you to do some things that might interfere with your memory.'

Attention and concentration

'First I'd like you to count out loud from 1 to 20.'_____
'Now could you count backwards from 20 to 1.'_____
'Next can I get you to spell the word WORLD for me?'_____ WORLD

—/5 'Now can you try to spell WORLD backwards for me?' _D_L_R_O_W

Memory recall

'Now what were those three words I asked you to remember for me?'

—/3 SPONTANEOUS RECALL: _____ MELBOURNE, _____ CRICKET, _____ BLUE
Optional: Cued recall (___ City, ___ Sport, ___ Colour)
Recognition (List four cities, four sports, four colours)

Language

'Sometimes as people get older they have trouble remembering words, the right word. Does that ever happen to you?'
'Well, let's see. What do you call this?'

—/1 ___ PEN (Optional more difficult items ___ Cap ___ Point)
—/1 ___ WATCH (Optional difficult items ___ Strap ___ Winder)
'Can I get you to repeat a sentence, exactly as I say it?'
—/1 NO IFS, ANDS OR BUTS _____
'Can I get you to do three things with this envelope?'
—/3 'PICK IT UP WITH YOUR LEFT HAND ___, FOLD THE ENVELOPE IN HALF ___ and PUT THE ENVELOPE ON THE FLOOR' ___
'Can you read what's written on the envelope and do what it says?'
—/1 'CLOSE YOUR EYES' (Written in large letters)
'Can you write a sentence for me on the back?'
—/1 SENTENCE (should contain subject and object and make sense)

Orientation

'Can you put your address on the envelope?'
—/5 NUMBER ___ , STREET _____ , SUBURB/CITY _____ , STATE _____ , COUNTRY _____ .
'Can you put today's date on the back?'
—/5 DATE _____ , MONTH _____ , YEAR _____ , DAY _____ , SEASON _____ .

Visuospatial skills

'Can you make a COPY of this figure for me?'
—/1
—/30 *Total score:* Probable cognitive impairment < 24
Definite cognitive impairment < 17

Fig. 8.2 *A practical adaptation of the mini-mental state examination*   ADAPTED FROM M.F. FOLSTEIN, S.E. FOLSTEIN AND P.R. McHUGH, MINI-MENTAL STATE J PSYCH RESEARCH, 1975, 12:189

- ears: simple hearing test; auroscopic examination
- oral cavity, including teeth and gums
- neck especially thyroid
- lungs: consider peak flow meter
- pulse and blood pressure (repeat)
- heart; breasts
- abdomen; hernial orifices
- spine
- lower limbs: joints; circulation; feet including nails

- gait
- men: rectal examination; scrotum and testes
- women: cervical smear if appropriate

The mini-mental status examination

Evidence of memory difficulty remains the best single indicator of dementia and should always be evaluated by formal memory testing. However, memory problems may be due to factors other than dementia, and demonstrating failure in other areas of cognitive functioning (language, spatial ability, reasoning) is necessary to confirm the diagnosis of dementia.[6] A number of screening tests are available but the mini-mental status examination depicted in Figure 8.2 can be used.

Laboratory investigations

The laboratory tests should be selected according to the evaluation of the patient and to costs versus potential benefits.

Recommended investigations for suspected dementia include:[8]

• renal function
• hepatic function
• thyroid function
• full blood screen
• blood glucose
• serum electrolytes (especially if on diuretics)
• urinalysis
• serum B_{12} and folate
• syphilis serology
• chest X-ray
• computerised tomography

Behavioural changes in the elderly

As general practitioners we are often called to assess abnormal behaviour in the elderly patient, with the question being asked, 'Is it dementia?' or 'Is it Alzheimer's, doctor?'

There are many other causes of behavioural changes in people over the age of 65 years and dementia must be regarded as a diagnosis of exclusion. The clinical presentation of some of these conditions can be virtually identical to early dementia.

The clinical features of early dementia include:

• poor recent memory
• impaired acquisition of new information
• mild anomia (cannot remember names)
• personality change, e.g. withdrawn, irritable
• minimal visuospatial impairment, e.g. tripping easily
• inability to perform sequential tasks

The differential diagnosis for behavioural changes apart from dementia include several other common and important problems (which must be excluded) and can be considered under a mnemonic for dementia.[7]

D	drugs and alcohol depression
E	ears eyes
M	metabolic, e.g. hyponatraemia diabetes mellitus hypothyroidism
E	emotional problems, e.g. loneliness
N	nutrition: diet, e.g. Vitamin B group deficiency, teeth problems
T	tumours ⎫ trauma ⎭ of CNS
I	infection
A	arteriovascular disease → cerebral insufficiency

All these conditions should be considered with the onset of deterioration in health of the elderly person. Even apparently minor problems such as the onset of deafness (e.g. wax in ears), visual deterioration (e.g. cataracts), diuretic therapy, poor mastication and diet, urinary tract intercurrent infection, boredom and anxiety can precipitate abnormal behaviour.

Elder abuse

It is important to keep in mind the possibility of abuse of the elderly, especially where there is a family history of abuse of members. The issue is as important as child and spouse abuse. Over 1 million elderly people are estimated to be the victims of physical or psychological abuse each year in the United States.[3] We should keep in mind the occasional possibility of Munchausen's syndrome by proxy.

Depression and dementia

The main differential diagnosis of dementia is depression, especially major depression, which is termed pseudodementia. The mode of onset is one way in which it may be possible to distinguish between depression and dementia. Dementia has a slow and surreptitious onset that is not clear-cut, while depression has a more definable and clear-cut onset that may be precipitated by a specific incident. Patients with dementia have no insight while those with depression have insight, readily give up tasks, complain bitterly and become distressed by their inability to perform their normal enjoyable tasks.

In response to cognitive testing, the typical response of the depressed patient is 'don't know', while making an attempt with a near miss typifies the patient with dementia (see Table 8.1).

Table 8.1 *Comparison of dementia and pseudodementia (commonly severe depression)*

	Dementia	Pseudodementia
Onset	Insidious	Clear cut, often acute
Course over 24 hours	Worse in evening or night	Worse in morning
Insight	Nil	Present
Orientation	Poor	Reasonable
Memory loss	Recent > remote	Recent = remote
Responses to mistakes	Agitated	Gives up easily
Response to cognitive testing (questions)	Near miss! Difficulty understanding	'Don't know' Slow and reluctant but understands words (if co-operative)

It is vital to detect depression in the elderly as they are prone to suicide. 'Nothing to look back on with pride and nothing to look forward to.' The middle-aged and elderly may not complain of depression, which can be masked. They may present with somatic symptoms or delusions.

Dementia (chronic organic brain syndrome)

The incidence of dementia increases with age, affecting about 1 person in 10 over 65 years and 1 in 5 over 80 years. The important causes of dementia are:

- degenerative cerebral diseases including Alzheimer's disease (60%)
- vascular (15%)
- alcohol excess[8]

The characteristic feature is impairment of memory. Abstract thinking, judgment, verbal fluency and the ability to perform complex tasks also become impaired. Personality may change, impulse control may be lost and personal care deteriorates.[8]

The DSM-III (R) criteria for dementia are presented in Table 8.2 and clinical clues suggesting dementia in Table 8.3.

The many guises of dementia can be considered in terms of four major symptom groups.[6]

1. Deficit presentations: due to loss of cognitive abilities, including
   - forgetfulness
   - confusion and restlessness
   - apathy (usually a late change)
   - self-neglect with no insight
   - poor powers of reasoning and understanding
2. Unsociable presentations: based on personality change, including
   - uninhibited behaviour

- risk taking and impulsive behaviour
- suspicious manner
- withdrawn behaviour

3. Dysphoric presentations: based on disturbed mood and personal distress, including
   - depression (hopeless and helpless)
   - irritability with emotional outbursts
   - lack of co-operation
   - insecurity
4. Disruptive presentations: causing distress and disturbance to others, including
   - aggressive, sometimes violent, behaviour
   - agitation with restlessness

The problem occasionally results in marked emotional and physical instability. It is sad and difficult for relatives to watch their loved ones develop aggressive and antisocial behaviour, such as poor table manners, poor personal cleanliness, rudeness and a lack of interest in

Table 8.2 *DSM-III (R) criteria for dementia*

Diagnosis of dementia requires evidence of:

A Memory impairment

B At least one of the following:
  1. Abstract thinking impairment
  2. Impaired judgment
  3. Disturbed higher cortical functions:
     - Language = aphasia
     - Motor actions = apraxia
     - Recognition = agnosia
     - Constructional difficulties

C Personality change

D Disturbance significantly interferes with work, social interactions or relationships

E Not due to delirium or other disorders, e.g. major depression

Source: Diagnostic and Statistical Manual (3rd edn Revised). Washington, DCA: American Psychiatric Association, 1987.

Table 8.3 *Clinical clues suggesting dementia*

1. Patient presentations
   - new psychological problems in old age
   - ill-defined and muddled complaints
   - uncharacteristic behaviour
   - relapse of physical disorders
   - recurrent episodes of confusion

2. Problems noted by carers
   - 'not themselves'—change in personality, e.g. humourless
   - domestic accidents, especially with cooking and heating
   - unsafe driving
   - false accusations
   - emotional, irritable outbursts
   - tendency to wander
   - misplacing or losing items, e.g. keys, money, tablets, glasses
   - muddled on awakening at night

3. Mental state observations
   - vague, rambling or disorganised conversation
   - difficulty dating or sequencing past events
   - repeating stock phrases or comments
   - playing down obvious, perhaps serious, problems
   - deflecting or evading memory testing

Source: After McLean[6]

others. Sometimes severe problems such as violent behaviour, sexual promiscuity and incontinence will eventuate.

There is always the likelihood of accidents with household items such as fire, gas, kitchen knives and hot water. Accidents at the toilet, in the bath and crossing roads may be a problem, especially if combined with failing sight and hearing. Such people should not drive motor vehicles.

Without proper supervision they are likely to eat poorly, neglect their bodies and develop medical problems such as skin ulcers and infections. They can also suffer from malnutrition and incontinence of urine or faeces.

Management of suspected dementia

Exclude reversible or arrestable causes of dementia.
- full medical history (including drug and alcohol intake)
- mental state examination
- physical examination
- investigations (see page 413)

Management of dementia

There is no cure for dementia—the best that can be offered to the patient is tender loving care.

Education, support and advice should be given to both patient and family. Multidisciplinary evaluation and assistance are needed. Regular home visits by caring sympathetic people are important. Such people include relatives, friends, general practitioners, district nurses, home help, members of a dementia self-help group, religious ministers and meals on wheels. The sufferers tend to manage much better in the familiar surroundings of their own home and this assists in preventing behaviour disturbance.

Special attention should be paid to organising memory aids such as lists, routines and medication, and to hygiene, diet and warmth. Adequate nutrition, including vitamin supplements if necessary, has been shown to help.

Associated problems [8]

Depression can occur early in dementia and requires intervention. Demented patients are vulnerable to superimposed delirium which is often due to:
- urinary tract infection
- other febrile illness
- prescribed medication
- drug withdrawal

Delirium should be suspected if a stable patient becomes acutely disturbed.

Medication [8]

Demented patients often do not require any psychotropic medication. Antidepressant drugs can be prescribed for depression. Tacrine appears to be ineffective but donepezil (5–10 mg/day) and rivastigmine (6–12 mg/day) appear to delay progression of dementia to a modest extent.

To control psychotic symptoms or disturbed behaviour probably due to psychosis:

olanzapine 2.5–10 mg (o) daily

or

risperidone 0.5–2 mg (o) daily

To control symptoms of anxiety and agitation use:

oxazepam 15 mg (o) 1 to 4 times daily

but benzodiazepines should be used only for short periods as they tend to exacerbate cognitive impairment in dementia.

Paraphrenia

Paraphrenia is that condition where the symptoms and signs of paranoid psychosis appear for the first time in the elderly. In this non-psychotic mental illness, the patient, who is usually an elderly female, presents with paranoid delusions such as a feeling of being watched or persecuted. These are usually associated with visual and hearing problems.

Falls in the elderly

Falls in the elderly are a major problem as 30% of people over the age of 65 experience at least one fall per year with 1 in 4 of these having significant injury. About 5% of falls result in fracture.[9]

The main causes are:

- neurological, e.g. cerebrovascular disease
- sensory impairment, e.g. visual, vestibular
- cardiovascular, e.g. postural hypotension
- musculoskeletal, e.g. arthritis, foot disorders
- cognitive and psychological conditions, e.g. dementia, delirium
- medication/drug related, e.g. sedatives, alcohol
- physiological changes, e.g. gait disorders
- environmental factors, e.g. slipping or tripping
- combinations of the above

The most significant clinical risk factors for falls have been shown to be visual impairment, impaired general function, postural hypotension, hearing impairment, drug usage especially sedatives, decreased lower limb strength, and impaired balance and gait.

Assessment

The history should embrace the above causes and risk factors. In particular a description of the fall by a witness, the perceived dysfunction at the time of the fall and whether there was loss of consiousness is particularly important.

The physical examination should include cardiac function, neurological status including the mini-mental function test and the musculo-skeletal system including assessment of gait. The 'get up and go' test (Table 8.4) is useful.

As special investigations (especially for those proving difficult to evaluate) consider full blood examination and ESR, blood sugar, urea and electrolytes, thyroid function tests, cardiac investigations e.g. ambulatory ECG monitoring, ambulatory blood pressure monitoring, vestibular function testing, and CT scans or MRI scan.[10]

Management and prevention

Steps should be taken to correct any medical disorders and risk factors. It is appropriate to refer to a multidisciplinary team including occu-

Table 8.4 *The 'get up and go' test: A brief test of postural competence*

1. Get up from chair without use of arms.
2. Observe normal gait and 360° turn.
3. Carry out the Romberg test (slight push with eyes closed).
4. Observe tandem walking (heel toe, straight line).

pational therapists and physiotherapists. Assessment of circumstances in the home is very helpful. This may lead to reducing environmental hazards and providing walking aids.

Adverse drug reactions

Ageing is associated with increased rates of adverse drug reactions.[1] The rate of adverse drug reactions for a single medication rises from about 6% at age 20 years to about 20% at age 70 years.

For less than six medications taken concurrently the rate of adverse drug reactions is about 6%. For greater than six medications taken concurrently the rate of adverse drug reactions jumps to 20%.[1]

Factors predisposing to adverse drug reactions in the elderly[1]

Most adverse drug reactions in the elderly are entirely predictable. Most are merely an extension of the pharmacological action of the drug, e.g. all antihypertensives will reduce blood pressure and have the capacity to cause hypotension and falls in a person with impaired baroreceptor function or poor homeostasis in their vascular tree. Very few adverse reactions are idiosyncratic or unexpected.

The five mechanisms of adverse drug reactions in the elderly are:

1. *Drug–drug interaction*
   e.g. beta-blockers given concomitantly with digoxin increases the risk of heart block and bradycardia.

   Alcohol used in combination with antidepressants increases the risk of sedation.

2. *Drug–disease interaction*
   e.g. in the presence of renal impairment, tetracyclines carry an increased risk of renal deterioration.

3. *Age-related changes leading to increases in drug plasma concentration*
Decreased renal excretion can extend the half-life of medication, leading to accumulation and toxicity.

4. *Age-related changes leading to increased drug sensitivity*
e.g. there is some suggestion that the pharmacological response to warfarin, narcotics and benzodiazepines is increased in the elderly. Conversely the pharmacological response to insulin, theophylline and beta adrenergic blocking agents is thought to be decreased.

5. *Patient error*
Multiple medications can lead to patient error. The incidence and prevalence of dementia also increases with age.

Increasing the number of simultaneous medications increases the risk for all five mechanisms of adverse drug reactions.

In a study on adverse drug reaction in elderly patients the drugs most frequently causing admission to hospital were:[11]

• digoxin
• diuretics
• antihypertensives (including beta-blockers)
• psychotropics and hypnotics
• analgesics and NSAIDs

The same study showed that drugs regularly prescribed without revision were:

• barbiturates
• benzodiazepines
• antidepressants
• antihypertensives
• beta-blockers
• digoxin
• diuretics

Drug regimens should be kept as simple as possible to aid compliance and avoid or minimise drug interactions.

The elderly may need much lower doses of anxiolytics and hypnotics than younger patients to produce the same effect, thus rendering them more susceptible to adverse effects and toxicity. The elderly are especially liable to accumulate the longer-acting benzodiazepines.

In particular, any drug or combination of drugs with anticholinergic properties, e.g. tricyclic antidepressants, antiparkinsonian agents, antihistamines, phenothiazines and some cold remedies, can precipitate a central anticholinergic syndrome.[8]

Starting medications[8]

The starting dose of a drug in the aged[8] should be at the lower end of recommended ranges. Dosage increments should be gradual and reviewed regularly.

That is, start low, go slow and monitor frequently. It is important to individualise doses for the elderly.

References

1. Harris E. *Prescribing for the ageing population.* Update Course Proceedings Handbook, Melbourne: Monash University Medical School, 1992.

2. Sloane PD, Slatt LM, Baker RM. *Essentials of family medicine.* Baltimore: Williams and Wilkins, 1988, 49–56.

3. Mold JW. Principles of geriatric care. American Health Consultants. Primary care reports. 1996, 2(1):2–9.

4. Lang D. Home visits to the elderly. Aust Fam Physician, 1993; 22:264.

5. Ellard J. How to irritate and confuse your elderly patients—20 simple rules. Mod Med Aust, 1990; 7:66–68.

6. McLean S. Is it dementia? Aust Fam Physician, 1992; 21:1762–1776.

7. Turnbull JM. *Dementia and depression in the elderly.* California: AUDIO DIGEST family practice, 1993; 41:10.

8. Mashford ML (Chairman). *Psychotropic drug guidelines* (3rd edn). Victorian Medical Postgraduate Foundation, 1996–97, 77–79.

9. Hindmarsh JJ, Estes H. Falls in older persons: Causes and intervention. Arch Int Med, 1989; 149: 2217.

10. Quail GG. An approach to the assessment of falls in the elderly. Aust Fam Physician, 1994; 23:873–883.

11. Briant RH. Medication problems of old age. Patient Management, 1988; 5:27–31.

9
Prevention in general practice

—

When meditating over a disease, I never think of finding a remedy for it, but, instead, a means of preventing it.

Louis Pasteur 1884

Definitions[1]

Prevention may be defined as the means of promoting and maintaining health or averting illness.

It is concerned with removal or reduction of risks, early diagnosis, early treatment, limitation of complications, including those of iatrogenic origin, and maximum adaptation to disability.

The promotion of health concerns helping well people to learn healthy behaviours and to accept responsibility for their own well-being.

A preventive attitude implies that the doctor understands and can utilise the preventive potential in each primary care consultation by an 'opportunistic approach'. In addition to the traditional management of both presenting and continuing problems, the doctor takes the opportunity to modify the patient's health-seeking behaviour, to provide education about the illness, and to promote health by relating the patient's present condition to previous unhealthy behaviour.

Primary prevention

Primary prevention includes action taken to avert the occurrence of disease. As a result there is no disease. Primary preventive strategies include:

1. education to bring about changes in lifestyle factors known to be associated with diseases, e.g. smoking cessation, healthily balanced diets, reduction in alcohol intake, exercise
2. sterilisation of surgical instruments and other medical equipment
3. eradication as with vector control of mosquitoes to prevent malaria
4. immunisation against infective diseases
5. sanitation, keeping our water supplies clean and disposing efficiently of sewage and industrial wastes
6. legislation to ensure that some of these primary preventive measures are carried out.

Secondary prevention

Secondary prevention includes actions taken to stop or delay the progression of disease.

The term is usually applied to measures for the detection of disease at its earliest stage, i.e. in the presymptomatic phase, so that treatment can be started before irreversible pathology is present. The early recognition of hypertension through routine testing (screening) of patients allows treatment during the presymptomatic phase of the illness process. Screening for cervical cancer allows the treatment of cervical dysplasia, a premalignant condition. Other examples include mammography and endoscopy for polyps of the large bowel.

Tertiary prevention

Tertiary prevention includes the management of established disease so as to minimise disability.

The term is usually applied to the rehabilitation process necessary to restore the patient to the best level of adaptation possible when there has been damage of an irreversible nature. A patient who has suffered a stroke because of hypertension may be restored to a useful lifestyle with appropriate rehabilitation.

Relationship between types of prevention

It can be seen that there is a clearer demarcation between primary and secondary prevention than between secondary and tertiary prevention, although the latter term is particularly useful in dealing with the elderly and the handicapped. Conceptually, curative medicine falls within the definitions of secondary and tertiary prevention while public health measures are mainly concerned with primary prevention. Prevention is really wider than medical practice but because of the success of public health practices in the past, more attention is now being focused on prevention by doctors (see Fig. 9.1).[2]

As general practitioners our role in prevention is twofold:

1. First, we can recognise the preventable factors that are involved in an illness process and determine appropriate interventions.
2. Second, we can act to implement the preventive measure. In cases where the responsibility rests with the individual or the community, doctors can support prevention through education, applying political pressure or working with community agencies.

The practice of preventive medicine by the doctor

What is preventable?

The first step in the implementation of prevention is to define which specific diseases can be prevented and to what extent, given certain restraints such as human resources, technology and the cost to the community. All diseases have a potential preventability but it may be unrealistic to try to achieve this.

Diseases that can be prevented can be grouped according to their aetiology. They fall into the following broad categories:

- genetic disorders
- conditions occurring during pregnancy and the puerperium
- developmental disorders
- accidents
- infections
- addictions
- behavioural disorders
- occupational disorders
- premature vascular disease
- neoplasms

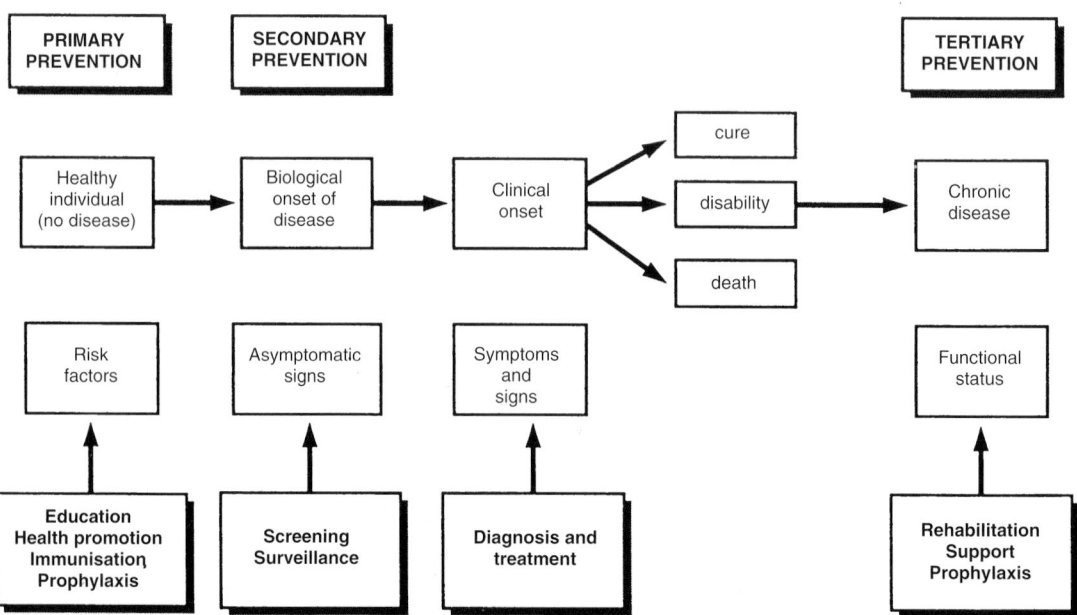

Fig. 9.1 *The phases of prevention in relation to the natural history of disease*

- handicap in the disabled
- certain 'other' diseases, e.g. diverticular disease

Mortality is the only reliable index by which the outcome of preventive activities can be judged. Conditions can be ranked in importance as causes of premature death according to the 'person years of life lost before 70 years' as follows:[1]

Accidents, poisoning and violence	29%
Neoplasms	19%
Circulatory diseases	17%
Perinatal conditions	10%
Congenital conditions	7%

This gives quite a different perspective to prevention and explains why the efforts of public health authorities and practising doctors do not always coincide.

The interventions available to us in medical practice are as follows:
1. educational—health promotion, health education and illness education
2. screening
3. surveillance
4. interventional care—immunisation, behaviour modification and drug prophylaxis
5. Rehabilitation

Optimal opportunities for prevention

Primary prevention *par excellence* can be practised in general practice under the opportunities provided by the following clinical circumstances:

- antenatal care
- postnatal care
- advising people travelling overseas
- visits by infants with their parents
- times of crisis or potential crisis
- the premarital check-up

The Royal College of General Practitioners (UK) has identified the seven most important opportunities for prevention as:
1. family planning
2. antenatal care
3. immunisation
4. fostering the bonds between mother and child
5. discouragement of smoking

6. detection and management of raised BP
7. helping the bereaved

Mortality and morbidity considerations

An understanding of the mortality and morbidity patterns in the modern human being is essential to the planning of preventive programs. The great infectious diseases of the past, such as tuberculosis, syphilis, smallpox, influenza, diphtheria and streptococcal infections, have been largely contained but other diseases have become prominent as life expectancy increases. The great modern diseases are atherosclerosis (hardening of the arteries), malignant disease (cancer), HIV infection and iatrogenesis (doctor-induced illness).

These diseases and the common causes of mortality (Table 9.1) act as a focus for our energies in addressing preventive programs.

It is worth focusing on the changes in disease indices during the past generation in order to evaluate the effect of preventive and health promotion programs during this period (Table 9.2).[3] The messages are to harness and promote with renewed vigour those strategies that are working, such as prevention of death from coronary artery disease and motor vehicle accidents, and to re-evaluate those important areas such as Aboriginal mortality, HIV infection, cancer, suicide and asthma which are bad news!

A global strategy for good health

The World Health Organisation defines good health as 'a state of dynamic harmony between the body, mind and spirit of a person and the social and cultural influences which make up his or her environment'.

A considerable amount of epidemiological information has emerged to support what

Table 9.1 *Common causes of deaths in Australia*

Circulatory disease		
Ischaemic heart disease	25% }	
Cerebrovascular disease	10% }	35%
Malignant disease		27%
Respiratory disease		8%
Accidents, poisoning and violence		6%
Digestive disease		3%

Source: Australian Institute of Health & Welfare, 1996.

Table 9.2 *Apparent changes in disease indices 1960–1988*

Improvements	No change or deterioration
Overall mortality	Aboriginal mortality
Heart attack	(minor improvement)
Stroke	Cancers
Unintentional injuries/	—pancreas
poisonings	—breast
—motor vehicle	—skin
—drownings	—lung (women)
—falls	—prostate
—occupational injury	AIDS
Most infectious diseases	Alcohol-related diseases
Cancer of lung (men)	Drug abuse
Cervical cancer (women)	Asthma
Cancer of stomach	Senile dementia
Unintentional pregnancies	STDs
Violence/homicide	Suicide in the young
Pregnancy complications	Cirrhosis
Congenital abnormalities	Musculoskeletal disorders
Dental health	
Perinatal complications	
Chronic bronchitis	

Source: G. Egger, R. Spark and J. Lawson, *Health promotion strategies and methods*, McGraw-Hill, Sydney, 1990, 2–3.

general practitioners have known for a long time—that a common-sense healthy lifestyle not only promotes good health but also reduces the risk of the main causes of mortality and morbidity in this country, including cardiovascular disease and cancer.

The common theme for virtually all disease is to follow the guidelines below.

Diet

- Keep to ideal weight.
- Take a high-fibre diet.
- Eat more fruits and vegetables, breads and cereals (preferably wholegrain).
- Eat fish at least twice a week.
- Eat less saturated fat, refined sugar and salt.
- Avoid 'fast foods' and deep-fried foods.
- Do not eat animal meat every day and then eat small portions.
- Always trim fat off meat.
- Use olive oil for cooking in preference to polyunsaturated oils.
- Drink more water.
- Limit caffeine intake: 0–3 drinks a day (maximum).
- Check plasma cholesterol and if elevated aim to reduce it with diet.

Lifestyle and mental health

- Do not smoke.
- Do not imbibe alcohol or, if one must, limit it to no more than two standard drinks a day— reserve alcohol for special occasions and to only one occasion in the day.
- Take regular exercise, e.g. 30 minutes per day for 3 days per week.
- Practise relaxation.
- Partake in ample recreational activities.
- Encourage a circle of friends who can offer emotional support.
- Give expression to feelings rather than suppressing them.
- Discuss problems regularly with someone with a listening ear.

Behaviour modification

Lifestyle habits that have developed over many years can be very difficult to change even when the individual is well motivated to change. There are a variety of instructional, motivational and behavioural techniques that can be used to initiate a lifestyle change program; GPs should be aware of these and use the resources of a multidisciplinary team to give support to motivated people who as a rule find behaviour modification difficult.

Vascular disease

Risk factors for vascular disease (atherosclerosis) are:

- hypertension
- smoking
- high cholesterol
- diabetes
- obesity
- sedentary lifestyle
- stress
- alcohol excess
- poor diet
- family history

The preceding guidelines for good health, if followed, will help prevent the development of cardiovascular and cerebrovascular disease.

It is worth noting that the death rate from coronary heart disease is about 70% higher for smokers than for non-smokers and for very heavy smokers the risk is almost 200% higher. It has been shown that the incidence of heart disease falls in those who have ceased smoking.

Of particular interest is the UK study that showed high-dose vitamin E (400–800 IU daily) was cardioprotective and reduced the incidence of myocardial infarction in angina patients.[4]

Malignant disease

Primary prevention of cancer is an important objective and there is a need to focus on this vital factor as much as on secondary prevention. The interesting statistics on the 5-year survival rate for specific cancers are shown in Table 9.3.

That environmental factors are involved in the aetiology of colorectal cancer and other cancers is indicated by wide variations in incidence between different countries.

Suspicion falls on diet and there is epidemiological evidence implicating diets high in animal fats and low in insoluble fibre, fruits and vegetables, and also high alcohol consumption. It is noted that there are higher incidence rates in people migrating from low- to high-risk countries, e.g. Japanese to Hawaii[5] and Greeks and Italians to Australia.[6]

Studies in the United States indicate that at least 35% of all cancer deaths are related to diet. Obese individuals have increased risk of colon, breast and uterine cancers. High-fat diets are a risk factor for prostate, breast and colon cancers. Salt-cured, smoked and nitrate-cured foods increase the risk of upper GI cancers. Foods rich in vitamin A and folate (dark green and deep yellow vegetables and fruits) and vitamin C and cruciferous vegetables (cabbage, brussels sprouts, broccoli and cauliflower) are all considered to have protective effects for various cancers.[7] Photochemicals (plant chemicals) exist in these foods and in other vegetables and fruit that have a cancer-protective effect.[8]

Overall, diet, smoking, alcohol and occupational exposures (5%) appear to account for over 73% of all cancer mortality.[7]

Doll and Peto[9] consider that environmental factors are responsible for 80–90% of cancers and estimate that diet is a major factor in the cause of cancer in 40% of men and 60% of women.

The role of immunity in cancer

The development of a number of cancers appears to be related to a depression of the individual's immune system, particularly in relation to cellular immunity, in a similar way (albeit on a different scale) to the effect of HIV infection. Studies have shown that the immune system is adversely influenced by:[10]

- stress, especially bereavement
- depression
- ageing
- drugs
- pollutants
- cigarette smoke
- inappropriate diet
- alcohol
- radiation

On the other hand, a protective effect on the immune system is provided by:

- food antioxidants (Table 9.4)
- tranquillity
- meditation

Food antioxidants (Table 9.4) appear to protect against free radicals that can suppress immunity. Free radicals, which are usually a toxic form of oxygen containing an odd number of electrons, are produced by a variety of toxins as mentioned above.[10,11,12] Apart from the possible toxicity to immunity from free radicals, they may also damage body tissues such as the liver in alcoholics as well as increasing susceptibility to degenerative diseases.[13]

In some instances malignancies appear to undergo unpredictable remissions with patients following an optimal diet, taking antioxidants,

Table 9.3 *Cancer prognosis: 5-year survival*

Cancer	USA (whites) 1960–63 %	USA (whites) 1983–88 %	Australia 1960 %	South Australia 1977–90 %
Lung	8	13	10	12
Bowel	40	58	35	55
Breast	63	79	60	75
Pancreas	1	3	2	4
Stomach	11	16	10	20

Source: Statistics provided by Dr Graham Giles, Anti Cancer Council of Victoria

Table 9.4 *Food antioxidants*

Vitamin A, esp. beta-carotene
Vitamin C
Vitamin E
Ubidecarenone (coenzyme Q10)
Selenium
Zinc
Manganese   } nutrient
Copper   } co-factors

Source: After Sali[10]

changing their lifestyle and practising meditation. However, Bury in a review of the literature
of antioxidant nutrients concludes that 'high
intake of antioxidant nutrients from food sources
appears to offer some health advantage but
claims for any therapeutic benefit of antioxidant
supplements are premature and scientificially
unjustified at present'.[14]

Diet certainly appears to be a most important
factor in the primary prevention of disease. If
immune deficient diseases can respond in such a
way, imagine what a powerful primary preventive
force such a lifestyle represents for all disease.

Asthma and other respiratory diseases

The death rate and morbidity rate for asthma
and other respiratory diseases is unacceptable
and much of it can be prevented.[15] A recent
report claims that at an estimated cost of $585
to $720 million per year the cost of asthma to
the Australian community compares with the
total cost of coronary artery disease ($623
million).[15] The report also claimed that there is
evidence that a significant proportion of diagnosed asthmatics are currently receiving treatment that does not provide the best possible
control of the disease.

Prevention means being better informed and
treating such an 'irritable' disease as bronchial
asthma aggressively. It means focusing on better
assessment and monitoring (e.g. home use of the
mini peak flow meter), better delivery of medication to the airways (e.g. use of spacers
attached to inhalers and/or use of pumps and
nebulisers) and appropriate management of
the cause (inflammation of the bronchial tree)
by the use of inhaled corticosteroids or
sodium chromoglycate as first-line treatment for

significant asthma. Following the six-step asthma
management plan (Table 9.5) of the National
Asthma Campaign would certainly promote prevention in this fickle disease.

The protective effect for asthma and COAD
of vitamin C, fish oils, low-salt diet and other
natural antioxidants is highlighted by Sridhar.[16]

Table 9.5 *The six-step asthma management plan (National Asthma Campaign: Australia)*

1. Establish the severity of the asthma.
2. Achieve best lung function.
3. Maintain best lung function—avoid trigger factors.
4. Maintain best lung function—follow an optimal medication program.
5. Develop an action plan.
6. Educate and review regularly.

Periodic health examination

Since 86% of the population visit a general practitioner at some stage of the year,[3] and these
people visit about five times each year (on
average), GPs are in an ideal position to develop
strategies for a periodic health examination. An
emphasis should be placed on the history in
addition to the physical examination and related
basic investigations.

As for any smooth-running quality professional
program, it is important to be organised with prepared practice staff, checklists and record
systems. The Royal Australian College of General
Practitioners has developed a College Record
System, which has several leaflets covering all
approaches to the patient 'check-up'.[17]

The following guidelines for the periodic
health examination are adapted from those recommended by the Preventive and Community
Medicine Committee of the RACGP.[17] This represents appropriate screening at the front line of
primary health care.

Aims of screening

In practice, screening is not only to detect
disease at its earliest stage, but also to find individuals at risk or those with established disease
who are not receiving adequate care. There are
three levels at which screening can be applied
in general practice:

1. 'well' individuals with risk factors that predispose to disease, e.g. obesity, uncomplicated
essential hypertension, hyperlipidaemia

2. asymptomatic individuals with signs of early disease or illness, e.g. developmental dysplasia of the hip, ectopic testis, glaucoma, bacteriuria of pregnancy, carcinoma *in situ* of cervix
3. symptomatic individuals whose irreversible abnormalities are unreported but the effects can be controlled or assisted, e.g. visual defects, deafness, mental handicap.

The history[17]

An appropriate history will allow the recognition of certain risk factors that may foreshadow future disease. Though established patients will have a previously acquired database, their history should be reviewed and updated. It is recommended that the following items be included in history taking in the appropriate age groups.

Family history. In particular, cardiovascular disease, some cancers (breast, bowel, melanoma with dysplastic naevi), diabetes, asthma, genetic disorders and bowel disease will alert the doctor to specific risk factors (and psychological factors) for these patients.

Suicide and accidents. Consider the risk factors predisposing to suicide and accidents, which are the major preventable causes of death in children and young adults.

Substance abuse. Tobacco and alcohol are the major causes of preventable death in adults, although other drugs contribute to a lesser extent. Counselling by general practitioners, about smoking in particular, has been shown to be effective.

Exercise and nutrition. These factors have a role to play in preventing cardiovascular disease and to a lesser extent in blood pressure control, cancer, diabetes and constipation. They have an even greater role to play in improving general well-being and preventing morbidity.

Occupational health hazards. Consider these in working adults, as occupational health hazards can significantly contribute to morbidity and mortality, e.g. exposure to toxic substances, unsafe work practices.

Physical functioning, home conditions and social supports. Consider these in elderly people, as physical function and social supports are of crucial importance in determining whether they can care for themselves—intervention can prevent accidents and death.

Sexuality/contraception. Sexually transmitted diseases are all preventable, as are unwanted pregnancies. Opportunities should be sought to ask young people, in particular, about their sexuality, and to counsel them. The question 'Do you have any concerns about sex?' is very useful in this context.

Osteoporosis. Osteoporosis affects nearly a third of all postmenopausal women, most of whom suffer osteoporotic fractures. Fractures of the femoral neck have a particularly poor prognosis, with up to a third of these women dying within 6 months, and many more requiring continuing nursing home care. Bone loss accelerates at the time of the menopause, and can be reduced by hormone replacement therapy.

Women at risk of osteoporosis are short, slim, Caucasian; they drink coffee and alcohol, smoke, eat a high-protein and high-salt diet, and don't exercise.

Masquerades in general practice. It is worth considering the 'masquerades' (Chapter 15, Tables 15.4 and 15.5), which may present as undifferentiated illness, as a means of following the important medical principle of early detection of disease: engendering a certain awareness.

Primary masquerades to consider are:
- depression
- diabetes mellitus
- drug problems
- anaemia
- thyroid disorders, especially hypothyroidism
- urinary tract infection
- vertebral (spinal) dysfunction

Hypothyroidism has been estimated to exist in up to 15% of women aged 60 and above, and searching for clues may elicit subtle symptoms and signs previously attributed to ageing.

Relationships and psychosocial health. Consider the mental health of patients, particularly the elderly, by enquiring about how they are coping with life, how they are coping financially, about their peace of mind and how things are at home. Focus on the quality of their close relationships, e.g. husband–wife, father–son, mother–daughter, employer–employee. Enquire about losses in their life, especially family bereavements.

Examination screening specific to children[17]

Childhood health record books provide an excellent opportunity for communication between different health care givers; parents should be provided with the record books and encouraged to bring them to every visit. Various recommendations for screening are made under the following headings.

Height/weight/head circumference. Record height from age 3 and weight at regular intervals to age 5 years. Record head circumference at birth and then up to 6 months. The adequacy of a child's growth cannot be assessed on one measurement and serial recordings on growth charts are recommended. Head circumference recordings may provide further data about a child's growth.

Hips. Screen for congenital dislocation at birth, 6–8 weeks, 6–9 months and 12–24 months.

The flexed hips are abducted, checking for movement and a 'clunk' of the femoral head forwards (the test is most likely to be positive at 3–6 weeks and usually negative after 8 weeks). Shortening or limited abduction is also abnormal. Ultrasound examination is more sensitive than the clinical examination especially up to 3 to 4 months. Observe gait when starting to walk.

Strabismus. Strabismus should be sought in all infants and toddlers by occlusion testing (not very sensitive), examining light reflexes and questioning parents, which must be taken very seriously. Amblyopia can be prevented by early recognition and treatment of strabismus by occlusion and surgery. Early referral is essential.

Visual acuity. At birth and 2 months, eyes should be inspected and examined with an ophthalmoscope with a 3+ lens at a distance of 20–30 cm to detect cataracts and red reflexes. At 9 months gross vision should be determined by assessing ability to see common objects. Visual acuity should be formally assessed at school entry using Sheridan Gardiner charts.

Hearing. Hearing should be tested by distraction at 9 months; also by pure tone audiometry at 1000 and 4000 hertz when child is 4 years (pre-school entry) and 12 years.

Note: Formal audiological evaluation should be carried out at any time if there is clinical suspicion or parental concern. No simple screening test is very reliable for sensori-neural or conductive deafness.

Testes. Screen at birth, and 6–8 weeks, 6–9 months and 3 years for absence or maldescent. Those who have been treated for maldescent have a higher risk of neoplastic development in adolescence.

Dental assessment/fluoride. Advise daily fluoride drops or tablets, if water supply is not fluoridated. Children's teeth should be checked regularly, particularly if a school dental service is not available. Advice should be given on sugar consumption, especially night-time bottles, and tooth cleaning with fluoride toothpaste to prevent plaque.

Scoliosis. Screening of females by the forward flexion test, which is carried out around 12 years of age, is of questionable value because of poor sensitivity and specificity.

Congenital heart disease. The heart should be auscultated at birth, in the first few days, at 6–8 weeks and on school entry.

Femoral pulses. Testing for absence of femoral pulses or delay between brachial/femoral pulses at birth and 8 weeks will exclude coarctation of the aorta. Refer the child immediately if concerned.

Speech and language. A child's speech should be intelligible to strangers by 3 years. It is related to hearing.

Screening for adults[17]

The following recommendations apply for adults.

Weight. Weight should be recorded at least every few years. Obesity is a major reversible health risk for adults contributing to many diseases, e.g. heart disease, diabetes, arthritis. Body Mass Index (BMI) should ideally be between 20 and 25.

$$\text{BMI} = \frac{\text{Wt (kg)}}{\text{Ht (m)}^2}$$

Abdominal obesity is a major risk factor for adults. The waist/hip circumference ratio is regarded as a useful predictor of cardiac disease. Recommended waist/hip ratios are:

males   < 0.9
females < 0.8

Blood pressure. Blood pressure should be recorded at least every 1–2 years on all people 16 years and over. There is no dispute that control of blood pressure results in reduced mortality from cerebrovascular accidents and, to a lesser extent, heart disease, renal failure and retinopathy.

Cholesterol. All adults aged 18 and over should have a 5-yearly estimation of serum cholesterol. Total cholesterol is adequate for screening purposes. HDL levels give additional information. The National Heart Foundation recommends keeping cholesterol levels below 4.5–5.0 mmol/L for high risk patients and 6.0 mmol/L for lower risk population. Formost, dietary modification is sufficient to achieve these levels; some may require drug treatment.

Carcinoma of the cervix. Women aged 18–70 who have ever been sexually active should have a Pap smear every 2 years. Those over 70 who have never been screened should have two successive tests before screening is ceased. After consideration of the relative risks to the individual woman, she and her physician may choose to increase the interval between smears, but the interval should not be greater than 3 years.

Risk factors include:
- all women who are or ever have been sexually active
- early age at first sexual intercourse
- multiple sexual partners
- genital wart virus infection
- cigarette smoking

Carcinoma of the breast. Mammography should be performed at least every 2 years on women aged 50–70 years. It is not useful for screening prior to age 40 years due to difficulty in discriminating malignant lesions from dense tissue. There is insufficient evidence of long-term benefit to recommend screening in the 40–50 age group. Mammography must not be used alone to exclude cancer if a lump is palpable. Such lesions require a complete appraisal since, even in the best hands, mammography still has a false negative rate of at least 10%.

Colorectal cancer. A history should be taken, with specific enquiry as to family history of adenomas or colorectal cancer, past history of inflammatory bowel disease and rectal bleeding. Rectal examination should be performed as part of an examination. Faecal occult blood testing (FOBT) is now recommended for screening for people over 50 years without symptoms and with average or slightly above average risk.

Should a positive history be elicited, then the following are recommended:
- past history or large bowel cancer or colonic adenomas—colonoscopy
- past or present history of ulcerative colitis—colonoscopy with biopsies
- familial polyposis, Gardner's syndrome—sigmoidoscopy or colonoscopy

Prophylactic colectomy needs consideration in some.

Apart from annual FOBT screening the NH&MRC currently recommends 5-yearly colonoscopy for people from 50 years of age if there is a family history of either two first-degree relatives diagnosed at any age or one first-degree relative diagnosed under the age of 55 years.

Skin cancer. All patients should be informed regularly about the need for protection of the skin from solar radiation, using clothing and sunscreens, and avoiding exposure during midday hours.

Skin cancer, which is increasing in incidence, is common in Australia, particularly in more northern areas. Squamous cell carcinoma, and melanoma in particular, may be lethal. Detection and treatment of early lesions prevents mortality and morbidity. Prevention of skin cancer by reduction of sun exposure should be taught to all patients.

Oral hygiene/cancer. Patients should be counselled about cessation of smoking and alcohol consumption, and dental hygiene should be taught. The oral cavity should be inspected annually in patients over the age of 40.

Although oral cancer has a relatively low incidence, premalignant lesions may be detected by inspection of the oral cavity. Its incidence is highest in elderly people with a history of heavy smoking or drinking. Poor dental hygiene may result in poor nutrition, particularly among the elderly.

Immunisation

Basic diseases (diphtheria, tetanus, polio, whooping cough, measles, mumps, hepatitis B, rubella) should be covered. Children and adolescents should be immunised according to the routine NH&MRC recommendation.

Age	Immunisation
Birth	Hepatitis B
2 months	Triple antigen, Hib, Hepatitis B and Polio vaccine
4 months	Triple antigen, Hib, Hepatitis B and Polio vaccine
6 months	Triple antigen, Hib and Polio vaccine
12 months	Measles/mumps/rubella, Hib and Hepatitis B
18 months	Triple antigen
4–5 years (prior to school entry)	Triple antigen, measles/mumps/rubella and Polio vaccine
15–19 years (prior to leaving school)	Adult diphtheria/tetanus and Polio vaccine

Special considerations. While not part of the routine schedule, the NH&MRC endorses hepatitis B vaccine for all infants and preadolescents (3 doses). It also advises against injections into the buttock (challenged by many), preferring the anterolateral thigh for children under 12 months with the deltoid region being an alternative in older children and adults. Do not postpone immunisation for minor illnesses such as mild URTI. Acellular pertussis vaccine, which will eventually become a standard component of triple antigen, is available for infants having a previous reaction.

All adults should receive an Adult Diphtheria & Tetanus (ADT) booster *each* 10 years.

All women of child-bearing years should have their rubella antibody status reviewed.

The general immunisation schedule is presented in Table 9.6.

Paracetamol prophylaxis. Consider giving 15 mg/kg paracetamol liquid to children within a 30-minute period before the injection and then a further dose in 2 to 4 hours, to reduce the side effects of the vaccines.

Influenza. Influenza immunisation is recommended on an annual basis for persons of all ages with chronic debilitating diseases, especially chronic cardiac, pulmonary, renal and metabolic diseases, persons over 65 years of age, Aboriginal and Torres Strait Islander adults over 50 years of age and persons receiving immuno-

Table 9.6 *NH&MRC standard vaccination schedule*

Initial courses			
Diphtheria, tetanus and pertussis	Intramuscular	Triple antigen	2, 4, 6, 18 months
Poliomyelitis	Oral	Sabin	2, 4, 6 months
Measles, mumps and rubella	Subcutaneous	MMR	12 months
Haemophilus Influenzae b	Intramuscular	various	varies by vaccine: from 2 months or at 18 months; usually 2, 4, 6, 18 months
Hepatitis B	Intramuscular	HBsAg subunit	0, 2, 4, 12 months
Booster doses			
Diphtheria, tetanus and pertussis	Intramuscular	Combined diph/tetanus (CDT)	4–5 years or prior to school entry
Poliomyelitis	Oral	Sabin	as above and 15–19 years
Measles, mumps and rubella	Subcutaneous	MMR	4–5 years
Hepatitis B	Intramuscular	HBsAg subunit	consider at 5 years after initial course (depends on blood tests)
Diphtheria and tetanus	Intramuscular	Adult diph/tetanus (ADT)	15–19 years or prior to school leaving, then every 10 years

suppressant therapy. Health care personnel may wish to consider it for their own use.

Pneumococcal disease. This should be considered for the same risk groups as influenza vaccine. Those at higher risk of fatal pneumococcal infection, e.g. post splenectomy or Hodgkin's disease, should receive a booster every 5 years.

Hepatitis A. Immunisation is recommended for:
• certain occupational groups at risk, e.g. health workers, child care workers, sewerage workers
• non-immune homosexual men
• those with chronic liver disease
• recipients of blood products
• travellers to hepatitis A endemic areas

Hepatitis B. Immunisation is recommended routinely for all children and for individuals of all ages who, through work or lifestyle, may be exposed to hepatitis B and have been shown to be susceptible. Such groups would include health care personnel, personnel and residents of institutions, prisoners and prison staff, persons with frequent and/or close contact with high-risk groups, and persons at increased risk due to their sexual practices. Household contacts of any of the above groups should be considered for immunisation. Booster doses may be considered after 5 years for those at high risk. A blood test 3 months after the third dose should be considered for such people.

Haemophilus influenza type b. Hib immunisation is recommended for all children, especially those in child care. It is ideal to achieve immunity by the age of 18 months and preferably commencing at 2 months. Risk factors for Hib disease include day care attendance, presence of ill siblings under 6 years of age in the home and household crowding.

Q fever. People at reasonable risk from Q fever, particularly abattoir workers, should be given this vaccine, which is virtually 100% effective.

Measles–mumps–rubella. Both females and males should be immunised against measles, mumps and rubella at the age of 12 months using the trivalent vaccine. All should also be re-immunised during the years between age 10 and 16.

References

1. Piterman L, Sommer SJ. *Preventive care.* Melbourne: Monash University, Department of Community Medicine, Final Year Handbook, 1993, 75–85.
2. Silagy C. Prevention in general practice. In: McNeil J et al. eds, *A textbook of preventive medicine*, Melbourne: Edward Arnold, 1990, 269–277.
3. National Health Strategy. *The future of general practice.* Issues paper No. 3. Canberra: AGPS, 1992, 54–169.
4. Stephens NG, Parsons A, Schofield P et al. Randomised controlled trial of vitamin E in patients with coronary disease: Cambridge Heart Antioxidant Study (CHAOS). Lancet, 1996; 347:781–786.
5. Locke FB, King H. Cancer mortality risk among Japanese in the United States. National Cancer Institute, 1980; 65:1149.
6. Potter JD, McMichael AJ. Diet and cancer of the colon and rectum: A case control study. National Cancer Institute, 1986; 76:557–69.
7. Rakel RE. *Essentials of family practice.* Philadelphia: Saunders, 1993, 126–127.
8. Editorial. Position of the American Dietetic Association: Photochemicals and functional foods. J Am Diet Assoc, 1993; 93:493–496.
9. Doll R, Peto R. *The causes of cancer.* New York: Oxford University Press, 1981, 1197–1219.
10. Sali A. Strategies for cancer prevention. Aust Fam Physician, 1987; 16:1603–1613.
11. Beisel WR. Single nutrients and immunity. Am J Clin Nutrition, 1982; 35(supp):147–148.
12. Meyskens FZ, Prasad KN. *Vitamins and cancer: Human cancer prevention by vitamins and micronutrients.* Clifton: Humana Press, 1986, 3–478.
13. Dormandy TL. An approach to free radicals. Lancet, 1983; 2:1010–1014.
14. Bury R. *Clinical applications of antioxidant nutrients.* Department of Human Services, Victoria, 1996, 26.
15. Antic R. *Report on the cost of asthma in Australia.* Melbourne: National Asthma Campaign, 1992,14–33.
16. Sridhar MK. Editorial. Nutrition and lung health. BMJ, 1995; 310:75–76.
17. Royal Australian College of General Practitioners. *Guidelines for preventive activities in general practice* (4th edn). Melbourne: RACGP, 1996.

10
Health promotion and patient education

Never believe what a patient tells you his doctor said.

Sir William Jenner (1815–98)

Health promotion[1]

Health promotion is the motivation and encouragement of individuals and the community to see good health as a desirable state that should be maintained by the adoption of healthy practices. It is also the process of helping people obtain their optimal health.

For those who feel healthy, the message may have little meaning, but it is reinforced by contact with others who become ill, particularly within the family.

Health education

Health education is the provision of information about how to maintain or attain good health.

There are many methods including the advertising of health practices; the provision of written information, e.g. about diet and exercise, immunisation, accident prevention and the symptoms of disease; and methods to avoid disease, e.g. sexually transmitted disease.

Illness education

A great deal of so-called 'health' education is in reality information about the cause of particular illnesses. Clearly the medical practitioner is in a pre-eminent position to provide his or her patients with specific information about the cause of an illness at the time either individually or to the family. This educative strategy has a preventive objective that is often the modification of help-seeking behaviour.

Every consultation is an opportunity to provide information about the condition under care and this can be reinforced in written, diagrammatic or printed form. Patients' own X-rays can be similarly used to illustrate the nature of the problem.

Health promotion in general practice

General practitioners are ideally placed to undertake health promotion and prevention, mainly due to opportunity.

There are several reasons for this health promotion role:

- Population access: over 80% of the population visit a GP at least once a year.[2]
- On average, people visit a GP about five times each year.
- GPs have a knowledge of the patient's personal and family health history.
- The GP can act as leader or co-ordinator of preventive health services in his or her local area.
- The GP can participate in community education programs.
- GPs should undertake opportunistic health promotion—the ordinary consultation can be used not just to treat the presenting problem, but also to manage ongoing problems, co-ordinate care with other health professionals, check whether health services are being used

appropriately and undertake preventive health activities.[2]

Opportunistic health promotion

The classic model by Stott and Davis (Table 3.1) highlights the opportunities for health promotion in each consultation.[3] Since the consultation is patient-initiated, it is the doctor who needs to be the initiator of preventive health care. The potential in the consultation involves reactive and proactive behaviour by the doctor (Fig. 10.1).[4]

Reactive professional behaviour deals only with the presenting complaint. It may be performed with skill but if the practitioner is only trained to perform reactively then the opportunity for preventive and promotive health care will be lost.

Proactive behaviour is defined as professional behaviour that is necessary for the patient's well-being, but it is performed not merely as a response to the presenting problem and it is initiated by the doctor.[4] It includes health promotion, preventive care and screening and the early detection of disease before it becomes symptomatic. Other aspects of proactive care are seen in Figure 10.1.

Proactive behaviour also includes:[4]

- continuing care of a previously treated problem, e.g. rechecking blood pressure, checking diabetic control, follow-up bereavement counselling
- co-ordination of care by organising referral to appropriate agencies or specialists and maintaining adequate medical records
- The modification of abnormal or inappropriate help-seeking behaviour: e.g. the person who never attends is at risk from 'silent disease'; the too frequent attender wastes resources and serious illness may be overlooked

This mix of reactive and proactive behaviour is not appropriate in every consultation. It requires counselling skills and training in the delivery of quality general practice.

Methods

- Being informed and updated by maintaining continuing medical education, especially in preventive roles.
- Using health promotional material for patient education:
  — handouts
  — waiting room posters
  — waiting room video systems.

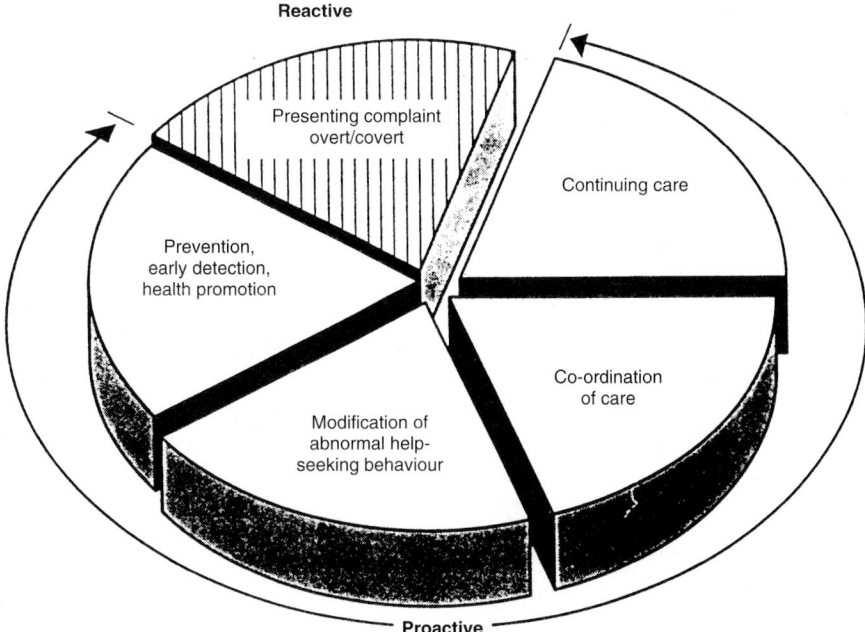

Fig. 10.1 *The potential in every general practice consultation*   REPRODUCED WITH PERMISSION FROM M. SALES

- Having an efficient medical record system.
- Operating a patient register and recall system.
- Encouraging regular health checks for at-risk groups.
- Providing regular advice on:
  — nutrition
  — exercise
  — stress management
  — weight control.
- Providing personal health records to the parents of newborn babies.

Health goals and targets

Health goals and targets as determined by the Health Targets and Implementation Committee[5] were set in three areas—population groups, major causes of illness and death, and risk factors (Table 10.1). The targets are to achieve significant results by the year 2000 and are expanded under the following headings. The four prime targets are cardiovascular disease, cancer, accident prevention and mental health.

1. Population groups[2,5]

The socioeconomically disadvantaged

Goal
- To reduce significantly differences in death rates, illness and the prevalence of health risk factors between socioeconomically advantaged and disadvantaged Australians.

Table 10.1 *Health promotion areas in which goals and targets have been set*

Population groups
The socioeconomically disadvantaged, Aborigines, migrants, women, men, older people, children and adolescents.

Major causes of illness and death
Heart disease and stroke, cancers (including lung, breast, cervical and skin cancer), injury, communicable diseases, musculoskeletal disease, diabetes, disability, dental disease, mental illness, asthma.

Risk factors
Drugs (including tobacco smoking, alcohol misuse, pharmaceutical misuse or abuse, illicit drugs and substance abuse), nutrition, physical inactivity, high blood pressure, high blood cholesterol, occupational health hazards, unprotected sexual activity, environmental health hazards.

Source: Health Targets and Implementation Committee[5]

Aborigines

Goal
- To reduce significantly the gap in health status between Aborigines and the rest of the Australian population.

Migrants

Goals
- To ensure that the health advantage of migrants on arrival in Australia is not eroded by the adoption of less healthy lifestyles or environments.
- To ensure that the special health needs of refugees on arrival in Australia are met.

Women

Goal
- To improve the overall health and well-being of Australian women.

Target
- To be determined as part of the National Women's Health Policy.

Men

Goals
- To improve the overall health and well-being of Australian men.
- To reduce the incidence of premature death among Australian men, especially in lower socioeconomic groups.

Older people

Goal
- To reduce the percentage of older Australians with health problems that preclude their independence.

Children and adolescents

Goal
- To reduce preventable illness, injury and death among Australian children and adolescents.

2. Major causes of sickness and death

Heart disease and stroke

Goal
- To reduce avoidable illness and premature death from heart disease and stroke.

Targets
- By the year 2000 to achieve a significant reduction in:
  — the death rate from heart disease
  — the death rate from stroke

— the prevalence of smokers (15% or less)
— the proportion of adults who persistently have a diastolic blood pressure of greater than 90 millimetres of mercury
— the prevalence of plasma cholesterol levels of 6.5 millimoles per litre or more in people aged 25–64 years
— the mean fasting plasma cholesterol level from 5.6 millimoles per litre to 4.8 millimoles per litre or less in people aged 25–64 years
— the prevalence of overweight and obesity in people aged 25–64 years
— the contribution of fat to dietary energy
— dietary sodium intake to 100 millimoles (2.3 grams) or less per day.
• To increase participation in sufficient activity to achieve and maintain physical fitness and health.

Lung cancer
Goal
• To reduce the incidence of death from lung cancer.

Breast cancer
Goal
• To reduce illness and death from breast cancer.
Target
• To increase participation in breast cancer screening to 70% or more of eligible women.

Cervical cancer
Goal
• To reduce the incidence of death from cervical cancer.
Targets
• To increase triennial participation in Pap smear screening of women aged 18–69 years.
• To establish organised population-based cervical neoplasia screening programs in each state and territory.

Skin cancer
Goals
• To reduce illness and death from melanoma and other skin cancers through early detection.
• To reduce the incidence of all forms of skin cancer through protection against ultraviolet exposure.
Targets
• To reduce exposure to ultraviolet radiation.

• To reduce exposure to ultraviolet radiation for people at high risk of skin cancer.

Injury
Goal
• To reduce preventable death and disability from injury and poisoning.
Targets
• To reduce:
— the death rate from drowning to 2 per 100 000 per annum or less in children aged 1–4 years
— fractures related to playground equipment
— the incidence of poisoning severe enough to require hospitalisation
— the incidence of burns and scalds that are severe enough to require hospitalisation
— the incidence of injury severe enough to require medical attention
— death and injury due to motor vehicle accidents in children aged 0–4 years
— the incidence of motor vehicle injury, including whiplash, due to rear-end collisions involving passenger cars
— illness and death due to alcohol-related motor vehicle accidents

Communicable diseases
Goals
• To reduce the incidence of death and disability caused by communicable diseases for which immunisation is available.
• To eradicate measles, hepatitis B and rubella embryopathy.
• To minimise illness due to communicable diseases not preventable through immunisation by promoting accurate diagnosis and effective infection control procedures.
Targets
• To ensure that evidence of a completed immunisation schedule is used as a condition of primary school enrolment, with exemptions being granted for defined medical, personal or religious reasons.
• To eradicate indigenous measles.
• To ensure use of a combined measles/mumps/rubella (MMR) vaccine in all immunisation programs for children.
• To increase immunity against rubella to 90% or more of women aged 15 to 34 years.
• To increase participation in screening for hepatitis B surface antigen just before childbirth, of individuals at a high risk of being infected.

- To ensure that hepatitis B immunoglobulin and a complete course of vaccination is given to all newborn infants of women identified as carriers.
- To increase vaccination against hepatitis B of newborn infants in populations which have 10% or more of their individuals identified as carriers.
- To ensure that a contingency plan for the control of epidemics of Australian encephalitis and other mosquito-transmitted diseases is developed.
- To ensure that maps of the mosquito breeding sites associated with the spread of viral diseases are prepared.
- To ensure that knowledge of the avoidance of sexually transmitted diseases is gained by adolescents aged 15 years.

Musculoskeletal diseases

Goal
- To reduce the prevalence of musculoskeletal diseases.

Diabetes

Goal
- To reduce preventable illness, handicap and premature death due to diabetes.

Targets
- To establish a national database to record the incidence of diabetes and its complications.
- To slow down the increase in the prevalence of diabetes in Australia.

Disability

Goal
- To reduce the proportion of handicapped people having insufficient social, emotional and physical support to maintain independence.

Dental disease

Goals
- To reduce the incidence of dental disease.
- To reduce inequalities in dental health status.

Mental illness

Goal
- To reduce the levels of psychiatric illness and psychosocial problems.

Asthma

Goal
- To reduce illness and death from asthma.

3. Risk factors

Drugs

Goal
- To minimise the harmful effects of drugs.

Tobacco smoking

Goals
- To prevent the onset of smoking in non-smokers, especially children.
- To reduce the number of smokers.
- To reduce the exposure of smokers to tobacco-derived carcinogens.
- To reduce involuntary exposure to tobacco smoke.

Targets
- To reduce the prevalence of smokers to 15% or less.
- To reduce the difference in the prevalence of smokers between upper white and lower blue collar men.
- To reduce the prevalence of regular smokers in adolescents aged 15 years.
- To introduce regulations to prohibit the sale of tobacco products to minors in all states and territories.
- To introduce legislation or regulations to prohibit smoking on government controlled or regulated public transport and associated buildings in all states and territories.
- To ensure that all government buildings are smoke-free.
- To ensure that all enclosed public spaces are smoke-free.

Alcohol misuse

Goals
- To reduce the incidence and prevalence of alcohol dependence and other alcohol-related problems.
- To reduce consumption of alcohol per capita.

Pharmaceutical misuse or abuse

Goals
- To reduce the incidence of misuse of pharmaceuticals.
- To ensure appropriate use of pharmaceutical drugs.

Target
- To develop a comprehensive medicinal drug policy pursuant to the recommendations of the World Health Organisation Conference of Experts on the Rational Use of Drugs.

Illicit drugs and substance abuse

Goal

• To reduce the use of illicit drugs and substance abuse.

Nutrition

Goal

• To reduce the incidence and prevalence of diet-related health disorders.

Targets

• To reduce the prevalence of overweight and obesity in people aged 25–64 years.
• To reduce the contribution of fat to dietary energy.
• To reduce the contribution of refined sugars to dietary energy.
• To reduce dietary sodium intake to 100 millimoles (2.3 grams) per day or less.
• To reduce the contribution of alcoholic beverages to dietary energy.
• To increase dietary fibre intake to 30 grams per day or more.
• To increase the level of breast-feeding at 3 months of life.

Physical inactivity

Goal

• To increase participation by adults in sufficient activity to achieve and maintain physical fitness and health.

Target

• To increase participation in sufficient activity to achieve and maintain physical fitness and health.

High blood pressure

Goal

• To reduce the incidence and prevalence of high blood pressure.

Targets

• To reduce the proportion of adults who persistently have a diastolic blood pressure greater than 90 millimetres of mercury.
• To increase the proportion of adults who have had their blood pressure accurately measured within the last 2 years.

High blood cholesterol

Goal

• To reduce the incidence and prevalence of high blood cholesterol levels.

Targets

• These targets are based on the work of the Better Health Commission Cardiovascular Taskforce.

Occupational health hazards

Goals

• To reduce the incidence of occupational illness, injury and death.
• To provide all workers with a safe and healthy working environment.

Unprotected sexual activity

Goal

• To reduce the number of unwanted pregnancies among teenagers.

Target

• To reduce both the birth rate and total pregnancy rate for females aged 15 years or less.

Environmental health hazards

Goal

• To increase protection against and reduce exposure to environmental hazards posing a threat to health.

Targets

• To ensure an adequate supply of good quality drinking water to the whole population.
• To reduce the number of deaths and injuries caused by the use of hazardous chemicals in the home.
• To safely dispose of the intractable chemical wastes at present stored in Australia.

Psychosocial health promotion

The preceding health goals and targets focus mainly on physical illness and do not emphasise mental health. However, this area represents an enormous opportunity for anticipatory guidance. It includes the important problems of stress and anxiety, chronic pain, depression, crisis and bereavement, sexual problems, adolescent problems, child behavioural problems, psychotic disorders and several other psychosocial problems.

Time spent in counselling, giving advice, stressing ways of coping with potential problems such as suicide and deterioration in relationships is rewarding. GPs need to pay more attention to promoting health in this area, which at times can be quite complex.

Patient education

Evidence has shown that intervention by general practitioners can have a significant effect on patients' attitudes to a change to a healthier lifestyle. If we are to make an impact on improving the health of the community, we must encourage our patients to take responsibility for their own health and thus change to a healthier lifestyle. They must be supported, however, by a caring doctor who follows the same guidelines and maintains a continuing interest. Examples include modifying diet, cessation of smoking, reduction of alcohol intake and undertaking exercise.

In an American survey of 360 patients, 90% reported wanting a pamphlet at some or all of their office visits. Overall, 67% reported reading or looking through and saving pamphlets received, 30% read or looked through them and then threw them away, and only 2% threw them away without review. Only 11% of males and 26% of females reported ever asking a doctor for pamphlets. More patients desire pamphlets than are receiving them.[6]

Patient educational materials have been shown to have a beneficial effect. Giving patients a handout about tetanus increased the rate of immunisation against tetanus among adults threefold.[7] An educational booklet on back pain for patients reduced the number of consultations made by patients over the following year and 84% said that they found it useful.[8] The provision of systematic patient education on cough significantly changed the behaviour of patients to follow practice guidelines and did not result in patients delaying consultation when they had a cough lasting longer than 3 weeks or one with 'serious' symptoms.[9]

There is no evidence that patient education has a harmful effect. Patient education about drug side effects has been shown not to have any detectable adverse effects.[10]

One form of patient education is giving handouts (either prepared or printed from a computer at the time of the consultation) to the patient as an adjunct to the verbal explanation which, it must be emphasised, is more important than the printed handout.

The patient education leaflets should be in non-technical language and focus on the key points of the illness or problem. The objectives are to improve the quality of care, reduce costs and encourage a greater input by patients in the management of their own illness. In modern society where informed consent and better education about health and disease is expected, this information is very helpful from a medicolegal viewpoint.

The author has produced a book called *Patient Education*, which has a one-page summary of each of 197 common medical conditions.[11] The concept is to photocopy the relevant problem or preventive advice and hand it to the patient or relative. Over the years the greatest demand (following a survey of requests for prints of the sheets) has been for the following (in order):

- exercises for your back (Fig. 10.2)
- backache (Fig. 10.3)
- exercises for your neck
- your painful neck
- exercises for your knee
- breast-feeding and milk supply
- how to lower cholesterol
- breast self-examination
- testicular self-examination
- vaginal thrush
- menopause
- anxiety
- coping with stress
- depression
- bereavement

Summary

Recommended target areas for health promotion in general practice include:

- nutrition
- weight control
- substance abuse and control
  — smoking
  — alcohol
  — other drugs
- exercise practices
- appropriate sleep, rest and recreation
- safe sexual practices
- promotion of self-esteem and personal growth
- stress management

Important health promotion recommendations are to encourage patients:[12]

- to cease smoking
- to reduce alcohol intake to safe levels
  — women no more than two standard drinks per day
  — men no more than three standard drinks per day

Fig. 10.2 *Patient education leaflet (diagrammatic part only): exercises for your lower back*

Right	Wrong

Fig. 10.3 *Patient education leaflet on backache (diagrammatic part only): rules of care for sitting, lying, lifting and bending*

— three alcohol-free days per week
- to limit caffeine intake to three drinks per day
- to increase regular physical activity
  — 30 minutes per day for 3 days per week, sufficient to produce a sweat
- to reduce fasting plasma cholesterol to 4.8 mmol per litre
- to have a diastolic BP of less than 90 mm of mercury
- to have a body mass index of between 20 and 25

$$BMI = \frac{(weight\ in\ kg)}{(height\ in\ metres)^2}$$

- to reduce fat, refined sugar and salt intake in all food

- to increase dietary fibre to 30 grams per day
- to build up their circle of friends who offer emotional support
- to express their feelings rather than suppress them
- to discuss their problems regularly with some other person
- to work continuously to improve their relationships with people
- not to drive a car when angry, upset or after drinking
- to have a 2-yearly Pap smear
- to avoid casual sex
- to practise safe sex
- to have an HIV antibody check before entering a relationship

References

1. Piterman L, Sommer SJ. *Preventive care*. Melbourne: Monash University, Department of Community Medicine, Final Year Handbook, 1993; 75–85.

2. National Health Strategy. *The future of general practice*. Issues paper No 3. Canberra: AGPS, 1992; 54–169.

3. Stott N, Davis R. The exceptional potential in each primary care consultation. JR Coll Gen Pract, 1979; 29: 201–5.

4. Sales M. Health promotion and prevention. Aust Fam Physician, 1989; 18:18–21.

5. Health Targets and Implementation (Health for All) Committee. *Health for all Australians*. Canberra: AGPS, 1988.

6. Shank JC, Murphy M, Schulte-Mowry L. Patient preferences regarding educational pamphlets in the family practice center. Fam Med, 1991; 23(6):429–32.

7. Cates CJ. A handout about tetanus immunisation: Influence on immunisation rate in general practice. BMJ, 1990; 300(6727):789–90.

8. Roland M, Dixon M. Randomised controlled trial of an educational booklet for patients presenting with back pain in general practice. JR Coll Gen Pract, 1989; 39(323):244–6.

9. Rutten G, Van Eijk J, Beek M, Van der Velden H. Patient education about cough: Effect on the consulting behaviour of general practice patients. Br J Gen Pract, 1991; 41(348):289–92.

10. Howland JS, Baker MG, Poe T. Does patient education cause side effects? A controlled trial. J Fam Pract, 1990; 31(1): 62–4.

11. Murtagh J. *Patient education* (2nd edn). Sydney: McGraw-Hill, 1996.

12. Fisher E. The botch of Egypt: Prevention better than cure. Aust Fam Physician, 1987; 16:187.

11

Whole person approach to management

—

Never forget that it is not a pneumonia, but a pneumonic man who is your patient.

Sir William Gull (1816–90)

The management of the whole person, or the holistic approach, is an important approach to patient care in modern medicine. Whole person diagnosis is based on two components:[1]

1. the disease-centred diagnosis
2. the patient-centred diagnosis

The disease-centred consultation is the traditional medical model based on the history, examination and special investigations, with the emphasis on making a diagnosis and treating the disease. The disease-centred diagnosis, which is typical of hospital-based medicine, is defined in terms of pathology and does not focus significantly on the feelings of the person suffering from the disease.

The patient-centred consultation not only takes into account the diagnosed disease and its management but also adds another dimension—that of the psychosocial hallmarks of the patient (Table 11.1) including details about:[1]

- the patient as a person
- emotional reactions to the illness
- the family
- the effect on relationships
- work and leisure
- lifestyle
- the environment

Dimensions to whole person management

In the diagnostic model presented in Chapter 15 the fifth and final question is: 'Is the patient trying to tell me something else?' and this self-posed question should be scrutinised and answered in most instances. This presupposes being tuned in to the patient, watching for cues and listening.

An efficient medical record system also helps the process, since following a set routine generally ensures that important facets of the patient's psychosocial history are not omitted.

The answer to the above question takes into account the patient's:

- feelings
- fears or concerns
- expectations of the doctor
- future aspirations

Such an approach may determine whether there is a 'hidden agenda' in the presentation and whether various stressors including interpersonal conflicts are significant factors in the illness.

Illustrative case history

The patient. John R, aged 47, bus driver.
Disease-centred problem. Low back pain for 5 months, after sudden onset of left sciatica (now settled) and low back pain (see Fig. 11.1).

Table 11.1 *Whole person diagnosis and management*

WHOLE PERSON DIAGNOSIS AND MANAGEMENT

Disease-centred diagnosis
• aetiology of disease

Patient-centred diagnosis
• significance of illness to patient
• effect on family and relationships
• effect on work and income
• psychological effects
  — stress and anxiety
  — abnormal illness/behaviour
  — sleep
  — depression
• effect on sexuality
• effect on attitudes and spirituality

Disease-centred management
• rest
• drugs
• intervention
• surgery
• other invasive techniques

Patient-centred management
• psychological support
• appropriate reassurance
• patient education
• empowering self-responsibility
• anticipatory guidance/special hazards
• prevention
• health promotion
• lifestyle recommendations/modifications
  — diet/nutrition
  — exercise
  — alcohol
  — smoking
  — stress management
• family and social supports
• self-help groups
• alternative options
• consultation and referral
• follow-up

Back pain analysis

History of injury: Yes—lifting a large suitcase out of the bus.

Site and radiation: Low lumbar—central and unilateral (left), left buttock.

Type of pain: Dull ache (severe at times). Has changed from a throbbing burning pain to a deep ache.

Onset: Present after sitting for long periods and provoked by various activities such as gardening and lifting.

Offset: Fluctuates throughout day — better with restricted activity.

Aggravation: Sitting, car travel, coughing and sneezing, soft beds, sex and more strenuous activity.

Relief: Walking, gentle activity, swimming, massage.

Associations: Stiffness in the back, headache, tiredness, insomnia.

Current management of the problem: Visited another doctor at first, then an allied health professional; referred to a consultant who diagnosed a disc prolapse, and considered surgical removal of the disc was the only appropriate treatment. Patient has 'played a waiting game' and is taking analgesics only.

Past history: Haemorrhoidectomy, mild episodes of back pain, appendicectomy.

Family history: Non-insulin dependent diabetes, coronary artery disease.

Drug history: Piroxicam 20 mg daily (prescribed by consultant); OTC analgesics; allergic to penicillin and indomethacin; alcohol—average 4 standard drinks a day; smoking—20 cigarettes a day.

Fig. 11.1 *Mr JR: site of low back pain and illustration of painful limitation of movement on direction of movement diagram*

Physical examination

General: Overweight middle-aged man with stiff gait.

Examination of lumbar spine

Inspection: Gait and movement—stiff, cautious.
Posture—normal, no muscle spasm.

Palpation: Tender over spinous process L4, over the L4–L5 interspinous space, and unilaterally to left between L4 and L5.

Movement: Restricted left lateral flexion and forward flexion (Fig. 11.1).

General: Lower limbs normal. No neurological abnormalities.
Urine analysis: NAD

Investigations

(Past) plain X-ray—slight narrowing L4–L5 disc, minimal degenerative changes in facet joints.

CT scan—mild spondylosis (facet joints) and L4–L5 disc degeneration: nerve roots unaffected.

Disease-centred diagnosis
L4–L5 disc degeneration

Disease-centred management
• back brace
• piroxicam 20 mg daily
• codeine and paracetamol compound tablets prn

Patient-centred problems

A more detailed history about the effect of the back disorder on the patient revealed the following:

• humiliation about being on workers' compensation
• boredom and frustration leading to irritable behaviour ('not like me')
• anxious about his future, particularly occupation
• fears of being a cripple 'in a wheelchair'
• conflicts with family members
• concern about reduction of sexual performance
• anger with lack of response from medical management
• anger with lack of interest in his problem
• concerns about something more serious (he admitted to a fear of cancer)
• feelings of depression: unable to cope, sleep disturbance
• concern about taking drugs, especially NSAIDs

Patient-centred physical examination (additional)
General: Tense and anxious man looking older than his years, senile arcus.
Cardiovascular examination: Blood pressure $^{165}/_{100}$.
Weight: 85 kg.
Height: 1.67 metres.
Body mass index: 30.5

Problem list
- chronic back pain
- hypertension
- obesity
- anxiety
- depression
- concerns about
  - — serious disease
  - — future employment
  - — finances
  - — sexual performance
  - — drug taking
- family disruption
- problem drinking
- nicotine excess
- NIDDM risk
- ischaemic heart disease risk

Discussion
JR (a real patient) is representative of many patients encountered in general practice with the common problem of chronic back pain. His case serves to illustrate the importance of managing the whole person.

Approaches to management
Psychological support
Factors that make patients feel supported and generate their confidence in the doctor include:
- showing an interest in all aspects
- examining the problematic area
- performing a more thorough examination
- picking up 'cues' and drawing attention to them

It is noteworthy just how impressed some patients are when they are physically examined. It is appreciated particularly by those who say: 'The other doctor did not get me to take off my clothes nor examine me'.

Support includes acting as the patient's advocate during the complex process of coping with the red tape of workers' compensation formalities, examinations by other doctors and any medicolegal issues.

Appropriate reassurance
Reassurance should be given from an appropriate knowledge base. It should be emphasised to the patient that on the law of averages the chronic back pain should eventually resolve and the patient can look forward to resuming a relatively normal life.

The patient should also be reassured that he does not have malignancy or a physically crippling disorder.

Explanation, basic counselling and patient education
One of the most important features of management is careful and appropriate explanation including the reasons for the pain and why it is self-perpetuating. A useful approach is that given on page 42, whereby the explanation is that the main triggering factor (the prolapsed disc) has basically resolved but the central nervous system is still registering the pain, analogous to a 'phantom limb'. The development of anxiety and depression has caused continuing overactivity of the pain pathways, which need to be 'switched off' by the various treatments that will be given.

Explore various concerns including the effect of his illness on his family relationships and sexual activity, and provide counselling as necessary. The patient should then be handed suitable patient education material as presented in Figure 10.3 and encouraged to undertake an exercise program (Fig. 10.2). Education about the problems of anxiety, depression and lifestyle factors should also be addressed.

Empowering self-responsibility
Emphasise to the patient that he must take the responsibility for his own health and rehabilitation. This involves an active program of exercises and swimming, taking preventive measures and following recommendations about health promotion. It also involves dedication to restoration of ideal weight since his obesity (BMI > 30) would be contributing to his back pain.

Medication
Explain tactfully that since there is no clinical evidence of inflammation, his NSAIDs can be ceased.

Because he is depressed with an anxiety component and insomnia, an antidepressant can be prescribed to be taken at night (see explanation for the patient on page 41). He can be assured that not only will this help his psychological state but it should help 'shut the pain pathway gate' and reverse the overactivity of the nervous system.

Patient education including patient education handouts about possible side effects and how to cope with them would be appropriate.

Prevention and health promotion

The patient should be informed in a supportive way that he has the following risk factors:

- family history of cardiovascular disease
- family history of diabetes
- hypertension (related to obesity, NSAIDs, alcohol excess and smoking)
- smoking
- obesity
- possible hypercholesterolaemia (senile arcus noted)
- stress and anxiety

It would be important to stress (despite the fact that he might not be receptive during a depressed state) that for the sake of his future health it was time to change his lifestyle to try to reverse the risk factor process.

Advice on the prevention of recurrence of his back problem is important with advice on daily activities, lifting, bending and so on. The use of a brace is not generally recommended as dependency on the supportive device tends to lead to aggravation of the chronicity of the back.

Lifestyle recommendation

In JR's case, and indeed for many patients, he should receive advice, education, guidelines and support in the basic lifestyle factors, namely:

- diet control
  — weight reduction
  — low fat/cholesterol diet
  — high fibre
  — alcohol restriction
- smoking
- exercise and suitable physical activities
- interesting hobbies
- relaxation techniques

Family support and counselling

It would be ideal to include Mrs JR in the next consultation or, better still, arrange a home visit to discuss the role the family can take in his rehabilitation. Explanations and seeking family support would be very helpful.

Other positive suggestions would be to encourage Mrs JR to perform massage (as instructed) on the aching back and co-operate with his diet and other lifestyle issues, and to assess the state of the bed and the chairs as a possible aggravation factor for the back pain.

Anticipatory guidance and special hazards

Possible problems for JR include aggravation of his back pain by inappropriate physical and emotional stressors, marital break-up, loss of job and even suicide. These issues should be diplomatically discussed with the patient in a positive way. It is to be hoped that the interest, encouragement and support he receives can help avert these serious problems.

Recommended treatment for JR

- attention to lifestyle factors
- antidepressant medication
- referral for therapy
  — hydrotherapy
  — mobilisation
  — active exercises
- therapeutic massage

Alternative options

There are many alternative therapies that can be used to help alleviate his painful condition. It is important for GPs to keep abreast of these therapies and their relative success rate based on scientific evidence. (Where known, the relative success rate, based on research by the author, is indicated.[2]) If the response is slow, one or more of these treatment modalities can be selected and the patient referred to a reputable therapist experienced in the therapy.

- spinal mobilisation and manipulation (64%)
- manipulation under general anaesthesia (34%)
- transcutaneous electrical nerve stimulation (TENS)
- acupuncture
- biofeedback
- meditation
- facet joint injections (20%)
- nerve blockage (48% after 6 months)
- epidural injections
- neurofasciotomy (42%)
- radiofrequency denervation (65%)
- electrotherapy
  for superficial heating
  — radiant heat lamps
  — infra-red lamps
  for deep heating
  — short-wave diathermy
  — ultrasound

Consultation and referral

One of the skills of a responsible general practitioner is to sum up his or her own limitations with a particular problem and consult with and/or refer to a colleague if it is in the patient's best interests. Effective communication and advice is only a phone call away. Patients with a chronic illness should be referred to an expert in the discipline to satisfy patient, family and GP that everything possible is being attempted to help the patient. Patients and their families often judge us by the quality of the referral process and its outcome; so considerable thought has to be given to the most outstanding consultant for that particular problem at a given time. The GP should remain in charge of the team and direct management.

JR could be referred to medical consultants such as an orthopaedic surgeon, an orthopaedic physician or a rheumatologist. It would be inappropriate to refer him to a psychiatrist in the early stage of his pain but if a psychological problem intervened and complicated management (as in this case) referral should be strongly considered. As a rule depression and anxiety can be managed well by a caring family doctor.

Probably the best option for a patient like JR is referral to a pain clinic that is staffed by a multidisciplinary team of specialists including psychiatrists, social workers, physiotherapists, occupational therapists and other medical specialists. They look at the total problem and the whole person. As a patient similar to JR said after attending a pain clinic: 'For the first time all my problems—physical, psychological, drug dependency and other disturbed fragments of my life—have been dealt with by the whole team'.

Follow-up
Careful instructions to ensure follow-up visits by the patient is important as there is a tendency for some dissatisfied and emotional patients to seek attention elsewhere and thus get on the chronic disorder 'merry-go-round'.

Outcome
JR gradually improved, presumably because depression had complicated the problem. The aphorism 'acute pain = acute anxiety and chronic pain = depression' applied to JR and relief of his depression, combined with supportive measures such as physiotherapy, hydrotherapy, physical therapy and strong psychological support from his family and GP, provided the 'holistic' approach to healing.

The holistic approach to management[3]

In a healing profession obsessed with interventionism, invasive technology and drug management, the general practitioner has an obligation to his or her patients to use natural healing methods wherever possible and be very discerning and conservative with investigatory medicine.

Patients appreciate natural remedies and taking responsibility for their own management wherever possible and appropriate. Examples include relative rest, exercise, swimming, stress management, meditation, spiritual awareness, antioxidant therapy (e.g. vitamin C, vitamin E, selenium), weight control, optimal healthy nutrition, avoidance of toxins (e.g. illicit drugs, nicotine, caffeine and alcohol) and sexual fulfilment.

Underlying a successful outcome is motivation, and the healing factor of the physician in being the motivator, teacher and facilitator should never be underestimated.

References

1. Carson N. The diagnostic process. In: Department of Community Medicine Final Year Handbook, Melbourne: Monash University, 1990, 9–25.

2. Murtagh J. Back pain in general practice. Melbourne: Monash University, 1988, MD thesis. 160–165.

3. Hetzel R. *The new physician: Tapping the potential for true health.* Melbourne: Houghton Mifflin, 1991.

12
Travel and tropical medicine

—

If you can't peel it, boil it or cook it—don't eat it.

Anon

Emporiatics—the science of travel medicine

With over 400 million international trips being taken annually the health problems faced by travellers are considerable and variable depending on the countries visited and the lifestyle adopted by the traveller.[1] There is evidence that many travellers are receiving inaccurate predeparture travel advice.[2] Travellers to North America, Europe and Australasia are usually at no greater risk of getting an infectious disease than they would be at home, but those visiting the less developed tropical and subtropical countries of Africa, Central and South America and South-East Asia are at significant risk of contracting infectious diseases.

Problems range in complexity from the most frequent and usually benign problems, such as traveller's diarrhoea, to more exotic and potentially fatal infections such as malaria, Japanese encephalitis and HIV. It must also be remembered that in some countries with volatile political changes there is the possibility of injury, incarceration or being left stranded. Travel means transport and thus the potential for accidents and crippled body and bank balance. Insurance for such contingencies is as important as preventive health measures.

Key facts and checkpoints

- The main diseases facing the international traveller are traveller's diarrhoea (relatively mild) and malaria, especially the potentially lethal chloroquine-resistant falciparum malaria (CRFM).
- Most cases of traveller's diarrhoea are caused by enterotoxigenic *Escherichia coli* (*E.coli*)—up to 75%.
- Enteroinvasive *E.coli* (a different serotype) produces a dysentery-like illness similar to *Shigella*.
- Traveller's diarrhoea is contracted mainly from contaminated water and ice used for beverages, washing food or utensils or cleaning teeth.
- One bite from an infected mosquito during a single overnight stop in a malaria area can result in a possible lethal infection.
- Infections transmitted by mosquitoes include malaria, yellow fever, Rift Valley fever, Japanese encephalitis and dengue fever. Preventing their bites is excellent prevention.
- Every year over 500 Australians catch malaria while travelling overseas.
- Malaria is a dusk-till-dawn risk only, but bites from daytime mosquitoes can cause dengue.
- CRFM is steadily increasing, as is resistance to newer antimalarials.
- It is important for general practitioners to consult a Travel Medicine Database to obtain specific information about 'at risk' countries.

Principles of pretravel health care

- Advise the patient to plan early—at least 8 weeks beforehand.
- Advise a dental check.
- Allow adequate time for consultation, e.g. 30–45 minutes.
- Individualise advice.
- Provide current information.

- Provide written as well as verbal advice.
- Provide a letter concerning existing medical illness and treatment.
- Encourage personal responsibility.

Gastrointestinal infections

The commonest problem facing travellers is traveller's diarrhoea but other important diseases caused by poor sanitation include hepatitis A, and worm infestations such as hookworm and schistosomiasis.

Contamination of food and water is a major problem especially in Third World countries.

Reputable soft drinks, such as Coca-Cola, should be recommended for drinking. Indian-style tea, in which the milk is boiled with tea, is usually safe, but tea with added milk is not. The food handlers can be infected and the water used to wash food may be contaminated.

Traveller's diarrhoea

Traveller's diarrhoea is a special problem in Mexico, Nepal, India, Pakistan, Latin America, the Middle East and central Africa and its many colourful labels include 'Bali Belly', 'Gippy Tummy', 'Rangoon Runs', 'Tokyo Trots' and 'Montezuma's Revenge'. It occurs about 6–12 hours after taking infected food or water.

The illness is usually mild and lasts only two or three days. It is unusual for it to last longer than five days. Symptoms include abdominal cramps, frequent diarrhoea with loose watery bowel motions and possible vomiting. Very severe diarrhoea, especially if associated with the passing of blood or mucus, may be a feature of a more serious bowel infection such as amoebiasis.

Most traveller's diarrhoea is caused by an enterotoxigenic *E. coli*. Travellers are infected because they are exposed to slightly different types or strains of *E. coli* from the ones they are used to at home.[3]

The possible causes of diarrhoeal illness are listed in Table 12.1.

Treatment
Refer to Figure 12.1.[3]

| Mild diarrhoea |

- Maintain fluid intake—cordial or diluted soft drink.
- Antimotility agents (judicious use: if no blood in stools)
  loperamide (Imodium) 2 caps statim then 1 after each unformed stool (max: 8 caps/day)

or

diphenoxylate with atropine (Lomotil) 2 tablets statim
then 1–2 (o) 8 hourly.
Imodium is the preferred agent.

| Moderate diarrhoea |

- Attend to hydration.
- Patient can self-administer antibiotic—e.g. norfloxacin 400 mg bd for 3 days, or ciprofloxacin; use co-trimoxazole in children.
- Avoid Lomotil or Imodium.

Table 12.1 *Causes of diarrhoea in travellers*

	Causative organism	*Type of illness*
Bacteria	Escherichia coli	Traveller's diarrhoea
	Shigella species	Dysentery
	Salmonella species	Typhoid fever, food poisoning
	Campylobacter jejuni	Traveller's diarrhoea, dysentery
	Vibrio cholerae	Cholera
	Yersinia enterocolitica	Traveller's diarrhoea
	Aeromonas hydrophilia	Traveller's diarrhoea
	Staphylococcus aureus (toxin)	Food poisoning
	Clostridium perfringens	Food poisoning
	Bacillus cereus	Food poisoning
Viruses	Rotavirus	Children's diarrhoea
	Norwalk virus	Traveller's diarrhoea
Protozoa parasites	Cryptosporidium	
	Entamoeba histolytica	Amoebiasis
	Giardia lamblia	Giardiasis
	Strongyloides stercoralis	Strongyloidiasis
Chemicals	Capsicum (chilli)	

Fig. 12.1 *Algorithm for adult travellers with acute diarrhoea* AFTER LOCKE[3]

Severe diarrhoea (patient toxic and
febrile)

- ? Admit to hospital.
- Attend to hydration—use an oral hydrate solution, e.g. Gastrolyte or WHO formulation.
- Avoid Lomotil and Imodium.
- Antibiotic: norfloxacin or ciprofloxacin.

Note: There is increasing resistance to doxycycline and co-trimoxazole, especially in South-East Asia.

Persistent diarrhoea

Any travellers with persistent diarrhoea after visiting less developed countries, especially India and China, may have a protozoal infection such as amoebiasis or giardiasis. If the patient has a fever and mucus or blood in the stools, suspect amoebiasis. Giardiasis is characterised by abdominal cramps, flatulence, and bubbly, foul-smelling diarrhoea persisting beyond 2 to 4 days.

Treatment
Giardiasis: tinidazole or metronidazole
Amoebiasis: metronidazole or tinidazole
Patient can self-administer these drugs and carry them if visiting areas at risk, but they can have a severe adverse reaction with alcohol.

Preventive advice

The following advice will help prevent diseases caused by contaminated food and water. These 'rules' need only be followed in areas of risk such as Africa, South America, India and other parts of Asia.

- Purify all water by boiling for 10 minutes. Adding purifying tablets is not so reliable, but if the water cannot be boiled some protection is provided by adding Puratabs (chlorine) or iodine (2% tincture of iodine), which is more effective than chlorine—use 4 drops iodine to 1 litre of water and let it stand for 30 minutes.

- Do not use ice. Drink only boiled water (supplied in some hotels) or well-known bottled beverages (mineral water, 7-up, Coca-Cola, beer).
- Avoid fresh salads or raw vegetables (including watercress). Salads or uncooked vegetables are often washed in contaminated water. Bananas and fruit with skins are safe once you have peeled and thrown away the skin but care should be taken with fruit that may possibly be injected with water.
- Be wary of dairy products such as milk, cream, ice-cream and cheese.
- Avoid eating raw shellfish and cold cooked meats.
- Avoid food, including citrus fruits, from street vendors.
- Drink hot liquids wherever possible.
- Use disposable moist towels for hand washing.

The golden rule is: *If you can't peel it, boil it or cook it—don't eat it.*

Malaria

General aspects:

- Travellers to all tropical countries are at some risk.
- Malaria is endemic in 102 countries;[4] 2.3 billion people are at risk.
- The risk is very low in the major cities of Central and Southern America and South-East Asia but can be high in some African cities.
- Malaria is either benign (vax, ovale) or malignant (falciparum).
- Resistance to many drugs is increasing:
  - The lethal *Plasmodium falciparum* is developing resistance to chloroquine and the antifolate malarials (Fansidar and Maloprim).[4]
  - Resistance is now reported to mefloquine.
  - CRFM is common in South-East Asia, Papua New Guinea, northern South America and parts of Africa.
- Chloroquine is still effective against *P. ovale* and *P. vivax* (the most common forms).
- The long-awaited vaccine will make all the complex drug management much simpler. However, it still appears to be many years away despite considerable research.
- Patients who have had splenectomies are at grave risk from *P. falciparum* malaria.
- People die from malaria because of delayed diagnosis, delayed therapy, inappropriate therapy and parasite–host factors.
- Practitioners should follow updated recommended guidelines, e.g. NH&MRC, WHO.

Malaria risk assessment

The risk of catching malaria is increased by:

- being in a malaria area, especially during and after the wet season
- a prolonged stay in a malaria area, especially rural areas, small towns and city fringes
- sleeping in unscreened rooms without mosquito nets over the bed
- wearing dark clothing with short-sleeved shirts and shorts
- taking inappropriate drug prophylaxis

Malarial prevention

Travellers should be advised that malaria may be prevented by following two simple rules:

- avoid mosquito bites; and
- take antimalarial medicines regularly

In order to avoid mosquito bites, travellers are advised to:

- keep away from rural areas after dusk
- sleep in air-conditioned or properly screened rooms
- use insecticide sprays to kill any mosquitoes in the room or use mosquito coils at night
- smear an insect repellent on exposed parts of the body; an effective repellent is diethyl-m-toluamide (Muskol, Repellem, Rid)
- use mosquito nets (tuck under mattress; check for tears)
- impregnate nets with permethrin (Ambush) or deltamethrin
- wear sufficient light-coloured clothing, long sleeves and long trousers, to protect whole body and arms and legs when in the open after sunset
- avoid using perfumes, cologne and after shave lotion (also attracts insects)

Important considerations in malaria prophylaxis

1. Minimise exposure to mosquitoes and avoid bites.
2. Know areas of risk:
   - tropical South America (southern Mexico to northern half South America)
   - tropical Africa (sub-Sahara to northern South Africa)
   - Nile region including Egypt
   - Southern Asia especially tropical areas

Table 12.2   *Common drugs used for malarial prophylaxis*

	Adult dosage	Children's dose	Comments
Chloroquine	300 mg base (2 tabs) same day each week 2 wk before, during, 4 wk after exposure	5 mg base/kg up to maximum adult dose	Only antimalarial approved for pregnancy Aggravates psoriasis Beware of retinopathy
Doxycycline	100 mg each day, 1–2 days before, during, 2–4 weeks after	> 8 years only 2 mg/kg/day up to 100 mg	Photosensitivity reactions
Mefloquine	250 mg (1 tab) same day each week, 1 week before, during, 2 weeks after	Not recommended < 45 kg > 45 kg as for adults	Side effects: dizziness, 'fuzzy' head, blurred vision Beware of beta-blockers
Proguanil	200 mg (2 tabs) same day each week 1 day before, during, 4 weeks after	< 1 year: ¼ tablet 1–4 years: ½ tablet 5–8 years: 1 tablet 9–14 years: 1½ tablet > 14 years: adult	Safe in lactation and pregnancy (give folic acid) Side effects: GIT disturbances, headache, dizziness, rash

3. Know areas of widespread chloroquine resistance:
   - Asia, tropical South America (rare north of Panama Canal), sub-Sahara, East Africa
4. Consider several factors:
   - intensity of transmission
   - season and length of stay
   - itinerary   urban—hotel
               urban—non-hotel
               rural—housing
               rural—backpacking
   - resistance patterns
   - host factors — age
               — pregnancy
               — associated illness
               — compliance
5. Know the antimalarial drugs (Table 12.2).
6. Balance risk benefit of drug prophylaxis: drug side effects versus risk of CRFM.
7. Visiting areas of CRFM does not automatically require the use of potentially harmful drugs.[1]

8. Those at special risk are pregnant women, young children and the immunocompromised. Advise against travel.
9. No drugs give complete protection.

Drug prophylaxis

Guidelines

- Accommodation in large air-conditioned hotels in most cities of South-East Asia (dusk–dawn) for < 2 weeks: no prophylaxis required.
- For low-risk travel (urban: dusk–dawn) in areas of high resistance for < 2 weeks: chloroquine adequate; use a treatment course of mefloquine if necessary (Table 12.3).
- For short- and long-term travel to rural areas of high resistance, e.g. South-East Asia including Thailand, Kenya, Tanzania, Ecuador, Venezuela, Brazil: doxycycline daily alone or mefloquine (once a week).

Table 12.3   *Drugs used for chloroquine-resistant malaria (presumptive breakthrough where professional medical care unavailable)[5]*

	Adult dose	Children's dose
Mefloquine	750 mg (3 tablets) statim, then 500 mg after 6–8 hours or 1000 mg statim	only recommended if weight > 45 kg (as for adults)
Pyrimethamine/sulfadoxine (Fansidar)	3 tablets as a single dose	2–11 months: ¼ tablet 1–3 years: ½ tablet 4–8 years: 1 tablet 9–14 years: 2 tablets > 14 years: 3 tablets

Summary of recommendations
1. CSFM area: chloroquine
2. CRFM area:
     mefloquine 250 mg/week
           or
     doxycycline 100 mg/day
3. Multidrug-resistant area
   doxycycline 100 mg/day

   for stays > 8 weeks
         chloroquine
               +
         doxycycline 50–100 mg/day
Standby treatment: mefloquine + Fansidar[5]
CSFM = chloroquine-sensitive falciparum
            malaria
CRFM = chloroquine-resistant falciparum
            malaria

Specific infectious diseases and immunisation

Protection from many types of infection is available through immunisation. All travellers should be immunised against tetanus, polio and diphtheria and measles. Protection against tetanus requires an initial course of three injections followed by a booster every 10 years.

Vaccinations are required for special circumstances. Yellow fever vaccination is a legal requirement for any travellers returning from a yellow fever endemic area. Cholera is not usually required.

Some travellers may be exposed to tuberculosis, hepatitis, plague, rabies, typhoid, typhus, and meningococcal infection. Immunisation against these is available and recommended for those at risk. Smallpox has now been eradicated from the world and therefore smallpox vaccination is no longer required for any traveller.

Japanese B encephalitis presents as a special problem to the traveller.

Table 12.4 outlines a summary of recommendations to consider.[6]

Compulsory immunisations

The two vaccinations that may be required before visiting 'at risk' areas are meningococcus and yellow fever.

Yellow fever

Yellow fever is a serious viral infection spread by mosquitoes and, like malaria, is a tropical

Table 12.4 *Summary of preventive measures and vaccinations*

All travellers, all destinations
   Tetanus toxoid and diphtheria booster
   if > 10 years since last dose
   if > 5 years for Third World travel
   give CDT < 8 years ADT > 8 years

All travellers to developing countries free of malaria
   Tetanus toxoid booster
   Polio immunisation if > 10 years
   Measles immunisation (consider MMR)
   Yellow fever (if compulsory)
   Preventive measures against:
   • gastrointestinal infections
   • sexually transmitted diseases
   • mosquito bites

Travellers to developing and other countries at high risk of infection
   As above plus:
   Malaria prophylaxis
   Hepatitis A-vaccine or immunoglobulin
   Hepatitis B
   Typhoid
   Tuberculosis (BCG if Mantoux -ve)
   Other vaccinations: consider
   • meningococcus (required in some countries)
   • Japanese B encephalitis
   • rabies
   • typhus
   • plague
   • anthrax
   • cholera

disease. Yellow fever vaccination is essential for travel to or through equatorial Africa and northern parts of South America, and for re-entry to Australia from those countries.

One injection only is required and the immunisation is valid for 10 years. Children aged less than 9 months should not be given this vaccine. It should not be given within 3 weeks of cholera vaccine.

Note: It is important to check specific country requirements in the World Health Organisation book on vaccination requirements.[8]

According to WHO a certificate against yellow fever is the only certificate that should be required for international travel. The requirements of some countries are in excess of International Health Regulations. However, vaccination against yellow fever is strongly recommended to all travellers who intend to visit places other than the major cities in the countries where the disease occurs in humans.

Meningococcal infection

Meningitis due to this organism is a contagious lethal disease. It is common in Nepal, Mongolia,

Vietnam and parts of Africa and Asia, especially in the dry season. Travellers trekking through the Kathmandu valley of Nepal and those attending the Haj pilgrimage to Saudi Arabia are at special risk and should have the vaccine. However, some countries require immunisation for entry. A booster is required after 3 years.

Voluntary immunisation

Precautions against the following diseases are recommended for those travellers who may be at special risk.

Hepatitis A, B, E
Hepatitis A is a common problem in rural areas of developing countries. There is a declining level of antibodies to hepatitis A in developed countries and adults are at special risk; so 1 or 2 doses of hepatitis A vaccine should be given. If there is insufficient time a single injection of human immunoglobulin (IG) can give protection for 3 to 6 months. It is safe for all age groups but children under 8 years should not need it. A blood test for hepatitis A antibodies should be carried out to determine a person's immunity.

Prevention
• The rules of avoiding contaminated food and water apply (as for traveller's diarrhoea).

Hepatitis B is endemic in South-East Asia, South America and other developing countries. Vaccination is recommended especially for people working in such countries, particularly those in the health care area or those who may expect to have sexual or drug contact. If patients have a 'negative' HBV core IgG titre, then vaccination would be worthwhile (3 doses: 0, 1 and 6 months). Hepatitis E has a high mortality rate in pregnant women.

Typhoid
Typhoid immunisation is not required for entry into any country but is recommended for travel to Third World countries where the standards of sanitation are low. It should be considered for travellers to smaller cities, and village and rural areas in Africa, Asia, Central and South America and Southern Europe.

The parenteral (subcutaneous) vaccine can be used but the new Typhim Vi vaccine or the oral vaccine, which have fewer side effects, are generally preferred. The oral vaccine, which is given as a series of four capsules, appears to afford protection for about 5 years but is contraindicated in the immunocompromised.

Cholera
Cholera vaccination is not officially recommended by the World Health Organisation (WHO) because it has only limited effectiveness. It is advisable for health care workers or others at risk entering an endemic area. Cholera is given in two injections 7 to 28 days apart. It is not recommended in children under 5 years or pregnant women.

Japanese B encephalitis
This mosquito-borne flavivirus infection presents a real dilemma to the traveller and doctor because it is a very severe infection (mortality rate 20–40%) with high infectivity and high prevalence in endemic countries. The vaccine is prone to give anaphylaxis and is unlicensed in Australia and the United States. It may be obtained only in very restricted circumstances but can be obtained more readily abroad.

The disease is prevalent during summer in the region bound in the west by Nepal and Siberian Russia and in the east by Japan and Singapore, especially in Nepal, Burma, Korea, Vietnam, Thailand, China, eastern Russia and the lowlands of India. Rice paddies and pig farms are areas of risk. The usual preventive measures against mosquito bites are important.

Rabies
Rabies vaccination is recommended for some international aid workers or travellers going to rabies-prone areas for long periods. The vaccination can be effective after the bite of a rabid animal; so routine vaccination is not recommended for the traveller. Affected animals include dogs, cats, monkeys and feral (wild) animals. A traveller who sustains a bite or scratch or even is licked by an animal in countries at risk should wash the site immediately with soap or a detergent, and then seek medical help. The prebite vaccination does not remove the need for postexposure vaccination.

Typhus
Typhus is transmitted to humans by bites from lice, fleas or ticks. Immunisation against typhus is desirable for doctors, nurses, and agricultural and technical advisers whose work takes them

to remote areas of Bolivia, Burundi, Ethiopia, Mexico, Rwanda and mountainous regions of Asia. A booster injection should be given at 12 months if the traveller is still in an area of risk.

Plague

Plague is still prevalent in rodents in several countries such as Vietnam, Brazil, Peru, Ecuador, Kenya and Malagasy Republic. Although not compulsory, vaccination is recommended for those engaged in field operations in plague areas and rural health workers who may be exposed to infected patients. Two doses are given to adults (3 to children < 12 years) and a booster every 6 months.

Special problems

Prevention of sexually transmitted diseases

Casual sexual contacts place the traveller at risk of contracting a serious, perhaps fatal, sexually transmitted disease (STD). The common STDs especially prevalent in South-East Asia and Africa are non-specific urethritis, gonorrhoea (especially penicillin-resistant strains), hepatitis B, and syphilis. HIV infection is a rapidly increasing problem, with heterosexual transmission common in Africa and in South-East Asia. Unusual STDs such as lymphogranuloma venerum, chancroid and donovanosis are encountered more commonly in tropical developing countries. A practical rule is to assume that all 'at risk' travellers are both ignorant and irresponsible and advise accordingly.

Prevention
Abstinence or take your partner
(condoms and diaphragms do not give
absolute protection)

Drugs

Possession of and trafficking in drugs is very hazardous and many people are held in foreign prisons for various drug offences. The penalty for carrying drugs can be death!

Countries that currently may enforce the death penalty are Burma, Indonesia, Malaysia, Singapore, Thailand and Turkey. Travellers should be warned about taking cannabis while in a foreign country, as it can cause profound personality changes in the user.

Drug addicts should under no circumstances travel. Young travellers should be wary about accepting lifts or hitchhiking in countries 'at risk'.

Problems in the returned traveller

- Most will present within 2 weeks except HIV infection.
- Common infections encountered are giardiasis, amoebiasis, hepatitis A, B or E, gonorrhoea or *Chlamydia trachomatis*, malaria and helminthic infestations.
- An important non-infected problem requiring vigilance is deep venous thrombosis and thromboembolism.
- The asymptomatic traveller may present for advice about an illness acquired or about exposure (without illness) such as rabies, malaria, schistosomiasis and sexually transmitted diseases.

Exposure to STDs

If a patient has had unprotected intercourse and is at definite risk of acquiring an STD such as penicillin-resistant gonorrhoea or NSU, the following may be appropriate:[1]

ceftriaxone 250 mg IM (as a single dose)
doxycycline 100 mg (o) for 10 days.

Gastrointestinal symptoms

Mild diarrhoea

- stool microscopy and culture
- look for and treat associated helminthic infestation, e.g. roundworms, hookworms.

Moderate or prolonged (> 3 weeks) diarrhoea

Usually due to *Giardia lamblia*, *Entamoeba histolytica*, *Campylobacter jejuni*, salmonella, *Yersinia enterocolitica* or Cryptosporidium.

- stool examination (3 fresh specimens)
  — microscopy
  — wet preparation
  — culture
- treat pathogen (see guidelines under diarrhoea pp. 92–93)

Non-pathogens such as *E.coli* and *Endolimax nana* are often reported but do not treat specifically.

Note: Consider exotic causes such as schistosomiasis, strongyloidiasis and ciguatera in unusual chronic post-travel 'gastroenteritis'.

Persistent abdominal discomfort

This common syndrome includes bloating, intestinal hurry and borborygmi, and often follows an episode of diarrhoea. Usually no pathogens are found on stool examination. However, giardiasis can be difficult to detect and an empirical course of tinidazole (2 g statim) is worthwhile. Any persistent problem then is a type of post-infective bowel dysfunction or irritable bowel. Reassurance is important.

Fever

- Causes range from mild viral infections to potentially fatal cerebral malaria (Table 12.5) and meningococcal septicaemia.
- The common serious causes are malaria, typhoid, hepatitis (especially A and B), dengue fever and amoebiasis.
- Most deaths from malaria have occurred after at least 3 or 4 days of symptoms that may be mild. Death can occur within 24 hours. Factors responsible for death from malaria include delayed presentation, missed or delayed diagnosis (most cases), no chemoprophylaxis and old age.
- Refer immediately to a specialist unit if the patient is unwell.
- Be vigilant for meningitis and encephalitis.
- Be vigilant for amoebiasis—can present with a toxic megacolon, especially if antimotility drugs given.
- If well but febrile:
  First line screening tests
  — full blood examination and ESR
  — thick and thin films
  — liver function tests
  — urine for micro and culture
- Refer immediately if malaria is proven or if fever persists after a further 24 hours.

Malaria

See Figure 12.2.
- incubation period: *P. falciparum* 7–14 days; others 12–40 days
- most present within 2 months of return
- can present up to 2 or more years
- can masquerade as several other illnesses

Symptoms

- high fever, chills, rigor, sweating, headache
- usually abrupt onset
- can have atypical presentations, e.g. diarrhoea, abdominal pain, cough

Table 12.5 *Fever and malaise in the returned traveller: diagnostic strategy model*

Note: *All fever in a returned traveller is malaria until proved otherwise!*

Q. *Probability diagnosis*
A. Viral respiratory illness, e.g. influenza
   Hepatitis (may be subclinical)
   Gastroenteritis

Q. *Serious disorders not to be missed*
A. Malaria
   Typhoid
   Japanese B encephalitis
   Meningococcal meningitis
   Melioidosis
   Amoebiasis (liver abscess)
   HIV infection

Q. *Pitfalls (often missed)*
A. Ascending cholangitis
   Infective endocarditis
   Dengue fever
   Lyme disease
   Bronchopneumonia
   Ross River fever
   Rarities
      Legionnaires' disease
      Schistosomiasis
      African trypanosomiasis
      Yellow fever
      Rift Valley fever
      Spotted fever
      Lasa fever

Note: Three causes of a dry cough (in absence of chest signs) are malaria, typhoid, amoebic liver abscess.

Q. *Seven masquerades checklist*
A. Drugs   √ (reaction to antimalarials)
   Urinary infection   √

> *Investigations (if no obvious cause)*
> - Full blood examination
> - Thick and thin blood films
> - Blood culture
> - Liver function tests
> - Urine—micro and culture
> - Stool—micro and culture
> - ESR
> - New malaria tests

Other features

- Beware of modified infection.
- Must treat within 4 days.
- Typical relapsing patterns often absent.
- Thick smear allows detection of parasites (some laboratories are poorly skilled with thick films).
- Thin smear helps diagnose malaria type.

Typical features

headache
malaise
fever/chills
prostration
sweating
myalgia

T	P	BP	R
↑↑	↑	N↓	N↑

hepatomegaly

Other possible features

cerebral problems
• delirium
• convulsions
• coma
anaemia
jaundice
vomiting

postural hypotension

cough

splenomegaly

abdominal
pain
diarrhoea

arrhythmia

dark urine
(blackwater fever)

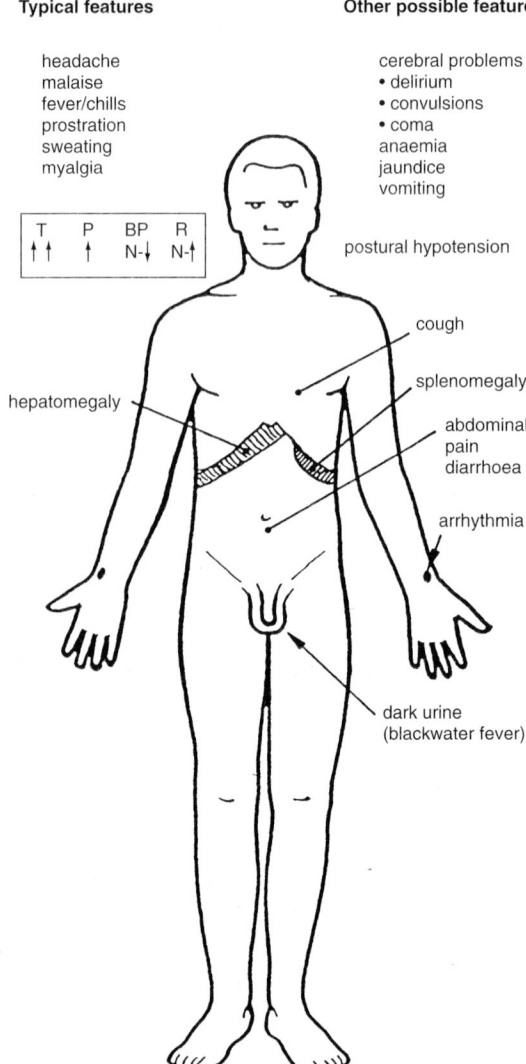

Fig. 12.2 *Clinical features of malaria*

If index of suspicion high, repeat the smear ('No evidence of malaria' = 3 negative daily thick films). Monocytosis is a helpful diagnostic clue. Newer tests e.g. PCR tests and ICT card tests show promise. Cerebral malaria and blackwater fever are severe and dramatic.

<hr>

Treatment

• admit to hospital with infectious disease expertise
• supportive measures including fluid replacement

• *P. vivax, P. ovale, P. malariae*[4,7]
(check G₆PD first)

Correction: (check G_6PD first)
chloroquine 4 tabs (o) statim, then 2 tabs in 6 hours,
then 2 tabs on day 2 and day 3
+
primaquine 15 mg (o) daily for 14 days
• *P. falciparum*[4,7]
uncomplicated:
quinine sulphate 600 mg (o) 8 hourly, 7 days
+
doxycycline 100 mg (o) daily, 7 days
or
Fansidar, 3 tablets on day 3
or (alone as alternative to above)
mefloquine (for breakthrough dose)
complicated:
quinine dihydrochloride 20 mg/kg IV (over 4 hours)
then after 4-hour gap 10 mg/kg IV 8 hourly until improved
then
quinine (o) 7 days + Fansidar statim
Note: Check for hypoglycaemia.
Beware if antimalarial use in previous 48 hours.

Typhoid fever
Incubation period 10–14 days.

Clinical presentation

• insidious onset
• headache prominent
• dry cough
• fever gradually increases in 'stepladder' manner over 4 days or so
• abdominal pain and constipation (early)
• diarrhoea and rash (late)

| *Diagnosis* | on suspicion → blood culture serology not very helpful |
| *Treatment* | ciprofloxacin |

Dengue fever
Also known as 'breakbone' fever, it is widespread in SE Pacific and endemic in Queensland.

Features

• mosquito-borne viral infection
• incubation period 5–6 days
• abrupt onset fever, malaise, headache, pain behind eyes, severe backache

- severe aching of muscles and joints
- fever subsides for about 2 days then returns
- maculopapular rubelliform rash on limbs → trunk
- generalised erythema with 'islands of sparing'
- the rare haemorrhagic form is very severe; may present with shock
- later severe fatigue and depression (prone to suicide)

Diagnosis	specific serology
Treatment	is symptomatic with supportive follow-up
Prevention	avoid mosquito bites—no vaccine available

Japanese B encephalitis and meningococcal meningitis

Consider these serious infections in a patient presenting with headache, fever and malaise before neurological symptoms such as delirium, convulsions and coma develop.

Other tropical infections

Travellers to tropical or subtropical areas are at risk of more unusual infections. Most of these infections are contracted through contaminated food and water, insect bites and walking barefoot on contaminated soil. The risk of such infections is highest in rural areas of countries other than Europe, North America and Australasia.

African trypanosomiasis (sleeping sickness)

Clinical features

- incubation period about 3 weeks
- fever, headache and a skin chancre or nodule
- lymphadenopathy, hepatosplenomegaly

Diagnosis	demonstrating trypomastigotes in peripheral blood smear or chancre aspirate
Treatment	• suramin IV • infectious disease consultation essential
Prevention	Avoid bites of the tsetse fly. If visiting areas of East, Central and West Africa, especially the 'safari game parks', travellers should use insect repellent and wear protective light-coloured clothing including long sleeves and trousers.

Cutaneous leishmaniasis

This may be encountered in travellers and servicemen and servicewomen returning from the Middle East, especially the Persian Gulf. The protozoa is transmitted by a sandfly and has an average incubation period of 9 weeks. The key clinical finding is an erythematous papule. Diagnosis is made by performing a punch biopsy and culturing tissue in a special medium. Treatment for extensive lesions is with high dosage ketoconazole for 1 month. Smaller lesions should be treated topically with 15% paromomycin and 12% methyl benzethonium chloride ointment applied bd for 10 days.[8] A special vaccine is available in some Middle Eastern countries, e.g. Israel.

Schistosomiasis (bilharzia)

The first clinical sign is a local skin reaction at the site of penetration of the parasite (it then invades liver, bowel and bladder). This site is known as 'swimmer's itch'. Within a week or so there is a generalised allergic response usually with fever, malaise, myalgia and urticaria. A gastroenteritis-like syndrome can occur (nausea, vomiting, diarrhoea) and respiratory symptoms, particularly cough. Clinical findings, such as trypanosomiasis, include lymphadenopathy and hepatosplenomegaly.

The infestation is caused by parasite organisms (schistosomes) whose eggs are passed in human excreta, which contaminates watercourses (notably stagnant water) and irrigation channels in Egypt, other parts of Africa, South America, some parts of South-East Asia and China. Freshwater snails are the carriers (vectors).

Diagnosis	detecting eggs in the stools, the urine or in a rectal biopsy
Treatment	praziquantel
Prevention	Travellers should be warned against drinking from, or swimming and wading in, dams, watercourses or irrigation channels, especially in Egypt and other parts of Africa.

Hookworm and strongyloidiasis

Hookworm and *Strongyloides* are parasites that are acquired by walking barefoot (or wearing thongs or sandals) on earth contaminated by faeces. The larvae penetrate the skin, travel through the lungs and settle in the small intestine. The first sign is local irritation or 'creeping eruption' at the point of entry known as 'ground itch', which is often unnoticed. This subsides within 2 days or so and is followed 1–2 weeks later by respiratory symptoms, which may be associated with bronchitis and bronchopneumonia. Eventually a severe and chronic anaemia may develop. Hookworm infection is the commonest cause of iron deficiency anaemia in the world. Strongyloidiasis, which usually does not present with anaemia, is an important pathogen since it remains undetected for decades and presents as a severe infection such as septicaemia when the host becomes immunocompromised for any reason.

Diagnosis	detecting larvae or ova in the stool

Treatment (adults)	• Hookworm—mebendazole 100 mg bd for 3 days • Strongyloidiasis — thiabendazole 1.5 g bd for 2 days (or more) • Adverse effects are common. Beware of these drugs in pregnancy and children.

Prevention	Travellers should be warned to wear shoes and socks in endemic areas to prevent entry of the larvae into the skin of the feet.

Cutaneous larva migrans

Cutaneous larva migrans (creeping eruption) should be suspected in any pruritic, erythematous lesion with a serpiginous eruption on the skin, especially the hands and feet of a person from a subtropical or tropical area. It is caused by the larvae of dog or cat hookworms penetrating and migrating throughout human skin, the larva always being just ahead of the lesion it causes. The diagnosis is based on the classic clinical appearance and by eosinophilia. Biopsy is usually not indicated. The problem is usually self-limiting.

Diagnosis	clinical (characteristic appearance), eosinophilia (biopsy usually not indicated)

Treatment	• albendazole or thiabendazole[7] • antihistamines for pruritus *Note:* This is usually a self-limiting problem.

Prevention	As for hookworm. Moist sandy soil contaminated with dog or cat faeces is a common source.

Cutaneous myiasis

Myiasis, which refers to the infestation of body tissues by the larvae (maggots) of flies, often presents as itchy 'boils'. Primary myiasis invariably occurs in travellers to tropical areas such as Africa whereby the fly can introduce the larvae into the skin, or it can be due to secondary invasion of pre-existing wounds. Close inspection of lesions may reveal part or all of the larva. The simplest treatment is lateral pressure and tweezer extraction.

Trichuriasis (whipworm)

This common tropical parasite is sometimes seen in northern Australia. When the eggs are ingested with food, the larvae hatch in the small intestine and develop into adult worms, 3 to 5 cm long, which attach by means of their whip-like end to the mucosa of the large intestine. The majority of infected persons are asymptomatic but in heavy infection, abdominal cramps, diarrhoea, distension, nausea and vomiting and even rectal prolapse may develop.

Diagnosis	identifying characteristic eggs in faecal smears

Treatment	oral mebendazole or albendazole

Scrub typhus

Scrub typhus is found in South-East Asia, northern Australia and the western Pacific. It is caused by *Rickettsia tsutsugamushi*, which is transmitted by mites.

Features

• abrupt onset febrile illness with headache and myalgia
• a black eschar at the site of the bite with regional and generalised lymphadenopathy

- short-lived macular rash
- can develop severe complications, e.g. pneumonitis, encephalitis

| Diagnosis | serological assays and micro-immunofluorescence |

| Treatment | doxycycline 100 mg bd for 7–10 days. |

Queensland tick typhus

Queensland tick typhus, which is caused by *Rickettsia australis*, is directly related to a tick bite. The symptoms are almost identical to scrub typhus, although less severe, and the treatment is identical.

Melioidosis

This serious disease with a high mortality is caused by the Gram-negative bacillus, *Pseudomonas pseudomallei*, a soil saprophyte that infects humans mainly by penetrating through skin wounds, especially abrasions. It is mostly acquired while wading in rice paddies. It is mainly a disease of Third World countries and occurs between 20° North and 20° South of the equator, mainly in South-East Asia and including Northern Australia. It may manifest as a focal infection or as septicaemia with abscesses in the lung, kidney, liver or spleen. It presents with fever, cough and myalgia. It is called the 'Vietnamese time bomb' because it can present years after the initial infection in Vietnamese war veterans.

| Diagnosis | blood culture, swabs from focal lesions, haemagglutination test |

| Treatment (adults)[7] | ceftazidime 2g IV, 6–8 hourly
   + either
co-trimoxazole 320/1600 mg (o) or IV, 12 hourly
   or
doxycycline 100 mg (o) or IV, 12 hourly
all for at least 14 days
   followed by
oral co-trimoxazole or doxycycline bd for 3 months |

| Prevention | Traumatised people with open wounds (especially diabetics) in endemic areas (tropical South-East Asia) should be carefully nursed. |

Ciguatera

This is a type of fish food poisoning caused by eating tropical fish, especially large coral trout and large cod, in tropical waters, e.g. the Caribbean and tropical Pacific. The problem is caused by a type of poison that concentrates in the fish after they feed on certain micro-organisms around reefs. Ciguatera poisoning presents as a bout of 'gastroenteritis' (vomiting, diarrhoea and stomach pains) and then symptoms affecting the nervous system such as muscle aching and weakness, paraesthesia and burning sensations of the skin, particularly of the fingers and lips. There is no cure for the problem but it can be treated with gammaglobulin. It is unwise to eat large predatory reef fish, especially their offal (mainly the liver).

Pregnancy and travel

Most international airlines do not allow passengers to travel after the thirty-sixth week of pregnancy and may require a doctor's certificate after twenty-eight weeks. Air travel is contraindicated in the last month of pregnancy and until the seventh day after delivery. The past obstetric history should be taken into account. The same health risks apply except that most antimalarial tablets and vaccinations are not recommended. Only chloroquine is definitely safe. Live vaccinations (measles, rubella, influenza) are generally contraindicated[9] but the WHO considers it safe to have polio vaccine. Administration of killed or inactivated vaccines, toxoids and polysaccharides is permitted during pregnancy. Yellow fever vaccine is considered safe after the sixth month. As a general rule pregnancy and travel to Third World countries do not mix and pregnant women should be advised not to travel to these countries.

Tetanus immunisation is important as protection is passed on to the child during early infancy. Immunoglobin can be safely given as prevention against hepatitis.

The antimalarial drugs chloroquine, quinine and proguanil may be given to pregnant women but all others mentioned in Table 12.2 are contraindicated.

Children and travel

Although children including infants are good travellers and adapt well, their resistance, especially to heat and infections, is lower. A child can suffer from acute dehydration very rapidly.[9] Air travel is not recommended for infants of less than 7 days or premature infants.

The change in atmospheric pressure on landing can cause distressing ear pain, so taking a bottle during descent is recommended.

In tropical areas it is important to keep children well hydrated and they should wear loose cotton clothing. A good guide to the health of children is the amount and colour of their urine. If it is scanty and concentrated they are not getting sufficient fluid.

Most vaccines (diphtheria, tetanus, poliomyelitis, BCG) can safely be given in the first few weeks of life. Measles is common overseas and it is worthwhile considering it even under 12 months. Yellow fever vaccine should not be given under 12 months. Hence the importance of protection against mosquito bites. Malaria prophylaxis is important. Chloroquine, proguanil and quinine may be given safely to infants. However, as a rule young children should be discouraged from travel.

Air travel

Air travel is safe and comfortable, but jet lag and air sickness are problems that face many travellers.

Jet lag

This is the uncomfortable aftermath of a long flight in which the person feels exhausted and disoriented, and has poor concentration, insomnia and anxiety. The problem on arrival is poor concentration and judgment during the daytime.

Other symptoms that may occur include anorexia, weakness, headache, blurred vision and dizziness.

Jet lag is a feature of flying long distances east–west or west–east through several time zones, causing the person's routine daily rhythm of activity and sleep to get out of phase. The worst cases appear to be in those travelling eastbound from England to Australia. It can occur with travel in any direction, but the north–south flights are not so bothersome.

Factors influencing jet lag

Personal factors. These include age, state of health, tolerance to change, preparation for the long trip and, very importantly, the emotional and mental state.

General factors. Noise, vibration, air humidity and sitting still for long periods can influence jet lag.

Specific factors. Duration of the flight, time of departure, and changes in climate and culture at the destination affect the severity of jet lag. The problem is aggravated by:

- stress of the pretrip planning
- last minute rushing and anxiety
- lack of sleep during the trip
- overeating and excessive alcohol during the flight
- smoking

How to minimise the problem (advice to patients)

Before the flight

- Allow plenty of time for planning.
- Plan a stopover if possible.
- If possible arrange the itinerary so that you are flying into the night.
- Ensure a good sleep the night before flying.
- Ensure a relaxed trip to the airport.
- Take along earplugs if noise (75–100 decibels) is bothersome.

During the flight

- *Fluids.* Avoid alcohol and coffee. Drink plenty of non-alcoholic drinks such as orange juice and mineral water.
- *Food.* Eat only when hungry and even skip a meal or two. Eat the lighter, more digestible parts of your meals and avoid fatty foods and rich carbohydrate foods.
- *Dress.* Women should wear loose clothes (e.g. long skirts, comfortable jeans, light jumpers) and avoid girdles or restrictive clothing. Wear comfortable (not tight) shoes and take them off during flight.
- *Smoking.* Reduce smoking to a minimum. Non-smokers should seek a non-smoking zone.
- *Sleep.* Try to sleep on longer sections of the flight (give the movies a miss). Close the blinds, wear special eye masks and ask for a pillow. Sedatives such as temazepam (Euhypnos or Normison) or antihistamines can help sleep.
- *Activity.* Try to take regular walks around the aircraft and exercise at airport stops. Keep feet up when resting, and exercise by flexing the major muscles of the legs. Avoid resting the calves of legs against the seat for long periods.

Rest without napping during daylight sectors.
- *Special body care.* Continually wet the face and eyes. A wetting agent such as hydromellose 0.5% eye drops can help those with a tendency to sore eyes.

At the destination

Take a nap for 1–2 hours if possible.

Wander around until you are tired and go to bed at the usual time. It is good to have a full day's convalescence and avoid big decision making soon after arrival. Allow about three days for adjustment after the London to Australia flight.

Who is fit to fly?

Patients with these problems should avoid flying:[9]

- upper airways congested by infection, including influenza
- acute gastroenteritis
- severe respiratory disease (emphysema, chronic bronchitis, pneumothorax)
- unstable heart failure
- severe anaemia (below 8 g/dL)
- pregnancy beyond 200 days (28 weeks) (up to 36 weeks if necessary)
- previous violent or unpredictable behaviour
- within 4 weeks of a myocardial infarction
- within 14 days of a cerebrovascular accident
- within 14 days of major surgery
- brain tumour or recent skull fracture
- recent eye surgery
- severe or poorly controlled hypertension
- poorly controlled epilepsy

Special precautions are required by travellers with the following problems:

- *Colostomy.* Patients should wear a large colostomy bag and take extra bags.
- *Varicose veins.* Such patients should wear supportive stockings and exercise frequently.
- *Plaster casts.* Those with broken limbs in plaster should be careful of swelling.
- *Pacemakers.* Those with pacemakers may have a problem with X-rays at some overseas airports. Mention it to security officials before passing through security equipment.
- *Epilepsy.* Medication should be increased on the day of travel.
- *Diabetics.* Diabetics should discuss their therapy and control with their doctor. They should carry sweets.

Travel sickness

Almost everyone is sick when sailing on rough seas. However, some people, especially children, suffer sickness from the effect of motion on a boat, in a car or in a plane. The larger the boat, plane or car, the less the likelihood of sickness; travel by train rarely causes sickness. Nearly all children grow out of the tendency to have travel sickness, but many adults remain 'bad' sailors.

The problem is caused by sensitivity of the semicircular canals of the inner ear. They are affected by the movement and vibration of travel. Some people have sensitive inner ear canals and are prone to sickness, especially on certain types of journeys (e.g. winding roads through hills) and in certain vehicles.

The main symptoms of travel sickness are nausea, vomiting, dizziness, weakness and lethargy. Early signs are pallor and drowsiness, and sudden silence from an active, talkative child.

How to minimise the problem

1. Keep calm and relaxed before and during travel. With children avoid excitement and apprehension about the travelling. Encourage activities such as looking at distant objects; discourage activities such as reading and games that require close visual concentration.
2. Lie down, if possible, because this rests the inner ear canals and reduces the urge to vomit. If travelling by car, stop regularly for breaks. Passengers should use the front seat if possible.
3. Do not have a large meal a few hours before the journey or during it; avoid milk and fried or greasy foods. Do not travel with an empty stomach: have a light simple meal about an hour before and do not drink too much. Glucose drinks such as lemonade are suitable, as are glucose sweets and biscuits while travelling.

Medication for travel sickness

Many medicines are available for travel sickness. They include hyoscine, various antihistamines and other phenothiazine derivatives, all of which can cause drowsiness; although a problem to drivers, this sedative effect may be helpful for children or for those travelling long distances by plane.

Phenothiazine derivatives that provide appropriate anti-labyrinthine activity include prochlorperazine (Stemetil), promethazine hydrochloride (Phenergan) and promethazine theoclate (Avomine).

Combination antihistamine and hyoscine preparations for travel sickness include Trava-calm and Benacine (Table 12.6).

Hyoscine comes in tablet form, either alone or in combination and in the now popular adhesive patches.

Recommended medications

> *Car travel: adult passengers and children*

- Dimenhydrinate (Andrumin, Dramamine)
  or
  Promethazine theoclate (Avomine)
  or
  Hyoscine (Kwells)

Table 12.6 *Medication to consider for motion sickness*

Drug (genre)	Brand names and formulations	Dosage	
		Adults	**Children**
Antihistamines			
Dimenhydrinate	Andrumin 25 mg, 50 mg	50 mg statim then 4 hourly prn (max 300 mg/24 hours)	avoid < 2 years 2–6 years: 6.25 mg
	Dramamine 25 mg, 50 mg syrup 12.5 mg/5 mL		6–8 years: 12.5 mg 8–12 years: 25 mg > 12 years: 50 mg tds (max 3–4 doses/24 hours)
Pheniramine	Avil, 10 mg, 50 mg syrup 3 mg/mL	25–50 mg tds	infants 10 mg bd < 10 years: 10 mg tds > 10 years: 10–20 mg tds
	Fenamine 50 mg syrup 3 mg/mL		
Promethazine theoclate	Avomine 25 mg	25 mg statim or nocte for long journeys	< 5 years: ¼ tab 5–10 years: ½ tab > 10 years: 1 tab
Promethazine hydrochloride	Phenergan 10 mg, 25 mg syrup 1 mg/mL	25 mg bd	1–5 years: 5 mg bd 5–12 years: 10 mg bd
Related phenothiazines			
Prochlorperazine	Stemetil 5 mg suppositories 5 mg, 25 mg	5–15 mg tds	0.2 mg/kg bd or tds < 10 kg: avoid
Hyoscine			
Hyoscine hydrobromide	Kwells 0.3 mg tab	1–2 tab statim then 1 tab 4–6 hour prn (max 4/24 hours)	2–7 years: ¼ tab > 7 years: ½ tab (max 4 doses/24 hours)
	Scop 1.5 mg transdermal	1 patch per 72 hours	avoid < 10 years
Combinations			
Hyoscine (0.2 mg) + dimenhydrinate (50 mg) + caffeine (20 mg)	Travacalm	1–2 tabs statim (max 4/24 hours)	< 2 years: avoid 2–3 years: ¼ tab 4–7 years: ¼–½ tab 8–13 years: ½–1 tab (max 4 doses/24 hours)

General rules All tablets should be taken 30–60 minutes before departure and repeated 4–6 hourly as necessary (aim for maximum of 4 doses per 24 hours). Antihistamines should be used less frequently and some may be used once a day. Take care with drowsiness, pregnancy, the elderly and prostatic problems. Common adverse effects are drowsiness, irritability, dry mouth, dizziness and blurred vision which are compounded by alcohol, antidepressants and tranquillisers. Hyoscine overdosage (from skin discs) can include confusion, memory loss, giddiness and hallucinations.

These preventive oral preparations should ideally be taken 30–60 minutes before the trip and can be repeated 4–6 hourly during the trip (maximum 4 tablets in 24 hours).
- Hyoscine dermal discs (Scop)
  One of these adhesive patches should be applied to dry unbroken hairless skin behind the ear, 5–6 hours before travel and left on for 3 days. Wash the hands thoroughly after applying and removing the disc—be careful of accidental finger-to-eye contact.

| Sea travel |

Sea travel generally poses no special problems apart from motion sickness and the possibility of injuries in the aged. The larger the ship the less likely the problem. Those prone to sea sickness are advised to take antiemetics 60 minutes before sailing and for the first 2 days at sea until they obtain their 'sea legs'. However, the use of hyoscine transdermal delivery systems is recommended for convenience.

Severe sea sickness. The standard treatment is promethazine (Phenergan) 25 mg IM injection. If injections are not possible prochlorperazine (Stemetil) suppositories can be used.

The aged. Generally the elderly travel well but should take safeguards to avoid falls. The Chief Surgeon on P & O's ship *Canberra* recommends that elderly people should bring the following:

- a letter from their doctor stating diagnosis and medication
- a spare set of spectacles
- a spare set of dentures
- a walking stick (if appropriate)

Altitude sickness[10]

High altitudes pose special problems for people who live at low altitude, especially if they have heart and lung disease. The severity depends on altitude, the speed of ascent, the temperature and level of activity. The high altitudes of Africa (Kilimanjaro, Kenya), India, Nepal (Himalayas), Rockies of Canada and the United States, and South America provide such problems. It is usually safe to trek under 2500 metres altitude but problems may occur over 3000 metres.

Forms
1. acute mountain sickness (mild $\rightarrow$ severe)
2. high-altitude pulmonary oedema
3. high-altitude cerebral oedema

Clinical features
- usually within 8–24 hours of exposure
- frontal headache (worse in morning and when supine)
- malaise, fatigue, anorexia, nausea, insomnia

More severe: fluid retention, dyspnoea, vomiting, dry cough, dizziness.

Serious: marked dyspnoea, neurological symptoms and signs

Management

| Prevention | • careful acclimatisation with gradual ascent[10]
• spend 2–3 days at intermediate altitudes
• ascent rate less than 300 metres per day above 3000 metres
• ample fluid intake
• acetazolamide (Diamox) 250 mg 8 hourly the day before ascent; continue 3–6 days (deaths from mountain sickness have still occurred while on this drug) |

| Treatment | • immediate (urgent and rapid) descent to below 2000 metres
• oxygen
• dexamethasone e.g. 4 mg, 6 hourly |

Travellers' medical kit

If a person intends to travel for a long time the following represents a comprehensive medical kit. It should not be regarded as an alternative to seeking appropriate medical help if it is available. Typical examples of general items are included in brackets.

Materials
- bandaids and elastoplast dressing strip
- bandages (2 cotton gauze, 2 crepe $\times$ 10 cm)
- pocket torch

- steristrips or 'butterfly strips' (to patch small cuts)
- sterile gauze and cotton wool
- thermometer
- scissors and tweezers
- safety pins

Topical items
- antifungal cream
- chlorhexidine/cetrimide antiseptic cream (Savlon)
- insect repellent containing diethyl-m-toluamide (Muskol, Repellem or Rid)
- insecticide spray
- mosquito net repellent solution: permethrin (Ambush—ICI)
- nasal spray or drops
- Stingose spray (for bites and stings)
- Strepsils
- UV antisunburn cream

Medication checklist
Those items marked with * usually require a prescription.
```
*  Antibiotics— norfloxacin 400 mg (6 tablets
                  for 3 days)
              — co-trimoxazole (for children)
   Antacid tablets—for heartburn or indigestion
*  Antimalarials—where appropriate
*  Diamox tablets for acute mountain sickness
*  Fasigyn 2 g or Flagyl 2.4 g—for amoebiasis or
   giardiasis
   Laxative (Senokot)
*  Imodium or Lomotil—for diarrhoea
   Motion sickness tablets (Avomine, Kwells or
   Phenergan)
   Paracetamol tablets—for fever or pain
*  Sleeping tablets (temazepam, promethazine)
   Rehydration mixture (Gastrolyte).
```

General tips for the traveller
Checklist for 'at risk' countries
- 'If you can't peel, boil or cook it, don't eat it.'
- Boil or purify water, avoid dairy products, ice-cream, shellfish, food left in open, salads, watercress, ice and recooked or reheated food.
- Never walk around barefoot at night in snake areas (and use a torch).
- Always shake your shoes before putting them on.
- Never wear nylon items in hot tropical areas.

- Never bathe, wade or drink in rivers, lakes or harbours unless you know they are bilharzia-free.
- Keep yourself well covered after dark and use a mosquito net.
- Use insect repellent on skin frequently.
- Use an insecticide spray in your bedroom.
- Seek medical help if bitten by an excited dog, after washing bite.

Other tips
- Organise a dental check before departure.
- Arrange stopovers on a long flight (if possible).
- Take along a spare pair of spectacles and adequate medication.
- Arrange health and travel insurance.
- Check out your nearest embassy/consulate when visiting remote areas or politically unstable countries.
- Consider a traveller's medical kit.
- Never carry a parcel or luggage through Customs to oblige a stranger or recent acquaintance.
- Abstain from sex with a stranger.
- Have a credit card that allows a quick cash advance or an airline ticket purchase (for many countries a policy of 'if you get sick, then get out' is necessary).
- Most death and injury among travellers is caused by motor accidents. Avoid buses in India (and elsewhere)—trains are safer.

References
1. Oldmeadow M. *Travel medicine*. Melbourne: Monash University. Proceedings of Update Course for General Practitioners, 1991, 4.
2. Grayson L, McNeill J. Preventive health advice for Australian travellers to Bali. Med J Aust, 1988; 149: 462–466.
3. Locke DM. Traveller's diarrhoea. Aust Fam Physician, 1990; 19:194–203.
4. Currie B. Malaria. In: MIMS Disease Index (2nd edn). Sydney: IMS Publishing, 1996, 293–296.
5. Hudson B. Travel medicine. In: MIMS Disease Index (2nd edn). Sydney: IMS Publishing, 1996, 521–530.
6. Munro R, Macleod C. Recommendations for international travellers. Mod Med Aust, August 1991, 50–57.

7. Mashford L et al. Antibiotic guidelines. Victorian Medical Postgraduate Foundation (9th edn). 1996/97; 60–90.

8. Amichai B, Finkelstein E et al. Think cutaneous leishmaniasis. Aust Fam Physician, 1993; 22:1213–1217.

9. World Health Organisation. International Health for Travellers, 1996.

10. McDonnell L. Altitude sickness. Aust Fam Physician, 1990; 19:205–208.

13

Research in general practice

—

*Not the possession of truth, but the effort of struggling
to attain it brings joy to the researcher.*

Goffhold Lassing (1729–81)

Effective research is the trademark of the medical profession. When confronted with the great responsibility of understanding and treating human beings we need as much scientific evidence as possible to render our decision making valid, credible and justifiable.

Research can be defined as 'a systematic method in which the truth of evidence is based on observing and testing the soundness of conclusions according to consistent rules'[1] or, to put it more simply, 'research is organised curiosity',[2] the end point being new and improved knowledge.

In the medical context the term 'research' tends to conjecture bench-type laboratory research. However, the discipline of general practice provides a fertile research area in which to evaluate the morbidity patterns and the nature of common problems in addition to the processes specific to primary health care.

There has been an excellent tradition of research conducted by general practitioners. Tim Murrell in his paper 'Nineteenth century masters of general practice'[3] describes the contributions of Edward Jenner, Caleb Parry, John Snow, Robert Koch and James MacKenzie, and notes that 'among the characteristics they shared was their capacity to observe and record natural phenomena, breaking new frontiers of discovery in medicine using an ecological paradigm'.

This tradition was carried into the 20th century by GPs such as William Pickles, the first president of the Royal College of General Practitioners, Keith Hodgkin and John Fry, all of whom meticulously recorded data that helped to establish patterns for the nature of primary health care. In Australia the challenge was taken up by such people as Clifford Jungfer, Alan Chancellor, Charles Bridges-Webb, Kevin Cullen and Trevor Beard in the 1960s,[4] and now the research activities of the new generation of general practitioners, academic based or practice based, have burgeoned and are flourishing.

The aim of this chapter is to present a brief overview of research and in particular to encourage general practitioners, either singly or collectively, to undertake research—simple or sophisticated—and also to publish their work. The benefits of such are well outlined in John Howie's classic text *Research in general practice*[5].

Why do research?

The basic objective of research is to acquire new knowledge and justification for decision making in medical practice. Research provides a basis for the acquisition of many skills, particularly those of critical thinking and scientific methodology. The discipline of general practice is special to us with its core content of continuing, comprehensive, community-based primary care, family care, domiciliary care, whole person care and preventive care. To achieve credibility and parity with our specialist colleagues we need to research this area with appropriate methodology and to clearly define the discipline. There is no area of medicine that involves such a diverse range and quantity of decisions each day as general practice, and therefore patient management needs as much evidence-based rigour as possible.

Our own patch, be it an isolated rural practice or an industrial suburban practice, has its own microepidemiological fascination. Thus it provides a unique opportunity to find answers to questions and make observations about that particular community.

There are also personal reasons to undertake research. The process assists professional development, encouraging clear and critical thinking, improvement of knowledge and the satisfaction of developing new skills and opening horizons.

This writer undertook many small studies on common everyday problems during 10 years in country practice to determine the most effective treatments for which no or minimal evidence in the literature could be found. Many of these recommendations for problems such as tennis elbow, cold sores, aphthous ulcers, ingrown toenails, hiccoughs, back pain, nightmares, temporomandibular dysfunction and warts appear in this text. Although the numbers were relatively small it was a useful study to compare treatments for about ten or twenty cases to test hypotheses and allow trends to emerge. The results from a large controlled trial would, of course, take precedence over these recommendations if they differed. However, the exercise, albeit limited, added immense interest to one's practice, which at times can be tedious without such scholarly challenges.

An important reason to undertake research is to conform with quality assurance processes that are now being expected of practitioners. The significant processes evaluating our accountability for quality control include audits of our own records, studies of critical incidents and morbidity studies.

Who should do research?

Any general practitioner searching for answers to questions and who has the opportunities should undertake research. Research is largely opportunistic and for some may be an impulsive reaction to a fascinating observation and in others a carefully conceived plan.

It can be undertaken in solo practice where the ability for personalised supervision of outcomes in patients is unique but where double-blind controlled trials are nigh impossible.

Research can be collaborative, and in fact this is an excellent way to get started. This can occur in a group practice.

Practitioners with computer skills and information technology at their fingertips are ideally placed to undertake research. Many general

practitioners who have started 'small' have progressed to great heights of research activity, especially using their computer skills. In the process of posing questions and eventually finding the answers they frequently refer to the experience as 'good fun'.

Asking questions

We often ask questions during the course of managing patients and such questions can form the basis of a research project, however simple.

Typical questions might be:

- 'Is all night-time cough in children due to asthma?'
- 'Is suicide in adolescent males precipitated by sexual problems?'
- 'Is cancer precipitated by stress or unhappiness?'
- 'Is recurrent migraine caused by cervical dysfunction?'
- 'Is there any significant difference in response to various antibiotics to treat otitis media in children presenting in general practice?'
- 'Does the distribution of leaflets by the receptionist in the waiting room lead to increased immunisation rates or Pap smears?'
- 'Are my patients satisfied with the services they receive?'
- 'Does the provision of patient information leaflets for the management of hypertension (or diabetes) lead to better compliance?'

Research on what?

General practice has its own unique characteristics including illness content, processes, epidemiology, health services, quality assurance and doctor–patient relationships. The special contact with patients provides opportunities to evaluate the patient's perspective on health service delivery, psychosocial issues and communication skills. The old saying 'dig where you are' is relevant to all of us. General practitioners invariably develop their own special interests and this is a logical area in which to conduct research. Conducting a morbidity and prescribing survey in a practice is a simple and fascinating study. If the results are added to a wider study invaluable information about the nature of general practice is obtained.[5,6,7]

The development of the International Classification of Health Problems in Primary Care and the International Classification of Process in Primary Care by the World Organisation of

National Colleges and Assemblies of General Practice and the World Health Organisation has greatly assisted the process of morbidity studies. This information is now presented in the publication International Classification of Primary Care (ICPC).[8]

Research in general practice obviously covers many clinical areas studied by other groups but we may ask different types of questions, study different populations and use different methodologies, especially qualitative methods.

It would be logical to conduct research on those common problems requiring continuing care by the GP. These include:

- alcohol problems
- allergic disorders, e.g. asthma, allergic rhinitis
- anxiety and depression
- arthritis
- chronic back pain and neck pain
- cancer
- cardiovascular disorders
- diabetes mellitus
- epilepsy
- hypertension
- migraine and other headache

Special opportunities such as the observation that certain diseases or conditions are linked with specific circumstances present frequently in primary care. An example is the observation that a group of farmers who presented to their rural practitioner over a period of time with lymphosarcoma were all exposed to a specific herbicide to control blackberry growth on their farms. This led to further statewide investigations of this association, which indicated a significant link between the agent and the disease.

Understanding terminology
Validity and reliability

- An ideal method of collecting research material is one that is valid.
- A valid method is one that measures what it claims to measure.
- A reliable method is one that produces repeatable results.

Validity refers to the 'true' answer, which must be relevant, complete and accurate. Three significant questions that evaluate validity are:[9]

- Is the study useful or is the result inconclusive?
- Do you accept the results of this study as applied to the source population?

- Do the results apply to the population in which you would be interested?

Internal validity refers to the adequacy of the study methods in reference to the study population, while *external validity* refers to the generalisability of the results to the general population.

Reliability refers to the stability of question-and-answer response and is most successfully measured by testing and then retesting (repeatedly). The most frequently used method of testing for repeatability is to repeat application of the test.

Sensitivity, specificity and predictive values

Sensitivity and specificity, which are integral to validity, are important considerations in decision making in medicine, particularly in choosing appropriate investigations for disease diagnoses. The method of calculation of sensitivity and specificity, and predictive values is summarised in Figure 13.1.

The *sensitivity* of a test depends on the proportion of people with the characteristic (disease) in whom the test is positive (that is, percentage positive with disease). The ultimate sensitive test is one that detects all true positive cases.

The *specificity* of a test depends on the proportion of people without the characteristic (disease) in whom the test is negative (that is, percentage negative of healthy people). The ultimate specific test is one that detects all the truly negative (disease-free) cases.

A clinical example of sensitivity and specificity is presented in Table 13.1.

Table 13.1 *The predictability of signs and symptoms for carpal tunnel syndrome*[10]

	Sensitivity %	Specificity %
Paraesthesia	97	4
Waking at night	91	14
Anaesthesia	57	61
Phalen's test	58	54
Tinel's test	42	63
Two point discrimination test	6	98

	Test positive	Test negative		
Condition present	A True positive	C False negative	A + C	Sensitivity $\dfrac{A}{A+C}$ %
Condition absent	B False positive	D True negative	B + D	Specificity $\dfrac{D}{B+D}$ %
	Positive predictive value $\dfrac{A}{A+B}$ %	Negative predictive value $\dfrac{D}{C+D}$ %		

Sensitivity: How often a test shows pathology when it is present
Specificity: How often a test is normal when no pathology present
Positive predictive value: Indicates the likelihood of the patient having disease when the test is positive
Negative predictive value: Indicates the likelihood of the patient having disease when the test is negative

Fig. 13.1 *Definitions of sensitivity, specificity and predictive values*

Predictive values that are useful indices of validity can be expressed as positive and negative values. Consider the example of a patient presenting with haematuria. In general practice the positive predictive value for carcinoma as the cause would be less than 5% but about 50% in the inpatient hospital setting.

Incidence and prevalence

It is easy to confuse the meanings of these two terms:

• *Incidence* refers to the number of new cases of a disease (or factor of interest) occurring in a defined population within a specified period of time.
• *Prevalence* refers to the total number of individuals who have the disease (or factor of interest) at a particular time or during a particular period in the population at risk of having the disease at this time.

Example: the prevalence of multiple sclerosis in temperate climates is 1 in 1 to 2000 compared with 1 in 10 000 in the tropics. The incidence of multiple sclerosis in the Australian state of Victoria (population 4 400 000) is 8 per 100 000 per year.

Bias

This is any effect occurring during the investigation that tends to produce results that depart systematically from the true values. Varieties of bias include *measurement bias* (e.g. fault with a sphygmomanometer recording blood pressure), *confounding bias* (e.g. influence of alcohol on a study investigating the association between stress and hypertension) and *selection bias* (e.g. using hospital outpatients in a community-based study).

Confounding

This is a situation in which a measure of the effect of exposure on risk is distorted by the association of exposure with other (known or unknown) factors that influence the outcome.[1] A confounder is a factor that distorts the apparent magnitude of the effect of a study on risk.

Chance

One must question the probability that the results favouring the experimental intervention could have occurred by chance; therefore, we resort to statistical help in the form of a probability statement or significance level.

How is the research undertaken?

'Getting started' can be quite difficult for the beginner. However, assistance that should be accessed is available from several sources including individual GPs with research experience, university departments of general practice and the RACGP research committee. It is appropriate to seek out a suitable supervisor for the study. A chronological method follows.

1. *The idea.* We start with an idea or question, which needs to be interesting, relevant, significant and answerable.[9] It may be appropriate to develop a hypothesis at this stage.

2. *Floating the idea.* The next step is to discuss the idea with colleagues or an appropriate accessible authority.

3. *Literature search.* This is a review of the literature, for example a Medline search or checking with a central research 'bank'.

4. *Preparing a plan.* This can be a short written plan outlining the methodology for the study.

5. *Evaluation of the plan.* The next step is to contact a supervisor or appropriate authority to evaluate the study plan, which may be referred to a reference group or research committee.

6. *Development of a protocol*:

   (a) Prepare background; outline objectives and develop a hypothesis.
   (b) Select target population using clear criteria and appropriate numbers.
   (c) Design the research:
       qualitative or quantitative?
       questionnaire/s
   (d) Assess internal validity
   (e) Consider statistical implications early:
       — number of patients
       — method for data analysis
   (f) Recruit subjects and assistants.
   (g) Assess the time frame.
   (h) Assess the ethical considerations → ethics approval committee.

7. *Pilot study and timetable.* Consider a preliminary pilot study and project timetable.

8. *Seek funding.* Solicit advice for appropriate funding bodies.

9. *The study.* Conduct the study.

10. *Publication.* Prepare for publication.

Research design

Hypothesis development

The reasoning process of the researcher is based on the null hypothesis—that is, an experimental group does not differ from a control 'normal' group in outcome. The question to consider is: 'What is the probability that results from the experimental intervention would have occurred by chance?' The answer is based on a probability statement: 'The probability that the positive results occurred by chance is less than 5% $(P<0.05)$'.[11]

Selecting a representative sample of appropriate size

Two basic components of subject selection are sample size and sample representativeness. The latter should be selected in a well-controlled manner.

A common question is: 'What is the ideal size of the sample?' There is no fixed answer but it must be adequate to produce statistically meaningful results.

Recruitment of patients is a particular skill and often hard work, but it is easier if the researcher has a large pool of patients with whom he or she enjoys a good relationship. A useful rule is to aim to approach $3n$ patients if you wish to work with a sample size of n.

Some guidelines for choosing the sample size are:[11]

- the more the individuals in the population differ, the larger the required sample
- the more planned comparisons, the larger the size
- larger sample sizes allow detection of smaller differences

Types of research[1]

The two broad categories of research in general practice are qualitative research, which is based on observation and talking with people, and quantitative research, which is based on measurement and analysis of data collection.

Qualitative research

This research is basically concerned with evaluating human behaviour from the subjects' perspective. It is based on close observation and is expressed in a descriptive way.

The methods used are:

- interviews
- focus groups
- participation observation
- document analysis

Qualitative research is an excellent method for generating hypotheses and can lead to quantitative research.

Quantitative research

Quantitative research is research based on the collection of data in numerical quantities. It is concerned with hypothesis testing, reliability and validity. It can be classified broadly as observational, which includes case control, cross-sectional and cohort studies, and experimental, which includes the classic controlled trial.[12]

- *Case control (or retrospective) study* is an observational study in which people with a disease (cases) are compared with those without it (control group).
  —Examples: Patients with mesotheliomas were investigated for exposure to asbestos or other agents; the mothers of children born with birth defects were investigated for an association with drug intake during pregnancy.
- *Cross-sectional or prevalence study* follows a correlation approach using existing data bases. It is a survey of the frequency of disease, risk factors or other characteristics in a defined population at one particular time.
  —Example: The prevalence of diabetes mellitus (diagnosed and undiagnosed) was investigated in an Aboriginal community living in a particular area of metropolitan Sydney.
- *Cohort (or prospective) study* is also referred to as 'follow up'. The study follows a group (cohort) of individuals with a specified characteristic or disease over a period of time. Comparisons may be made with a control group.
  —Example: 120 patients with chronic sciatica were followed over 10 years to determine the outcome of their pain and neurological deficit. These were compared with a matched group who had undergone laminectomy.

- *Clinical controlled trial* is an experimental study that tests for hypothesised outcomes. An intervention is conducted on a randomly selected group of people and compared with a matched control group not subject to the specific intervention. The objective is to establish a causal relationship between the intervention and the hypothesised outcome. The ideal scientific trial is a double-blind trial. This is the typical study when assessing the outcome of a drug trial as compared with placebo.

Literature search

A comprehensive search of the literature on a particular subject is fundamental to commencing a study. The first issue is to determine if a particular study has already been done or whether it has a different emphasis. A cross-check with the RACGP or other relevant institute's databank is also worthwhile.

An appropriate starting point is a search such as Medlars or Medline search, which can be conducted by your medical library. It is important to carefully choose the correct key words in order to focus and economise the search. It may also be worthwhile reviewing the indexes of *Family Medicine Literature Index* (FAMLI) published by the College of Family Physicians of Canada or the *British Journal of General Practice*.

The review will provide a stimulus for more detailed knowledge and lateral thinking on the subject. Should a research project be pursued, it is essential to undertake a critical review of the literature rather than just summarising conclusions of previous studies and quoting the author's conclusions or quotations.

Writing a paper for publication

Writing papers with a view to publication, especially in refereed prestigious journals, is a skill that can be acquired by practising a set format.

Getting started is the first difficult hurdle. An original, interesting, credible and challenging paper will invariably be accepted for publication. It is important to follow the guidelines for authors found in the relevant journals.

Key guidelines or 'clichés' to follow include:

- Have crystal clear objectives.
- Small is beautiful (around 1500 words).
- Practice makes perfect.
- Prefer the familiar word to the unfamiliar.
- A picture is worth a thousand words.

- Statistics shouldn't lie.
- Take a test run: consider peer review.
- Keep it simple and comprehensible.

In his book *How to write and publish papers in medical sciences* Edward J. Huth[13] writes:

Before sitting down to write, or even plan a paper in detail, you need to answer five questions:
- *What do I have to say?*
- *Is the paper worth writing?*
- *What is the right format for the message?*
- *What is the audience for the message?*
- *What is the right journal for the paper?*

Getting started

It is recommended that the writer has a simplified system such as answering the following for each research article.[13,14]

1. How did I get into this in the first place?   *Introduction*
2. What did I do?   *Methods*
3. What did I find out?   *Results and*
4. So what?   *Discussion*

The anatomy of a paper

Abstract/Summary

This is critical to the overall impression conveyed by the paper. An interesting precise summary can virtually captivate the reader. Ideally it should be 50 to 100 words (maximum 150–200). A useful tip is to study abstracts found in the Medlars (or other) computerised reference system (CRD). It is surprising how many papers are submitted without an abstract—a fact that irritates editors. The best form of abstract is the structured abstract, which is ideal for a research paper.

Introduction

The introduction should be brief and interesting. A useful strategy is the inclusion of an appropriate quotation, especially from a celebrated scholar such as Osler or Hippocrates. It should include a concise literature review (based on CRD) where appropriate. The introduction should outline the aims of the study and raise questions.

Methods

This section should be readily followed by readers, especially those wishing to repeat the methodology. There should be sufficient detail by which to judge the validity of the study and its findings. Subheadings in methods include subjects (description of these and how sample was selected), study design, instrumentation (describe study instruments, any pilot-testing, reliability and validity) and data analysis.

Results

The purpose of this section is to present the data outcome without interpretation. The results section can be crucial to the success of the paper for it provides the opportunity for creativity and flair. The paper can be made visually appealing with graphs of various types, tables and simple but expressive line drawings. The assistance of a computer expert and access to special graphic effects is a bonus.

Discussion

The discussion should be incisive, relevant and honest. Avoid calling this section the summary or conclusion. Discuss and compare findings with relevant research as presented in the introduction. Try to answer the questions posed in the study with a neat synthesis and 'take home' message for the reader.

Discussions have a propensity to be too long, muddled and inconclusive. Summarise the research findings, generalise results to the larger population of interest, draw conclusions based on the findings and suggest issues for further research.

References

Use a genuine reference list in preference to a bibliography or 'further reading'. The reference list should be honest and very accurate. Keep the list brief—long lists impress very few. Up to 25 references is optimal. References are the biggest problem for subeditors for they tend to be sloppy or omitted. Other authors become upset by lack of proper acknowledgment in a reference list. Personal communication and unpublished material are not acceptable as references.

Most journals use the Vancouver style of referencing with references being numbered consecutively in the order in which they are mentioned in the text.

Acknowledgments

This is not to be overlooked, especially if illustrative material is produced. Copyright rules do apply; so permission of both the author and the publisher is necessary to reproduce figures or tables. This is the author's responsibility—not the editor's.

What are the publications of general practice research?

Any medical journal, generalist or specialist, can be approached but chances of publication are greatest in journals that almost exclusively publish general practice research. These include *Australian Family Physician, Family Practice, Journal of Family Practice, Family Medicine, British Journal of General Practice, Archives of Family Medicine, Family Practice Research Journal* and *Journal of the American Board of Family Practice*.

Critical appraisal of published research

The objective of critically appraising a paper is to determine if the methods and results of the research have significant validity to produce useful information. The appraisal starts with a careful review of the abstract, which ideally should be presented in a structured format.

The critical questions are as follows:
1. What were the objectives of the study?
2. Were the ethical aspects properly followed?
3. What was the study design?
4. Were there any potential problems associated with the design?
5. Were all the patients who entered the study properly accounted for at its conclusion?
6. What were the important results?
7. How would you interpret and explain these results?

Recommended reading

Research methods for primary care series
Volume 1: Norton P, et al. *Primary care research*. Newbury Park: Sage, 1992.
Volume 2: Stewart M et al. *Tools for primary care research*. Newbury Park: Sage, 1992.
Volume 3: Crabtree B, Miller W. *Doing qualitative research*. Newbury Park: Sage, 1992.

General
Armstrong D et al. *Research methods for general practice*. Oxford: Oxford Medical Publications, 1990.
Howie JGR. *Research in general practice* (2nd edn). London: Chapman & Hall, 1992.

Sacket DR, Haynes RB, Guyatt GH, Tugwell P. *Clinical epidemiology: A basic science for clinical medicine* (2nd edn). Boston: Little, Brown. 1991.

References

1. Schattner P. Introduction to research and research designs. In: Piterman L ed, *Introduction to research in family medicine MFM 2006*, 1996, 2–7.
2. Eimerl T. Organised curiosity. J Coll Gen Pract, 1960; 3(1): 246–252.
3. Murrell TGC. Nineteenth century masters of general practice. Med J Aust, 1991; 155: 785–792.
4. Anderson NA, Bridges-Webb C, Chancellor A. *General practice in Australia*. Sydney: Sydney University Press, 1986, 124–130.
5. Howie JGR. *Research in general practice* (2nd edn). London. Chapman & Hall, 1992, 12–14.
6. Bridges-Webb C. The Australian general practice morbidity and prescribing survey, 1969–1976. Med J Aust (Supplement) 1976; 2:5–20.
7. Bridges-Webb C, Britt H, Miles DA et al. Morbidity and treatment in general practice in Australia 1990–1991, Med J Aust, 1992; 157:51–57.
8. Lamberts H, Wood M. *ICPC: International Classification of Primary Care*. Oxford: Oxford University Press, 1987.
9. Silagy CA, Schattner P eds. *An introduction to general practice research*. Melbourne: Department of Community Medicine, Monash University, 1990.
10. Buch-Jaeger N, Foucher G. Carpal tunnel syndrome: Validity of clinical signs. Journal Hand Surgery, 1994; 19B:72–74.
11. Rakel RE. *Essentials of family practice*. Philadelphia: WB Saunders Company, 1993, 182–191.
12. Fowkes FGR, Fulton PM. Critical appraisal of published research: Introductory guidelines. BMJ, 1991; 302:1136–1140.
13. Huth E. *How to write and publish papers in the medical sciences*. Philadelphia: Isipress, 1982.
14. Saltman D. Medical writing. Aust Fam Physician, 1987; 673–676.

PART 2

DIAGNOSTIC PERSPECTIVE IN GENERAL PRACTICE

———

14

Inspection as a clinical skill

—

More mistakes, many more, are made by not looking than by not knowing

Sir William Jenner (1815–98)

General practitioners have an ideal opportunity to practise the art of careful observation and to notice all the signs and features characteristic of a patient from the time seen in the waiting room until the physical examination. We should be 'like Sherlock Holmes' in our analysis of the patient and accept the challenge of being astute diagnosticians and proud members of a noble profession.

It is important to stand back (so to speak) and look at the patient's general appearance and demeanour. We should be assessing their mood and affect as much as their physical appearance. The first assessment to make is 'Does the patient look sick?'

First impressions

The first impression of the patient is always striking in some way and we should discipline ourselves to be as analytical as possible.

A rapid inspection from a trained observer may be all that is necessary to allow the observer to pinpoint specific disorders such as anaemia, hyperthyroidism, jaundice, acromegaly and alcohol abuse. Such 'spot' diagnosis is not justifiable unless the original signs are supported by further examination, which must be comprehensive.

The following observations should therefore be made:

1. facial characteristics
2. abnormalities of the head and neck
3. examination of the mouth
4. character and distribution of hair
5. examination of the skin (in general)
6. height and weight
7. posture and gait
8. genitalia
9. examination of extremities (hands, feet, nails, etc.)

Physiognomy

Physiognomy, which is the art of judging character from the features of the face, flourished in the Middle Ages. According to Addison, 'everyone is in some degree a master of that art which is physiognomy; and naturally forms to themselves the character of a stranger from the features of the face'. In reality, all doctors use a physiognomical approach to diagnose many medical conditions although we may not be as expert at the art as we should be.

The face is a person's most immediate means of communicating with others; it is a shield and banner, a mask and a mirror. It reveals mental faculties and emotional turmoil. It is the first perspective gained of patients as they walk into the consulting room.

The face as a mirror of disease

A fascinating aspect of the art of clinical medicine is the clinical interpretation of the patient's facies. Not only are specific skin lesions common on the face but the face may also mirror endocrine disorders and organ failure such as respiratory, cardiac, renal and liver failure.

Jaundice may be masked by the natural colour of the cheeks but the yellow conjunctivae will be distinctive. A marked plethoric complexion may be seen in chronic alcoholics (alcohol may produce a pseudo-Cushing's syndrome), in Cushing's disease or in polycythaemia. Thickening of the subcutaneous tissues may be seen in chronic alcoholism, acromegaly and myxoedema, and the puffiness of the eyelids in the latter condition may simulate the true subcutaneous oedema of renal disease.

An individual's personality and mood rarely fail to leave an impression on the facial characteristics. This is partly due to the alteration in facial lines and wrinkles, which may become modified in anger, irritability, anxiety and stress. More profound changes occur with mental disease. Various CNS diseases such as Parkinson's disease and myopathies can affect facial expression, e.g. the immobile face of the patient with Parkinson's disease.

The appearance of the eyes can also be very significant and may reflect underlying systemic disease.

Diagnostic facies

Acromegalic

The enlarged characteristic face is due to a large supraorbital ridge that causes frontal bossing, a broad nose and a prominent broad and square lower jaw. Other features include an enlarged tongue and soft tissue swelling of the nose, lips and ears.

Alcoholic (due to chronic use)

It is important to recognise the characteristic changes as early as possible—a plethoric face, thickened 'greasy' skin, telangiectasia, suffused conjunctivae and rosacea. Other features may include rhinophyma, parotid swelling and characteristic changes to the lips and corners of the mouth.

Bird-like (systemic sclerosis: CREST syndrome)

The bird-like features, beaking of the nose, limitation of mouth opening, puckering or furrowing of the lips and a fixed facial expression, are due to binding down of facial skin. Other features include telangiectasia on the face and hands.

Chipmunk (thalassaemia major)

There is bossing of the skull, hypertrophy of the maxillae (which tends to expose the upper teeth), prominent malar eminences and depression of the bridge of the nose. The major haemoglobinopathies cause hyperplasia of the skull and facial bones because of an increase in the bone marrow cavity.

Cushingoid

The face has a typical 'moon shape', plethora, hirsutism (more obvious in women), acne.

Facial nerve palsy

Features include unilateral drooping of the corner of the mouth and flattening of the nasolabial fold.
UMN type: the forehead movement is spared.
LMN type: e.g. Bell's palsy, Ramsay Hunt syndrome: lack of forehead muscle tone.

Obese

The distinguishing feature from the 'moon face' of Cushing's disease is the general roundness and uniform fatness of the face.

Thyrotoxic (hyperthyroidism)

The prominent eyes (sclera may not be covered by the lower eyelid) and conjunctivitis are features of the thyrotoxic patient. The thyroid stare (a frightened expression) may also be present.

Myxoedemic (hypothyroidism)

The face usually has an apathetic look and is 'puffy' with possible periorbital oedema. There is broadening of the lower part of the face. The skin (not the sclera) may appear yellow (due to hypercarotenaemia) and is generally dry and coarse. Other features may include thin, coarse, listless hair and loss or thinning of the outer third of the eyebrows. The tongue is usually enlarged and the patient speaks with a 'thickened', croaking, slow speech.

Marfanoid (Marfan's syndrome)

The typical tall stature, arachnodactyly and chest deformities, combined with the facial features of a subluxation of the lens of the eye and high arched palate, help to pinpoint the diagnosis.

Mongoloid (Down syndrome)

The facial features include a flat profile, with crowded features, a round head, dysplastic low-set ears, protruding tongue, mongoloid slant of the eyes with epicanthic folds, mouth hanging open and peripheral silver iris spots (Brushfield's spots).

Mitral (mitral valve disease, especially mitral stenosis)

This is typically shown in flushed or rosy cheeks with a bluish tinge due to dilatation of the malar capillaries. It is associated with pulmonary hypertension.

Myotonic (dystrophia myotonia)

Typical features include frontal baldness, expressionless triangular facies, partial ptosis, cataracts and temporal muscle atrophy.

Myopathic (myopathy/myasthenia gravis)

Facial characteristics include an expressionless, 'tired' looking face with bilateral ptosis.

Pagetic (Paget's disease)

The main feature is skull enlargement, notably of the frontal and parietal areas (the head circumference is usually greater than 55 cm, which is abnormal)—the 'hat doesn't fit any more' hallmark. Other features include increased bony warmth and deafness.

Parkinsonian

Characteristic is the mask-like facies with lack of facial expression and fixed unblinking stare. There is immobility of the facial muscles.

Turner's syndrome

The facial characteristics include ptosis—'fish-like' mouth, small chin (micrognathia), low-set ears and deafness. Cardiac lesions include co-arctation of aorta and pulmonary stenosis. Webbing of the neck is the classic sign.

Specific characteristics

Various facial signs may be present. The causes of these signs are listed below.

Butterfly 'rash'

- SLE   Erythema, scaling with a discrete red advancing edge on the cheeks and bridge of the nose. The sharp border, lack of pustules and adherent scale make it differ from rosacea.

- Rosacea   Papules, pustules and telangiectasia on an erythematous background on cheeks, forehead and chin.
- Erysipelas   Painful, erythematous, indurated skin infection with a well-defined raised edge.
- Seborrhoeic   Red and scaly rash involving eyebrows, eyelids, naso-labial folds.
  dermatitis
- Photosensitivity   Erythematous on areas that are exposed to sun
  eruptions

Chloasma/melasma

Increased browning pigmentation, usually confined to symmetrical areas of the cheeks. Caused by drugs:

- combined oral contraceptive pill
- hydroxychloroquine (Plaquenil)
- diphenylhydrazine

Malar flush

- mitral stenosis
- pulmonary stenosis
- rosacea
- SLE
- mesenteric adenitis

Spider naevi

- pregnancy
- liver disease
- vitamin B deficiency, in normal people

Enlarged tongue

- acromegaly
- hypothyroidism
- amyloidosis

Cataracts

- senility
- corticosteroid therapy
- diabetes
- hypoparathyroidism
- dystrophia myotonia
- trauma
- ocular disease, e.g. glaucoma

Telangiectasia

- systemic sclerosis
- CREST syndrome
- liver disease, e.g. alcoholism

Cyanosis

Cyanosis is a bluish discolouration of the skin and mucous membranes due to deoxygenated haemoglobin concentrated in the superficial blood vessels. It is classified as central or peripheral.

Central

Cyanosis is present in parts of the body with good circulation such as the lips and tongue. The areas feel warm. The main causes are pulmonary disease, pulmonary oedema, cyanotic congenital heart disease (right to left shunt), respiratory depression, polycythaemia.

Peripheral

Cyanosis is in the extremities such as the outer surface of the lips, nose and ears. The areas feel cold. The main causes are peripheral vascular disease, cardiac failure, exposure to cold, left ventricular failure and all causes of central cyanosis.

Clubbing of fingers

Features

- Loss of usual angle between base of nail and nail fold.
- Curvature in two planes.
- Increased sponginess in base of nail.
- Increased convexity of nail.
- Mainly caused by respiratory disease.

Causes

1. Lung disease
   (a) carcinoma
   (b) bronchiectasis
   (c) cystic fibrosis
   (d) abscess/empyema
   (e) pulmonary fibrosis
2. Heart disease
   (a) bacterial endocarditis
   (b) cyanotic congenital heart disease
3. Liver disease
   (a) cirrhosis
4. Gastrointestinal disease
   (a) ulcerative colitis
   (b) Crohn's disease
   (c) coeliac disease
5. Congenital disease

Increased pigmentation

Increased pigmentation is not common but if obvious in areas exposed to the sun look for 'hidden' areas such as the inner aspect of the forearms. Causes include those listed below.

Increased melanocyte-stimulating hormone (MSH)

- Addison's disease
- Cushing's disease
- Ectopic ACTH syndrome

Metabolic

- Hyperthyroidism
- Haemochromatosis
- Cirrhosis of the liver
- Porphyria
- Chronic renal failure
- Malnutrition/malabsorption
- Pregnancy

Drugs

- Oral contraceptive pill
- Psoralens
- Photochemotherapy (PUVA)
- Arsenic, gold, silver
- Phenothiazines
- Antimalarials (chloroquine/hydroxychloroquine)
- Dapsone
- Antibiotics (busulphan, bleomycin)
- Amiodarone

Tumours

- Lymphomas
- *Acanthosis nigricans*
- Metastatic melanoma

15

A safe diagnostic strategy

—

For most diagnoses all that is needed is an ounce of knowledge, an ounce of intelligence, and a pound of thoroughness.

Anon
Lancet 1951

The discipline of general practice is probably the most difficult, complex and challenging of the healing arts. Our field of endeavour is at the very front line of medicine and as practitioners we shoulder the responsibility of the early diagnosis of very serious, perhaps life-threatening, illness in addition to the recognition of anxiety traits in our patients.

The teaching of our craft is also an exciting challenge and presupposes that we have a profound comprehension of our discipline.

Our area is characterised by a wide kaleidoscope of presenting problems, often foreign to the classical textbook presentation and sometimes embellished by a 'shopping list' of seemingly unconnected problems or vague symptoms—the so-called undifferentiated illness syndrome.[1] Common undifferentiated symptoms include tiredness or fatigue, sleeping problems, anxiety and stress, dizziness, headache, indigestion, anorexia and nausea, sexual dysfunction, weight loss, loss of interest, flatulence, abdominal discomfort and chest discomfort.[2] It is important, especially in a busy practice, to adopt a fail-safe strategy to analyse such presenting problems. Such an approach is even more important in a world of increasing medical litigation and specialisation.

To help bring order to the jungle of general practice problems the author has developed a simple model to facilitate diagnosis and reduce the margin of error.

The basic model

The use of the diagnostic model requires a disciplined approach to the problem with the medical practitioner quickly answering five self-posed questions. The questions are contained in Table 15.1.

Table 15.1 *The diagnostic model for a presenting problem*

1. What is the probability diagnosis?
2. What serious disorders must not be missed?
3. What conditions are often missed (the pitfalls)?
4. Could this patient have one of the 'masquerades' in medical practice?
5. Is this patient trying to tell me something else?

This approach, which is based on considerable experience, requires the learning of a predetermined plan which, naturally, would vary in different parts of the world but would have a certain universal application in the so-called developed world.

Each of the above five questions will be expanded.

1. The probability diagnosis

The probability diagnosis is based on the doctor's perspective and experience with regard to prevalence, incidence and the natural history of disease. General practitioners acquire first-hand epidemiological knowledge about the patterns of illness apparent in individuals and in the community, which enables them to view illness from a perspective that is not available to doctors in any other disciplines. Thus, during the medical interview, the doctor not only is gathering information, allocating priorities and making hypotheses, but also is developing a probability diagnosis based on acquired epidemiological knowledge.

2. What serious disorders must not be missed?

While epidemiological knowledge is a great asset to the general practitioner it can be a disadvantage in that he or she is so familiar with what is common that the all-important rare cause of a presenting symptom may be overlooked. On the other hand, the doctor in the specialist clinic, where a different spectrum of disease is encountered, is more likely to focus on the rare at the expense of the common cause. However, it is vital, especially working in the modern framework of a litigation-conscious society, not to miss serious, life-threatening disorders.

To achieve early recognition of serious illness the general practitioner needs to develop a 'high index of suspicion'. This is generally regarded as largely intuitive, but this is probably not so, and it would be more accurate to say that it comes with experience.

The serious disorders that should always be considered 'until proven otherwise' include malignant disease, acquired immunodeficiency syndrome (AIDS), coronary disease and life-threatening infections such as meningitis, Haemophilus influenza b infections, septicaemia and infective endocarditis (Table 15.2).

Myocardial infarction or ischaemia is extremely important to consider because it is so potentially lethal and at times can be overlooked by the busy practitioner. It does not always manifest as the classical presentation of crushing

Table 15.2 *Serious 'not to be missed' conditions*

Neoplasia, especially malignancy

HIV infection/AIDS

Asthma

Severe infections, especially:
- meningoencephalitis
- septicaemia
- epiglottitis
- infective endocarditis

Coronary disease
- myocardial infarction
- unstable angina
- arrhythmias

Imminent or potential suicide

Intracerebral lesions, e.g. SAH

Ectopic pregnancy

---

central pain but can present as pain of varying severity and quality in a wide variety of sites. These sites include the jaw, neck, arm, epigastrium and interscapular region. Coronary artery disease may manifest as life-threatening arrhythmias that may present as palpitations and/or dizziness. A high index of suspicion is necessary to diagnose arrhythmias.

3. What conditions are often missed?

This question refers to the common 'pitfalls' so often encountered in general practice. This area is definitely related to the experience factor and includes rather simple non-life-threatening problems that can be so easily overlooked unless doctors are prepared to include them in their diagnostic framework.

Classic examples include smoking or dental caries as a cause of abdominal pain; allergies to a whole variety of unsuspected everyday contacts; foreign bodies; occupational or environmental hazards as a cause of headache, respiratory discomfort or malaise; and faecal impaction as a cause of diarrhoea. We have all experienced the 'red face syndrome' from a urinary tract infection whether it is the cause of fever in a child, lumbar pain in a pregnant woman or malaise in an older person. The dermatomal pain pattern caused by herpes zoster prior to the eruption of the rash (or if only a few sparse vesicles erupt) is a real trap.

Menopausal symptoms can also be overlooked as we focus on a particular symptom. Some important pitfalls are given in Table 15.3.

4. The masquerades

It is important to utilise a type of fail-safe mechanism to avoid missing the diagnosis of these disorders. Some practitioners refer to consultations that make their 'head spin' in confusion and bewilderment, with patients presenting with a 'shopping list' of problems. It is in these patients that a checklist is useful. Consider the apparently neurotic patient who presents with headache, lethargy, tiredness, constipation, anorexia, indigestion, shortness of breath on exertion, pruritus, flatulence, sore tongue and backache. In such a patient we must consider a diagnosis that links all these symptoms, especially if the physical examination is inconclusive; this includes iron deficiency anaemia, depression, diabetes mellitus, hypothyroidism and drug abuse.

Table 15.3 *Classic pitfalls*

Abscess (hidden)
Allergies
Candida infection
Chronic fatigue syndrome
Coeliac disease
Domestic abuse including child abuse
Drugs (see Table 15.4)
Herpes zoster
Faecal impaction
Foreign bodies
Giardiasis
Haemochromatosis
Lead poisoning
Malnutrition (unsuspected)
Menopause syndrome
Migraine (atypical variants)
Paget's disease
Pregnancy (early)
Seizure disorders
Tourette's syndrome
Urinary infection

A century ago it was important to consider diseases such as syphilis and tuberculosis as the great common masquerades, but these infections have been replaced by iatrogenesis, malignant disease, alcoholism, endocrine disorders and the various manifestations of atherosclerosis, particularly coronary insufficiency and cerebrovascular insufficiency.

If the patient has pain anywhere it is possible that it could originate from the spine; so the possibility of spinal pain (radicular or referred) should be considered as the cause for various

Table 15.4 *The seven primary masquerades*

1. Depression
2. Diabetes mellitus
3. Drugs
   • iatrogenic
   • self-abuse
     — alcohol
     — narcotics
     — nicotine
     — others
4. Anaemia
5. Thyroid and other endocrine disorders
   • hyperthyroidism
   • hypothyroidism
6. Spinal dysfunction
7. Urinary infection

pain syndromes such as headache, arm pain, leg pain, chest pain, pelvic pain and even abdominal pain. The author's experience is that spondylogenic pain is one of the most underdiagnosed problems in general practice.

A checklist that has been divided into two groups of seven disorders is presented (Tables 15.4 and 15.5). The first list, 'the seven primary masquerades', represents the more common disorders encountered in general practice; the second list includes less common masquerades although some, such as Epstein-Barr mononucleosis, can be

Table 15.5 *The seven other masquerades*

1. Chronic renal failure
2. Malignant disease
   • lymphomas
   • lung
   • caecum/colon
   • kidney
   • multiple myeloma
   • ovary
   • metastasis
3. HIV infection/AIDS
4. Baffling bacterial infections
   • syphilis
   • tuberculosis
   • infective endocarditis
   • the zoonoses
   • chlamydia infections
   • atypical pneumonias e.g. Legionnaires
   • others
5. Baffling viral (and protozoal) infections
   • Epstein–Barr mononucleosis
   • TORCH organisms, e.g. cytomegalovirus
   • hepatitis A,B,C,D,E
   • mosquito-borne infections
     — malaria
     — Ross River fever
     — others
6. Neurological dilemmas
   • Parkinson's disease
   • Guillain-Barré syndrome
   • seizure disorders
   • multiple sclerosis
   • myasthenia gravis
   • space-occupying lesion of skull
   • migraine and its variants
   • others
7. Connective tissue disorders and the vasculitides
   • Connective tissue disorders
     — SLE
     — systemic sclerosis
     — dermatomyositis
     — overlap syndrome
   • Vasculitides
     — polyarteritis nodosa
     — giant cell arteritis/polymyalgia rheumatica
     — granulomatous disorders

Neoplasia, especially malignancy of the so-called 'silent areas', can be an elusive diagnostic problem. Typical examples are carcinoma of the nasopharynx and sinuses, ovary, caecum, kidney and lymphoietic tissue. Sarcoidosis is another disease that can be a real masquerade (p. 459).

As a practical diagnostic ploy, the author has both lists strategically placed on the surgery wall immediately behind the patient. The lists are rapidly perused for inspiration should the diagnosis for a particular patient prove elusive.

Is the patient trying to tell me something?

The doctor has to consider, especially in the case of undifferentiated illness, whether the patient has a 'hidden agenda' for the presentation.[3] Of course, the patient may be depressed (overt or masked) or may have a true anxiety state. However, a presenting symptom such as tiredness may represent a 'ticket of entry' to the consulting room. It may represent a plea for help in a stressed or anxious patient. We should be sensitive to patients' needs and feelings, and as listening, caring, empathetic practitioners provide the right opportunity for the patient to communicate freely.

Deep sexual anxieties and problems, poor self-esteem, and fear of malignancy or some other medical catastrophe are just some of the reasons patients present to doctors. The author has another checklist (Table 15.6) to help identify the psychosocial reasons for a patient's malaise.

In the author's experience of counselling patients and families the number of problems caused by interpersonal conflict is quite amazing and makes it worthwhile specifically exploring the quality of close relationships, such as those of husband–wife, mother–daughter and father–son.

Table 15.6 *Underlying fears or image problems that cause stress and anxiety*

1. Interpersonal conflict in the family
2. Identification with sick or deceased friends
3. Fear of malignancy
4. STDs especially AIDS
5. Impending 'coronary' or 'stroke'
6. Sexual problem
7. Drug-related problem
8. Crippling arthritis
9. Financial woes
10. Other abnormal stresses

Identification and transference of illness, symptoms and death, in particular, are important areas of anxiety to consider. Patients often identify their problems with relatives, friends or public personalities who have malignant disease. Other somatoform disorders and the factitious disorders, including the fascinating Munchausen's syndrome, may be obvious or extremely complex and difficult to recognise.

The bottom line is that patients are often desperately searching for security and we have an important role to play in helping them.

Some examples of application of the model

Hiccough

Summary of diagnostic strategy model for abnormal hiccough

1. Q. *Probability diagnosis*
   A. Food and alcohol excess
      Psychogenic/functional
      Postoperative
      • gastric distension
      • phrenic nerve irritation

2. Q. *Serious disorders not to be missed*
   A. Neoplasia
      • CNS
      • neck
      • oesophagus
      • lung
      Subphrenic abscess
      Myocardial infarction/pericarditis
      CNS disorders, e.g. CVA, infection

3. Q. *Pitfalls*
   A. Alcohol excess
      Smoking
      Aerophagy
      GIT disorders
      • oesophagitis
      • peptic ulcer
      • hiatus hernia
      • cholecystitis
      • hepatomegaly
      Rarities
      Sudden temperature change
      Neck cysts and vascular abnormalities

4. Q. *Seven masquerades checklist*
   A. Depression   –
      Diabetes   –
      Drugs   √
      Anaemia   –

Thyroid disease	–
Spinal dysfunction	possible
UTI	–

5. *Q. Is the patient trying to tell me something?*
   A. Emotional causes always to be considered.

Halitosis

Summary of diagnostic strategy model

1. *Q. Probability diagnosis*
   A. Dietary habits
      Orodental disease
      Dry mouth, e.g. on waking
      Smoking/alcohol

2. *Q. Serious disorders not to be missed*
   A. Malignancy:
      lung, oropharynx, larynx, stomach, nose, leukaemia
      Pulmonary tuberculosis
      Quinsy
      Lung abscess
      Blood dyscrasias/leukaemia
      Uraemia
      Hepatic failure

3. *Q. Pitfalls*
   A. Nasal and sinus infection
      Systemic infection
      Appendicitis
      Bronchiectasis
      Hiatus hernia

Rarities
Pharyngeal and oesophageal diverticula
Sjögren's syndrome
Scurvy

4. *Q. Seven masquerades checklist*
   A.

Depression	√	
Diabetes	√	acetone
Drugs	√	
Anaemia	–	
Thyroid disease	–	
Spinal dysfunction	–	
UTI	–	

5. *Q. Is the patient trying to tell me something?*
   A. Possible manifestation of psychogenic disorder.

References

1. Murtagh J. Common problems: A safe diagnostic strategy. Aust Fam Physician, 1990; 19:733–742.

2. Frith J, Knowlden S. Undifferentiated illness. Med J Aust, 1992; 156:472–476.

3. Levenstein JH, McCracken EC, McWhinney IR et al. The patient-centred method. I. A model for the doctor–patient interaction in family medicine. Fam Practice, 1986; 3:24–30.

16

Depression

—

I am ignorant and impotent and yet, somehow or other, here I am, unhappy, no doubt, profoundly dissatisfied . . . In spite of everything I survive.

Aldous Huxley (1894–1963)

Depressive illness, which is probably *the* greatest masquerade of general practice, is one of the commonest illnesses in medicine and is often confused with other illnesses. It is a very real illness that affects the entire mind and body. Unfortunately, there is a social stigma associated with depression and many patients tend to deny that they are depressed.

It is a useful working rule to consider depression as an illness that seriously dampens the five basic activities of humans:

• energy for activity
• sex drive
• sleep
• appetite
• ability to cope with life

Many episodes of depression are transient and should be regarded as normal but 10% of the population have significant depressive illness. The lifetime risk of being treated for depression is approximately 12% for men and 25% for women.[1]

Classifications

• Affective or mood disorders refer to those conditions in which there is a disturbance of affect or mood.
• The DSM-IV classification divides the disorder into the depressive disorders and bipolar disorders (both manic and depressive episodes).
• The depressive disorders include major depression, adjustment disorders with depressive mood, and dysthymia.

— Major depression includes those disorders with one or more major depressive episodes.[1]
— Dysthymia refers to long-standing (2 years or more) depression of mild severity ('neurotic depression').[1]
— Adjustment disorder with depressed mood is a less severe form of depression without sufficient criteria for major depression. It is very common and occurs in response to identifiable stressors ('reactive depression', e.g. loss of employment). Its duration is usually no longer than 6 months.

Major depression

The patient can experience many symptoms, both physical and mental. The DSM-IV diagnostic criteria for depression are outlined in the following boxed section.

These criteria can be extended to include:

• a feeling of not being able to cope with life
• continual tiredness

DSM-IV diagnostic criteria
for major depression
At least five of the following symptoms for 2 weeks
(criterion 1 or 2 essential)

1. Depressed mood
2. Loss of interest or pleasure
3. Significant appetite or weight loss or gain (usually poor appetite)
4. Insomnia or hypersomnia (usually early morning waking)
5. Psychomotor agitation and retardation
6. Fatigue or loss of energy
7. Feelings of worthlessness or excessive guilt
8. Impaired thinking or concentration; indecisiveness
9. Suicidal thoughts/thoughts of death

- loss of sense of humour
- tension and anxiety
- irritability, anger or fearfulness
- somatic symptoms such as headache, constipation, indigestion, weight loss, dry mouth and unusual pains or sensations in the chest or abdomen

The symptoms may vary during the day, but are usually worse on waking in the morning. Some patients have psychotic features, usually only delusions but sometimes also hallucinations, and may be misdiagnosed as schizophrenic.

In practice the DSM-IV classification seems too rigid and the experienced doctor has to consider the global constellation of symptoms. Better management follows early diagnosis and intervention before the formal criteria for major depression develop.

Important points

- The essential feature of depression is mood change which can vary in intensity from despondency to intense despair.[1]
- The other major feature is loss of interest or pleasure, including loss of interest in family, hobbies, sexual activity and personal appearance.

Minor depression

Minor depression is basically a condition where fluctuations of symptoms occur with some vague somatic symptoms and a transient lowering of mood that can respond to environmental influences. Suicidal feelings are fleeting, and delusions and hallucinations are absent. These patients usually respond in time to simple psychotherapy, reassurance and support. However, care should be taken lest they move into major depression.

Masked depression

This is a difficult yet common type of depression in practice and tends to be misdiagnosed. Patients do not complain of the classic symptoms and tend to deny depression, which is perceived as a social stigma and a sign of weakness. They usually have multiple minor complaints of the 'ticket of entry' type. Mood changes may be elicited only after careful questioning.

The classic affective features of depression are masked by a complex of somatic complaints.

Such symptoms include fatigue; anorexia; weight loss; menstrual changes; unusual sensations in the abdomen, chest or head; bodily aches and pain; dry mouth; and difficulty in breathing.

If depression is not considered many fruitless, expensive and distressing investigations may be performed. According to Davies,[2] nearly half of patients with depressive illness report to the doctor with complaints that suggest physical illness. The family doctor has to suspect masked depression in a patient with a multitude of physical complaints or with complaints that do not fit any definite pattern of organic disease.

The differential diagnoses of depression are presented in Table 16.1.

An Australian study on masked depression concluded:[3]

It must be stressed that the masking of the depressive state occurs on the doctor's side as well as the patient's, and an awareness that this may be so leads us to recommend that, once organic lesions have been excluded, there is a place for the use of an adequate therapeutic trial of antidepressants.

The following additional points were made by a panel of psychiatrists at a symposium entitled 'Depression: Masked or Missed?' in Dallas, Texas:[4]

- Some patients dismissed as 'crocks' may go on to suicide if their depression is not treated.

Table 16.1 *Differential diagnoses of depression*

Psychiatric conditions
- anxiety disorder
- schizophrenia
- drug and alcohol abuse
- dementia

Organic disorders
- malignancy, e.g. lung, pancreas, lymphoma
- hypothyroidism
- hyperparathyroidism
- other endocrine disorders, e.g. Cushing's, Addison's
- anaemia, especially pernicious anaemia
- postinfective states, e.g. Epstein–Barr mononucleosis
- cerebrovascular disease
- Parkinson's disease
- congestive cardiac failure
- systemic lupus erythematosus
- drugs (which may cause depression)
  — antihypertensives
  — benzodiazepines e.g. diazepam
  — antiparkinson drugs
  — corticosteroids
  — cytotoxic agents
  — NSAIDs
  — oral contraceptives/progestogen

- Masked depression would be missed much less frequently if the physician would look beneath symptoms that do not quite ring true.
- The patient with the 'tired blood syndrome' deserves something other than an iron tonic.
- Depression frequently accompanies organic diseases that are associated with nausea and other illness.
- A complete work-up may help to rule out organic disease but may result in iatrogenic disease if pursued overzealously.
- Alcoholism should be suspected as a cause of depression.

Depression in the elderly

Severe depression affects 1–2% of the elderly population while 10% have significant depression affecting their life. Milder depression can affect a further 20%. Depression can have bizarre features in the elderly and may be misdiagnosed as dementia or psychosis. Agitated depression is the most frequent type of depression in the aged.[1] Features may include histrionic behaviour, delusions and disordered thinking.

Depression is often missed in the elderly because it is atypical and less expressive, and patients tend to be ashamed and reluctant to admit it. Four key guidelines help diagnosis:

- Are you basically satisfied with your life?
- Do you feel that your life is empty?
- Are you afraid that something bad is going to happen to you?
- Do you feel happy most of the time?

A useful clue is a change in sleep pattern; so a request for sleeping tablets may lead to the prescription for a more sedating antidepressant. Medical illness is an important precipitant of depression in the elderly. Tricyclic antidepressants have to be used with caution in the elderly and most have some contraindications to their use. ECT has a useful place in treatment of severe cases.

Depression in children

Sadness is common in children but depression, although not as common, does occur and is characterised by feelings of helplessness, worthlessness and despair. Parents and doctors both tend to be unaware of depression in children.[5]

Major depression in children and adolescents may be diagnosed using the same criteria as for adults, namely loss of interest in usual activities and the presence of a sad or irritable mood, persisting for 2 weeks or more.[6] The other constellation of depressive symptoms including somatic complaints may be present. Examples include difficulty in getting to sleep, not enjoying meals, poor concentration and low self-esteem. It can present as antisocial behaviour or as a separation anxiety, e.g. school refusal. Although suicidal thoughts are common, suicide is rare before adolescence. Depressed adolescents are a serious suicide risk. Referral of these patients to an experienced child psychiatrist is advisable.

The diagnostic approach

Depression can be associated with many illnesses but it is important to realise that the somatic symptoms may be the presentation of depressive illness and thus 'undifferentiated illness' is a feature. The patient tends to complain of aches and pains, gastrointestinal symptoms and other similar symptoms rather than emotional problems.

There is a relationship between anxiety and depression so that many depressed patients are agitated and anxious—a feature that may mask the underlying depression.[7]

Questions to assess level of depression
- What do you think is the matter with you?
- Do you think that your feelings are possibly caused by nerves, anxiety or depression?
- Can you think of any reason why you feel this way?
- Do you feel down in the dumps?
- Do you feel that you are coping well?
- Do you have any good times?
- Has anything changed in your life?
- How do you sleep? Do you wake early?
- What time of the day do you feel at your worst?
- Where would you put yourself between 0 and 100%?
- Have you felt hopeless?
- Do you brood about the past?
- What is your energy like?
- What is your appetite like?
- Are you as interested in sex as before?
- Do you feel guilty about anything?
- Do you feel that life is worthwhile?
- Has the thought of ending your life occurred to you?
- Do you cry when no one is around? (especially for children)

Depression scales

Consider the use of depression scales, for example:

- Hamilton Depression Inventory
- Beck Depression Scale
- General Health Questionnaire

Management

Important considerations from the outset are:

- Is the patient a suicide risk?
- Does the patient require inpatient assessment?
- Is referral to a specialist psychiatrist indicated?

If the symptoms are major and the patient appears in poor health or is a suicide risk, referral is appropriate.

The basic treatments are:

- Psychotherapy, including education, reassurance and support. All patients require minor psychotherapy. More sophisticated techniques such as cognitive or behavioural therapy may be used for selected patients. Cognitive therapy basically involves teaching patients new ways of positive thinking, which have to be relevant and achievable for the patient. Patients need to be able to recognise their own negative cognitions including their anxieties and worries.
- Pharmacological agents.
- Electroconvulsive treatment.

Note: Reassurance and support are needed for all depressed patients.

Useful guidelines

- Mild depression: psychotherapy alone may suffice but keep medication in mind.
- Moderate to severe depression: psychotherapy plus antidepressants is recommended.
- Reassurance and support are needed for all depressed patients.

Explanatory supportive notes for patients and relatives[8]

Most people feel unhappy or depressed every now and again, but there is a difference between this feeling and the illness of depression.

Depression is a very real illness that affects the entire mind and body. People cannot seem to lift themselves out of their misery or 'fight it themselves'. Superficial advice like 'snap out of it' is unhelpful, because the person has no control over it.

What is the cause?

The cause is somewhat mysterious, but it has been found that an important chemical is present in smaller amounts than usual in the nervous system. It is rather like a person low in iron becoming anaemic.

Depression can follow a severe loss, such as the death of a loved one, a marital separation or financial loss. On the other hand it can develop for no apparent reason, although it may follow an illness such as glandular fever or influenza, an operation or childbirth. Depression is seen more commonly in late adolescence, middle age (both men and women), retirement age and in the elderly.

What is the treatment?

The basis of treatment is to replace the missing chemicals with antidepressant medication. Antidepressants are not drugs of addiction and are very effective but take about two weeks before an improvement is noticed. Alcohol can interact with the tablets; so it is important not to drink and drive. If the person is very seriously depressed and there is a risk of suicide, admission to hospital will most likely be advised. Other more effective treatments can be used if needed. The depressed person needs a lot of understanding, support and therapy. Once treatment is started, the outlook is very good (an 80% cure rate).

Important points

- Depression is an illness.
- It is more common than realised.
- It just happens; no one is to blame.
- It affects the basic functions of energy, sex, appetite and sleep.
- It can be lethal if untreated.
- It can destroy relationships.
- The missing chemical needs to be replaced.
- It responds well to treatment.

Recommended reading

Paul Hauck, *Overcoming depression*. The Westminster Press, London, 1987.

Antidepressant medication

The initial choice of an antidepressant depends on the age and sex of the patient, prior response to medication, safety in overdosage and the side-effect profile. All antidepressants are equally efficacious. The tricyclics and tetracyclics have been the first-line drugs but the newer drugs, the selective serotonin reuptake inhibitors and moclobemide (a reversible monoamine oxidase inhibitor (MAOI) antidepressant) are equally effective, are better tolerated, have a wider safety margin[6] and are now considered first-line drugs.

Tricyclic antidepressants[6]

I. amitriptyline and imipramine
   - the first generation tricyclics
   - the most sedating: valuable if marked anxiety and insomnia
   - strongest anticholinergic side effects, e.g. constipation, blurred vision, prostatism
II. clomipramine, desipramine, dothiepin, doxepin, nortriptyline
   - less sedating and anticholinergic activity
   - nortriptyline is the least hypotensive of the tricyclics

Dosage: 50–75 mg (o) nocte, increasing every 2 to 3 days to 150 mg (o) nocte by day 7.

If no response after 2 to 3 weeks, increase by 25–50 mg daily at 2 to 3 week intervals (depending on adverse effects) to 200–250 mg (o) nocte. Trial for 6 weeks.

General adverse effects

- dry mouth, weight gain, constipation, sedation
- glaucoma, urinary retention, tremor
- confusion and delirium in the elderly (caution in the elderly)
- sexual dysfunction
- postural hypotension
- cardiac conduction impairment (caution in heart disease)
- lowered seizure threshold

Tetracyclic antidepressants[6]

Mianserin 30–60 mg (o) nocte increasing to 60–120 mg (o) nocte by day 7

Adverse effects

- sedation, lethargy, dizziness, polyarthritis, dry mouth, headache
- neutropenia (reversible) especially > 65 years (uncommon)
- less anticholinergic effects than tricyclics
- fewer cardiovascular side effects

Selective serotonin reuptake inhibitors
e.g. fluoxetine, paroxetine, sertraline, fluvoxamine, citalopram

- Fluoxetine and paroxetine 20 mg (o) mane

This dose is usually sufficient for most patients. If no response after 2 to 3 weeks, increase by 20 mg at 2 to 4 week intervals to 40–80 mg (o) daily in divided doses.

- Sertraline, 50 mg (o) daily, starting dose; can increase to 200 mg daily.
- Fluvoxamine, 50 mg (o) bd, starting dose; can increase to 200 mg daily.
- Citalopram 20 mg (o) daily, up to 60 mg (max).

These new drugs have a similar efficacy profile to the tricyclics. They do not appear to cause weight gain, interact with alcohol or cause serious cardiovascular effects.

Adverse effects

Nausea, nervousness, fatigue, agitation, diarrhoea, headaches, insomnia. Possible effects include sexual dysfunction, mainly ejaculatory disturbances, allergic reactions and hypomania (in some manic depressives).

They should not be used with MAOIs or the tricyclics.

Moclobemide

Moclobemide 150 mg (o) bd. If no response after 2 to 3 weeks, increase by 50 mg daily to maximum 300 mg (o) bd.

- This is a reversible MAOI, which is less toxic than the irreversible MAOIs.
- It has minimal interaction with tyramine-containing foodstuffs, so that no dietary restrictions are necessary.
- Adverse effects include nausea, headache, agitation, dizziness and insomnia.
- The irreversible MAOIs, which should be reserved for second-line MAOI therapy, include phenelzine and tranylcypromine.

Serotonin noradrenaline reuptake inhibitors

The first of the SNRIs to be released is venlafaxine. It is recommended for major depression where other therapy is inappropriate. The starting dose is 37.5 mg (o) bd increasing to 75 mg bd after 2 weeks if necessary.

Side effects appear to include nausea, dizziness, insomnia and sexual dysfunction, giving the drug a similar side-effect profile to the SSRIs. It should not be used concomitantly with MAOIs and various 'wash-out periods' from other antidepressants are required.

5-HT$_2$ receptor blockers

Nefazodone is the first of the serotonin type 2 (5-HT$_2$) receptor blockers. It is recommended for the treatment of major depressive disorders and is effective for depression associated with anxiety. The usual dose is 300–600 mg (o) daily in two equally divided doses. The starting dose is 50 mg bd for 1 week and then 100 mg bd for week 2.

Reported adverse effects include asthenia, dry mouth, nausea, constipation, somnolence and dizziness.

Notes about antidepressants[6]

- Tricyclics can be given once daily (usually in the evening).
- There is a delay in onset of action of 1–2 weeks after a therapeutic dose (equivalent to 150 mg imipramine at least) is reached.
- Each drug should have a clinical trial at an adequate dose for at least 4–6 weeks before treatment is changed.
- The SSRIs are probably now the first-line drugs of choice and the tricyclics second-line.
- Consider referral if there is a failed (adequate) trial.
- Full recovery may take up to 6 weeks or longer (in those who respond).
- Continue treatment at maintenance levels for at least 6 to 9 months.[1] There is a high risk of relapse.
- For a second episode use antidepressants for 3 to 5 years.
- MAOIs are often the drugs of choice for neurotic depression or atypical depression.[1]

The serotonin syndrome[9]

This is a dangerous adverse reaction related to the use of the SSRIs and is most likely to occur with the combined use of MAOI drugs and other agents. The diagnosis is based on three criteria:

- Symptoms must coincide with the introduction or dose increase of a serotonergic agent.
- Other causes such as infection, substance abuse or withdrawal must be excluded.
- At least three of the symptoms or signs attributed to the syndrome must be present, i.e.
  — mental status/behaviour changes, e.g. agitation, confusion, hypomania, seizures
  — altered muscle tone, e.g. tremor, shivering, myoclonus
  — autonomic instability, e.g. hypertension, tachycardia, fever, diarrhoea

The offending agents should be withdrawn immediately and supportive therapy initiated.

Electroconvulsive therapy

Electroconvulsive therapy (ECT) is safe, effective and rapidly acting.[1,6,10]

Indications

- psychotic depression, for example delusions, hallucinations
- melancholic depression unresponsive to antidepressants
- substantial suicide risk
- ineffective antidepressant medication
- severe psychomotor depression
  — refusal to eat or drink
  — depressive stupor
  — severe personal neglect

Immediate referral for hospital admission is necessary in most of these circumstances. The usual course is 6–8 treatments over 3 weeks. All antidepressants can be used in combination with ECT and after ECT to prevent relapse.

Recurrent depression

Lifelong antidepressant therapy may have to be considered. Lithium is an alternative medication for long-term use.

Suicide

The risk of suicide is a concern in all depressed patients. Between 11% and 17% of people who have suffered a severe depressive disorder at any time will eventually commit suicide.[10] Referral for hospital admission should be arranged for patients who are at great risk for suicide. There is a distinction between patients who are determined to suicide and those who attempt suicide (parasuicide).

Risk factors for suicide include:

- male sex
- older age > 55 years
- adolescents
- young adults 15–25 years
- immigrant status
- isolation/living alone
- recent divorce, separation or bereavement
- recent loss of employment or retirement
- family history of psychiatric illness (including suicide)
- impulsive, hostile personality

Table 16.2 *SAD PERSONS Index: Suicide risk assessment*

Risk factor	Criteria	Score
Sex	Male	1
Age	< 20 years; > 45 years	1
Depression	Major, e.g. depressed mood	2
Psychiatric history	Previous attempts	1
Excessive drug use	Ethanol or other drug abuse	1
Rationality loss	Psychosis, severe depression	2
Separated	Loss of spouse or other single	1
Organised plan	Determined suicide plan	2
No supports	No community back-up; generally isolated	1
Sickness	Chronic illness	1

Score > 7 = high suicide risk

- previous suicide attempt
- severe depression
- financial difficulties
- alcohol or other substance abuse
- psychosis
- early dementia
- physical illness, especially if chronic pain

A useful suicide risk assessment is the SAD PERSONS (mnemonic) index (Table 16.2). A score greater than 7 represents a very high risk that demands careful attention including referral to an acute psychiatric service.

If there is concern about suicide risk and treatment is supervised outside hospital, provide closer supervision and considerable support, and prescribe drugs that are less toxic in overdosage, e.g. mianserin or fluoxetine. If tricyclics are prescribed, useful guidelines are that dangerous medical complications occur with an equivalent dosage of 1000 mg (40 tablets) of imipramine and a high risk of death with 2000 mg (80 tablets).[6]

When to refer[1]

- Uncertainty about diagnosis
- Inpatient care obviously necessary
- Severe depression
- Inability to cope at home
- Psychotically depressed (with delusions or hallucinations)
- Substantial suicide risk
- Failure of response to routine antidepressant therapy
- Associated psychiatric or physical disorders
- Difficult problem in the elderly—where diagnosis including 'dementia' is doubtful
- Children with apparent major depression

References

1. Burrows GD. Depressive disorders. In: MIMS Disease Index (2nd edn). Sydney: IMS Publishing, 1996, 139–141.

2. Davies B. *An introduction to clinical psychiatry.* University of Melbourne, 1977, 76–77.

3. Serry DK, Serry M. Masked depression and the use of antidepressants in general practice. Med J Aust, 15 February 1969, 35–37.

4. Depression: Masked or missed? Patient Care, Oct 1972, 1(3):6–14.

5. Robinson MJ. *Practical paediatrics* (2nd edn), Melbourne: Churchill Livingstone, 1990, 552–553.

6. Moulds RFW. *Psychotropic drug guidelines* (3rd edn), Melbourne: Victorian Medical Postgraduate Foundation, 1996/7, 107–118.

7. Davis A, Bolin T, Ham J. *Symptom analysis and physical diagnosis* (2nd edn), London: Bailliere Tindall, 1990, 983.

8. Murtagh J. *Patient education* (2nd edn). Sydney: McGraw-Hill, 1996, 146.

9. Keltner N. Serotonin syndrome: A case of fatal SSRI/MAOI interaction. Perspectives in Psychiatric Care, 1994; 30(4):26–31.

10. Kumar PJ, Clark ML. *Clinical medicine* (2nd edn), London: Bailliere Tindall, 1990, 983.

11. Rogers I. *Guidelines for the management of common emergencies in the emergency department* (2nd edn). Auckland Hospital, 1996, 43.

17
Diabetes mellitus

—

Diabetes comes from a Greek word meaning 'to pass or flow through' (i.e. excessive urination) and mellitus means 'sweet'.

There are two main types of diabetes (see Table 17.1).

- Type I is known as juvenile onset diabetes or insulin dependent diabetes mellitus (IDDM).
- Type II is known as maturity onset diabetes or non-insulin dependent diabetes mellitus (NIDDM).

The two key tasks

The main objectives for the GP in the optimal management of the diabetic patient, in order to prevent complications are:

1. achieve strict glycaemic control (as measured by plasma glucose and HbAlc)
2. achieve blood pressure control (≤ 140/90 mmHg, supine)

Key facts and checkpoints

- The prevalence of diabetes is about 3% of the adult population (includes about 1% undiagnosed).[1]
- A further 3% will have impaired glucose tolerance.[1]
- About 30% of these people will develop clinical diabetes within 10 years.[1]
- Many type II diabetics are asymptomatic.
- Diabetes can exist for years before detection and complications may be evident.
- Type II diabetes is not a mild disease. About one-third of those surviving 15 years will require insulin injections to control symptoms or complications.[2] Complications occur in type II diabetes as well as in type I.
- There are several causes of secondary diabetes that are very uncommon (see Table 17.2).

Clinical features

The classical symptoms of uncontrolled diabetes are:

- polyuria
- polydipsia
- loss of weight (type I)
- tiredness and fatigue
- propensity for infections, especially of the skin and genitals (vaginal thrush)

The young insulin dependent diabetic typically presents with a brief 2–4 week history of the classic triad of symptoms:

| Thirst |
| Polyuria |
| Weight loss |

Other symptoms are:

- vulvovaginitis
- pruritus vulvae } due to *Candida albicans*
- balanitis
- nocturnal enuresis (type I)
- blurred vision/visual changes

Symptoms of complications (may be presenting feature)

Table 17.1 *Clinical differentiation between type I and type II diabetes*

	Type I IDDM	Type II NIDDM
Relative frequency (approx)	15%	85%
Peak age incidence	10–30 years	> 40 years
Age of onset	usually < 20	> 40
Onset	rapid	insidious
Weight at onset	low (thin)	high (obese)
Ketoacidosis	yes	no
Familial	weak	strong
Insulin status	deficient	resistant
Complications	yes	yes

Note: These are generalisations and the clinical features may vary, e.g. type II may be thin and have a rapid onset; type I may exhibit a weak genetic link.

- staphylococcal skin infections
- polyneuropathy
  - tingling or numbness in feet
  - pain (can be severe if present)
- impotence
- arterial disease
  - myocardial ischaemia
  - peripheral vascular disease

The clinical examination should follow the guidelines under the heading 'Examinations' in Table 17.5 (p. 146).

Diagnosis of diabetes

Diabetes is diagnosed as follows:[3]

1. If symptomatic (at least two of polydipsia, polyuria, frequent skin infections or frequent genital thrush).

Table 17.2 *Causes of secondary diabetes*

Endocrine disorders
- Cushing's syndrome
- acromegaly
- phaeochromocytoma

Pancreatic disorders
- haemochromatosis
- chronic pancreatitis

Drug-induced diabetes (transient)
- thiazide diuretics
- oestrogen therapy (high dose—not with low-dose HRT)
- corticosteroids

Other transient causes
- gestational diabetes
- medical or surgical stress

- fasting venous plasma glucose (VPG) ≥ 7.0 mmol/L
- random VPG (at least 2 hours after last eating) ≥ 11.1 mmol/L

2. If asymptomatic:
At least 2 separate elevated values, either fasting, 2 or more hours postprandial, or the 2 values from an oral glucose tolerance test (OGTT).

Note: If random or fasting VPG lies in uncertain range (5.5–11.0 mmol/L) in either a symptomatic patient or a patient with risk factors (over 50 years, overweight, blood relative with NIDDM or high blood pressure) perform an OGTT. The cut-off point for further testing has now been reduced to 5.5 mmol/L.[4]

The OGTT should be reserved for true borderline cases and for gestational diabetes. A screening test at 26–30 weeks gestation is recommended.

The diagnostic criteria after a 75 g load of glucose are:

Venous plasma glucose	Fasting	2 hours later
Normal	< 5.5	< 7.0
Impaired tolerance	5.5–7.8	≥ 7.0–11.1
Diabetes	> 7.0	> 11.1
Gestational diabetes	> 5.5	≥ 7.0

Urinalysis is unreliable in diagnosis since glycosuria occurs at different plasma glucose values in patients with different renal thresholds.

Management principles

- Provide detailed and comprehensive patient education, support and reassurance.
- Achieve control of presenting symptoms.
- Achieve blood pressure control ($\leqslant$ 140/90 mmHg supine).
- Emphasise the importance of the diet: good nutrition, adequate complex carbohydrates, restricted fats and sugars.
- Promptly diagnose and treat urinary tract infection.
- Treat and prevent life-threatening complications of ketoacidosis or hyperosmolar coma.
- Treat and prevent hypoglycaemia in those having insulin and oral hypoglycaemic agents.
- Organise self-testing techniques, preferably blood glucose monitoring.
- Detect and treat complications of diabetes—neuropathy, nephropathy, retinopathy, vascular disease.
- Beware of the deadly quartet (syndrome X):[5]
  1. upper truncal obesity
  2. dyslipidaemia
     ↑ triglycerides
     ↓ HDL cholesterol
  3. glucose intolerance, i.e. NIDDM
  4. hypertension
  These are all risk factors for coronary atherosclerosis.

Monitoring techniques

- blood glucose estimation (fasting and postprandial)
- urine glucose (of limited usefulness)
- urine ketones (for type I diabetes)
- glycosylated haemoglobin (HbAlc) (essential to know glycaemic control)
- microalbuminuria (regarded as an early and reversible sign of nephropathy)
- blood pressure
- serum lipids

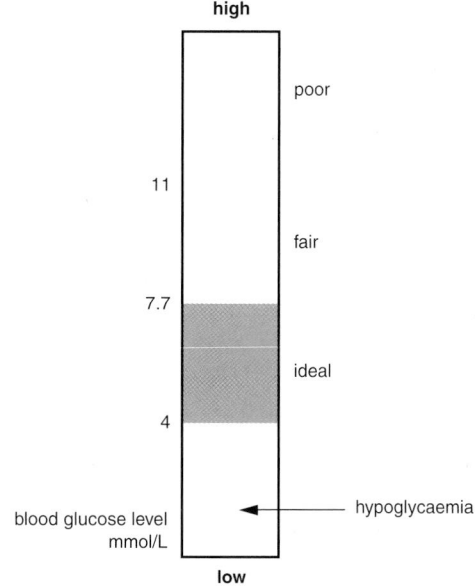

Fig 17.1 *Control guidelines for diabetic management*

- renal function (serum urea/creatinine)
- ECG

Control guidelines are summarised in Figure 17.1 and Table 17.3.

Blood glucose monitoring at home

This can be done using visual strips or a glucose meter (glucometer). Patients should be advised about the most appropriate glucometer to obtain.

| Method |

- Obtain capillary blood by pricking the finger with a lancet.
- Place a large drop of blood to cover both colour strips (avoid smearing).
- At 60 seconds blot off excess blood with tissue paper. (Time can vary from 30 to 60 seconds depending on the brand used.)

Table 17.3 *Suggested guidelines for glycaemic control (plasma glucose mmol/L)*

	Ideal	Acceptable (fair)	Suboptimal or unacceptable
Before meals (fasting)	< 6	6–7.7	> 7.7
After meals (2 hours postprandial)	< 7.7	7.7–11	> 11
Glycohaemoglobin (HbAlc) %*	< 7	6–7.7	> 11

* HbAlc is an index of the mean plasma glucose levels over the preceding 2–3 months (assume a reference range of 4.5–8%). The reference ranges vary in different laboratories.

- The strip is read by comparing the colour with a colour chart or by using an electronic meter (glucometer).

How often and when?

- Type I diabetes:
  — twice a day (at least once)
  — four times a day (before meals and before bedtime) at first and for problems
  — may settle for 1–2 times a week (if good control)
- Type II diabetes:
  — twice a day (fasting and 2–3 hours postprandial)
  — if good control—once a week or every 2 weeks

Note:
- Capillary blood glucose is approximately 7% higher than venous blood.
- Glucometer error is usually ± 5%.

Glycosylated haemoglobin

Glycosylated haemoglobin is abnormally high in diabetics with persistent hyperglycaemia and is reflective of their metabolic control. The major form of glycohaemoglobin is haemoglobin Alc, which normally comprises 4–6% of the total haemoglobin.[5] Glycohaemoglobins have a long half-life and its measure reflects the mean plasma glucose levels over the past 2–3 months and hence provides a good method of assessing overall diabetic control. It should be checked every 3–6 months.

Insulin dependent diabetes mellitus

The three main objectives of the treatment of IDDM are:[5]

1. Maintain good health, free from the problems of hyperglycaemia and hypoglycaemia.
2. Achieve proper growth and maturation for children and protect the foetus and mother in a mother with IDDM.
3. Prevent, arrest or delay long-term macrovascular and microvascular complications.

Insulin regimens for type I diabetes

The most commonly used insulin injection preparations are the 'artificial' human insulins. Insulins are classified according to their time course of action:

- rapid-acting and short duration—lispro insulin
- short-acting—neutral (regular, soluble)

- intermediate-acting—isophane (NPH) or lente
- long-acting—ultralente
- mixed short/intermediate—biphasic (neutral + isophane)

Starting insulin[2]

It is important to use the simplest regimen for the patient and to provide optimal education about its administration and monitoring. Full replacement of insulin is achieved by using 2, 3 or 4 injections per day.

1. *The pre-mixed 2 injection system:* Give twice daily, before breakfast and before evening meal.
   e.g. Mixtard 30/70, Humulin 30/70 (the most common)
   Typical starting dose: 0.3 IU/kg/day—for a 70 kg person use 10 units bd
2. *3 injections per day*
   Short-acting insulin before breakfast and lunch
   Intermediate- or long-acting insulin before evening meal
3. *4 injections (basal-bolus) system:*
   Short-acting insulin before breakfast, lunch and dinner
   Intermediate-acting insulin at bedtime

Insulin requirements often vary significantly even in the same individual under different lifestyle conditions. The new rapid-acting analogues can be taken with meals.

Methods of giving insulin injections

When: Get the patient to develop a set routine such as eating meals on time and giving the injection about 30 minutes before the meal.

Where: Into subcutaneous tissue—the best place is the abdomen (Fig. 17.2). It is advisable to keep to one area such as the abdomen and avoid injections into the arms, near joints and the groin. The injection should be given at a different place each time, keeping a distance of 3 cm or more from the previous injection. This reduces the risk of the development of lipodystrophy.

How: Pinch a large area of skin on the abdomen between the thumb and fingers and insert the needle straight in. After withdrawing the needle, press down firmly (do not rub or massage) over the injection site for 30 seconds.

Fig 17.2 *Method of giving insulin injections; use the abdomen*

Guidelines for the patient[6]

The proper injection of insulin is very important to allow your body, which lacks natural insulin, to function as normally as possible. You should be very strict about the way you manage your insulin injections and have your technique down to a fine art.

Common mistakes:

- poor mixing technique when mixing insulin
- wrong doses (because of poor eyesight)
- poor injection technique—into the skin or muscle rather than the soft, fatty layer
- not taking insulin when you feel ill

Drawing up the insulin

Make sure your technique is checked by an expert. You may be using either a single insulin or a mixed insulin. A mixed insulin is a combination of shorter and longer acting insulin and is cloudy.

Rules for mixing

- Always draw up clear insulin first.
- Do not permit any of the cloudy insulin to get into the clear insulin bottle.
- Do not push any of the clear insulin into the cloudy insulin bottle.

Golden rules

- Take your insulin every day, even if you feel ill.
- Do not change your dose unless instructed by your doctor or you are competent to do so yourself.

Problems

Injection sites should be inspected regularly because lipo-hypertrophy or lipo-atrophy can occur.

Type II (NIDDM) diabetes

First-line treatment: • diet therapy (especially if obese) • exercise program

Most symptoms improve dramatically within 1 to 4 weeks on diet and exercise.[2] The secret to success is patient compliance through good education and supervision. The role of a diabetic education service, especially with a dietician, can be invaluable. If unsatisfactory control persists after 3–6 months, consider adding an oral hypoglycaemic agent (Table 17.4).

One of the sulfonylureas is usually selected: they are effective and have a low side-effect profile. They should be introduced with care and in a low dose in the elderly. Metformin, which has moderate antidiabetic potential, has less tendency to cause weight gain and is often used for obese patients. It tends to cause diarrhoea. Metformin can be added to a sulfonylurea.

When oral hypoglycaemics fail (secondary failure) the new agent acarbose can be added (it is also very effective first line). The classic symptoms of hyperglycaemia may be present but more commonly patients experience general disability. Approximately 30% of NIDDM patients eventually require insulin even after years of successful oral therapy.

The importance of diet

Type I patients often require three meals and sometimes regular snacks each day.

Type II patients usually require less food intake and restriction of total food intake.

Principles of dietary management

- Keep to a regular nutritious diet.
- Achieve ideal body weight.
- Reduce calories (kilojoules)
  — added sugar
  — dietary fat.
- Increase proportions of vegetables, fresh fruit, cereal foods.
- Special diabetic foods are not necessary.
- Qualitative diets, rather than quantitative diets (such as 'exchanges' or 'portions'), are now used.

Table 17.4 *Commonly prescribed oral hypoglycaemic agents*

Drug	Duration of action (hours)	Maximum effective daily dose	Notes
Sulfonylureas			Hypoglycaemia most common side effect.
Tolbutamide	6–10	1 g, tds	Shorter acting sulfonylurea, e.g. tolbutamide, is preferred in elderly.
Gliclazide	6–12	160 mg, bd	Longer acting potent ones cause troublesome hypoglycaemia in elderly.
Glipizide	6–12	20 mg, bd	Others: weight gain (common), rash and GIT (rare).
Glibenclamide	16–24	10 mg, bd	
Chlorpropamide	24–72	500 mg, mane	
Biguanides			Usually reserved for obese but now first line.
Metformin	6–10	1 g, tds or 850 mg, bd	Side effects: GIT disturbances e.g. diarrhoea. Avoid in cardiac, renal and hepatic disease. Lactic acidosis can be a serious complication.
Thiazolidinediones			
Rosiglitazone		4–8 mg	Oedema, hepatic effects

Patient education

The following handout is helpful to patients:

The importance of diet

All diabetics require a diet in which refined carbohydrate and fat intake is controlled. The objectives of the diet are:

- to keep to ideal weight (neither fat nor thin)
- to keep the blood sugar level as near normal as possible

This is achieved by:

- eating good food regularly (not skimping)
- spacing the meals throughout the day (three main meals and three snacks) for many type I diabetics
- cutting down fat to a minimum
- avoiding sugar and refined carbohydrates (e.g. sugar, jam, honey, chocolates, sweets, pastries, cakes, soft drinks)
- eating a balance of more complex carbohydrates (starchy foods such as wholemeal bread, potatoes and cereals)
- eating a good variety of fruit and vegetables
- cutting out alcohol or drinking only a little

The importance of exercise

Exercise is very beneficial to your health. Exercise is any physical activity that keeps you fit. Good examples are brisk walking (e.g. 2 km per day), jogging, tennis, skiing and aerobics. Aim for at least 30 minutes three times a week, but daily exercise is ideal. Go slow when you start and increase your pace gradually.

> **Good advice**
> - Exercise is important.
> - Do not get overweight.
> - A proper diet is the key to success.
> - A low-fat, no-sugar diet is needed.
> - Do not smoke.
> - Minimise alcohol.
> - Take special care of your feet.
> - Self-discipline will help make your life normal.
> - Join a diabetic-support organisation.

Psychosocial considerations

The psychological and social factors involving the patient are very influential on outcome. Considerable support and counselling is necessary to help both patient and family cope with the 'distress' of the diagnosis and the discipline required for optimal control of their blood glucose. Reasons for poor dietary compliance and insulin administration must be determined and mobilisation of a supportive multidisciplinary network (where practical) is most helpful. The general practitioner should be the pivot of the team. Joining a self-support group can be very helpful.

Foot care

Foot problems are one of the commonest complications that need special attention; so prevention is the appropriate approach. Pressure sores can develop on the soles of the feet from corns, calluses, ill-fitting footwear, and stones and nails. Minor injuries such as cuts can become a major problem through poor healing. Infection of the wound is a major problem. The patient's footwear must be checked.

Advice to the diabetic patient

1. Keep your diabetes under good control and do not smoke.
2. Check your feet daily. Report any sores, infection or unusual signs.
3. Wash your feet daily:
   - Use lukewarm water (beware of scalds).
   - Dry thoroughly, especially between the toes.
   - Soften dry skin, especially around the heels, with lanoline.
   - Applying methylated spirits between the toes helps stop dampness.
4. Attend to your toenails regularly:
   - Clip them straight across.
   - Do not cut them deep into the corners or too short across.
5. Wear clean cotton or wool socks daily; avoid socks with tight elastic tops.
6. Exercise the feet each day to help the circulation in them.

How to avoid injury

- Wear good-fitting, comfortable leather shoes.
- The shoes must not be too tight.
- Do not walk barefoot, especially out of doors.
- Do not cut your own toenails if you have difficulty reaching them or have poor eyesight.
- Avoid home treatments and corn pads that contain acid.
- Be careful when you walk around the garden and in the home.
- Do not use hot water bottles or heating pads on your feet.
- Do not test the temperature of water with your feet.
- Take extra care when sitting in front of an open fire or heater.

Complications of diabetes

Complications may occur in both type I and type II diabetes even with early diagnosis and treatment (Fig. 17.3). Insulin dependent diabetics still have a significantly reduced life expectancy. The main causes of death are diabetic nephropathy and vascular disease (myocardial infarction and stroke).

Diabetes causes both macrovascular and microvascular complications but microvascular disease is specific to diabetes. Complications are illustrated in Figure 17.3. Special attention should be paid to the 'deadly quartet' associated with type II diabetes.

Microvascular disease

The small vessels most affected from a clinical viewpoint are the retina, nerve sheath and renal glomerulus. In younger patients it takes about 10 to 20 years after diagnosis for the problems of diabetic retinopathy, neuropathy and nephropathy to manifest.

Nephropathy

Prevention of diabetic nephropathy is an essential goal of treatment. Early detection of the yardstick, which is microalbuminurea, is important as the process can be reversed with optimal control. The dipstick method is unreliable. Screening is done simply by an overnight collection (10–12 hours) of all urine including the first morning sample. It is sent to the laboratory to determine the albumin excretion rate. Microalbuminurea is 20–200 µg/minute (2 out of 3 positive collections).

ACE inhibitors should be used for evidence of hypertension.

Neuropathy

The following types of neuropathy may occur:

- sensory polyneuropathy
- isolated mononeuropathy and multiple mononeuropathy
  - isolated peripheral nerve lesions, e.g. median nerve
  - cranial nerve palsies, e.g. III, VI
  - amyotrophy
- autonomic neuropathy, especially postural hypotension and impotence

The pain of neuropathy can be treated with capsaicin cream and/or oral carbamazepine.

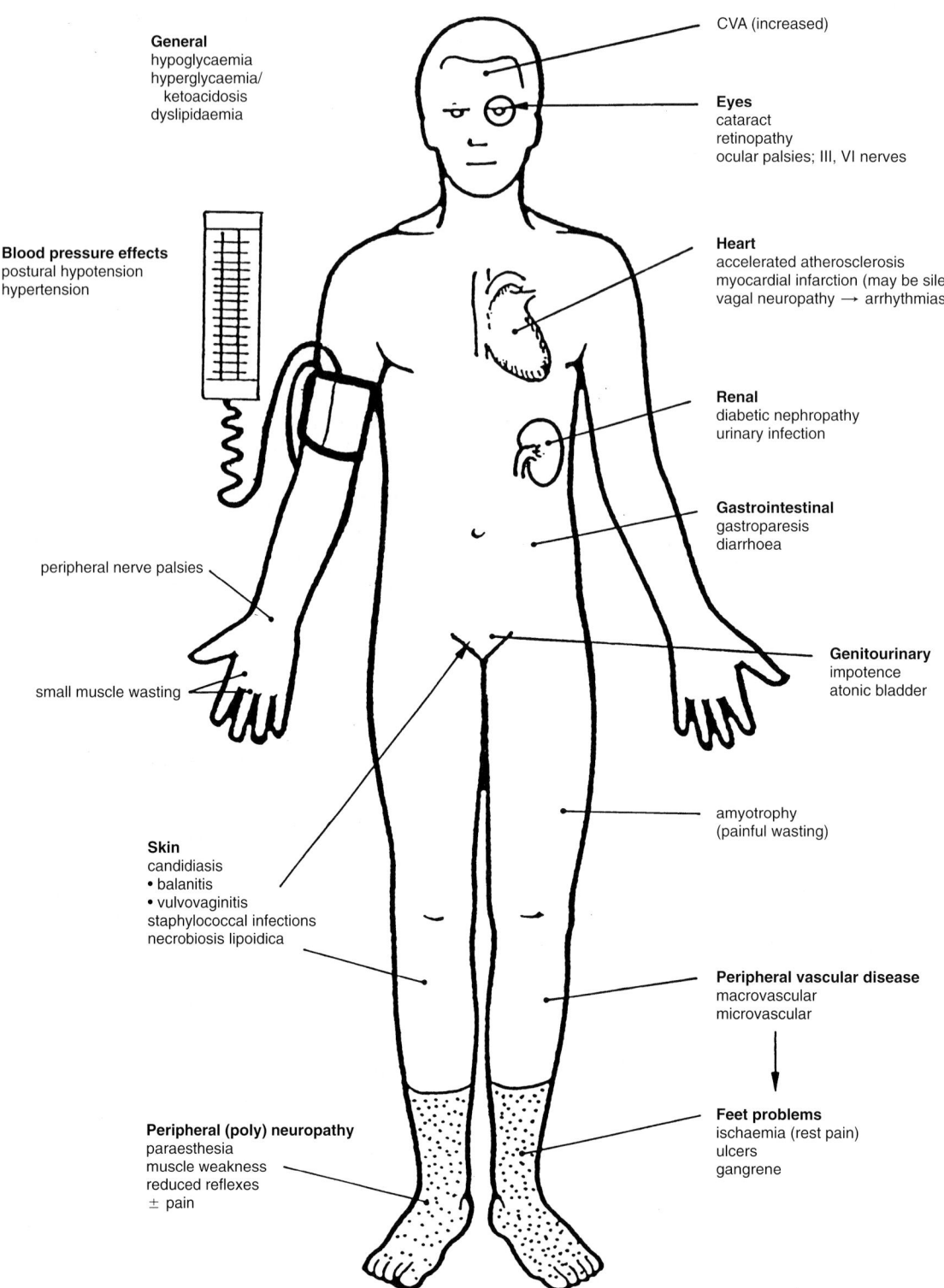

General
hypoglycaemia
hyperglycaemia/
 ketoacidosis
dyslipidaemia

CVA (increased)

Eyes
cataract
retinopathy
ocular palsies; III, VI nerves

Blood pressure effects
postural hypotension
hypertension

Heart
accelerated atherosclerosis
myocardial infarction (may be silent)
vagal neuropathy → arrhythmias

Renal
diabetic nephropathy
urinary infection

Gastrointestinal
gastroparesis
diarrhoea

peripheral nerve palsies

small muscle wasting

Genitourinary
impotence
atonic bladder

amyotrophy
(painful wasting)

Skin
candidiasis
• balanitis
• vulvovaginitis
staphylococcal infections
necrobiosis lipoidica

Peripheral vascular disease
macrovascular
microvascular

Peripheral (poly) neuropathy
paraesthesia
muscle weakness
reduced reflexes
± pain

Feet problems
ischaemia (rest pain)
ulcers
gangrene

Fig 17.3 *The complications of diabetes*

Infections

Poorly controlled diabetics are prone to infections, especially:

- skin — mucocutaneous candidiasis, e.g. balanitis, vulvovaginitis
  — staphylococcal infections, e.g. folliculitis
- urinary tract — cystitis (women)
  — pyelonephritis and perinephric abscess
- lungs — pneumonia: staphylococcal, strep. pneumonia, others
  — tuberculosis

Hypoglycaemia

Hypoglycaemia[5] occurs when blood glucose levels fall to less than 3.0 mmol/L. It is more common with treated IDDM but can occur in NIDDM on oral hypoglycaemic drugs, notably sulfonylureas (biguanides hardly ever cause hypoglycaemia).

Clinical variations

1. Classic warning symptoms: sweating, tremor, palpitations, hunger, perioral paraesthesia. Usually treated with refined carbohydrate, e.g. glucose.
2. Rapid loss of consciousness, usually without warning—hypoglycaemic unawareness is less common.
3. Coma: stuporose, comatose or 'strange' behaviour.

For mild cases give something sweet by mouth, followed by a snack.

Treatment of severe cases or patient unconscious

| Treatment of choice |

- 10–25 mL 50% Dextrose IV
  (instil rectally using the nozzle of the syringe if IV access difficult)

or

| Alternative |

- 1 mL glucagon IM

Admit to hospital if concerned (rarely necessary). Ascertain cause of the hypoglycaemia and instruct the patient how to avoid a similar situation in the future.

Diabetic ketoacidosis

This life-threatening emergency requires intensive management. It usually occurs during an illness (e.g. gastroenteritis) when insulin is omitted.

Clinical features

- develops over a few days, but may occur in a few hours in 'brittle' diabetics
- preceding polyuria, polydipsia, drowsiness
- vomiting and abdominal pain
- hyperventilation—severe acidosis (acidotic breathing)
- ketonuria

Management

- Arrange urgent hospital admission.
- Give 10 units rapid-acting insulin IM (not SC).
- Commence IV infusion of normal saline.

Treatment errors and pitfalls[2]

- Avoid prescribing oral hypoglycaemic agents prematurely. Allow a reasonable trial of diet and exercise for NIDDM patients, especially if they are overweight.
- Review the need for continued oral therapy after 3 months of treatment.
- Glucose tolerance tests should be avoided if the diagnosis can be made on the basis of symptoms and fasting or random blood sugar (a glucose load carries a risk of hyperosmolar coma).
- Keep an eye on the development of ketones in IDDM patients by checking urinary ketones and if present watch carefully because diabetic ketoacidosis is a life-threatening emergency.

When to refer[2]

- Type I diabetic patients for specialist evaluation and then 1 to 2 yearly review.
- Type II diabetic patients:
  — all young patients
  — those requiring education
  — those requiring insulin
  — those with complications
- For ophthalmological screening: every 1 to 3 years to inspect retina.
- Diabetics with treatable complications, including:
  — retinopathy
  — nephropathy
  — neuropathy

Shared care

The management of the diabetic patient provides an ideal opportunity for shared care between a co-operative team comprising the patient, the general practitioner and the specialist diabetic team. The objective is to encourage patients to attend their own doctor for primary care and be less reliant on hospital outpatient services or the diabetic clinics. A well co-ordinated arrangement with good communication strategies provides optimal opportunities for the ongoing education of the patient, the general practitioner and the specialist diabetic team.

Table 17.5   *Type I (IDDM): A follow-up program*[5]

1. *History*
   Smoking and alcohol use
   Symptoms of hypoglycaemia, hyperglycaemia
   Check symptoms relating to eyes, circulation, feet*
2. *Examinations*
   Weight, height; BMI
   Blood pressure—standing and lying
   Examine heart*
   Carotid and peripheral pulses*
   Eyes
   • visual acuity (Snellen chart)
   • ? cataracts
   • optic fundi (or ophthalmologist referral)*
   • ? diabetic retinal photography
   Tendon reflexes and sensation for peripheral neuropathy*
   Skin (general)
   Foot examination including footwear*
   Check injection sites
   Urine examination: protein, ketones, glucose, nitrites
3. *Biochemistry*
   Blood glucose
   Glycosylated haemoglobin
   Urea and creatinine
   Lipids
   Urine microalbumin* (overnight collections)
4. *Education on self-management*
   Diet—or dietary review by dietician
      Self-monitoring of blood glucose. Check patterns of use of blood glucose test strips and examine test profiles.
   Exercise program
5. *Review insulin regimen and dose*
6. *Consider other specialist referrals*
7. Schedule review appointment—forgetting to do this is a frequent cause of failure to return.

Items marked * comprise a program for detection of long-term complications. They should be conducted annually, commencing 5 years after diagnosis.

Practice tips

• For every diagnosed diabetic there is an undiagnosed diabetic; so vigilance for diagnosing diabetes is important.
• Follow-up programs should keep to a prepared format. A format that can be used for IDDM is presented in Table 17.5. This can be modified for NIDDM.
• Hyperglycaemia is a common cause of tiredness. If elderly type II diabetic patients are very tired, think of hyperglycaemia and consider giving insulin to improve their symptoms.
• The management of the diabetic patient is a team effort involving family members, a nurse education centre, podiatrists, domiciliary nursing service, general practitioner and consultant.
• If a diabetic patient (particularly IDDM) is very drowsy and looks sick, consider first the diagnosis of ketoacidosis.
• Foot care is vital: always examine the feet when the patient comes in for review.
• Treat associated hypertension with ACE inhibitors or a calcium channel blocker (also good in combination).
• Use a team approach and encourage joining special support groups (e.g. Diabetes Australia).

References

1. Phillips P. *Diabetes*. CHECK Programme, unit 236. Melbourne: RACGP, 1991, 5–20.
2. Welborn TA. Diabetic mellitus. In: MIMS Disease Index (2nd edn). Sydney: IMS Publishing, 1996, 149–152.
3. Nankervis A, Farrance I, Clague A. Revised criteria for diagnosis of diabetes. Med J Aust, 1993; 158:566–567.
4. Welborn T et al. *National diabetic study. Metabolism, Clinical and Experimental.* 1997.
5. Cohen M. Management of insulin dependent diabetes. Aust Fam Physician, 1990, 19:1201–1214.
6. Murtagh J. *Patient education* (2nd edn). Sydney: McGraw-Hill, 1996, 151 (Diabetes: Insulin injections).
7. Murtagh J. *Patient education* (2nd edn). Sydney: McGraw-Hill, 1996, 150 (Diabetes: Foot care for diabetics).
8. Kumar PJ, Clark ML. *Clinical medicine* (2nd edn). London: Bailliere Tindall, 1990, 835–845.

18
Drug problems

—

A custome loathsome to the eye, hateful to the nose, harmeful to the braine, dangerous to the lungs and the blacke stinking fume thereof, neerest resembling the horrible Stigian smoke of the bottomless pit.

James I (1566–1625)
On smoking

Drug-related problems are true masquerades in family practice. This includes prescribed drugs, over the counter drugs and social or illegal street drugs. It is important therefore that all prescribing doctors maintain a high index of suspicion that any clinical problem may be associated with their treatment of the patient.

Adverse drug reactions

An adverse drug effect is defined as 'any unwanted effect of treatment from the medical use of drugs that occurs at a usual therapeutic dose'. Almost every drug can cause an adverse reaction, which must be elicited in the history. Any substance that produces beneficial therapeutic effects may also produce unwanted, adverse or toxic effects. The severity of the reaction may range from a mild skin rash or nausea to sudden death from anaphylaxis. A study has shown that the incidence of adverse reactions increases from about 3% in patients 10–20 years of age to about 20% in patients 80–89 years of age.[1]

Reactions can be classified in several ways, e.g. side effects, overdosage, intolerance, hypersensitivity and idiosyncrasy. However, a useful classification of unwanted effects is divided into type A and type B.

Type A reactions are the most common and involve *Augmented pharmacology*, i.e. they are caused by unwanted, albeit predictable, effects of the drug.

Examples

• constipation due to verapamil
• blurred vision and urinary outflow problems due to tricyclic antidepressants
• hyperuricaemia due to thiazide diuretics

Type A reactions are dose-dependent.

Type B reactions are by definition *Bizarre*. The reactions are unpredictable from known properties of the drug. Examples include hepatotoxicity and blood dyscrasias.

Golden rules for prevention of adverse effects

Before prescribing any drug the prescriber should consider the following rules:

1. Is the drug really necessary?
2. What will happen if it is not used?
3. What good do I hope to achieve?
4. What harm may result from this treatment?

Common adverse effects

There is an extensive list of clinical problems caused by drugs as side effects or interactions that are highlighted throughout this book. Common side effects include:

CNS	malaise, drowsiness, fatigue/tiredness, headache, dizziness
CVS	palpitations, peripheral oedema, hypotension
GIT	nausea, vomiting, dyspepsia, change in bowel habit (diarrhoea, constipation)
Skin	rash, pruritus, flushing
Psychiatric/ Emotional	insomnia, irritability, anxiety, depression, agitation

Drugs that commonly produce adverse effects

Antimicrobials	• penicillin/cephalosporins
	• sulphonamides
	• tetracyclines
	• streptomycin
	• ketoconazole
Anticonvulsants	• carbamazepine
	• phenobarbitone
	• phenytoin
	• sodium valproate
Antidepressants	• tricyclics
	• MAO inhibitors
Anti-inflammatories and analgesics	• aspirin/salicylates
	• codeine/morphine, etc.
	• NSAIDs
	• gold salts
Antihypertensive agents	• (several)
Cardiac agents	• digoxin
	• quinidine
	• amiodarone
	• other antiarrhythmics
Diuretics	• thiazides
	• frusemide
Tranquillisers	• phenothiazines
	• benzodiazepines
	• barbiturates
	• chlordiazepoxide
Other drugs include	• cytotoxics
	• hormones
	• allopurinol
	• warfarin

Nicotine

'Smoking is good for you', according to an old Arab proverb. 'The dogs will not bite you because you smell so bad; thieves will not rob you at night because you cough in your sleep and you will not suffer the indignities of old age because you will die when you are relatively young.'

Tobacco smoking is the largest single, preventable cause of death and disease in Australia. It has been estimated to have caused approximately 20 000 deaths in 1991, over six times the number of deaths from road accidents.[2] Diseases attributed to smoking are summarised in Figure 18.1.

Getting patients to quit

Several studies have highlighted the value of opportunistic intervention by the family doctor.

It is important not only to encourage people to quit but also to organise a quitting program and follow-up. In Australia 80% of smokers (representing about 30% of the adult population) have indicated that they wish to stop smoking. Point out that it is not easy and requires strong will power. As Mark Twain said, 'Quitting is easy—I've done it a thousand times.'

Methods

• Educate patients about the risks to their health and the many advantages of giving up smoking, and emphasise the improvement in *health*, *longevity*, *money savings*, *looks* and *sexuality*.
• The extent of nicotine dependence can be assessed using a questionnaire (based on the Fagerstrom Test) and scoring system.[3]

Facts to point out

• Advantages
 — Food tastes better.
 — Sense of smell improves.
 — Exercise tolerance is better.
 — Sexual pleasure is improved.
 — Bad breath improves.
 — Risk of lung cancer drops: after 10–15 years of quitting it is as low as someone who has never smoked.
 — Early COAD can be reversed.
 — Decreases URTIs and bronchitis.
 — Chance of premature skin wrinkling and stained teeth is less.
 — Removes effects of passive smoking on family and friends.
 — Removes problem of effects on pregnancy.
• Ask them to keep a smoker's diary.
• If they say no to quitting, give them motivational literature and ask them to reconsider.
• If they say yes, make a contract (example below).

A contract to quit

'I .... agree to stop smoking on ....
I understand that stopping smoking is the single best thing I can do for my health and that my doctor has strongly encouraged me to quit.'

............................(Patient's signature)

............................(Doctor's signature)

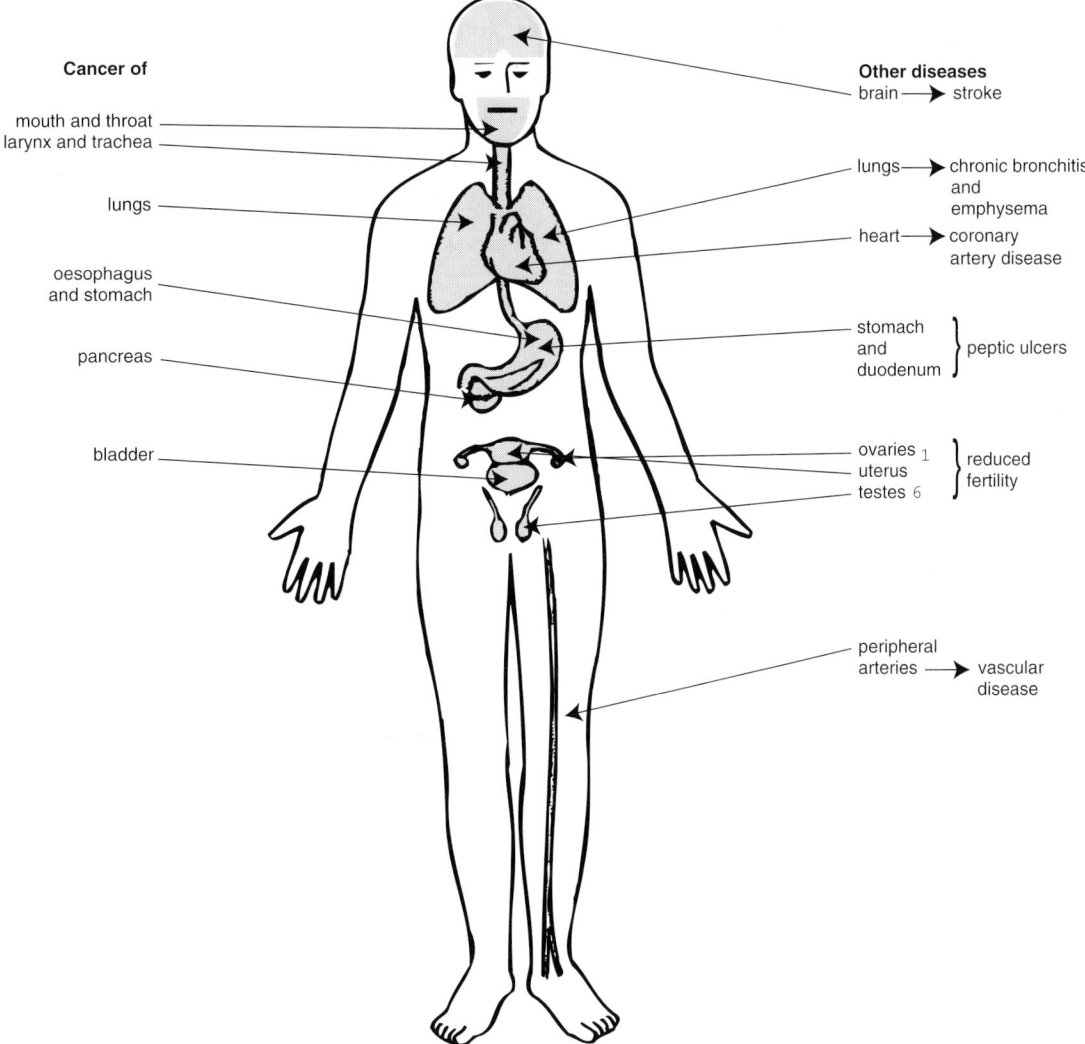

Fig. 18.1 *Possible serious adverse effects of nicotine smoking*

• These motivated patients will require educational and behavioural strategies to help them cope with quitting. Ongoing support by their GP is very important.
• Organise joining a support group.
• Arrange follow-up (very important), at least monthly, especially during first 3 months.
• *Going 'cold turkey'* (stopping completely) is preferable but before making the final break it can be made easier by changing to a lighter brand, inhaling less, stubbing out earlier and reducing the number. Changing to cigars or pipes is best avoided.

Quitting tips (advice to patient)
• Make a definite date to stop (e.g. during a holiday).

After quitting
• Eat more fruit and vegetables (e.g. munch carrots, celery and dried fruit).
• Foods such as citrus fruit can reduce cravings.
• Chew low-calorie gum and suck lozenges.
• Increase your activity (e.g. take regular walks instead of watching TV).
• Avoid smoking situations and seek the company of non-smokers.

- Drink more water and avoid substituting alcohol for cigarettes.
- Be single-minded about not smoking—be determined and strong.
- Take up hobbies that make you forget smoking (e.g. water sports).
- Put aside the money you save and have a special treat. You deserve it!!

Withdrawal effects

The initial symptoms are restlessness, cravings, hunger, irritability, poor concentration, headache, tachycardia, insomnia, increased cough, tension, depression, tiredness and sweating. After about 10 days most of these effects subside but it takes about three months for a smoker to feel relatively comfortable with not smoking any more. Nicotine replacement therapy certainly helps patients cope.

Pharmacological treatment

Nicotine replacement therapy, which should be used in conjunction with an educational support program, has been proved to be effective and is available as chewing gum, inhaler or transdermal patches (the preferred method). Ideally the nicotine should not be used longer than 3 months.

Nicotine gum[3]

This is available as 2 mg and 4 mg.

- Low dependence (less than 10 cigarettes per day): use non-pharmacological methods rather than replacement
- Moderate dependence (10–14 cigarettes per day): 2 mg
- High dependence (> 15 per day): 4 mg initially, changing to 2 mg after 4–6 weeks.

Useful points

- Chew each piece slowly for about 30 minutes.
- Ensure all the nicotine is utilised.
- Chew at least 6 pieces per day, replacing at regular intervals (not more than 1 piece per hour)
- Use for 3 months, weaning off before the end of this period.

Transdermal nicotine[3]

This is available as 16-hour or 24-hour nicotine patches in three different strengths. The patients should stop smoking immediately on use.

Recommendations

- Moderate dependence: 14 mg patch; change to 7 mg patch after 4–6 weeks
- High dependence: 21 mg patch; change to 14 mg patch after 4–6 weeks

Apply to non-hairy, clean, dry section of skin on upper outer arm or upper chest and leave in place for 24 hours. Rotate sites with a 7-day gap for reuse of a specific site.

Contraindications

These are pregnancy and breast-feeding, children, severe myocardial ischaemia, arrhythmias or recent CVA.

Adverse reactions

- Gum: hiccoughs, orodental problems, jaw pain, gastrointestinal including exacerbation of peptic ulcer
- Patches: local reaction, sleep disturbances (use 16-hour patch for this)
- Both: nervousness, sweating, dry mouth, dyspepsia, abdominal cramps, angina and arrhythmias

Alcohol

Excessive drinking of alcohol can cause several clinical manifestations. Identification of the alcohol-affected person is complicated by the tendency of some to hide, underestimate or understate the extent of their intake.

In order to diagnose and classify alcohol-dependent people, the family doctor has to rely on a combination of parameters that include clinical symptoms and signs, available data on quantity consumed, clinical intuition, personal knowledge of the social habits of patients, and information (usually unsolicited) from relatives, friends or other health workers.

A checklist of pointers to the adverse effects of chronic alcohol abuse is presented in Table 18.1. In a study by the author the outstanding clinical problems are the psychogenic disorders (anxiety, depression and insomnia) and hypertension.[4] Susceptibility to work and domestic accidents were also significant findings.

The challenge to the family doctor is early recognition of the alcohol problem. This is achieved by developing a special interest in the problem and a knowledge of the early clinical and social

Table 18.1   *Checklist of pointers of alcohol abuse*

Psychosocial features
- concern about drinking by self, family or others
- heavy drinking—more than six glasses per day
- early morning drinking
- reaching for the bottle when stressed
- regular hotel patron
- skipping meals/poor diet
- cancelling appointments
- increased tolerance to alcohol
- alcohol-related accidents
- frequent drinking during working day
- marital problems
- behavioural problems in children
- driving offences
- criminal offences
- financial problems
- absenteeism from work / loss of job
- heavy smoking

Clinical features
- characteristic facies
- hand tremor
- alcohol foetor by day
- morning nausea and vomiting
- traumatic episodes
- dyspepsia—gastritis/ulcer
- obesity
- palpitations
- impotence
- insomnia/nightmares
- anxiety/depression
- hypertension
- hepatomegaly
- gout
- pancreatitis
- personal neglect, 'vagabond' look

pointers, and being ever alert to the tell-tale signs of alcohol dependence (refer to Chapter 106).

Hard addictive street drugs

There are several psychotropic substances that are used for their effects on mood and other mental functions. Many of the severe problems are due to withdrawal of the drug. Symptomatic behaviour common to the hard addictive drugs includes:

- rapid disappearance of clothing, personal belongings from home
- signs of unusual activity around hang-outs and other buildings
- loitering in hallways or in areas frequented by addicts
- spending unusual amounts of time in locked bathrooms
- inability to hold a job or stay in school
- rejection of old friends
- using the jargon of addicts

Newer drugs include 'crack', which is a cocaine base where the hydrochloride has mostly been removed, usually in a microwave oven. Crack can be inhaled or smoked. It is the crude form of methamphetamine, a derivative of amphetamine.

A summary of the effects of 'hard' street drugs is presented in Table 18.2.

Narcotic dependence

This section will focus on heroin dependence.

Typical profile of a heroin-dependent person[5]
- Male or female: 16–30 years.
- Family history: often severely disrupted, e.g. parental problems, early death, separation, divorce, alcohol or drug abuse, sexual abuse, mental illness, lack of affection.
- Personal history: low threshold for toleration, unpleasant emotions, poor academic record, failure to fulfil aims, poor self-esteem.
- First experiments with drugs are out of curiosity, and then regular use follows with loss of job, alienation from family, finally moving into a 'drug scene' type of lifestyle.

Methods of intake
1. Oral ingestion
2. Inhalation — intranasal
              — smoking
3. Parenteral — subcutaneous
              — intramuscular
              — intravenous

Withdrawal effects
These develop within 12 hours of ceasing regular usage. Maximum withdrawal symptoms usually occur between 36 and 72 hours.
- anxiety and panic
- irritability
- chills and shivering
- excessive sweating
- 'gooseflesh' (cold turkey)
- loss of appetite, nausea (possibly vomiting)
- lacrimation/rhinorrhoea
- tiredness/insomnia
- muscle aches and cramps
- abdominal colic
- diarrhoea

Table 18.2 *Illicit substance abuse: A summary of hallmarks*

Drug	Physical symptoms	Look for	Dangers
LSD	Severe hallucinations. Feelings of detachment. Incoherent speech. Cold hands and feet. Vomiting. Laughing and crying.	Cube sugar with discolouration in centre. Strong body odour. Small tube of liquid.	Suicidal tendencies. Unpredictable behaviour. Chronic exposure causes brain damage. LSD causes chromosomal breakdown.
Amphetamines	Aggressive or overactive behaviour. Giggling. Silliness. Euphoria. Rapid speech. Confused thinking. No appetite. Extreme fatigue. Dry mouth. Shakiness.	Jars of pills of varying colours. Chain smoking.	Death from overdose. Hallucinations. Methamphetamines sometimes cause temporary psychosis.
Barbiturates	Drowsiness. Stupor. Dullness. Slurred speech. Drunk appearance. Vomiting.	Pills of various colours.	Death from overdose or as a result of withdrawal. Addictions. Convulsions.
Narcotics (a) opiates, e.g. heroin	Stupor/drowsiness. Marks on body. Watery eyes. Loss of appetite. Bloodstain on shirt sleeve. Running nose.	Needle or hypodermic syringe. Cotton. Tourniquet—string. Rope, belt, burnt bottle, caps or spoons. Glassine envelopes.	Death from overdose. Mental deterioration. Destruction of brain and liver. Hepatitis. Embolisms.
(b) cocaine	Similar effects to amphetamines—muscle pains, irritability, paranoia, hyperactive, jerky movements.	Powder: in microwave ovens	Death from overdose— sudden death from arrhythmias. Seizures, mental disorders. Severe respiratory problems.
Phencyclidine (angel dust)	Lack of co-ordination. Feeling of increased physical strength. Hallucinations. Mood disorders.	White powder. Tablets— unbranded. Syringes. Smoked in conjunction with marijuana.	Suicidal tendencies. Death from overdose. Mental disorder. Self-injury.
Marijuana	Initial euphoria. Floating feeling. Sleepiness. Wandering mind. Enlarged eye pupils. Lack of co-ordination. Craving for sweets. Changes of appetite.	Strong odour of burnt leaves. Small seeds in pocket lining. Cigarette paper. Discoloured fingers.	Inducement to take stronger narcotics. Recent medical findings reveal that prolonged usage causes cerebral lesions.
Glue sniffing	Aggression and violence. Drunk appearance, slurred speech. Dreamy or blank expression.	Tubes of glue, glue smears. Large paper or plastic bags or handkerchiefs.	Lung/brain/liver damage. Death through suffocation or choking.

A secondary abstinence syndrome is identified[5] at 2 to 3 months and includes irritability, depression and insomnia.

Complications
Medical

• Acute heroin reaction: respiratory depression—may include fatal cardiopulmonary collapse. There is an alarming increase in opioid deaths (including methadone).

• Injection site: scarring, pigmentation, thrombosis, abscesses, ulceration (especially with barbiturates).
• Distal septic complications: septicaemia, infective endocarditis, lung abscess, osteomyelitis, ophthalmitis.
• Viral infections: hepatitis B, hepatitis C, HIV infection.
• Neurological complications: transverse myelitis, nerve trauma.
• Physical disability: malnutrition.

Table 18.3 *A street drug dictionary*

Amphetamines or uppers
- Benzedrine: roses, beanies, peaches
- Dexedrine: dexies, speed, hearts
- Methedrine: meth, crystals, white light
- Drinamyl: purple hearts, goof balls

Hallucinogens

LSD: acid, blue cheer, strawberry fields, barrels, sunshine, pentagons, purple haze, peace pills, blue light.
Cannabis (Indian hemp)
1. Hashish (the resin):   hash, resin
2. Marijuana (from leaves):   pot, tea, grass, hay, weed, locoweed, Mary Jane, rope, bong, jive, Acapulco gold.
      Cigarettes: reefers, sticks, muggles, joints
      Smoking pot: blow a stick, blast a joint, blow, get high, get stoned

Narcotics

Morphine: Morph, Miss Emma
Heroin: H, Big H, Big Harry, GOM (God's own medicine), crap, junk, dynamite (high-grade heroin),
      lemonade (low-grade heroin)
      Injection of dissolved powder: mainlining, blast, smack
      Inhalation of powder: sniffing
Cocaine: coke, snow, lady of the streets, nose candy, toot, snort, crack
H & C: speed balls

Miscellaneous

Barbiturates: devils, barbies, goof balls

Social

Alienation from family, loss of employment, loss of assets, criminal activity (theft, burglary, prostitution, drug trafficking).

Management

Management is complex because it includes the medical management not only of physical dependence and withdrawal but also of the individual complex social and emotional factors. The issue of HIV prevention also has to be addressed. Patients should be referred to a treatment clinic and then a shared care approach can be used. The treatments include cold turkey with pharmacological support, acupuncture, megadoses of vitamin C, methadone substitution and drug-free community education programs.

Methadone maintenance programs that include counselling techniques are widely used for heroin dependence. Acute toxicity requires injections of naloxone.

The natural history of the opiate dependence indicates that many patients do grow through their period of dependence and, irrespective of treatments provided, a high percentage become rehabilitated by their mid-thirties.

Cannabis (marijuana)

Cannabis is a drug that comes from a plant called *Cannabis sativa* or the Indian hemp plant.

It contains a chemical called tetrahydrocannabinol, which makes people get 'high'. It is commonly called marijuana, grass, pot, dope, hash or hashish. Other slang terms are Acapulco Gold, ganga, herb, J, jay, hay, joint, reefer, weed, locoweed, smoke, tea, stick, Mary Jane and Panama Red. Marijuana comes from the leaves, while hashish is the concentrated form of the resinous substances from the head of the female plant and can be very strong (it comes as a resin or oil). The drug is usually smoked as a leaf (marijuana) or a powder (hashish), or hashish oil is added to a cigarette and then smoked. The effects of taking cannabis depend on how much is taken, how it is taken, how often, whether it is used with other drugs and on the particular person. The effects vary from person to person. The effects of a small to moderate amount include:

- feeling of well-being and relaxation
- decreased inhibitions
- woozy, floating feeling
- lethargy and sleepiness
- talkativeness and laughing a lot
- red nose, gritty eyes and dry mouth
- unusual perception of sounds and colour
- nausea and dizziness
- loss of concentration
- looking 'spaced out' or drunk

- lack of co-ordination
- a new form called 'skunk' or 'mad weed' causes paranoia

The effects of smoking marijuana take up to 20 minutes to appear and usually last 2 to 3 hours and then drowsiness follows. The main problem is habitual use with the development of dependence, although dependence (addiction) is worse than originally believed.

Long-term use and addiction

The influence of 'pot' has a severe effect on the personality and drive of the users. They lose their energy, initiative and enterprise. They become bored, inert, apathetic and careless. A serious effect of smoking pot is loss of memory. Some serious problems include:

- crime
- lack of morality—scant respect for others and their property
- respiratory disease (more potent than nicotine for lung disease): causes COAD, laryngitis and rhinitis
- often prelude to taking hard drugs
- becoming psychotic (resembling schizophrenia): the drug appears to unmask an underlying psychosis

Withdrawal

Sudden withdrawal produces insomnia, night sweats, nausea, depression, myalgia, irritability and maybe anger and aggression.

Management

The best treatment is prevention. People should either not use it or limit it to experimentation. If it is used, people should be prepared to 'sleep it off' and not drive.

Anabolic steroids

The apparent positive effects of anabolic steroids include gains in muscular strength (in conjunction with diet and exercise) and quicker healing of muscle injuries. However the adverse effects, which are dependent on the dose and duration, are numerous.

Adverse effects in women are:

- masculination—male pattern beard growth
- suppression of ovarian function
- changes in mood and libido
- hair loss

In adult men, adverse effects are:

- feminisation: enlarged breasts, high-pitched voice

Table 18.4 *Prohibited classes of substances with examples International Olympic Committee Medical Commission 1998*

Classes	Examples
A. Stimulants	Amiphenazole, amphetamines, caffeine (above 12 μg/mL in urine), cocaine, ephedrine, mesocarb, terbutaline,* salmeterol,* salbutamol,* pseudoephedrine, phenylpropanolamine
B. Narcotics**	Diamorphine (heroin), methadone, morphine, pethidine, pentazocine
C. Anabolic agents	Methandienone, nandrolone, stanozolol, testosterone, oxandrolone, DHEA
D. Diuretics	Acetazolamide, frusemide, hydrochlorothiazide, triamterene, indapamide, spironolactone (and related substances)
E. Peptide and glycoprotein hormones and analogues	Growth hormone, corticotrophin, chorionic gonadotrophin, erythropoietin *Note*: masking agents such as probenecid are banned
Classes subject to certain restrictions	
A. Alcohol	Restricted in certain sports (refer to regulations)
B. Marijuana	Restricted in certain sports (refer to regulations)
C. Local anaesthetics	Most agents permissible except cocaine: route restricted to local or intra-articular injection
D. Corticosteroids	Route of administration restricted to topical inhalation, local or intra-articular injection
E. Beta-blockers	Restricted in certain sports

* permitted by inhaler only but with permission
** codeine, dextromethorphan, dextropropoxyphene, dihydrocodeine, diphenoxylate and pholcodeine are permitted

Table 18.5 *Guidelines for treatment of specific conditions*
International Olympic Committee Medical Code 1996

Asthma	Allowed	Salbutamol inhaler, salmeterol inhaler, terbutaline inhaler
	Banned	Sympathomimetic products, e.g. ephedrine, pseudoephedrine, isoprenaline, systemic beta-2 agonists
Cough	Allowed	All antibiotics, steam and menthol inhalations, cough mixtures containing antihistamines, pholcodine, dextromethorphan, dihydrocodeine
	Banned	Sympathomimetic products, e.g. ephedrine, phenylpropanolamine
Diarrhoea	Allowed	Diphenoxylate, loperamide, products containing electrolytes, e.g. Gastrolyte
	Banned	Products containing opioids, e.g. morphine
Hayfever	Allowed	Antihistamines, nasal sprays containing a corticosteroid or antihistamine, sodium cromoglycate preparations
	Banned	Products containing ephedrine, pseudoephedrine
Pain	Allowed	Aspirin, codeine, dihydrocodeine, ibuprofen, paracetamol, all NSAIDs
	Banned	Products containing opioids, e.g. morphine, or caffeine
Vomiting	Allowed	Domperidone, metoclopramide

- acne
- testicular atrophy and azoospermia
- libido changes
- hair loss

Severe effects with prolonged use include:

- liver function abnormalities including hepatoma
- tumours of kidneys, prostate
- heart disease

In prepubescent children there can be premature epiphyseal closure with short stature.

Drugs in sport

It is important for general practitioners to have a basic understanding of drugs that are banned and those that are permissible for elite sporting use. The guidelines formulated by the International Olympic Committee (IOC) Medical Commission are generally adopted by most major sporting organisations.[7] Tables 18.4 and 18.5 provide useful guidelines. The IOC's list of prohibited drugs is regularly revised. Banned classes of drugs include stimulants, narcotics, anabolic agents, diuretics and various hormones. Banned methods include blood doping (the administration of blood, red blood cells and related blood products) and pharmaceutical, chemical and physical manipulation (substances or methods that alter the integrity and validity of the urine testing).

Restricted drugs include alcohol, marijuana, local anaesthetics, corticosteroids and beta-blockers. Practitioners can check the guidelines and provide written notification to the relevant authority.

References

1. Kumer PJ, Clark ML. *Clinical medicine* (2nd edn). London: Bailliere Tindall, 1990, 733–740.
2. Holman CDJ. *The quantification of drug-caused morbidity and mortality in Australia.* Canberra: Commonwealth Department of Community Services and Health, 1988.
3. Mashford ML (chairman). *Cardiovascular drug guidelines* (2nd edn). VMPF Therapeutics Committee, 1995/6, 53–58.
4. Murtagh JE. Alcohol abuse in an Australian community. Aust Fam Physician, 1987; 16:20–25.
5. Jagoda J. *Drug dependence and narcotic abuse: Clinical consequences.* Course Handbook: Melbourne: Monash University of Community Medicine, 1987, 66–71.
6. Goldman L. *Handbook on alcohol and other drug problems for medical practitioners.* Canberra: Australian Government Publishing Service, 1991, 35.
7. International Olympic Committee. *List of prohibited classes of substances and prohibited methods.* Lausanne; IOC, 1996.

19

Anaemia

—

Anaemia is a label, not a specific diagnosis. Anaemia is defined as a haemoglobin (Hb) below the normal reference level for the age and sex of that individual. It is regarded as a masquerade because the problem can develop surreptitiously and the patient may present with many seemingly undifferentiated symptoms before the anaemia is detected. Once identified, a cause must be found.

Key facts and checkpoints

- In Australia, most people with anaemia will have iron deficiency ranging from up to 5% for children to 20% for menstruating females.[1]
- The remainder will mainly have anaemia of chronic disease.
- The incidence of haemoglobinopathy traits, especially thalassaemia, is increasing in multicultural Western societies.
- If a patient presents with precipitation or aggravation of myocardial ischaemia, heart failure or intermittent claudication, consider the possibility of anaemia.
- The serum ferritin, which is low in iron-deficiency anaemia, is probably the best test to monitor iron-deficiency anaemia as its level reflects the amount of stored iron.
- Normal reference values for peripheral blood are presented in Table 19.1.

Table 19.1 *Normal reference values for peripheral blood—adults*

	Male	Female
Haemoglobin g/L	130–180	115–165
Red cells × 10^{12}/L	4.5–6	4–5.5
PCV (haematocrit)	40–53	35–47
MCV (fL)	80–95 to 100	
Platelets × 10^9/L	150–400	
White cell count × 10^9/L	4–11	
Neutrophils	2.5–7.5	
Lymphocytes	< 4.5	
Monocytes	< 0.8	
Eosinophils	< 0.44	
Reticulocytes %	0.5–2	
ESR mm/hour	< 20	

Reproduced with permission from Dr M. Gribble[2]

Clinical features of anaemia

Patients with anaemia may be asymptomatic. When symptoms develop they are usually non-specific.

Symptoms
- tiredness/fatigue
- muscle weakness
- headache
- lack of concentration
- faintness/dizziness
- dyspnoea on exertion
- palpitations
- angina on effort
- intermittent claudication

Signs
Non-specific signs
- pallor
- tachycardia
- systolic flow murmur

If severe
- ankle oedema
- cardiac failure

Specific signs
- jaundice—haemolytic anaemia
- koilonychia (spoon-shaped nails)—iron deficiency anaemia

History

The history may indicate the nature of the problem:

- iron deficiency: inadequate diet, pregnancy, GIT loss, menorrhagia, NSAID and anticoagulant ingestion
- folate deficiency: inadequate diet especially with pregnancy and alcoholism, small bowel disease
- Vitamin B_{12} deficiency: previous gastric surgery, ileal disease or surgery, pernicious anaemia, selective diets, e.g. vegetarians, fad
- haemolysis: abrupt onset anaemia with mild jaundice

Classification of anaemia

The various types of anaemia are classified in terms of the red cell size—the mean corpuscular volume (MCV).

- microcytic — MCV $\leq$ 80 fL
- macrocytic — MCV $>$ 98 fL
- normocytic — MCV 80–98 fL

Note: Upper limit of MCV varies from 95–100 depending on age and laboratory.

Table 19.2 outlines a classification of some of the more common causes of anaemia encountered in general practice. There can be an interchange of disorders between the above groups, e.g. the anaemia of chronic disorders (chronic infection, inflammation and malignancy) can occasionally be microcytic as well as normocytic; the anaemia of hypothyroidism can be macrocytic in addition to the more likely normocytic; the anaemia of bone marrow disorder or infiltration can also be occasionally macrocytic.

Microcytic anaemia — MCV $\leq$ 80 fL

The main causes of microcytic anaemia are iron deficiency and haemoglobulinopathy, particularly thalassaemia. Consider lead poisoning.

Iron-deficiency anaemia

Iron deficiency is the most common cause of anaemia worldwide. It is the big cause of microcytic anaemia with the main differential diagnosis of microcytic anaemia being a haemoglobinopathy such as thalassaemia.

Key features

- microcytic anaemia
- serum ferritin low (NR: 20–200 µg/L)
- serum iron low
- increased transferrin
- reduced transferrin saturation
- response to iron therapy

Non-haematological effects of chronic iron deficiency

- angular stomatitis
- glossitis
- oesophageal webs
- atrophic gastritis
- brittle nails and koilonychia

Important causes[1]

Blood loss

- menorrhagia
- gastrointestinal bleeding, e.g. carcinoma, haemorrhoids, peptic ulcer, GORD, NSAID therapy
- frequent blood donations
- malignancy

Increased physiological requirements

- prematurity, infant growth
- adolescent growth
- pregnancy

Malabsorption

- coeliac disease
- postgastrectomy

Dietary

- inadequate intake
- special diets, e.g. fad, vegetarianism

Investigations

Investigations are based on the history and physical examination including the rectal examination. If GIT bleeding is suspected the faecal occult blood is not considered very valuable but appropriate investigations include gastroscopy and colonoscopy, small bowel biopsy and small bowel enema.

Table 19.2 *Selected causes and investigations of anaemia*

Causes/ classification	Primary diagnostic feature	Secondary investigations
Microcytic (MCV < 80 fL)		
Iron deficiency	s.Fe ↓; s.ferr ↓; transferrin ↑	Therapeutic trial of iron; GIT evaluation for blood loss
Haemoglobinopathy e.g. thalassaemia	s.Fe N; s.ferr N or ↑	Haemoglobin investigation
Sideroblastic anaemia (hereditary)	s.Fe N; s.ferr N or ↑	Bone marrow examination
Occasionally microcytic		
Anaemia of chronic disease (sometimes microcytic)	s.Fe ↓; s.ferr N or ↑; transferrin ↓	Specific for underlying disorder
Macrocytic (MCV > 98 fL)		
(a) With megaloblastic changes		
Vitamin B_{12} deficiency	s.B_{12} ↓; rc/Fol N or ↑	IF antibody assay; Schilling test
Folate deficiency	s.B_{12} N; rc.Fol ↓	Usually none
Cytotoxic drugs	Appropriate setting; s.B_{12}N; rc.Fol N	None
(b) Without megaloblastic changes		
Liver disease/alcoholism	Appropriate setting; uniform macrocytosis; s.B_{12}N; rc.Fol N	Liver function tests
Myelodysplastic disorders (including sideroblastic anaemia)	Specific peripheral blood findings; s.B_{12}N; rc.Fol N	Bone marrow examination
Normocytic (MCV 80–98 fL)		
Acute blood loss/occult	Isolated anaemia; Retic ↑	Dictated by clinical findings
Anaemia of chronic disease [1]	Appropriate setting; Retic ↓	s.Fe ↓ and s.ferr N or ↑
Haemolysis	Specific red cell changes; Retic ↑	s.Bil and s.LDH ↑; s.hapt ↓; specific tests for cause
Chronic renal disease	Isolated anaemia; Retic ↓	Renal function
Endocrine disorders	Appropriate setting; isolated anaemia; Retic ↓	Specific endocrine investigation

Abbreviations: MCV = mean corpuscular volume; s.Fe = serum iron; s. ferr = serum ferritin; s.B_{12} = serum vitamin B_{12}; rc.Fol = red cell folate; IF = intrinsic factor; Retic = reticulocyte count; s.Bil = serum bilirubin; s.LDH = serum lactate dehydrogenase; s.hapt = serum haptoglobin; N = normal; ↓ = reduced; ↑ = elevated
Source: Adapted from Anaemia, MIMS Disease Index,[1] with permission of MIMS Australia, a division of MediMedia Australia Pty Limited

Haemological investigations: Typical findings

- microcytic, hypochromic red cells
- anisocytosis (variation in size), poikilocytosis (shape)
- low serum iron
- raised iron-binding capacity
- serum ferritin low (the most useful index)

The state of the iron stores is assessed by considering the serum iron, the serum ferritin and the serum transferrin in combination. Typically, in iron deficiency, the serum iron and ferritin are low and the transferrin high, but the serum iron is also low in all infections—severe, mild and even subclinical—as well as in inflammatory states, malignancy and other chronic conditions. Serum ferritin estimations are spuriously raised in liver disease of all types, chronic inflammatory conditions and malignancy; and transferrin is normally raised in pregnancy. Since each of these estimations can be altered in conditions other than iron deficiency, all three quantities have to be considered together to establish the iron status.[2]

Treatment

- Correct the identified cause.
- Diet—iron-rich foods, vitamin C rich foods (see Table 19.3).
- Iron preparations
  — oral iron
  — parenteral iron is probably best reserved for special circumstances
  Response
  — Anaemia responds after about 2 weeks and is usually corrected after 2 months.[1]
  — Oral iron is continued for 3 to 6 months to replenish stores.

Table 19.3 *Optimal adult diet for iron deficiency*

Adults should limit milk intake to 500 mL a day while on iron tablets.

Avoid excess caffeine, fad diets and excess processed bread.

Eat ample iron-rich foods (especially protein).

Protein foods
- Meats—beef (especially), veal, pork, liver, poultry
- Fish and shellfish, e.g. oysters, sardines, tuna
- Seeds, e.g. sesame, pumpkin
- eggs, especially egg yolk

Fruits
- Dried fruit, e.g. prunes, figs, raisins, currents, peaches
- Juices, e.g. prune, blackberry
- Most fresh fruit

Vegetables
- Greens, e.g. spinach, silver beet, lettuce
- Dried peas and beans, e.g. kidney beans
- Pumpkin, sweet potatoes

Grains
- Iron-fortified breads and dry cereals
- Oatmeal cereal

For better iron absorption, add foods rich in vitamin C, e.g. citrus fruits, cantaloupe, brussel sprouts, broccoli, cauliflower.

— Monitor progress with regular serum ferritin.

— A serum ferritin > 50 μg/L generally indicates adequate stores

Failure of iron therapy

Consider:

— poor compliance

— continuing blood loss

— malabsorption, e.g. severe coeliac disease

— incorrect diagnosis, e.g. thalassaemia minor, chronic disease

— bone marrow infiltration

Thalassaemia

This inherited condition is seen mainly (although not exclusively) in people from the Mediterranean basin, the Middle East, north and central India and South-East Asia including south China. The heterozygous form is usually asymptomatic; patients show little if any anaemia and require no treatment. The condition is relatively common in people from these areas. The homozygous form is a very severe congenital anaemia

needing lifelong transfusional support, but is comparatively rare, even among the populations prone to thalassaemia.[2]

The key to the diagnosis of the heterozygous thalassaemia minor is significant microcytosis quite out of proportion to the normal Hb or slight anaemia, and confirmed by finding a raised Hb A2 on Hb electrophoresis. DNA screening analysis is becoming available. The importance of recognising the condition lies in distinguishing it from iron-deficiency anaemia, for iron does not help thalassaemics and is theoretically contraindicated. Even more importantly it lies in recognising the risk that, if both parents have thalassaemia minor, they run a one in four chance of having a baby with thalassaemia major in every pregnancy, with devastating consequences for both the affected child and the whole family.

Treatment of thalassaemia major is transfusion to a high normal Hb with packed cells plus desferrioxamine.

Haemoglobin E

This Hb variant is common throughout South-East Asia.[2] It has virtually no clinical effects in either the homozygous or heterozygous forms, but these people have microcytosis, which must be distinguished from iron deficiency; moreover, if the Hb E gene is combined with the thalassaemia gene, the child may have a lifelong anaemia almost as severe as thalassaemia major. Both genes are well established in the South-East Asian populations in Australia as well as in their own countries.

Macrocytic anaemia — MCV $>$ 98 fL
Alcohol and liver disease

Each individually, or in combination, leads to macrocytosis with or without anaemia. The importance of this finding lies in its often being the first indication of alcohol abuse, which can so frequently go unnoticed unless there is a firm index of suspicion. Chronic liver disease due to other causes may also be late in producing specific clinical symptoms.

Drug toxicity

Cytotoxic drugs, anticonvulsants in particular, and various others (see Table 19.4) may cause macrocytosis. It is of little clinical significance and does not need correction unless associated with anaemia or other cytopenia.

Table 19.4 *Drugs causing macrocytosis*[2]

Alcohol	
Cytotoxics/ immunosuppressants	Azathioprine Methotrexate 5.fluororacil
Antibiotics	Co-trimoxazole Pyrimethamine (incl. Fansidar and Maloprim) Zidovudine
Anticonvulsants	Phenytoin Primidone Phenobarbitone

Myelodysplastic syndromes

These conditions have been recognised under a variety of names, such as 'refractory anaemia' and 'preleukaemia', for a long time, but only relatively recently have they been grouped together. They are quite common in the elderly but may be seen in any age group (refer Table 19.2).

These conditions frequently present as a macrocytic anaemia with normal serum B$_{12}$ and red cell folate, and are unresponsive to these or any other haematinics; they are usually associated with progressive intractable neutropenia or thrombocytopenia or both, and progress slowly but relentlessly to be eventually fatal, terminating with infection, haemorrhage or, less often, acute leukaemia.

Vitamin B$_{12}$ deficiency (pernicious anaemia)

Although well recognised, this is a much less common cause of macrocytosis than the foregoing conditions. It is usually caused by lack of intrinsic factor due to autoimmune atrophic changes and by gastrectomy. Anaemia does not develop for about three years after total gastrectomy. B$_{12}$ deficiency may also be seen together with other deficiencies in some cases of malabsorption and Crohn's disease.

Vitamin B$_{12}$ is found only in foods of animal origin and consequently very strict vegetarians may eventually develop deficiency. The clinical features are anaemia (macrocytic), weight loss and neurological symptoms especially a polyneuropathy. The serum Vitamin B$_{12}$ is below the normal level.

Replacement therapy[1]

• Vitamin B$_{12}$ (1000 μg) IM injection; body stores (3–5 mg) are replenished after 10–15 injections given every 2 to 3 days.

• maintenance with 1000 μg injections every third month

Folic acid deficiency

The main cause is poor intake associated with old age, poverty and malnutrition, usually associated with alcoholism. It may be seen in malabsorption and regular medication with antiepileptic drugs such as phenytoin.[3] It is rarely, but very importantly, associated with pregnancy, when the demands of the developing foetus together with the needs of the mother outstrip the dietary intake—the so-called 'pernicious anaemia of pregnancy' which, if not recognised and treated immediately, can still be a fatal condition. Unlike Vitamin B$_{12}$, folic acid is not stored in the body to any significant degree and requirements have to be satisfied by the daily dietary intake.

Replacement therapy

Oral folate 5 mg/day, to replenish body stores (5–10 mg) in about four weeks.

Normocytic anaemia[2] (anaemias without change in the MCV)

Acute haemorrhage

This is the most common cause of normocytic anaemia and is usually due to haematemesis and/or melaena.

Chronic disease

Chronic inflammation. Intercellular iron transport within the marrow is suppressed in inflammation so that, despite normal iron stores, the developing red cells are deprived of iron and erythropoiesis is depressed. If the inflammation is shortlived, the fall in Hb is not noticeable but, if it continues, an anaemia may develop that responds only when the inflammation subsides.

Malignancy. Anaemia may develop for the same reasons that apply to chronic inflammation.

Renal failure

This is often associated with anaemia due to failure of erythropoietin secretion and is unresponsive to treatment, other than by alleviating the insufficiency or until erythropoietin is administered.

Haemolysis

Haemolytic anaemias are relatively infrequent. The more common of the congenital ones are hereditary spherocytosis and deficiencies of the red cell enzymes, pyruvate kinase and G_6PD, although most cases of G_6PD deficiency haemolyse only when the patient takes oxidant drugs such as sulphonamides or eats broad beans—'favism'.

Acquired haemolytic anaemias include those of the newborn due to maternal haemolytic blood group antibodies passing back through the placenta to the foetus, and adult anaemias due to drug toxicity or to acquired autoantibodies. About half of the latter are 'idiopathic' and half associated with non-Hodgkin's lymphomas, and the anaemia may be the presenting sign of lymphoma. Some of these antibodies are active only at cool temperatures—cold agglutinin disease; others act at body temperature and are the more potent cause of autoimmune haemolytic anaemia.

Bone marrow replacement

This may be due to foreign tissue such as carcinomatous metastases or fibrous tissue as in myelofibrosis; it may also be due to overgrowth by one or other normal elements of the bone marrow as in chronic myeloid leukaemia, chronic lymphocytic leukaemia and lymphoma as well as by acute leukaemic tissue. A leukoerythroblastic picture, in which immature red and white cells appear in the peripheral blood, is often seen when the marrow is replaced by foreign tissue.

Anaemia in children

Haemoglobin reference range:
- Infant   term (cord blood):   135–195 g/L
             3–6 months: 95–135 g/L
- Child   1 year: 105–135 g/L
             3–6 years: 105–140 g/L
             10–12 years: 115–145 g/L

Important causes of anaemia in childhood include iron-deficiency anaemia (quite common), thalassaemia major, sickle-cell anaemia and drug-induced haemolysis. Consider one of the haemoglobinopathies in children of Mediterranean, South-East Asian, Arabic or African–American descent, especially with family history, normal ferritin or anaemia resistant to iron therapy. Investigate with Hb electrophoresis.

Drugs that can cause haemolysis (the film will have reticulocytosis, spherocytosis and frag-

mented red cells) include some antibiotics, e.g. sulfamethoxazole, antimalarials and some anti-inflammatories.

Think of anaemia in adolescents, especially females with a rapid growth spurt at the menarche and a relatively poor diet.

Iron deficiency in children[4]

- Iron deficiency is present in up to 10–30% of children in high-risk groups.
- It is often subclinical and anaemia develops in relatively few.
- It can lead to reduced cognitive and psychomotor performance (even without anaemia).
- High-risk groups include those infants < 6 months who are premature and/or with low birth weight; toddlers 6–36 months with a diet high in cows milk and low in iron-containing foods; those exclusively breast-fed after 6 months; those with delayed introduction of solids; those with general poor food intake; and those with lack of Vitamin C in diet.
- Possible symptoms include irritability, lethargy, minor behavioural changes.

Prevention

- Introduce iron-containing solids early—at 4 to 5 months.
- Avoid cows milk in first 12 months.
- Avoid excessive cows milk up to 24 months.
- Use iron-fortified formulas and cereals.

Important sources of iron

Infant milk formulas, meat, especially red meat (also fish and chicken), green vegetables especially legumes, dried fruit, juices, fortified cereals.

Treatment

Treatment is mainly with ferrous gluconate (1 mL/kg of 300 mg/5 mL mixture). Continue for 3 months after Hb has normalised.

Practice tips

- Iron-deficiency anaemia is blood-loss anaemia until proved otherwise.
- Blood-loss anaemia is usually due to menorrhagia or gastrointestinal loss until proved otherwise.
- A therapeutic trial of iron (without investigations) is indefensible.

- Intramuscular injections of iron can tattoo so use with care: an IM iron dose is not 'stronger' than an oral iron dose.

Haemochromatosis

This is a condition in which the total body iron is increased to 20–60 g (normal 4 g). The excess iron is deposited in and damages several organs.
- liver → cirrhosis (one-third develop a hepatoma)
- pancreas → 'bronze' diabetes
- skin → bronze or leaden grey colour
- heart → restrictive cardiomyopathy
- pituitary → hypogonadism: impotence etc.
- joints → arthralgia (esp. hands); chondro-calcinosis

It may be primary (hereditary—autosomal recessive) or secondary (e.g. chronic haemolysis,↑ dietary iron, multiple transfusions).

Symptoms: (maybe) extreme lethargy, polyuria & poly-dipsia, arthralgia, loss of libido

Signs: (look for) hepatomegaly, very tanned skin, cardiac arrhythmias

Diagnosis: *Iron studies*
increased serum transferrin saturation
increased serum ferritin > 1000 µg/L
CT or MRI—↑ iron deposition in liver
liver biopsy (if LFT enzymes abnormal)
genetic studies: HFE gene—a C282 Y mutation
Screen first degree relatives (s. ferritin & s. transferrin saturation)
Note: FBE & ESR are normal

Manage-ment: weekly venesection 500 mL (250 mg iron) until serum iron levels normal (may take at least 2 years) then every 3–4 months to keep s. ferritin (< 100 µg/L) and iron normal.
Life expectancy is normal if treated before cirrhosis or diabetes develops.
Normal diet

References

1. Van Der Weyden M. Anaemia. In: MIMS Disease Index (2nd edn). Sydney: IMS Publishing, 1996, 26–29.
2. Gribble M. Haematology. CHECK Unit 188. Melbourne: CHECK Programme, 1987, 3–2.
3. Kumer PJ, Clark ML. *Clinical medicine* (2nd edn). London: Bailliere Tindall, 1990, 297–307.
4. Efron D et al. *Paediatric handbook* (5th edn). Melbourne: Blackwell Science, 1996, 142–146.

20

Thyroid and other endocrine disorders

—

It would indeed be rash for a mere pathologist to venture forth on the uncharted sea of the endocrines, strewn as it is with the wrecks of shattered hypotheses, where even the most wary mariner may easily lose his way as he seeks to steer his bark amid the glandular temptations whose siren voices have proved the downfall of many who have gone before.

William Boyd (1885–1969)

Thyroid disorders can be a diagnostic trap in family practice and early diagnosis is a real challenge. A family practice of 2500 patients can expect one new case of thyroid disorder each year and ten 'cases' in the practice with a slight preponderance of hyperthyroid patients compared with hypothyroid patients.[1] The diagnosis of an overactive or underactive thyroid can be difficult as the early clinical deviations from normality can be subtle.

The clinical diagnosis of classical Graves' disease is usually obvious with the features of exophthalmos, hyperkinesis and a large goitre but if the eye and neck signs are absent it can be misdiagnosed as an anxiety state. Elderly patients may present with only cardiovascular signs such as atrial fibrillation and tachycardia or with unexplained weight loss.

The hypothyroid patient can be very difficult to diagnose in the early stages, especially if the patient is being seen frequently. Hypothyroidism often has a gradual onset with general symptoms such as constipation and lethargy, and the diagnosis is usually made late by which time the disorder is quite florid in manifestation.

If suspected, serum thyroid-stimulating hormone (TSH) should be requested.

Other endocrine disorders are relatively uncommon and therefore difficult to diagnose in

the early stages of development. Certain symptoms (Table 20.1) alert one to the possibility of an endocrine disorder.

Tests for thyroid disorders

Thyroid function tests

Advances in technology have allowed the biochemical assessment of thyroid function to change dramatically in recent years with the introduction of the serum free thyroxine (T_4) and the monoclonal TSH assays. With the highly sensitive TSH assays it is now possible to distinguish suppressed TSH levels (as in hyperthyroidism) from low but normal levels of TSH in the euthyroid state. However, the new assays are not foolproof and require interpretation in the context of the clinical picture. The serum TSH is the most sensitive index of thyroid function and is the preferred test for suspected thyroid dysfunction.

Serum tri-iodothyronine (T_3) measurement and serum free thyroxine (T_4) can be useful in suspected T_3 toxicosis where serum T_4 may be normal, and for monitoring patients with treated thyroid dysfunction.

The relative values are summarised in Table 20.2.

Thyroid autoantibodies

Raised autoantibodies (antimicrosomal or antithyroid peroxidase) are suggestive of Hashimoto's disease (autoimmune thyroiditis).

Fine needle aspiration

This is the single most cost-effective investigation in the diagnosis of thyroid nodules. It is the best

Table 20.1 *Symptoms related to the endocrine system*

Psychogenic changes
- depression
- anxiety
- psychosis

Constitutional symptoms
- tiredness, lethargy
- weakness

Sexual dysfunction
- menstrual dysfunction, e.g. amenorrhoea
- loss of libido
- loss of pubic hair
- hirsutism

Diabetogenic symptoms
- polyuria/polydipsia

Glycaemia fluctuations
- hypoglycaemia
- hyperglycaemia

Weight changes
- weight loss
- weight gain

Cardiac changes
- heart rate disturbances
- myocardial ischaemia

Skeletal changes
- osteoporosis
- bone pain

Muscle changes

Skin changes
- pigmentation
- vitiligo
- coarse dry skin
- striae

Blood pressure fluctuations
- postural hypotension
- hypertension

Gastrointestinal
- anorexia
- nausea
- constipation
- diarrhoea

Tongue enlargement
- hypothyroidism, myxoedema, acromegaly

way to assess a nodule for malignancy. Care needs to be taken in the interpretation of the cytology results in conjunction with an experienced cytologist/pathologist.

Thyroid isotope scan

The scan may help in the differential diagnosis of thyroid nodules. A functioning nodule is said to be less likely to be malignant than a non-functioning nodule (cyst, colloid nodule, haemorrhage and carcinoma are not functioning).

Thyroid ultrasound

A thyroid ultrasound is usually more sensitive in the detection of thyroid nodules. A multinodular goitre may be diagnosed on ultrasound while the clinical impression may be that of a solitary nodule (the other nodules not being palpable clinically). A multinodular goitre is said to be less likely to be malignant than a solitary thyroid nodule. An ultrasound allows for follow-up of thyroid nodule(s) to note if there are any changes in size over a period of time and to then discuss appropriate intervention with the patient. It can also differentiate a solid from a cystic mass.

High resolution ultrasound is better than CT in assessing glandular texture.

CT scan

CT scan of the thyroid may be used particularly to determine if there is significant compression in the neck from a large multinodular goitre with retrosternal extension. Again follow-up CT scans may allow one to determine the progression or otherwise of such a goitre.

Table 20.2 *Summary of thyroid function tests*

	TSH thyroid-stimulating hormone	T_4 free thyroxine	T_3 tri-iodothyronine
Hypothyroidism			
• primary	↑*	↓*	N or ↓ (not useful)
• secondary (pituitary dysfunction)	N or ↓	↓	N or ↓
Hyperthyroidism	↓*	↑	↑*
Sick euthyroid	N or ↓	N or ↓	N or ↓

Note: Results similar to hyperthyroidism can occur with acute psychiatric illness.
  * Main tests

Hypothyroidism (myxoedema)

Hypothyroidism, which is relatively common, is more prevalent in elderly women (up to 5%).[2] The term *myxoedema* refers to the accumulation of mucopolysaccharide in subcutaneous tissues. The early changes are subtle and can be misdiagnosed, especially if only a single symptom is dominant.

Patients at risk include:

- previous Graves' disease
- autoimmune disorders, e.g. rheumatoid arthritis
- Down syndrome
- Turner's syndrome
- drug treatment: lithium, amiodarone
- previous thyroid surgery
- previous radioactive ablation of the thyroid

Clinical features

The main features are:

- constipation
- cold intolerance
- lethargy
- physical slowing
- mental slowing
- huskiness of voice
- puffiness of face and eyes
- pallor
- loss of hair

Physical examination

See Figure 20.1. The main signs are:

- sinus bradycardia
- delayed reflexes (normal muscular contraction, slow relaxation)
- coarse, dry and brittle hair
- dry, cool skin
- obesity
- goitre

Other diverse presentations of thyroid disorders are given in Table 20.3.

Hashimoto's disease (autoimmune thyroiditis)

Hashimoto's disease, which is an autoimmune thyroiditis, is the commonest cause of bilateral non-thyrotoxic goitre in Australia. Features are:

- bilateral goitre
- classically described as firm and rubbery
- patients may be hypothyroid or euthyroid

Diagnosis is confirmed by a strongly positive antithyroid microsomal antibody titre and/or fine needle aspiration cytology.[3]

Hashimoto's disease may present as postpartum hypothyroidism. The hypothyroidism may resolve in 6–12 months or may be permanent.[3]

Laboratory diagnosis of hypothyroidism

Thyroid function tests (Table 20.2).

T_4—subnormal
TSH—elevated

If T_4 low and TSH low or normal, consider pituitary dysfunction (secondary hypothyroidism) or sick euthyroid syndrome.

Other abnormal tests

- serum cholesterol elevated
- anaemia—usually normocytic
  —may be macrocytic
- ECG—sinus bradycardia, low voltage, flat T waves

Management principles

Confirm the diagnosis; provide appropriate patient education; and refer the patient where appropriate.

Exclude co-existing hypoadrenalism and ischaemic heart disease before T_4 replacement.

Note: Treatment as primary hypothyroidism when hypopituitarism is the cause may precipitate adrenal crisis.

Thyroid medication

Thyroxine 100–150 µg daily (once daily)

Note: Start with low doses (25–50 µg daily) in elderly and ischaemic heart disease.
Avoid overdosage.

Monitor TSH levels monthly at first. As euthyroidism is achieved, monitoring may be less frequent, e.g. 2–3 months. When stable on optimum dose of T_4, monitor every 2–3 years.

Special treatment considerations

- *Ischaemic heart disease*
  Rapid thyroxine replacement can precipitate myocardial infarction, especially in the elderly.
- *Pregnancy and postpartum*
  Continue thyroxine during pregnancy; watch for hypothyroidism (an increased dose of T_4 may be required).
- *Elective surgery*
  If euthyroid—can stop thyroxine for one week.
  If subthyroid—defer surgery until euthyroid.
- *Myxoedema coma*
  Urgent hospitalisation under specialist care is required.
  Intensive treatment is required, which may involve parenteral T_4 or T_3.

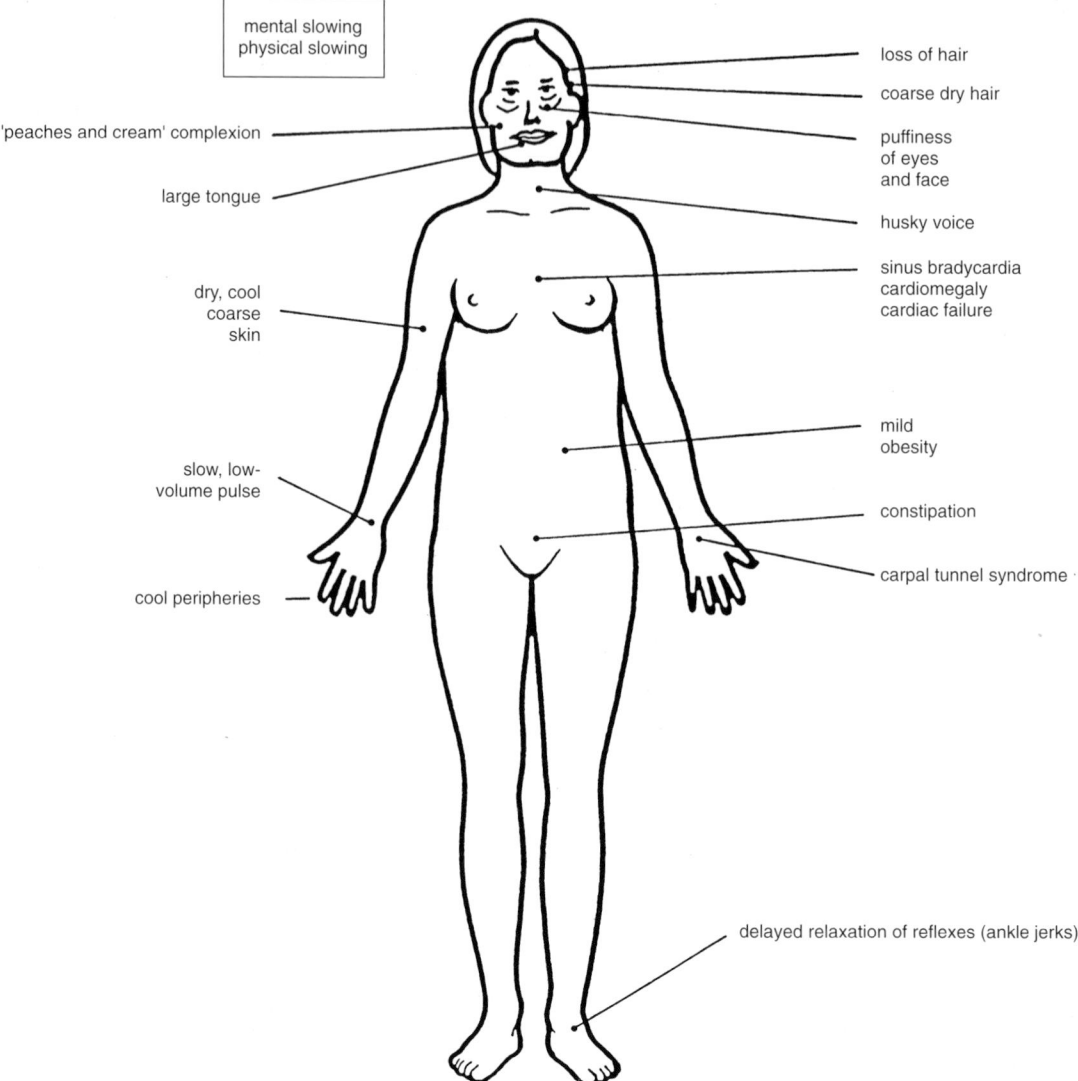

mental slowing
physical slowing

loss of hair

coarse dry hair

'peaches and cream' complexion

puffiness
of eyes
and face

large tongue

husky voice

dry, cool
coarse
skin

sinus bradycardia
cardiomegaly
cardiac failure

slow, low-
volume pulse

mild
obesity

constipation

cool peripheries

carpal tunnel syndrome

delayed relaxation of reflexes (ankle jerks)

Fig. 20.1 *Clinical features of hypothyroidism*

Neonatal hypothyroidism

Misdiagnosing this serious condition leads to failure to thrive, retarded growth and poor school performance. If untreated it leads to permanent intellectual damage (cretinism). The clinical features of the newborn include coarse features, dry skin, supra-orbital oedema, jaundice, harsh cry, slow feeding and umbilical hernia. It is detected by routine heel prick blood testing. Thyroxine replacement should be started as soon as possible, preferably before 14 days of age.

When to refer[2]

- Doubt about diagnosis, diagnostic tests or optimum replacement dosage
- Apparent secondary hypothyroidism, severe illness and associated ischaemic heart disease
- Concurrent autoimmune disease
- Hypothyroidism with goitre, postpartum and in the neonate
- Myxoedema coma

Table 20.3 *Various diverse presentations of thyroid disorders[2]*

	Hypothyroidism	Hyperthyroidism
General	Lethargy, tiredness Dry skin Husky voice	Weakness Sweaty skin, especially hands
Psychiatric	Depression Dementia Psychosis (myxoedema madness)	Anxiety/irritability Hyperkinesis Psychosis
Musculoskeletal	Myofibrositis Myalgia Joint effusions	Muscle weakness Proximal myopathy
Skin	Dry cool skin Vitiligo	Warm, thin, soft, moist skin Vitiligo Pretibial myxoedema
Cardiovascular	Ischaemia Cardiomegaly Pericardial effusion Bradycardia Hyperlipidaemia	Tachycardia Atrial fibrillation Heart failure Systolic hypertension
Endocrine	Galactorrhoea Goitre Infertility	Goitre Gynaecomastia
Gynaecological	Menstrual irregularity Menorrhagia (mainly) Oligomenorrhea	Oligomenorrhea
Neurological	Neuropathy Nerve entrapment e.g. carpal tunnel Ataxia	Periodic paralysis Tremor
Haematological	Anaemia	–
Emergency	Myxoedema coma Postanaesthetic hypoventilation	Thyroid crisis
Other	Reduced libido Weight gain Cold intolerance	Reduced libido Eye signs Fever (uncommon) Premature grey hair Weight loss

Hyperthyroidism

Hyperthyroidism (thyrotoxicosis) is also relatively common and may affect up to 2% of women, who are affected 4 to 5 times more often than men.

Causes of thyrotoxicosis[4,5]
- Graves' disease (typical symptoms with a diffuse goitre and eye signs)
- autonomous functioning nodules
- subacute thyroiditis (de Quervain's thyroiditis)—viral origin
- excessive intake of thyroid hormones—thyrotoxicosis factitia

Important notes
- The classic symptoms may be lacking in elderly patients who may have only cardiovascular manifestations, e.g. unexplained heart failure or cardiac arrhythmias.
- Care has to be taken not to dismiss hyperthyroidism as severe anxiety.

Clinical features
- loose bowel motions
- heat intolerance
- sweating of hands
- muscle weakness
- weight loss despite normal or increased appetite

- emotional lability, especially anxiety
- palpitations

Physical examination

See Figure 20.2. Signs are:
- agitated restless patient
- warm and sweaty hands
- fine tremor
- goitre
- proximal myopathy

Eye signs
- lid retraction (small area of sclera seen above iris)
- lid lag
- exophthalmos
- ophthalmoplegia

Investigations
- T_4 (and T_3) elevated
- TSH suppressed
- radioisotope scan

The isotope scan enables a diagnosis of Graves' disease to be made when the scan shows uniform increased uptake. Increased irregular uptake would suggest a toxic multinodular goitre, while there is poor or no uptake with de Quervain's thyroiditis and thyrotoxicosis factitia.

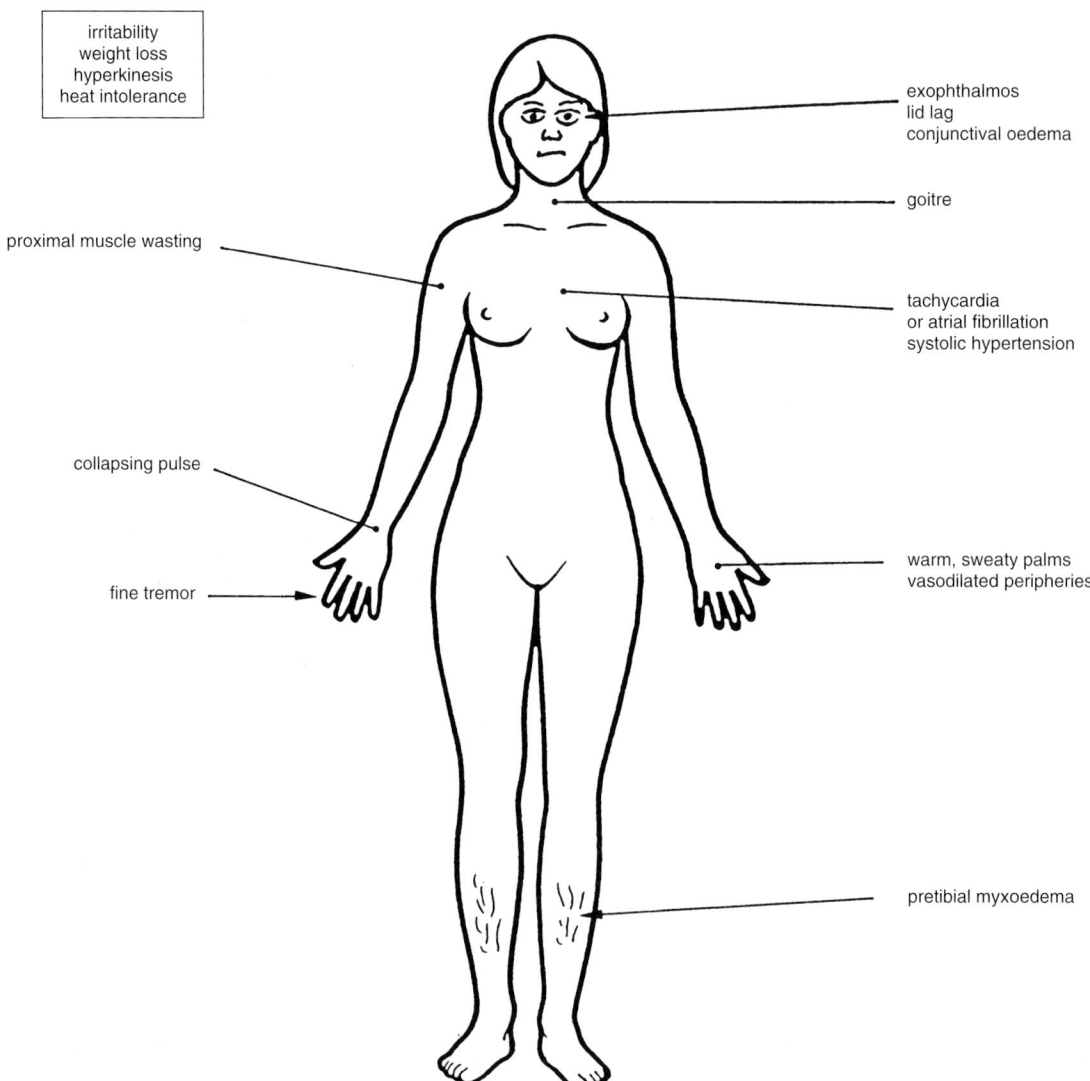

irritability
weight loss
hyperkinesis
heat intolerance

exophthalmos
lid lag
conjunctival oedema

goitre

proximal muscle wasting

tachycardia
or atrial fibrillation
systolic hypertension

collapsing pulse

warm, sweaty palms
vasodilated peripheries

fine tremor

pretibial myxoedema

Fig. 20.2 *Clinical features of hyperthyroidism*

Management principles
- Establish the precise cause before initiating treatment.
- Educate patients and emphasise the possibility of development of recurrent hyperthyroidism or hypothyroidism and the need for lifelong monitoring.

Treatment modalities[5,6]
- radioactive iodine therapy (I_{131})
- thionamide antithyroid drugs (initial doses)
  — carbimazole 10–45 mg (o) daily
  — propylthiouracil 200–600 mg (o) daily
- adjunctive drugs
  — beta-blockers (for symptoms in acute florid phase)
  — lithium carbonate (rarely used when there is intolerance to thionamides)
  — Lugol's iodine: mainly used prior to surgery
- surgery
  — subtotal thyroidectomy
                  or
  — total thyroidectomy

Treatment of Graves' disease
There is no ideal treatment, and selection of antithyroid drugs, radioiodine or surgery depends on many factors including age, size of goitre, social and economic factors and complications of treatment.

Guidelines[4,5]
- Younger patients with small goitres and mild case—18-month course antithyroid drugs.
- Older patients with small goitres—as above or radioiodine (when euthyroid).
- Large goitres or moderate to severe cases—antithyroid drugs until euthyroid, then surgery.
- In Australia (as in the USA) I_{131} is being increasingly used.

Treatment of autonomous functioning nodules
Control hyperthyroidism with antithyroid drugs, then surgery or I_{131}. Long-term remissions on antithyroid drugs in a toxic nodular goitre are rare.

Treatment of subacute thyroiditis[6]
Hyperthyroidism is usually transient and follows a surge of thyroxine after a viral-type illness. Symptoms include pain and/or tenderness over the goitre (especially on swallowing) and fever. In the acute phase treatment is based on rest, analgesics (aspirin 600 mg (o) 4–6 hourly) and soft foods. Rarely, when pain is severe, corticosteroids may be used. Antithyroid drugs are not indicated but beta-blockers can be used to control symptoms.

Thyroid crisis
Clinical features are marked anxiety, weakness, hyperpyrexia, tachycardia (> 150 per minute), heart failure and arrhythmias. It is usually precipitated by surgery or an infection in an undiagnosed patient.

It requires urgent intensive hospital management with antithyroid drugs; IV saline infusion, IV corticosteroids, anti-heart failure and anti-arrhythmia therapy.

When to refer[4]
- Doubt about the diagnosis
- Severe hyperthyroidism, especially if there is coexisting thyrocardiac disease
- Pregnant patients with hyperthyroidism
- Progression of exophthalmos

Thyroid carcinoma
The main presentations are a painless nodule, a hard nodule in an enlarged gland or lymphadenopathy with thyroid enlargement. Papillary carcinoma is the most common malignancy. Although rare compared with non-malignant lesions (such as colloid nodules, cysts, haemorrhage and benign adenomas), it is important not to miss carcinoma because of the very high cure rate with treatment. This involves total thyroidectomy, ablative I_{131} treatment, thyroxine replacement and follow-up with serum thyroglobulin measurements and thallium scanning. Fine needle aspiration is the investigation of choice.

Adrenal cortex disorders
It is worth keeping in mind the uncommon disorders of the adrenal cortex, which can also be difficult to diagnose in the early stages, namely:
- chronic adrenal insufficiency (Addison's disease)—deficiency of cortisol and aldosterone
- Cushing's syndrome—cortisol excess
- primary hyperaldosteronism (refer Chapter 111)

Addison's disease

Clinical features
- lethargy/excessive fatigue
- anorexia and nausea
- diarrhoea/abdominal pain
- weight loss
- dizziness/funny turns
  — hypoglycaemia (rare)
  — postural hypotension (common)
- hyperpigmentation, especially mucous membranes of mouth and hard palate.

If Addison's disease remains undiagnosed, wasting leading to death may occur. Severe dehydration can be a feature.

Diagnosis
- elevated serum potassium, low serum sodium
- low plasma cortisol (fails to respond to synthetic ACTH)

Addisonian crisis

An Addisonian crisis develops because of an inability to increase cortisol in response to stress, which may include intercurrent infection, surgery or trauma.

Clinical features
- nausea and vomiting
- acute abdominal pain
- severe hypotension progressing to shock
- weakness, drowsiness progressing to coma

Urgent management
- establish IV line with IV fluids
- hydrocortisone sodium succinate 200 mg IV
- arrange urgent hospital admission

Cushing's syndrome

The four main causes are:
- iatrogenic—chronic corticosteroid administration
- pituitary ACTH excess
- adrenal tumour
- ectopic ACTH or (rarely) corticotrophin-releasing hormone (CRH) from non-endocrine tumours, e.g. oat cell carcinoma of lung

The clinical features are caused by the effects of excess cortisol and/or adrenal androgens.

Clinical features
- proximal muscle wasting and weakness
- central obesity, buffalo hump
- Cushing's facies: plethora, moon face, acne

- hirsutism
- abdominal striae
- thin skin, easy bruising
- hypertension
- hyperglycaemia
- menstrual changes, e.g. amenorrhoea
- osteoporosis
- psychiatric changes, especially depression

Diagnosis (apart from iatrogenic cause)
- cortisol excess (plasma or 24-hour urinary cortisol)
- dexamethasone suppression test
- serum ACTH
- radiological localisation
  — MRI for ACTH-producing pituitary tumours
  — CT scanning for adrenal tumours

Other endocrine disorders

Acromegaly

Symptoms suggestive of acromegaly include:
- excessive growth of hands (increased glove size)
- excessive growth of tissues, e.g. nose, lips, face
- excessive growth of feet (increased shoe size)
- increased size of jaw and tongue
- general: weakness, sweating, headaches
- sexual changes including amenorrhoea and loss of libido
- disruptive snoring (most have sleep apnoea)

Diagnosis[6]
- plasma growth hormone excess
- elevated insulin-like growth factor 1
- CT scanning pituitary
consider associated diabetes

Hypopituitarism

This rare disorder should be considered with:
- a history of postpartum haemorrhage
- symptoms of hypothyroidism
- symptoms of adrenal insufficiency
- symptoms suggestive of a pituitary tumour

Primary hyperparathyroidism

Hyperparathyroidism is caused by an excessive secretion of parathyroid hormone and is usually due to a parathyroid adenoma. The classic clinical features of hyperparathyroidism are due to the effects of hypercalcaemia. Rarely, a parathyroid crisis in a misdiagnosed patient may result in death from severe hypercalcaemia.

Clinical features

- Renal   — polyuria with nocturia (and thirst)
                            — renal colic
- Musculoskeletal   — aching legs, especially shins
                            — muscle aching
                            — muscle weakness
                            — back pain
- Gastrointestinal   — anorexia, nausea
                            — constipation
- Psychiatric   — depression
                            — personality changes

> *Classic mnemonic*: bones, moans, stones, abdominal groans

Diagnosis

- exclusion of other causes of hypercalcaemia
- serum parathyroid hormone (elevated)

Hypercalcaemia

Suspect hypercalcaemia if there is weakness, tiredness, malaise, anorexia, nausea or vomiting, constipation, thirst, polyuria, drowsiness, dizziness, muscle aches and pains, visual disturbances. Measure urea and electrolytes (especially calcium), creatinine, albumin.

Primary hyperparathyroidism and neoplasia especially lung, breast (with metastases to bone) account for over 90% of cases.

Diabetes insipidus

Impaired secretion of vasopressin (antidiuretic hormone) from the posterior pituitary leads to polyuria, nocturia and compensatory polydipsia resulting in the passage of 3 to 20 L of dilute urine per day. There are several causes of diabetes insipidus (DI), the commonest being postoperative (hypothalamic-pituitary) which is usually transient only. Other causes of cranial DI include congenital tumours, infections and infiltrations. In nephrogenic DI the renal tubules are insensitive to vasopressin. Differential diagnoses include compulsive (psychogenic) water drinking and the syndrome of secretion of inappropriate antidiuretic hormone (SIADH), which is caused by cancer (e.g. lung, lymphomas, kidney, pancreas), pulmonary disorders, various intracranial lesions and drugs such as carbamezepine and many antipsychotic agents.

The treatment of DI is desmopressin, usually given twice daily intranasally.

Hypoparathyroidism

Hypoparathyroidism, which is uncommon, causes hypocalcaemia. Causes include congenital deficiency (di George's syndrome), idiopathic (autoimmune) hypoparathyroidism and postoperative thyroidectomy and parathyroidectomy. The main features are neuromuscular hyperexcitability, tetany and neuropsychiatric manifestations.

Two important signs of hypocalcaemia are Trousseau's sign and Chvostek's sign.

Treatment involves careful adjustments in dosage of calcitriol and calcium to correct hypocalcaemia and avoid hypercalcaemia (the latter may lead to renal impairment).

References

1. Fry J. *Common diseases* (4th edn). Lancaster: MTP Press Limited, 1985, 358–361.
2. Stockigt J, Topliss DJ. Hypothyroidism. In: MIMS Disease Index (2nd edn). Sydney: IMS Publishing, 1996, 267–269.
3. Yuen R. Common thyroid conditions. Current therapeutics, 1992; 10:23–29.
4. Yuen R. *Endocrinology 1*. RACGP: CHECK Programme, unit 243,1992, 2–5.
5. Hales I. Thyrotoxicosis. In: MIMS Disease Index. Sydney: IMS Publishing, 1991–92, 541–543.
6. Moulds RFW. *Therapeutic guidelines: Endocrinology*. Melbourne: Therapeutic Guidelines Limited, 1997, 53–91.

21
Spinal dysfunction

—

The spine is an ordered series of bones running down your back. You sit on one end of it, sometimes too hard with ill effect, and your head sits on the other. Poor spine—what a load.

Anon, 19th century

Spinal or vertebral dysfunction can be regarded as a masquerade mainly because the importance of the spine as a source of various pain syndromes has not been emphasised in medical training. Practitioners whose training and treatment are focused almost totally on the spine may swing to the other extreme and some may attribute almost every clinical syndrome to dysfunction of spinal segments. The true picture lies somewhere in between.

The diagnosis is straightforward when the patient is able to give a history of a precipitating event such as lifting, twisting the neck or having a motor vehicle accident, and can then localise the pain to the midline of the neck or back. The diagnostic problem arises when the pain is located distally to its source, whether it is radicular (due to pressure on a nerve root) or referred pain. The problem applies particularly to pain in anterior structures of the body.

If a patient has pain anywhere it is possible that it could be spondylogenic and practitioners should always keep this in mind.

The various syndromes caused by spinal dysfunction will be presented in more detail under neck pain, thoracic back pain and lumbar back pain.

Cervical spinal dysfunction[1]

The cervical spine is the origin of many confusing clinical problems such as headache, migraine-like headache, arm pain, facial pain, periauricular pain, anterior chest pain and even visual dysfunction and dizziness. If the cervical spine is overlooked as a source of pain (such as in the head, shoulder, arm, upper chest—anterior and posterior—and around the ear or face) the cause of the symptoms will remain masked and mismanagement will follow.

Dysfunction of the cervical spine can cause many unusual symptoms such as headache and vertigo, a fact that is often not recognised. Despite teaching to the contrary from some lecturers, the cervical spine is a common cause of headache, especially dysfunction of the facet joints at the C1–2 and C2–3 levels. The afferent pathways from these levels share a common pathway in the brain stem as the trigeminal nerve, hence the tendency for pain to be referred to the head and the face (see p. 526).

Manipulation of the cervical spine can be a dramatically effective technique, but it should be used with care and never used in the presence of organic disease and vertebrobasilar insufficiency. It should, therefore, be given only by skilled therapists. Two groups at special risk from quadriplegia are those with rheumatoid arthritis of the neck and Down syndrome, because of the instability of the odontoid process.

Thoracic spinal dysfunction

The most common and difficult masquerades related to spinal dysfunction occur with disorders of the thoracic spine (and also the low cervical spine) which can cause vague aches and pains in the chest, including the anterior chest.

Pain in the thoracic spine with referral to various parts of the chest wall and upper abdomen is common in all ages and can closely mimic the symptoms of visceral disease such as angina pectoris and biliary colic. If a non-cardiac cause of chest pain is excluded then the possibility of referral from the thoracic spine should be considered in the differential diagnosis. People of all ages can experience thoracic problems and it is surprisingly common in young people, including children.

Pain of thoracic spinal origin may be referred anywhere to the chest wall, but the commonest sites are the scapular region, the paravertebral region 2–5 cm from midline and, anteriorly, over the costochondral region.

Thoracic pain of lower cervical origin[2]
The clinical association between injury to the lower cervical region and upper thoracic pain is well known, especially with 'whiplash' injuries. It should be noted that the C4 dermatome is in close proximity to the T2 dermatome.

The T2 dermatome appears to represent the cutaneous areas of the lower cervical segments, as the posterior primary rami of C5,6,7,8 and T1 innervate musculature and have no significant cutaneous innervation.

The pain from the lower cervical spine can also refer pain to the anterior chest, and mimic coronary ischaemic pain. The associated autonomic nervous system disturbance can cause considerable confusion in making the diagnosis.

The medical profession tends to have a blind spot about various pain syndromes in the chest, especially the anterior chest and upper abdomen, caused by the common problem of dysfunction of the thoracic spine. Doctors who gain this insight are amazed at how often they diagnose the cause that previously did not enter their 'programmed' medical minds.

Physical therapy to the spine can be dramatically effective when used appropriately. Unfortunately, many of us associate it with quackery. It is devastating for patients to create doubts in their minds about having a 'heart problem' or an 'anxiety neurosis' when the problem is spinal and it can be remedied simply (Chapter 34).

Lumbar spinal dysfunction
The association between lumbar dysfunction and pain syndromes is generally easier to correlate. The pain is usually located in the low back and referred to the buttocks or the backs of the lower limbs. Problems arise with referred pain to the pelvic area, groin and anterior aspects of the leg. Such patients may be diagnosed as suffering from inguinal or obturator hernial and nerve entrapment syndromes.

Typical examples of referral and radicular pain patterns from various segments of the spine are presented in Figure 21.1.

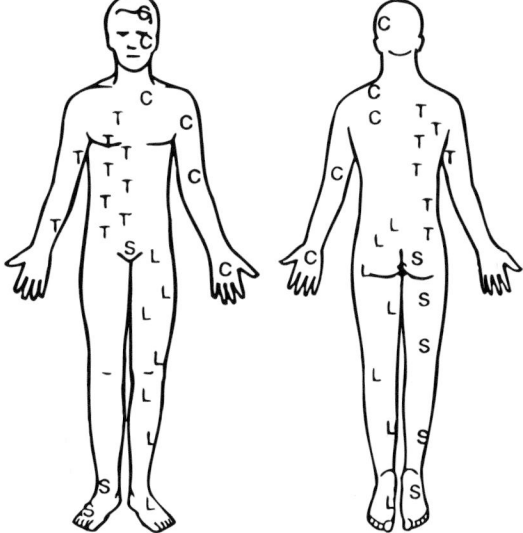

C = cervical; T = thoracic; L = lumbar; S = sacral

Fig 21.1 *Examples of referred and radicular pain patterns from the spine (one side shown for each segment)*

References
1. Murtagh J. *Cautionary tales*. Sydney: McGraw-Hill,1992, 36–130.
2. Kenna C, Murtagh J. *Back pain and spinal manipulation* (2nd edn). Oxford: Butterworth Heinemann, 1997, 213–218.

22

Urinary tract infection

—

Experience has taught them, as mine has me, that one must listen to reason and agree with Hippocrates, Galen, Avicenna and many others, ancient and modern, that there is no surer way to determine the temperaments and constitutions of people of either sex than to look at the urine.

Davach de La Riviere, 18th century
The Mirror of Urines

Urinary tract infection (UTI) is a common problem affecting all ages and accounts for approximately 1% of all attendances in general practice. It is very common in sexually active women but uncommon in men and children.

Organisms causing UTI in the community are usually sensitive to most of the commonly used antibiotics. The important decision to make is whether to proceed with further investigation of the urinary tract. The morbidity of urinary infections in both children and adults is well known but it is vital to recognise the potential for progressive renal damage, ending in chronic renal failure. The main task in the prevention of chronic pyelonephritis is the early identification of patients with additional factors, such as reflux or obstruction, which could lead to progressive renal damage.

Key facts and checkpoints

- Screening of asymptomatic women has shown that about 5% have bacterial UTI.[1]
- About 1% of neonates and 1–2% of schoolgirls have asymptomatic bacteriuria.[2]
- About one-third of women have been estimated to have symptoms suggestive of cystitis at some stage of their life.

- The vast majority of these women have anatomically normal renal tracts, are at no significant risk from the UTI and respond quickly to simple therapy. The prevalence of underlying abnormalities is estimated at around 4%.[3]
- UTIs are largely caused by organisms from the bowel that colonise the perineum and reach the bladder via the urethra. In many young women infections are precipitated by sexual intercourse. Ascending infection accounts for 93% of UTIs.
- Haematogenous infection can occur sometimes, especially with the immunocompromised patient.
- All males and females less than 5 years presenting with a UTI require investigation for an underlying abnormality of the urinary tract.
- In the presence of a normal urinary tract there is no evidence that UTI leads to progressive renal damage.

UTI as a masquerade

Urinary tract infection can be regarded as a masquerade when it presents with a constitutional problem or general symptoms, without symptoms suggestive of a urinary infection such as frequency, dysuria and loin pain. This applies particularly to infants and young children and the elderly but is not uncommon in adult women and in pregnancy. Acute UTI may occasionally present as acute abdominal pain.

In infants and children, presenting nonspecific symptoms include:

- fever
- failure to thrive
- vomiting
- abdominal pain
- diarrhoea

In the elderly:

- confusion
- behaviour disturbance
- fever of undetermined origin

Classification and clinical syndromes

Sterile pyuria

This is defined as the presence of pus cells but a sterile urine culture.[2] The common causes of sterile pyuria are:

- contamination of poorly collected urine specimens
- urinary infections being treated by antibiotics
- analgesic nephropathy
- staghorn calculi
- bladder tumours
- tuberculosis

Asymptomatic bacteriuria

This is defined as the presence of a significant growth of bacteria in the urine, which has not produced symptoms requiring consultation.[1] On close questioning many patients admit to mild urinary symptoms.

- This is common only in sexually active women, the elderly and those with urinary tract abnormalities. UTI can exist without any symptoms.[1]
- These patients are more likely to have a past history of symptomatic UTI or to develop symptoms in the future than subjects with sterile urine.[1]
- During pregnancy, asymptomatic bacteriuria leads to acute clinical UTI in up to 30% of women.

Symptomatic bacteriuria

This is defined as the presence of frequency, dysuria and loin pain alone or in combination, together with a significant growth of organisms on urine culture.[2]

The clinical differentiation between cystitis or lower UTI and renal or upper UTI cannot be made accurately on the basis of symptoms, except in those patients with well-defined loin pain and/or tenderness.

Acute cystitis (dysuria–frequency syndrome)[1]

- Inflammation of the bladder and/or urethra is associated with dysuria (pain or scalding with micturition) and/or urinary frequency.

- In severe cases, haematuria may be present, and the urine may have an offensive smell.
- Constitutional symptoms are minimal or absent.
- Other causes of dysuria and frequency include urethritis, prostatitis and vulvovaginitis, all of which can normally be distinguished clinically.

Acute pyelonephritis[1]

- Acute bacterial infection of the kidney produces loin pain and constitutional upset, with fever, rigor, nausea and sometimes vomiting.
- The symptoms of acute cystitis are often also present.
- The differential diagnosis includes causes of the acute abdomen such as appendicitis, cholecystitis and acute tubal or ovarian diseases. The presence of pyuria and absence of rebound tenderness are helpful in distinction.

The clinical manifestations of UTI are summarised in Figure 22.1.

Uncomplicated urinary tract infection

This is cystitis occurring in the uninstrumented non-pregnant female without structural or neurological abnormalities.

Urethral syndrome

The urethral syndrome (sometimes termed abacterial cystitis) is that where the patient presents with dysuria and frequency but does not show a positive urine culture.[3]

- 30–40% of adult women with urinary symptoms have this syndrome.[3]
- Many actually have bacterial cystitis but a negative culture.
- The organisms may be anaerobic or fastidious in their culture requirements.
- The organisms may include *Ureaplasma*, *Chlamydia* and viruses.
- The urine may have antiseptic contamination or residual antibiotic.
- The infection may be undergoing spontaneous resolution at the time of the culture.

Interstitial cystitis[3]

This is an uncommon but important cause of the urethral syndrome.

- The classical symptoms are frequency day and night and a dull suprapubic ache relieved briefly by bladder emptying.
- The feature is small haemorrhages on distension of the bladder.

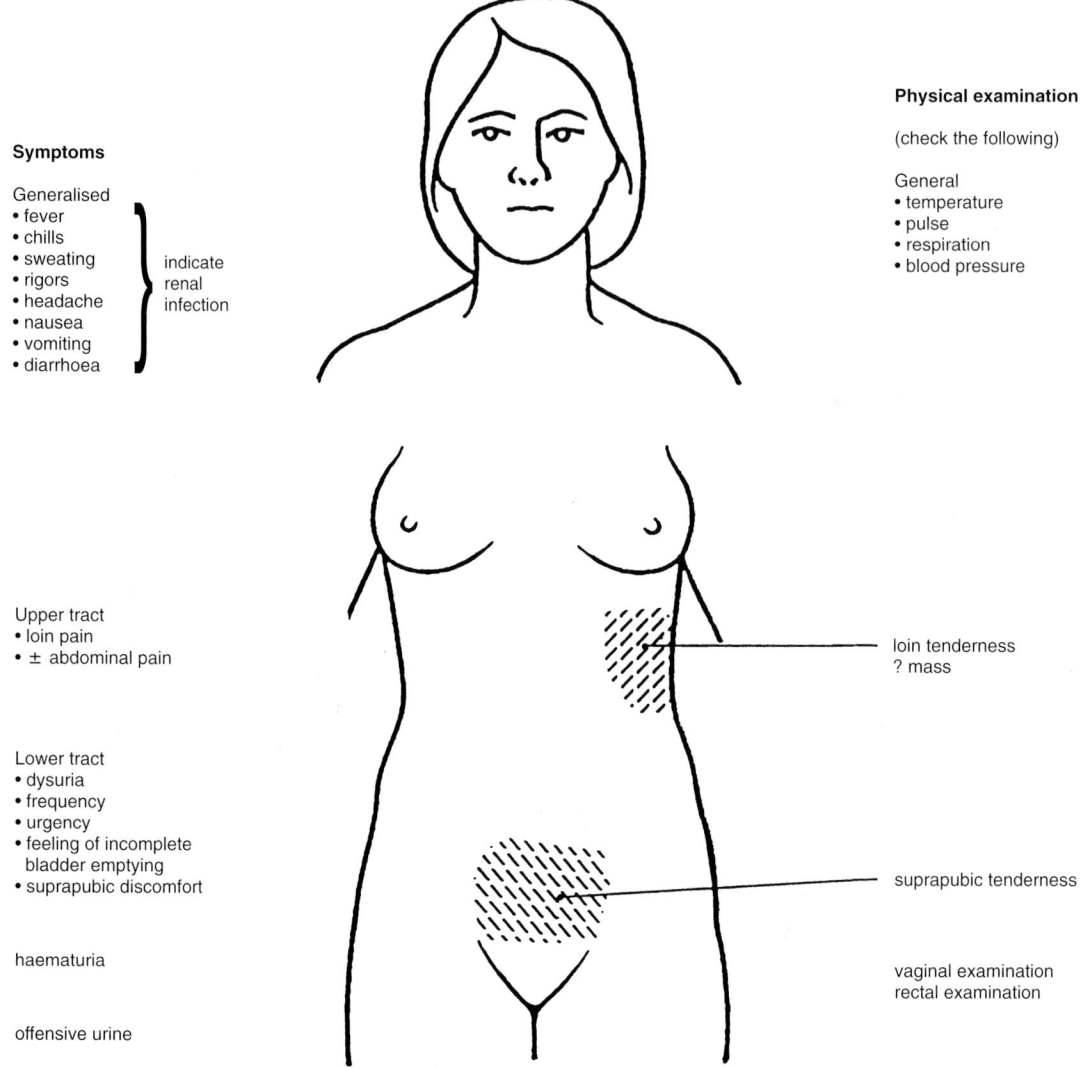

Symptoms

Generalised
• fever
• chills
• sweating
• rigors
• headache
• nausea
• vomiting
• diarrhoea
} indicate renal infection

Upper tract
• loin pain
• ± abdominal pain

Lower tract
• dysuria
• frequency
• urgency
• feeling of incomplete
  bladder emptying
• suprapubic discomfort

haematuria

offensive urine

Physical examination

(check the following)

General
• temperature
• pulse
• respiration
• blood pressure

loin tenderness
? mass

suprapubic tenderness

vaginal examination
rectal examination

Fig. 22.1 *Clinical manifestations of urinary tract infection*

Laboratory diagnosis

The laboratory diagnosis of UTI depends on careful collection, examination and culture of urine.

Collection of urine[1]

It is best to collect the first urine passed in the morning, when it is highly concentrated and any bacteria have been incubated in the bladder overnight. Preferably the urine should be taken to the laboratory immediately, but it can be stored for up to 24 hours at 4°C to prevent bacterial multiplication.

• *Midstream specimen of urine (MSU).* This is best collected from a full bladder, to allow at least 200 mL of urine to be passed before collection of the MSU. It is important that the urine flow is continuous, and the container is moved in and out of the stream collecting at least 20 mL.
  — In women, a tampon should first be inserted and the vulva washed with clean water (to avoid contamination with vaginal and vulval organisms). The labia are then held apart with the fingers to prevent contact with the urinary stream while the specimen is collected.

— In males, the foreskin (if present) is retracted and the glans washed with clean water.

- *Catheter specimen of urine (CSU).* In women who have difficulty with collecting an uncontaminated MSU (as is commonly the case in the elderly, the infirm and the grossly obese), a short open-ended catheter can be inserted and a specimen collected after 200 mL has flushed the catheter.

- *Suprapubic aspirate of urine (SPA).* This is an extremely reliable way to detect bacteriuria in neonates and in patients where UTI is suspected but cannot be confirmed because of low colony counts or contamination in an MSU. Under local anaesthetic, a needle (lumbar puncture needle in adults) is inserted into the very full bladder about 1 cm above the pubic symphysis, and 20 mL is collected by a syringe. Any organisms in an SPA specimen indicate UTI.

Dipstick testing

The reagents in dipstick testing are generally sensitive but have to be interpreted with care. 'Leucocyte esterase dipsticks' are useful in detecting pyuria and give a good guide to infection with a specificity of 94–98% (2–6% false positive) and 74–96% sensitivity (4–26% false negatives).[4] Positive nitrite dipsticks give a useful guide to the presence of bacteria. Unexplained haematuria detected by 'dipstick' analysis needs investigation.

Microscopic examination

The urine is examined under a microscope to detect pyuria (more than ten pus cells—WBCs—per high-powered field) but should be examined in a counting chamber to calculate the number of WBCs/mL of urine. In the counting chamber pyuria is > 8000 WBC/mL in phase contrast microscopy. Pyuria is a very sensitive sign of UTI. Vaginal squames and debris indicate contamination.

Culture of the urine

The nature and number of organisms present in the urine are the most useful indicators of UTI.[1]

- Most common are enteric organisms. *Escherichia coli* is responsible for about 90% of UTIs with other Gram-negative organisms (*Klebsiella* sp and *Proteus* sp) and Gram-positive cocci (*Streptococcus faecalis* and staphylococci) also occurring.

- Infections due to organisms other than *E.coli*, e.g. *Pseudomonas* sp, are suggestive of an underlying renal tract abnormality.

- If $> 10^5$ colony forming units (cfu) per mL of bacteria are present in an MSU, it is highly likely that the patient has a UTI.

- On the other hand, it is most important to realise that up to 30% of women with acute bacterial cystitis have less than 10^5 cfu/mL in the MSU. For this reason, it is reasonable to treat women with dysuria and frequency even if they have $<10^5$ cfu/mL of organisms in an MSU.

Management

- The indications for investigation of urinary tract infections are presented in Table 22.1.
- Appropriate antimicrobial therapy can be expected to cure 80–90% of uncomplicated UTIs.
- Optimal treatment includes:
  — high fluid intake
  — complete bladder emptying, especially at bedtime or after intercourse
  — urinary alkalinisation for severe dysuria

Table 22.1 *Investigation of urinary tract infections*

Investigations are indicated in:
- all children
- all males
- all women with:
  — acute pyelonephritis
  — recurrent infections
  — confirmed sterile pyuria
  — other features of renal disease

Basic investigations include:
- MSU—microscopy and culture (post-treatment)
- Renal function tests: plasma urea and creatinine
- Intravenous urogram (IVU) and/or ultrasound

Special considerations:
- In children: micturating cystogram
- In adult males: consider prostatic infection studies if IVU normal
- In severe pyelonephritis: ultrasound or IVU (urgent) to exclude obstruction
- In pregnant women: ultrasound to exclude obstruction

Acute uncomplicated cystitis

Advice to women (especially if recurrent attacks):

- Keep yourself rested.
- Drink a lot of fluid: 2–3 cups of water at first and then 1 cup every 30 minutes.

- Try to empty your bladder completely each time.
- Gently wash or wipe your bottom from front to back with soft, moist tissues after opening your bowels (for prevention in recurrent attacks).
- Use analgesics such as paracetamol for pain.
- Make the urine alkaline by using sodium citro-tartrate (4 g orally 6 hourly)—not if taking nitrofurantoin.

Antimicrobial regimen (for non-pregnant women)[5]
Multiple dose therapy preferred to single dose therapy.

- use for 5 days in women (trimethoprim—3 days).
- use for 10 days in women with known UT abnormality.
  — trimethoprim 300 mg (o) daily for 3 days
        or
  — cephalexin 500 mg (o) 12 hourly
        or
  — amoxycillin/potassium clavulanate 250/125 mg (o) 8 hourly (preferred agent)
        or
  — norfloxacin 400 mg (o) 12 hourly for 3 days (if resistance to above agents proven)
- Follow-up: MSU 3 weeks later.

Note: • Avoid using important quinolones—norfloxacin or ciprofloxacin—as first-line agents
  • Co-trimoxazole is not first line because it has no advantage over trimethoprim and has more side effects.

Treatment of men[5]
Use any one of the regimes for non-pregnant women, but use for a minimum of 14 days. The dose of cephalexin is 250 mg (o) 6 hourly.

Acute pyelonephritis
Mild cases can be treated with oral therapy alone using double the dosage of drugs recommended for uncomplicated cystitis, except for trimethoprim when the same dosage is recommended. Norfloxacin (400 mg (o) 12 hourly) is used if resistance to these drugs is proven.

For severe infection with suspected septicaemia admit to hospital and treat initially with parenteral antibiotics for 2 to 5 days after taking urine for microscopy and culture and blood for culture.

amoxycillin 2 g IV 6 hourly[5]
plus
gentamicin 5–7 mg/kg/day, single daily dose

Follow with oral therapy for a total of 14 days therapy. Drug levels of gentamicin require monitoring. Gentamicin can be replaced with IV cefotaxime or ceftriaxone if desired.

All patients should be investigated for an underlying urinary tract abnormality.

Recurrent or chronic urinary tract infections
Recurrent infections occur as a relapse of a previously treated infection or because of reinfection, often with differing organisms. Persistent (chronic) UTIs indicate that the organism is resistant to the antimicrobial agents employed or that there is an underlying abnormality such as a renal stone or a chronically infected prostate in the male patient. Such infections may be treated with prolonged courses of an appropriate antibiotic or removal of the focus of infection.

In men and children an anatomical abnormality is usual, while recurrent cystitis in women often occurs despite a normal tract. In men, instruction on perineal hygiene, more frequent bladder emptying and postintercourse voiding may assist in the prevention of reinfection.

Treatment of recurrent or chronic UTI[5]
A 10 to 14 day course of
- amoxycillin/potassium clavulanate (250/125 mg) (o) 8 hourly
        or
- trimethoprim 300 mg (o) once daily
  or (if proven resistance to above agents)
- norfloxacin 400 mg (o) 12 hourly
        or
- hexamine hippurate 1 g (o) bd

Prophylaxis for recurrent UTI[5]
In some female patients a single dose of a suitable agent after intercourse is adequate but, in more severe cases, courses may be taken for 6 months or on occasions longer.

- nitrofurantoin (macrocrystals) 50 mg (o) nocte
        or
- trimethoprim 150 mg (o) nocte
        or
- norfloxacin 200–400 mg (o) nocte (if proven resistance to others)

Asymptomatic bacteriuria

- In neonates and preschool children, treat and investigate for evidence of vesicoureteral reflux.
- In men less than 60 years old, treat and investigate, especially for chronic prostatitis.
- In women, give single dose therapy and investigate only those in whom UTI persists or recurs.
- In pregnant women, treat because of the risk of developing pyelonephritis (up to 40% risk).
- School-age children and elderly men and women (over 60 years) probably do not require treatment if their urinary tracts are normal.
- In patients with long-term indwelling catheters treatment is not usually required or useful.
- Prophylaxis should be given for recurrent asymptomatic bacteriuria in pregnant women, in patients with associated renal tract abnormality, and in those undergoing genitourinary instrumentation or surgery or intermittent catheterisation.

Urinary tract infection in children

UTI in infants and very young children is often renal in nature and may be associated with generalised symptoms such as fever, vomiting, diarrhoea and failure to thrive. Symptoms of dysuria and frequency appear only after the age of 2 years when the child is able to indicate the source of the discomfort. In a girl or boy (rare presentation) with symptoms of dysuria and frequency an underlying abnormality is likely to be present with a reported incidence of vesicoureteric reflux as high as 40% and scarred kidneys (reflux nephropathy) in 27%.[3]

Thus the early detection of children with vesicoureteric reflux and control of recurrent renal infection could prevent the development of scars, hypertension and chronic renal failure. Radiological investigation of children with UTIs shows normal kidneys in approximately 66% and reflux in approximately 33%.

Antimicrobial treatment for acute cystitis in children[5]

Treatment should be continued for 5 to 10 days.
- trimethoprim 6 mg/kg (maximum 300 mg) orally, daily (suspension is 50 mg/5 mL)

or

- cephalexin 10 mg/kg (maximum 250 mg) orally 6 hourly

or

- co-trimoxazole 4/20 mg/kg, orally bd

or

- amoxycillin/potassium clavulanate 10/2.5 mg/kg (maximum 250/125 mg) orally 8 hourly

Norfloxacin and ciprofloxacin should be avoided routinely in children.

Check MSU in 3 weeks.

Urinary infections in the elderly

The typical settings in which UTIs occur in the elderly are in the frail, those who are immobilised, and those with faecal incontinence and inadequate bladder emptying. The presenting symptoms may be atypical, especially with upper UTI where fever of undetermined origin and behaviour disturbances may be a feature. In men obstructive uropathy from prostatism should be excluded by ultrasound.

Uncomplicated infections should be treated the same way as for other age groups but no antimicrobial treatment is recommended for asymptomatic bacteriuria.

Urinary infections in pregnancy

UTI in pregnant women requires careful surveillance. Asymptomatic bacteriuria should always be excluded during early pregnancy because it tends to develop into a full-blown infection. Acute cystitis is treated for 10 to 14 days with any of the following antimicrobials: cephalexin, amoxycillin/potassium clavulanate or nitrofurantoin (if a beta-lactam antibiotic is contraindicated). The dosages are the same as for other groups. Asymptomatic bacteriuria should be treated with a week-long course.

Genitourinary tuberculosis

The genitourinary tract is involved in 3–5% of cases of tuberculosis.[6] The genital and urinary tracts are often involved together as a result of miliary spread.

The commonest presenting complaints are dysuria and frequency, which can be severe. Other symptoms include strangury when the bladder is severely affected, loin pain and haematuria. Routine urine culture shows sterile pyuria.

Diagnosis is made on specific culture for mycobacterium, or biopsy of bladder lesions or the typical X-ray appearance of distorted calyces and medullary calcification. Treatment is with antituberculosis drugs.

Common treatment errors[1]

- Not treating women with dysuria and frequency merely because there are $< 10^5$ cfu/mL in an MSU
- Overtreating women with acute cystitis and normal urinary tracts; single-dose therapy is effective in 70–80% of cases, and overtreatment often leads to vaginal candidiasis or antibiotic-induced diarrhoea
- Using single-dose therapy in patients with known anatomical abnormalities
- Failing to consider chronic prostatic infection in men with recurrent UTI and a normal IVU

When to refer

- It is wise to refer all patients with urinary tract abnormalities to a nephrologist or urologist for advice on specific management.
- Refer also if the simple methods outlined above do not control recurrent UTI.
- Refer males with urinary infections that are not clearly localised to the prostate.
- Refer patients with impaired renal function.

Practice tips

- Most symptomatic UTIs are acute cystitis occurring in sexually active women with anatomically normal urinary tracts.
- A clinical diagnosis based on experience, plus positive nitrite dipstick test and the finding of

pyuria by office microscopy will generally enable immediate curative treatment.
- A 3-day course of trimethoprim 300 mg daily for 3 days is a suitable first choice for acute uncomplicated cystitis in women.
- Avoid overinvestigation of patients in whom there is a low likelihood of demonstrating structural abnormalities.
- In males the prostate is the most common source of recurrent UTI.
- Urinary tract infection is commonly associated with microscopic haematuria (occasionally macroscopic haematuria).
- Persisting haematuria should be investigated.
- Due to the rising level of *E. coli* resistance, amoxycillin is no longer recommended unless susceptibility of the organism is proven.[5]

References

1. Becker GJ. Urinary tract infection. In: MIMS Disease Index (2nd edn). Sydney: IMS Publishing, 1996, 545–547.
2. Heale W. *Renal disease*. CHECK Programme. Melbourne: RACGP, 1987, 1–20.
3. Kincaid-Smith P, Larkins R, Whelan G. *Problems in clinical medicine*. Sydney: MacLennan & Petty, 1990, 280–283.
4. Sloane P, Slatt M, Baker R. *Essentials of family medicine*. Baltimore: Williams and Wilkins, 1988, 162–168.
5. Mashford ML. *Antibiotic guidelines* (9th edn). Melbourne: VMPF Therapeutics Committee, 1996–97, 30–35.
6. Bullock N, Sibley G, Whitaker R. *Essential urology*. Edinburgh: Churchill Livingstone, 1989, 126–129.

23
Malignant disease

—

Cancers of the tongue and mouth begin with a small hard lump, and sometimes with a little sore; both of which are attended with pricking pains, and they spread in the same manner with cancerous sores in other parts. It is so great an evil, that the slightest suspicion of it occasions very great uneasiness.

William Heberden (1701–1801)

The terms *malignancy, cancer* and *neoplasia* are usually used interchangeably. The differences between a malignant tumour and a benign tumour are summarised in Table 23.1.

Table 23.1 *Different characteristics of benign and malignant tumours*

Benign	Malignant
Well differentiated	Undifferentiated
Non-invasive	Invasive
Slow growth	Rapid growth
Not anaplastic	Anaplastic
Not metastatic	Metastatic

Malignant disease accounts for 1 in 8 deaths of people under 35 years in Australia and 1 in every 4 (25%) of deaths in those over 45 years.[1] Cancer is the only major cause of death in Australia that is increasing in both sexes. At current rates about 1 in 3 males and 1 in 4 females will develop a cancer, excluding non-melanoma skin cancers, by the age of 75.[1]

The six most common causes of death from cancer in Australia are cancer of the lung, bowel, breast, prostate, lymphoma and pancreas.

Neoplasia, especially malignancy of the silent areas, can present as undifferentiated illness and be a real masquerade. The so-called 'silent' malignancies that pose a special problem include carcinoma of the ovary, kidney, caecum

and ascending colon, liver (hepatoma), melanoma and haematological tissue.

This chapter will focus on the general features of these malignancies.

Acute emergency problems that can develop with various malignancies include spinal cord compression, malignant effusions, disseminated intravascular coagulation and hypercalcaemia.

Cancer in children

Although uncommon in children under 15 years, cancer is the second most common cause of death in this age group. The most common cancers (in order) are leukaemias, especially acute lymphocytic leukaemia (34%), brain tumours especially astrocytoma (20%), lymphomas especially non-Hodgkin's (13%), neuroblastoma, Wilms' tumour, soft tissue tumours especially rhabdomyosarcoma and bone tumours.

Survival has improved dramatically in recent decades, indicating the value of early diagnosis and referral for expert treatment.

Clinical manifestations

The clinical manifestations of malignancy are usually due to:

- pressure effects of the growth
- infiltration or metastases in various organs, e.g. liver, brain, lungs, bone, blood vessels
- systemic symptoms including paraneoplastic effects

Systemic symptoms

These can be divided into general non-specific effects and paraneoplastic syndromes, which are the remote effects caused by the tumour.

Undifferentiated general symptoms
- tiredness/fatigue/weakness
- anorexia and nausea
- weight loss

Paraneoplastic effects
The paraneoplastic effects or syndromes are very important clinically because they may provide an early clue to the presence of a specific type of cancer, in addition to the possible lethal effect of the metabolic or toxic effect, e.g. hyponatraemia. These effects include:

- ectopic hormone production
- skin abnormalities
- metabolic effects
  — fever/sweats
  — weight loss
- haematologic disorders
  — anaemia
  — erythrocytosis
  — coagulation disorder
  — others
- neuropathies and CNS abnormalities
- collagen vascular disorders

A summary of various paraneoplastic syndromes is presented in Table 23.2.

Table 23.2 *Paraneoplastic syndromes and associated tumours: more common examples*

Hormone excess syndrome	Tumour
Cushing's	Lung, kidney, adrenal, thymoma, pancreas
ACTH	Lung, kidney, thymoma, thyroid
Gonadotrophins	Lung, choriocarcinoma, hepatoma

Other syndromes	Tumour
Hypercalcaemia	Lung, breast, kidney, multiple myeloma, prostate, pancreas, adrenal, hepatoma
Fever	Kidney, hepatoma, lymphoma, pancreas, thymoma
Neurologic	Lung, breast, thymoma, Hodgkin's, prostate
Coagulopathy	Lung, breast, hepatoma, prostate, pancreas
Thrombophlebitis	Kidney, pancreas, prostate
Polycythaemia	Kidney, hepatoma
Dermatomyositis	Lung, breast, pancreas

Clinical approach
A history of constitutional symptoms that are often quite undifferentiated (often bizarre) may provide the clue to the possibility of an underlying malignancy. An occupational history may be relevant to the clinical problem (see Table 23.3).

Tumour markers
A tumour marker is an abnormal characteristic that is specific for a particular type of malignancy, e.g. the Philadelphia chromosome for chronic myeloid leukaemia. Other examples include human chorionic gonadotrophin (HCG) (elevated in trophoblastic tumours and germ cell neoplasms of the testes and ovaries) and the oncofetal antigens—carcino-embryonic antigen (CEA) and alpha fetoprotein (AFP).

CEA and AFP are not specific markers but are elevated in certain tumours and are very useful in monitoring tumour activity.

Tumour markers, some of which are yet unidentified, would appear to have an important role in future diagnosis and management of malignant disease. The most valuable are those associated with testis cancer — AFP and beta HCG. Markers may be an adjunct to diagnosis of certain malignancies including CEA for bowel cancer and CA–125 for ovarian cancer.

Lung cancer
Apart from non-melanoma skin cancer, lung cancer is the most common cancer in Australia both in terms of incidence and death, accounting for at least 20% of cancer deaths.[1] In the United States it accounts for 35% of cancer deaths in men and 21% of deaths in women. Only 10–25% are asymptomatic at the time of diagnosis but lung cancer can cause an extraordinary variety of clinical symptoms and signs with a reputation for several paraneoplastic syndromes.

The paraneoplastic syndromes include hypercalcaemia, Cushing's syndrome, carcinoid syndrome, dermatomyositis, visual loss progressing to blindness from retinal degeneration, cerebellar degeneration and encephalitis.

The presentation of cough and chest pain renders it less of an 'occult' malignancy than several other types.

Table 23.3 *Occupational causes of cancer*

Agent	Occupation	Cancer
Arsenic	Chemical industry	Lung, skin, liver
Asbestos	Insulation worker	Mesothelioma
Benzene	Glue worker, varnisher	Leukaemia
Soot, coal tar	Chimney sweep	Skin
Radiation	Mining, watch dials	Various
Ultraviolet light	Farmer, sailor	Skin
Vinyl chloride	PVC manufacturing	Liver (angiosarcoma)

Renal tumours

The most important tumours of the kidney are adenocarcinoma (80% of all renal tumours)[2] and nephroblastoma (Wilms' tumour).

Adenocarcinoma

Adenocarcinoma of the kidney has a great diversity of presenting symptoms, including:

- general symptoms of neoplasia
- haematuria (60%)
- loin pain (40%)
- loin mass
- signs of anaemia
- left supraclavicular lymphadenopathy
- varicocele
- hypertension
- symptoms of metastases (to liver, lungs, brain, bones)
  — respiratory symptoms
  — neurological symptoms and signs
  — bone pain
  — pathological fracture (vertebral collapse)
- urinalysis: 67% positive for blood

The classic triad of symptoms (in 10–15% of patients) is:[2]

- haematuria
- loin pain
- palpable kidney mass

Wilms' tumour

Wilms' tumour is responsible for 10% of all childhood malignancies. Clinical features include:[2]

- peak incidence 2–3 years
- general symptoms of neoplasia
- palpable mass 80%
- abdominal pain 30%
- haematuria 25%

Early diagnosis with nephrectomy and chemotherapy leads to a very favourable prognosis.

Ovarian cancer

Ovarian cancer has the highest mortality rate of all the gynaecological cancers because the majority of patients present in the late stage of the disease. It is usually asymptomatic prior to the development of metastases. Epithelial tumours are the most common of malignant ovarian tumours. They are uncommon under 40 years of age and the average age of diagnosis is 50 years.[3]

The most common presentation is abdominal swelling (mass and/or ascites). Non-specific symptoms, which may be present for a long time before diagnosis, include abnormal uterine bleeding, weight loss, abdominal discomfort, reduced capacity for food, anorexia, nausea and vomiting.

Carcinoma of caecum and ascending colon

Malignancy in this area is more likely to present with symptoms of anaemia without the patient noting obvious blood in the faeces or alteration of bowel habit.

The leukaemias

The leukaemias are caused by an acquired malignant transformation in the stem cell in the haemopoietic system. Acute leukaemia has a rapidly fatal course if untreated, while chronic leukaemia has a variable chronic course with an inevitable fatal outcome. See Figure 23.1. The main features of each type are as follows.

Acute leukaemia

Symptoms
- general constitutional, e.g. malaise
- symptoms of anaemia

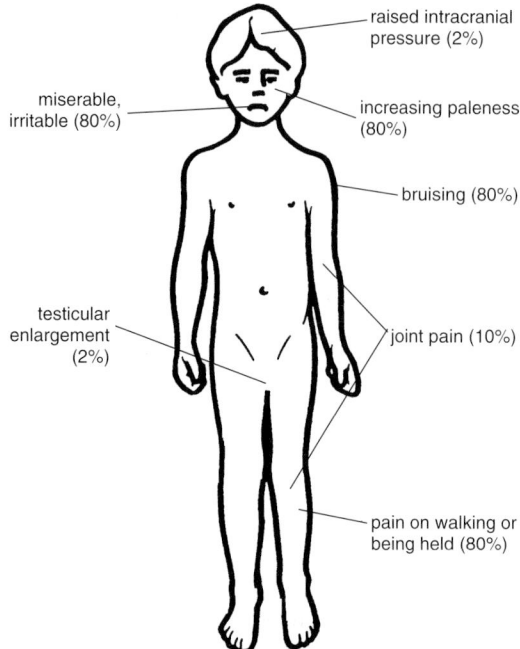

Labels on figure:
- raised intracranial pressure (2%)
- miserable, irritable (80%)
- increasing paleness (80%)
- bruising (80%)
- testicular enlargement (2%)
- joint pain (10%)
- pain on walking or being held (80%)

Fig 23.1 *Clinical features of a child with leukaemia*[4]

- susceptibility to infection, e.g. sore throat, mouth ulceration, chest infection
- easy bruising and bleeding, e.g. epistaxis, gingival bleeding
- bone pain (notably in children with ALL) and joint pain
- symptoms due to infiltration of tissues with blast cells, e.g. gingival hypertrophy in AML

Signs
- pallor of anaemia
- petechiae, bruising
- gum hypertrophy/gingivitis/stomatitis
- signs of infection
- variable enlargement of liver, spleen and lymph nodes
- bone tenderness, especially sternum and liver

Diagnosis
- FBE and film
  — normochromic/normocytic anaemia
  — pancytopenia with circulatory blast cells
  — platelets: usually reduced
- Bone marrow examination

Chronic myeloid leukaemia
Main clinical features
- a disorder of middle age
- insidious onset

- constitutional symptoms: malaise, weight loss, fever
- symptoms of anaemia
- splenomegaly (very large)
- priapism
- gout
- markedly elevated white cell count (granulocytes)
- marked left shift in myeloid series
- presence of Philadelphia chromosome

Chronic lymphocytic leukaemia
Main clinical features
- a disorder of late middle age and elderly
- insidious onset
- constitutional symptoms: malaise, weight loss, fever
- lymphadenopathy—neck, axilla, groin (80%)
- moderately enlarged spleen and liver (about 50%)
- mild anaemia
- lymphocytosis $> 15 \times 10^9$/L
- 'mature' appearance of lymphocytes

The lymphomas

Lymphomas, which are malignant tumours of lymphoid tissue, are classified as Hodgkin's disease and non-Hodgkin's lymphoma on the basis of histological appearance of the involved lymph tissue.

Hodgkin's disease
Clinical features
- painless (rubbery) lymphadenopathy, especially cervical nodes
- constitutional symptoms, e.g. malaise, weakness, weight loss
- fever and drenching night sweats
- pruritus
- alcohol-induced pain in any enlarged lymph nodes
- possible enlarged spleen and liver

Diagnosis is by lymph-node biopsy with histological confirmation.

Non-Hodgkin's lymphomas
Non-Hodgkin's lymphomas are a heterogeneous group of cancers of lymphocytes derived from the malignant clones of B or T cells.

Main clinical features
- painless lymphadenopathy—localised or wide-spread
- constitutional symptoms possible, especially sweating
- pruritus is uncommon
- extra nodal sites of disease, e.g. skin, GIT
- possible enlarged liver and spleen
- possible nodular infiltration of skin, e.g. mycosis fungoides

Diagnosis is by lymph-node biopsy.

Multiple myeloma

Multiple myeloma is regarded as a disease of the elderly, the mean age of presentation being 60 years.[4] The classic presenting triad in an older man is anaemia, back pain and elevated ESR.

Main clinical features
- bone pain, e.g. backache (in more than 80% of patients)
- bone tenderness
- weakness, tiredness
- recurrent infections
- symptoms of anaemia
- bleeding tendency
- replacement of bone marrow by malignant plasma cells

Diagnostic criteria
The presence of:[4]
- paraprotein in serum
- Bence-Jones protein in urine
- bony lytic lesions

Carcinoid syndrome

Hormone secretion by carcinoid cells causes the characteristic carcinoid syndrome long before local growth or metastatic spread of the tumour is apparent.

The syndrome
Classic triad: skin flushing (especially face), diarrhoea (with abdominal cramps), valvular heart disease
Other features: wheezing, telangiectasia, hypotension
Sites of tumours: ileum, stomach, bronchi

Potentially curable malignant tumours

Several tumours are curable by chemotherapy even in the advanced stage. Such tumours are as follows.

Haematological tumours
- some lymphomas
- Hodgkin's disease
- acute lymphatic leukaemia
- acute myeloid leukaemia

Solid tumours
- choriocarcinoma
- testicular carcinoma
- neuroblastoma
- Wilms' tumour
- Burkitt's tumour
- embryonal rhabdomyosarcoma
- small cell lung cancer

Tumours curable by adjuvant chemotherapy
- breast cancer (especially up to stage 2)
- osteogenic cancer
- soft tissue cancer
- colorectal cancer

Metastatic tumours

It is very helpful for the practitioner to have a working knowledge of possible primary sources of tumour when metastatic lesions are detected in various organs.

Common sites of metastatic presentation are the lymph nodes, liver, lung, mediastinum and bone. Other sites include the brain, bone marrow, peritoneum, retroperitoneum, skin and the spinal cord.

These important sites (listed below) are followed by likely primary sources with the most likely listed first.
- *Liver.* Colon, pancreas, liver, stomach, breast, lung, melanoma
- *Lung and mediastinum.* Breast, lung, colon, kidney, testes, cervix/uterus, Hodgkin's disease, melanoma
- *Bone.* Breast, prostate, lung, Hodgkin's disease, kidney, thyroid, melanoma
- *Brain.* Breast, lung, colon, lymphoma, kidney, melanoma, prostate

- *Skin.* Lung, colon, melanoma, Kaposi's sarcoma
- *Lymph nodes*:
  - *High cervical.* Hodgkin's disease, lymphoma, squamous cell carcinoma, oropharynx, nasopharynx
  - *Low cervical.* Lung, stomach, lymphoma, Hodgkin's disease, oropharynx, larynx, skin, tongue
  - *Axillary.* Breast, lung, lymphoma
  - *Inguinal.* Lymphoma, ovary, uterus, vulva, prostate, skin
- *Retroperitoneum.* Lymphoma, Hodgkin's disease, ovary, uterus, testes, prostate

It is important to keep in mind those malignancies that are potentially curable and refer as soon as possible.

Prevention

Preventive measures for malignant disease are addressed in more detail in Chapter 9. The significant decrease in deaths from cancer of the stomach in this country in recent years is probably reflected in our improved diet with more fresh fruit and vegetables. Important preventive measures include an appropriate healthy diet, no smoking, sun protection and perhaps safe sex measures. Of concern is the rapid increase in incidence of prostate cancer, chronic myeloid leukaemia, myeloma and non-Hodgkin's lymphoma.

References

1. Australia's Health 1990. Canberra: Australian Institute of Health, 1990, 57–64.
2. Bullock N, Sibley G, Whitaker Q. *Essential urology.* Edinburgh: Churchill Livingstone, 1989, 202–208.
3. Dalrymple C. Ovarian cancer: A sinister and silent disease. Mod Med Aust, July 1992, 26–37.
4. Vowels MR. Common presentations and management of leukaemia in childhood. Aust Fam Physician, 1994; 23: 1519–1521.
5. Kumer PJ, Clark ML. *Clinical medicine* (2nd edn). London: Bailliere Tindall, 1990, 349–351.

24

Human immunodeficiency virus infection – could it be HIV?

—

The verdict for him too was death, not the inevitable death that horrified and yet was tolerable because science was helpless before it, but the death which was inevitable because the man was a little wheel in the great machine of a complex civilisation.

W. Somerset Maugham (1874–1965)
Of Human Bondage

HIV, the cause of the well-known AIDS, can rightly be included as one of the clinical masquerades of modern medicine. Public health measures in the Western world have limited the spread of the disease, particularly in Australia where the incidence of new cases has remained relatively constant in the past 10 years. By contrast the incidence in Africa and Asia continues to rise at an alarming rate. The introduction of combination treatment with the protease inhibitors in November 1995 has changed the previously understood natural history of the disease and has given rise to renewed hope that HIV will become a chronic manageable disease.

The benefit of early diagnosis has become even more impressive since the discovery that HIV is not a latent infection throughout most of its course. Soon after initial infection, an explosive replication of HIV occurs, which is brought under control by the immune system in 6 to 8 weeks as the host-versus-virus interaction reaches an active and dynamic equilibrium. This dynamic situation continues throughout a person's lifetime, with as many as 10 billion new virions produced and up to 2 billion CD_4 lymphocytes destroyed and replaced daily. Clinical immunodeficiency develops when the body's ability to replace CD_4 cells is finally exhausted, resulting in further uncontrolled viral replication. It has taken over a decade to get this understanding of the dynamics of HIV infection. Viral load assays based on molecular techniques have revolutionised our understanding of the natural history of HIV disease. These advances make it imperative to make the diagnosis early in the course of the disease in order to start combination treatment to lessen the viral load.

The general practitioner is central in prevention, diagnosis, counselling, monitoring and management of HIV disease. The GP must be alert to the benefits of early diagnosis as summarised in Table 24.1

Key facts and checkpoints

- HIV is a retrovirus with two known strains that cause a similar spectrum of syndromes: HIV_1 and HIV_2.
- Always consider HIV in those at risk: enquire about history of STDs, injection of illicit drugs, past blood transfusions, sexual activities and partners.
- About 50% of patients develop an acute infective illness similar to glandular fever within weeks of acquiring the virus (the HIV seroconversion illness).[2] The main features are fever, lymphadenopathy, lethargy and possibly sore throat, and a generalised rash.
- If these patients have a negative infectious mononucleosis test, perform an HIV antibody,

Table 24.1 *The benefits of early HIV diagnosis*

To individual patients
Prolongation of the asymptomatic period
Delayed disease progression
Prevention of opportunistic infections
Optimal maintenance of health through patient education and counselling
Cures are only likely with early intervention

To the cohort of HIV-positive individuals
Monitoring of advances in treatment
Increased participation in research and clinical trials
Development of new services to meet changing patient needs

To the community
Documentation of changes in epidemiology
Reduced high-risk activities
Contact tracing
Control of HIV transmission

To the doctors
Time to influence the course of disease
Time to counsel the patient

Source: Penny R. Could it be HIV? 2. Benefits of early diagnosis of HIV infection. Med J Aust, 1993; 158:35–36 © Copyright 1993, *The Medical Journal of Australia*—reproduced with permission

which may have to be repeated in four weeks or so if negative.
- Patients invariably recover to enter a long period of good health for five years or more.[1]
- Pneumocystitis pneumonia is the commonest presentation of AIDS.
- Approximately 15–25% of HIV-positive children are infected from HIV-infected mothers.[3]
- Infants born to these mothers may develop the disease within a few months, with 30% affected by the age of 18 months.
- The time for the onset of AIDS in HIV-affected adults varies from 2 months to 20 years or longer; the median time is around 10 years.
- In family practice the most common presentation of HIV-related illness is seen in the skin/oral mucosa.[4]
- HIV antibody testing is a two-stage process: ELISA test for screening is followed by another method, e.g. Western blot, if ELISA is positive.
- The seroconversion period from acquiring HIV infection to a positive antibody test varies between individuals: this period is known as the 'window period'.
- All HIV infected patients require regular monitoring for immune function and viral load. The viral load test monitors viral activity.
- The level of immune depletion is best measured by the CD_4 positive T lymphocyte (helper

T cell) count—the CD_4 cell count. The cut-off points for good health and severe disease appear to be 500/μL and 200/μL respectively.[1]

Occurrence and transmission

HIV can be isolated from blood, tissues, semen, saliva, breast milk, cervical and vaginal secretions and tears of infected persons. HIV is transmitted in semen, blood and vaginal fluids, transplanted organs and breast milk through:
- unprotected sexual intercourse (anal or vaginal) and in rare cases oral sex with an infected person
- infected blood entering the body (through blood transfusion or by IV drug users sharing needles/syringes)
- needle-stick injury
- artificial insemination, organ transplantation
- infected mothers (to babies during pregnancy, at birth or in breast milk)

Infection with HIV can occur via the vagina, rectum or open cuts and sores, including any on the lips or in the mouth. Social (non-sexual) contact and insect vectors have not been implicated in transmission.

Clinical manifestations[5]

There are a multiplicity of clinical findings in HIV infection (Fig. 24.1). The clinical stages of HIV disease are summarised in Table 24.2.[6]

Acute (seroconversion illness)

At least 50% of patients have an acute illness associated with seroconversion. The illness usually occurs within 6 weeks of infection and is characterised by fever, night sweats, malaise, severe lethargy, anorexia, nausea, myalgia, arthralgia, headache, photophobia, sore throat, diarrhoea, lymphadenopathy, generalised maculoerythematous rash and thrombocytopenia. Neurological manifestations including meningoencephalitis and peripheral neuritis are commonly observed. Acute HIV infection should be considered in the differential diagnosis of illnesses resembling glandular fever. This illness is self-limiting and usually revolves within 1 to 3 weeks. However, chronic lethargy, depression and irritability may persist after the acute illness. Non-specific viraemic sequelae such as mucosal ulceration, desquamation, exacerbation of seborrhoea and recurrences of herpes simplex may occur (see Fig. 24.1).

Table 24.2 *Clinical stages of HIV disease*[6]

Clinical stage	Common clinical features	CD$_4$count
Seroconversion illness (self-limited 1–3 weeks)	Fever, headache (may have aseptic meningitis), sore throat, maculopapular rash, lymphadenopathy, splenomegaly; Atypical lymphocytes on FBE	Transient decrease, commonly followed by a return to near normal levels
Asymptomatic	Headaches Persistent generalised lymphadenopathy	Usually > 300/µL Gradual decrease of 50–80/µL
Symptomatic—early	Oral and vaginal candidiasis, oral hairy leukoplakia, seborrhoeic dermatitis, psoriasis, recurrent varicella-zoster infection, cervical dysplasia, unexplained fever, sweats, weight loss, diarrhoea, tuberculosis	Usually 150–500/µL
—late	PCP, Kaposi's sarcoma, oesophageal candidiasis, cerebral toxoplasmosis, lymphoma, HIV-1 associated dementia complex, cryptococcal meningitis	Usually < 150/µL
Advanced	CMV retinitis, cerebral lymphoma, *Mycobacterium avium* complex (MAC) infection	Usually < 50/µL

Reproduced with permission[6]

Acute illness may be accompanied by neutropenia, lymphopenia, thrombocytopenia, and mildly elevated ESR with serum transaminases. During recovery a lymphocytosis may occur with appearance of atypical mononuclear cells and an inversion of the CD$_4$+:CD$_8$+ ratio due to elevation of CD$_8$+cells.

Differential diagnoses are given in Table 24.3.

Table 24.3 *Differential diagnoses of primary HIV infection*

Epstein-Barr mononucleosis

Syphilis: secondary

TORCH organisms
• toxoplasmosis
• rubella
• cytomegalovirus
• herpes simplex

Disseminated gonococcal infection

Hepatitis A,B,C,D or E

Influenza

Other virus infections

AIDS—defining conditions

The original US Centers for Disease Control (CDC) classification has been modified with time to provide a more simplified scheme for defining AIDS. The HIV/AIDS case surveillance system simply specifies a list of clinical conditions associated with the late stages of HIV infection as being 'AIDS-defining'.[7]

The AIDS-defining conditions are:

• candidiasis of bronchi, trachea or lungs
• candidiasis, oesophageal
• cervical cancer, invasive
• coccidioidomycosis, disseminated or extra-pulmonary
• cryptococcosis, extrapulmonary
• cryptosporidiosis, chronic intestinal (> 1 month's duration)
• cytomegalovirus disease (other than liver, spleen, or nodes)
• cytomegalovirus retinitis (with loss of vision)
• encephalopathy, HIV-related
• herpes simplex: chronic ulcer(s) (> 1 month's duration); or bronchitis, pneumonitis or oesophagitis
• histoplasmosis, disseminated or extrapulmonary
• isosporiasis, chronic intestinal (> 1 month's duration)
• Kaposi's sarcoma
• lymphoma, Burkitt's (or equivalent term)
• lymphoma, immunoblastic (or equivalent term)
• lymphoma, primary, of brain
• *Mycobacterium avium* complex of *M. Kansasii*, disseminated or extrapulmonary

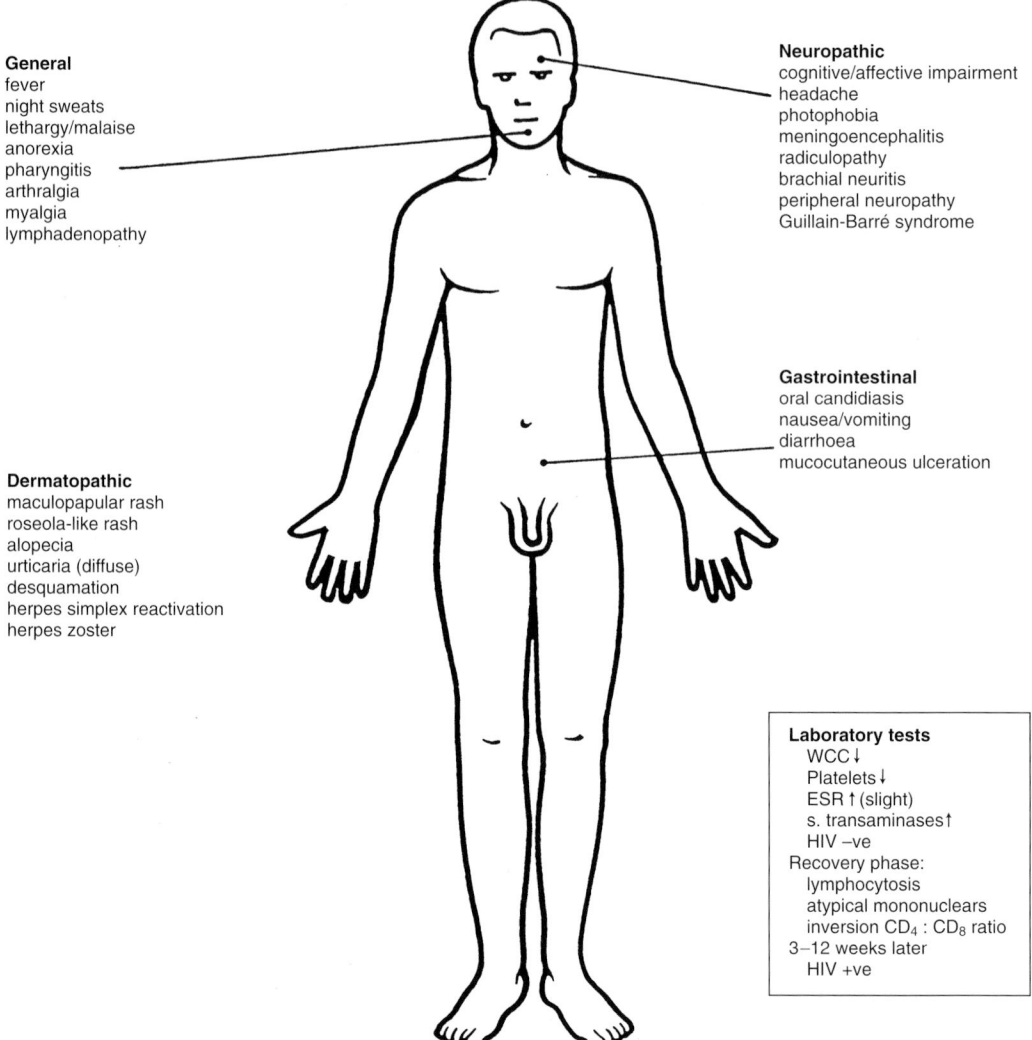

General
fever
night sweats
lethargy/malaise
anorexia
pharyngitis
arthralgia
myalgia
lymphadenopathy

Neuropathic
cognitive/affective impairment
headache
photophobia
meningoencephalitis
radiculopathy
brachial neuritis
peripheral neuropathy
Guillain-Barré syndrome

Gastrointestinal
oral candidiasis
nausea/vomiting
diarrhoea
mucocutaneous ulceration

Dermatopathic
maculopapular rash
roseola-like rash
alopecia
urticaria (diffuse)
desquamation
herpes simplex reactivation
herpes zoster

Laboratory tests
WCC↓
Platelets↓
ESR↑ (slight)
s. transaminases↑
HIV −ve
Recovery phase:
lymphocytosis
atypical mononuclears
inversion CD$_4$: CD$_8$ ratio
3–12 weeks later
HIV +ve

Fig. 24.1 *Possible clinical features of primary HIV infection*

- *Mycobacterium tuberculosis*, any site (pulmonary or extrapulmonary)
- *Mycobacterium*, other species or unidentified species, disseminated or extrapulmonary
- *Pneumocystis carinii* pneumonia
- *Salmonella* septicaemia, recurrent
- toxoplasmosis of brain
- wasting syndrome due to HIV

The Australian AIDS surveillance case definition does not refer to the CD$_4$ cell count although in the United States AIDS is also defined by CD$_4$ cell count of < 200/μL, regardless of clinical condition.

Common clinical presentations of HIV infection

Fever
This is of unknown origin.

Weight loss
This is usually severe and muscle wasting.

Respiratory
- sinusitis
- non-productive cough, increasing dyspnoea and fever: due to opportunistic pneumonias

More than 50% of patients present with pneumocystitis pneumonia which may have an abrupt or insidious onset.[6] With the insidious type of onset, examination and chest X-ray are often normal early. Many other agents, e.g. CMV, cryptococcosis and TB, can be responsible. Exclusion of pneumocystitis pneumonia is important as this condition carries a high mortality if untreated.

Gastrointestinal
- chronic diarrhoea (many causes) with weight loss or dehydration

Neurological
- headache
- progressive dementia (HIV encephalopathy)
- ataxia due to myelopathy
- seizures
- mononeuritis
- Guillain–Barré type mononeuropathy
- toxoplasma encephalitis
- cryptococcal meningitis
- peripheral neuropathy
- progressive visual loss (CMV retinitis)
- CNS lymphoma

Oral cavity
- aphthous ulcers
- angular chelitis
- periodontal/gingival disease
- tonsillitis
- oral candidiasis
- oral hairy cell leukaemia (frequently mistaken for candidiasis but affects lateral border of tongue)

Genitourinary
- cervical dysplasia
- vaginal candidiasis
- various STDs, e.g. HSV, HPV

Skin
- impetigo
- warts
- herpes simplex
- shingles, especially multidermatomal
- seborrhoeic dermatitis
- cutaneous mycoses
- Kaposi's sarcoma (painless red-purple lesions on any part of the body including palms, soles, oral cavity and other parts of the GIT)

Figure 24.2 presents the chronology of HIV-induced disease correlated with time since infection and CD_4 cell levels.

Investigations and diagnosis[6]
The laboratory investigation of AIDS covers three broad areas:
1. Tests for HIV infection:
   e.g. enzyme linked immunosorbent assay (ELISA); Western blot technique (used for confirmation)
2. Tests of immune function:
   - CD_4^+ lymphocyte counts—the strongest predictor of possible clinical manifestations of HIV infection
   - Low CD_4^+ cells (counts < 500 cells/μL) = defective cell immunity[1,5]
   - Counts < 200 cells/μL = severe immunodeficiency
3. Viral load: a measure of serum level of RNA of HIV virus—correlates with progression to AIDS and death
4. Tests for opportunistic infections and other problems:
   e.g. other STDs, EBV, CMV, hepatitis, Mantoux test

Management
Patients with HIV infection require considerable psychosocial support, counselling and regular assessment from a non-judgmental caring practitioner.

The holistic approach to life
Most people with HIV infection will take 'natural therapies'. This should be viewed as being complementary with the management suggested by the GP, and the patient should be encouraged to tell his or her doctors of the alternative medicines being taken. Anecdotal reports suggest that 75% of people with HIV regularly use 'natural therapies,'[8] and in the setting of the long-term nature of the condition it is important for doctors to be supportive and create a climate of acceptance around these practices.

Positive lifestyle factors include:
- a very healthy balanced diet: high fruit and vegetable intake, pure fruit juices, high fibre, low fat, high complex carbohydrates
- toxic avoidance: processed foods, caffeine, illicit drugs, alcohol, cigarettes

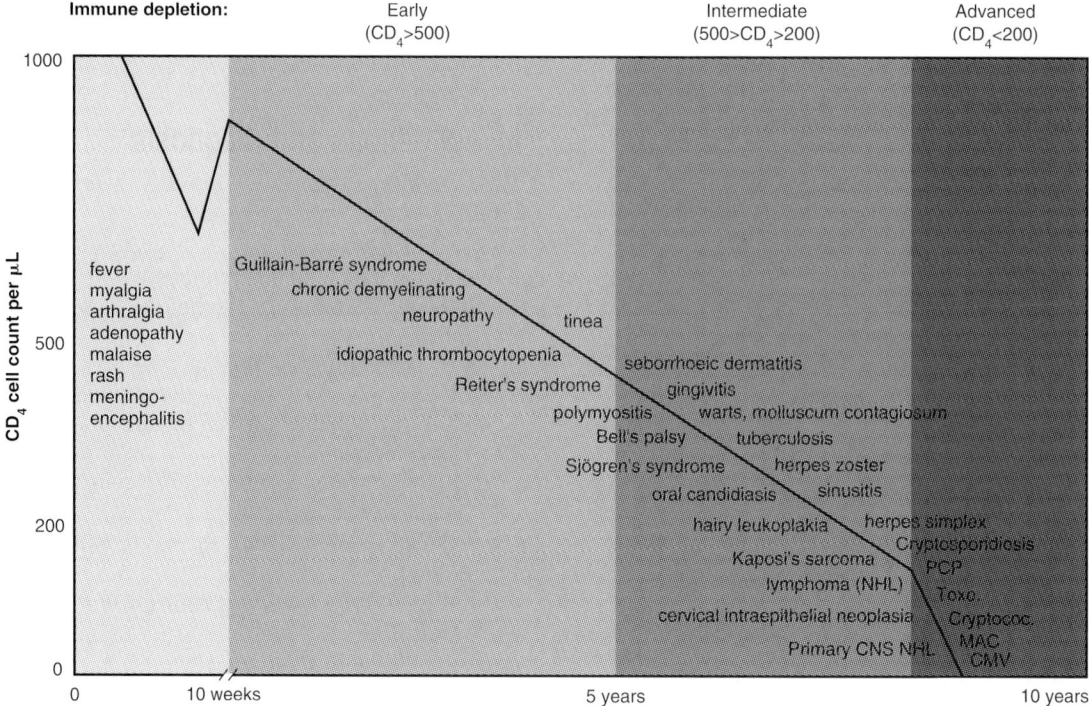

Fig 24.2 *Chronology of HIV-induced disease correlated with time since infection* G.J. STEWARD, COULD IT BE HIV? 1. THE CHALLENGE: CLINICAL DIAGNOSIS OF HIV, *THE MEDICAL JOURNAL OF AUSTRALIA*, 1993, 158:31–34 © COPYRIGHT 1993 *THE MEDICAL JOURNAL OF AUSTRALIA*. REPRODUCED WITH PERMISSION

- relaxation and meditation (reduction of and self-monitoring of stress levels)
- appropriate sleep and exercise
- consider supplementary antioxidants
- support groups and continuing counselling

Medication[8]

Optimal antiretroviral therapy now depends on the use of combinations of drugs. Monotherapy is no longer accepted practice. Refer to Table 24.4 for the summary of recommendations of the drugs for use in HIV infection. Viral resistance is the limiting factor, no matter how potent an individual drug may be at reducing viral load initially. The trials of combined zidovudine and lamivudine demonstrated both a more sustained decrease in plasma viral load than either drug did alone, and a more delayed development of viral resistance. There are now many antiretroviral drugs available for use in Australia (Table 24.5) and clinicians have a much wider scope of treatments available. However, many questions remain about combination therapy and further trials using viral load as a clinical endpoint should provide pointers for treatment.

Currently the use of 3 drugs is favoured. Subcutaneous injections of interleukin-2 have been shown to boost immunity.

The HIV test: the role of the family doctor

The astute general practitioner will use the opportunity of a request for an HIV test to explore preventive and sexual health issues. A full sexual history and drug history must incorporate the three C's of counselling, confidentiality and consent in the pretest interview.

Many HIV-positive patients have described how the results left them bewildered and devastated, especially with an unexpected positive result. Part of the reason given was the lack of any form of pretest counselling.

Initial consultation

- First establish why the patient is presenting 'now' for the test.
- Explore the 'hidden component' of the patient's consultation.

Table 24.4 *Summary of recommendations for the use of antiretroviral medication in HIV*

- Combination therapy is now standard best practice.
- Measurement of HIV-RNA viral load should be used to monitor risk of clinical progression, and to gauge effectiveness of therapy.
- Treatment is recommended when the patient is symptomatic, and when plasma HIV-RNA values exceed 5000–30 000 copies/mL, or when CD_4 count is below 500×10^6 cells/L.
- With mild to moderate immunodeficiency, treatment should be initiated with a two-drug combination of nucleoside RT inhibitors (e.g. AZT/DDC, AZT/3TC, D4T/3TC) or with 2 nucleoside and 1 non-nucleoside RT inhibitor (e.g. AZT/DDI/nevirapine).
- With moderate to severe immunosuppression or high viral loads, a three-drug combination (including a protease inhibitor) should be used.
- A change in treatment should be considered when the viral load returns to within 70% (0.5 log) of pretreatment values, or when there is a consistent fall in CD_4 count, or when new symptoms develop.
- A new regimen should include one or more (preferably two) new drugs that the patient has not previously used, and that are not cross resistant with the previous drugs.

Reproduced with permission[8]

- Take a full sexual, medical and drug-taking history. It is recognised that this can be embarrassing for both the doctor and the patient, but those experienced in this process advise the following approach:
    Establish a supportive, non-judgmental atmosphere. Encourage disclosure of history and patterns of partners and sexual practices in a gender-neutral situation. Make no assumptions about sexual preferences; they will be indicated by the patient as the history evolves, provided you allow this to happen; this will take time.
- Non-judgmental matter-of-fact questions such as 'Have you injected yourself with drugs?' and (to a male patient) 'Do you have sex with men?' may permit honest disclosure.
- Stress the importance of disclosure of prior, known infections with STDs. Assess the patient's risk for an STD.
- Assess the patient's coping strategies and social network.

Pretest counselling

- Give information on the test (what it tells and does not tell).
- Explain about the false negative and 'window period'.
- Give appropriate information about HIV disease and other STDs.
- Dispel any myths about transmission of infection.
- Give preventive advice on safer practices (sex and IV drugs).
- Assess the possible coping mechanisms of the patient.
- Assess the patient's social support networks and interpersonal bonds.
- Reassure about confidentiality. This is a legal requirement.
- Discuss who to tell: informing sexual contacts.
- Offer tests other than STDs.

Finally

- Discuss how patient 'will cope with the test'.
- Discuss legal requirements (check with state laws).
- Advise of need for informed consent (not only for HIV test but other STDs).
- Make arrangements to discuss the test results.

Consider the useful question: 'How would your behaviour change, if at all, as a result of having this test today?'

Test result (about 2 weeks later)

This must be given in consultation (whether positive or negative): avoid the telephone.

Table 24.5 *Currently available antiretroviral drugs*

Nucleoside analogue RT* inhibitors	Non-nucleoside analogue RT inhibitors	Protease inhibitors
• zidovudine (AZT) • didanosine (DDI) • zalcitabine (DDC) • stavudine (D4T) • lamivudine (3TC)	• nevirapine • delavirdine	• saquinavir • indinavir • ritonavir • nelfinavir

* RT = reverse transcriptase
Reproduced with permission[8]

The negative test result

- Provide reassurance.
- Emphasise the safe sex information.
- Counter any suggestion that current risk-taking behaviour is safe.
- Retest if in high-risk category or known HIV contact or in a 'window period' of 12 weeks.
- A test in 3 months helps rule out recent acquisition.
- Maintain confidentiality.

The positive test result

Good pretest history taking, risk assessment and counselling will make the task of informing the patient of a positive test result a lot easier. Being able to inform the patient of an improved prognosis due to combination drug therapy is also of assistance in breaking the news. Be warm and open. Many patients want to be touched for reassurance. The words 'you are not dying' can be firmly stated a few times. Educate the patient about the difference between HIV infection and the acquired immunodeficiency syndrome. Discuss with the patient who he or she is going to tell the result and help the patient decide on the most supportive friend. Ask the patient what he or she is going to do after the consultation and make an appointment for the next day. Give the patient an HIV support line number for overnight telephone support if required. Discuss the issue of contact tracing briefly and in more depth at the next consultation, because sexual contacts should be notified.

Start immediate post-test counselling and education. Emphasise that HIV-positive does not equal AIDS and need not lead to it in the short term.

Interview and full clinical assessment

- Assessment of general health
- Particular assessment of prior psychiatric history and confirm prior STDs and drugs
- Evidence of EBV (glandular fever), hepatitis B, HIV illness (acute seroconversion illness)
- Further counselling and discussion of specific problems
- Assessment of bonds and relationships with regard to support

Examination—to set a base level

- Full examination; skin, CNS—especially fundi, chest, abdomen and genitals; urine and lung function test
- Monitor temperature and weight

Blood tests—to set a base level and check immune status

- Repeat HIV antibody test (to eliminate possibility of error)
- CD_4 cells with FBE and a differential WCC
- viral load test
- G_6PD screen for enzyme deficiency
- Serology for syphilis (RPR), hepatitis B, toxoplasmosis, cytomegalovirus
- Test for gonorrhoea and chlamydia, herpes and thrush (if indicated)

Encourage a holistic approach to health maintenance and enhancement. Explore their feelings, anxieties, fears and confidentiality concerns. Reinforce safer practices.

The second post-positive result consultation (1–2 weeks later)

- Give results of repeat HIV test and base-line tests.
- Explore patient's understanding, feelings, coping abilities and spiritual issues (if appropriate).
- Some of the common questions that patients with HIV infection ask are:
  - Am I going to get sick?
  - How long will I live for?
  - Are there any treatments available?
  - Is there a cure around the corner?
  - What is going to happen to me?
  - Should I tell my friends?
  - Should I tell my family?
  - What are the social and legal issues?

It is worth pre-empting these questions and having ready appropriate answers for that particular patient.

- Give appropriate reassurance: prognosis may be much better, in respect of long remission, than appreciated.
- Discuss support systems.
- Check personal prophylaxis (safer sex and needle-sharing habits).
- Reinforce lifestyle strategies and suggest how patients can help themselves: give case examples.
- Recommend meditation and appropriate literature.
- Provide appropriate referrals (if needed):
  - specialist counsellors
  - self-help and support groups
  - meditation classes

- Advise patients about their legal and ethical responsibilities not to pass on the infection to others.
- Organise contact tracing.
- Address the difficult issue of telling sexual partners.
- If the patient is unwilling to inform sexual partners or is uncertain of who they may be, then contact-tracing organisations run through state government offices are of assistance in tracing sexual partners who may be at risk.
- If a patient refuses to inform a sexual partner of the risk then the doctor may disclose this information to the patient's partner in the following circumstances: if there is a clear risk of transmission; if the patient has been given education and counselling and this has been ignored; or if the doctor in the case has sought advice from colleagues and institutional ethics committee and before disclosure discussed it with the medical defence organisation. The doctor then should provide the patient with written advice that the patient must notify the partner, and if the patient still refuses to do so then the doctor has the right to do so.
- Discuss 'safer sex' guidelines. Condom usage is essential to prevent further viral loading and this needs to be explained, as well as the reason of protecting others.

Continuing maintenance consultations

- Provide appropriate support, encouragement and counselling.
- Frequency depends on CD_4 cell count (e.g. 3 to 6 monthly).
- Examination:
  — Check general condition, temperature and weight.
  — Look for unusual lung infection, diarrhoea, skin lesions, tongue and oropharynx, fevers, wasting and neurological signs.
  — Examine for signs of cytomegalovirus retinitis.
  — Look for early signs of AIDS-related dementia.
- Tests
  — CD_4 cell count and syphilis serology
  — viral load test
  — chest X-ray and induced sputum (if cough, SOB), faeces microculture if diarrhoea persists, Candida mouth swabs and herpes swabs appropriately
- Treat intercurrent illness (Table 24.6).

Contact tracing

Contacts of HIV-positive patients should be traced and offered testing with counselling.[5] Patients with HIV infection must be advised of the risk they pose to seronegative sexual partners. A person who has HIV or is at risk of HIV infection must not make any blood, semen or tissue donation. Because of the probable association between genital ulcerative disease and HIV transmission, the effective management of STDs is part of the general strategy for HIV control.

Prevention of HIV infection

1. *Counselling the person at risk re 'safer practices'*

No effective vaccine has been developed. Modification of behaviour is the only valid strategy for prevention of HIV infection. Education programs to encourage sexual practices that reduce the exchange of genital secretions (safe sex) may achieve risk reduction for sexually active individuals. Condoms provide a barrier if used properly and consistently but may be too easily damaged to offer reliable protection during anal intercourse. A water-based lubricant such as KY gel or Lubafax should be used: oil-based lubricants such as Vaseline weaken condoms.

Discuss alternative sex practices including touching, cuddling, body-to-body rubbing and mutual masturbation.

Emphasise the importance of being in control with drug taking, IV usage, safe sex practices and the needle-exchange program.

2. *Health professionals*

Care should be exercised whenever blood samples are taken or sharps have been used. Advise safe disposal of sharps and other disposables and appropriate sterilisation of material. Gloves should be worn for all invasive procedures. Management of needle-stick injuries and other at-risk exposures is described in Chapter 116.

Community education

Educating the community in a non-emotional, responsible way about AIDS should be a priority. While the personal, community and global benefits of effective AIDS education are

Table 24.6   *General practice treatment of HIV-related dermathopathy*

Dermatoses	Treatment
Common	
Oral candidiasis	miconazole oral gel or amphotericin lozenges or nystatin lozenges
Hairy leukoplakia on tongue	no treatment or aciclovir
Seborrhoeic dermatitis, e.g. nasolabial folds, hairy areas	miconazole 2% or ketoconazole 2% hydrocortisone 1% (if very itchy)
Itchy folliculitis	oral antihistamines miconazole +hydrocortisone topical
Less common	
Perianal herpes simplex	Mild: topical aciclovir cream (if available) Betadine or silver nitrate Severe: aciclovir 200 mg 5 times daily
Molluscum contagiosum	needle incision then Betadine or liquid nitrogen
Candidal angular stomatitis	clotrimazole or miconazole cream
Herpes zoster	Mild: menthol in flexible collodion Severe: refer for IV aciclovir
Severe tinea pedis	topical clotrimazole or miconazole ketoconazole 200 mg (o) daily

Source: After Pohl[4]

generally acknowledged, the fear of addressing such a sensitive issue sometimes results in failure to act.[9] AIDS education in schools in particular can be an important strategy. People with HIV infection would be appropriate resource educators and the use of videos would be a most appropriate medium for education.

When to refer[11]

Most patients with HIV disease need referral to a specialist or clinic that can manage the patient expertly and sympathetically.

Referral should take place at the time of:
- onset of a life-threatening opportunistic infection
- the need to initiate antiretroviral drug therapy
- administration of prophylactic pentamidine aerosol therapy
- serious psychological problems related to HIV-positive status.

References

1. Stewart GJ. The challenge: the clinical diagnosis of HIV. Med J Aust, 1993, 158: 31–34.
2. Boyle MJ, McMurchie M, Tindall B, Cooper D. HIV seroconversion illness. Med J Aust, 1993; 158:42–44.
3. Kumar P, Clark M. *Clinical medicine* (2nd edn). London: Bailliere Tindall, 1990, 68–73.
4. Pohl M. Managing HIV patients in general practice. Patient Management, June 1989; 49–61.
5. NH&MRC. *Handbook on sexually transmitted diseases.* Canberra: Department of Community Services and Health, 1990, 1–55.
6. McCoy R. Alarm bells. When to worry about your patient with HIV. Aust Fam Physician, 1997; 26:803–809.
7. Kaldor JM, Crofts N. Epidemiological surveillance for HIV and AIDS. Med J Aust, 1996; 165:268–271.

8. Bradford D. Update on issues for HIV management. Aust Fam Physician, 1997; 26:812–817.

9. World Health Organisation report. *AIDS prevention through health promotion*. Geneva: WHO, 1991, 68–73.

10. Mashford ML (Chairman). *Antibiotic guidelines* (9th edn). VMPF Therapeutics Committee, 1996–97, 82–86.

11. Bradford DL. Acquired immune deficiency syndrome. In: MIMS Index (2nd edn). Sydney: IMS Publishing, 1996, 1–5.

Acknowledgment
Part of this text, including clinical manifestations, prevention and contact tracing is reproduced from the *Handbook on sexually transmitted diseases*.[5] Commonwealth of Australia copyright, reproduced by permission.

25

Baffling viral and protozoal infections

—

Our lot is a perilous age . . . but where shall we fly to escape from pestilences that come and pestilences that do not come, from ships that bring us yellow fever, from cattle diseases that can only be exterminated by exterminating the cattle, from infectious patients whose pulses must be felt with a pair of tongs and their chests explored with tarred stethoscopes.

Jacob Bigelow 1860

Almost any infection, especially if subacute or insidious in its onset, can be baffling and can belong to the 'fever of undetermined origin' group of infections. Syphilis and tuberculosis were the great mimics of the past. Now malaria and Epstein-Barr mononucleosis can be regarded as important mimics. Epstein-Barr mononucleosis (syn: infectious mononucleosis, glandular fever) can be a perennial baffler and can be confused with HIV infection in its primary clinical phase. Any of the febrile diseases can be confusing before declaring themselves with classical symptoms such as the jaundice of hepatitis or the rash of dengue fever, or before serological tests become positive.

Viral and protozoal infections that can present as masquerades include:

- HIV infection (especially primary)
- Epstein-Barr mononucleosis (EBM)
- TORCH organisms
  — toxoplasmosis
  — rubella
  — cytomegalovirus (CMV)
  — herpes simplex virus
- Hepatitis A,B,C,D,E

- Mosquito-borne infections
  — malaria
  — dengue fever
  — yellow fever
  — Japanese encephalitis
  — Ross River fever

The TORCH organisms (TORCH being an acronym for toxoplasmosis, rubella, cytomegalovirus and herpes) are well known for their adverse intrauterine effects on the foetus. Three are viral (toxoplasmosis is a Protozoa) and the first three of these foetal pathogens are acquired by passage across the placenta. Most of these organisms are noted for being opportunistic infections in immunocompromised patients, especially in later stage HIV infection.

The mosquito-borne infections are mainly viral, apart from the Protozoa causing malaria, and are of particular significance in travellers returning from endemic areas.

Four similar clinical presentations

The four infections (EMB, primary HIV, CMV and toxoplasmosis) produce almost identical clinical presentations and tend to be diagnosed as glandular fever or pseudoglandular fever. It is important for the first contact practitioner to consider all four possibilities, especially keeping in mind the possibility of HIV infection.

A worthwhile approach is to make a provisional diagnosis based on the clinical variations as presented in Table 25.1.

Screening tests are:

- Full blood count, especially WCC

Table 25.1 *Clinical features differentiating HIV, EBV, CMV and toxoplasmosis infections (all can present with a similar illness)*

Feature	EBV infection	HIV infection	CMV infection	Toxoplasmosis
Onset	Insidious	Acute	Insidious	Insidious or acute
Fever	A feature Intermittent	A feature	Quotidian (afternoon spikes)	Low grade
Fatigue/malaise	Common	Common, severe	Common	Common
Tonsillar hypertrophy	Common	Mild enlargement	Uncommon	Uncommon
Exudative pharyngitis	Common	Rare	Rare	Occurs
Mucocutaneous ulcers	Rare	Common	Unknown	Unknown
Skin rash	About 5%	Common	About 5%	About 10%
Jaundice	About 8%	Rare	Uncommon	Uncommon
Diarrhoea	Unknown	Occurs	Unknown	Unknown
Cervical lymphadenopathy	Common	Common	Uncommon	Common (a feature)
Hepatomegaly	About 8%	Rare	Common	Occasional
Splenomegaly	About 50%	Rare	About 50%	Up to 30%
Atypical lymphocytes	In 80–90%	In < 50%	Common	Uncommon

- Paul Bunnell test (for heterophil antibodies)
- Serological test for cytomegalovirus (specific antibodies)
- Serological test for toxoplasmosis (specific antibodies)
- HIV antibody test (ELISA)

Epstein-Barr mononucleosis

Epstein-Barr mononucleosis (infectious mononucleosis, glandular fever) (EBM) is a febrile illness caused by the herpes (Epstein-Barr) virus. It can mimic diseases such as HIV primary infection, streptococcal tonsillitis, viral hepatitis and acute lymphatic leukaemia. There are three forms: the febrile, the anginose (with sore throat) and the glandular (with lymphadenopathy).

It may occur at any age but usually between 10 and 35 years, commonest in 15–25 year old age group.

The typical clinical features are presented in Table 25.2 and Figure 25.1.

Epidemiology

EB mononucleosis has an annual incidence of 4–5 new cases in a population of 2500.[3] It usually affects people in their late teenage years or early twenties. It is endemic in most countries. Subclinical infection is common in young children.

The incubation period is at least one month but data are insufficient to define it accurately.

Epstein-Barr virus is excreted in oropharangeal secretions during the illness and for some months (sometimes years) after the clinical infection. EBM has a low infectivity and isolation is not necessary. It is apparently transmitted only by close contact such as kissing and sharing drinking vessels.

Progress of the primary infection is checked partly by specific antibodies (which might prevent cell-to-cell spread of the virus) and partly by a cellular immune response, involving cytotoxic T cells, which eliminates the infected cells. This response accounts for the clinical picture. The virus is never eliminated from the body.

Second attacks and fatalities do occur and there is a possible association between EBM and lymphoma.[3]

The rash

The rash of EBM is almost always related to antibiotics given for tonsillitis. The primary rash, most often non-specific, pinkish and maculopapular (similar to that of rubella), occurs in about 5% of cases only.

The secondary rash is most often precipitated by one of the penicillins, especially ampicillin or

Table 25.2 *Clinical features of EBM[1,2]*

Symptoms

- slow onset malaise 1–6 weeks
- fever
- myalgia
- headaches, anorexia
- blocked nose—mouth breathing
- nasal quality to voice
- sore throat (85%)
- nausea ± vomiting
- rash—primary 5%
- dyspepsia

Clinical findings

- exudative pharyngitis (84%)
- petechiae of palate (not pathognomonic) (11%)
- lymphadenopathy, especially posterior cervical
- rash—maculopapular
- splenomegaly (50%)
- jaundice ± hepatomegaly (5–10%)
- clinical or biochemical evidence of hepatitis

amoxycillin. About 90–100% of patients prescribed ampicillin or amoxycillin will be affected; up to 50% of those given penicillin will develop the rash. It can be extensive and sometimes has a purplish tinge.

The complications of EB mononucleosis are presented in Table 25.3 and the differential diagnoses in Table 25.4.

Laboratory diagnosis

The following confirm the diagnosis of EB mononucleosis.

- White cell count shows absolute lymphocytosis.
- Blood film shows atypical lymphocytes.
- Paul Bunnell test for heterophil antibody is positive (although positivity can be delayed or absent in 10% of cases).
- Diagnosis confirmed (if necessary) by EBV-specific antibodies, viral capsule antigen (VCA) antibodies—IgM, IgG.

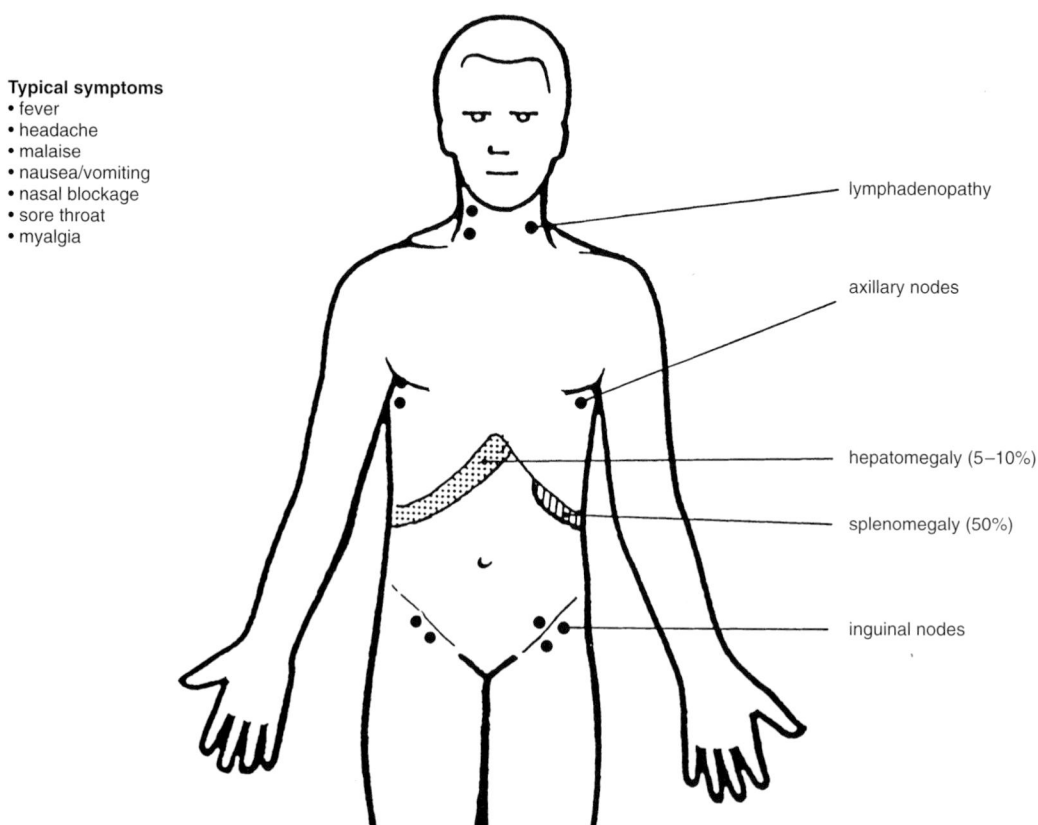

Typical symptoms
- fever
- headache
- malaise
- nausea/vomiting
- nasal blockage
- sore throat
- myalgia

lymphadenopathy

axillary nodes

hepatomegaly (5–10%)

splenomegaly (50%)

inguinal nodes

Fig. 25.1 *Clinical features of Epstein-Barr mononucleosis*

Table 25.3 *Complications of EB mononucleosis*[1]

Common
- antibiotic-induced skin rash
- prolonged debility
- hepatitis
- depression

Rare

Cardiac
- myocarditis
- pericarditis

Haematological
- agranulocytosis
- haemolytic anaemia
- thrombocytopenia

Respiratory tract
- upper airway obstruction (lymphoid hypertrophy)

Miscellaneous
- ruptured spleen

Neurological
- cranial nerve palsies, especially facial palsy
- Guillain-Barré syndrome
- meningoencephalitis
- transverse myelitis

Table 25.4 *Differential diagnoses of EB mononucleosis*[1]

Other agents that cause typical EBM syndrome
- HIV infection (acute initial illness)
- cytomegalovirus
- toxoplasmosis

Exudative tonsillitis resembling EBM
- acute streptococcal pharyngitis
- adenovirus infection
- diphtheria (unlikely in Australia)

Hepatitis A,B,C,D,E

Lymphadenopathy, fever and splenomegaly
- lymphoma
- leukaemia

Complications of EBM without other manifestations
- encephalitis

Others
- drug reaction
- influenza

However culture for Epstein-Barr virus and tests for specific virus antibodies are not done routinely.

False positives for Paul Bunnell test:
- hepatitis
- Hodgkin's disease
- acute leukaemia

Prognosis
EBM usually runs an uncomplicated course over 6–8 weeks. Major symptoms subside within 2–3 weeks. Patients should be advised to take about 4 weeks off work.

Treatment
- supportive measures (no specific treatment)
- rest (the best treatment) during the acute stage, preferably at home and indoors
- aspirin or paracetamol to relieve discomfort
- gargle soluble aspirin or 30% glucose to soothe the throat
- advise against alcohol, fatty foods, continued activity especially contact sports (risk of splenic rupture)
- ensure adequate hydration
- corticosteroids for:
  — neurological involvement
  — thrombocytopenia
  — threatened airway obstruction

Post-EBM malaise
Some young adults remain debilitated and depressed for some months. Lassitude and malaise may extend up to a year or so.

Cytomegalovirus infection
Cytomegalovirus (CMV) has a worldwide distribution and causes infections that are generally asymptomatic. The virus (human herpes virus 5) may be cultured from various sites of healthy individuals. It has its most severe effects in the immunocompromised, especially those with AIDS, and also in recipients of solid organ transplants and bone marrow grafts; 90% of AIDS patients are infected with CMV and 95% have disseminated CMV at autopsy. CMV infection can be an important development following massive blood transfusion, including those given to infants. The incubation period of CMV ranges from 20 to 60 days and the illness generally lasts about 2 to 6 weeks.[4]

Clinical features
Three important clinical manifestations are described.

1. Perinatal disease

Intrauterine infection may cause serious abnormalities in the foetus including CNS involvement (microcephaly, hearing defects, motor disturbances), jaundice, hepatosplenomegaly, haemolytic anaemia and thrombocytopenia. Up to 30% of CMV-affected infants have mental retardation.[5]

2. Acquired CMV infection

In healthy adults CMV produces an illness similar to Epstein-Barr mononucleosis with fever, malaise, arthralgia and myalgia, generalised lymphadenopathy and hepatomegaly. However, cervical lymphadenopathy and exudative pharyngitis are rare.

The infection may be spread by blood transfusion, and CMV should be suspected on clinical grounds in a patient with a febrile illness resembling EBM following major surgery such as open heart surgery or renal transplantation and where extensive transfusion has been necessary.

The fever often manifests as quotidian intermittent fever spiking to a maximum in the mid-afternoon and falling to normal each day (Fig. 25.2). There is often a relative lymphocytosis with atypical lymphocytes but the heterophil antibody test is negative. Liver function tests are often abnormal. Specific diagnosis can be made by demonstrating rising antibody titres. The virus can be isolated from the urine and blood.

Fig. 25.2 *Cytomegalovirus infection: typical quotidian intermittent fever pattern*

3. CMV disease in the immunocompromised host

Disseminated CMV infection occurs in the immune-deficient person, notably HIV infection causing opportunistic severe pneumonia, retinitis (a feature of AIDS), encephalitis and diffuse involvement of the gastrointestinal tract.

Treatment

In the patient with normal immunity no treatment apart from supportive measures is required, as the infection is usually self-limiting. In immunosuppressed patients various antiviral drugs such as ganciclovir and foscarnet have been used with some benefit.

Toxoplasmosis

Toxoplasmosis, which is caused by *Toxoplasma gondii*, an obligate intracellular protozoan, is worldwide, albeit a rare infection. The definitive host in its life cycle is the cat (or pig or sheep) and the human is an intermediate host. However, clinical toxoplasmosis is very uncommon. Infection in humans usually occurs through eating foodstuffs contaminated by infected cat faeces. Its main clinical importance is an opportunistic infection.

The five major clinical forms of toxoplasmosis are:[6]

1. asymptomatic lymphadenopathy (the commonest)
2. lymphadenopathy with a febrile illness, similar to EB mononucleosis
3. acute primary infection: a febrile illness similar to acute leukaemia or EB mononucleosis; a rash, myocarditis, pneumonitis, chorioretinitis and hepatosplenomegaly can occur
4. neurological abnormalities: includes headache and neck stiffness, sore throat and myalgia
5. congenital toxoplasmosis: this is a rare problem but if it occurs it typically causes CNS involvement and has a poor prognosis

In the immunocompromised, clinical forms 3 and 4 are typical features with meningoencephalitis being a serious development.

Diagnosis

Diagnosis is by serological tests, which are sensitive and reliable.

Treatment

Patients with a mild illness or with asymptomatic infection require no treatment. Children under 5 years may be treated to avoid the possible occurrence of chorioretinitis. Symptomatic patients are treated with pyrimethamine plus sulphadiazine. Spiramycin is usually used in pregnant patients.

Malaria

Malaria, a protozoal infection, is an important masquerade and mimic. The diagnosis requires a high index of suspicion in a traveller returning from an endemic area (see p. 99 for more details).

In humans malaria is caused by four species of plasmodium:

- *Plasmodium vivax* and *P. ovale*—tertian malaria
- *P. falciparum*—malignant tertian malaria
- *P. malariae*—quartan malaria

Some clinical features

- It has an incubation period of 7 to 40 days.
- Most present within 2 months of returning from malaria area.
- It can present after 2 or more years.
- It is an acute febrile illness with headache.
- It can have atypical presentations such as gastrointestinal symptoms (diarrhoea, nausea, vomiting, abdominal pains), dry cough and arthralgia
- Typical relapsing patterns may be absent.

Special notes

- Beware of treatment-modified infection.
- Early diagnosis is essential as it must be treated within 4 days.

Diagnosis

Diagnosis is with thick and thin smears. Two or three blood samples should be taken each day for 3 to 4 days and found to be negative before a patient is declared malaria-free. The presence of monocytosis is a helpful diagnostic pointer.

Amoebiasis

Amoebiasis can be diagnosed in a sick traveller returning from an endemic area with severe diarrhoea characterised by blood and mucus. Complications include fulminating colitis, amoebomas (a mass of fibrotic granulation tissue) in the bowel and liver abscess.

Amoebic liver abscess

Clinical features

- high swinging fever
- profound malaise and anorexia
- tender hepatomegaly
- effusion or consolidation of base of right chest

There is often no history of dysentery, and jaundice is unusual. Diagnosis is by serological tests for amoeba and by imaging (CT scan). Treatment is with metronidazole and by percutaneous CT guided aspiration.

Dengue fever

Also known as 'breakbone fever', dengue is an arthropod-borne viral disease found mainly in Asia and Africa (see pp. 100–101). The features are the acute onset of fever, headache, retrobulbar pain, severe backache and aching of muscles and joints. Lymphadenopathy, petechiae on the soft palate and skin rashes may occur.

The diagnosis of dengue is based on clinical suspicion and also viral isolation by tissue culture in sera obtained early in the disease. Severe fatigue and depression (with suicidal risk) is a feature of convalescence. The patients are managed symptomatically and with support and reassurance.

Japanese encephalitis

This viral illness is also acquired overseas, especially in South-East Asia and the Far East. The onset is heralded by severe rigors, fever, headache and malaise. The encephalitic stage is marked by fever, neck rigidity and neurological signs such as altered consciousness and convulsions. Coma can follow. Diagnosis is by specific antibody detection. Treatment is symptomatic.

Yellow fever

This viral illness, acquired in the tropical areas of Africa and South America, can have a variety of presentations. If yellow fever is mild it resembles influenza. However, the typical clinical features are a febrile illness—(high fever, headache, flushed face, arthralgia, GIT symptoms, relative bradycardia (Faget's sign))— followed by apparent recovery and then the classical features of fever, deepening jaundice, proteinuria and bleeding from the gums.

Ross River fever

Epidemic polyarthritis or Ross River virus, which is an alpha virus, occurs in all states of Australia. It is most prevalent in mosquito-prone areas (especially during the summer) and in tropical and temperate coastal regions and inland riverine areas.[7] Subclinical infection is common with variable clinical manifestations.

Clinical features

- all age groups especially 20–30 years
- incubation period 3–21 days (usually 7–11)

Major symptoms

- polyarthritis (75% of patients), mainly fingers, wrists, feet, ankles and knees
- maculopapular rash—widespread, often 'subtle', mainly trunk and limbs
- myalgia

Other symptoms

- pyrexia (mild)
- headache
- nausea
- fatigue with exercise

Signs (which may be present) include joint swelling (mainly hands and feet), tenosynovitis around the wrists and ankles (poor prognostic sign), the rash and mild lymphadenopathy.

Outcome

In many patients the illness resolves within 2 to 4 weeks and most feel normal within 3 months, but some with a more severe arthritis can enter a chronic phase lasting 18 months or more.

Diagnosis

Diagnosis is by antibody testing of serum. The differential diagnosis includes other viral infections that cause arthritis such as hepatitis B, rubella, Barmah Forest virus (a mosquito-borne virus) and dengue, and early rheumatoid arthritis and rheumatic fever.

Treatment

Treatment is symptomatic with bed rest and simple analgesics such as aspirin. NSAIDs are used for more severe cases. Oral corticosteroids are effective but should be avoided if possible.

Deadly infections (worldwide)

The World Health Organisation in its 1996 report[8] estimated that the leading cause of approximately 50 million deaths in the world in 1995 was infectious diseases, which accounted for about one-third or 17 million deaths. Other figures included diseases of the circulatory system (15 million deaths including ischaemic heart disease—7.2 million—and stroke—4.6 million) and cancer 6.2 million deaths (approximately 12%).

The report indicated that nearly 50 000 people are dying every day from infectious diseases such as cholera, malaria and tuberculosis. At least 30 new infections have emerged in the past 20 years, and for many of them there is no treatment, cure or vaccine. These include rotavirus (which causes infant diarrhoea), *Legionella pneumophila*, *Lyme borreliosis* (Lyme disease), the Wantaan virus (which can cause a fatal haemorrhagic fever), HIV and hepatitis E and C.

The report also said that until recently the struggle for control over infectious diseases had seemed almost over, with smallpox eradicated and six other diseases, including polio, leprosy and guinea-worm disease, singled out for eradication within a few years. However, half the

Table 25.5 *The world's deadliest infectious diseases*

Infectious disease	Cause	Annual deaths
1. Acute lower respiratory infections (mostly pneumonia)	Bacterial or viral	4 400 000 (approx. 4 m children)
2. Diarrhoeal diseases	Bacterial or viral	3 100 000
3. Tuberculosis	Bacterial	3 100 000
4. Malaria	Protozoal	2 100 000
5. Hepatitis B	Viral	1 100 000
6. HIV/AIDS	Viral	1 100 000
7. Measles	Viral	1 000 000
8. Neonatal tetanus	Bacterial	460 000
9. Pertussis	Bacterial	355 000
10. Intestinal worm disease		135 000

Source: World Health Organisation 1995 figures

world's 5.72 billion were at risk of many infectious diseases since many that seemed under control such as tuberculosis and malaria were becoming more prevalent. Some such as yellow fever and cholera were striking in new regions. Other infections were resistant to drugs and virtually untreatable. The previously almost forgotten diseases such as yersinia (the plague) had re-emerged.

The deadly haemorrhagic fevers that have broken out in isolated endemics include the zoonotic African diseases—Ebola haemorrhagic fever, Marburg haemorrhagic fever and Lassa fever. These are caused by filoviruses and for most no specific treatment is available.

Another serious infection that emerged sporadically was the so called 'flesh eating' Streptococcus A infection, which was a particularly virulent strain causing localised destruction of soft tissue.

The lessons to be learned include careful surveillance, attention to prevention especially with effective immunisation programs, rational antibiotic prescribing and care with travelling to developing tropical countries.

Prion transmitted diseases

Prions are proteinaceous infectious particles devoid of nucleic acid that can present with a wide spectrum of clinical neurological manifestations. The feature is transmissible spongiform encepalopathy with Creutzfeld–Jakob disease being the classic example. Transmission is from contaminated human tissue eg. corneal graft, cadaver pituitary human gonadotrophin or eating contaminated beef.

Classical clinical features:
- progressive dementia (starts with memory loss)
- myoclonus
- fatigue and somnolence
- variable neurological features eg. ataxia

References

1. Dwyer D. Mononucleosis syndrome. In: MIMS Disease Index (2nd edn). Sydney: IMS Publishing, 1996, 317–320.
2. Mead M, Patterson H. *Tutorials in general practice*. London: Pitman, 1983; 3–4.
3. Fry J. *Common diseases*: Lancaster: MTP Press, 1992, 85–90.
4. Wilson J et al. *Harrison's principles of internal medicine* (12th edn). New York: McGraw Hill, 1991, 613–695.
5. Tierney LM et al. *Current medical diagnosis and treatment* (35th edn). Stamford: Appleton & Lange, 1996, 1165–1167.
6. Kumar PJ, Clark ML. *Clinical medicine* (2nd edn). London: Bailliere Tindall, 1990, 83–84.
7. Whitby M. Ross River fever. In: MIMS Disease Index (2nd edn). Sydney: IMS Publishing, 1996, 452–453.
8. WHO. Annual Report, Geneva, May 1996.

26
Baffling bacterial infections

—

In its beginning the malady is easier to cure but difficult to detect, but later it becomes easy to detect but difficult to cure.

Niccolo Machiavelli (1469–1527)
On tuberculosis

Bacterial infections can present diagnostic brain-teasers, and a high index of suspicion is needed to pinpoint the diagnosis. Many are rarely encountered, thus making diagnosis more difficult yet demanding vigilance and clinical flexibility.

The list includes:

- syphilis
- tuberculosis
- infective endocarditis
- the zoonoses, e.g. brucellosis, Lyme disease
- clostridial infections
  — tetanus
  — gas gangrene
  — puerperal infection
  — botulism
- hidden suppuration
  — abscess
  — osteomyelitis
- mycoplasma infections
  — atypical pneumonia
- *Chlamydia* infections
  — psittacosis
  — non-specific arthritis
  — pelvic inflammatory disease
  — trachoma
  — atypical pneumonia
- legionnaires' disease

Chlamydia and rickettsial organisms have been confirmed as being small bacterial organisms.

Syphilis

Although syphilis is uncommon in the general population it is extremely common in certain Aboriginal groups and is frequently acquired from homosexual activity or sexual contacts overseas.[1]

It presents either as a primary lesion or through the chance finding of positive syphilis serology. Family physicians should be alert to the various manifestations of secondary syphilis, which can cause difficulties in diagnosis. Congenital syphilis is rare where there is general serological screening of antenatal patients.

Clinical manifestations[2]

Primary syphilis
The primary lesion or chancre usually develops at the point of inoculation after an incubation period averaging 21 days. The chancre is typically firm, painless, punched out and clean. The adjacent lymph nodes are discretely enlarged, firm and non-suppurating. Anorectal changes may occur in homosexual men.

Untreated, early clinical syphilis usually resolves spontaneously within 4 weeks, leading to latent disease which may proceed to late destructive lesions.

Secondary syphilis
The interval between the appearance of the primary chancre and the onset of secondary manifestations varies from 6 to 8 weeks. Constitutional symptoms including fever, headache, malaise and general aches and pains may precede or accompany the signs of secondary syphilis.

The most common feature of the secondary stage of infection is a rash, which is present in about 80% of cases. The rash is typically a symmetrical, generalised, coppery red maculo-papular eruption on face, palms and soles and is neither itchy nor tender. It can resemble any skin disease except those characterised by vesicles. Other features may be:

- condylomata lata, which are broad-based, moist, warty or papular growths occurring in skin folds or creases
- patchy alopecia (scalp, outer third of eyebrow)
- oral, pharyngeal or vulvovaginal ulcers or 'mucous patches', which are round lesions with a greyish-white base edged by a dull red areola which may coalesce to produce a serpiginous ulcer—the 'snail-track ulcer'
- lymphadenopathy characterised by firm, enlarged painless nodes typically involving inguinal, suboccipital, posterior cervical, axillary and preauricular groups.

Latent syphilis

Positive serology in a patient without symptoms or signs of disease is referred to as latent syphilis and is the commonest presentation of syphilis in Australia today. Possibly because of the wide-spread use of antibiotics the infection often proceeds to the latent stage without a recognised primary or secondary stage.

Late syphilis

Tertiary manifestation of syphilis, which is very rare, may be 'benign' with development of gummas (granulomatous lesions) in almost any organ, or more serious with cardiovascular or central nervous system involvement. Benign gummatous disease is rare but cardiovascular disease and neurosyphilis occasionally occur. Careful management and follow-up of patients with early or latent disease is essential to prevent late sequelae.

Late syphilis should be excluded in any patient with aortic incompetence or dilatation of the ascending arch of the aorta. Syphilis should be excluded as the cause of dementia, person-ality change, multifocal neurological disorders, nerve deafness, pupillary abnormalities, retinal disease or uveitis.

Think of syphilis

Syphilis should not be overlooked as a cause of oral or anorectal lesions. The diagnosis of syph-ilis depends on a detailed history, careful clinical examination and specific examinations.

Underlying these approaches is the need to think of the possibility of syphilis for concurrent STDs.

Syphilis and HIV infection[2]

HIV and syphilis are commonly associated. In patients with AIDS and syphilis, standard regimens for syphilis are not always curative. Seronegative syphilis has been reported in patients with HIV infection. Lymphadenopathy in a patient with HIV infection may be due to coexisting secondary syphilis.

Diagnostic tests

Dark field examination[2]

Spirochaetes can be demonstrated by micro-scopic examination of smears from early lesions using dark-field techniques and provide an immediate diagnosis in symptomatic syphilis. Antibiotics or antiseptics should not be used until satisfactory examination has been com-pleted. Dark-field examination has relatively low sensitivity and is not suitable for oral lesions. The direct fluorescent antibody techniques (FTA–ABS) can be used on this smear.

Serology

Serological tests provide indirect evidence of infection, and the diagnosis of asymptomatic syphilis relies heavily on these tests. The two main types of tests are:

- Reagin tests (VDRL and RPR)—not specific for syphilis but useful for screening
- Treponemal tests (TPHA, FTA–ABS)—specific tests, with the latter being sensitive and widely used.

Treatment: refer to Chapter 98.

Tuberculosis

Tuberculosis, caused by *Mycobacterium tubercu-losis*, still has a worldwide distribution with a very high prevalence in Asian countries where 60–80% of children below the age of 14 years are affected.[3] This has special implication in Australia where large numbers of Asian migrants are settling. The WHO estimates that one-third of the world's population is infected by the tubercle bacillus.

Tuberculosis can be a mimic of other diseases and a high level of suspicion is necessary to consider the diagnosis, especially if there are extrapulmonary manifestations. There may be no symptoms or signs, even in advanced disease.

Primary infection
The primary infection usually involves the lungs. The focus is usually subpleural in the upper to mid zones and is almost always accompanied by lymph node involvement.

Erythema nodosum may accompany the primary infection. Primary TB is symptomless in most cases although there may be a vague illness associated with a cough. In most people this pulmonary focus heals but leaves some surviving tubercle bacilli, even if it becomes calcified.

Progressive primary tuberculosis
If the immune response is inadequate, progressive primary TB develops, with constitutional and pulmonary symptoms. Rarely haematogenous spread can occur to the lungs ('miliary tuberculosis'), to the pleural space (tuberculosis pleural effusion) or to extrapulmonary sites such as the meninges and bone.

Post-primary or adult-type pulmonary TB
Most cases of TB in adults are due to reactivation of disease some years later and not to reinfection. The factors causing this include poor social living conditions with malnutrition, diabetes and other factors lowering natural immunity such as immunosuppressant drugs, corticosteroids, lymphoma and HIV infection (later stage).

Reactivated pulmonary TB
This usually presents with constitutional symptoms of poor health and night sweats, and a cough that is initially dry but may become productive and be bloodstained (see p. 383). Sometimes the infection will be asymptomatic.

Extrapulmonary TB
The main sites of extrapulmonary disease (in order of frequency in Australia) are the lymph nodes (the commonest, especially in young adults and children), genitourinary tract (kidney, epididymis, Fallopian tubes), pleura and pericardium, the skeletal system (arthritis and oestomyelitis with cold abscess formation), central nervous system (meningitis and tuberculomas), the eye (choroiditis, iridocyclitis), the skin (lupus vulgaris), and the adrenal glands (Addison's

disease), gastrointestinal tract (ileocaecal area and peritoneum).

These sites are illustrated in Figure 26.1.

Miliary tuberculosis
This disorder follows diffuse dissemination of tubercle bacilli via the bloodstream and is fatal without treatment. It can occur within 3 years of the primary infection or much later because of reactivation.

Diagnosis of TB
A high index of suspicion is critical for the diagnosis of TB.
- Mantoux test (a guide only)
- chest X-ray; CT scan if doubtful
- sputum for stain (acid fast bacilli)
- sputum for culture (takes about 6 weeks but important)
- immunochromatographic fingerprick test (new and promising)
- biopsies on lesions/lymph nodes ⎫ may be
- fibre optic bronchoscopy to ⎬ necessary
  obtain sputum ⎭
- consider HIV studies

Tuberculin (Mantoux) testing and BCG vaccination
A tuberculin (Mantoux) test should be performed prior to BCG vaccination in all individuals over 6 months of age. (It is read at 48–72 hours.)

If area of induration:
- < 5 mm—negative (*Note*: may be negative in presence of very active pulmonary infection)
- 5–10 mm: typical of past BCG vaccination
- > 5 mm—significant in immunocompromised, close contacts and HIV infection
- > 10 mm—positive = tuberculosis infection (active or inactive)
- > 15 mm—highly significant for 'normal' people

The BCG vaccination should be given if reaction < 5 mm induration.

BCG recommended for:
- Aboriginal and Torres Strait Islander neonates in regions of high incidence
- neonates born to patients with leprosy
- children < 5 years travelling for long periods to countries of high TB prevalence

BCG considered for:
- neonates in household with immigrants or visitors recently arrived from countries of high

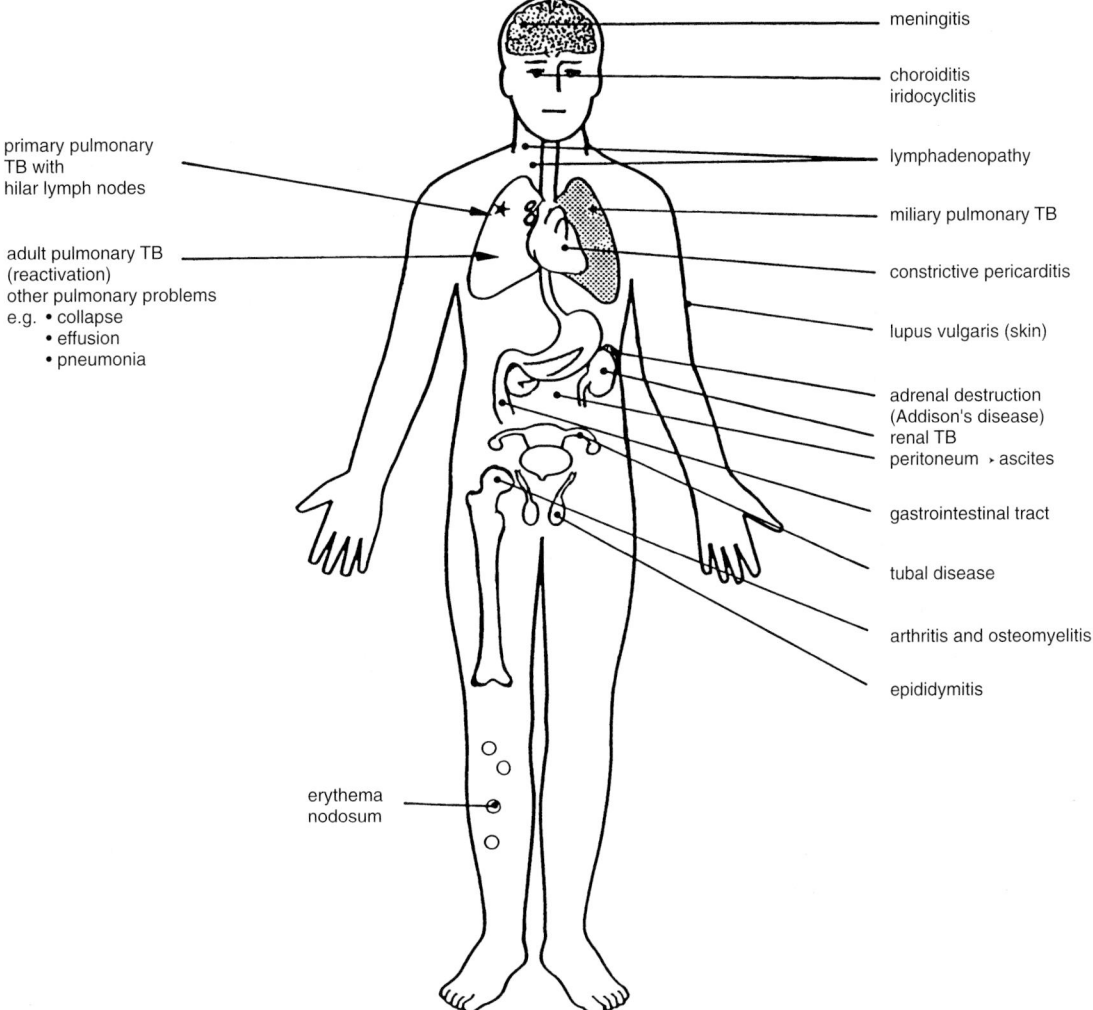

Fig. 26.1 *Pulmonary and extrapulmonary distribution of tuberculosis: the primary infection starts in the lung and then spread can occur throughout the body, especially to lymph nodes*

prevalance e.g. South-East Asia (*Note*: tuberculin test not necessary for neonates < 14 days)
- children and adolescents < 16 years with continued exposure to active TB patient and where isonizid therapy contraindicated
- others at increased risk (and where value of BCG vaccine uncertain), e.g. health care workers, travellers > 5 years with significant exposure

BCG contraindicated for:
- tuberculin reactions > 5 mm
- immunocompromised or malignancies involving bone marrow lymphatics
- high-risk HIV infection
- significant fever or intercurrent illness
- generalised skin diseases including keloid tendency
- pregnancy
- previous infection

Treatment

The current antimicrobial treatment is to use 4 antituberculous drugs (rifampicin + isoniazid + pyrazinamide + ethambutol) for 2 months then rifampicin + isoniazid for 4 months. The usual precautions with adverse reactions are required. Pyridoxine 25 mg daily is recommended for adults on isoniazid.

Infective endocarditis

Infective endocarditis can be a difficult problem to diagnose but must be considered in the differential diagnosis of fever, especially in patients with a history of cardiac valvular disorders. It is caused by microbial infection of the cardiac valves or endocardium. Previously referred to as bacterial endocarditis, the term *infective endocarditis* is preferred because not all the infecting organisms are bacteria.

It may present as a fulminating or acute infection but more commonly runs an insidious course and is referred to as subacute (bacterial) endocarditis. Its incidence is increasing, probably due to the increasing number of elderly people with degenerative valve disease, more invasive procedures, IV drug use and increased cardiac catheterisation.[4]

Predisposing factors

- past history of endocarditis
- rheumatically abnormal valves
- congenitally abnormal valves
- mitral valve prolapse
- calcified aortic valve
- congenital cardiac defects, e.g. VSD, PDA
- prosthetic valves
- IV drug use
- central venous catheters
- temporary pacemaker electrode catheters

Note: Only about 50% of patients with infective endocarditis have previously known heart disease.[4]

Responsible organisms

- *Streptococcus viridans* (50% of cases)
- *Streptococcus bovis*
- *Enterococcus faecalis*
- *Staphylococcus aureus* (causes 50% of acute form)
- *Candida albicans/Aspergillus* (IV drug users)
- *Staphylococcus epidermidis*
- *Coxiella burnetti* (Q fever)

Presentations

- Acute endocarditis
- Subacute endocarditis
- Prosthetic endocarditis

Infective endocarditis without cardiac murmur is frequently seen in IV drug users who develop infection on the tricuspid valve.

Warning signs for development of endocarditis

- change in character of heart murmur
- development of a new murmur
- unexplained fever and cardiac murmur = infective endocarditis (until proved otherwise)
- a febrile illness developing after instrumentation (e.g. urethral dilatation) or minor and major surgical procedures, e.g. dental extraction, tonsillectomy, abortion
- the 'classic tetrad' of clinical features[4]
  — signs of infection
  — signs of heart disease
  — signs of embolism
  — immunological phenomena

There is a significant high mortality and morbidity from infective endocarditis which is often related to a delay in diagnosis.

| A golden rule |

Culture the blood of every patient who has a fever and a heart murmur.

Clinical features

The classic clinical features are summarised in Figure 26.2.

The patients are often elderly, appear pale and ill, with intermittent fever, and complain of vague aches and pains. The full clinical presentation takes time to develop. A febrile illness of 1 to 2 weeks duration is a common presentation.

Investigation

This includes:

- full blood count and ESR: ESR ↑, anaemia and leucocytosis
- urine: proteinuria and microscopic haematuria
- blood culture: positive in about 75%[4]
  — at least 3 sets of samples (aerobic and anaerobic culture)
- echocardiography: to visualise vegetations
- chest X-ray
- ECG

Consider renal function tests and C-reactive protein.

Management

The patient should be referred because optimal management requires close co-operation between physician, microbiologist and cardiac surgeon.

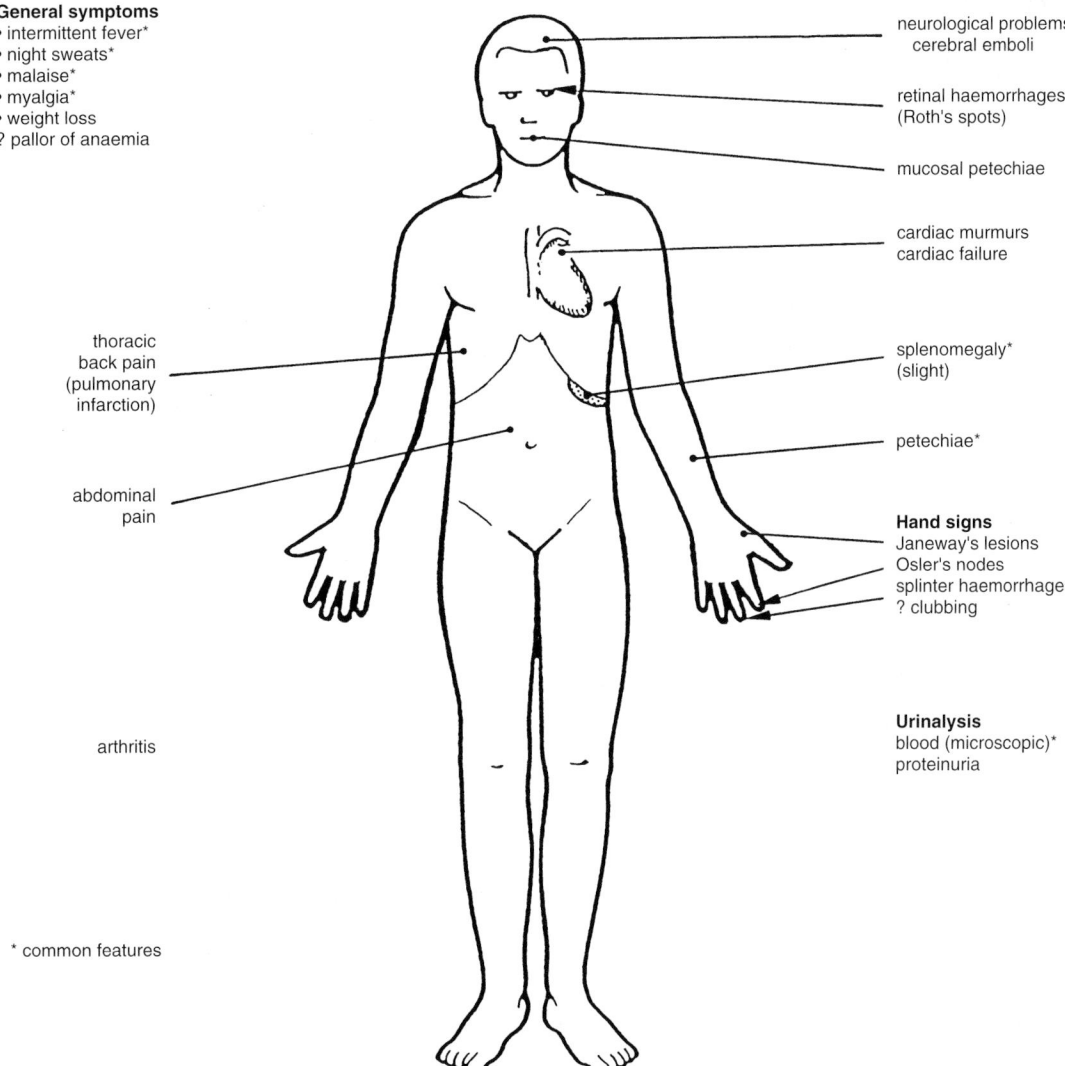

General symptoms
• intermittent fever*
• night sweats*
• malaise*
• myalgia*
• weight loss
? pallor of anaemia

neurological problems
cerebral emboli

retinal haemorrhages
(Roth's spots)

mucosal petechiae

cardiac murmurs
cardiac failure

thoracic
back pain
(pulmonary
infarction)

splenomegaly*
(slight)

petechiae*

abdominal
pain

Hand signs
Janeway's lesions
Osler's nodes
splinter haemorrhages
? clubbing

Urinalysis
blood (microscopic)*
proteinuria

arthritis

* common features

Fig. 26.2 *Infective endocarditis: possible clinical features*

Any underlying infection should be treated, e.g. drainage of dental abscess. Bactericidal antibiotics are chosen on the basis of the results of the blood culture and antibiotic sensitivities. Four blood cultures should be sent to the laboratory within the first hour of admission and treatment should seldom be delayed longer than 24 hours.

Antimicrobial treatment[5,6]
There are two important principles of management:

• Treatment must be given intravenously for at least 2 weeks.
• Treatment is prolonged—usually 4 to 6 weeks.

Consultation with an infectious disease physician or clinical microbiologist should be sought. Once cultures have been taken, prompt empirical antimicrobial treatment should be commenced, especially in fulminating infection suspected to be endocarditis. Benzylpenicillin, gentamicin and flucloxacillin/dicloxacillin are recommended,

e.g.   benzylpenicillin 1.8 g IV, 4 hourly
                   plus
       flucloxacillin/dicloxacillin 2 g IV,
       4 hourly
                   plus
       gentamicin 2 mg/kg IV, 8 hourly

Prevention of endocarditis

Antibiotic prophylaxis[6,7,8]

Low-risk patients (no prosthetic valves or previous attack of endocarditis):

- amoxycillin 3 g (50 mg/kg up to adult dose) orally, 1 hour beforehand (if not on long-term penicillin), then 1.5 g (o) at 6 hours

    or

- (amoxy) ampicillin 1 g (50 mg/kg up to adult dose) IV just before procedure commences or IM 30 minutes before if having a general anaesthetic, followed by 500 mg, 6 hours later.

If hypersensitive to penicillin: vancomycin or teicoplanin or clindamycin.

  High-risk patients (prosthetic valves or previous attacks of endocarditis), having dental procedures, oral surgery or upper respiratory tract surgery, GIT or GU surgery, cardiac catheterisation or temporary pacemaker insertion:

- (amoxy) ampicillin 1 g IV or IM (as above) with 500 mg, 6 hours later

    plus

- gentamicin 1.5 mg/kg (2.5 mg/kg in children to maximum dose 80 mg) IV (just before) or IM (30 minutes before).

If hypersensitive to penicillin: vancomycin or teicoplanin plus gentamicin.

Zoonoses

Zoonoses are those diseases and infections that are naturally transmitted between vertebrate animals and humans (see Table 26.1). Zoonotic diseases (which are not restricted to farming communities) can present as a mild illness but are prolonged in duration and can have debilitating sequelae.[10] There is a long list of diseases, which vary from country to country, and includes plague, rabies, scrub typhus, Lyme disease, tularaemia, hydatid disease, orf, anthrax, erysipeloid, listeriosis, campylobacteriosis and ornithosis (psittacosis).

Diagnosis of zoonoses[9]

If a zoonosis is overlooked in the differential diagnosis, many will remain undiagnosed and untreated.

Fever and sweats (influenza-like illness)

Any patient with undiagnosed fever should be questioned about exposure to animals, recent

Table 26.1 *Major zoonoses in Australia*

Zoonosis	Organism/s	Animal host	Mode of transmission	Main presenting features
Q fever	*Coxiella burnetti*	Various wild and domestic animals	• Inhaled dust • Animal contact • Unpasteurised milk	Fever, rigors, myalgia, headache, dry cough
Leptospirosis	*Leptospira pomona*	Various domestic animals	• Infected urine contaminating cuts or sores	Fever, myalgia, severe headache, macular rash
Brucellosis	*Brucella abortus*	Cattle	• Contamination of cuts or sores by animal tissues • Unpasteurised milk	Fever (undulant), sweats, myalgia, headache, lymphadenopathy
Lyme disease	*Borrelia burgdorferi*	Marsupials (probable)	• Tick bites	Fever, myalgia, arthritis, backache, doughnut-shaped rash
Psittacosis	*Chlamydia psittaci*	Birds: parrots, pigeons, ducks, etc.	• Inhaled dust	Fever, myalgia, headache, dry cough
Bovine tuberculosis	*Mycobacterium bovis*	Cattle	• Unpasteurised milk	Fever, sweats, weight loss, cough (as for human pulmonary TB)
Listeriosis	*Listeria monocytogenes*	Various wild and domestic animals	• Unpasteurised milk or cheese • Contaminated vegetables • Person to person	Mild febrile illness (in most): meningoencephalitis in those susceptible (neonates, pregnancy, elderly etc.)

travel both in and out of Australia, animal bites, cat scratches, consumption of raw milk, mosquito and tick bites, pets and occupation.

Rash
Consider rickettsial illness such as leptospirosis, Q fever, Lyme disease.

Cough or atypical pneumonia
Consider Q fever, psittacosis, bovine TB.

Arthralgia/arthritis
Consider Lyme disease, Ross River fever.

Meat workers
Consider Q fever, leptospirosis, orf, anthrax.

Papular/pustular lesions
Consider orf, anthrax (black).

Brucellosis

Brucellosis (undulant fever, Malta fever) has diminished in prevalence since the campaign to eradicate it from cattle. Entry is mainly by the mouth, or abraded or cut skin.

Features of acute brucellosis
- incubation period 1–3 weeks
- insidious onset: malaise, headache, weakness
- the classic fever pattern is undulant (refer to p. 500).

Possible:

- lymphadenopathy
- hepatomegaly
- spinal tenderness
- splenomegaly (if severe)

Complications such as epididymo-orchitis, oesteomyelitis and endocarditis can occur. Localised infections in sites such as bones, joints, lungs, CSF, testes and cardiac valves are possible but uncommon.

Symptoms of chronic brucellosis are virtually indistinguishable from the 'chronic fatigue syndrome' and can present with FUO.

Diagnosis
- blood cultures (positive in 50% during acute phase)[6]
- Brucella agglutination test (rising titre)

Treatment[11]
- Adults: doxycycline 100 mg (o) bd for 6 weeks

          plus either

         rifampicin 600 mg (o) daily for 6 weeks

            or

        gentamicin 5–7 mg/kg/day IV daily for 2 weeks
- Relapses do occur.

Prevention and control
Involves eradication of brucellosis in cattle, care handling infected animals and pasteurisation of milk. No vaccine is currently available for use in humans.

Q fever

Q fever is a zoonosis due to *Coxiella burnetti*. It is the most common abattoir-associated infection in Australia and can also occur in farmers and hunters. Rash is not a major feature but can occur if the infection persists without treatment.

Clinical features
- incubation period 1–3 weeks
- sudden onset fever, rigors and myalgia
- dry cough (may be pneumonia in 20%)[9]
- petechial rash (if persisting infection)

Persistent infection may cause pneumonia or endocarditis so patients with valvular disease are at risk of endocarditis. It is a rare cause of hepatitis. The acute illness may resolve spontaneously. Untreated chronic infection is usually fatal.

Diagnosis
- Serodiagnosis is by complement fixation tests.

Treatment
- doxycycline 100 mg (o) bd for 5–7 days
- for endocarditis: prolonged course doxycycline plus clindamycin or rifampicin
- Children: > 8 same antibiotics according to weight

        < 8 co-trimoxazole (instead of doxycycline)

Prevention
The disease can be prevented in abattoir workers by using Q fever vaccine.

Leptospirosis

Leptospirosis follows contamination of abraded or cut skin or mucous membranes with leptospira-infected urine of many animals including pigs, cattle, horses, rats and dogs. In Australia it is almost exclusively an occupational infection[9] of farmers and workers in the meat industry. Early diagnosis is important to prevent it passing into the immune phase.

Clinical features
- incubation period 3–20 days (average 10)
- fever, myalgia
- severe headache
- macular rash: conjunctivitis

Some may develop the immune phase (after an asymptomatic period of 1–3 days) with aseptic meningitis or jaundice and nephritis (icterohaemorrhagic fever, Weil's disease) with a significant mortality.

Diagnosis
- high or rising titre of antibodies: can be cultured

Treatment[10]
- doxycycline 100 mg (o) bd for 5–7 days

  or

  benzylpenicillin 900 mg IV, 6 hourly for 5–7 days

Lyme disease

Lyme disease (known as *Lyme borreliosis*) was first described in 1975 and named after the town Lyme in Connecticut (US). It is widespread in the United States and is now appearing in Europe, Asia and Australia. Very infective, it is caused by a spirochaete, *Borrelia burgdorferi*, and transmitted by Ixodes ticks, so that people living and working in the bush are susceptible. It has been reported in deer farmers. Lyme disease presents in three phases.

Stages of Lyme disease

Stage 1

- *Erythema migrans*—a characteristic pathognomonic rash, usually a doughnut-shaped well-defined rash about 6 cm in diameter at the bite site (Fig. 26.3).

- ± a flu-like illness: malaise, fever, myalgia, arthralgia, backache.

Stage 2 (weeks or months later)

- Neurological problems, e.g. limb weakness, muscle pain, aseptic meningitis, painful radiculopathies, cranial nerve palsies, e.g. Bell's palsy.
- Cardiac problems: arrhythmias, myocarditis.

Stage 3

- Arthritis (weeks or months later). In children it can be mistaken for juvenile chronic arthritis. In adults, it usually affects one or two joints, especially the knee joints. A LIMP syndrome (localised intermittent musculoskeletal pain) is described, which is severe pain without significant findings on examination.

Diagnosis
- Clinical pattern especially rash of *erythema migrans*. Serology to demonstrate Lyme antibodies, which take about 6 weeks to develop from the onset of the disease.

Treatment
- A typical regime for adults is doxycycline 100 mg bd for 21 days (the earlier the diagnosis the more effective the treatment).

Psittacosis

Most patients are bird fanciers. Psittacosis accounts for 1–5% of hospital admissions for pneumonia. The disease may follow a low-grade course over several months but can have a dramatically acute presentation.

Clinical features
- incubation period 1–2 weeks
- fever, malaise, myalgia
- headache
- cough
- minimal chest signs
- splenomegaly (sometimes)

Mortality can be as high as 20% if untreated.

Diagnosis
- serology—rising antibody

Treatment
- tetracycline or erythromycin

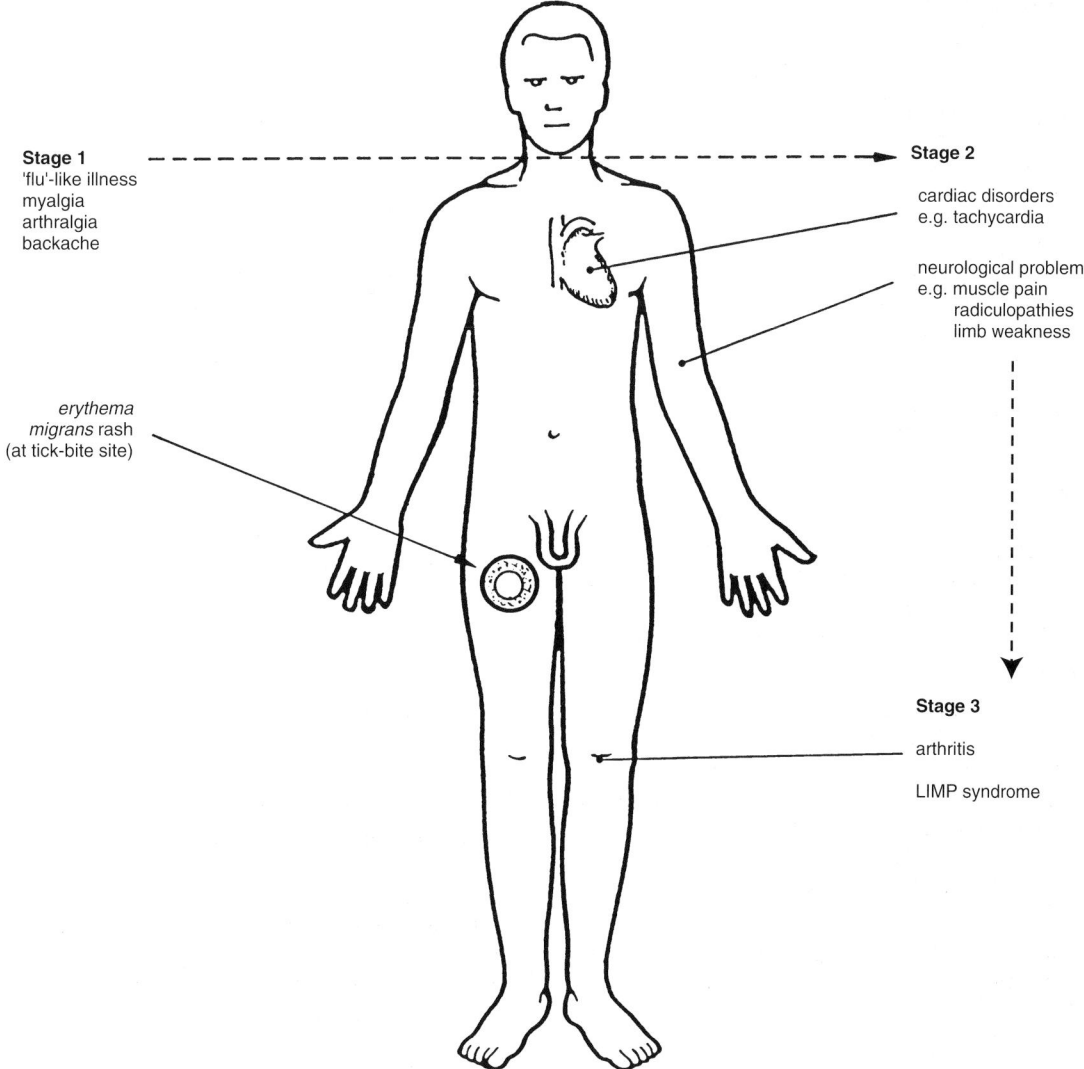

Stage 1
'flu'-like illness
myalgia
arthralgia
backache

Stage 2

cardiac disorders
e.g. tachycardia

neurological problems
e.g. muscle pain
    radiculopathies
    limb weakness

*erythema
migrans* rash
(at tick-bite site)

Stage 3

arthritis

LIMP syndrome

Fig. 26.3 *Lyme disease: clinical features*

Listeriosis

Listeriosis is caused by *Listeria monocytogenes*, a bacterium widespread in nature that can contaminate food and has been found in many fresh and processed foods, e.g. dairy products especially unpasteurised milk, soft cheese, processed meats and smoked seafood. Its significance lies in the mortality rate in high-risk groups such as pregnant women, the immuno-compromised, frail aged, and very young but especially neonates and foetuses. Babies may be stillborn or aborted.

Clinical features
It may be subclinical but possible presentations include:
* influenza-like illness (usually mild)
* food poisoning (atypical)
* meningitis especially infants, elderly
* septicaemia (in susceptible)
* pneumonia (in susceptible)

Diagnosis
* microscopy or isolation of organism from infected site
* serological tests available

Treatment
Amoxycillin 1 g (o) 8 hourly for 10–14 days[12]

Other zoonoses

- mosquito-transmitted infections—Murray Valley encephalitis, Ross River virus, Barmah Forest virus
- infections from bites and scratches—cat scratch disease, rat bite fever
- hydatid disease, orf, milker's nodules
- toxoplasmosis, histoplasmosis, hookworm

Clostridial diseases

Tetanus
This sometimes misdiagnosed bacterial infection (*Clostridium tetani*) can appear from one day to several months after the injury, which can be forgotten. A total of 10–20% of patients with tetanus have no identifiable wound of entry.[13]

Clinical features
- prodrome: fever, malaise, headache
- trismus (patient cannot close mouth)
- risus sardonicus (a grin-like effect from hypertonic facial muscles)
- opisthotonos (arched trunk with hyperextended neck)
- spasms, precipitated by minimal stimuli

Differential diagnosis: phenothiazine toxicity, strychnine poisoning, rabies

Management
- Refer immediately to expert centre.
- Intubate and ventilate if necessary.

Gas gangrene
Gas gangrene (clostridial myonecrosis) is caused by entry of one of several clostridia organisms into devitalised tissue such as exists following severe trauma to a leg.

Clinical features
- sudden onset of pain and swelling in the contaminated wound
- brownish serous exudate
- gas in the tissue on palpation or X-ray
- prostration and systemic toxicity
- circulatory failure ('shock')

Management
- Refer immediately to surgical centre
- Start benzylpenicillin 2.4 g IV, 4 hourly.

Botulism
Botulism is food poisoning caused by the neurotoxin of *Clostridium botulinum*. From 12 to 36 hours after ingesting the toxin from canned, smoked or vacuum-packed food (e.g. home-canned vegetables or meat) visual problems such as diplopia suddenly appear. General muscle paralysis and prostration quickly develop.

Pneumonia

Surprisingly the initial presentation of pneumonia can be misleading, especially when the patient presents with constitutional symptoms such as fever, malaise and headache rather than respiratory symptoms. A cough, although usually present, can be relatively insignificant in the total clinical picture. This problem applies particularly to atypical pneumonia but can occur with bacterial pneumonia, especially lobar pneumonia (refer to pp. 379–80).

The atypical pneumonias
Clinical features
- fever, malaise
- headache
- minimal respiratory symptoms, non-productive cough
- signs of consolidation absent
- chest X-ray (diffuse infiltration) incompatible with chest signs

Causes
Mycoplasma pneumoniae—the commonest:
- adolescents and young adults
- treat with tetracycline, e.g. doxycycline 100 mg bd for 10 days

Legionella pneumophila (legionnaires' disease):
- related to cooling systems in large buildings
- incubation 2–10 days

Diagnostic criteria include:
- prodromal-like illness
- a dry cough, influenza, confusion or diarrhoea
- lymphopenia with marked leucocytosis
- hyponatraemia

Patients can become very prostrate with complications—treat with erythromycin.

Chlamydia psittaci (psittacosis)
• treat with doxycycline 100 mg bd for 10 days
Coxiella burnetti (Q fever)

References

1. Hart G. Syphilis. In: MIMS Disease Index (2nd edn). Sydney: IMS Publishing, 1996, 493–496.

2. NH & MRC. *Handbook on sexually transmitted diseases*. Canberra: Department of Community Services and Health, 1990, 23–29.

3. Kumar PJ, Clark ML. *Clinical medicine* (2nd edn). London: Bailliere Tindall, 1990, 41–42.

4. Oakley C. Infective endocarditis. Medicine International, 1986; 21: 872–878.

5. Mashford ML. *Antibiotic guidelines* (9th edn). Melbourne: Victorian Postgraduate Medical Foundation, 1996, 28–33.

6. Speed B. Endocarditis, infective. In: MIMS Disease Index (2nd edn). Sydney: IMS Publishing 1996, 167–169.

7. Mashford ML. *Antibiotic guidelines* (9th edn). Melbourne: Victorian Postgraduate Medical Foundation, 1996, 92–96.

8. Kumar PL, Clark ML. *Clinical medicine* (2nd edn). London: Bailliere Tindall, 1990, 30–65.

9. Benn R. Australian zoonoses. Current Therapeutics, July 1990, 31–40.

10. Scott J. Zoonoses. Current therapeutics. April 1995, 42–45.

11. Mashford ML. *Antibiotic guidelines* (9th edn). Melbourne: Victorian Postgraduate Medical Foundation, 1996, 133–134.

12. National Health and Medical Research Council Statement. Listeria, advice to medical practitioners, 1992.

13. Wilson J et al. *Harrison's principles of internal medicine* (12th edn), New York, 1991, chapter 105 (tetanus).

Acknowledgment

Part of this text, on the clinical manifestations of syphilis, is reproduced from the *Handbook on sexually transmitted diseases*[2]. 'Commonwealth of Australia, copyright reproduced by permission'.

27
Chronic renal failure

—

I have never yet examined the body of a patient dying with dropsy attended by albuminous urine, in whom some obvious derangement was not discovered in the kidneys.

Richard Bright 1827

Chronic renal failure (CRF) is defined as a severe reduction in nephron mass over an extended period of time resulting in uraemia.[1] It is not common but can present surreptitiously and be a real master of disguise in clinical practice. Asymptomatic CRF may be discovered on routine health screening, as a chance finding in hospitalised or hypertensive patients, or during follow-up of patients with known renal disease.[2]

Key facts and checkpoints

- At least 50 to 60 people per million of the population are treated for end-stage renal failure (ESRF) each year.
- Two-thirds of these are under 60 years of age.
- Approximately one-third have glomerulonephritis, 2–18% analgesic nephropathy, 10% diabetes mellitus, 7% polycystic kidney disease, 6% reflux nephropathy and 4% hypertension. (Table 27.1)[3]
- The commonest cause of nephritis leading to renal failure in Australia is IgA nephropathy.
- In children the incidence of chronic renal failure is quite low (1 to 2 per million of the population).[3]
- Warmer climates, poorer living conditions and certain genetic predispositions are associated with a higher prevalence of renal failure.
- Renal failure should be considered in the diagnosis of patients with:

  — unexplained anaemia
  — unexplained poor health
  — unusually high analgesic intake[3]
- Uraemic symptoms are non-specific and usually are not recognised until the creatinine clearance is less than 20% of normal.
- CRF is characterised by the accumulation of uraemic toxins and a deficiency of renal hormones that cause dysfunction of organs other than kidneys.
- This interaction can cause phosphate retention, secondary hyperparathyroidism and bone disorders such as osteomalacia.
- It is possible to identify stages of renal failure (Table 27.2).

Table 27.1 *Significant causes of chronic renal failure*

Chronic glomerulonephritis

Reflux nephropathy

Diabetes mellitus

Polycystic kidneys

Hypertension

Obstructive nephropathy
- bilateral ureteric obstruction
- bladder outflow obstruction
  — prostatic enlargement
  — urethral stenosis

Lupus nephritis

Renal artery stenosis

Gout

Amyloidosis

Hypercalcaemia

Drugs

Table 27.2 *Stages of renal failure*

Stage and % of kidney function	Biochemistry (for 60–75 kg patient)	Symptoms and signs	Recommended action

1. 50–100%	• Normal blood tests
	• Abnormal urine tests
		• Nil obvious
		• Deterioration renal function with:
		  — nephrotoxic antibiotics
		  — ACE inhibitors
		  — NSAIDs
			• Dietary manipulation
			• Strict control BP
			• Specialist referral

2. 20–50%	• S creatinine ↑ from 0.1→ 0.4 mmol/L • Other tests normal	• ↑ blood pressure • Urine abnormalities	• As above
3. 10–20%	• S creatinine ↑ 0.4 → 0.8 mmol/L • Possible ↑ uric acid, phosphate, HCO_3	• Nocturia • Mild malaise	• Adjust medication to control abnormal electrolytes • Consider dialysis

4. <10%	• S creatinine ↑ to 0.9 mmol/L
	• ↑ K^+, HCO_3
	• Anaemia
		• Multiple see Fig. 27.1	• Probably dialysis
			• Treat:
			  — renal bone disease
			  — nutrition
			  — anaemia

5. <5%	• S creatinine >0.9 mmol/L • Anaemia	• Multiple severe symptoms • Impaired conscious state • Cardiorespiratory dysfunction	• Dialysis • Treatment for end stage renal failure

Important clinical associations

The possibility of CRF should be monitored in patients with:

• diabetes mellitus
• hypertension
• severe gout
• a history of urinary tract abnormality
  e.g. vesico-ureteric reflux
      bladder outflow obstruction

The possibility of CRF should be considered and investigated in patients presenting with:

• unexplained poor health
• hypertension
• anaemia
• pruritus
• hyperparathyroidism
• pericarditis
• urinary tract symptoms or signs
  e.g. proteinuria
     haematuria
     oedema
     nocturia
     loin pain
     prostatic obstruction

• neurological disturbances
  e.g. confusion
     coma
     peripheral neuropathy
     seizures

Patients with CRF may present with features of acute renal failure with the intervention of complicating factors such as:

• drug toxicity
• infection
• fluid imbalance

Urgent treatment of the following conditions, which can lead to rapid renal failure, is essential:

• progressive nephritis
• systemic lupus erythematosus
• vasculitides
  e.g. polyarteritis nodosa
     Wegener's granulomatosis

The clinical approach
History
A hallmark of early stage CRF is a non-specific history and examination, and the diagnosis is

very difficult in the absence of a known past history of renal disease. The diagnosis can be established only by renal function tests. Symptoms from CRF are rare unless the creatinine clearance is less than 20% of normal and only become common when less than 10% of normal.

In patients with chronic renal disease, symptomatic uraemia may be precipitated by prerenal factors such as fluid loss from vomiting or diarrhoea, infection, antibiotic therapy especially tetracyclines, or increasing hypertension.

Symptoms and signs

The symptoms and signs of CRF are summarised in Figure 27.1.

The common early presenting symptoms are generally non-specific and referable to the gastrointestinal tract, presumably due to the formation of ammonia in the upper GIT.

Such symptoms include:

• anorexia
• nausea
• vomiting
• tiredness
• lethargy

If a patient presents with these symptoms and has a sallow appearance due to combination of anaemia and brownish pigmentation, then CRF should be highly suspected.

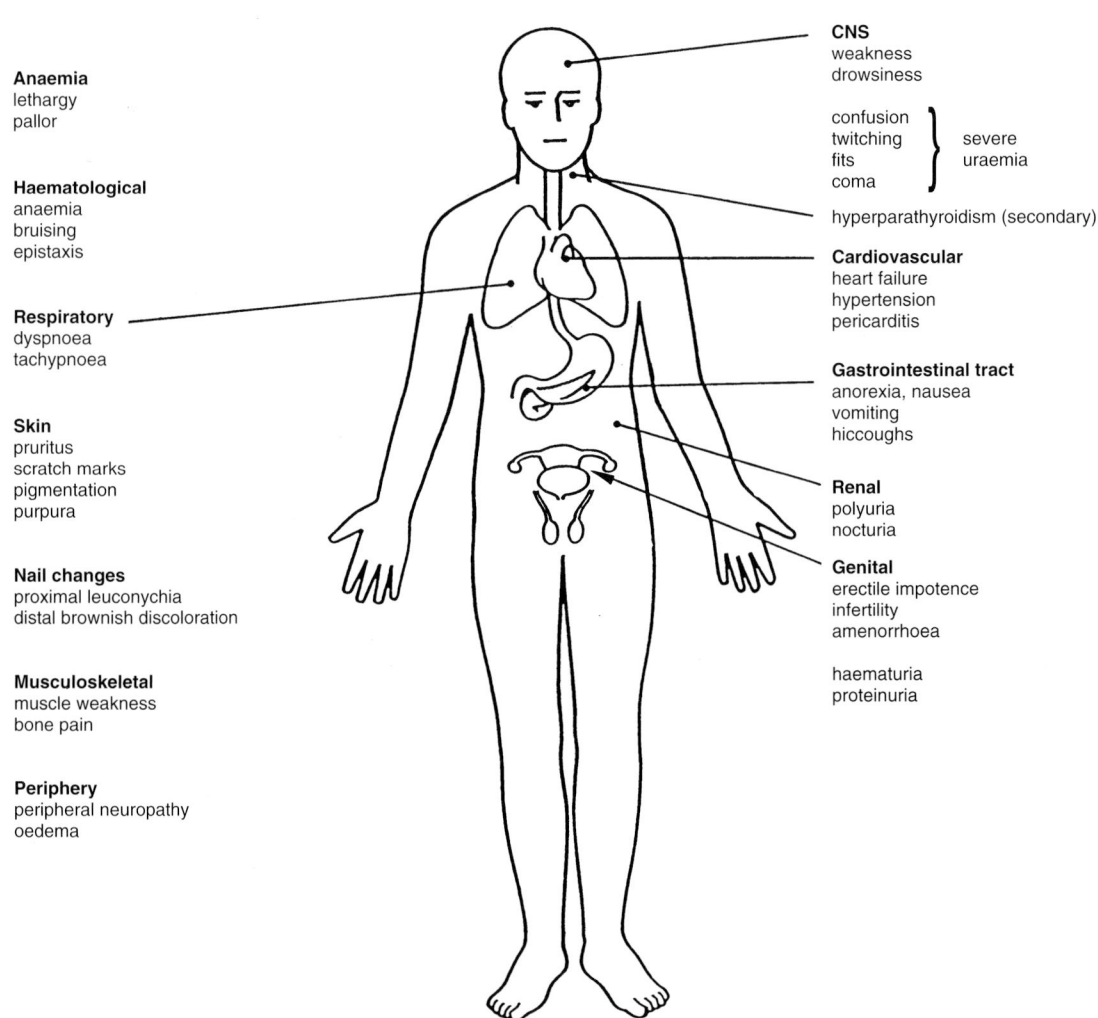

Anaemia
lethargy
pallor

Haematological
anaemia
bruising
epistaxis

Respiratory
dyspnoea
tachypnoea

Skin
pruritus
scratch marks
pigmentation
purpura

Nail changes
proximal leuconychia
distal brownish discoloration

Musculoskeletal
muscle weakness
bone pain

Periphery
peripheral neuropathy
oedema

CNS
weakness
drowsiness

confusion ⎫
twitching ⎬ severe
fits ⎭ uraemia
coma

hyperparathyroidism (secondary)

Cardiovascular
heart failure
hypertension
pericarditis

Gastrointestinal tract
anorexia, nausea
vomiting
hiccoughs

Renal
polyuria
nocturia

Genital
erectile impotence
infertility
amenorrhoea

haematuria
proteinuria

Fig 27.1 *Clinical features of chronic renal disease*

Physical examination

General inspection of the patient with CRF will usually reveal a sallow complexion with yellow–brown pigmentation in the skin, which is often dry and pruritic. The patient's mental state should be noted. The respiratory and pulse rates are usually rapid because of anaemia and metabolic acidosis. Other findings may include bruising, uraemic foetor, reduced mental status, pericarditis and peripheral neuropathy. The abdomen should be carefully palpated especially in the renal areas. A rectal examination is indicated to detect prostatomegaly or other rectal or pelvic pathology. Ophthalmoscopic examination may show hypertensive or diabetic retinopathy. Urinalysis should test glucose, blood and protein. Proteinuria should be confirmed with a 24-hour urine protein estimation.

Investigations

Renal function tests (most appropriate for the general practitioner):

- plasma urea
- plasma creatinine
- creatinine clearance (more precise)

Plasma electrolytes

- sodium, potassium, chloride, bicarbonate
- calcium and phosphate

Consider:

- magnesium, urate, glucose
- lipids
- prescribed drug level
- cardiac studies
- full blood ? anaemia

Determination of underlying cause

- imaging of urinary tract—ultrasound
- immunological tests
- renal biopsy

Chronic renal failure in children

The incidence of CRF in children is about 2 per million of the total population per year. The commonest causes include chronic glomerulonephritis, obstructive nephropathy and reflux nephropathy. Identification of structural renal abnormalities by obstetric ultrasound and early investigation of urinary tract infections may decrease the incidence of CRF. Dialysis and transplantation are normally considered for children over 2 years of age with end-stage CRF. For children under 2 years there are complex ethical, psychological and technical problems.[4] Nevertheless the prognosis for such treatment is poor.

Monitoring CRF

The most important test in identifying and monitoring CRF is the plasma creatinine level. The normal range is about 40–120 micromols per litre (0.04–0.12 mmol/L) but the laboratory will indicate their appropriate reference level. A more precise estimate can be made by checking the creatinine clearance.

Management

The patient should be referred to an appropriate specialist as early as possible. The underlying disease and any abnormalities causing progressive renal damage must be corrected where possible. The management of CRF is based on the team approach involving specialists and paramedical personnel. The patient is usually faced with years of ongoing care so that an empathic support team based around the patient's general practitioner is very important to the patient who will require considerable psychosocial support.

Optimum treatment includes:

- regular review
- good blood pressure control (the most effective way to slow progression)
- keeping plasma phosphate levels in normal range
- maintaining effective fluid and electrolyte balance
- prompt treatment of intercurrent illness
- judicious use of drugs
- avoiding treatment errors, especially with drugs
  - avoid potassium-sparing diuretics
  - other drugs that may cause problems include digoxin, tetracyclines, gentamicin, NSAIDs, nitrofurantoin and ACE inhibitors
- rapid treatment of complications, especially salt and water depletion and acute urinary infection
- diet: low protein, sodium and potassium
- treating anaemia with human recombinant erythropoietin.

Blood pressure control

- no added salt diet (with care)
- drug control: none of the antihypertensive agents are specifically contraindicated but

those eliminated mainly by the kidney (e.g. ACE inhibitors, atenolol, sotalol) should be given in lower dosage. ACE inhibitors should not be used in presence of renal artery stenosis; loop diuretics, e.g. frusemide, are effective in larger doses (thiazide diuretics are ineffective).[3]

Hyperphosphataemia control

- balanced nutrition to reduce dietary phosphate
- protein restriction
- calcium carbonate (to bind phosphate)

Dialysis

Dialysis is indicated when all other methods fail. About two-thirds of patients receive haemodialysis and one-third are on continuous ambulatory peritoneal dialysis.

Transplantation

Transplantation is the treatment of choice for failure except where contraindicated such as with active tuberculosis and perhaps the elderly. However, a critical shortage of donors remains a problem.

When to refer

- Haematuria is an indication of active disease and such patients should be referred immediately for investigation. Oliguria makes this even more urgent.

- Any patient with impaired renal function should be investigated and a management plan formulated.
- Patients with creatinine clearance of less than 20 mL/min (plasma creatinine > 0.05 mmol/L) are best followed in a renal clinic. Diabetic patients warrant specialist referral when the plasma creatinine is at 0.2 mmol/L.[3]

References

1. Tally N, O'Connor S. *Clinical examinations* (2nd edn). Sydney: Maclennan & Petty, 1992, 195–209.
2. Kumar PJ, Clark M. *Clinical medicine* (2nd edn). London: Bailliere Tindall, 1990, 475–478.
3. Dawborn JK. Chronic renal failure. In: MIMS Disease Index (2nd edn). Sydney: IMS Publishing, 1996, 442–443.
4. Robinson MJ. *Practical paediatrics* (2nd edn). Melbourne: Churchill Livingstone, 1990, 441–442.
5. Kincaid Smith P, Larkins R, Whelan G. *Problems in clinical medicine*. Sydney: Maclennan & Petty, 1990, 319–324.

28

Connective tissue disorders and the vasculitides

—

In its more aggravated forms diffuse scleroderma is one of the most terrible of all human ills. Like Tithonus to 'wither slowly' and like him to be 'beaten down and marred and wasted', until one is literally a mummy, encased in an ever shrinking, slow contracting skin of steel, is a fate not pictured in any tragedy.

Sir William Osler 1898

The connective tissue disorders and the vasculitides are groups of diseases that are difficult to classify because their causation is generally unknown. They all cause joint and soft tissue inflammation and multiple other possible manifestations that create diagnostic difficulties.

It is convenient to consider a working classification of joint pain (Table 28.1) that includes apparent joint pain (arthralgia), as some of the inflammatory disorders cause problems in the soft tissues around joints, e.g. giant cell arteritis and hydroxyapatite crystalopathy of the tendons around the shoulder joint.

Vasculitis is, in fact, a condition common to the connective tissue disorders and to the so-called vasculitides.

Connective tissue disorders

The connective tissue disorders or diseases comprise three distinct conditions, namely systemic lupus erythematosus, systemic sclerosis and polymyositis/dermatomyositis (Fig. 28.1).[1]

Mixed connective tissue disorder is that disease which includes features of all three disorders and is sometimes referred to as 'overlap' syndrome.

Common features include:

- arthralgia or arthritis
- multisystem involvement
- vasculitis
- immunological abnormalities

Systemic lupus erythematosus

Systemic lupus erythematosus (SLE) is the commonest of the connective tissue disorders. It is a multisystem autoimmune disorder with a wide variety of clinical features that are due to vasculitis (Fig. 28.2). Arthritis is the commonest clinical feature of SLE (90% of cases). Milder manifestations outnumber more severe forms.

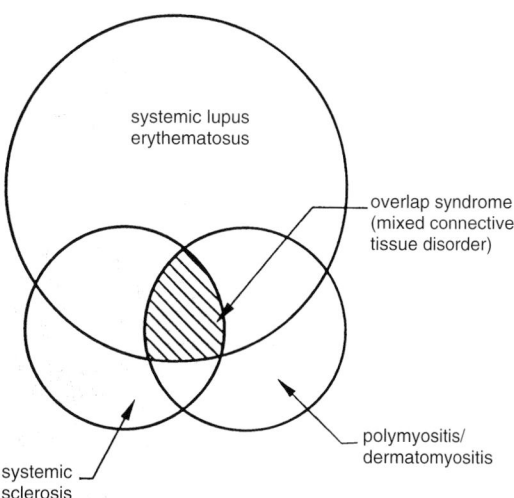

Fig. 28.1 *The connective tissue disorders*

Table 28.1   *A classification of rheumatological pain*

Hyperacute (red hot) joints	Crystals	• urate: gout • calcium pyrophosphate • hydroxyapatite
	Pus	e.g. staphylococcal septic arthritis
Inflammation of joints	Symmetrical	e.g. rheumatoid arthritis
	Asymmetrical	e.g. spondylo-arthropathies
Non-inflammatory joint disorder • osteoarthritis	Typical	Primary, e.g. in hands
	Atypical	e.g. post-trauma haemochromatosis
Joint and soft tissue inflammation	Connective tissue disorders	• SLE • systemic sclerosis • polymyositis/dermatomyositis
	Vasculitides	• polyarteritis nodosa • giant cell arteritis • polymyalgia rheumatica
Non-articular (soft tissue) inflammation	Generalised	e.g. fibrositis
	Localised	e.g. plantar fasciitis epicondylitis

Source: After Dr Stephen Hall

Features
• prevalence about 1 in 1000 of population
• mainly affects women in 'high oestrogen' period (90% of cases)
• peak onset between 15 and 40 years
• fever, malaise, tiredness common
• multiple drug allergies
• problems with OCP and pregnancy

Criteria for classification of SLE
(SLE = 4 or more of these 11 criteria)
• Malar (butterfly) rash
• Discoid rash
• Photosensitivity
• Arthritis
• Oral ulcers
• Serositis (pleurisy or pericarditis)
• Renal disorders (proteinuria or casts)
• Neurological disorders (intractable headache, seizures or psychosis)
• Haematological disorders (haemolytic anaemia, leucopenia, lymphopenia or thrombocytopenia)
• Immunological disorders (positive LE cells, anti-DNA, anti-Sm or false positive syphilis serology)
• Positive antinuclear antibody

Diagnostic tests
• ESR—elevated in proportion to disease activity
• antinuclear antibodies (ANA)— positive in 95%
• double stranded DNA antibodies— 90% specific for SLE but present in only 60% } the key tests
• rheumatoid factor—positive in 50%
• LE test—inefficient and not used

The diagnosis cannot be made on blood tests alone. Supportive clinical evidence is necessary.

Management[2]
• appropriate explanation, support and reassurance, use of sunscreens
• refer to consultant for shared care
• drug treatments
— mild: NSAIDs (for arthralgia)

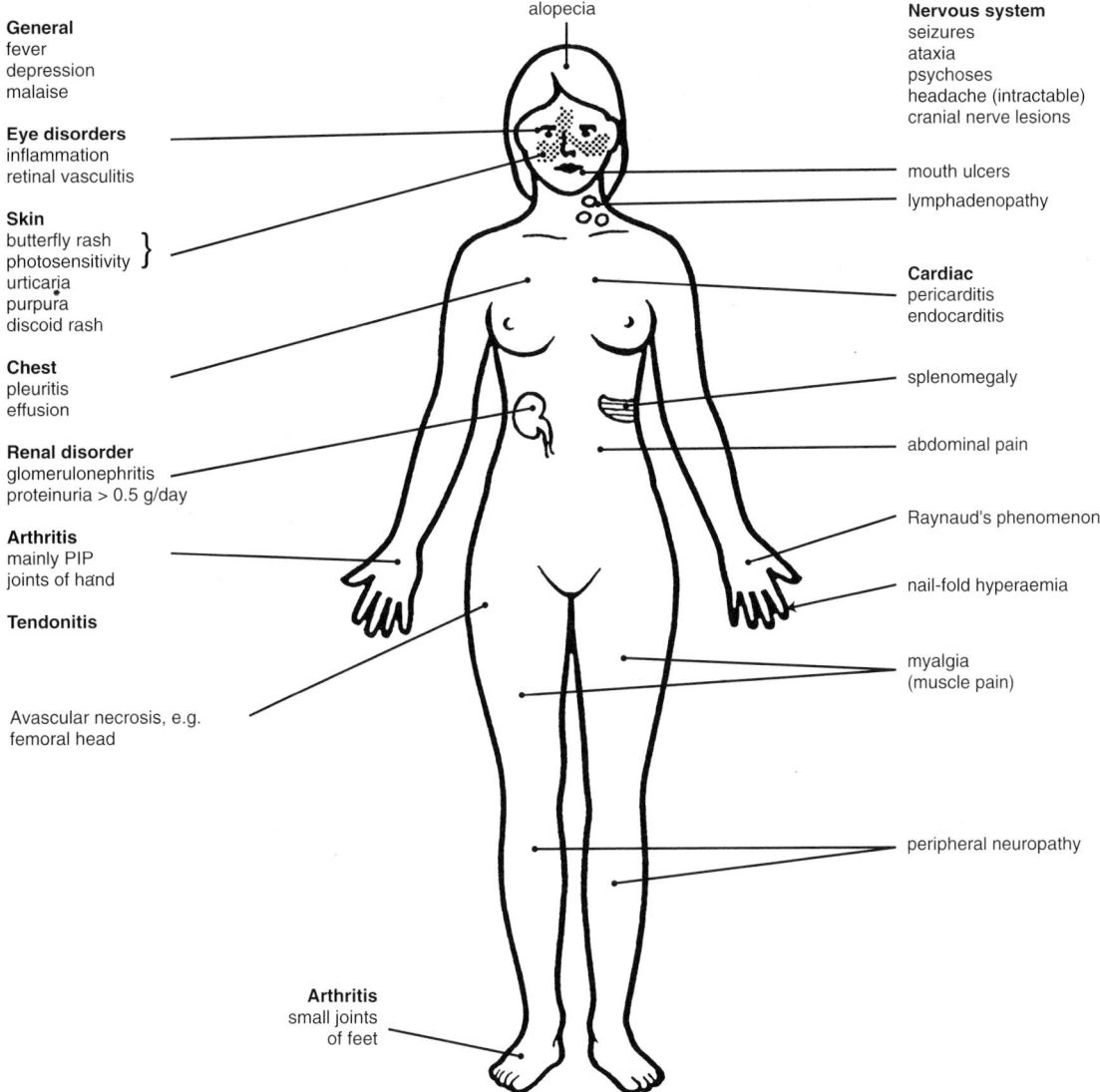

General
fever
depression
malaise

Eye disorders
inflammation
retinal vasculitis

Skin
butterfly rash
photosensitivity }
urticaria
purpura
discoid rash

Chest
pleuritis
effusion

Renal disorder
glomerulonephritis
proteinuria > 0.5 g/day

Arthritis
mainly PIP
joints of hand

Tendonitis

Avascular necrosis, e.g.
femoral head

alopecia

Nervous system
seizures
ataxia
psychoses
headache (intractable)
cranial nerve lesions

mouth ulcers
lymphadenopathy

Cardiac
pericarditis
endocarditis

splenomegaly

abdominal pain

Raynaud's phenomenon

nail-fold hyperaemia

myalgia
(muscle pain)

peripheral neuropathy

Arthritis
small joints
of feet

Fig. 28.2 *Clinical features of SLE*

— moderate (esp. skin, joint serosa involved):
— severe:

low-dose antimalarials, e.g. hydroxychloroquine up to 6 mg/kg once daily corticosteroids are the mainstay immunosuppressive drugs, e.g. azathioprine

• avoid drugs in those in clinical remission and with normal complement levels
• other treatments such as plasma exchange and immunosuppressive regimens available for severe disease

Systemic sclerosis (scleroderma)

It can present as a polyarthritis affecting the fingers of the hand in 25% of patients, especially in the early stages. Soft tissue swelling produces a 'sausage finger' pattern. Systemic sclerosis mainly affects the skin, presenting with Raynaud's phenomenon in over 85% (Fig. 28.3).

Features
• females/males 3:1
• a progressive disease of multiple organs

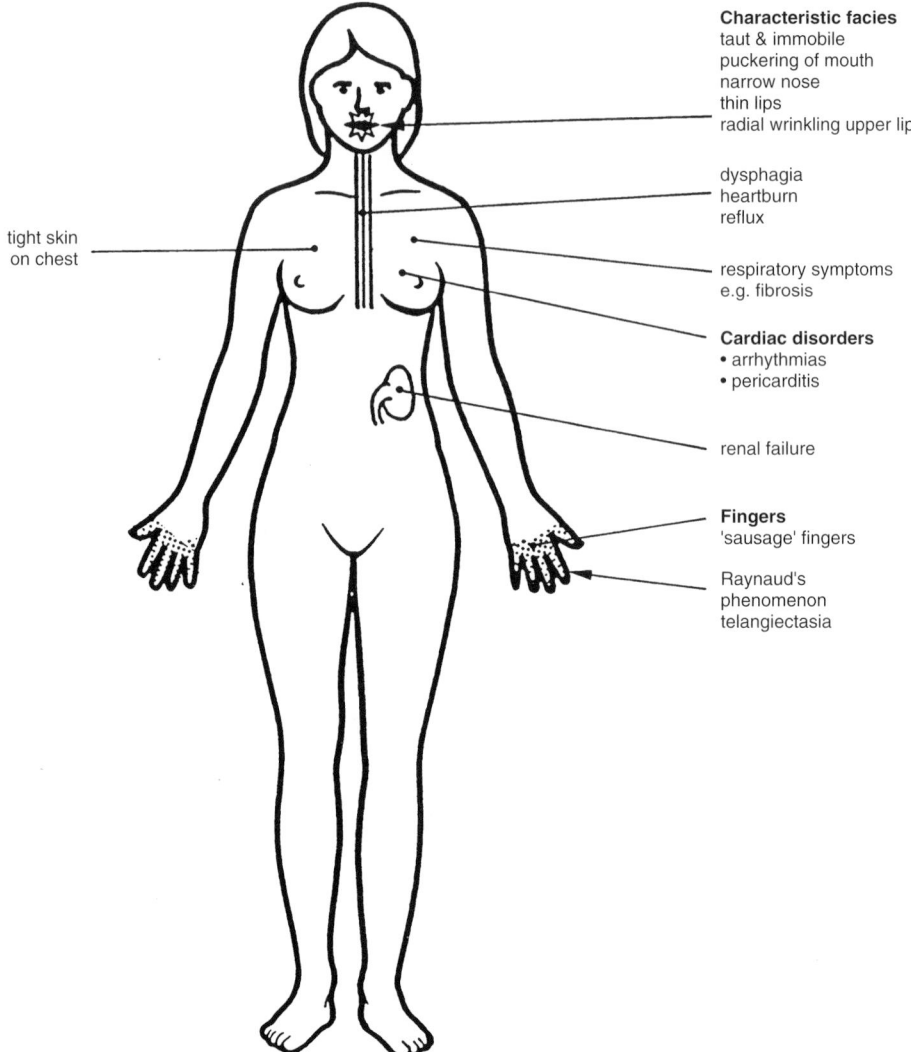

Fig. 28.3 *Clinical features of systemic sclerosis*

- Raynaud's phenomenon
- stiffness of fingers and other skin areas
- 'bird-like' facies (mouth puckered)
- dysphagia and diarrhoea (malabsorption)
- respiratory symptoms
- cardiac symptoms: pericarditis, etc.
- look for tight skin on chest (Roman breastplate)

Diagnostic tests[3]
- ESR may be raised
- normocytic normochromic anaemia may be present
- antinuclear antibodies—up to 90% positive (relatively specific)
- rheumatoid factor—positive in 30%

- anticentromere Abs—specific (positive in 90% with limited disease and 5% with diffuse)
- antitopoisomerase I (anti-Scl-70) antibody is specific but only positive in 20–40%
- skin biopsy—increase in dermal collagen

Management
- refer to consultant for shared care
- empathic explanation, patient education
- analgesics and NSAIDs for pain
- avoid vasospasm (no smoking, beta-blockers, ergotamine): nifedipine may help Raynaud's
- treat malabsorption if present; skin emollients
- D-penicillamine can help if significant systemic or cutaneous involvement[4]

Localised scleroderma

- morphoea—plaques of erythema with violaceous periphery, feels hard; mainly on trunk
- linear—may be 'en coup de sabre' (a sabre stroke)

Polymyositis and dermatomyositis

Polymyositis is an uncommon systemic disorder whose main feature is symmetrical muscle weakness and wasting involving the proximal muscles of the shoulder and pelvic girdles.

Polymyositis + associated rash = dermatomyositis

Clinical features

- any age group
- peak incidence 40–60 years
- female to male ratio 2:1
- muscle weakness and wasting proximal limb muscles
- main complaint is weakness
- muscle pain and tenderness in about 50%
- arthralgia or arthritis in about 50% (resembles distribution of rheumatoid arthritis)
- dysphagia in about 50% due to oesophageal involvement
- Raynaud's phenomenon
- consider associated malignancy: lung and ovary

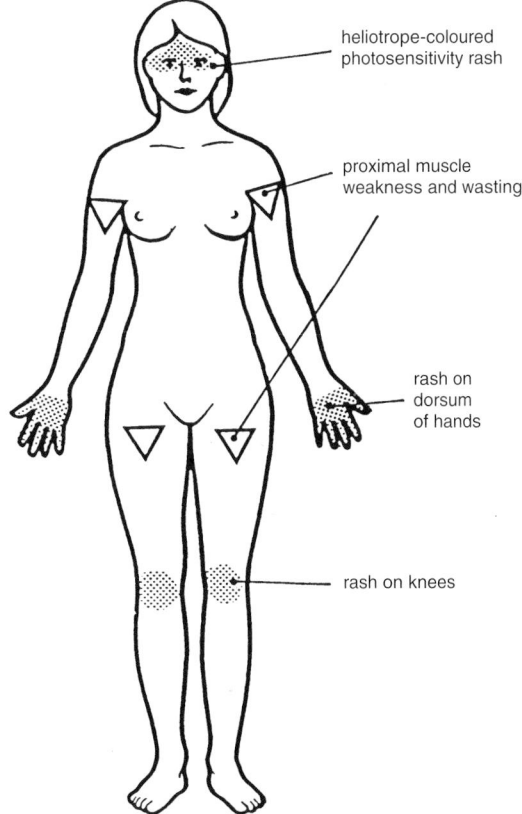

Fig. 28.4 *Clinical features of polymyositis/dermatomyositis*

The rash

The distinctive rash shows features of photosensitivity. There is violet discolouration of the eyelids, forehead and cheeks, and possible erythema resembling sunburn and periorbital oedema. There is a characteristic rash on the hands especially the fingers and nail folds. The knees and elbows are commonly involved.

The main features are summarised in Figure 28.4.

Diagnosis

- muscle enzyme studies (serum creatine kinase and aldolase)
- biopsies—skin and muscle
- EMG studies—show characteristic pattern

Teatment includes corticosteroids and cytotoxic drugs. Early referral is appropriate.

The vasculitides

The vasculitides or vasculitis syndromes are a heterogeneous group of disorders involving inflammation and necrosis of blood vessels, the clinical effects and classification depending on the size of the vessels involved.

Small vessel vasculitis is the common type encountered in practice. Medium vessel vasculitis includes polyarteritis nodosa and large vessel vasculitis includes giant cell arteritis.

Small vessel vasculitis

This is associated with many important diseases such as rheumatoid arthritis, SLE, bacterial endocarditis, Henoch-Schönlein purpura and hepatitis B. Skin lesions are usually associated with these disorders and the most common presentation is painful, palpable purpura such as occurs with Henoch-Schönlein purpura.

Rarer causes

The major vasculitides are polyarteritis nodosa (PN), polymyalgia rheumatica (PR), and giant cell arteritis (GCA), and Wegener's granulomatosis (WG). Unfortunately, many of these patients die

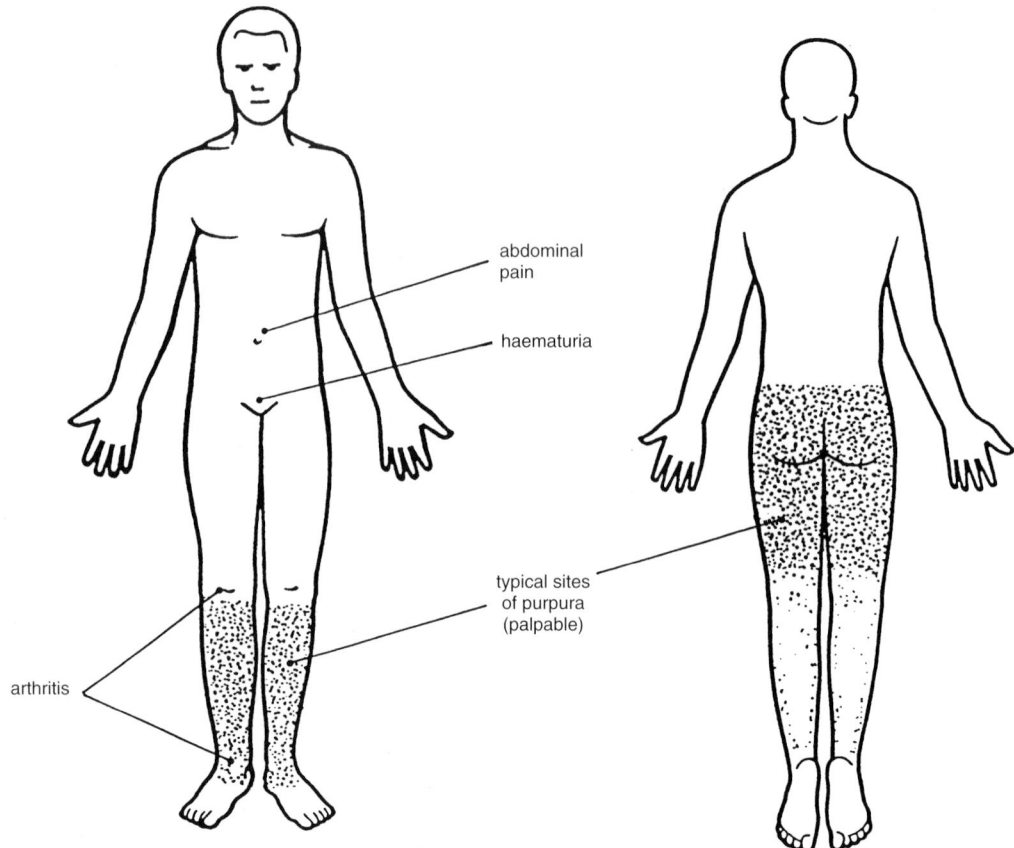

Fig. 28.5 *Henoch-Schönlein purpura: typical distribution*

or become terminally ill before the diagnosis is suspected.

Henoch-Schönlein purpura

More details are presented about this disorder on page 335.

Clinical features

- all ages, mainly in children
- rash mainly on buttocks and legs (Fig. 28.5)
- can occur on hands, arms and trunk
- arthritis: mainly ankles and knees
- abdominal pain (vasculitis of GIT)
- haematuria (reflects nephritis)

Polyarteritis nodosa

The hallmark of polyarteritis nodosa is necrotising vasculitis of large arteries leading to skin nodules, infarctive ulcers and other serious manifestations (Fig. 28.6). The cause is unknown but associations are found with drug abusers (especially adulterated drugs), B cell lymphomas, other drugs and hepatitis B surface antigen. It should be suspected in any multisystemic disease of obscure aetiology.

Clinical features

- young to middle-aged men
- constitutional symptoms: fever, malaise, myalgia, weight loss
- migratory arthralgia or polyarthritis
- subcutaneous nodules along arterial lines
- livedo reticularis and skin ulcers
- renal impairment and hypertension
- cardiac disorders: arrhythmia, failure, infarction
- diagnosis confirmed by biopsy or angiogram
- ESR raised
- treatment with corticosteroids and immunosuppressants
- death is usually from renal disease

General
malaise
weight loss
fever

Cardiac
myocardial infarction
arrhythmia
heart failure

Lungs
pleurisy
asthma

Renal
glomerulonephritis

nodules

hypertension

livedo reticularis

arthritis

ulcer

Fig. 28.6 *Clinical features of polyarteritis nodosa*

Polymyalgia rheumatica and giant cell arteritis

The basic pathology of this very important disease complex is giant cell arteritis (synonyms: temporal arteritis; cranial arteritis). The clinical syndromes are polymyalgia rheumatica and temporal arteritis. The clinical manifestations of polymyalgia rheumatica invariably precede those of temporal arteritis of which there is about a 20% association. The diagnosis is based on clinical grounds. No definite cause has been found.

Clinical features of polymyalgia rheumatica

- pain and stiffness in proximal muscles of shoulder and pelvic girdle, cervical spine (Fig. 28.7)
- symmetrical distribution
- typical ages 60–70 years (rare < 50)
- both sexes: more common in women
- early morning stiffness
- may be systemic symptoms: weight loss, malaise, anorexia
- painful restriction of movement of shoulders and hips
- signs may be absent later in day

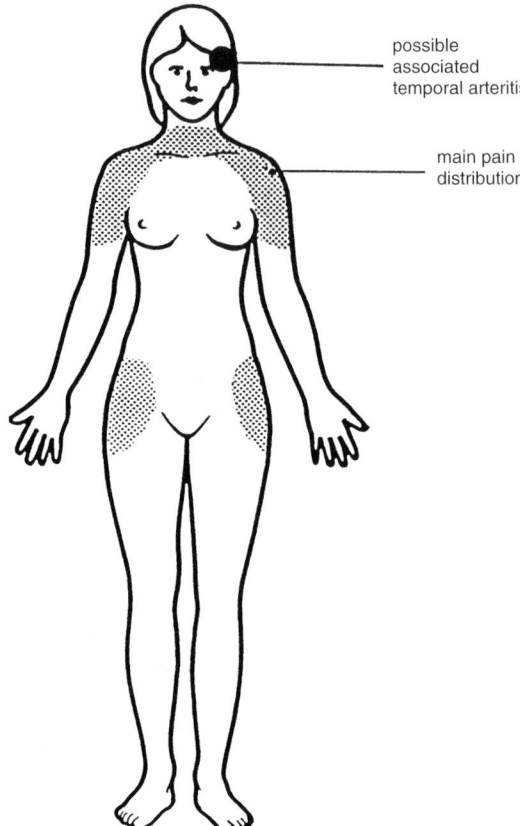

possible
associated
temporal arteritis

main pain
distribution

Fig. 28.7 *Polymyalgia rheumatica: typical sites of areas of pain and stiffness*

Clinical features of temporal arteritis
• headache—unilateral, throbbing
• temporal tenderness
• loss of pulsation of temporal artery
• jaw claudication
• biopsy of artery (5 cm) is diagnostic

Investigation
• no specific test for polymyalgia rheumatica
• ESR—extremely high, around 100
• C-reactive protein—elevated
• mild anaemia (normochromic, normocytic)

Treatment

Prednisolone

• Starting dose
  — temporal arteritis   60 mg
  — polymyalgia rheumatica   15 mg
• Taper down gradually to the minimum effective dose (often < 5 mg daily) according to

the clinical response and the ESR. Aim for treatment for 2 years: relapses are common.
Other drugs:
azathioprine or methotrexate can be used as steroid sparing agents.

Wegener's granulomatosis
In this rare granulomatous vasculitis of unknown cause there is a classic triad: upper respiratory tract granuloma, fleeting pulmonary shadows (nodules) and glomerulonephritis. Without treatment it is invariably fatal and sometimes the initial diagnosis is that made at autopsy. It is difficult to diagnose, especially as the patient (usually young to middle-aged) presents with a febrile illness and respiratory symptoms, but early diagnosis is essential.

Clinical features
• adolescence to elderly, mean age 40–45
• constitutional symptoms (as for PN)
• lower respiratory symptoms, e.g. cough, dyspnoea
• upper respiratory symptoms: rhinorrhoea, epistaxis, sinus pain
• polyarthritis
• renal involvement—usually not clinically apparent
• chest X-ray points to diagnosis—multiple nodes, cavitations
• antineutrophil antibodies are a useful diagnostic marker (not specific)
• diagnosis confirmed by biopsy, usually an open lung biopsy
• better prognosis with early diagnosis and treatment with cyclophosphamide.

References
1. Kumer PJ, Clark ML. *Clinical medicine* (2nd edn). London: Bailliere Tindall, 1990, 392–399.
2. Ryan PFJ. Systemic lupus erythematosus. In: MIMS Disease Index (2nd edn). Sydney: IMS Publishing, 1996, 497–499.
3. Randell P. Scleroderma. In: MIMS Disease Index (2nd edn). Sydney: IMS Publishing, 1996, 458–460.
4. Steen VD et al. D-penicillamine therapy in progressive systemic sclerosis. Annals of Internal Medicine, 1982; 97:652–659.

29
Neurological dilemmas

—

The disease is of long duration; to connect, therefore, the symptoms which occur in its later stages with those which mark its commencement, requires a continuance of observation of the same case, or at least a correct history of its symptoms, even for several years.

James Parkinson (1755–1824)
An essay on the shaking palsy

In general practice there are many neurological problems that present a diagnostic dilemma with some being true masquerades for the non-neurologist. This applies particularly to various seizure disorders, space-occupying lesions in the cerebrum and the cerebellum, demyelinating disorders, motor neurone disorders and peripheral neuropathies.

The most common pitfall that occurs with neurological disorders is misdiagnosis, and the most common reason for misdiagnosis is an inadequate history. Failure to appreciate the neurological meaning of points elicited during the history is another reason for misdiagnosis.

Some very important neurological disorders are presented in this section: Parkinson's disease, which is common and can be easily misdiagnosed especially when the classic 'pill rolling' tremor is absent or mild; multiple sclerosis (MS), because it is difficult to diagnose initially; and acute idiopathic demyelinating polyneuropathy (Guillain-Barré syndrome), because it can be rapidly fatal if misdiagnosed. MS can masquerade as almost anything—'If you don't know what it is, think of MS.'

Another brain teaser for the family doctor is to diagnose accurately the various types of epilepsy. The most commonly misdiagnosed seizure disorders are complex partial seizures or atypical generalised tonic clonic seizures (see Chapter 50).[1] Even more difficult is the differentiation of real seizures from pseudo- or non-epileptic seizures.

Diplopia

The onset of diplopia (double vision) in adults is often acute, very distressing and invariably easy to diagnose. It can be divided into two distinct types: uniocular (confined to one eye) or binocular, which usually results from extraocular muscular imbalance or weakness. The type of binocular diplopia—vertical, horizontal or oblique—provides clues in identifying the affected muscle.

Causes of uniocular diplopia
- early cataract (common in older patient—usually in dim light and at night)
- dislocated lens
- severe astigmatism
- psychogenic/functional

Causes of binocular diplopia
- ocular nerve palsies (3, 4 or 6)
  consider: — CVA or TIA
  — tumour (orbital or intracerebral)
  — aneurysm
  — diabetes mellitus
  — arteritis
  — head injury
  — ophthalmoplegic migraine (transient)
- muscle tethering, e.g. blow-out orbital fracture
- concussion
- multiple sclerosis (recurrent diplopia)
- myasthenia gravis ⎫ multiple muscle
- hyperthyroidism ⎭ movement

Office tests

Test for double vision with each eye occluded. If diplopia persists it is uniocular. If, however, double vision disappears when either eye is covered, there is a defect of one of the muscles moving the eyeball. Determine whether diplopia occurs in any particular direction of gaze. It is most marked when moved in the direction of action of the weak muscle. Ask patient to follow your finger, red pin or penlight with both eyes and move it in an H pattern.

- 3rd nerve—eye turned out: divergent squint
- 6th nerve—failure to abduct: convergent squint

See Figure 29.1.

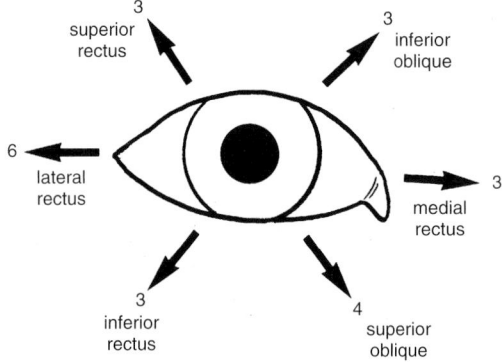

Fig. 29.1 *Direction of movement of the right eye indicating the responsible extra-ocular muscles and cranial nerves (3 = oculomotor, 4 = trochlear, 6 = abducens)*

Laboratory test

ESR (consider arteritis)

Note: • Exclude 3rd and 6th nerve palsies as they may be secondary to life-threatening conditions.
• Refer urgently if diplopia is binocular, of recent onset and persistent.

Motor weakness

Muscle weakness is a common feature of many disorders ranging from neurogenic and myogenic disorders to metabolic and psychiatric. It is very important clinically to be able to differentiate upper motor neurone (UMN) signs from lower motor neurone (LMN) signs (Table 29.1).

Upper motor neurone lesions

UMN signs occur when a lesion has interrupted a neural pathway at a level above the anterior

Table 29.1 *Clinical differences between a lower motor neurone lesion and an upper motor neurone lesion*

Manifestation	UMN	LMN
Weakness	Present	Present
Wasting	Absent or mild	Marked
Power	Reduced	Reduced
Tone	Usually increased (spastic paralysis) ± clonus	Absent or decreased (flaccid paralysis)
Fasciculations	Absent	May be present
Reflexes	Brisk tendon reflexes Abdominal absent Extensor plantar response	Absent or diminished

horn cell.[2] Examples include lesions in motor pathways in the cerebral cortex, internal capsule, brainstem or spinal cord.

Clinical examples include stroke (thrombosis, embolism or haemorrhage in the brain), tumours of the various pathways, and demyelinating disease such as multiple sclerosis and infection, for example HIV.

Lower motor neurone lesions

LMN signs occur when a lesion interrupts peripheral neural pathways from the anterior horn cell, that is, the spinal reflex arc.

Clinical examples include peripheral neuropathy, Guillain-Barré syndrome, motor neurone disease, poliomyelitis and a thickened peripheral nerve, e.g. leprosy.

Note: A spinal cord lesion causes LMN signs at the level of the lesion and UMN signs below that level.

Neurogenic and myogenic muscle weakness

It is also important to distinguish between weakness caused by neurological conditions, especially those causing LMN lesions and muscular disorders. The features are compared in Table 29.2.

Tremor

Tremor is an important symptom to evaluate correctly. A list of causes is presented in Table 29.3. A common pitfall in patients presenting with

Table 29.2 *Muscle weakness: main clinical differences between neurogenic and myogenic lesions*[3]

Myogenic weakness	Neurogenic weakness
Reflexes often present despite severe weakness	Reflexes often absent despite minimal weakness
Weakness out of proportion to wasting	Wasting out of proportion to weakness
Sensation normal	± sensory changes
No fasciculation	Fasciculation a feature

Table 29.3 *Causes of tremor*

- Physiological
- Benign essential (familial) tremor
- Senile
- Anxiety, including hyperventilation
- Hyperthyroidism
- Toxic, e.g. alcohol, liver failure, uraemia
- Drugs, e.g. lithium, narcotic withdrawal
- Parkinson's disease
- Drug-induced parkinsonism
- Cerebellar disease
- Cerebral tumour (frontal lobe)
- Alzheimer's dementia
- Wilson's disease
- Miscellaneous, e.g. red-nucleus lesion, hypoglycaemia

tremor is for Parkinson's disease to be diagnosed as benign essential tremor and for benign essential tremor to be diagnosed as Parkinson's disease, but the clinical distinction is not always easy and it must be remembered that as many as 20% will experience both concurrently.

Tremors can be classified as follows:

Resting tremor—Parkinsonian

The tremor of Parkinson's disease is present at rest. The hand tremor is most marked with the arms supported on the lap and during walking. The characteristic movement is 'pill-rolling' where movement of the fingers at the metacarpophalangeal joints is combined with movements of the thumb. The resting tremor decreases on finger-nose testing but a faster action tremor may supervene. The best way to evoke the tremor is to distract the patient, such as focusing attention on the left hand with a view to 'examining' the right hand or by turning the head.

Action or postural tremor

This fine tremor is noted by examining the patient with the arms outstretched and the fingers apart. The tremor may be rendered more obvious if a sheet of paper is placed over the dorsum of the hands. The tremor is present throughout movement, being accentuated by voluntary contraction.

Causes include:

- essential tremor (also called familial tremor or benign essential tremor)
- senile tremor
- physiological
- anxiety/emotional
- hyperthyroidism
- alcohol
- drugs, e.g. drug withdrawal (e.g. heroin, cocaine, alcohol), amphetamines, lithium, sympathomimetics (bronchodilators), sodium valproate, heavy metals (e.g. mercury), caffeine, amiodarone
- phaeochromocytoma

Intention tremor (cerebellar disease)

This coarse oscillating tremor is absent at rest but exacerbated by action and increases as the target is approached. It is tested by 'finger-nose-finger' touching or running the heel down the opposite shin, and past pointing of the nose is a feature. It occurs in cerebellar lobe disease and with lesions of cerebellar connections.

Flapping (metabolic tremor)

A flapping or 'wing-beating' tremor is observed when the arms are extended with hyperextension of the wrists. It involves slow, coarse and jerky movements of flexion and extension at the wrists.

Note: Flapping (asterixis) is not strictly a tremor.

Causes
- Wilson's disease
- hepatic encephalopathy
- uraemia
- respiratory failure
- lesions of the red nucleus of the midbrain (the classic cause of a flap)

Essential tremor

Essential tremor, which is probably the most common movement disorder, has been variously called benign, familial, senile or juvenile tremor.

However, it is not always benign and there is no family history in about half the cases.

Features

- autosomal dominant disorder (variable penetrance)
- often begins in early adult life, even adolescence
- begins with a slight tremor in one hand and spreads to other with time
- may involve head (titubation), chin and tongue and rarely trunk and legs
- interferes with writing (not micrographic), handling cups of tea and spoons, etc.
- tremor most marked when arms held out (postural tremor)
- tremor exacerbated by anxiety
- may affect speech if it involves bulbar musculature
- relieved by alcohol
- can swing arm and gait normal

Triad of features

- positive family history
- tremor with little disability
- normal gait

Distinguishing essential tremor from Parkinson's disease

This is not always easy as a postural tremor can be present in Parkinson's disease although the hand tremor is most marked at rest with the arms supported on the lap. Parkinsonian tremor is slower at 4–6 Hz while essential tremor is much faster at around 8–13 Hz.

A most useful way to differentiate the two causes is to observe the gait. It is normal in essential tremor but in Parkinson's there may be loss of arm swing and the step is usually shortened.

Management of essential tremor

Most patients do not need treatment and all that is required is an appropriate explanation.[1] If necessary, use propranolol (first choice) or primidone[4]. A typical starting dose of propranolol is 40 mg bd; many require 120–240 mg/day.[4] If the tremor is only intrusive at times of increased emotional stress, intermittent use of benzodiazepines, e.g. lorazepam, 30 minutes before exposure to the stress may be all that is required. Modest alcohol intake, e.g. a glass of scotch, is very effective.

Parkinson's disease

One of the most important clinical aspects of Parkinson's disease, which has a slow and insidious onset, is the ability to make an early diagnosis. Sometimes this can be very difficult especially when the tremor is absent or mild, as occurs with the atherosclerotic degenerative type of parkinsonism. The lack of any specific abnormality on special investigation leaves the responsibility for a diagnosis based on the history and examination. As a general rule of thumb the diagnosis of Parkinson's disease is restricted to those who respond to levodopa—the rest are termed parkinsonism.

Key facts and checkpoints

- Parkinson's disease is a most common and disabling chronic neurological disorder.
- The prevalence in Australia is 100–120 per 100 000.[5]
- The mean age of onset is between 58 and 62.[5]
- The incidence rises sharply over 70 years of age.[5]
- The classic triad of Parkinson's disease (Fig. 29.2) is:
  — tremor
  — rigidity
  — bradykinesia (poverty of movement)
- Hemi-parkinsonism can occur; all the signs are confined to one side and thus must be differentiated from hemiparesis. In fact most Parkinson's disease starts unilaterally.
- Always consider drug-induced parkinsonism. The usual drugs are phenothiazines, butyrophenones and reserpine. Tremor is uncommon but rigidity and bradykinesia may be severe. Refer to Table 29.4.

Physical signs

- Power, reflexes and sensation are usually normal.
- The earliest abnormal physical signs to appear are loss of dexterity of rapid alternating movements and absence of arm swing, in addition to increased tone with distraction.
- Frontal lobe signs such as grasp and glabellar taps (only allow 3 blinks) are more common with parkinsonism.

Note: There is no laboratory test for Parkinson's—it is a clinical diagnosis. Hypothyroidism and depression, which also cause

masked facies

staring expression

slow, monotonous speech

failure
to swing
arm

pill-rolling
tremor
at rest

slow and shuffling gait
short steps

Fig. 29.2 *Basic clinical features of Parkinson's disease*

slowness of movement, may cause confusion with diagnosis.

The Steele-Richardson syndrome (parkinsonism, mild dementia and vertical gaze dysfunction) is worth considering.

Principles of management

- Provide appropriate explanation and education.
- Explain that Parkinson's disease is slowly progressive, and is improved but not cured by treatment. It does not usually shorten life.
- Support systems are necessary for advanced Parkinson's disease.
- Walking sticks with appropriate education into their use may be necessary to help prevent falls and constant care is required, so that admission to a nursing home for end-stage disease may be appropriate.

Pharmacological management

Avoid postponing treatment. It should be commenced as soon as symptoms interfere with working capacity or the patient's enjoyment of life. This will be apparent only if the correct questions are asked as the patient may accept impaired enjoyment without appreciating that it is due to Parkinson's disease. Start low, e.g. Sinemet 100/25 (½ tab bd). The dosage should be tailored so that the patient neither develops side effects nor is on an inadequate dose of medication without significant therapeutic benefit (Table 29.5).

The older drugs such as anticholinergics and amantadine have minimal usage in modern management as levodopa, which basically counters bradykinesia, is the best drug and the baseline of treatment. With the onset of disability (motor disturbances) levodopa in combination with a decarboxylase inhibitor (carbidopa or benserazide) in a 4:1 ratio should be introduced. Levodopa therapy does not significantly improve tremor but improves rigidity, dyskinesia and gait disorder. Consider benzhexol or benztropine if tremor is the feature.

Pergolide can be used in treatment, especially with the levodopa 'on–off' phenomenon (fluctuations throughout the day). It appears to be most effective when used in combination. The major side effects of pergolide are similar to levodopa. Dyskinesia and nausea are less problematic but severe psychiatric disturbances are more common with bromocriptine. It should therefore be used with caution in patients with a history of confusion or dementia. Selegiline promises to be an effective first-line drug. If there is associated pain, depression or insomnia, the tricyclic agents, e.g. amitriptyline, can be effective.

Treatment strategy

Mild (minimal disability):

- levodopa preparation (low dose)
  e.g. levodopa 100 mg + carbidopa 25 mg (½ tab bd—increase gradually as necessary to 1 tab (o) tds)
- amantadine 100 mg (o) bd may help the young or the elderly for up to 12 months
- selegiline (can postpone need for L-dopa)

Moderate[10] (independent but disabled, e.g. writing, movements, gait):

- levodopa preparation
- add if necessary—pergolide or selegiline
  pergolide 50 µg (o) bd, gradually increasing to 1.5 mg (max) bd
  selegiline 2.5 mg (o) daily, increasing to 5 mg (max) bd

Table 29.4 *Parkinson's disease: symptoms and signs (a checklist)*

General	• Tiredness • Lethargy • Restlessness
Tremor	• Present at rest • Slow rate—4 to 6 cycles per second • Alternating, especially arms • Pill-rolling (severe cases) *Note:* may be absent or unilateral
Rigidity	• 'Cogwheel' • Lead pipe
Bradykinesia/hypokinesia	• Slowness of initiating a movement • Difficulty with fine finger tasks • Micrographia (Fig. 29.3) • Masked facies • Relative lack of blinking • Impaired convergence of eyes • Excessive salivation (late) • Difficulty turning over in bed and rising from a chair • Slow monotonous speech/dysarthria
Gait disorder	• No arm swing on one or both sides • Start hesitation • Slow and shuffling • Short steps (*petit pas*) • Slow turning circle • 'Freezing' when approaching an obstacle • Festination
Disequilibrium	• Poor balance • Impaired righting reflexes • Falls (usually late)
Posture	• Progressive forward flexion of trunk • Flexion of elbow at affected side
Autonomic symptoms	• Constipation (common) • Postural hypotension • Depression (early)
Psychiatric	• Progressive dementia in 30–40% usually after 10 years[5]

Severe   (disabled, dependent on others):
• levodopa (to maximum tolerated dose) + pergolide or selegiline
• consider antidepressants

Long-term problems

After 3–5 years of levodopa treatment side effects may appear in about one half of patients:[5]
• involuntary movements—dyskinesia (use lower dose + pergolide)
• end of dose failure (reduced duration of effect to 2–3 hours only)
• 'on-off' phenomenon (sudden inability to move with recovery in 30–90 minutes)
• early morning dystonia, e.g. clawing of toes (due to disease—not a side effect); management of motor problems summarised in Table 29.6.

Advanced disease[10]

• Apomorphine can be used for severe akinesia not responsive to levodopa:
apomorphine 600 µg to 6 mg (mean 3.4 mg) SC
• For nausea and vomiting side effects:
domperidone 20 mg (o) tds
• Better control may also be achieved with:
amantadine 100 mg (o) bd

Fig. 29.3 *Micrographia, one of the signs of Parkinson's disease*

Table 29.5 *Anti-parkinson drugs*

Agent	Main side effects
Amantadine	• Nausea and vomiting • Ankle oedema • Livedo reticularis
Anticholinergic agents • benzhexol • benztropine • biperiden • orphenadrine • procyclidine	• Dryness of mouth • Confusion in elderly • Contraindicated in glaucoma and prostatism • Other anticholinergic effects, e.g. constipation
Bromocriptine	• Nausea and vomiting • Dizziness, fatigue • Psychiatric disturbances • Pleuropulmonary changes
Levodopa Levodopa + benserazide Levodopa + carbidopa	• Nausea and vomiting • Involuntary dyskinetic movements • Psychiatric disturbances • On–off phenomena • End of dose failure
Pergolide	• Nausea • Hypotension • Confusion • Dyskinesia • Sleep disturbances
Selegiline	• Dry mouth • Nausea • Dizziness, fatigue
Apomorphine (SC injection)	• Nausea • Psychosis • Dyskinesia

Table 29.6 *Management of motor problems in treated Parkinson's disease*[7]

Motor problem	Management
End of dose failure	• Dosages closer together • Slow-release preparations • MAO-B inhibitor, e.g. selegiline • Dopaminergic agonist, e.g. pergolide
'On-off' phenomenon	• Subcutaneous apomorphine for 'off' phase (1 hour action) with domperidone (o) to prevent vomiting • Levodopa and ascorbic acid solution
Loss of efficacy	• Increase levodopa dose as high as possible • Dopaminergic agonist, e.g. pergolide
Peak dose dyskinesia	• Decrease levodopa dose • MAO-B inhibitor, if efficacy lost • Dopaminergic agonist, e.g. pergolide
Early morning dystonia	• Slow release levodopa • Dopaminergic agonists, e.g. pergolide
Nocturnal akinesia	• Slow release levodopa • Dopaminergic agonist

Contraindicated drugs
• phenothiazines
• butyrophenones

Surgical treatment

The indication for surgery (stereotactic thalamotomy)[6] is the presence of tremor or rigidity not responding to chemical therapy. It is more appropriate for younger patients with a unilateral tremor.[10] The success rate of surgery is at least 80%. It alleviates tremor and rigidity but does not prevent progression of bradykinesia, dysarthria or dementia. This is a very effective treatment that has often been overlooked but should never be forgotten.

When to refer

If the diagnosis is unclear at the time of initial presentation, it is appropriate either to review the patient at a later date or to refer the patient for more neurological assessment.

Once diagnosed or highly suspected it is best to refer to establish the diagnosis and to seek advice on initiation of treatment. Patients and families usually prefer this approach. In the initial years before motor fluctuations develop, management could be performed by the general practitioner according to an overall plan developed in liaison with a neurological colleague. When fluctuations develop and end-stage diseases manifest (e.g. gait disorders) specialist supervision is appropriate.[1]

Practice tips

- Levodopa is the gold standard for therapy.
- Longer acting levodopa preparations may reduce the 'end of dose' failure effect but remember the possible need for a 'kick start' with short-acting preparations, e.g. first thing in the morning.
- Ensure that a distinction is made between drug-induced involuntary movements and the tremor of Parkinson's disease.
- Keep the dose of levodopa as low as possible to avoid these drug-induced involuntary movements.
- In the elderly with a fractured hip always consider Parkinson's disease (a manifestation of disequilibrium).
- Remember the balance of psychosis and Parkinson's disease in treatment.
- Keep in mind the 'sundown' effect—patients often go psychotic as the sun goes down.
- Don't fail to attend to the needs of the family, who often suffer in silence.
- Bromocriptine and pergolide should be used very cautiously in the elderly because of possible acute psychotic reactions.

Multiple sclerosis

Multiple sclerosis (MS) is the most common cause of progressive neurological disability in the 20–50 year age group.[8] Early diagnosis is difficult because MS is characterised by widespread neurologic lesions that cannot be explained by a single anatomical lesion, and the various symptoms and signs are subject to irregular exacerbations and remissions. The most important issue in diagnosis is the need for a high index of suspicion.

MS is a primary demyelinating disorder with demyelination occurring in plaques throughout the white matter of the brain, brainstem, spinal cord and optic nerves. The clinical features depend on their location.

Clinical features
(See Fig. 29.4.)
- more common in females
- peak age of onset is in the fourth decade
- transient motor and sensory disturbances
- upper motor neurone signs
- symptoms develop over several days but can be sudden
- monosymptomatic initially in about 80%
- multiple symptoms initially in about 20%
- common initial symptoms include:
  — visual disturbances of optic neuritis
    • blurred vision or loss of vision in one eye (sometimes both)
    • central scotoma with pain on eye movement (looks like unilateral papilloedema)
  — diplopia (brainstem lesion)
  — weakness in one or both legs, paraparesis or hemiparesis
  — sensory impairment in the lower limbs and trunk
    • numbness, paraesthesia
    • band-like sensations
    • clumsiness of limb (loss of position sense)
    • feeling as though walking on cotton wool
  — vertigo (brainstem lesion)
- subsequent remissions and exacerbations that vary from one individual to another
- there is a progressive form especially in women around 50 years

Neurological examination
The findings depend on the site of the lesion or lesions and include optic atrophy, weakness, hyper-reflexia, extensor plantar responses, nystagmus (two types: cerebellar or ataxic), ataxia, inco-ordination and regional impairment of sensation.

Symptoms causing diagnostic confusion
- bladder disturbances, including retention of urine and urgency
- 'useless hand' due to loss of position sense
- facial palsy
- trigeminal neuralgia
- psychiatric symptoms

In established disease common symptoms are fatigue, impotence and bladder disturbances.

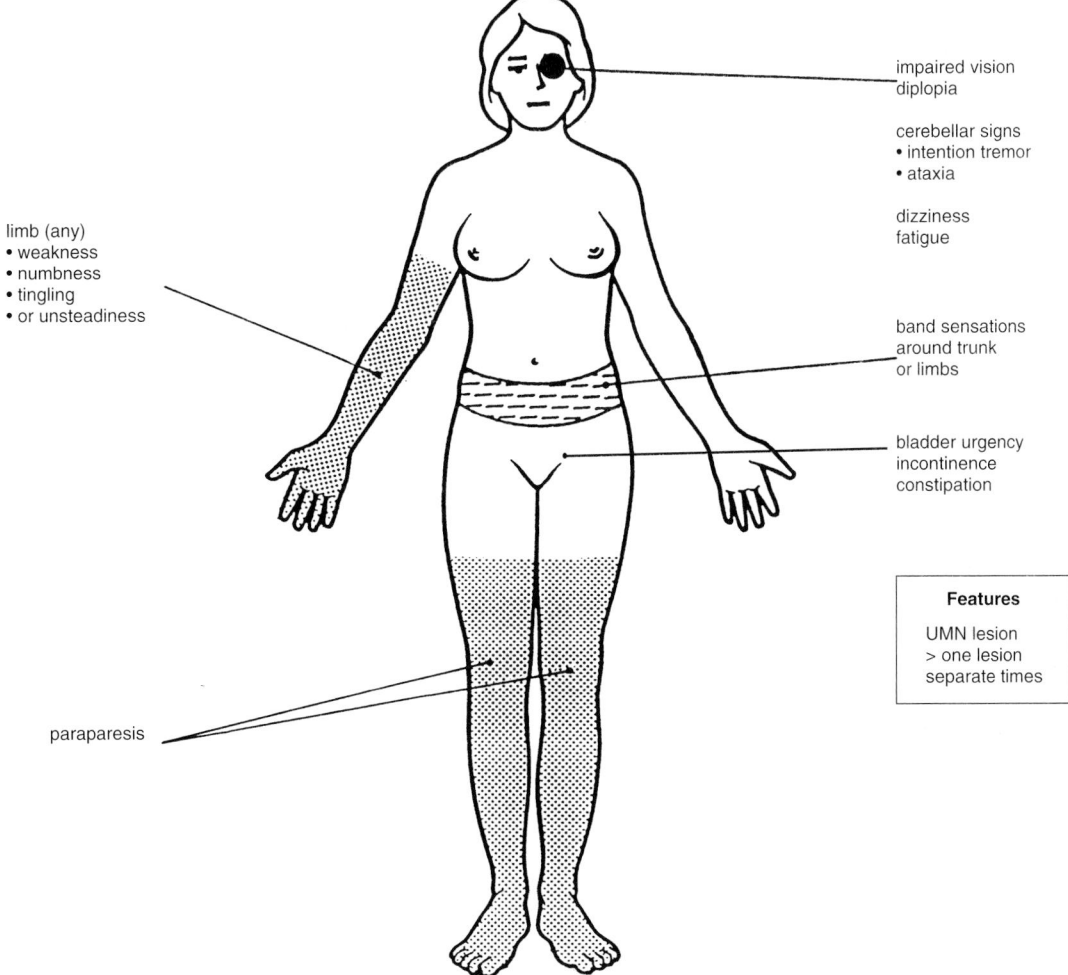

impaired vision
diplopia

cerebellar signs
• intention tremor
• ataxia

dizziness
fatigue

limb (any)
• weakness
• numbness
• tingling
• or unsteadiness

band sensations
around trunk
or limbs

bladder urgency
incontinence
constipation

Features

UMN lesion
> one lesion
separate times

paraparesis

Fig. 29.4 *Basic clinical signs in multiple sclerosis*

Diagnosis

The diagnosis is clinical and depends on the following determinants:

- Lesions are invariably UMN.
- Lesions affect the CNS white matter.
- >1 part of CNS is involved, although not necessarily at time of presentation.
- Episodes are separated in time (it is possible to make a diagnosis with the first episode).

Other neurological diseases such as infections (e.g. encephalitis), malignancies, spinal cord compression, spinocerebellar degeneration and others must be excluded.

Investigations

- Lumbar puncture: oligoclonal IgG detected in CSF in 90% of cases[8] (only if necessary)

- Visual evoked potentials: abnormal in about 90% of cases
- CT scan: rarely demonstrates MS lesions but useful in excluding other pathology
- MRI scan: usually abnormal, demonstrating MS lesions in about 90% of cases[8]

Course and prognosis

- The course is variable and difficult to predict. An early onset (< 30) is usually 'benign' while a late onset (≥ 50) is often 'malignant'.
- MS follows a classical history of relapses and remissions in 80–85% of patients.[9]
- The rate of relapse is about once in 2 years.
- About 20% have a progressive course from the onset with a progressive spastic paraparesis (applies mainly to late-age onset).

- The average duration of MS is about 30 years from diagnosis to death.[8]
- A benign course occurs in about 40% of patients with 10–20% never suffering major disability.
- The median time to needing a walking aid is 15 years.[10]
- The likelihood of developing MS after a single episode of optic neuritis is about 60%.

Management principles

- All patients should be referred to a neurologist for confirmation of the diagnosis, which must be accurate.
- Explanation about the disease and its natural history should be given.
- Acute relapses require treatment if causing significant disability.
- Depression and anxiety, which are common, require early treatment.

Relapses
Mild relapses
Mild symptoms such as numbness and tingling require only confirmation, rest and reassurance.

Moderate relapses[10]
For symptoms that are unpleasant or disabling use a short course of high-dose prednisolone.

- prednisolone 75 mg (o) once daily for 4 days, then 50 mg (o) daily for 4 days, then 25 mg (o) daily for 4 days

Severe relapses or attacks[10,11]
These attacks include optic neuritis, paraplegia or brainstem signs. Admit to hospital for IV therapy:

- methylprednisolone 1 g in 200 mL saline by slow IV injection (3 hours) daily for 3 to 5 days

Observe carefully for cardiac arrhythmias.

Drugs to prevent relapses[11]
Interferon beta-1b (SC injection) and beta-1a (IM injection) are effective (but expensive) for those with frequent and severe attacks. Copolymer-1 is still under evaluation.

Drugs to reduce progression[10,12]
Current recommended treatment given under careful supervision:

- methotrexate 7.5 mg (o), on 1 day each week
  +
- folic acid 5 mg (o), 3 days after each methotrexate dose

Immunosuppression can also be given with cyclophosphamide or azathioprine.[13]

Treatment of symptoms[10]
Spasticity
- physiotherapy
- baclofen 10–25 mg (o) nocte
- for continuous drug therapy:
  — baclofen 5 mg (o) tds, increasing to 25 mg (o) tds
    +
  — diazepam 2–10 mg (o) tds

Paroxysmal, e.g. neuralgias
- carbamazepine or clonazepam

See references 10 and 12 for treatment of other symptoms.

Acute idiopathic demyelinating polyneuropathy (Guillain-Barré syndrome)

Guillain-Barré syndrome is the best known of the peripheral neuropathies that have an acute onset, and it is potentially fatal. Early diagnosis of this serious disease by the family doctor is crucial as respiratory paralysis may lead to death. The underlying pathology is segmental demyelination of peripheral nerves and nerve roots.

Clinical features
- paraesthesia or pain in the limbs
- weakness in the limbs (usually symmetrical)
- both proximal and distal muscles affected
- facial and bulbar paralysis
- weakness of extraocular muscles (rarely)
- reflexes depressed or absent
- variable sensory loss but rare

Within 3–4 weeks the motor neuropathy, which is the main feature, progresses to a maximum disability, possibly with complete quadriparesis and respiratory paralysis.[14]

Investigations
- CSF protein is elevated; cells are usually normal.
- Motor nerve conduction studies are abnormal.

Management

- Respiratory function (vital capacity) should be measured regularly (2–4 hours at first).
- Tracheostomy and artificial ventilation may be necessary.
- Physiotherapy to prevent foot and wrist drop and other general care should be provided.
- Plasmapheresis is the mainstay of treatment.
- IV immunoglobulin is also effective.[13]
- Corticosteroids are not generally recommended.

Outcome

About 80% of patients recover without significant disability. Approximately 5% relapse.[14]

Myasthenia gravis

Myasthenia gravis (MG) is an acquired autoimmune disease that usually affects muscle strength. Patients have fluctuating symptoms and variable distribution of muscle weakness. All degrees of severity ranging from occasional mild ptosis to fulminant quadriplegia and respiratory arrest can occur.[15] (See Table 29.7.)

Table 29.7   *Clinical classification of acquired myasthenia gravis (MG)*

Group I	Ocular MG
Group IIA	Mild generalised MG
IIB	Moderate to severe MG
Group III	Acute severe (fulminating) MG with respiratory muscle weakness
Group IV	Late (chronic) severe MG

Clinical features

- painless fatigue with exercise
- weakness also precipitated by emotional stress, pregnancy, infection, surgery
- variable distribution of weakness:
  - ocular • ptosis (60%) and diplopia
    - ocular myasthenia only remains in about 10%
  - bulbar: weakness of chewing, swallowing, speech, whistling and head lolling
  - limbs (proximal and distal)
  - generalised
  - respiratory: breathlessness, ventilatory failure

Note: The classical MG image is 'the thinker'— the hand used to hold the mouth closed and the head up.

Diagnostic tests

- serum anti-acetylcholine receptor antibodies
- electrophysiological tests if antibody test negative
- CT scan and chest X-ray to detect thymoma
- edrophonium test still useful

Management principles[15]

- Detect possible presence of thymoma with CT or MR scan of thorax. If present, removal is recommended.
- Thymectomy is recommended early for generalised myasthenia, especially in all younger patients with hyperplasia of the thymus, even if not confirmed preoperatively.
- Plasmapheresis is useful for acute crisis or where temporary improvement is required or patients are resistant to treatment.
- Avoid drugs that are relatively contraindicated.
- Pharmacological agents:
  - anticholinesterase drugs, e.g. pyridostigmine, neostigmine or distigmine: should be used only for mild to moderate symptoms
  - corticosteroids: useful for all grades of MG; should be introduced slowly

Practice tips

- The combination of ocular and facial weakness should alert the family doctor to the possibility of a neuromuscular disorder, especially MG or mitochondrial myopathy.[15] Look for weakness and fatigue.
- Beware of facioscapulohumeral dystrophy.
- Ptosis may develop only after looking upwards for a minute or longer.
- Smiling may have a characteristic snarling quality.

Ptosis

It is worth remembering that the four major causes of ptosis are:

1. 3rd cranial nerve palsy:
   ptosis, eye facing 'down and out', dilated pupil, sluggish light reflex
2. Horner's syndrome:
   ptosis, miosis (constricted pupil), ipsilateral loss of sweating
3. Mitochondrial myopathy:
   progressive external ophthalmoplegia or limb weakness, induced by activity
4. Myasthenia gravis:
   ptosis and diplopia

Dystonia

Definition

Dystonias are sustained or intermittent abnormal repetitive movements or postures resulting from alterations in muscle tone. The dystonic spasms may affect one (focal) or more (segmental) parts of the body or the whole body (generalised).

Key points

- Misdiagnosis is common as transient symptoms may be mistaken for an emotional or psychiatric disorder. Many cases take years to diagnose.
- Dystonias are often regarded as nervous tics.
- The cause is thought to be disorders of the basal ganglia of the brain, but mainly there is no known specific cause.
- Neuroleptic and dopamine receptor blocking agents (e.g. levodopa, metoclopramide) can induce a severe generalised dystonia, e.g. oculogyric crisis, which is treated with benztropine 1–2 mg IM or IV.[16]

Focal dystonias

- *Blepharospasm* is a focal dystonia of the muscles around the eye resulting in uncontrolled blinking, especially in bright light.
- *Oromandibular dystonia* affects the jaw, tongue and mouth resulting in jaw grinding movements and grimacing. Proper speech and swallowing may be disrupted.
- *Meige's syndrome* is a combination of blepharospasm and oromandibular dystonia.

    Note: It must be differentiated from the buccal-lingual-facial movements of tardive dyskinesia.

- *Hemifacial spasms* involves involuntary, irregular muscle contractions and spasms affecting one side of the face. It usually starts with twitching around the eye and then spreads to involve all the facial muscles on one side. It is usually due to irritation of the facial nerve in its intracranial course and surgical intervention may alleviate this problem.
- *Writer's cramp, typist's cramp, pianist's cramp, golfer's cramp* are all occupational focal dystonias of the hand and/or forearm initiated by performing these skilled acts.

- *Cervical dystonia or spasmodic torticollis* is a focal dystonia of unilateral cervical muscles. It usually begins with a pulling sensation followed by twisting or jerking of the head, leading to deviation of the head and neck to one side. In early stages patients can voluntarily overcome the dystonia.
- *Laryngeal or spastic dystonia* is focal dystonia of laryngeal muscles resulting in a strained, hoarse or creaking voice. It may lead to inability to speak in more than a whisper.

Treatment of focal dystonias

The current treatment for focal or segmental (spread to an adjacent body region) dystonias is localised injection of purified botulinum A toxin into the affected muscle groups. The dosage is highly individualised and needs to be repeated at intervals of 3 and 6 months. The injections have to be given with great caution.

Tics

Motor and vocal tics are a feature of Tourette's disorder. If socially disabling treat with:

- haloperidol 0.25 mg (o) nocte, very gradually increasing to 2 g (max) daily[10]

References

1. Iansek R. *Pitfalls in Neurology.* Proceedings of Monash University Medical School Update Course, 1992, 40–44.
2. Talley NJ, O'Connor S. *Clinical examination* (3rd edn). Sydney: Maclennan & Petty, 1996, 391–392.
3. Berkow R. *The Merck manual* (16th edn). Rahway, NJ: Merck & Co, 1992, 1432–1433.
4. Morris JGL. *Essential tremor.* In: MIMS Disease Index (2nd edn). Sydney: IMS Publishing, 1996, 179–180.
5. Selby G, Herkes G. Parkinson's disease. In: MIMS Disease Index (2nd edn). Sydney: IMS Publishing, 1996, 395–398.
6. Selby G. Stereotactic surgery. In: Koller WC ed, *Handbook of Parkinson's disease.* New York: Marcel Dekker Inc., 1987, 421–435.
7. Iansek R. Parkinson's disease. Current Therapeutics, 1995; 36 (10); 55–63.

8. McLeod JR. Multiple sclerosis. In: MIMS Disease Index (2nd edn). Sydney: IMS Publishing, 1996, 321–323.

9. Matthews B. Multiple sclerosis. Medicine International, 1988; 48:1961–1967.

10. Moulds RFW (Chairman). *Therapeutic guidelines: Neurology* (1st edn). Melbourne: Therapeutic Guidelines, 1997; 79–137.

11. Burnham JA et al. The effect of high-dose steroids on MRI gadolinium enhancement in acute demyelinating lesions. Neurology, 1993; 43: 655–661.

12. Jacobs L et al. Advance in specific therapy for multiple sclerosis. Curr Opin Neurol, 1994; 7: 250–254.

13. Milanese C et al. A double blind study on azathioprine in the treatment of multiple sclerosis. J Neurology, 1993; 240:295–298.

14. Pollard J. Neuropathy, peripheral. In: MIMS Disease Index (2nd edn). Sydney: IMS Publishing, 1996, 346.

15. McLeod JG. Peripheral neuropathy. Medicine International, 1988; 48: 1980–1984.

16. Darveniza P. Myasthenia gravis. In: MIMS Disease Index (2nd edn). Sydney: IMS Publishing, 1996, 324–326.

PART 3

PROBLEM SOLVING
IN GENERAL PRACTICE

30
Abdominal pain

—

A great fit of the stone in my left kidney: all day I could do but three or four drops of water, but I drunk a draught of white wine and salet oyle, and after that, crabs' eyes in powder with the bone in the carp's head and then drunk two great draughts of ale with buttered cake; and I voyded with an hour much water and a stone as big as an Alexander seed. God by thanked!

John Dee 1594

Abdominal pain represents one of the top 15 presenting symptoms in primary care[1] and varies from a self-limiting problem to a life-threatening illness requiring immediate surgical intervention. Abdominal pain can be considered to be acute, subacute, chronic or recurrent. It can embrace all specialties including surgery, medicine, gynaecology, geriatrics and psychiatry. For acute abdominal conditions it is important to make a rapid diagnosis in order to reduce morbidity and mortality. Most cases require surgical referral (Table 30.1). Lower abdominal pain in women adds another dimension to the problem and will be presented in a separate chapter.

Table 30.1 *Surgical causes of the acute abdomen*

Process	Organ involved	Disorder
Inflammation	Bowel	Inflammatory bowel disease
	Appendix	Appendicitis
	Gall bladder	Cholecystitis
	Pancreas	Pancreatitis
	Fallopian tube	Salpingitis
	Colonic diverticulae	Diverticulitis
Perforation	Duodenum	Perforated duodenal ulcer
	Stomach	Perforated gastric ulcer
	Colon (diverticula or carcinoma)	Faecal peritonitis
	Gall bladder	Biliary peritonitis
	Appendix	Appendicitis
Obstruction	Gall bladder	Biliary colic
	Small intestine	Acute small bowel obstruction
	Large bowel	Acute large bowel obstruction
	Ureter	Ureteric colic
	Urethra	Acute urinary retention
	Mesenteric artery occlusion	Intestinal infarction
Haemorrhage	Fallopian tube	Ruptured ectopic pregnancy
	Spleen or liver	Ruptured spleen or liver (haemoperitoneum)
	Ovary	Ruptured ovarian cyst
	Abdominal aorta	Ruptured AAA
Torsion (ischaemia)	Sigmoid colon	Sigmoid volvulus
	Ovary	Torsion ovarian cyst
	Testes	Torsion of testes

Key facts and checkpoints

- The commonest causes of the acute abdomen in two general practice series were: *Series 1* acute appendicitis (31%) and the colics (29%); *Series 2* acute appendicitis (21%), the colics (16%), mesenteric adenitis (16%).[3] The latter study included children.
- As a general rule upper abdominal pain is caused by lesions of the upper GI tract and lower abdominal pain by lesions of the lower GI tract.
- Colicky midline umbilical abdominal pain (severe) → vomiting → distension = small bowel obstruction.
- Midline lower abdominal pain → distension → vomiting = large bowel obstruction.
- If the acute abdomen has a surgical cause, the pain nearly always precedes the vomiting.
- Mesenteric artery occlusion must be considered in an elderly person with arteriosclerotic disease or in patients with atrial fibrillation presenting with severe abdominal pain or following myocardial infarction.
- Up to one-third of presentations of abdominal pain are considered to be non-specific, whereby no specific cause is found.

A diagnostic approach

A summary of the separate diagnostic models for acute abdominal pain and chronic abdominal pain are presented in Tables 30.2 and 30.3.

Probability diagnosis

The most common causes of acute abdomen are acute appendicitis, acute gastroenteritis, an irritable bowel syndrome, the various 'colics' and ovulation pain (mittelschmerz). Mesenteric adenitis is common in children. The various causes of chronic or recurrent abdominal pain are presented in Table 30.3. A study on chronic abdominal pain[4] showed that the commonest reasons (approximate percentages) were: no discoverable causes (50%), minor causes including muscle strains (16%), irritable bowel syndrome (12%), gynaecological causes (8%), peptic ulcers and hiatus hernia (8%).

Serious disorders not to be missed

Most of the causes of the acute abdomen are serious and early diagnosis is mandatory to reduce mortality and morbidity. It is vital not to misdiagnose a ruptured ectopic pregnancy,

Table 30.2 *Acute abdominal pain (adults): diagnostic strategy model*

Q. *Probability diagnosis*
A. Acute gastroenteritis
   Acute appendicitis
   Mittelschmerz/dysmenorrhoea
   Irritable bowel syndrome

Q. *Serious disorders not to be missed*
A. Cardiovascular
   - myocardial infarction
   - ruptured AAA
   - dissecting aneurysm aorta
   - mesenteric artery occlusion
   Neoplasia
   - large or small bowel obstruction
   Severe infections
   - acute salpingitis
   - peritonitis
   - ascending cholangitis
   - intra-abdominal abscess
   Ectopic pregnancy
   Small bowel obstruction
   Sigmoid volvulus
   Perforated ulcer

Q. *Pitfalls (often missed)*
A. Acute appendicitis
   Myofascial tear
   Pulmonary causes
   - pneumonia
   - pulmonary embolism
   Faecal impaction (elderly)
   Herpes zoster
   Rarities
   - porphyria
   - lead poisoning
   - haemochromatosis
   - sickle cell disease
   - tabes dorsalis

Q. *Seven masquerades checklist*
A. Depression   √
   Diabetes   √
   Drugs   √
   Anaemia   sickle cell
   Thyroid disease   —
   Spinal dysfunction   √
   UTI   √

Q. *Is the patient trying to tell me something?*
A. May be very significant.
   Consider Munchausen's syndrome, sexual dysfunction and abnormal stress.

which causes lower abdominal or suprapubic pain of sudden onset, or the life-threatening vascular causes such as a ruptured or dissecting aortic aneurysm, mesenteric artery occlusion and myocardial infarction (which can present as epigastric pain).

Perforated ulcers and strangulated bowel, such as volvulus of the sigmoid and entrapment of the the small bowel in a hernial orifice or around

Table 30.3 *Chronic or recurrent abdominal pain (adult): diagnostic strategy model*

Q. *Probability diagnosis*
A. Irritable bowel syndrome
   Mittelschmerz/dysmenorrhoea
   Peptic ulcer/gastritis

Q. *Serious disorders not to be missed*
A. Cardiovascular
   • mesenteric artery ischaemia
   • abdominal aortic aneurysm
   Neoplasia
   • carcinoma bowel/stomach
   • carcinoma pancreas
   • ovarian tumours
   Severe infections
   • hepatitis
   • recurrent PID

Q. *Pitfalls (often missed)*
A. Food allergies
   Lactase deficiency
   Constipation
   Chronic pancreatitis
   Crohn's disease
   Endometriosis
   Diverticulitis
   Rarities
   • uraemia
   • lead poisoning
   • Crohn's diease
   • porphyria
   • sickle cell disease
   • Addison's disease

Q. *Seven masquerades checklist*
A. Depression   √
   Diabetes   —
   Drugs   √
   Anaemia   —
   Thyroid disease   —
   Spinal dysfunction √
   UTI   √

Q. *Is the patient trying to tell me something?*
A. A strong possibility: consider hypochondriasis, anxiety, sexual dysfunction.

adhesions, also demand an early diagnosis.

There are some important 'red flag' symptoms and signs[1] of abdominal emergencies demanding urgent attention:

• collapsing at toilet (points to intra-abdominal bleeding)
• light-headedness
• progressive intractable·vomiting
• progressive abdominal distension
• progressive intensity of pain
• prostration

Signs

• pallor and sweating
• hypotension
• atrial fibrillation or tachycardia
• fever
• rebound tenderness and guarding
• decreased urine output

Dangers of misdiagnosis

• ectopic pregnancy → rapid hypovolaemic shock
• ruptured aortic aneurysm → rapid hypovolaemic shock
• gangrenous appendix → peritonitis/pelvic abscess
• perforated ulcer → peritonitis
• obstructed bowel → gangrene

Pitfalls

A very common pitfall is misdiagnosing acute appendicitis, especially in the elderly, in children, in pregnancy and in those on steroids, where the presentation may be atypical. Early appendicitis presents typically with central abdominal pain that shifts to the right iliac fossa (RIF) some 4 to 6 hours later. This causes confusion early on. It can cause diarrhoea with abdominal pain, especially if a pelvic appendix, and can be misdiagnosed as acute gastroenteritis.

Disaccharidase deficiencies such as lactase deficiency are associated with cramping abdominal pain, which may be severe. The pain follows some time, maybe hours, after the ingestion of milk and is accompanied by the passage of watery stool. The association with milk may be unrecognised by the patient.

Herpes zoster, especially in the elderly patient with unilateral abdominal pain in the dermatomal distribution, is a trap. Referred pain from conditions above the diaphragm such as myocardial infarction, pulmonary embolism and pneumonia can be misleading. The rare general medical causes such as diabetes ketoacidosis, acute porphyria, Addison's disease, lead poisoning, tabes dorsalis, sickle cell disease, haemochromatosis and uraemia often create a diagnostic dilemma and should be kept in mind.

Specific pitfalls

• Misdiagnosing a ruptured ectopic pregnancy in the patient on contraception or with a history of normal menstruation or where the brownish vaginal discharge is mistaken for a normal period
• Failing to examine hernial orifices in a patient with intestinal obstruction

- Misleading temporary improvement (easing of pain) in perforation of gangrenous appendix or perforated peptic ulcer
- Overlooking a perforation in the elderly or in patients taking corticosteroids, because of relative lack of pain
- Overlooking acute mesenteric artery obstruction in an elderly patient with colicky central abdominal pain
- Attributing abdominal pain, frequency and dysuria to a urinary infection when the cause could be diverticulitis, pelvic appendicitis, salpingitis or a ruptured ectopic pregnancy

Seven masquerades checklist

Depression, diabetes, drugs, spinal dysfunction and urinary tract infection can all cause abdominal pain although the pain may be more subacute or chronic. Abdominal pain and even tenderness can accompany diabetic ketoacidosis. Drugs that can cause abdominal pain are listed in Table 30.4.

Spinal dysfunction of the lower thoracic spine and thoracolumbar junction can cause referred pain to the abdomen (Fig. 30.1). The pain is invariably unilateral, radicular in distribution, and related to activity. It can be confused with intra-abdominal problems such as biliary disease (right-sided), appendicitis and Crohn's disease (right side), diverticular disease (left-sided) and pyelonephritis.

Psychogenic considerations

Psychogenic factors can be most relevant especially in recurrent or chronic abdominal pain where no specific cause can be identified in most cases.[5] Bain and Spaulding found that 40%

Table 30.4 *Drugs to consider as a cause of abdominal pain*

Alcohol
Antibiotics, e.g. erythromycin
Aspirin
Corticosteroids
Cytotoxic agents
Tricyclic antidepressants, e.g. imipramine
Iron preparations
Nicotine
NSAIDs
Sodium valproate
Phenytoin

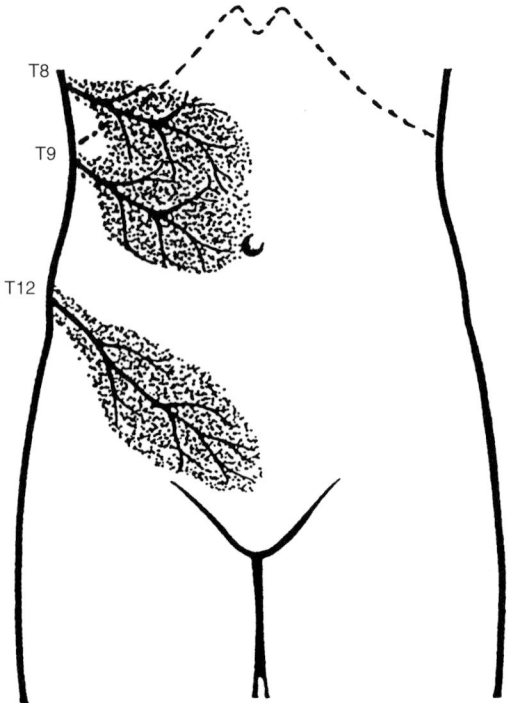

Fig 30.1 *Referred pain patterns to the anterior abdominal wall from dysfunction of the thoracic spine via anterior cutaneous branches of the nerve roots (right side). Note the possibility of confusion with biliary pain, appendicitis and inguinal disorders*

of presenting adult abdominal pain had non-structural causes with 28% having psychiatric diagnoses and 6% spastic colon. They noted that 'psychological disturbances are often fairly easy to identify if care is taken to obtain the personal history and to assess the patient's personality, but the diagnostic terms used to describe psychological disturbances lack precision'.

The clinical approach

History

The urgency of the history will depend on the manner of presentation, whether acute or chronic. Pain has to be analysed according to its quality, quantity, site and radiation, onset, duration and offset, aggravating and relieving factors and associated symptoms and signs.

Special attention has to be paid to:

- anorexia, nausea or vomiting
- micturition
- bowel function
- menstruation
- drug intake

Key questions

Point to where the pain is and where it travels to.
Questions to ask:

- What type of pain is it: is it constant or does it come and go?
- How severe would you rate it from 1 to 10?
- Have you ever had previous attacks of similar pain?
- What else do you notice when you have the pain?
- Do you know of anything that will bring on the pain? Or relieve it?
- What effect does milk, food or antacids have on the pain?
- Have you noticed any sweats or chills or burning of urine?
- Are your bowels behaving normally? Have you been constipated or had diarrhoea or blood in your motions?
- Have you noticed anything different about your urine?
- What medications do you take?
- How much aspirin do you take?
- Are you smoking heavily or taking heroin or cocaine?
- How much alcohol do you drink?
- How much milk do you drink?
- Have you travelled recently?
- What is happening with your periods? Is it mid-cycle or are your periods overdue?
- Does anyone in your family have bouts of abdominal pain?
- Do you have a hernia?
- What operations have you had for your abdomen?
- Have you had your appendix removed?

Physical examination

A useful checklist for conducting the examination is:

- general appearance
- oral cavity
- vital parameters: temperature, pulse, BP, respiratory rate
- chest: check heart and lungs for upper abdominal pain (especially if absent abdominal signs)
- abdomen: inspection, palpation, percussion and auscultation.

The abdominal examination should be performed with the patient lying flat and the abdomen uncovered from xiphisternum to groin. Ask the patient to breathe through the mouth during the examination. Consider the following:

- inguinal region (including hernial orifices) and femoral arteries
- rectal examination: mandatory
- vaginal examination (females): for suspected problems of the fallopian tubes, uterus or ovaries
- thoracolumbar spine (if referred spinal pain suspected)
- urine analysis: white cells, red cells, glucose and ketones, porphyrins
- special clinical tests
  — Murphy's sign (a sign of peritoneal tenderness with acute cholecystitis)
  — iliopsoas and obturator signs

Guidelines

Palpation: palpate with gentleness—note any guarding or rebound tenderness

- guarding indicates peritonitis
- rebound tenderness indicates peritoneal irritation (bacterial peritonitis, blood). Feel for maximum site that corresponds to focus of the problem.

Patient pain indicator: the finger pointing sign indicates focal peritoneal irritation; the spread palm sign indicates visceral pain.

Atrial fibrillation: consider mesenteric artery obstruction.

Tachycardia: sepsis and volume depletion.

Tachypnoea: sepsis, pneumonia, acidosis.

Pallor and 'shock': acute blood loss.

Physical signs may be reduced in the elderly, grossly obese, severely ill and patients on corticosteroid therapy.

Investigations

The following investigations may be selected:

- haemoglobin—anaemia with chronic blood loss, e.g. peptic ulcer, carcinoma, oesophagitis
- blood film—abnormal red cells with sickle cell disease
- white cell count—leucocytosis with appendicitis (75%),[2] acute pancreatitis, mesenteric adenitis (first day only), cholecystitis (especially with empyema), pyelonephritis
- ESR—raised with carcinoma, Crohn's disease, abscess, but non-specific
- C reactive protein (CRP)—use in diagnosing infection, inflammation, e.g. pancreatic
- liver function tests—hepatobiliary disease
- serum amylase—if raised to greater than 5 times normal upper level acute pancreatitis is

most likely; also raised partially with most intra-abdominal disasters, e.g. ruptured ectopic, perforated peptic ulcers, ruptured empyema of gall bladder, ruptured aortic aneurysm
- pregnancy tests—urine and serum β HCG: for suspected ectopic
- urine:
  - blood: ureteric colic (stone or blood clot), urinary infection
  - white cells: urinary infection, appendicitis (bladder irritation)
  - bile pigments: gall bladder disease
  - porphobilinogen: porphyria (add Ehrlich's aldehyde reagent)
  - ketones: diabetic ketoacidosis
  - air (pneumaturia): fistula, e.g. diverticulitis, other pelvic abscess, pelvic carcinoma
- faecal blood—mesenteric artery occlusion, intussusception ('redcurrant jelly'), carcinoma colon, diverticulitis, Crohn's disease and ulcerative colitis

Radiology
The following tests can be considered according to the clinical presentation:
- plain X-ray abdomen (erect and supine): look for (Fig. 30.2)
  - renal/uteric stones—70% opaque[2]
  - biliary stones—only 10–30% opaque
  - air in biliary tree
  - calcified aortic aneurysm
  - marked distension sigmoid → sigmoid volvulus
  - distended bowel with fluid level → bowel obstruction

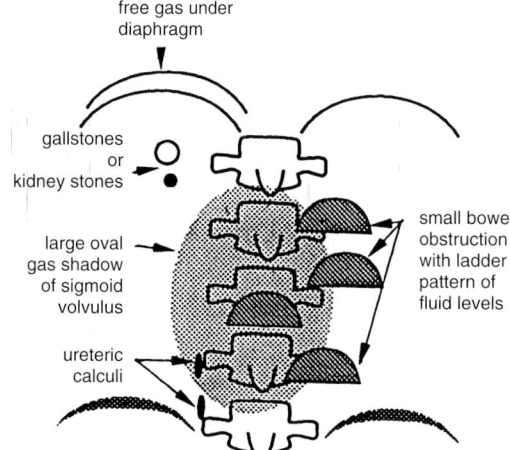

Fig. 30.2 *The acute abdomen: signs to watch for on plain abdominal X-ray*

- enlarged caecum with large bowel obstruction
- blurred right psoas shadow → appendicitis
- a senital loop of gas in LUQ → acute pancreatitis
- chest X-ray: air under diaphragm → perforated ulcer
- ultrasound: good for hepatobiliary system, kidneys and female pelvis: look for
  - gallstones
  - ectopic pregnancy
  - pancreatic pseudocyst
  - aneurysm aorta/dissecting aneurysm
  - hepatic metastases and abdominal tumours
  - thickened appendix
  - paracolic collection
- IVP
- contrast-enhanced X-rays, e.g. Gastrografin meal: diagnosis of bowel leakage
- barium enema
- HIDA nuclear scan—diagnosis of acute cholecystitis
- CT scan: gives excellent survey of abdominal organs including masses and fluid collection
- ERCP: shows bile duct obstruction and pancreatic disease
- MRI scan

Other tests:
- ECG
- endoscopy upper GIT
- sigmoidoscopy and colonoscopy

Diagnostic guidelines
General rules
- Upper abdominal pain is caused by lesions of the upper GIT.
- Lower abdominal pain is caused by lesions of the lower GIT or pelvic organs.
- Early severe vomiting indicates a high obstruction of the GIT.
- Acute appendicitis features a characteristic 'march' of symptoms: pain → anorexia nausea → vomiting.

Pain patterns
The pain patterns are presented in Figure 30.3. Colicky pain is a rhythmic pain with regular spasms of recurring pain building to a climax and fading. It is virtually pathognomonic of intestinal obstruction. Ureteric colic is a true colicky abdominal pain, but so-called biliary colic and renal colic are not true colics at all.

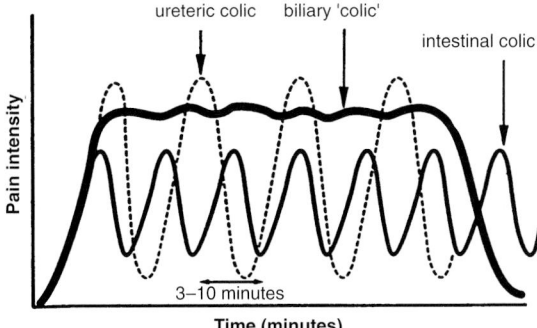

Fig. 30.3 *Characteristic pain patterns for various causes of 'colicky' acute abdominal pain*

Site of pain

Typical pain sites of abdominal pain (general guidelines only) are presented in Figures 30.4 and 30.5. Epigastric pain usually arises from disorders of the embryologic foregut such as the oesophagus, stomach and duodenum, hepatobiliary structures, pancreas and spleen. However, as some disorders progress the pain tends to shift from the midline to the right (gall bladder and liver) or left (spleen). Periumbilical pain usually arises from disorders of structures of the embryologic midgut, while structures from the hindgut tend to refer pain to the lower abdomen or suprapubic region.

Abdominal pain in children

Abdominal pain is a common complaint in children, especially recurrent abdominal pain, which is one of the most common complaints in childhood. The problem causes considerable anxiety in parents and it is important to differentiate the severe problems demanding surgery from non-surgical problems.

Acute abdominal pain

The causes of abdominal pain can be considered in the diagnostic model category.

1. Common causes/probability diagnosis
   - infantile colic
   - gastroenteritis (all ages)
   - mesenteri adenitis
2. Serious causes, not to be missed
   - intussusception (peaks at 6–9 months)
   - acute appendicitis (mainly 5–15 years)
   - bowel obstruction
3. Pitfalls
   - constipation
   - torsion of testes

Fig. 30.4 *Typical sites of various causes of acute abdominal pain*

chronic cholecystitis
biliary colic
hepatitis
hepatic congestion

peptic ulcer
oesophagitis/reflux
carcinoma stomach

chronic pancreatitis

irritable bowel syndrome

mesenteric artery ischaemia

diverticulitis
constipation

recurrent appendicitis
Crohn's disease

gynaecological disorders
• PID
• mittelschmerz
• ovarian tumours

Fig. 30.5 *Typical sites of various causes of chronic or recurrent abdominal pain*

- lactose intolerance
- peptic ulcer
- infections
  — mumps
  — tonsillitis
  — pneumonia
  — Epstein-Barr mononucleosis
  — urinary tract infection
Rarities
- Meckel's diverticulitis
- Henoch-Schönlein purpura
- sickle crisis
- lead poisoning
4. Seven masquerades checklist
  - diabetes mellitus
  - drugs
5. Psychogenic consideration
  - important cause

Infantile colic

This is the occurrence in a well baby of regular, unexplained periods of inconsolable crying and fretfulness, usually in the late afternoon and evening, especially between 2 weeks and 16 weeks of age. No cause for the abdominal pain can be found and it lasts for a period of at least 3 weeks. It is very common and occurs in about one-third of infants.

Typical features

- baby between 2 and 16 weeks old
- prolonged crying—at least 3 hours
- crying worst at around 10 weeks of age
- crying during late afternoon and early evening
- occurrence at least 3 days a week
- child flexing legs and clenching fists because of the 'stomach ache'
- normal physical examination

Management

Reassurance and explanation to the parents. Advice for the parents:
- Use gentleness (such as subdued lighting where the baby is handled, soft music, speaking softly, quiet feeding times).
- Avoid quick movements that may startle the baby.
- Make sure the baby is not hungry—underfeeding can make the baby hungry.
- If the baby is breast-fed, express the watery foremilk before putting the baby to the breast.
- Provide demand feeding (in time and amount).
- Make sure the baby is burped, and give posture feeding.
- Provide comfort from a dummy or pacifier.
- Provide plenty of gentle physical contact.
- Cuddle and carry the baby around (e.g. take a walk around the block).
- A carrying device such as 'snuggly' or 'Meh Tai Sling' allows the baby to be carried around at the time of crying.
- Make sure the mother gets plenty of rest during this difficult period.
- Do not worry about leaving a crying child for 10 minutes or so after 15 minutes of trying consolation.

Medication

Drugs are not generally recommended, but for very severe problems some preparations can be very helpful, e.g. simethicone preparations.

Intussusception

Intussusception is the diagnosis that should be foremost in one's mind with a child aged between 3 months and 2 years presenting with sudden onset of severe colicky abdominal pain, coming at intervals of about 15 minutes and lasting 2–3 minutes. Early diagnosis, within 24 hours of the onset, is essential, for after this time there is a significant rise in morbidity and mortality. It is due to telescoping of the segment of bowel into the adjoining distal segment, e.g. ileocaecal segment, resulting in intestinal obstruction.

Typical clinical features

See Figure 30.6.

- male babies > female
- age 6–12 months
- range: birth to school age, usually 5–24 months
- sudden onset acute pain with shrill cry
- vomiting
- pallor with attacks
- intestinal bleeding: redcurrant jelly (60%)[6]

Physical signs

- pale, anxious and unwell
- sausage-shaped mass in RUQ, especially during attacks (difficult)

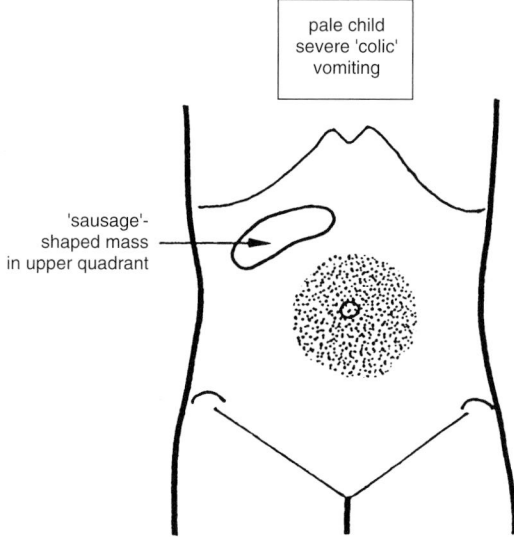

Fig. 30.6 *Typical features with pain distribution of acute intussusception*

- signe de dance, i.e. emptiness in RIF to palpation
- alternating high-pitched active bowel sounds with absent sounds
- rectal examination: ± blood

Diagnosis

- barium enema (avoid if dehydration, peritonitis or established bowel obstruction)

Treatment

- hydrostatic reduction by barium enema under radiological control or hydrostatic reduction with oxygen
- surgical intervention may be necessary

Differential diagnosis

- Acute gastroenteritis: can be difficult in those cases where there is some loose stool with intussusception and with blood and mucus without much watery stool in gastroenteritis. However, usually attacks of pain are of shorter duration, and there is loose watery stool, fever and no abdominal mass. If doubtful refer as possible intussusception.
- Impacted faeces can lead to spasms of colicky abdominal pain—usually an older child with a history of constipation.
- Other causes of intestinal obstruction, e.g. irreducible inguinal hernia, volvulus, intra-abdominal band.

Drugs

In any child complaining of acute abdominal pain, enquiry should be made into drug ingestion. A common cause of colicky abdominal pain in children is cigarette smoking (nicotine); consider other drugs such as marijuana, cocaine and heroin.

Acute appendicitis in children

This may occur at any age, being more common in children of school age and in adolescence, and uncommon under 3 years of age. Special problems of early diagnosis occur with the very young (less than 3 years) and in mentally retarded children, many of whom present with peritonitis.

Vomiting occurs in at least 80% of children with appendicitis and diarrhoea in about 20%. The temperature is usually only slightly elevated but in about 5% of cases it exceeds 39°C.[1]

In children the physical examination, especially eliciting abdominal (including rebound) tenderness, and the rectal examination demand considerable tact, patience and gentleness. Jumping or hopping induces pain.

A serious point of confusion can occur between pelvic appendicitis, causing diarrhoea and vomiting, and acute gastroenteritis. A particularly severe case of apparent gastroenteritis, especially if persistent, should be regarded as pelvic appendicitis until proved otherwise.

Mesenteric adenitis

This presents a difficult problem in differential diagnosis with acute appendicitis because the history can be very similar. At times the distinction may be almost impossible. In general, with mesenteric adenitis localisation of pain and tenderness is not as definite, rigidity is less of a feature, the temperature is higher, and anorexia, nausea and vomiting are also lesser features. The illness lasts about five days followed by a rapid recovery. Comparisons between the two are presented in Table 30.5 but if in any doubt it is advisable to consider the problem as acute appendicitis and perhaps proceed to laparotomy.

Mesenteric adenitis can sometimes present an anaesthetic risk and patients are usually quite ill in the immediate postoperative period.

Recurrent abdominal pain

Recurrent abdominal pain (RAP), three distinct episodes of abdominal pain over 3 or more months, occurs in 10% of school-aged children. In only 5–10% of children will an organic cause

be found so that in most the cause remains obscure.[8]

Organic causes

An organic cause, however, must be considered and excluded. Organic disease is more likely if:
- the pain is other than periumbilical
- the pain radiates rather than remains localised
- the pain wakens the child from sleep
- the pain is accompanied by vomiting
- the child is not completely well between attacks
- there is associated weight loss
- there is failure to thrive

Possible causes
- childhood migraine equivalent (pain with extreme pallor)
- lactose intolerance (symptoms related to milk ingestion)
- intestinal parasites (may disturb child about 60 minutes after falling asleep)

Investigations
- stool microscopy and culture
- urine analysis
- full blood count and ESR

Non-organic RAP

Typical clinical features:
- acute and frequent colicky abdominal pain
- pain localised to or just above umbilicus
- no radiation of pain
- pain lasts less than 60 minutes
- nausea frequent and vomiting rare

Table 30.5 *Comparison of the features of acute appendicitis and mesenteric adenitis in children (guidelines only)*

	Acute appendicitis	Mesenteric adenitis
Typical child	Older	Younger
Site of onset of pain	Midline Shifting to right	RIF Can be midline
Preceding respiratory illness	Uncommon	Invariable: URTI or tonsillitis
Anorexia, nausea, vomiting	+ +	±
Colour	Usually pale	Flushed: malar flush
Temperature	N or ↑	↑ ↑ → ↑ ↑ ↑
Abdominal palpation	Tender in RIF Guarding ± rigidity	Tender in RIF Minimal guarding Usually no rigidity
Rectal examination	Invariably tender	Often tender but lesser degree
Psoas and obturator tests	Usually positive	Usually negative

- diurnal (never wakes the child at night)
- minimal umbilical tenderness
- anxious child
- obsessive or perfectionist personality
- one or both parents intense about child's health and progress

Psychogenic factors

Although psychogenic factors are very relevant in individual cases there is scant hard evidence to support the widely held hypothesis[8] that such factors account for the vast majority of RAP. Some children will have obvious psychological problems or even be school avoidant, a common factor being family disruption.

Management options

- Give explanation, reassurance and support.
- Reassurance can only be given following a careful examination and thoughtfully chosen investigations.
- Emphasise that the disorder is common, and usually traverses childhood without ill effects.
- Identify any life stresses and provide insight therapy.
- Enquire about family structures and function, and school performance.
- Discourage identification with the sick role.
- Refer for psychological assessment and counselling if necessary.

Abdominal pain in the elderly

The elderly can suffer from a wide spectrum of disorders. Ischaemic events, emboli, cancer (in particular) and diverticulae of the colon are more common in old age; duodenal ulcer is less so. Those causes of abdominal pain that occur with more frequency include:

- vascular catastrophies
  - — ruptured abdominal aortic aneurysm
  - — mesenteric artery occlusion
- perforated peptic ulcer
- biliary disorders: bilary pain and acute cholecystitis
- diverticulitis
- sigmoid volvulus
- strangulated hernia
- intestinal obstruction
- carcinoma, especially of the large bowel
- herpes zoster, causing unilateral root pain
- constipation and faecal impaction

Problems arise with management because the pain threshold is raised (colic in particular is less severe) and there is an attenuated response to infection so that fever and leucocytosis can be absent. Non-specific signs such as confusion, anorexia and tachycardia might be the only systemic evidence of infection.

Specific causes of acute abdominal pain

Abdominal aortic aneurysm

An abdominal aortic aneurysm (AAA) may be asymptomatic until it ruptures or may present with abdominal discomfort and a pulsatile mass noted by the patient. There tends to be a family history and thus screening is appropriate in such families. Ultrasound screening is advisable in first-degree relatives over 50 years.

The risk of rupture is related to the diameter of the AAA and the rate of increase in diameter. The normal diameter of the abdominal aorta, which is palpated just above the umbilicus, is 10–30 mm, being 20 mm on average in the adult; an aneurysm is greater than 30 mm in diameter. Greater than 50 mm is significantly enlarged and is chosen as the arbitrary reference point to operate because of the exponential rise in risk of rupture with an increasing diameter. Refer all cases. The patency of a dacron graft after 5 years is approximately 95% (Fig. 30.7).

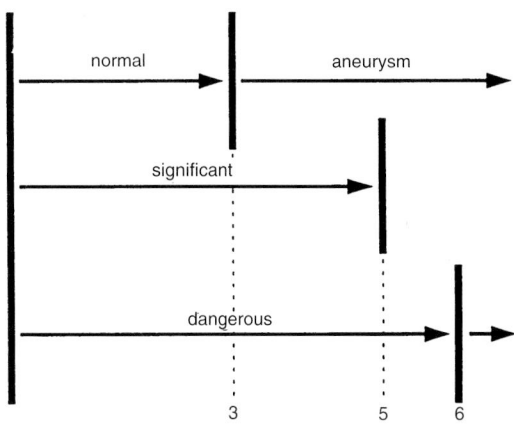

Diameter in cm

Fig. 30.7 *Guidelines for normal and abnormal widths of the abdominal aorta in adults (to exact scale)*

Investigations
- ultrasound (good for screening)
- CT scan (clearer imaging)
- MRI scan (best definition)

Rupture of aneurysm

This is a real surgical emergency in an elderly person who presents with acute abdominal and perhaps back pain with associated circulatory collapse (Fig. 30.8). The patient often collapses at toilet because they feel the need to defecate and the resultant Valsalva manoeuvre causes circulatory embarrassment.

The patient should be transferred immediately to a vascular surgical unit, which should be notified in advance. Two important emergency measures for the 'shocked' patient are intravenous access for plasma expanding fluid (a central venous line is best if possible) and the application of a MAST suit.

Mesenteric artery occlusion

Acute intestinal ischaemia arises from superior mesenteric artery occlusion either from an embolus or thrombosis in an atherosclerotic artery. Another cause is an embolus from atrial fibrillation. Necrosis of the intestine soon follows if intervention is delayed.

Typical clinical features
- abdominal pain—gradually becomes intense (Fig. 30.9)

Fig. 30.8 *Typical pain distribution of a ruptured aortic abdominal aneurysm*

Fig. 30.9 *Typical pain distribution of mesenteric arterial occlusion*

- profuse vomiting
- watery diarrhoea—blood in one-third of patients (later)
- patient becomes confused

Signs
- localised tenderness, rigidity and rebound over infarcted bowel (later finding)
- absent bowel sounds (later)
- shock develops later
- tachycardia (may be atrial fibrillation and other signs of atheroma)

Investigations
- CRP: May be elevated intestinal alkaline phosphatase.
- X-ray (plain): Shows 'thumb printing' due to mucosal oedema on gas-filled bowel. CT scanning may be helpful while mesenteric arteriography is performed if embolus is suspected. However it is commonly only diagnosed at laparotomy.

Management
Early surgery may prevent gut necrosis but massive resection of necrosed gut may be required as a life-saving procedure. Early diagnosis (within a few hours) is essential.
Note:
- Mesenteric venous thrombosis can occur but usually in patients with circulatory failure.

- Inferior mesenteric artery occlusion is less severe and survival more likely.

Acute retention of urine

Acute retention of urine usually causes severe lower abdominal pain, which may not be apparent in a senile or demented person. Apart from the common cause of an enlarged prostate it can also result from bladder neck obstruction by faecal loading or other pelvic masses or anticholinergic drugs. It is often precipitated by extreme cold or an excess of alcohol.

Management
- Perform a rectal examination and empty rectum of any impacted faecal material.
- Catheterise with size 14 Foley catheter to relieve obstruction and drain.
- Have the catheter *in situ* and seek a urological opinion.
- If there is any chance of recovery, e.g. if the problem is drug-induced, withdraw drug, leave catheter in for 48 hours, remove and give trial of prazosin 0.5 mg bd.

Faecal impaction

Faecal impaction is encountered typically in the aged, bedridden, debilitated patient. It may closely resemble malignant obstruction in its clinical presentation.[9] Spurious diarrhoea can occur, which is known as 'faecal incontinence'.

Acute appendicitis

Acute appendicitis is mainly a condition of young adults but it affects all ages (although uncommon under 3 years). It is the commonest surgical emergency and special care has to be taken with the very young and the very old. The symptoms can vary because of the different positions of the appendix.

Typical clinical features
See Figure 30.10. Typical clinical features are:
- maximum incidence 20–30 years
- initial pain is central abdominal (sometimes colicky)
- increasing severity and then continuous
- shifts and localises to RIF within 6 hours
- may be aggravated by walking (causing a limp) or coughing
- sudden anorexia

localised RIF pain
anorexia, nausea, vomiting
guarding

First
central abdominal pain
(visceral pain)

Later
RIF pain (somatic pain)
McBurney's point

Fig. 30.10 *Typical pain distribution of acute appendicitis*

- nausea and vomiting a few hours after the pain starts

Signs
- patient looks unwell
- flushed at first, then pale
- furred tongue and halitosis
- may be febrile
- tenderness in RIF, usually at McBurney's point
- local rigidity and rebound tenderness
- guarding
- ± superficial hyperaesthesia
- ± psoas sign: pain on resisted flexion of right leg, on hip extension or on elevating right leg (due to irritation of psoas especially with retrocaecal appendix)
- ± obturator sign: pain on flexing patient's right thigh at the hip with the knee bent and then internally rotating the hip (due to irritation of internal obturator muscle)
- Rovsing's sign: tenderness in RIF while palpating in LIF

PR: tenderness to right, especially if pelvic appendix or pelvic peritonitis.

Variations and cautions
- abscess formation → localised mass and tenderness
- retrocaecal appendix: pain and rigidity less and may be no rebound tenderness; loin tenderness; positive psoas test
- pelvic appendix: no abdominal rigidity; urinary frequency; diarrhoea and tenesmus; very

tender PR; obturator tests usually positive
- elderly patients: pain often minimal and eventually manifests as peritonitis; can simulate intestinal obstruction
- pregnancy (occurs mainly during second trimester): pain is higher and more lateral; harder to diagnose; peritonitis more common
- perforation more likely in the very young, the aged and the diabetic

Investigations

Few investigations are of value:
- blood cell count shows a leucocytosis (75%) with a left shift
- CRP—elevated
- plain X-ray may show local distension, blurred psoas shadow and fluid level in caecum
- ultrasound shows a thickened appendix (80–90% accurate)
- CT scan can aid diagnosis
- laparoscopy

Management

Immediate referral for surgical removal.

Small bowel obstruction

The symptoms depend on the level of the obstruction (Table 30.6). The more proximal the obstruction the more severe the pain.

Main causes

- outside obstruction, e.g. adhesions (commonest cause, e.g. previous laparotomy), strangulation in hernia or pockets of abdominal cavity
- lumen obstructions, e.g. foreign body, trichobezoar, gallstones, intussusception, malignancy

Table 30.6 *Small bowel obstruction: difference between a high and a low obstruction*

	High	Low
Frequency of spasms	3–5 minutes	6–10 minutes
Intensity of pain	+ + +	+
Vomiting	Early, frequent Violent	Later Less severe
Content:	Gastric juices then green	Feculent (later)
Dehydration and degree of illness	Marked	Less prominent
Distension	Minimal	Marked

Typical clinical features

- severe colicky epigastric and periumbilical (mainly) pain (Fig. 30.11)
- spasms last about 1 minute
- spasms every 3–10 minutes (according to level)
- vomiting
- absolute constipation (nil after bowel emptied)
- no flatus
- abdominal distension (especially if lower SBO)

Signs

- patient weak and sitting forward in distress
- visible peristalsis, loud borborygmi
- abdomen soft (except with strangulation)
- tender when distended
- increased sharp tinkling bowel sounds
- dehydration rapidly follows, especially in children and elderly

PR: empty rectum, may be tender
Note: check all hernial orifices including umbilicus
X-ray: plain erect film confirms diagnosis 'step-ladder' fluid levels in 3–4 hours
Gastrografin follow through for precise diagnosis

Management

- IV fluids and bowel decompression with nasogastric tube
- laparotomy or hernia repair

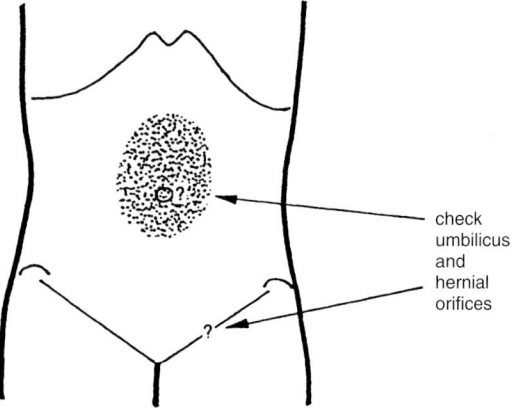

colicky central pain
vomiting
distension

check umbilicus and hernial orifices

Fig. 30.11 *Typical pain distribution of small bowel obstruction*

Large bowel obstruction

The cause is commonly colon carcinoma (75% of cases), especially on the left side, but it can occur in diverticulitis or in volvulus of the sigmoid colon (10% of cases) and caecum.[9] Sigmoid volvulus is more common in older men and has a sudden and severe onset. The pain is less severe than in SBO. Be wary of the non-surgical causes, simple constipation or acute pseudo-obstruction of the colon (Ogilvie's syndrome)

Typical clinical features
- sudden onset colicky pain (even with carcinoma)
- each spasm lasts less than 1 minute
- usually hypogastric midline pain (Fig. 30.12)
- vomiting may be absent (or late)
- constipation, no flatus

Signs and tests
- increased bowel sounds, especially during pain
- distension early and marked
- local tenderness and rigidity

PR: empty rectum; may be rectosigmoid carcinoma or blood. Check for faecal impaction.

X-ray: Distension of large bowel with separation of haustral markings, especially caecal distension.
Sigmoid volvulus shows a distended loop. Gastrografin enema confirms diagnosis.

Management
Surgical referral.

Perforated peptic ulcer

Perforation of a peptic ulcer can cause acute abdominal pain both with and without a prior history of peptic ulcer. It is an acute surgical emergency requiring immediate diagnosis. Consider a history of drugs, especially NSAIDs and H_2 antagonists. Perforated ulcers may follow a heavy meal. There is usually no back pain.

The maximal incidence is 45–55 years, most common in males, and a perforated duodenal ulcer is more common than a gastric ulcer.

Consider the clinical syndrome in 3 stages:
1. prostration
2. reaction (after 2–6 hours)—symptoms improve
3. peritonitis (after 6–12 hours)

Typical clinical features
See Figure 30.13. Typical clinical features are:
- sudden onset severe epigastric pain
- continuous pain but lessens for a few hours
- epigastric pain at first, and then generalised to whole abdomen
- pain may radiate to one or both shoulders (uncommon) or right lower quadrant
- nausea and vomiting (delayed)
- hiccough is a common late symptom

Fig. 30.12 *Typical pain distribution of large bowel obstruction*

Fig. 30.13 *Typical features of perforated peptic ulcer*

Signs

- patient lies quietly (pain aggravated by movement and coughing)
- pale, sweating or ashen at first
- board-like rigidity
- guarding
- maximum signs at point of perforation
- no abdominal distension
- contraction of abdomen (forms a 'shelf' over lower chest)
- bowel sounds reduced (silent abdomen)
- shifting dullness may be present
- pulse, temperature and BP usually normal at first
- tachycardia (later) and shock later (3–4 hours)
- breathing is shallow and inhibited by pain

PR: pelvic tenderness

X-ray: Chest X-ray may show free air under diaphragm (in 75%)—need to sit upright for prior 15 minutes.

Limited Gastografin meal can confirm diagnosis.

Special problems

- Beware of easing of pain as peritoneal fluid accumulates.
- Elderly patients may have minimal pain.
- Painless perforation can occur with steroids.
- Avoid giving morphine or pethidine until diagnosis confirmed.

Management

- pain relief
- drip and suction (immediate nasogastric tube)
- broad spectrum antibiotics
- immediate laparotomy after resuscitation
- conservative treatment may be possible, e.g. later presentation and Gastrografin swallow indicates sealing of perforation.

Ureteric colic

Renal colic is not a true colic but a constant pain due to blood clots or a stone lodged at the pelvic-ureteric junction; ureteric colic, however, presents as severe true colicky pain due to stone movement and ureteric spasm.

Typical clinical features

- maximum incidence 30–50 years (M > F)
- intense colicky pain: in waves, each lasting 30 seconds with 1–2 minutes respite

- begins in loin and radiates around the flank to the groin, thigh, testicle or labia (Fig. 30.14)
- usually lasts < 8 hours
- ± vomiting

Signs

- patient restless: may be writhing in pain
- pale, cold and clammy
- tenderness at costovertebral angle
- ± abdominal and back muscle spasm
- smoky urine due to haematuria

Diagnosis

- urine: microscopy; blood testing strip
- plain X-ray: most stones (75%) are radio-opaque (calcium oxalate and phosphate)
- intravenous pyelogram: confirms opacity, level of obstruction and kidney function
- ultrasound: to locate calculus and exclude obstruction

Management

If the diagnosis is in doubt (especially if narcotic addiction is suspected) get the patient to pass urine in the presence of an examiner and test for haematuria. While awaiting passage of urine, an indomethacin suppository may be tried for pain relief.

Fig. 30.14 *Ureteric colic: typical radiation of pain in left ureteric colic*

Routine treatment

- Pethidine 100 mg
  (average size adult)
  and
  metoclopramide 10 mg IM } IM injection
  or
  IV titration 50 mg
  (preferable)

- Avoid high fluid intake.
- Most cases settle and the patient can go home when pain relief is obtained and an intravenous pyelogram (IVP) arranged for the next day.
- Further pain can be alleviated by indomethacin suppositories but should be limited to two a day.
- An effective alternative treatment is diclofenac 75 mg IM injection then 50 mg (o) tds for 1 week.

Outcome and follow-up

- The calculus is likely to pass spontaneously if < 5 mm (90% < 4 mm pass spontaneously).[10]
- If > 5 mm intervention will usually be required by lithotripsy or surgery.
- If the patient passes the calculus, he or she should retrieve it and present it for analysis.
- A repeat IVP may be necessary if there is evidence of obstruction for more than 3 weeks.
- The cause of the 'stone' should be considered. Search for causes such as hyperparathyroidism, hypercalcaemia, hyperoxaluria.
- Fever with ureteric colic indicates an obstructed infected kidney.

Biliary pain

Abdominal pain can be produced by contraction of the biliary tree upon an obstructing stone or inspissated bile. Although the sterotyped patient is female, forty, fat, fair and fertile it can occur from adolescence to old age and in both sexes.

Typical clinical features

See Figure 30.15. Typical clinical features are:
- acute onset severe pain
- postprandial or at night (often wakes 2–3 am)
- constant pain (not colicky)
- lasts 20 minutes to 2–6 hours
- maximal RUQ or epigastrium
- may radiate to tip of right shoulder or scapula
- painful episode builds to a crescendo for about 20 minutes; may recede or last for hours
- some relief by assuming flexed posture
- ± nausea and vomiting with considerable retching

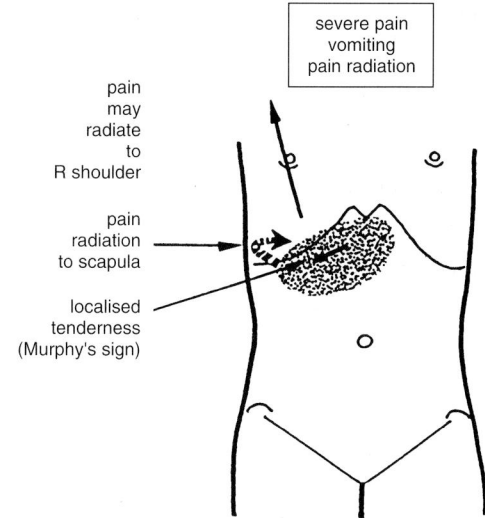

Fig. 30.15 *Typical site of pain of biliary colic and acute cholecystitis*

- often a history of biliary pain (may be mild) or jaundice
- often precipitated by a fatty meal

Signs

- patient anxious and restless, usually in a flexed position or rolling in agony
- localised tenderness (Murphy's sign) over fundus of gall bladder (on transpyloric plane)
- slight rigidity

Diagnosis

- abdominal ultrasound/DIDA
- CT-helical
- intravenous cholangiography if previous cholecystectomy
- LFTs may show elevated bilirubin and alkaline phosphatase

Management options

- pain relief
- gallstone dissolution or lithotripsy (in those unable to have surgery)
- cholecystectomy (main procedure)

Acute cholecystitis

Cholecystitis is associated with gallstones in over 90% of cases[11] and there is usually a past history of biliary pain. It occurs when a calculus becomes impacted in the cystic duct and inflammation develops. It is very common in the elderly. The acute attack is often precipitated by a large or fatty meal.

Typical clinical features
- steady severe pain and tenderness
- localised to right hypochondrium or epigastrium
- nausea and vomiting (bile) in about 75%
- aggravated by deep inspiration

Signs
- patient tends to lie still
- localised tenderness over gall bladder (positive Murphy's sign)
- muscle guarding
- rebound tenderness
- palpable gall bladder (approximately 15%)
- jaundice (approximately 15%)

Diagnosis
- ultrasound: gallstones but not specific for cholecystitis
- HIDA scan: demonstrates obstructed cystic duct—the usual cause
- WCC and CRP: can be elevated

Treatment
- bed rest
- IV fluids
- nil orally
- analgesics
- antibiotics
- cholecystectomy

Acute pancreatitis

With acute pancreatitis there may be a past history of previous attacks or a past history of alcoholism (35%) or gallstone disease (40–50%).

Typical clinical features
See Figure 30.16. Typical clinical features are:
- sudden onset of severe constant epigastric pain
- lasts hours or a day or so
- pain may radiate to back
- nausea and vomiting
- sweating and weakness

Signs
- patient is weak, pale, sweating and anxious
- tender in epigastrium
- lack of guarding, rigidity or rebound

severe pain
nausea & vomiting
relative lack abdominal signs

Fig. 30.16 *Typical pain distribution of acute pancreatitis*

- reduced bowel sounds (may be absent if ileus)
- ± abdominal distension
- fever, tachycardia

Diagnosis
- WCC—leucocytosis
- serum amylase (usually 5-fold increase)
- CRP—elevated
- serum glucose ↑, calcium ↓
- blood gases: pO_2
- LFTs: ? obstructive pattern
- plain X-ray, may be senital loop
- CT scan
- ultrasound better for detecting cysts and unsuspected gallstones

Management
- Arrange admission to hospital.
- Basic treatment is bed rest, nil orally, nasogastric suction (if vomiting), IV fluids and analgesics (pethidine, not morphine).
- may require ERCP if obstructive LFTs

Chronic pancreatitis
In contrast to acute pancreatitis the pain of chronic pancreatitis is milder but more persistent. The patient with this problem is often labelled as 'gastritis', 'ulcer' or 'neurotic' because of the indeterminate nature of the pain. Malabsorption and diabetes may result from pancreatitis and weight loss and steatorrhoea become prominent features.

Pain associated with carcinoma of the pancreas is indistinguishable from that of chronic pancreatitis but generally tends to be more severe and more prominent in the back. Use paracetamol or codeine for pain.

Acute diverticulitis

The patient with acute diverticulitis is usually over 40 years of age, with long-standing grumbling left-sided abdominal pain and constipation, but can have irregular bowel habit. It occurs in less than 10% of patients with diverticular disease.[2]

Typical clinical features
See Figure 30.17. Typical clinical features are:
- acute onset of pain in the left iliac fossa
- pain increased with walking and change of position
- usually associated with constipation

Signs
- tenderness, guarding and rigidity in LIF
- fever
- may be inflammatory mass in LIF

Investigations
- leucocytosis
- elevated ESR
- pus and blood in stools
- abdominal ultrasound/CT scan (especially)

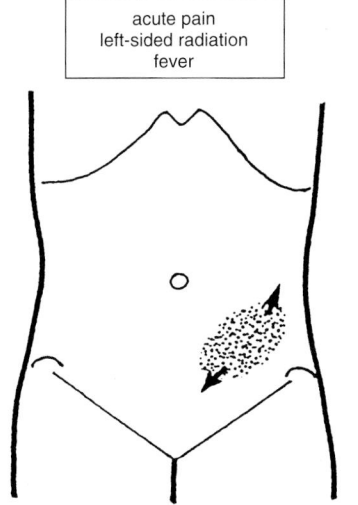

Fig. 30.17 *Typical pain distribution of acute diverticulitis*

Complications
- bleeding (can be profuse, especially in elderly)
- perforation (high mortality)
- abscess
- peritonitis
- fistula (bladder, vagina, small bowel)
- intestinal obstruction

Treatment
- antibiotics
- surgery for complications

Chronic or recurrent abdominal pain

Advances in technology have increased the opportunities for diagnosing chronic or recurrent abdominal pain[12] in adults:
- *Ultrasound.* This is the single most useful screening test. It can detect gallstones, pelvic pathology such as carcinoma of the ovary and retroperitoneal problems such as abdominal aneurysm and carcinoma of the pancreas.
- *Endoscopy.* This is the next most useful investigation. The history dictates whether it is gastroscopy or colonoscopy.

If the patient has 'red flag' symptoms (Table 30.7) and the above investigations are absent, consider the possibility of conditions such as carcinoma of the pancreas, carcinoma of the ovary, small bowel tumours, mesenteric ischaemia, Crohn's disease, metabolic disorders such as lactase deficiency, and rarer conditions as outlined in Table 30.3.

Other investigations that may help:
- CT scanning
- Laparoscopy: This may allow the identification of chronic adhesive obstruction, small bowel tumours or inflammation, or intra-abdominal malignancy.

Table 30.7 *Red flags for organic disease*[12]

Older patient
Nocturnal pain or diarrhoea
Progressive symptoms
Rectal bleeding
Fever
Anaemia
Weight loss
Abdominal mass
Faecal incontinence or urgency (recent onset)

Chronic appendicitis

It is possible to have recurrent episodes of sub-acute inflammation of the appendix. If suspected, laparoscopy performed during or soon after an attack is diagnostic.

Adhesions

There is no firm evidence that intra-abdominal adhesions are painful apart from complications such as bowel obstruction. Sometimes patients are 'cured' by laparoscopic divisions of adhesions.

Irritable bowel syndrome

See pp. 406–407.

At least 3 months of continuous or recurrent:
- cramping pain (relieved by defecation)
- central or left lower quadrant pain (more common) but can be at any site
- mucus in stool
- altered stool form or passage

Peptic ulcer (gastric or duodenal)

See p. 441.
- usually central epigastric pain
- burning pain
- relieved by antacids or food or milk
- DU: usually 2–3 hours after meals or wakes from sleep
  GU: may occur after meals but inconsistent relationship to eating

When to refer

- All cases of acute abdominal pain where urgent surgical intervention is required; special urgency and early diagnosis is important with:
  — ruptured ectopic pregnancy
  — ruptured abdominal aortic aneurysm
  — mesenteric artery occlusion
  — ruptured viscus
  — perforated peptic ulcer
  — strangulated obstructed bowel
  — intussusception
- All cases where the diagnosis is not apparent
- All cases where surgery is necessary
- Medical causes such as diabetic ketoacidosis and porphyria

Practice tips

- Special caution is required at the extremes of age when the symptoms and signs do not often reflect the seriousness of the underlying pathology.

- If an elderly patient presents with intense acute abdominal pain, inadequately relieved by strong parenteral injections, likely causes include mesenteric artery occlusion, acute pancreatitis and ruptured or dissecting aortic aneurysm.
- When an inflamed appendix ruptures, the abdominal pain improves for a significant period of time.
- A false sense of security can also occur with a perforated ulcer.
- Pus cells and red cells may be present in the urine with appendicitis when a pelvic appendix involves the bladder and a retrocaecal appendix involves the ureter.
- Consider diabetic ketoacidosis in a patient with abdominal pain, tenderness and rigidity and deep sighing respiration.

References

1. Sloane PD, Slatt LM, Baker RM. *Essentials of family medicine.* Baltimore: Williams and Wilkins, 1988, 135–141.
2. Sandler G, Fry J. Acute abdominal pain. In: *Early clinical diagnosis.* Lancaster: MTP Press, 1986, 137–176.
3. Murtagh J. *The anatomy of a rural practice.* Melbourne: Monash University Monograph, 1980, 34.
4. Sandler G, Fry J. Chronic abdominal pain. In: *Early clinical diagnosis.* Lancaster: MTP Press, 1986, 177–186.
5. Bain ST, Spaulding WB. The importance of coding presenting symptoms. Canadian Med Ass, 1967; 97(16):953–959.
6. Hodgkin K. *Towards earlier diagnosis* (5th edn). Edinburgh: Churchill Livingstone, 1985, 483–486.
7. Robinson MJ. *Practical paediatrics* (2nd edn). Melbourne: Churchill Livingstone, 1990, 526–531.
8. Feekery C. Recurrent abdominal pain. Aust Paed Review, 1991; 5:1–2.
9. Hunt P, Marshall V. *Clinical problems in general surgery.* Sydney: Butterworths, 1991, 193–243.
10. Farrell T. Emergency call. Aust Fam Physician, 1988; 17:467.
11. Tierney LM et al. *Current medical diagnosis and treatment.* Stamford: Appleton and Lange, 1996, 601.
12. Hugh TB. The investigation and management of recurrent or chronic abdominal pain. Mod Med Aust, 1995; 38(5):126–132.

31
Arthritis

—

Rheumatic disorders are common in old age: much of rheumatology is geriatric and much of geriatrics is rheumatology.

Dr Frank Dudley Hart[1] 1983

The clinical evaluation of the patient presenting with the complaint of arthralgia (painful joints) or arthritis (inflammation of the joints) can be a difficult and challenging exercise because it can be a presentation of many systemic disorders, some of which are rare. Important considerations are sex, age, the pattern of joint involvement (monoarticular or polyarticular), immediate and more remote history, family history and drug use—all of which may provide important diagnostic clues.

Key facts and checkpoints

- In a UK National Morbidity Survey rheumatic disease comprised just over 7% of all morbidity presenting to the family doctor.[2]
- The commonest cause was osteoarthritis, which affects 5–10% of the population.
- The same study indicated an episode rate for arthritis/arthralgia of 38.6 per 1000 population.
- The population incidence of rheumatoid arthritis is 2–3%.
- There should be no systemic manifestations with osteoarthritis.
- One-quarter of disability in elderly people is due to severe joint disease.
- Systemic diseases that may predispose to, or present with, an arthropathy include the connective tissue disorders, diabetes mellitus, a bleeding disorder, previous tuberculosis, the spondyloarthropathies such as psoriasis, SBE, hepatitis B, rheumatic fever, the various vasculitic or arteritic syndromes (the vasculitides) such as Wegener's granulomatosis, HIV infection; carcinoma of the lung, haemochromatosis, sarcoidosis, hyperparathyroidism, Paget's disease.
- The pain of inflammatory disease is worse at rest, e.g. on waking in the morning, and improved by activity.
- Gout and septic arthritis have a recognised cause and cure.
- Acute gout is almost exclusive to males: in women, it is usually seen only in those who are postmenopausal or on thiazide diuretics.

A diagnostic approach

A summary of the safety diagnostic model is presented in Table 31.1.

Probability diagnosis

The probability diagnoses for the patient presenting with arthritis are:

- osteoarthritis (mono or polyarthritis)
- viral arthritis (if acute and polyarthritis)

Osteoarthritis is very common in general practice. It may be primary, which is usually symmetrical, and can affect many joints. This clinical pattern is different from secondary osteoarthritis, which follows injury and other wear-and-tear causes.

Viral polyarthritis is more common than realised. It presents usually as a symmetric inflammation, mainly of the hands and feet, and is usually mild. It tends to terminate quickly and spontaneously without permanent damage to joints. It is caused by many viruses, including

267

Table 31.1 *Arthralgia: diagnostic strategy model*

Q. *Probability diagnosis*
A. Osteoarthritis
   Viral polyarthritis

Q. *Serious disorders not to be missed*
A. Rheumatoid arthritis
   Connective tissue disorders
   • SLE
   • systemic sclerosis
   • dermatomyositis
   Neoplasia
   • carcinoma bronchus
   • leukaemia
   HIV arthropathy
   Severe infections
   • rheumatic fever
   • endocarditis
   • tuberculosis
   • brucellosis
   • pyogenic arthritis
     — gonococcus
     — staphylococcus

Q. *Pitfalls (often missed)*
A. Fibromyalgia syndrome
   Polymyalgia rheumatica
   Crystal deposition
   • gout
   • pyrophosphate (pseudogout)
   Haemarthrosis
   Dengue fever
   Lyme disease
   Ross River virus
   Avascular necrosis

   Rarities
   Other vasculitides
   Haemochromatosis
   Sarcoidosis
   Hyperparathyroidism
   Familial Mediterranean fever
   Amyloidosis
   Pigmented villonodular synovitis

Q. *Seven masquerades checklist*
A. Depression   √
   Diabetes   √
   Drugs   √
   Anaemia   –
   Thyroid disease   √
   Spinal dysfunction   the spondyloarthropathies
   UTI   –

Q. *Is the patient trying to tell me something?*
A. Always a consideration with pain
   Psychogenic factors aggravate chronic arthritic conditions.

those causing influenza, mumps, rubella, varicella, hepatitis A and B, infectious mononucleosis, cytomegalovirus, parvovirus, Australian epidemic polyarthritis due to Ross River virus, and Barmah Forest virus.

Serious disorders not to be missed

These include rheumatoid arthritis, which can start as a monoarthritis; pyogenic arthritis, including gonococcus, staphylococcus and streptococcus infections; tuberculosis; rheumatic fever; and bacterial endocarditis.

It is important to be forever watchful for rheumatic fever. It presents typically as a migratory polyarthritis involving large joints sequentially, one becoming hot, red, swollen and very painful as the other subsides. It rarely lasts more than 5 days in any one joint.

A flitting polyarthritis can also occur with endocarditis in addition to a systemic upset and a cardiac murmur. Gonococcal infection may present in a single joint or as flitting polyarthritis, often accompanied by a rash. Brucellosis can cause arthritis and sacroiliitis and can be confused with the spondyloarthropathies.

HIV infection is becoming a great mimicker. It can present as a chronic oligoarticular asymmetrical arthritis.[3] It can also present as a rash very similar to psoriasis.

With the large influx of migrants from South-East Asia the possibility of tuberculosis presenting as arthritis should be kept in mind.

Connective tissue disorders may be involved. They include systemic lupus erythematosis, progressive systemic sclerosis (scleroderma), and dermatomyositis. It is most inappropriate to settle with a general diagnosis such as 'rheumatism' or 'arthritis' and where doubtful it is important to find the specific entity causing the problem.

In respect to malignant disease, arthralgia is associated with acute leukaemia, lymphoma and neuroblastoma in children and with carcinoma of the bronchus, which may cause hypertrophic osteoarthropathy especially of the wrist and ankle (not a true arthritis but simulates it). Occasionally polyarthritis may be the first feature of an occult neoplasm. Monoarticular metastatic disease may involve the knee (usually from lung or breast).

Pitfalls

There are several pitfalls, most of which are rare. A common pitfall is gout. This applies particularly to older women taking diuretics, whose osteoarthritic joints, especially of the hand, can be affected. The condition is often referred to as nodular gout and does not usually present as acute arthritis.

Fibromyalgia syndrome is a real puzzle (see p. 328) as it can mimic the connective tissue disorders in its early presentation—typically a woman in the third or fourth decade.

Another 'trap' is haemarthrosis in a patient with a bleeding disorder.

Infective causes that may be overlooked are dengue fever, especially in travellers returning from a tropical or subtropical area, and Lyme disease, which is now surfacing in many countries, especially where ticks are found.

There are many rare causes of arthritis. Sarcoidosis causes two forms: an acute benign form, usually in the ankles and knees, and a chronic form with long-standing sarcoidosis that involves joints (large or small) adjacent to underlying bone disease.

Then there are the uncommon vasculitides, which can cause confusion in diagnosis. This group includes polyarteritis nodosa, hypersensitive vasculitis, polymyalgia rheumatica/ giant cell arteritis, Wegener's granulomatosis, Henoch-Schönlein purpura and Behcet's syndrome.

Haemochromatoses can present with a degenerative arthropathy that characteristically affects the second or third metacarpophalangeal joints.[3]

Other rare causes of arthritis are erythema nodosum, serum sickness and Sjögren's syndrome.

General pitfalls
- Not searching beyond RA when an RA pattern polyarthritis may be part of another systemic disease
- Failing to search for some cause of arthritis other than osteoarthritis in a patient, especially an elderly patient, i.e. underdiagnosing; an important example of this is polymyalgia rheumatica
- Failing to consider the various drug interactions between NSAIDs, over the counter medications and other drugs used by the elderly
- Underdiagnosing and misdiagnosing through lack of appreciation of the many causes of arthritis, especially those presenting as part of a systemic disease

Seven masquerades checklist
- Depression—unlikely but complaints of arthralgia are possible
- Diabetes—occasionally causes an arthropathy

- Drugs—yes, a major consideration
- Anaemia—no
- Thyroid disease—possible
- Urinary infection—no
- Spinal dysfunction—only with the spondyloarthropathies

Drug-induced arthritis is the main feature of this important group of disorders. It usually affects the hands and is generally symmetrical. Drugs that cause arthritis are listed in Table 31.2.

Table 31.2 *Drug-induced arthralgia*

Commonest drugs inducing arthralgia
Note: Usually affects the hands and is symmetrical
Drugs inducing Lupus syndrome
• hydralazine
• procainamide
• antiepileptics, e.g. phenytoin
• chlorpromazine
• isoniazid
• methyldopa
Others
• co-trimoxazole
• amoxycillin
• mianserin
• carbimazole
• nitrofurantoin
• antihypertensives

Note: Diuretics, especially frusemide and thiazides, can precipitate gout.

Intravenous drug abuse may be associated with septic arthritis, hepatitis B and C, HIV-associated arthropathy, SBE with arthritis and serum sickness reactions.

Hyperthyroidism can uncommonly cause acropathy (clubbing and swelling of the fingers) and may present as pseudogout, while hypothyroidism can present with an arthropathy or cause proximal muscle pain, stiffness and weakness. Diabetes mellitus may cause an arthropathy that can be painless or mild to moderately painful.

The spondyloarthropathies may be a causative factor. They often present with an acute mono-arthritis particularly in teenagers some time before causing sacroiliitis and spondylitis.

Psychogenic considerations
Although 'arthralgia' is an uncommon complaint in psychoneurotic disorders, any pain syndrome can be a significant manifestation. The usual cause of arthralgia is inflammation in the joint, that is arthritis, but a functional cause is encountered from time to time.

Furthermore some patients who are unfortunate enough to acquire arthritis, especially the more serious disorders, certainly develop ongoing emotional and psychological problems that appear to aggravate their total problem.

So-called 'growing pains' of the lower limb are common in children, and the physical examination and investigations are normal. Parents need to be reassured that it is a benign condition while recognising that emotional factors may be quite significant. As Apley pointed out, 'physical growth is not painful, but emotional growth can hurt like hell'.[4]

The clinical approach

A priority is to determine whether or not the arthritis is caused by a primary rheumatic disorder or whether it is part of an underlying systemic disorder.

History

Very careful enquiry about the exact onset of the arthritis is important. This includes whether it was acute or insidious, and confined to specific joints or flitting as in rheumatic fever and sometimes in infective endocarditis. Is it a true polyarthritis or monoarthritis? Symmetrical or asymmetrical? It is also important to differentiate between arthralgia (pains in or around the joints) and arthritis (inflammation of the joints). Not all arthralgia is arthritis.

A family history is important because a positive family history is associated with conditions such as rheumatoid arthritis (rarely), ankylosing spondylitis, connective tissue disorders (rarely), psoriasis, gout, pseudogout and haemophilia.[5]

A very hot, red, swollen joint suggests either infection or crystal arthritis.

Key questions

- Can you carefully point out exactly where you feel the pain?
- Does the pain move from joint to joint or stay in the same joint?
- Are you aware of anything that brought on the pain?
- Does the pain disturb you at night?
- Do your joints feel very sore or stiff when you wake up in the morning?
- What effect does exercise or activity have on the pain or stiffness?

- Have you had an injury in the past to your painful joint(s)?
- Do you get pain over both your shoulders and upper arms?
- Have you got a skin rash? Is it new?
- Have you had a fever, sweats or chills?
- Do you get very tired, weak or out of sorts?
- Have you noticed any change in the colour of your urine?
- Have you had a sore throat?
- Have you had sinus trouble?
- Have you had acute pain in your big toe or in other joints before?
- Do you have a history of psoriasis?
- Do you have a history of rheumatic fever?
- Do you have pain in your neck or lower back or in other joints?
- Have you had any diarrhoea?
- Have you had a discharge from your penis?
- Have you had any problems wih your eyes?
- What drugs are you taking? Are you taking fluid tablets (diuretics)?
- How much alcohol would you drink a day?
- Have you been visiting the country or exposed to ticks or have you been to a deer farm?
- Have you travelled overseas recently?
- Have you been at risk of getting a sexually transmitted disease?
- Have you been drinking untreated milk recently?

Physical examination

A systematic examination of the affected joint or joints should be performed, looking for signs of inflammation, deformity, swelling and limitation of movement. Tenderness and warmth indicates inflammatory activity. Erythema indicates gouty arthritis or other crystalopathy, rheumatic fever or septic arthritis.

Joint swelling:

- acute (1–4 hours) with intense pain = blood, infection or crystals, e.g. gout
- subacute (1–2 days) and soft = fluid (synovial effusion)
- chronic and bony = osteoarthritis
- chronic and soft/boggy = synovial proliferation

A coarse crepitus suggests osteoarthritis. Each joint should be examined specifically. Inspection should note the presence of lumps or bumps such as Heberden's nodes on the osteoarthritic DIP joints of the hands, Bouchard's nodes on the osteoarthritic PIP joints of the hands, and rheumatoid nodules, which are the only pathognomonic finding of RA and gouty tophi. Signs that may be of diagnostic help are presented in Figure 31.1.

The specific inflamed joint or joints may give an indication of the disease process. Typical joints affected by various arthropathies are illustrated in Figure 31.2.

Investigations

Table 31.3 lists the many investigations that are used to reach a diagnosis.[6] Clinical acumen permits a judicious selection of specific tests rather than ordering an expensive battery.

It is important to keep in mind the many specific serological tests to detect infective causes of arthralgia. These include Australian epidemic polyarthritis, Lyme disease, rubella, brucella, hepatitis B, gonococcus, mycoplasma, HIV tests.

Plain X-ray is invaluable, although in some conditions radiological changes may be apparent only when the disease is well established. Typical X-ray changes for common conditions are presented in Figure 31.3. Arthrography has limited value in the diagnosis of polyarthritis but is very useful for specific joints such as the shoulder and the knee. Ultrasound examination for joints such as the shoulder and the hip can be very useful.

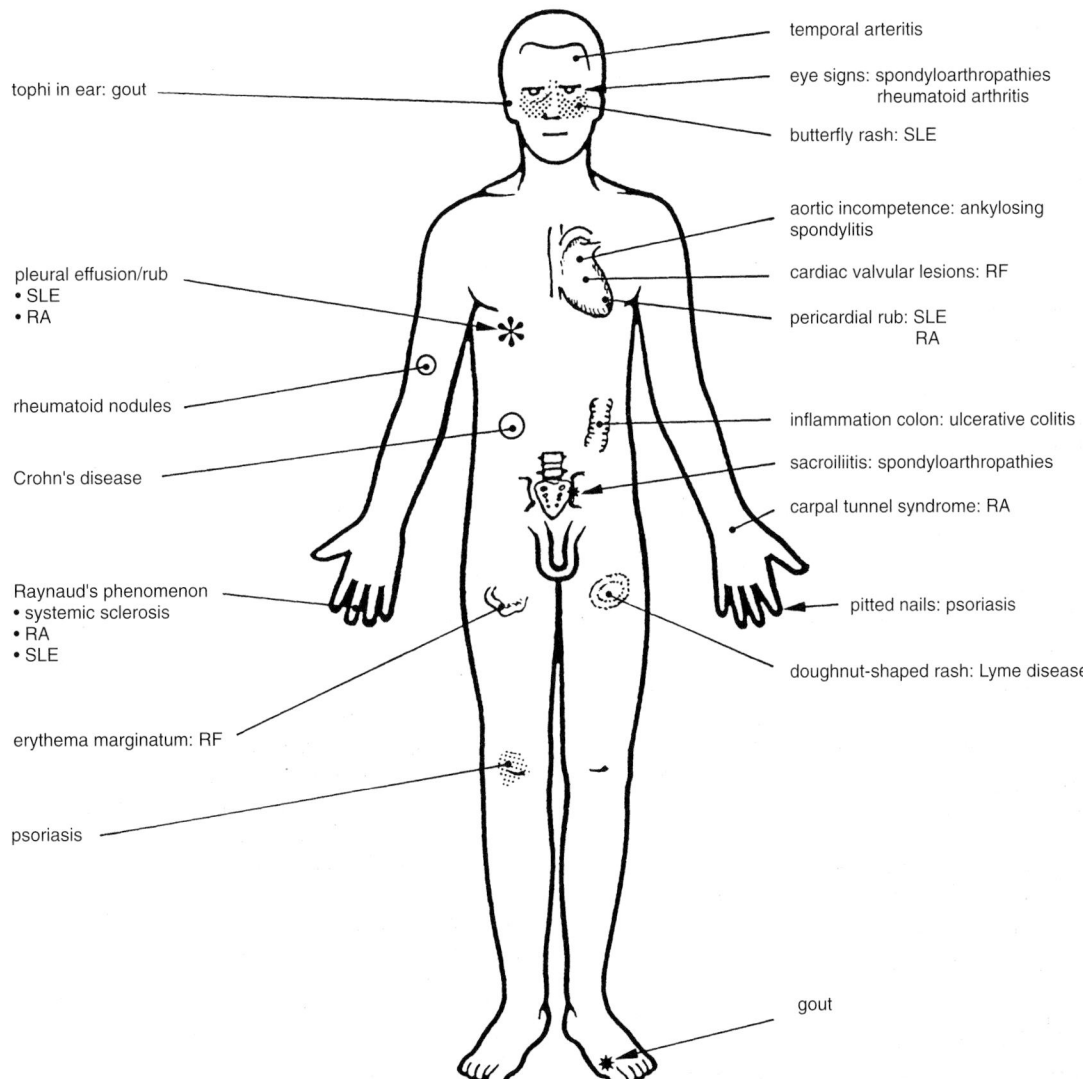

Fig. 31.1 *Physical examination: possible findings to consider in diagnosis*

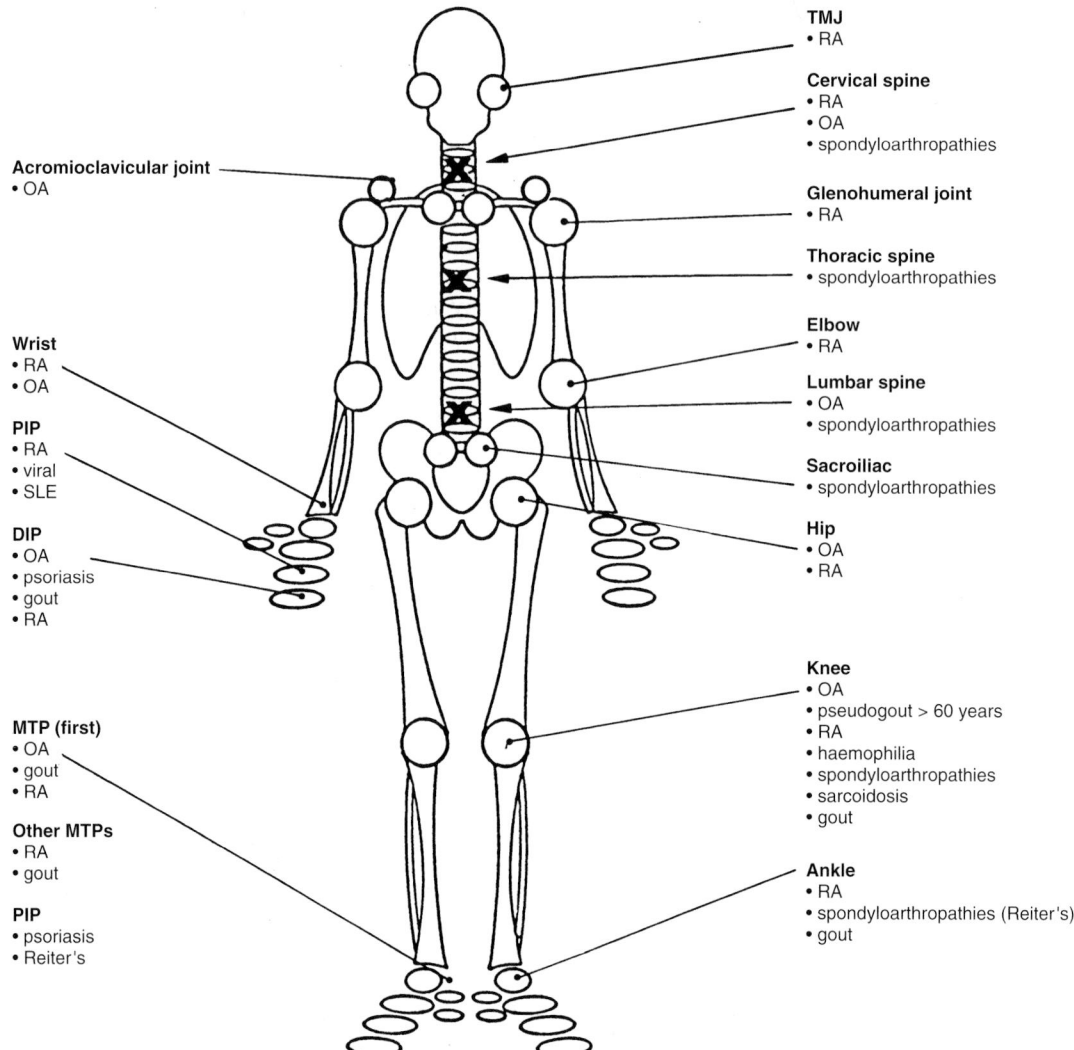

Fig. 31.2 *Joints typically affected by various arthropathies*

The various immunological tests for diagnosis of the connective tissue disorders are outlined with the description of each condition. Such screening tests include:
- rheumatoid factor
- antinuclear antibodies
- double stranded DNA antibodies

The LE cell test has been superseded by the antinuclear and ds DNA antibody tests.

Arthritis in children

Arthralgia (joint pain) is a common problem in childhood and, although arthritis is rare, the complaint demands considerable respect because of the many serious problems causing it. Arthritis may be part of an infectious disease such as rheumatic fever, rubella, mumps, cytomegalovirus infection, erythema infectiosum (human parvovirus), influenza or other viral infection, and is occasionally encountered with Henoch-Schönlein purpura. It is worth noting that underlying bone tumours can be present as joint pain if the tumour is adjacent to the joint. A checklist of causes is presented in Table 31.4.

Note: Acute-onset monoarticular arthritis associated with fever is septic until proven otherwise.

Table 31.3 *Investigations for arthritis*

Appropriate tests can be selected from the following:
- urine analysis: blood, protein, sugar
- synovial fluid: analysis, culture
- radiology—plain X-ray
- blood and other cultures
- haemoglobin and differential white cell count
- erythrocyte sedimentation rate (ESR)
- C-reactive protein
- serum uric acid, creatinine
- 24-hour urinary uric acid
- rheumatoid factor
- antinuclear antibody (screening test for SLE)
- double strand DNA antibodies
- HLA-B$_{27}$ (poor predictive value)
- various specific serological tests, e.g. Australian epidemic polyarthritis, rubella, Lyme disease, hepatitis B, Barmah Forest virus
- HIV serology
- antistreptolysin O titre
- streptococcal anti DNAse B
- streptococcal AHT
- arthroscopy and biopsy
- bone scan

Normal joint

Rheumatoid arthritis

cysts
joint destruction
subluxation
erosion joint margins
osteoporosis

Juvenile chronic arthritis

Juvenile chronic arthritis is defined as a chronic arthritis persisting for at least 3 months in one or more joints in a child less than 16 years of age.[4] It is rare, affecting only about one in 1000 children, but produces profound medical and psychosocial problems.

The commonest types of juvenile chronic arthritis are oligoarthritis affecting four or fewer joints (about 50%) and polyarthritis affecting five or more joints (about 40%). Systemic onset arthritis, previously known as Still's disease, accounts for about 10% of cases. It is usually seen in children under the age of 5 but can occur throughout childhood. The children present with a high remittent fever and coppery red rash, plus other features including lymphadenopathy, splenomegaly and pericarditis. Arthritis is not an initial feature but develops ultimately, usually involving the small joints of the hands, wrists, knees, ankles and metatarsophalangeal joints.

These children should be referred once the problem is suspected or recognised.

Rheumatic fever

Rheumatic fever typically occurs in children and young adults, the first attack usually occurring between 5 and 15 years of age.

Osteoarthritis

periarticular bone sclerosis

marginal osteophytes

loss of joint space

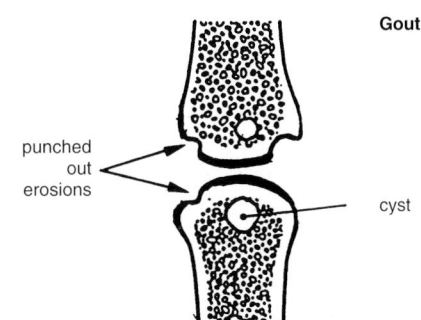

Gout

punched out erosions

cyst

Fig. 31.3 *X-rays for common arthritic conditions: typical changes*

Table 31.4 *Arthritis in children: causes to consider*

Infections
    Rheumatic fever
    Septic arthritis
    Meningococcaemia
    Osteomyelitis
    Reactive arthritis (post-infectious)
    Tuberculosis
    Viral infections, e.g. rubella, HIV
Inflammation—chronic arthritis
    Juvenile chronic arthritis
    • oligoarthritis
    • polyarticular (juvenile rheumatoid arthritis)
    • systemic disease (Still's disease)
    • juvenile ankylosing spondylitis
    Psoriatic arthritis
    Inflammatory bowel arthritis
Haematological disorders
    Thalassaemia
    Sickle-cell disease
    Haemophilia
Neoplasms
    Leukaemia
    Lymphoma
    Neuroblastoma
Orthopaedic conditions
    Perthes' disorder
    Slipped upper femoral epiphyses
    Chondromalacia
Others
    Henoch-Schönlein disorder
    Scurvy
    Traumatic arthritis
    Osteochondritis
    Psychogenic rheumatism
    Malignant tumour
    • bone
    • cartilage
    • synovium

Arthritis in perspective

Five per cent of all children complain of recurrent lower limb pain, which often awakens them from their sleep. There may be emotional factors involved and parents need appropriate reassurance. A careful history and physical examination are essential, and perhaps simple basic investigations may be appropriate. As Rudge[4] points out, we have to be vigilant against underdiagnosis, misdiagnosis and overdiagnosis.

Arthritis in the elderly

Osteoarthritis is very common with advancing age and for this reason care has to be taken not to simply attribute other causes of arthritis to osteoarthritis. Other musculoskeletal conditions

that become more prevalent with increasing age are:

• polymyalgia rheumatica
• Paget's disease of bone
• avascular necrosis
• gout
• pseudogout (pyrophosphate arthropathy)
• malignancy, e.g. bronchogenic carcinoma

Pseudogout

This crystal deposition arthropathy (chondrocalcinosis) is noted by its occurrence in people over 60 years. It usually affects the knee joint but can involve other joints.

Rheumatoid arthritis

Although it usually begins between the ages of 30 and 40 it can occur in elderly patients, when it often begins suddenly and dramatically. This is called 'explosive' RA and fortunately tends to respond to small doses of prednisolone and has a good prognosis.[7]

Rheumatic fever

Rheumatic fever (RF) is an inflammatory disorder that typically occurs in children and young adults following a group A streptococcus pyogenes infection. It is common in developing countries but uncommon in first world countries.

Clinical features

• young person 5–15 (can be older)
• acute onset fever, joint pains, malaise
• flitting arthralgia mainly in leg (knees, ankles) and elbows and wrists of the arm
• one joint settles as the other is affected
• may follow a sore thoat

However, the symptoms depend on the organs affected and arthritis may be absent.

Diagnosis

Based on   2 or more major criteria
                      or
              1 major + 2 or more minor criteria

in the presence of supporting evidence of preceding streptococcal infection.

Major criteria

• carditis
• polyarthritis
• chorea (involuntary abnormal movements)

- subcutaneous nodules
- erythema marginatum

Minor criteria
- fever
- previous RF or rheumatic heart disease
- arthralgia
- raised ESR/C-reactive protein
- ECG—prolonged PR intervals

Investigations
A selective combination of:

- throat swab
- ESR
- streptococcal ASOT
- streptococcal anti DNAse B
- streptococcal AHT
- C-reactive protein

Treatment
- rest in bed
- penicillin benzathine (pencillin 900 mg IM statim)
- high-dose aspirin
- corticosteroids for carditis
- prophylactic long-term penicillin

Osteoarthritis

Osteoarthritis (OA) is the most common type of arthritis, occurring in about 10% of the adult population and in 50% of those aged over 60.[8] It is a degenerative disease of cartilage and may be primary or secondary to causes such as trauma and mechanical problems, septic arthritis, crystalopathy or previous inflammatory disorders, or structural disorders such as SUFE and Perthes' disorder.

The arthritis
Primary OA is usually symmetrical and can affect many joints. Unlike other inflammatory disease the pain is worse on initiating movement and loading the joint, and eased by rest. OA is usually associated with pronounced stiffness, especially after activity, in contrast to RA.

Joints involved
In primary osteoarthritis all the synovial joints may be involved, but the main ones are:

- first carpometacarpal (CMC) joint of thumb
- first metatarsophalangeal (MTP) joint of great toe
- distal interphalangeal (DIP) joints of hands

Other joints that are affected significantly are the proximal interphalangeal joints, the knees, hips, acromioclavicular joints and joints of the spine, especially the facet joints of the cervical (C5-6, C6-7) and lumbar regions (L3-4, L4-5, L5-S1) (Fig. 31.4).

Clinical features
- pain: worse by the end of the day
         aggravated by use
         relieved by rest
         worse in cold and damp
- variable morning stiffness
- variable disability

Signs
- hard and bony swelling
- crepitus
- signs of inflammation (mild)
- restricted movements
- joint deformity

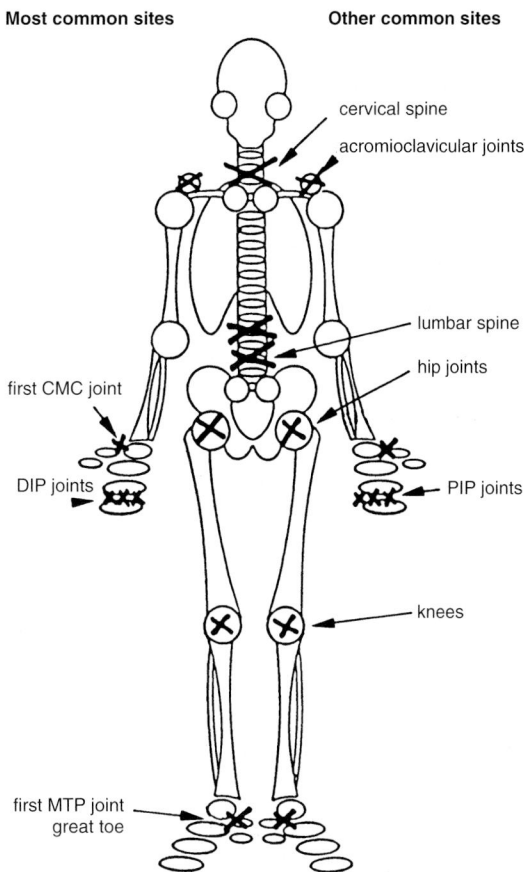

Most common sites   Other common sites

cervical spine

acromioclavicular joints

lumbar spine

hip joints

first CMC joint

DIP joints

PIP joints

knees

first MTP joint
great toe

Fig. 31.4 *Osteoarthritis: typical joint distribution*

Note: There should be no systemic manifestations.

Crystal arthropathy can complicate OA, especially in the fingers of people on diuretics, e.g. nodular gout.

Differentiation from an inflammatory arthropathy[9]

Osteoarthritis does not exhibit the typical inflammatory pattern. The clinical diagnosis is based on:
- gradual onset of pain after activity (worse towards the end of the day)
- the pattern of joint involvement
- the lack of soft tissue swelling
- the transient nature of the joint stiffness or gelling

Diagnosis

The diagnosis is clinical and radiological but the degree of changes on X-ray do not always parallel levels of symptoms.[8]

X-ray findings
- joint space narrowing with sclerosis of subchondral bone
- formation of osteophytes on the joint margins or in ligamentous attachments
- cystic areas in the subchondral bone
- altered shape of bone ends

Principles of management
- Provide explanation and reassurance including patient education handouts.
- Control pain and maintain function with appropriate drugs.
- Suggest judicious activity, exercise and physical therapy.
- Consider factors lowering the coping threshold, e.g. stress, depression, anxiety, overactivity.
- Refer for surgical intervention for debilitating and intractable pain or disability. Examples include OA of hip, knee, shoulder, first CMC joint of thumb, and first MTP joint where surgery is now very successful. Osteotomies still have a limited place for a varus or valgus deformity of the knee.

Optimal treatment
- *Explanation*. Provide patient education and reassurance that arthritis is not the crippling disease perceived by most patients.
- *Rest*. Rest during an active bout of inflammatory activity only; prolonged bed rest contraindicated.
- *Exercise*. A graduated exercise program is essential to maintain joint function. Aim for a good balance of relative rest with sensible exercise. It is necessary to stop or modify any exercise or activity that increases the pain.
- *Heat*. Recommended is a hot-water bottle, warm bath or electric blanket to soothe pain and stiffness. Advise against getting too cold.
- *Diet*. If overweight it is important to reduce weight to ideal level. Obesity increases the risk of osteoarthritis of the knee approximately fourfold and weight loss may slow progression;[10] otherwise, no specific diet has been proven to cause or improve OA. Some people claim that their arthritis is improved by having a nutritious balanced diet consisting of fish, rice and vegetables and avoiding meat, dairy produce, alcohol, pepper and spices.
- *Correction of predisposing factors and aids*. Apart from weight reduction the following may help:
  — walking stick
  — heel raise for leg length disparity
  — back brace
  — elastic or hinged joint support, e.g. knee
- *Physiotherapy*. Referral should be made for specific purposes such as:
  — correct posture and/or leg length disparity
  — supervision of a hydrotherapy program
  — heat therapy and advice on simple home heat measures
  — teaching and supervision of isometric strengthening
  — exercises, e.g. for the neck, back, quadriceps muscle
- *Occupational therapy*. Refer for advice on aids in the home, more efficient performance of daily living activities, protection of joints, and on the wide range of inexpensive equipment and tools.
- *Simple analgesics* (regularly for pain). Use paracetamol/acetaminophen (avoid codeine or dextroproproxyphene preparations, and aspirin if recent history of dyspepsia or peptic ulceration). Take before activity.
- *NSAIDs and aspirin*. These are the first-line drugs for more persistent pain or where there is evidence of inflammation, such as pain worse with resting and nocturnal pain. The risk versus benefit equation always has to be weighed carefully. As a rule, NSAIDs should be

avoided if possible. Significant risks of NSAIDs:
— gastric erosion with bleeding
— gastric ulceration
— depression of renal function
— hepatotoxicity

Note: Change to a suppository form will not necessarily render upper GI tract safe from irritation.

- *Intra-articular corticosteroids*. As a rule IA corticosteroids are not recommended but occasionally can be very effective for an inflammatory episode of distressing pain and disability on a background of tolerant pain, e.g. a flare-up in an osteoarthritic knee.
- *Viscosupplementation:* intra-articular hylans especially for OA of knee.
- *Contraindicated drugs*. For OA these include the immunosuppressive and disease-modifying drugs such as oral corticosteroids, gold, antimalarials and cytotoxic agents.

Rheumatoid arthritis

RA is the commonest chronic inflammatory polyarthritis and affects about 3% of the population. The disease can vary from a mild to a most severe debilitating expression. About 10–20% of patients have a relentless progression and require more aggressive drug therapy.[11]

The arthritis

RA generally presents with the insidious onset of pain and stiffness of the small joints of the hands and feet. The pain is persistent rather than fleeting and mainly affects the fingers where symmetrical involvement of the PIP joints produces spindling while the metacarpophalangeal joints develop diffuse thickening as does the wrist. In 25% of cases RA presents as arthritis of a single joint such as the knee,[7] a situation leading to confusion with Lyme disease or a spondyloarthropathy.

Joints involved

- hands: MCP and PIP joints, DIP joints (30%)
- wrist and elbows
- feet: MTP joints, tarsal joints (not IP joints), ankle
- knees (common) and hip (delayed—up to 50%)
- shoulder (glenohumeral) joints
- temporomandibular joints
- cervical spine

Refer to Figure 31.5.

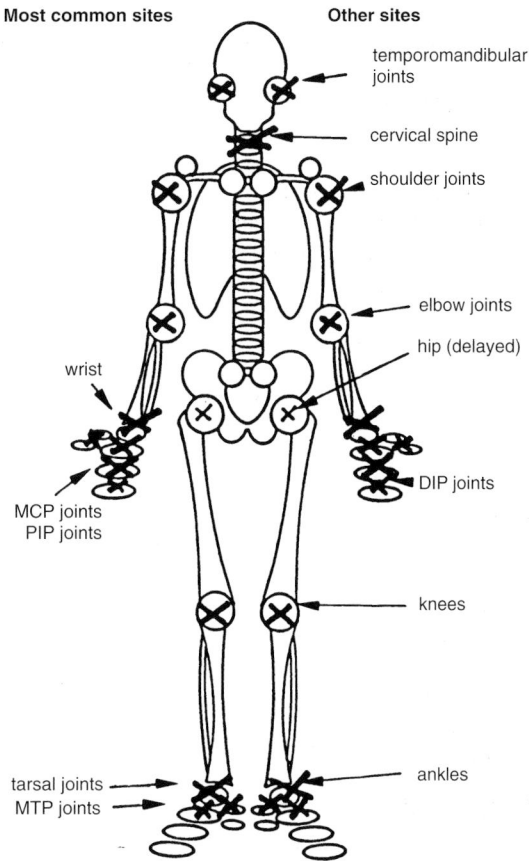

Most common sites · **Other sites**

temporomandibular joints
cervical spine
shoulder joints
elbow joints
hip (delayed)
wrist
DIP joints
MCP joints
PIP joints
knees
tarsal joints
MTP joints
ankles

Fig. 31.5 *Rheumatoid arthritis: typical joint distribution*

Clinical features

- insidious onset but can begin acutely (explosive RA)
- any age 10–75 years—peak 30–50 years but bimodal 25–50 (peak age) and 65–75
- women:men ratio 3:1
- joint pain — worse on waking, nocturnal pain, disturbed sleep
  — relieved with activity
- morning stiffness—can last hours
- rest stiffness, e.g. after sitting
- general: malaise, weakness, weight loss, fatigue
- disability according to involvement

Signs

- soft swelling (effusion and synovial swelling)
- warmth
- tenderness on pressure or movement
- limitation of movement
- muscle wasting
- later stages: deformity, subluxation, instability or ankylosing

The various possible extra-articular manifestations are summarised in Figure 31.6.

Investigations
- ESR usually raised according to active disease
- anaemia (normochronic and normocytic) may be present
- rheumatoid factor—positive in about 80–85%
- antinuclear antibodies—positive in 30%
- X-ray changes:
  — erosion of joint margin: 'mouse-bitten' appearance
  — loss of joint space (may be destruction)
  — juxta-articular osteoporosis
  — cysts
  — advanced: subluxation or ankylosing

Criteria for the diagnosis of rheumatoid arthritis are presented in Table 31.5.

Management principles[11]
- Give patient education support and appropriate reassurance. The diagnosis generally has distressful implications, and so the patient and family require careful explanation and support. It should be pointed out that the majority of patients have little or no long-term problems. Even in mild cases, continuing care and medical supervision is important.

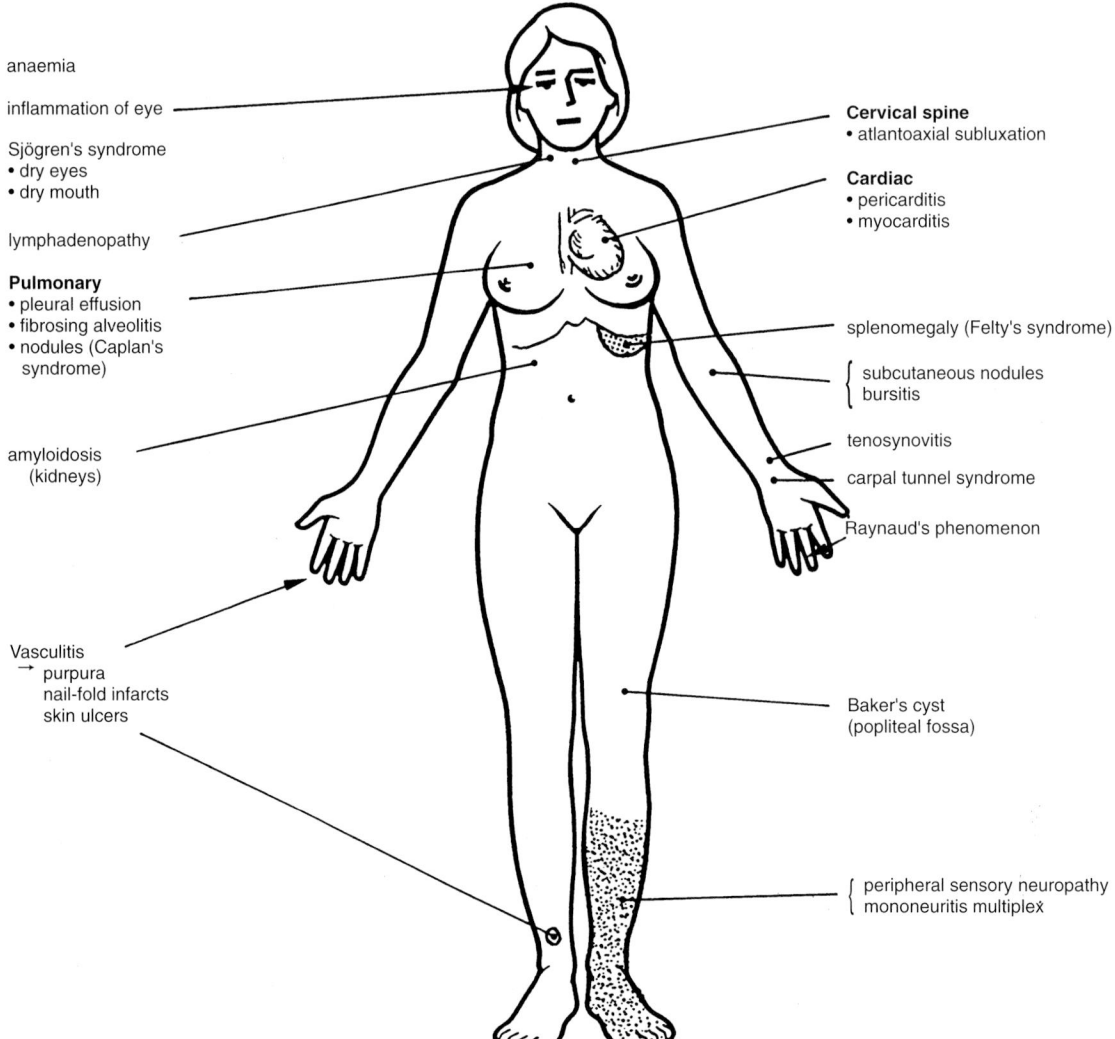

anaemia

inflammation of eye

Sjögren's syndrome
- dry eyes
- dry mouth

lymphadenopathy

Pulmonary
- pleural effusion
- fibrosing alveolitis
- nodules (Caplan's syndrome)

amyloidosis (kidneys)

Vasculitis
→ purpura
nail-fold infarcts
skin ulcers

Cervical spine
- atlantoaxial subluxation

Cardiac
- pericarditis
- myocarditis

splenomegaly (Felty's syndrome)

{ subcutaneous nodules
bursitis

tenosynovitis

carpal tunnel syndrome

Raynaud's phenomenon

Baker's cyst (popliteal fossa)

{ peripheral sensory neuropathy
mononeuritis multiplex

Fig. 31.6 *Rheumatoid arthritis: significant non-articular clinical manifestations*

Table 31.5 *American Rheumatism Association: criteria for the diagnosis of rheumatoid arthritis*

• **For classical RA**	**7 criteria needed**
• **For definite RA**	**5 criteria needed**
• **For probable RA**	**3 criteria needed**

1. Morning stiffness
2. Pain on motion or tenderness in at least one joint
3. Swelling of one joint, representing soft tissue or fluid
4. Swelling of at least one other joint (soft tissue or fluid) with an interval free of symptoms no longer than three (3) months
5. Symmetrical joint swelling (simultaneous involvement of the same joint, right and left)
6. Subcutaneous nodules over bony prominences, extensor surfaces or near joints
7. Typical X-ray changes that must include demineralisation in periarticular bone as an index of inflammation
8. Positive test for rheumatoid factor in the serum
9. Synovial fluid—a poor mucin clot formation on adding synovial fluid to dilute acetic acid
10. Synovial histopathology consistent with RA:
    (a) marked villous hypertrophy
    (b) proliferation of synovial cells
    (c) lymphocyte plus plasma cell infiltration in subsynovium
    (d) fibrin deposition within or upon microvilli
11. Characteristic histopathology of rheumatoid nodules biopsied from any site

• Use a team approach where appropriate, including a consultant referral for diagnosis and collaborative support.
• Fully assess the patient's functional impairment and impact on home life, work and social activity. Involve the family in decision making.
• Make judicious use of pharmaceutical agents. For serious cases consultant collaboration is essential.
• Review the patient regularly, continually assessing progress and drug tolerance.

Specific advice

• *Rest and splinting.* This is necessary where practical for any acute flare-up of arthritis.
• *Exercise.* It is important to have regular exercise especially walking and swimming. Have hydrotherapy in heated pools.
• *Referral.* Referring to physiotherapists and occupational therapists for expertise in exercise supervision, physical therapy and advice

regarding coping in the home and work is important.
• *Joint movement.* Each affected joint should be put daily through a full range of motion to keep it mobile and reduce stiffness.
• *Diet.* Although there is no special diet that seems to cause or cure RA there is evidence that avoiding animal fats (dairy products and some meats) and using fish oils is beneficial.[12] A nourishing well-balanced diet is common sense and obesity must be avoided.

Therapies used in the management of rheumatoid arthritis are presented in Table 31.6.

Pharmaceutical agents

• First line:	simple analgesics e.g. paracetamol aspirin NSAIDs
• Second line:	Disease-modifying agents e.g. hydroxychloroquine gold compounds (IM or orally) D-penicillamine sulphasalazine etanercept

Table 31.6 *Therapies used in the management of rheumatoid arthritis*

• Education (rest, literature, weight loss, joint protection advice)
• NSAIDs
• Simple analgesics
• DMARDs:*
  hydroxychloroquine
  sulphasalazine
  injectable gold
  D-penicillamine
  methotrexate
  oral gold
  azathioprine
  cyclophosphamide
  cyclosporin
• Physical therapy (hydrotherapy, isometric exercises)
• Occupational therapy (splints, aids and appliances)
• Corticosteroids:
  oral prednisolone
  intra-articular
  intravenous (steroid 'pulses')
  intramuscular
• Orthopaedic surgery:
  (synovectomy, joint replacement, arthrodesis, plastic hand surgery)
• Chiropody, footwear, insoles

*DMARDs = disease-modifying antirheumatic drugs
Source: After Reilly and Littlejohn[12]

- Third line: corticosteroids
  immunosuppressive agents
  e.g. methotrexate
  azathioprine
  cyclophosphamide
  cyclosporin

Standard initial drug therapy[21]

NSAIDs supplemented by paracetamol are suitable first-line agents. One of the disease-modifying drugs, either hydroxychloroquine or sulphasalazine, is usually used. If there is moderate to severe progressive disease an immunosuppressive drug, particularly methotrexate, is usually given. Such patients should be managed by a consultant.

Connective tissue disorders

The three connective tissue disorders have the common feature of arthritis or arthralgia. Refer to Chapter 28.

Systemic lupus erythematosus (SLE)

Arthritis is the commonest clinical feature of SLE (over 90%).[7] It is a symmetrical polyarthritis involving mainly small and medium joints, especially the proximal interphalangeal and carpal joints of the hand. It is usually non-erosive and non-deforming, although deformities of fingers and thumbs can occur due to laxity of ligaments, tendons and capsules causing joint instability.

The initial presentation is similar to rheumatoid arthritis. The fibromyalgia syndrome can cause confusion although it has a distribution confined mainly to the trunk, especially the back.

Investigations

The two main screening tests are:

- antinuclear antibodies—positive in 95%
- double-stranded DNA antibodies—specific for SLE but present in only 60%

Other screening tests are:

- ESR—elevated in proportion to disease activity
- rheumatoid factor—positive in 50%
- LE test—inefficient and not used

Drug treatment

- Mild—NSAIDs/aspirin ± hydroxychloroquine
- Moderate—low-dose antimalarials, e.g. hydroxychloroquine or chloroquine
- Moderate to severe—corticosteroids; immunosuppressive drugs, e.g. azathioprine

Systemic sclerosis

It can present as a polyarthritis affecting the fingers of the hand in 25% of patients, especially in the early stages. Soft tissue swelling produces a 'sausage finger' pattern. Systemic sclerosis mainly affects the skin, presenting with Raynaud's phenomenon in over 85%.

Investigations

- ESR may be raised
- normocytic normochronic anaemia may be present
- antinuclear antibodies—up to 90% positive
- rheumatoid factor—positive in 30%
- hypergammaglobulinaemia—50% positive
- antinucleolar and anticentromere ABs—specific (see p. 224).

Polymyositis and dermatomyositis

Arthralgia and arthritis occur in about 50% of patients and may be the presenting feature before the major feature of muscle weakness and wasting of the proximal muscles of the shoulder and pelvic girdles appear. The small joints of the hand are usually affected and it may resemble rheumatoid arthritis.

Crystal arthritis

Arthritis, which can be acute, chronic or asymptomatic, is caused by a variety of crystal deposits in joints. The three main types of crystal arthritis are monosodium urate (gout), calcium pyrophosphate dihydrate (CPPD) and calcium phosphate (usually hydroxyapatite).[13] Refer to Table 31.7.

Gout (monosodium urate crystal disease)

Gout is an abnormality of uric acid metabolism resulting in hyperuricaemia and urate crystal deposition. Urate crystals deposit in:

- joints—acute gouty arthritis
- soft tissue—tophi and tenosynovitis
- urinary tract—urate stones

Four typical stages of gout are recognised:

Stage 1	asymptomatic hyperuricaemia
Stage 2	acute gouty arthritis
Stage 3	intercritical gout (intervals between attacks)
Stage 4	chronic tophaceous gout and chronic gouty arthritis

Table 31.7 *Crystal-induced disease*

Crystals	Associated disease/syndrome	Typical joints or region affected

Monosodium urate	• Acute gout
	• Tophaceous gout
	• Asymptomatic
	• Chronic gouty arthritis
		Metatarsophalangeal joint of big toe
		Also: other foot joints
		     ankle
		     knee and patellar bursa
		     wrist
		     fingers

Calcium pyrophosphate dihydrate (CPPD)	• Acute pseudogout • Destructive arthropathy (like RA) • Asymptomatic (most common)	Knee, wrist In older people > 60 years M = F
Basic calcium phosphate	• Acute calcific periarthritis • Destructive arthropathy • Acute arthritis	Shoulder (supraspinatus)

Asymptomatic hyperuricaemia
• 10 times more common than gout[7]
• elevated serum uric acid (> 0.42 mmol/L in men, > 0.36 mmol/L in women)
• absence of clinical manifestations
• usually does not warrant treatment

Typical clinical features of gout
• mainly a disease of men
• onset earlier in men (40–50) than women (60+)[5]
• acute attack
  — excruciating pain in great toe
  — early hours of morning
• skin over joint—red, shiny, swollen and hot
• exquisitely tender to touch
• may be precipitated by
  — alcohol excess, e.g. binge drinking
  — surgical operation
  — starvation
  — drugs, e.g. frusemide, thiazide diuretics
• relief with colchicine, NSAIDs, corticosteroids
• can subside spontaneously (3 to 10 days) without treatment

The arthritis
Monoarthritis in 90% of attacks:
• MTP joint great toe—75%
• other joints—usually lower limbs
  — other toes
  — ankles
  — knees

Polyarticular onset is more common in old men and may occur in DIP and PIP joints of fingers. No synovial joint is immune.
  Refer to Figure 31.7.

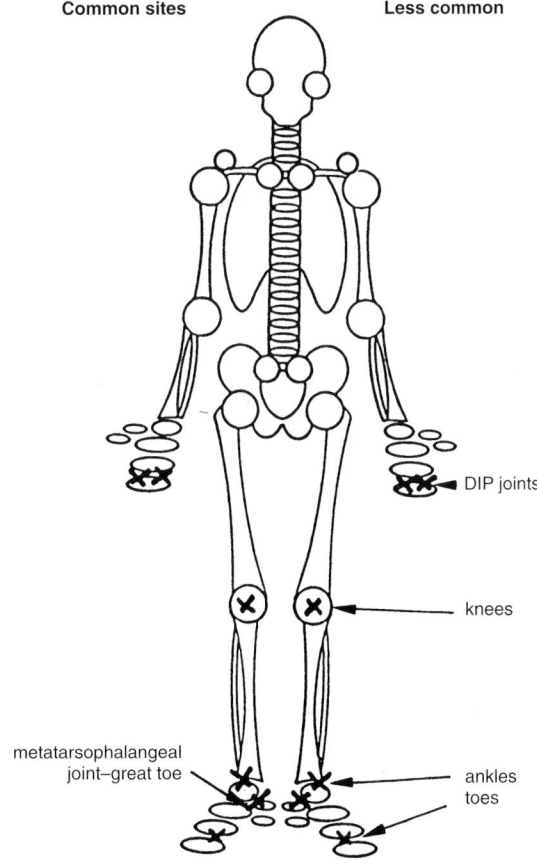

Fig. 31.7 *Gout: possible joint distribution*

Other features
• prone to recurrence
• tophi in ears, elbows (olecranon bursa), big toes, fingers, Achilles tendon (take many years)
• can cause patellar bursitis

Nodular gout

Develops in postmenopausal women with renal impairment on diuretic therapy who develop pain and tophaceous deposits around osteoarthritic interphalangeal (especially DIP) joints of fingers.[14]

Diagnosis

- elevated serum uric acid (up to 30% can be within normal limits with a true acute attack)[13]
- synovial fluid aspirate → typical uric acid crystals using compensated polarised microscopy; this should be tried first as it is the only real diagnostic feature
- X-ray: punched out erosions at joint margins

Management

For the acute attack, options include:

- NSAIDs, e.g. indomethacin 100 mg (o) statim, 75 mg 2 hours later, then 50 mg (o) tds for 24–48 hours, then 50–75 mg/day

  Note: Any other NSAID can be used. Add an antiemetic, e.g. metoclopramide 10 mg (o) tds.

- corticosteroids: intra-articular following aspiration and culture (gout and sepsis can occur together); a digital anaesthetic block is advisable. An oral course can be used: start with prednisolone 40 mg/day for 4 days then decrease gradually over 10 days
- corticotrophin (ACTH) IM in difficult cases, e.g. synthetic ACTH: tetracosactrin 1 mg IM
- colchicine (only if NSAIDs not tolerated): 0.5–1 mg (o) statim, then 0.5 mg (o) 3 or 4 times a day until pain relief (usually 24–48 hours) or diarrhoea develops (max: 6 mg/24 hours)

Note: Avoid aspirin.
Monitor renal function and electrolytes.

Long-term therapy

When acute attack subsides preventive measures include:

- weight reduction
- a normal, well-balanced diet
- avoidance of purine-rich food, e.g. organ meats (liver, brain, kidneys, sweetbread), tinned fish (sardines, anchovies, herrings), shellfish and game
- reduced intake of alcohol
- good fluid intake, e.g. water
- avoidance of drugs such as diuretics (thiazides, frusemide) and salicylates
- wearing comfortable shoes

Drug prophylaxis

Allopurinol (a xanthine oxidase inhibitor) is the drug of choice.
Dose: 100–300 mg daily
Indications:

- frequent acute attacks
- tophi or chronic gouty arthritis
- renal stones or uric acid nephropathy
- hyperuricaemia

Beware of renal insufficiency and elderly patients—use lower doses.

Method

- Commence 4 weeks after last acute attack.
- Start with 100 mg daily and increase by 100 mg daily after each month.
- Check uric acid level after 4 weeks: aim for level < 0.38 mmol/L
- Add colchicine 0.5 mg bd for 6 months (to avoid precipitation of gout) or indomethacin 50 mg bd.

The spondyloarthropathies

The spondyloarthropathies are a group of disorders with common characteristics affecting the spondyles (vertebrae) of the spine. It is appropriate to regard them as synonymous with the seronegative spondyloarthropathies in contradistinction to rheumatoid arthritis, which is seropositive and affects the cervical spine only. Apart from back pain this group tends to present with oligoarthropathy in younger patients.

Features[15]

- sacroiliitis with or without spondylitis
- enthesopathy, especially plantar fasciitis, Achilles tendinitis, costochondritis
- arthritis, especially larger lower limb joints
- extra-articular features, e.g. iritis, mucocutaneous lesions
- absent rheumatoid factor
- increased prevalence HLA-B_{27} antigen
- familial predisposition

The group of disorders

1. Ankylosing spondylitis
2. Reiter's syndrome/reactive arthritis
3. Inflammatory bowel disease (enteropathic arthritis)
4. Psoriatic arthritis
5. Juvenile chronic arthritis
6. Unclassified spondyloarthritis—partial features only

Ankylosing spondylitis

This usually presents with inflammatory back pain (sacroiliac joints and spine) and stiffness in young adults, and 20% present with peripheral joint involvement before the onset of back pain. It usually affects the girdle joints (hips and shoulders), knees or ankles. At some stage over 35% have joints other than the spine affected.

Key clinical features

- insidious onset of discomfort
- age less than 40 years
- persistence for > 3 months
- associated morning stiffness
- improvement with exercise or NSAIDs

Reactive arthritis (Reiter's syndrome)

This is a form of reactive arthropathy in which non-septic arthritis and often sacroiliitis develop after an acute infection with specific venereal or dysenteric organisms.

Reiter's syndrome = NSU + conjunctivitis ±
                   iritis + arthritis

Reactive arthritis = similar syndrome without ocular or mucocutaneous lesions

The arthritis tends to affect the larger peripheral joints especially the ankle (talocrural) and knees but the fingers and toes can be affected in a patchy polyarthritic fashion. Mucocutaneous lesions including keratoderma blennorrhagia and circinate balanitis may occur, although the majority develop peripheral arthritis only (see Fig. 31.8).

Enteropathic arthritis

Inflammatory bowel disease (ulcerative colitis, Crohn's disease and Whipple's disease) may rarely be associated with peripheral arthritis and sacroiliitis.

Psoriatic arthritis

Like Reiter's syndrome, this can develop a condition indistinguishable from ankylosing spondylitis. It is therefore important to look beyond the skin condition of psoriasis, for about 5% will develop psoriatic arthropathy. It can have several manifestations:

1. mainly DIP joints
2. identical RA pattern but RA factor negative
3. identical ankylosing spondylosis pattern with sacroiliitis and spondylitis
4. monoarthritis, especially knees
5. severe deformity or 'mutilans' arthritis

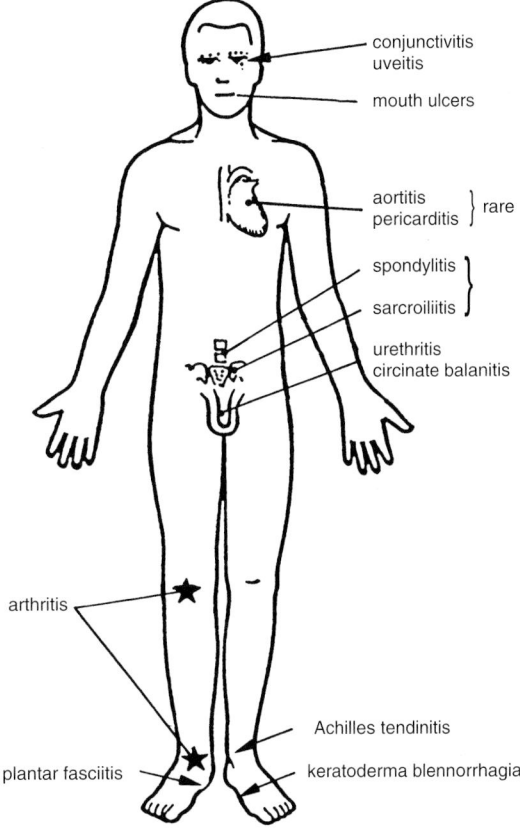

conjunctivitis
uveitis
mouth ulcers
aortitis
pericarditis } rare
spondylitis }
sarcroiliitis }
urethritis
circinate balanitis
arthritis
Achilles tendinitis
plantar fasciitis
keratoderma blennorrhagia

Fig. 31.8. *Possible clinical features of Reiter's disease*

Unclassified spondyloarthritis

Patients in this category seem to be the most frequently encountered in family practice. They clearly have a spondyloarthropathy but fail to meet the criteria for any one of the individual entities within the group. A typical patient is a young male in his third decade with a painful knee or other joint, unilateral (or bilateral) back pain with one of the entheseal problems, e.g. plantar fasciitis.

Investigations

- X-rays: Radiological sacroiliitis is central to the diagnosis. Changes include narrowing of SIJs, margin irregularity, sclerosis of periarticular bone and eventually bony fusion. Spondylitis usually follows.
- ESR: Most patients have an elevated ESR.
- HLA-B$_{27}$:   This test has low specificity and has limited value.

- Microbiology: In patients with a history of reactive arthritis cultures should be obtained from the urethra, faeces, urine and blood.[16]

Management principles

- Identify the most active elements of the disease and treat accordingly.
- Provide patient and family education with appropriate reassurance: this is vital. Stress that, although the disease is non-curable, treatment is effective and long-term prognosis generally good.
- Provide regular assessment and support.
- Give genetic counselling: e.g. in ankylosing spondylitis the risk to offspring is significant.
- Give advice regarding work, especially with posture.
- Refer for physiotherapy for exercises, postural exercises and hydrotherapy. Appropriate physiotherapy slows deterioration in spinal function.[17]
- Consider referral for occupational therapy.
- Pharmacological agents:
  — NSAIDs, e.g. indomethacin 75–200 mg daily to control pain, stiffness and synovitis
  — sulphasalazine (if NSAIDs ineffective)
  — intra-articular corticosteroids for severe monoarthritis and intralesional corticosteroids for enthesopathy.

Cautions

- Careful monitoring is required with NSAIDs and sulphasalazine.
- Systemic corticosteroids are not indicated.
- Immunosuppressants (low dose weekly methotrexate) may be needed for severe intractable problems with psoriasis and reactive arthritis.
- These conditions should be managed in collaboration with a consultant.
- Although phenylbutazone is the most effective NSAID, its side effects (esp. aplastic anaemia) are a major problem.

Lyme disease

Lyme disease (known as Lyme borreliosis) was first described in 1975 and named after the town of Lyme in Connecticut. It has spread to almost all the states of the United States and is appearing in Europe and Asia at an increasing rate.

Very infective, it is caused by a spirochete, *Borrelia burgdorferi*, and transmitted by *Ixodes* ticks, in particular the deer tick.

Diagnostic serology should be considered for patients with a history of tick bites, typical rash (a doughnut-shaped red rash about 6 cm in diameter) at the bite site, heart disorders (especially arrhythmias), unusual joint arthralgia or central nervous system disease. CNS disease includes muscle weakness of the limbs, muscular pain or evidence of meningitis. In children Lyme disease can be mistaken for juvenile chronic arthritis.

The arthralgia

The typical picture is that months (even years) after the tick bite up to 60% of patients will develop joint and periarticular pain (without objective findings), specific arthritis, mainly of the large joints such as the knee, and/or chronic synovitis.[18]

Treatment

Treatment is with penicillin, tetracycline or cephalosporins. If antibiotics are given early in the acute illness it tends to terminate abruptly.

The vasculitides

The vasculitides or vasculitis syndromes are a heterogeneous group of disorders involving inflammation and necrosis of blood vessels, the clinical effects and classification depending on the size of the vessels involved.

More common causes

These are the small vessel vasculitis effects associated with many important diseases such as rheumatoid arthritis, SLE, infective endocarditis, Henoch-Schönlein purpura and hepatitis B. Skin lesions and arthritis are usually associated with these disorders.

Rarer causes

The major vasculitides are polyarteritis nodosa, giant cell arteritis, polymyalgia rheumatica and Wegener's granulomatosis. Arthritis or limb girdle pain can be a component of the clinical presentation. The vasculitides are presented in more detail in Chapter 28.

When to refer

- Consider referring most severe true inflammatory disorders for diagnosis and initiation of

treatment, e.g. rheumatoid arthritis, spondyloarthropathy, connective tissue disorders and suspicion of a vasculitide
• Osteoarthritis
— generalised joint pain
— associated systemic symptoms
— deteriorating joint function

— intractable pain (especially at rest)
— if surgical procedure is contemplated[8]
• Rheumatoid arthritis
— persistent inflammation of a joint or joints
— patient ill and corticosteroids contemplated
— if a surgical procedure is contemplated

Table 31.8 *Diagnostic guidelines for arthritis*

Disorder	Sex ratio	Typical age	Typical common joints involved	Associated features
Osteoarthritis (generalised—primary)	FM 6:1	> 50	• DIP > PIP fingers • Base thumb (1st CMC) • 1st MTP joint • Cervical and lumbar spines • Hips and knees	• Pain worse in evenings, relieved by rest
Rheumatoid arthritis	FM 3:1	30–50	• PIP, MCP hands • Wrist • Base of toes (MTP joints) • Symmetrical	• Any joint: worse at rest, better with activity; morning stiffness • Constitutional symptoms • Carpal tunnel syndrome • Many other general effects
SLE	FM 9:1	15–35	• Symmetrical and variable • Small joints fingers • Often slight	• Constitutional symptoms • Fever • Adverse drug reactions • Any other system affected • Rash (80%) • Pleuritic symptoms (67%) • Raynaud's
Systemic sclerosis	FM 1	20–50	• Symmetrical • Polyarthritis fingers	• Raynaud's (90%) • Other skin changes • Dysphagia
Viral arthropathies (excluding HIV)	M = F	Children	• Transient • Usually PIP joints fingers	• Rash, fever
Ankylosing spondylitis	MF 3:1	18–30	• Sacroiliacs • Vertebral column esp. lumbar costovertebral • Also knees, hips or ankles	• Iridocyclitis • Chest dysfunction • Enthesopathy, e.g. plantar fasciitis
Psoriatic arthritis	M = F	Any age	• DIP joints—fingers and toes, sacroiliacs	• Psoriasis rash (pre-existing) • Pitted nails, 'sausage digits'
Enteropathic arthritis	M = F	Any age	• Lower extremity: knees, feet, ankles • hips: sacroiliacs	• Ulcerative colitis • Crohn's disease
Reactive arthritis: Genitourinary e.g. Reiter's Post-dysentery e.g. Salmonella	MF 20:1 M = F	15–30	As above	• Preceding dysentery or urethritis • Entheseal problems
Gout	MF 20:1	M 40–50 F > 60	• Big toe (MTP joint): any other possible esp. lower limb • DIP—osteoarthritis	• Tophi • Raised s. uric acid • Urate crystals in joints • Diuretics in elderly
Pseudogout	M = F	> 60 esp. > 70	• Knee	• Chondrocalcinosis • Pyrophosphate crystals in joint
Polymyalgia rheumatica	FM 3:1	> 60	• Morning stiffness and pain in girdles esp. shoulder • Joints normal or osteoarthritic	ESR ↑↑↑

- Spondyloarthropathies
  - initial referral for confirmation of diagnosis and initiation of treatment
  - disease unresponsive to conventional treatment
  - sudden deterioration in symptoms, esp. pain
  - onset of uveitis or other ocular complications
  - adverse drug reactions
- Undiagnosed arthritis in presence of constitutional symptoms
- Suspicion of a suppurative or serious infective condition, e.g. septic arthritis, endocarditis, brucellosis
- Children with evidence of juvenile arthritis, e.g. Still's disease

Practice tips

- Morning stiffness and pain, improving with exercise = rheumatoid arthritis.
- Flitting polyarthritis and fever = rheumatic fever; ? endocarditis; ? SLE.
- Polyarthritis (usually PIPs) and rash = viral arthritis or drug reaction.
- If rheumatoid arthritis involves the neck, beware of atlantoaxial subluxation and spinal cord compression.
- If the patient is young—think of SLE.
- If a patient returns from overseas with arthralgia, think of drug reactions, hepatitis, Lyme disease, but if the pain is intense consider dengue fever.
- Consider the possibility of Lyme disease in people with a fever, rash and arthritis who have been exposed to tick bites in rural areas.
- If a patient presents with Raynaud's phenomenon and arthritis, especially of the hands, consider foremost RA, SLE and systemic sclerosis.
- Avoid the temptation to apply on doubtful grounds a broad label such as arthritis or rheumatoid, or a precise diagnosis such as rheumatoid arthritis, and introduce drugs.[19] Table 31.8 (p. 285) presents the diagnostic guidelines.[20]

References

1. Hart FD. *Practical problems in rheumatology*. London: Dunitz, 1985, 77.
2. Cormack J, Marinker M, Morrel D. *Practice: A handbook of primary health care*. London: Kluwer-Harrop Handbooks, 1980; 3(61):1–12.
3. Lassere M, McGuigan L. Systemic disease presenting as arthritis—A diagnostic approach. Aust Fam Physician, 1991; 20: 1683–1714.
4. Rudge S. Joint pain in children: assessing the serious causes. Mod Med Aust, May 1990; 113–121.
5. Sandler G, Fry J. *Early clinical diagnosis*. Lancaster: MTP Press, 1986.
6. Nash PT, Webb J. Polyarticular and monoarticular arthritis. A diagnostic approach. Aust Fam Physician, 1986; 15: 1265–1275.
7. Kumer PJ, Clarke ML. *Clinical medicine* (2nd edn). London: Baillere Tindall, 1990; 382.
8. Muirden K. Osteoarthritis. In: MIMS Disease Index (2nd edn). Sydney: IMS Publishing, 1996, 365–367.
9. March LM. Osteoarthritis. Med J Aust, 1997; 166: 98–103.
10. Felson DT. Weight and osteoarthritis. J Rheumatol Suppl, 1995; 43:7–9.
11. Brooks P. Rheumatoid arthritis. In: MIMS Disease Index (2nd edn). Sydney: IMS Publishing, 1996, 446–449.
12. Reilly P, Littlejohn G. Current treatment concepts in arthritis. Aust Fam Physician, 1989; 18:1499–1509.
13. Hall S. Crystal arthritis: A clinician's view. Aust Fam Physician, 1991, 20: 1717–1724.
14. MacFarlane DG, Dieppe PA. Diuretic induced gout in elderly women. Br J Rheumatol, 1985; 24:155–159.
15. Creamer P, Edmonds J. Spondyloarthropathies. In: MIMS Disease Index (2nd edn). Sydney: IMS Publishing, 1996, 479–482.
16. Edmonds JP. Spondyloarthropathies. Med J Aust, 1997; 166: 214–218.
17. Vilitanen JV et al. Fifteen months follow up of intensive inpatient physiotherapy and exercise in ankylosing spondylitis. Clin Rheum, 1995; 14:413–419.
18. Tierney RM et al. *Current medical diagnosis and treatment* (35th edn). Stamford: Appleton and Lange, 1996, 1240–1242.
19. Kincaid-Smith P, Larkins R, Whelan G, eds. *Problems in clinical medicine*. Sydney: MacLennan and Petty, 1989, 391.
20. Hart FD. Early clinical diagnosis of 12 forms of arthritis. Mod Med Aust, March 1989, 34–40.
21. Mashford ML (Chairman). *Therapeutic guidelines* (3rd edn). Melbourne: Therapeutic Guidelines, 1997–1998, 74–88.

32
Anorectal disorders

—

Duncan ill with very bad piles—operated on last night, or, since that sounds alarming, lanced. Can't really sympathise with that particular disease, though the pain is terrible. Must laugh.

Virginia Woolf 1934
Diary entry

Anorectal problems are common in family practice and tend to cause anxiety in the patient that is often related to the fear of cancer. This fear may be well founded for many instances of rectal bleeding and lumps. It is important to keep in mind the association between haemorrhoids and carcinoma of the large bowel.

Anorectal problems include:

- pain
- lumps
- discharge
- bleeding
- pruritus

Common anorectal conditions are illustrated in Figure 32.1.

Anorectal pain

The patient may complain that defecation is painful or almost impossible because of anorectal pain.

Summary of causes
Pain without swelling:
- anal fissure
- anal herpes
- ulcerative proctitis
- proctalgia fugax
- solitary rectal ulcer

Painful swelling:
- perianal haematoma
- strangulated internal haemorrhoids
- abscess — perianal
  — ischiorectal

Anal fissure

Anal fissures cause pain on defecation and usually develop after a period of constipation (may be brief period) and tenesmus. Sometimes the pain can be excruciating, persisting for hours and radiating down the back of both legs. Anal fissures, especially if chronic, can cause minor anorectal bleeding (bright blood) noted as spotting on the toilet paper.

Examination
On inspection the anal fissure is usually seen in the anal margin, situated in the midline posteriorly (6 o'clock). The fissure appears as an elliptical ulcer involving the lower third of the anus from the dentate line to the anal verge.[1]

Digital examination and sigmoidoscopy are difficult because of painful anal sphincter spasm.

If there are multiple fissures Crohn's disease should be suspected. These fissures look different, being indurated, oedematous and bluish in colour.

In chronic anal fissures a sentinel pile is common and in long-standing cases a subcutaneous fistula is seen at the anal margin, with fibrosis and anal stenosis.[1]

Treatment
A trial of a high residue diet and avoidance of constipation (aim for soft bulky stools) may lead to resolution. A combined local anaesthetic and corticosteroid ointment applied to the fissure can provide relief and promote healing. Hot

Fig. 32.1 *Common anorectal conditions*

baths relax the internal anal sphincter. The most promising conservative treatment is the application of diluted glyceryl trinitrate ointment, e.g. Rectogesic, three times daily to the lower anal canal.[2]

Lateral internal sphincterotomy is indicated in patients with a recurrent fissure and a chronic fissure with a degree of fibrosis and anal stenosis. This surgical procedure is very effective. An alternative is injection of botulinum toxin into the sphincter.

Proctalgia fugax (levator ani spasm)

Main features:
- fleeting rectal pain
- varies from mild discomfort to severe spasm
- lasts 3–30 minutes
- often wakes patient at night
- a functional bowel disorder
- affects adults, usually professional males

Management
- explanation and reassurance
- salbutamol inhaler (2 puffs statim) worth a trial

Alternatives include glyceryl trinitrate spray for the symptom or prophylactic quinine sulphate before retiring.

Solitary rectal ulcer syndrome

These ulcers occur in young adults; they can present with pain but usually present as the sensation of a rectal lump causing obstructed defecation and bleeding with mucus. The ulcer, which is usually seen on sigmoidoscopy about 10 cm from the anal margin on the anterior rectal wall, can resemble carcinoma. Management is difficult and a chronic course is common. Treatment includes a high residue diet and the avoidance of constipation.

Perianal haematoma

A perianal haematoma is a purple tender swelling at the anal margin caused by rupture of an external haemorrhoidal vein following straining at toilet or some other effort involving a Valsalva manoeuvre. The degree of pain varies from a minor discomfort to severe pain. It has been described as the 'five day, painful, self-curing pile'.

Management

Surgical intervention is recommended, especially in the presence of severe discomfort. The treatment depends on the time of presentation after the appearance of the haematoma.

1. *Within 24 hours of onset.* Perform simple aspiration without local anaesthetic using a 19 gauge needle while the haematoma is still fluid.
2. *From 24 hours to 5 days of onset.* The blood has clotted and a simple incision under local anaesthetic over the haematoma with deroofing to remove the thrombosis is recommended. Removal of the haematoma reduces the chances of the development of a skin tag, which can be a source of anal irritation.
3. *Day 6 onwards.* The haematoma is best left alone unless it is very painful or (rarely) infected. Resolution is evidenced by the appearance of wrinkles in the previously stretched skin.

Follow-up

The patient should be reviewed in 4 weeks for rectal examination and proctoscopy, to examine for any underlying internal haemorrhoid that may predispose to further recurrence. Prevention includes an increased intake of dietary fibre and avoidance of straining at stool.

Strangulated haemorrhoids

A marked oedematous circumferential swelling will appear if all the haemorrhoids are involved. If only one haemorrhoid is strangulated proctoscopy will help to distinguish it from a perianal haematoma. Initial treatment is with rest and ice packs and then haemorrhoidectomy at the earliest possible time. It is best to refer for urgent surgery.

Perianal abscess

Clinical features

- severe, constant, throbbing pain
- fever and toxicity
- hot, red, tender swelling adjacent to anal margin
- non-fluctuant swelling

Careful examination is essential to make the diagnosis. Look for evidence of a fistula.

Treatment

Drain via a cruciate incision (with trimming of the corners) over the point of maximal induration. A drain tube can be inserted for 7 to 10 days.

Anorectal lumps

Anorectal lumps are relatively common and patients are often concerned because of the fear of cancer. A lump arising from the anal canal or rectum, such as internal haemorrhoids, tends to appear intermittently upon defecation, and reduce afterwards.[1] Common prolapsing lesions include second- and third-degree haemorrhoids, hypertrophied anal papilla, polyps and rectal prolapse. Common presenting lumps include skin tags, fourth-degree piles and perianal warts (Table 32.1).

Table 32.1 *Common anal lumps*

Prolapsing lumps
- 2nd- and 3rd-degree haemorrhoids
- rectal prolapse
- rectal polyp
- hypertrophied anal papilla

Persistent lumps
- skin tag
- perianal warts (condylomata accuminata)
- anal carcinoma
- 4th-degree haemorrhoids
- perianal haematoma
- perianal abscess

Skin tags

The skin tag is usually the legacy of an untreated perianal haematoma. It may require excision for aesthetic reasons, for hygiene or because it is a source of pruritus ani or irritation. A tag may be associated with a chronic fissure.

Method of excision

A simple elliptical excision at the base of the skin is made under local anaesthetic. Suturing of the defect is usually not necessary.

Perianal warts

It is important to distinguish the common viral warts from the condylomata lata of secondary syphilis. Local therapy includes the application of podophyllin every two or three days by the practitioner.

Internal haemorrhoids

Haemorrhoids or piles are common and tend to develop between the ages of 20 and 50. About one out of two Westerners suffers from them by the time 50 is reached.[3] Internal haemorrhoids are a complex of dilated arteries, branches of the superior haemorrhoidal artery and veins of the internal haemorrhoidal venous plexus (Fig. 32.2). The commonest cause is chronic constipation related to a lack of dietary fibre.

Anatomically there are three classical sites, namely 3, 7 and 11 o'clock (Fig. 32.3).

Clinical stages and pathology[3]

| Stage 1 | First-degree internal haemorrhoids: three bulges form above the dentate line. Bright bleeding is common. |

| Stage 2 | Second-degree internal haemorrhoids: the bulges increase in size and slide downwards so that the patient is aware of lumps when straining at stool, but they disappear upon relaxing. Bleeding is a feature. |

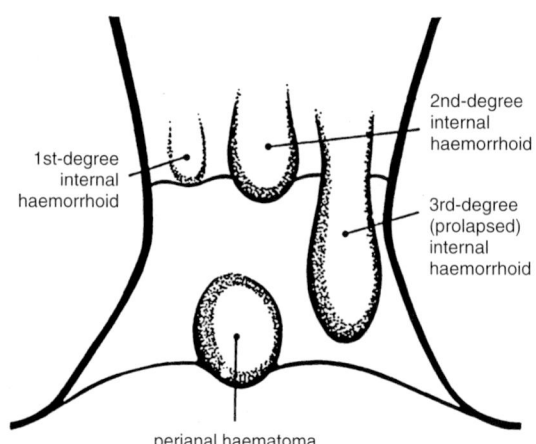

Fig. 32.2 *Classification of haemorrhoids*

1st-degree internal haemorrhoid

2nd-degree internal haemorrhoid

3rd-degree (prolapsed) internal haemorrhoid

perianal haematoma

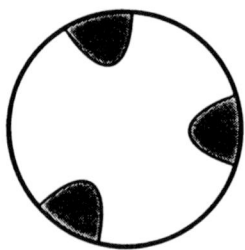

Fig. 32.3 *Three sites of primary haemorrhoids, looking into the anus from below*

| Stage 3 | Third-degree internal haemorrhoids: the pile continues to enlarge and slide downwards, requiring manual replacement to alleviate discomfort. Bleeding is also a feature. |

| Stage 4 | Fourth-degree internal haemorrhoids: prolapse has occurred and replacement of the prolapsed pile into the anal canal is impossible. |

Symptoms

Bleeding is the main and, in many people, the only symptom. The word 'haemorrhoid' means flow of blood. Other symptoms include prolapse, mucoid discharge, irritation/itching, incomplete bowel evacuation and pain.

Treatment

The treatment of haemorrhoids is based on four procedures: namely, injection, rubber band ligation, cryotherapy and sphincterotomy. Surgery is generally reserved for large strangulated piles. The best treatment, however, is prevention, and softish bulky faeces that pass easily prevent haemorrhoids. People should be advised to have a diet with adequate fibre by eating plenty of fresh fruit, vegetables, whole grain cereals or bran. They should complete their bowel action within a few minutes and avoid using laxatives.

Anal discharge

Anal discharge refers to the involuntary escape of fluid from or near the anus. The causes may be considered as follows.[3]

Continent

- anal fistula
- pilonidal sinus
- sexually transmitted diseases
  - — anal warts
  - — gonococcal ulcers
  - — genital herpes
- solitary rectal ulcer syndrome
- carcinoma of anal margin

Incontinent

- minor incontinence—weakness of internal sphincter
- severe incontinence—weakness of levator ani and puborectalis

Partial continence

- faecal impaction
- rectal prolapse

Rectal bleeding

Patients present with any degree of bleeding from a smear on the toilet tissue to severe haemorrhage. Various causes are presented in Figure 32.4.

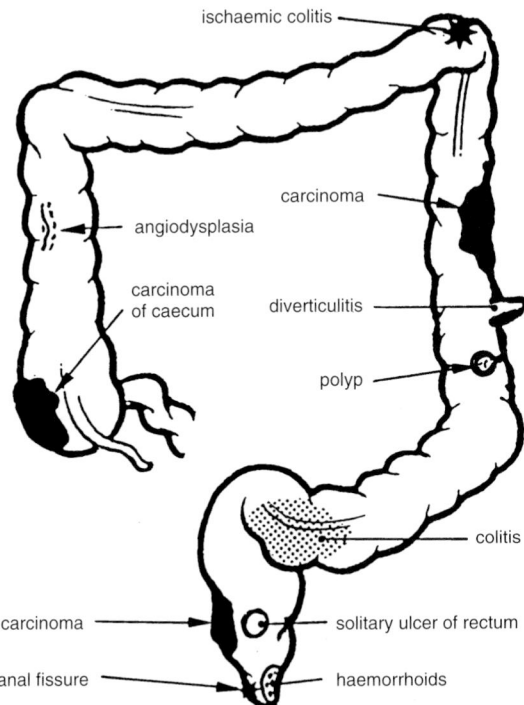

Fig. 32.4 *Various causes of rectal bleeding*

Local causes of bleeding include excoriated skin, anal fissure, a burst perianal haematoma and anal carcinoma. A characteristic pattern of bright bleeding is found with haemorrhoids. It is usually small non-prolapsing haemorrhoids that bleed.

The nature of the blood (e.g. bright red, dark red or black) and the nature of the bleeding (e.g. smear, streaked on stool, mixed with stool, massive) gives an indication of the source of the bleeding (Table 32.2). Black tarry (melaena) stool indicates bleeding from the upper gastrointestinal tract and is rare distal to the lower ileum. Patients with melaena should be admitted to hospital.

Frequent passage of blood and mucus indicates a rectal tumour or proctitis, whereas more proximal tumours or extensive colitis present different patterns.

Substantial haemorrhage, which is rare, can be caused by diverticular disease, angiodysplasia or more proximal lesions such as Meckel's diverticulum and even duodenal ulcers. Angiodysplasias are 5 mm collections of dilated mucosal capillaries and thick-walled submucosal veins, found usually in the ascending colon of elderly patients who have no other bowel symptoms. The site is identified by technetium-labelled red cell scan or colonoscopy.

The history should also include an analysis of any associated symptoms such as pain, diarrhoea or constipation, presence of lumps and a sensation of urgency or unsatisfied defecation. The latter symptoms point to a rectal cause. Associated change of bowel habit suggests a diagnosis of carcinoma of the rectum or left colon. Bleeding from right colon cancer is often occult, presenting as anaemia.

The examination includes a general assessment, anal inspection, digital rectal examination and proctosigmoidoscopy. Even if there is an anal lesion, proximal bleeding must be excluded in all cases by sigmoidoscopy[2] and by colonoscopy if there are any bowel symptoms or no obvious anal cause or a doubt about a lesion causing the symptoms.

Pruritus ani

Pruritus ani, which is itching of the anus, can be a distressing symptom that is worse at night, during hot weather and during exercise. It is seen typically in adult males with considerable inner drive, often at times of stress and in hot

Table 32.2 *Presentation and causes of rectal bleeding*[4]

Bright red blood in toilet separate from faeces	• Internal haemorrhoids
Bright red blood on toilet paper	• Internal haemorrhoids • Fissure • Anal carcinoma • Pruritus • Anal warts and condylomata
Blood and mucus on underwear	• 3rd-degree haemorrhoids • 4th-degree haemorrhoids • Prolapsed rectum • Mucosal prolapse • Prolapsed mucosal polyp
Blood on underwear (no mucus)	• Ulcerated perianal haematoma • Anal carcinoma
Blood and mucus mixed with faeces	• Colorectal carcinoma • Proctitis • Colitis, ulcerative colitis • Large mucosal polyp • Ischaemic colitis
Blood mixed with faeces (no mucus)	• Small colorectal polyps • Small colorectal carcinoma
Melaena (black tarry stools)	• Gastrointestinal bleeding (usually upper) with long transit time to the anus
Torrential haemorrhage (rare)	• Diverticular disease • Angiodysplasia
Large volumes of mucus in faeces (little blood)	• Villous papilloma of rectum • Villous papilloma of colon
Blood in faeces with menstruation (rare)	• Rectal endometriosis

Source: Orlay, G. *Office Proctology*, p. 11.[4] © Copyright 1987 George Orlay—reproduced with permission

weather when sweating is excessive. In children, threadworm infestation should be suspected. It may be part of general itching, such as with a skin disease, or localised whereby various anorectal disorders have to be excluded.

Physical signs

The skin changes can vary from minimal signs to marked pathology that can show linear ulceration, maceration or lichenification. Superficial skin changes can be moist and macerated or dry and scaly. Full anorectal examination is necessary.

Causes and aggravating factors

Psychological factors:

• stress and anxiety
• fear of cancer

Generalised systemic or skin disorders:

• eczema
• diabetes mellitus
• candidiasis

• psoriasis (look for fissures in natal cleft)
• antibiotic treatment
• worms: pinworm, threadworm
• diarrhoea causing excoriation

Local anorectal conditions:

• piles
• fissures
• warts

Zealous hygiene
Contact dermatitis:

• dyed or perfumed toilet tissue, soap, powder
• clothing

Excessive sweating:

• e.g. tight pantyhose in summer

Diagnostic approach

• urinalysis (? diabetes)
• anorectal examination
• scrapings and microscopy to detect organisms
• stool examination for intestinal parasites

Rules of treatment: patient education

1. *Scratching*. Stop—it's taboo! If you scratch at night, wear light cotton gloves to bed.
2. *Bathing*. Avoid hot water. Excessive showering and scrubbing is also bad for this condition. Use a cream such as bland aqueous cream or Cetaphil lotion or a mild soap substitute for cleaning rather than soap.
3. *Drying*. Keep the area as dry and cool as possible. After washing, dry gently and thoroughly with a soft towel or soft tissue: do not rub. Warm air from a hair drier is very useful.
4. *Bowel movements*. Keep bowels regular and smooth by eating plenty of high-fibre foods such as bran, fresh carrots and apples. Some doctors claim that your bowel actions should be so smooth and complete that toilet paper should hardly be necessary.
5. *Toilet*. Clean gently after bowel movements. Soft paper tissue (avoid pastel tints) may be used, and then clean with tufts of cotton wool with aqueous cream or bland soap and water. The best way is to use cotton wool in warm water.
6. *Soaps and powder*. Do not use perfumed soaps and talcum powder, including baby powder. Zinc powder, e.g. Curash, is suitable to keep the area dry and relieve itching.
7. *Clothing*. Wear loose clothing and underwear. In men, boxer shorts should be used in preference to jockey shorts. Cottons should be used. Let the air circulate in the area. At times a skirt but no underpants (in women) is desirable. Avoid pantyhose if possible.
8. *Topical creams*. Do not use ointments unless your doctor has prescribed them. If a cream has to be used, simple creams may be the most soothing (e.g. toilet lanoline).

Topical treatment

- Treat the cause (if known).
- Avoid local anaesthetics, antiseptics.

- Advise aqueous cream to wash anus (instead of soap).
- Most effective preparations (for short courses):

  hydrocortisone 1% cream

  or

  hydrocortisone 1% cream with clioquinol 3% or clotrimazole 1% (especially if dermatosis suspected)

If an isolated area and resistant, infiltrate 0.5 mL of triamcinolone intradermally. Fractionated X-ray therapy can be used if very severe.

Practice tips for pruritus ani

- Most cases of uncomplicated pruritus ani resolve with simple measures including explanation and reassurance.
- Otherwise prescribe hydrocortisone/clioquinol cream.
- Lifestyle stress and anxiety underlies most cases.
- In obese patients with intertrigo and excessive sweating strap the buttocks apart with adhesive tape.

References

1. Hunt P, Marshall V. *Clinical problems in general surgery*. Sydney: Butterworths, 1991, 311.
2. Lund JN, Scholefield JH. A randomised, prospective, double-blind, placebo-controlled trial of glyceryl trinitrate ointment in the treatment of anal fissure. Lancet, 1997, Jan 4; 11–13.
3. Ryan P. *A very short textbook of surgery* (2nd edn). Canberra: Dennis and Ryan, 1990, 37–42.
4. Orlay G. *Office proctology*. Sydney: Australasian Medical Publishing Company, 1987, 11–52.

33

Low back pain

—

Last Wednesday night while carrying a bucket of water from the well, Hannah Williams slipped upon the icy path and fell heavily upon her back. We fear her spine was injured for though she suffers acute pain in her legs she cannot move them. The poor wild beautiful girl is stopped in her wildness at last.

Francis Kilvert 1874

Low back pain accounts for at least 5% of general practice presentations. The most common cause is minor soft tissue injury, but patients with this do not usually seek medical help because the problem settles within a few days.

Most back pain in patients presenting to general practitioners is due to dysfunction of elements of the mobile segment, namely the facet joint, the intervertebral joint (with its disc) and the ligamentous and muscular attachments. This problem, often referred to as mechanical pain or traumatic joint derangement, will be described as vertebral dysfunction—a general term that, while covering radicular and non-radicular pain, includes dysfunction of the joints of the spine.

Key facts and checkpoints

- Back pain accounts for at least 5% of all presenting problems in general practice in Australia and 6.5% in Britain.[1]
- In the United States it is the commonest cause of limitation of activity under the age of 45.[2]
- Approximately 85% of the population will experience back pain at some stage of their lives, while 70% of the world's population will have at least one disabling episode of low back pain in their lives.[2]
- At least 50% of these people will recover within 2 weeks and 75% within 1 month, but recurrences are frequent and have been reported in 40–70% of patients.

- The most common age groups are the 30s, 40s and 50s, the average age being 45 years.
- The most common cause of back pain is a minor strain to muscles and/or ligaments, but people suffering from this type of back pain usually do not seek medical treatment as most of these soft tissue problems resolve rapidly.
- The main cause of back pain presenting to the doctor is dysfunction of the intervertebral joints of the spine due to injury, also referred to as mechanical back pain (at least 70%).
- The causes of this dysfunction are disorders of the facet joints and internal disruption of the intervertebral disc, the exact balance being uncertain.
- The second most common cause of back pain is spondylosis (synonymous with osteoarthritis and degenerative back disease). It accounts for about 10% of cases of low back pain.
- L5 and S1 nerve root lesions represent most of the cases of sciatica presenting in general practice. They tend to present separately but can occur together with a massive disc protrusion.
- An intervertebral disc prolapse has been proven in only 6–8% of cases of back pain.[2]

Causes of low back pain

To develop a comprehensive diagnostic approach, the practitioner should have a clear understanding of the possible causes of low back and leg pain and of the relative frequency of their clinical presentations. The major causes of low back pain in several hundred patients presenting to the author's general practice are summarised in Table 33.1.

Relevant causes are illustrated in Figure 33.1

Table 33.1   *Major causes of low back ± leg pain presenting in the author's general practice*

Patients	%
Vertebral dysfunction	71.8
Lumbar spondylosis	10.1
Depression	3.0
Urinary tract infection	2.2
Spondylolisthesis	2.0
Spondyloarthropathies	1.9
Musculoligamentous strains/tears	1.2
Malignant disease	0.8
Arterial occlusive disease	0.6
Other	6.4
	100.0

Anatomical and pathophysiological concepts

Recent studies have focused on the importance of disruption of the intervertebral disc in the cause of back pain. A very plausible theory has been advanced by Maigne[3] who proposes the existence, in the involved mobile segment, of a minor intervertebral derangement (MID). He defines it as 'isolated pain in one intervertebral segment, of a mild character, and due to minor mechanical cause'.

It is independent of radiological and anatomical disturbances of the segment. The most common clinical situation occurs where a vertebral level is found to be painful and yet to have a normal static and radiological appearance.

The MID always involves one of the two apophyseal joints in the mobile segment, thus initiating nociceptive activity in the posterior primary dermatome and myotome. The overlying skin is tender to pinching and rolling, while the muscles are painful to palpation and feel cord-like.

Maigne points out that the functional ability of the mobile segment depends intimately upon the condition of the intervertebral disc. Thus, if the disc is injured, other elements of the segment will be affected. Even a minimal disc lesion can produce apophyseal joint dysfunction which is a reflex cause of protective muscle spasm and pain in the corresponding segment, with loss of function (Figure 33.2).

In theory any structure with a nociceptive nerve supply may be a source of pain. Such structures include the ligaments, fascia and muscles of the lumbosacral spine, intervertebral joints, facet joints, dura-mater and sacroiliac joints.[4]

A diagnostic approach

A summary of the safety diagnostic model is presented in Table 33.2.

Probability diagnosis

The commonest cause of low back pain is vertebral dysfunction, which then has to be further analysed.

Table 33.2   *Low back pain: diagnostic strategy model*

Q.	*Probability diagnosis*
A.	Vertebral dysfunction esp. facet joint and disc Spondylosis (degenerative OA)
Q.	*Serious disorders not to be missed*
A.	Cardiovascular • ruptured aortic aneurysm • retroperitoneal haemorrhage (anticoagulants) Neoplasia • myeloma • metastases Severe infections • osteomyelitis • discitis • tuberculosis • pelvic abscess/PID Cauda equina compression
Q.	*Pitfalls (often missed)*
A.	Spondyloarthropathies • ankylosing spondylitis • Reiter's disease • psoriasis • bowel inflammation Sacroiliac dysfunction Spondylolisthesis Claudication • vascular • neurogenic Prostatitis Endometriosis
Q.	*Seven masquerades checklist*
A.	Depression √ Diabetes — Drugs — Anaemia — Thyroid disease — Spinal dysfunction √ UTI √
Q.	*Is this patient trying to tell me something?*
A.	Quite likely. Consider lifestyle, stress, work problems, malingering, conversion reaction

Note: Associated buttock and leg pain included.

Visceral and vascular
B—biliary disorders
U—penetrating duodenal ulcer
P—pancreatitis
R—renal disorders

aortic aneurysm (ruptured/dissecting)

retroperitoneal haemorrhage

female pelvic disorders
  e.g. endometriosis

prostatitis

abscess, e.g. pilonidal

arterial embolism

claudication of arterial occlusive disease

Musculoskeletal
Scheuermann's disorder

pathological fracture

metastatic disease

spondylolisthesis

disc disruption

facet joint dysfunction
spondylosis

sacroiliac dysfunction
sacroiliitis

trochanteric bursitis
gluteus medius bursitis

coccydynia

ischial bursitis

meralgia paraesthetica

neurogenic claudication

radicular pain ⎞ from
            ⎬ spinal
referred pain ⎠ dysfunction

radicular pain

Fig. 33.1 *Relevant causes of back pain with associated buttock and leg pain*

Muscle or ligamentous tears or similar soft tissue injuries are uncommon causes of back pain alone: they are generally associated with severe spinal disruption and severe trauma such as that following a motor vehicle accident.

In the lumbar spine most problems originate from either the apophyseal joints or the intervertebral discogenic joint, or from both simultaneously. The disc can cause pain, either intrinsically from internal disruption or extrinsically by pressure on adjacent pain-sensitive structures, leading to radicular pain (if the nerve root is involved) or non-radicular pain.

Degenerative changes in the lumbar spine (lumbar spondylosis) are commonly found in the older age group. This problem, and one of its complications, spinal canal stenosis, is steadily increasing along with the ageing population.

Serious disorders not to be missed

It is important to consider malignant disease, especially in an older person. It is also essential to consider infection such as acute osteomyelitis and tuberculosis, which is often encountered in recent immigrants, especially those from Asia. These conditions are considered in more detail under thoracic back pain. For pain or anaesthesia of sudden onset, especially when accompanied by neurological changes in the legs,

minor intervertebral disc disruption

E ← D ← C ← B ← A

Fig. 33.2 *Reflex activity from a MID in the intervertebral motion segment. Apart from the local effect caused by the disruption of the disc (A), interference can occur in the facet joint (B) and interspinous ligament (C) leading possibly to muscle spasm (D) and skin changes (E) via the posterior rami*   REPRODUCED FROM C. KENNA AND J. MURTAGH, *BACK PAIN AND SPINAL MANIPULATION*, BUTTERWORTHS, SYDNEY, 1989, WITH PERMISSION

consider cauda equina compression due to a massive disc prolapse and also retroperitoneal haemorrhage. It is important to ask patients if they are taking anticoagulants.

Pitfalls

The inflammatory disorders must be kept in mind, especially the spondyloarthropathies, which include psoriatic arthropathy, ankylosing spondylitis, Reiter's disease, inflammatory bowel

Table 33.3   *'Red flag' pointers to serious low back pain conditions*[5]

Age > 50 years
History of cancer
Temperature > 37.8°C
Constant pain—day and night
Weight loss
Significant trauma
Features of spondyloarthropathy
Neurological deficit
Drug or alcohol abuse
Use of anticoagulants
Use of corticosteroids
No improvement over 1 month
Possible cauda-equina syndrome
 • saddle anaesthesia
 • recent onset bladder dysfunction
 • severe or progressive neurological deficit

disorders such as ulcerative colitis and Crohn's disease, and reactive arthritis. The spondyloarthropathies are more common than appreciated and must be considered in the younger person presenting with features of inflammatory back pain, i.e. pain at rest, relieved by activity. The old trap of confusing claudication in the buttocks and legs, due to a high arterial obstruction, with sciatica must be avoided.

General pitfalls

• Being unaware of the characteristic symptoms of inflammation and thus misdiagnosing one of the spondyloarthropathies
• Overlooking the early development of malignant disease or osteomyelitis; if suspected, and an X-ray is normal, a radionuclide scan should detect the problem
• Failing to realise that mechanical dysfunction and osteoarthritis can develop simultaneously, producing a combined pattern
• Overlooking anticoagulants as a cause of a severe bleed around the nerve roots and corticosteroids leading to osteoporosis
• Not recognising back pain as a presenting feature of the drug addict.

'Red flag' pointers

There are several so called 'red flag' or precautionary pointers to a serious underlying cause of back pain. Such symptoms and signs should alert the practitioner to a serious health problem and thus guide selection of investigations, particularly plain films of the lumbar spine.[5]

Seven masquerades checklist

Of these conditions, depression and urinary tract infection have to be seriously considered. For the young woman with upper lumbar pain, especially if she is pregnant, the possibility of a urinary tract infection must be considered. These patients may not have urinary symptoms such as dysuria and frequency.

Depressive illness has to be considered in any patient with a chronic pain complaint. This common psychiatric disorder can continue to aggravate or maintain the pain even though the provoking problem has disappeared. This is more likely to occur in people who have become anxious about their problem or who are under excessive stress. Many doctors treat such patients with a therapeutic trial of antidepressant medication, for example, amitriptyline or doxepin.

Psychogenic considerations

The patient may be unduly stressed, not coping with life or malingering. It may be necessary to probe beneath the surface of the presenting problem.

A patient with low back pain following lifting at work poses a problem that causes considerable anguish to doctors, especially when the pain becomes chronic and complex. Chronic pain may be the last straw for patients who have been struggling to cope with personal problems; their fragile equilibrium is upset by the back pain. Many patients who have been dismissed as malingerers turn out to have a genuine problem. The importance of a caring, competent practitioner with an insight into all facets of his or her patient's suffering, organic and functional, becomes obvious. The tests for non-organic back pain are very useful in this context.

Nature of the pain

The nature of the pain may reveal its likely origin. Establish where the pain is worst— whether it is central (proximal) or peripheral. The following are general characteristics and guides to diagnosis:

- aching throbbing pain = inflammation, e.g. sacroiliitis
- deep aching diffuse pain = referred pain, e.g. dysmenorrhoea
- superficial steady diffuse pain = local pain, e.g. muscular strain
- boring deep pain = bone disease, e.g. neoplasia, Paget's disease

- intense sharp or stabbing (superimposed on a dull ache) = radicular pain, e.g. sciatica

A comparison of the significant features of the two most common types of pain—mechanical and inflammatory—is presented in Table 33.4.

The clinical approach

History

Analysing the history invariably guides the clinician to the diagnosis. The pain patterns have to be carefully evaluated and it is helpful to map the diurnal variations of pain to facilitate the diagnosis (Fig. 33.3).

It is especially important to note the intensity of the pain and its relation to rest and activity. In particular, ask whether the pain is present during the night, whether it wakes the patient, is present on rising or whether it is associated with stiffness.

Continuous pain present day and night is suggestive of neoplasia or infection. Pain on waking also suggests inflammation or depressive illness. Pain provoked by activity and relieved by rest suggests mechanical dysfunction while pain worse at rest and relieved by moderate activity is typical of inflammation. In some patients the coexistence of mechanical and inflammatory causes complicates the pattern.

Pain aggravated by standing or walking that is relieved by sitting is suggestive of spondylolisthesis. Pain aggravated by sitting (usually) and improved with standing indicates a discogenic problem.

Pain of the calf that travels proximally with walking indicates vascular claudication; pain in the buttock that descends with walking indicates neurogenic claudication. This latter problem is

Table 33.4 *Comparison of the patterns of pain for inflammatory and mechanical causes of low back pain*[6]

Feature	Inflammation	Mechanical
History	Insidious onset	Preciptating injury/previous episodes
Nature	Aching, throbbing	Deep dull ache, sharp if root compression
Stiffness	Severe, prolonged Morning stiffness	Moderate, transient
Effect of rest	Exacerbates	Relieves
Effect of activity	Relieves	Exacerbates
Radiation	More localised, bilateral or alternating	Tends to be diffuse, unilateral
Intensity	Night, early morning	End of day, following activity

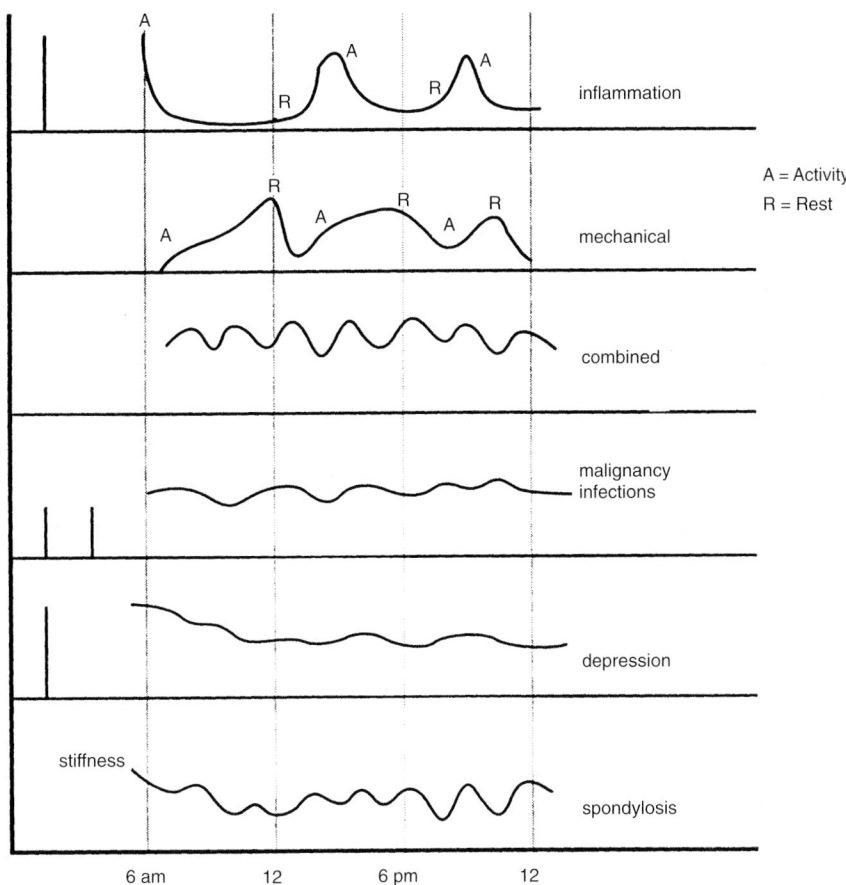

Fig. 33.3 *Typical daily patterns of pain for conditions causing back pain. Note conditions that can wake patients from sleep and also the combined mechanical and inflammatory patterns*

encountered more frequently in older people who have a tendency to spinal canal stenosis associated with spondylosis.

Key questions

- What is your general health like?
- Can you describe the nature of your back pain?
- Was your pain brought on by an injury?
- Is it worse when you wake in the morning or later in the day?
- How do you sleep during the night?
- What effect does rest have on the pain?
- What effect does activity have on the pain?
- Is the pain worse when sitting or standing?
- What effect does coughing or sneezing or straining at the toilet have?
- What happens to the pain in your back or leg if you go for a long walk?
- Do you have a history of psoriasis, diarrhoea, penile discharge, eye trouble or severe pain in your joints?
- Do you have any urinary symptoms?
- What medication are you taking? Are you on anticoagulants?
- Are you under any extra stress at work or home?
- Do you feel tense or depressed or irritable?

Physical examination

The basic objectives of the physical examination are to reproduce the patient's symptoms, detect the level of the lesion and determine the cause (if possible) by provocation of the affected joints or tissues. This is done using the time-honoured method of joint examination—look, feel, move and test function. The patient should be stripped to a minimum of clothing so that careful examination of the back can be made. A neurological examination of the lower limb should be performed if symptoms extend below the buttocks.

A useful screening test for a disc lesion and dural tethering is the slump test.[6]

The main components of the physical examination are:

1. Inspection
2. Active movements
   • forward flexion
   • extension   } to reproduce the patient's
   • lateral flexion (R & L) } symptoms
3. Provocative tests
4. Palpation (to detect level of pain)
5. Neurological testing of lower limbs (if appropriate)
6. Testing of related joints (hip, sacroiliac)
7. Assessment of pelvis and lower limbs for any deformity, e.g. leg shortening
8. General medical examination including rectal examination

Important landmarks

The surface anatomy of the lumbar region is the basis for determining the vertebral level. Key anatomical landmarks include the iliac crest, spinous processes, the sacrum and the posterior superior iliac spines (PSISs).

• The tops of the iliac crest lie at the level of the L4–L5 interspace (or the L4 spinous process).
• The PSISs lie opposite S2 (Fig. 33.4).

line projected from tops of iliac crests usually bisects L4–L5 interspace

posterior–superior iliac spine

sacral hiatus

coccyx

Fig. 33.4 *Surface anatomy and important landmarks of the lumbosacral spine*

Inspection

Inspection begins from the moment the patient is sighted in the waiting room. A patient who is noted to be standing is likely to have a significant disc lesion. Considerable information can be obtained from the manner in which the patient arises from a chair, moves to the consulting room, removes the shoes and clothes, gets onto the examination couch and moves when unaware of being watched.

The spine must be adequately exposed and inspected in good light. Patients should undress to their underpants; women may retain their brassiere and it is proper to provide them with a gown that opens down the back. Note the general contour and symmetry of the back and legs, including the buttock folds, and look for muscle wasting. Note the lumbar lordosis and any abnormalities such as lateral deviation. If lateral deviation (scoliosis) is present it is usually away from the painful side.

Note the presence of midline moles, tufts of hair or haemangioma that might indicate an underlying congenital anomaly such as spina bifida occulta.

Movements of the lumbar spine

There are three main movements of the lumbar spine. As there is minimal rotation, which mainly occurs at the thoracic spine, rotation is not so important. The movements that should be tested, and their normal ranges are as follows:

• extension (20°–30°) (Fig. 33.5a)
• lateral flexion, left and right (30°) (Fig. 33.5b)
• flexion (75°–90°: average 80°) (Fig. 33.5a)

Measurement of the angle of movement can be made by using a line drawn between the sacrum and large prominence of the C7 spinous process.

Palpation

Have the patient relaxed, lying prone, with the head to one side and the arms by the sides. The levels of the spinous processes are identified by standing behind the patient and using your hands to identify L4 and L5 in relation to the top of the iliac crests. Mark the important reference points.

Palpation, which is performed with the tips of the thumbs opposed, can commence at the spinous process of L1 and then systematically proceed distally to L5 and then over the sacrum and coccyx. Include the interspinous spaces as well as the spinous processes. When the thumbs

(a)

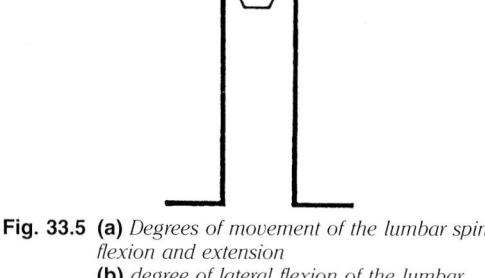

Extension

spinous process C7

20°–30° 80°

Flexion

sacrum

(b)

shoulder girdle

30° 30°

Fig. 33.5 **(a)** *Degrees of movement of the lumbar spine: flexion and extension*
(b) *degree of lateral flexion of the lumbar spine* REPRODUCED FROM C. KENNA AND J. MURTAGH, *BACK PAIN AND SPINAL MANIPULATION*, BUTTERWORTHS, SYDNEY, 1989, WITH PERMISSION

(or other part of the hand such as the pisiforms) are applied to the spinous processes, a firm pressure is transmitted to the vertebrae by a rocking movement for three or four 'springs'. Significant reproduction of pain is noted.

Palpation occurs at three main sites:
- centrally (spinous processes to coccyx)
- unilateral—right and left sides (1.5 cm from midline)
- transverse pressure to the sides of the spinous processes (R and L)

Provocation tests

Quadrant test
This test compresses the spinal joints, especially facet joints, on the painful side and can be used if active movements fail to reproduce the patient's pain. Stand behind the patient, place a hand on each shoulder and extend the lumbar spine to its limit. Ensuring the patient does not bend the knees, extend the spine to its limit, then laterally flex to the painful side, and then rotate to that side and apply some downwards pressure.

Slump test
The slump test is an excellent provocation test for lumbosacral pain and is more sensitive than the straight leg raising test. It is a screening test for a disc lesion and dural tethering. It should be performed on patients who have low back pain with pain extending into the leg, and especially for posterior thigh pain.

A positive result is reproduction of the patient's pain, and may appear at an early stage of the test (when it is ceased).

| *Method* |

1. The patient sits on the couch in a relaxed manner.
2. The patient then slumps forward (without excessive trunk flexion), and then places the chin on the chest.
3. The unaffected leg is straightened.
4. The affected leg only is then straightened (Fig. 33.6).
5. Both legs are straightened together.
6. The foot of the affected straightened leg is dorsiflexed.

Note: Take care to distinguish from hamstring pain. Deflexing the neck relieves the pain of spinal origin, not hamstring pain.

| *Significance of the slump test* |

- It is positive if the back or leg pain is reproduced.
- If positive, it suggests disc disruption.

Fig. 33.6 *The slump test: one of the stages*

- If negative, it may indicate lack of serious disc pathology.
- If positive, one should approach manual therapy with caution.

Neurological examination

A neurological examination is performed only when the patient's symptoms, such as pain, paraesthesia, anaesthesia and weakness, extend into the leg.

The importance of the neurological examination is to ensure that there is no compression of the spinal nerves from a prolapsed disc or from a tumour. This is normally tested by examining those functions that the respective spinal nerves serve, namely skin sensation, muscle power and reflex activity.

The examination is not daunting but can be performed quickly and efficiently in two to three minutes by a methodical technique that improves with continued use. The neurological examination consists of:

1. Quick tests
   — walking on heels (L5)
   — walking on toes (S1)
2. Dural stretch tests
   — slump test
   — straight leg raising (SLR)
3. Specific nerve root tests (L4, L5, S1)
   — sensation
   — power
   — reflexes

Main nerve roots

Refer to Figure 33.7.

L3: • femoral stretch test (prone, flex knee, extend hip)
  • motor—extension of knee
  • sensation—anterior thigh
  • reflex—knee jerk (L3, L4)

L4: • motor—resisted inversion foot
  • sensation—inner border of foot to great toe
  • reflex—knee jerk

L5: • motor—walking on heels
      —resisted extension great toe
  • sensation—middle three toes (dorsum)
  • reflex—nil

S1: • motor—walking on toes
      —resisted eversion foot
  • sensation—little toe, most of sole
  • reflex—ankle jerk (S1, S2)

Other examination

The method of examining the sacroiliac and hip joints is outlined in Chapter 59.

Investigations

Investigations for back pain can be classified into three broad groups: front-line screening tests; specific disease investigations; and procedural and preprocedural tests.

Screening tests

These are most important for the patient presenting with chronic back pain when serious disease such as malignancy, osteoporosis, infection or spondyloarthropathy must be excluded. The screening tests for chronic pain are:

- plain X-ray
- urine examination (office dipstick)
- erythrocyte sedimentation rate (ESR)
- serum alkaline phosphatase
- prostatic specific antigen (in males > 50)

Specific disease investigation

Such tests include:

- peripheral arterial studies
- HLA-B$_{27}$ antigen test for ankylosing spondylitis and Reiter's disease
- serum electrophoresis for multiple myeloma
- brucella agglutination test
- blood culture for pyogenic infection and bacterial endocarditis

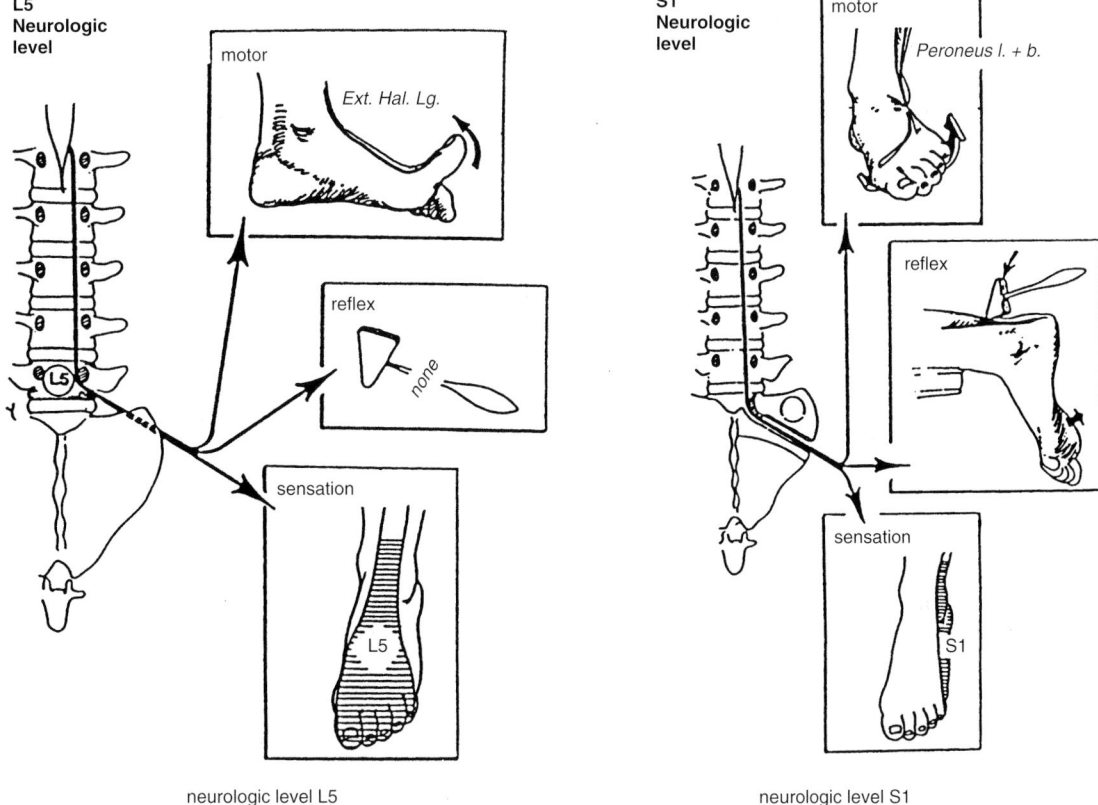

L5 Neurologic level

motor

Ext. Hal. Lg.

reflex

none

sensation

L5

neurologic level L5

S1 Neurologic level

motor

Peroneus l. + b.

reflex

sensation

S1

neurologic level S1

Fig. 33.7 *The main motor, sensory and reflex features of the nerve roots L5 and S1* REPRODUCED FROM S. HOPPENFELD, *PHYSICAL EXAMINATION OF THE SPINE AND EXTREMITIES*, APPLETON AND LANGE NORWALK, CT, USA, 1976, WITH PERMISSION

- bone scanning to demonstrate inflammatory or neoplastic disease and infections (e.g. osteomyelitis) before changes are apparent on plain X-ray
- tuberculosis studies
- X-rays of shoulder and hip joint
- electromyographic (EMG) studies to screen leg pain and differentiate neurological diseases from nerve compression syndromes
- radioisotope scanning
- technetium pyrophosphate scan of SIJ for ankylosing spondylitis
- selective anaesthetic block of facet joint under image intensification
- selective anaesthetic block of medial branches of posterior primary rami and other nerve roots

Procedural and preprocedural diagnostic tests

These tests should be kept in reserve for chronic disorders, especially mechanical disorders, that remain undiagnosed and unabated, and where surgical intervention is planned for a disc prolapse requiring removal.

Depending on availability and merit, such tests include:

- computerised tomography (CT scan)
- myelography or radiculography
- discography
- magnetic resonance imaging (MRI)

Summary of diagnostic guidelines for spinal pain

- Continuous pain (day and night) = neoplasia, especially malignancy or infection.
- The big primary malignancy is multiple myeloma.
- The big three metastases are from lung, breast and prostate.
- The other three metastases are from thyroid, kidney/adrenal and melanoma.
- Pain with standing/walking (relief with sitting) = spondylolisthesis.
- Pain (and stiffness) at rest, relief with activity = inflammation.

- In a young person with inflammation think of ankylosing spondylitis or Reiter's disease.
- Stiffness at rest, pain with or after activity, relief with rest = osteoarthritis.
- Pain provoked by activity, relief with rest = mechanical dysfunction.
- Pain in bed at early morning = inflammation, depression or malignancy/infection.
- Pain in periphery of limb
  = discogenic → radicular
  or vascular → claudication
  or spinal canal stenosis → claudication.
- Pain in calf (ascending) with walking = vascular claudication.
- Pain in buttock (descending) with walking = neurogenic claudication.
- One disc lesion = one nerve root (exception is L5–S1 disc).
- One nerve root = one disc (usually).
- Two or more nerve roots—consider neoplasm.
- The rule of thumb for the lumbar nerve root lesions is L3 from L2–L3 disc, L4 from L3–L4, L5 from L4–L5 and S1 from L5–S1.
- A large disc protrusion can cause bladder symptoms, either incontinence or retention.
- A retroperitoneal bleed from anticoagulation therapy can give intense nerve root symptoms and signs.

Back pain in children

The common mechanical disorders of the intervertebral joints can cause back pain in children, which must always be taken seriously. Like abdominal pain and leg pain, it can be related to psychogenic factors, so this possibility should be considered by diplomatically evaluating problems at home, at school or with sport.

Especially in children under the age of 10, it is very important to exclude organic disease. Infections such as osteomyelitis and tuberculosis are rare possibilities, and 'discitis' has to be considered. This painful condition can be idiopathic, but can also be caused by the spread of infection from a vertebral body. It has characteristic radiological changes.

Tumours causing back pain include the benign osteoid osteoma and the malignant osteogenic sarcoma. Osteoid osteoma is a very small tumour with a radiolucent nucleus that is sharply demarcated from the surrounding area of sclerotic bone. Although more common in the long bones of the leg, it can occur in the spine.

In older children and adolescents the organic causes of back pain are more likely to be inflammatory, congenital or from developmental anomalies and trauma.

A prolapsed intervertebral disc, which can occur (uncommonly) in adolescents, can be very unusual in its presentation. There is often marked spasm, with a stiff spine and lateral deviation, which may be out of proportion to the relatively lower degree of pain.

Spondylolisthesis can occur in older children, usually due to a slip of L5 or S1, because the articular facets are congenitally absent or because of a stress fracture in the pars interarticularis. It is necessary to request standing lateral and oblique X-rays.

Back pain in the elderly

Traumatic spinal dysfunction is still the most common cause of back pain in the elderly and may represent a recurrence of earlier dysfunction. It is amazing how commonly disc prolapse and facet joint injury can present in the aged. However, degenerative joint disease is very common and, if advanced, can present as spinal stenosis with claudication and nerve root irritation due to narrowed intervertebral foraminae.

Special problems to consider are malignant disease, degenerative spondylolisthesis, vertebral pathological fractures and occlusive vascular disease.

Acute back and leg pain due to vertebral dysfunction

Mechanical disruption of the vertebral segment or segments is the outstanding cause to consider, while the main serious clinical syndromes are secondary to disruption with or without prolapse of the intervertebral disc, usually L4–L5 or L5–S1.

Table 33.5 presents the general clinical features and diagnosis in acute back pain (fractures excluded) following vertebral dysfunction: the symptoms and signs can occur singly or in combination.

Fortunately, syndromes A and B are extremely rare but, if encountered, urgent referral to a surgeon is mandatory. Clinical features of the cauda equina syndrome are presented in Figure 33.8. Syndrome B can follow a bleed in patients taking anticoagulant therapy or be caused by a

Table 33.5 *Clinical features and diagnosis of vertebral dysfunction leading to low back and leg pain*[6]

Clinical features	Frequency	Diagnosis
Syndrome A (surgical emergency)	Very rare	Spinal cord (UMN) or cauda equina (LMN) compression
Saddle anaesthesia (around anus, scrotum or vagina) Distal anaesthesia Evidence of UMN or LMN lesion Loss of sphincter control or urinary retention Weakness of legs peripherally		
Syndrome B (probable surgical emergency)	Uncommon	Large disc protrusion, paralysing nerve root
Anaesthesia or paraesthesia of the leg Foot drop Motor weakness Absence of reflexes		
Syndrome C	Common	Posterolateral disc protrusion on nerve root or disc disruption
Distal pain with or without paraesthesia Radicular pain (sciatica) Positive dural stretch tests		
Syndrome D	Very common	Disc disruption or facet dysfunction
Lumbar pain (unilateral, central or bilateral) ± buttock and posterior thigh pain		

disc sequestration after inappropriate spinal manipulation.

Vertebral dysfunction with non-radicular pain

This outstanding common cause of low back pain is considered to be due mainly to dysfunction of the pain-sensitive facet joint. The precise pathophysiology is difficult to pinpoint but invariably is dysfunction of one of the spinal joints, most likely a facet joint of the MID as proposed by Maigne.

Typical profile[6]

Age: • Any age—late teens to old age, usually 22–55

History of injury: • Yes, lifting or twisting

Site and radiation: • Unilateral lumbar (may be central)
• Refers over sacrum, SIJ areas, buttocks

Type of pain: • Deep aching pain, episodic

Aggravation: • Activity, lifting, gardening, housework (vacuuming, making beds, etc.)

Relief: • Rest, warmth

Associations: • May be stiffness, usually good health

Physical examination (significant): • Localised tenderness—unilateral or central L4,L5 or S1 levels, may be restricted flexion, extension, lateral flexion

Diagnosis confirmation: • Investigation usually normal
Note: diagnosis made clinically

Management

• complete rest for 2 days (for acute pain only); otherwise, activity directed by degree of pain but normal activity encouraged from outset
• back education program
• analgesics
• exercise program and swimming (as tolerated)
• physical therapy—mobilisation, manipulation (for persistent problems) Refer to pages 1211–1212.

Radiculopathy

Radicular pain, caused by nerve root compression from a disc protrusion (most common cause) or tumour or a narrowed intervertebral

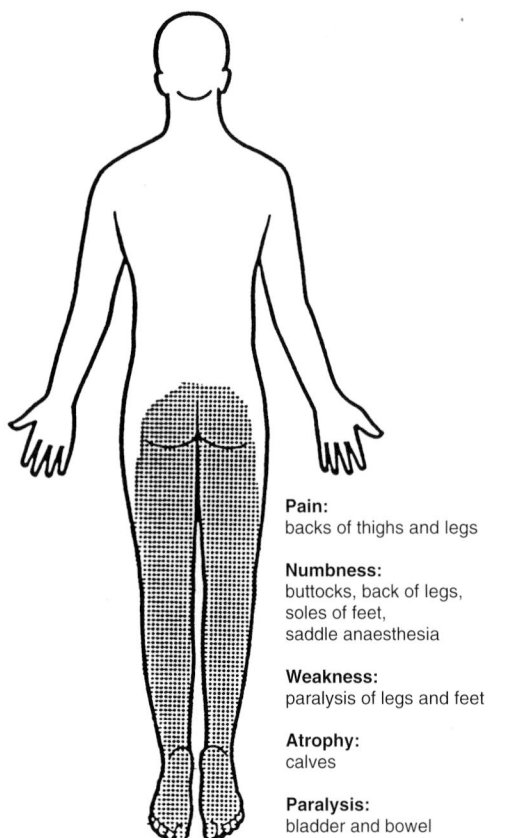

Pain:
backs of thighs and legs

Numbness:
buttocks, back of legs,
soles of feet,
saddle anaesthesia

Weakness:
paralysis of legs and feet

Atrophy:
calves

Paralysis:
bladder and bowel
urinary retention

Fig. 33.8 *Cauda equina syndrome due to massive prolapsed intervertebral disc*

foramina, typically produces pain in the leg related to the dermatome and myotome innervated by that nerve root. Leg pain may occur alone without back pain and vary considerably in intensity.

Typical profile of radicular pain (discogenic)

Age:	• Any age, usually middle-aged
History of injury:	• Yes, lifting or twisting • Can be spontaneous
Site and radiation:	• Unilateral low back, distal radiation along dermatome, tends to have a 'distal' emphasis
Type of pain:	• Deep aching or stabbing pain (episodic) develops soon after rising in morning • Has a 'travelling' nature

Aggravation:	• Activity, lifting, intercourse, sitting, bending, car travel, coughing, sneezing, straining
Relief:	• Rest, lying, standing
Associations:	• Distal paraesthesia ± numbness, stiffness
Physical examination (significant):	• Guarded and restricted movement • Loss of lumbar lordosis • Lateral deviation (scoliosis) • Restricted flexion, extension, lateral flexion

typically unilateral {	• SLR and slump test positive
	  ± specific muscle/myotomal weakness
	  ± reduced distal sensation
	  ± reduced ankle jerk (S1)

Diagnostic confirmation (for special reasons):	• CT scan, discogram, radiculogram, MRI or myelogram

The two nerve roots that account for most of these problems are L5 and S1. Most settle with time (6 to 12 weeks). The management is outlined at the end of this chapter and under 'Sciatica' (Chapter 60).

Spondylolisthesis

About 5% of the population have spondylolisthesis but not all are symptomatic. The pain is caused by extreme stretching of the interspinous ligaments or of the nerve roots. The onset of back pain in many of these patients is due to concurrent disc degeneration rather than a mechanical problem.

Typical profile[6]

Age:	• Any age; young adult if congenital, older person (over 50) if degenerative
History of injury:	• May precipitate problem
Site and radiation:	• Low lumbar • Radiates bilaterally or unilaterally into buttocks, hip, thighs and feet
Type of pain:	• Dull ache, episodic depending on activity
Onset:	• Onset usually midmorning after standing

Aggravation:	• Prolonged standing, walking, exercise
Relief:	• Sitting down, lying down
Associations:	• Paraesthesia in legs
	• Stiffness after exercise
	• May be associated discogenic lesion
Physical examination (significant):	• Stiff waddling gait
	• Increased lumbar lordosis
	• Flexed knee stance
	• Tender prominent spinous process of 'slipped' vertebrae
	• Limited flexion
	• Hamstring tightness or spasm
Diagnosis confirmation:	• Lateral X-ray (standing) (Fig. 33.9).

Management

It is amazing how this instability problem can be alleviated with excellent relief of symptoms by getting patients to follow a strict flexion exercise program for at least 3 months. The objective is for patients to 'splint' their own spine by strengthening abdominal and spinal muscles.

Extension of the spine should be avoided, especially hyperextension. Gravity traction might help. Recourse to lumbar corsets or surgery (for spinal fusion) should be resisted although it is appropriate in a few severe intractable cases.

stress fracture of the pars interarticularis

Fig. 33.9 *Spondylolisthesis: illustrating a forward shift of one vertebra on another*

Lumbar spondylosis

Lumbar spondylosis, also known as degenerative osteoarthritis or osteoarthrosis, is a common problem of wear and tear that may follow vertebral dysfunction, especially after severe disc disruption and degeneration.

Typical profile[6]

Age:	• Over 50 years
	• More common with increasing age
History of injury:	• Heavy manual work, trauma to spine, e.g. motor vehicle accident
Site and radiation:	• Low back pain
	• May radiate to buttocks
Type of pain:	• Dull nagging ache (often constant)
	• Acute episodes on chronic background
Aggravation:	• Heavy activity, bending
	• Limited tolerance of standing and sitting
Relief:	• Resting by lying straight, gentle exercise, hydrotherapy
Associations:	• Stiffness, especially in mornings
	• Stiffness with immobility
	• Generally good health
Physical examination	• All movements restricted
Diagnosis confirmation:	• X-ray

Stiffness of the low back is the main feature of lumbar spondylosis. Although most people live with and cope with the problem, progressive deterioration can occur leading to subluxation of the facet joints. Subsequent narrowing of the spinal and intervertebral foramen leads to spinal canal stenosis (Fig. 33.10).

Management

• basic analgesics (depending on patient response and tolerance)
• NSAIDs (judicious use)
• appropriate balance between light activity and rest
• exercise program and hydrotherapy (if available)

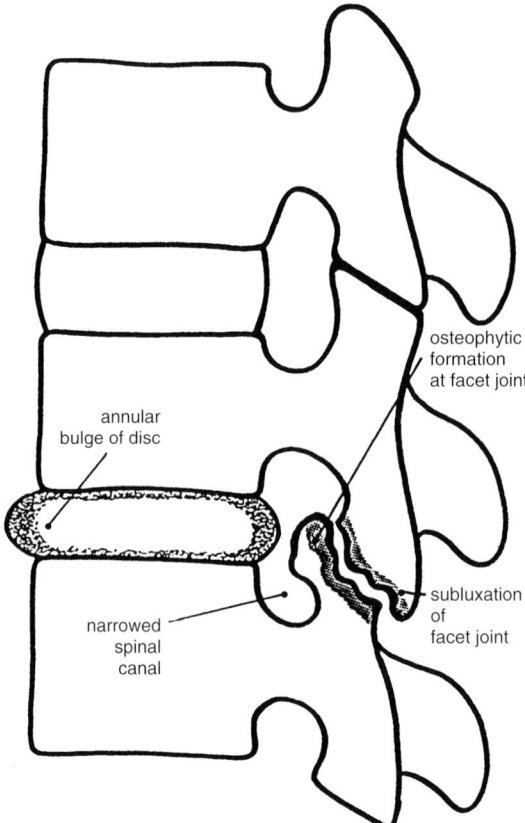

osteophytic formation at facet joint

annular bulge of disc

narrowed spinal canal

subluxation of facet joint

Fig. 33.10 *Lumbar spondylosis with degeneration of the disc and facet joint, leading to narrowing of the spinal canal and intervertebral foramen*

- regular mobilisation therapy may help
- consider trials of electrotherapy such as TENS and acupuncture

The spondyloarthropathies

The seronegative spondyloarthropathies are a group of disorders characterised by involvement of the sacroiliac joints with an ascending spondylitis and extraspinal manifestations such as oligoarthritis and enthesopathies (Figs. 33.11a, b, c) (refer Chapter 31). The pain and stiffness that are the characteristic findings of spinal involvement are typical of inflammatory disease; namely, worse in the morning, may occur at night and improves rather than worsens with exercise.

The main disorders in this group are ankylosing spondylitis, psoriatic arthritis, Reiter's disease, reactive spondyloarthropathies and the inflammatory bowel disorders. Hence the importance of searching for a history of psoriasis, diarrhoea, urethral discharge, eye disorders and episodes of arthritis in other joints. The following profile for ankylosing spondylitis serves as a typical clinical presentation of back pain for this group.

Typical profile of ankylosing spondylitis[6]

Age and sex:	• Young men 15–30 (rare onset after 40)
History of injury:	• None, unless coincidental
	• Has a slow insidious onset
Site and radiation:	• Low back, may radiate to both buttocks or posterior thigh (rare below knees)
	• Can alternate sides
Type of pain:	• Aching, throbbing pain of inflammation
	• Commonly episodic
Aggravation:	• Often worse at night (can wake patient), turning over in bed and rising in the morning
Relief:	• Activity including exercise
	• Patient may walk around during night for relief
Associations:	• Back stiffness, especially in morning
	• Pain and stiffness in thoracic or cervical spine
	• Pain and stiffness in thoracic cage
	• Peripheral joint pain (up to 50% of cases)
	• Iritis (up to 25% of cases)
Physical examination (significant):	• Absent lumbar lordosis
	• Lateral flexion limited first, then flexion and extension
	• Positive sacroiliac joint stress tests
	• Positive Schober's test
Diagnosis confirmation:	• X-ray of pelvis (sacroiliitis)
	• Bone scans and CT scans
	• ESR usually elevated
	• HLA-B$_{27}$ antigen positive in over 90% of cases (10% of population are positive)

Schober's test

This test is a useful objective means of measuring the mobility of the lumbar spine and is useful to

Fig. 33.11 **(a)** *Ankylosing spondylitis and psoriasis: main target areas on vertebral column and girdle joints*
(b) *Crohn's disease and ulcerative colitis: main target areas of enteropathies*
(c) *Reiter's disease: main target areas*

detect the spondyloarthropathies in younger patients.

Modified method
- Stand the patient erect and mark the spine in line with the dimples of Venus (the posterior superior iliac spines).
- Place another mark 10 cm above the first and a third mark 5 cm below the first mark.
- Ask the patient to bend forward, as if to touch the toes, to the point of maximal flexion.
- Finally, measure the distance between the upper and lower marks.

Interpretation
- Normal is > 5 cm increase in length.
- Less than 5 cm represents hypomobility, common in the inflammatory spinal disorders, severe spondylosis and intervertebral disc disorders.

Treatment
The earlier the treatment the better the outlook for the patient; the prognosis is usually good. The basic objectives of treatment are:

- prevention of spinal fusion in a poor position
- relief of pain and stiffness
- maintenance of optimum spinal mobility

The basic methods of management are:
- advice on good back care and posture
- general education and counselling
- exercise programs to improve the range of movement and maintain mobility
- referral to physiotherapist
- drug therapy, especially tolerated NSAIDs, preferably indomethacin in optimal dosage
- sulphasalazine—a useful second-line agent if the disease progresses despite NSAIDs

Malignant disease
It is important to identify malignant disease and other space-occupying lesions as early as possible because of the prognosis and the effect of a delayed diagnosis on treatment.

Typical profile[6]
Age: • Usually over 50, but the older the patient the greater the risk

History of injury:	• Usually insidious onset
Site and radiation:	• Localised pain anywhere in lumbar spine
	• Radiates into buttocks or legs (if nerve root involved)
Type of pain:	• Boring deep ache, can be referred or radicular, unrelenting continuous pain, getting worse
Aggravation:	• Movement
	• Specific activities such as lifting, gardening
Relief:	• Usually none
	• No response to treatment
Associations:	• Malaise, fatigue, weight loss
	• Muscular weakness
	• Night pain
Physical examination (significant):	• Flattened lumbar lordosis
	• Localised tenderness over vertebrae
	• All movements restricted and protective (if advanced)
	• Neurologically normal unless roots involved
	• More than one root may be involved
	• Major neurological signs incompatible with pain level
Diagnosis confirmation:	• X-ray
	• Serum alkaline phosphatase
	• ESR
	• Bone scan

With respect to the neurological features, more than one nerve root may be involved and major neurological signs may be present without severe root pain. The neurological signs will be progressive.

If malignant disease is proved and myeloma is excluded a search should be made for the six primary malignancies that metastasise to the spine (Fig. 33.12). If the bone is sclerotic consider prostatic secondaries, some breast secondaries or Paget's disease.

Non-organic back pain

Like headache, back pain is a symptom of an underlying functional, organic or psychological disorder.[5] Preoccupation with organic causation of symptoms may lead to serious errors in the assessment of patients with back pain. Any vulnerable aching area of the body is subject to aggravation by emotional factors.

Depressed patients are generally less demonstrative than patients with extreme anxiety and conversion disorders and malingerers, and it is easier to overlook the non-organic basis for their problem.

Typical profile[6]

Age:	• Any age, typical 30–50
History of injury:	• Yes—usually remote in the past; often motor vehicle accident
Site and radiation:	• Low back, central, often bilateral
	• May radiate to leg (may be bizarre pattern)
Type of pain:	• Variable, usually deep ache or burning
	• Continuous—acute or chronic
Aggravation:	• Work, especially housework, or manual work
	• Worse in mornings on waking
	• Stress and worry
Relief:	• Better in the evenings and on retiring
Associations:	• Headache
	• Fatigue, exhaustion, tiredness
	• Insomnia, inability to cope
	• Other aches and pains
Physical examination:	• Diffuse tenderness to palpation
	• Possible hyperactive reflexes

This profile is typical of the depressed patient with back pain. A trial of antidepressants for a minimum of 3 weeks is recommended and quite often a positive response with relief of backache eventuates.

Failure to consider psychological factors in the assessment of low back pain may lead to serious

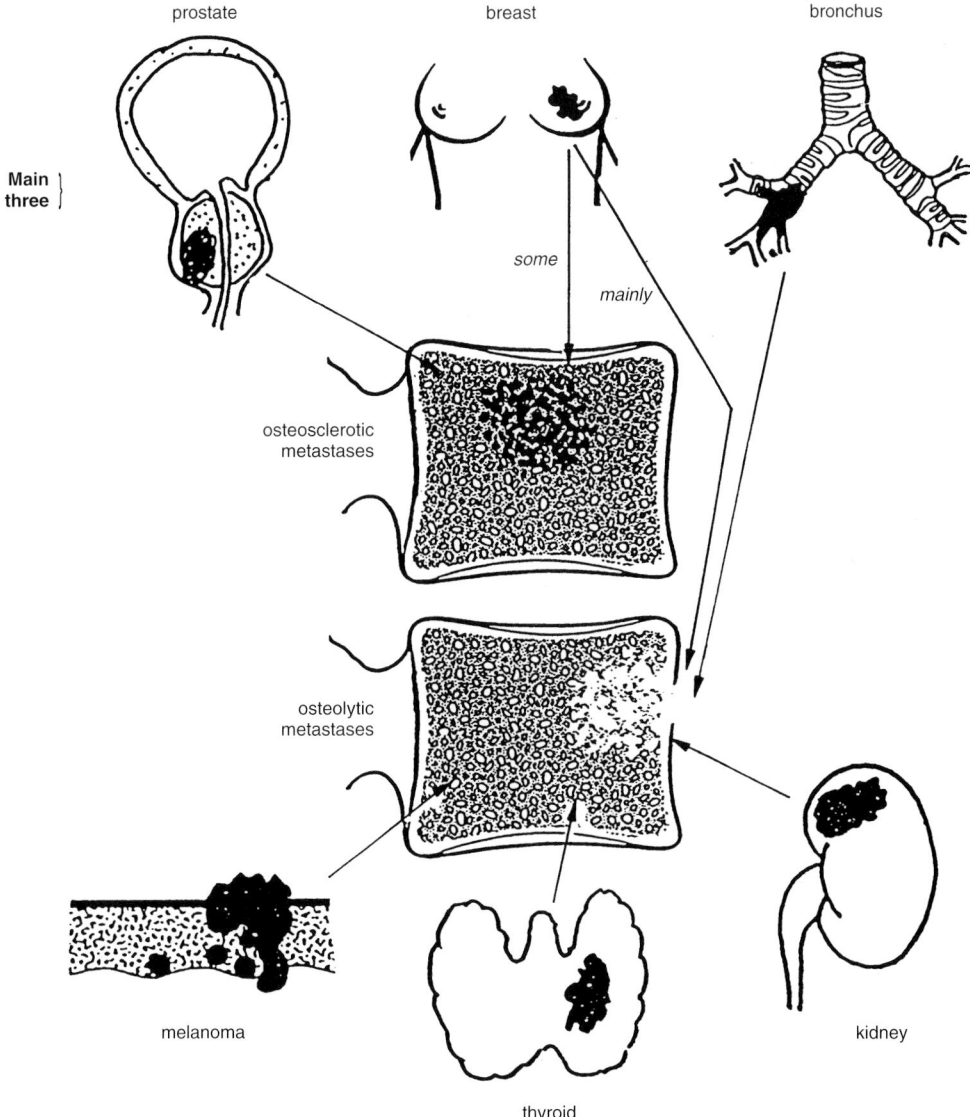

prostate

breast

bronchus

Main three }

some

mainly

osteosclerotic metastases

osteolytic metastases

melanoma

kidney

thyroid

Fig. 33.12 *Important primary malignancies metastasing to the spine. Note the difference between sclerotic and osteolytic metastases; multiple myeloma also causes osteoporotic lesions*

errors in diagnosis and management. Each instance of back pain poses a stimulating exercise in differential diagnosis. A comparison of organic and non-organic features is presented in Table 33.6.

Assessment of the pain demands a full understanding of the patient. One must be aware of his or her type of work, recreation, successes and failures; and one must relate this information to the degree of incapacity attributed to the back pain.

Patients with psychogenic back pain, especially the very anxious, tend to overemphasise their problem. They are usually demonstrative, the hands being used to point out various painful areas almost without prompting. There is diffuse tenderness even to the slightest touch and the physical disability is out of proportion to the alleged symptoms. The pain distribution is often atypical of any dermatome and the reflexes are almost always hyperactive. It must be remembered that patients with psychogenic back

Table 33.6 *Comparison of general clinical features of organic and non-organic based low back pain*[6,7]

	Organic disorders	Non-organic disorders
Symptoms		
Presentation	Appropriate	Often dramatic
Pain	Localised	Bilateral/diffuse Sacrococcygeal
Pain radiation	Appropriate Buttock, specific sites	Inappropriate Front of leg/whole leg
Time pattern	Pain-free times	Constant, acute or chronic
Paraesthesia/anaesthesia	Dermatomal Points with finger	May be whole leg Shows with hands
Response to treatment	Variable Delayed benefit	Patient often refuses treatment
		Initial improvement (often dramatic) then deterioration (usually within 24 hours)
Signs		
Observation	Appropriate Guarded	Overreactive under scrutiny Inconsistent
Tenderness	Localised to appropriate level	Often inappropriate level Withdraws from probing finger
Spatial tenderness (Magnuson)	Consistent	Inconsistent
Active movements	Specific movements affected	Often all movements affected
Axial loading test	No back pain (usually)	Back pain
SLR 'distraction' test	Consistent	Inconsistent
Sensation	Dermatomal	Non-anatomical 'sock' or 'stocking'
Motor	Appropriate myotome	Muscle groups, e.g. leg 'collapses'
Reflexes	Appropriate May be depressed	Brisk hyperactive

pain—for example, depression and conversion disorders—do certainly experience back pain and do not fall for the traps set for the malingerer.

Tests for non-organic back pain

Several tests are useful in differentiating between organic and non-organic back pain (e.g. that caused by depression or complained of by a known malingerer).

Magnuson's method (the 'migratory pointing' test)

1. Request the patient to point to the painful sites.
2. Palpate these areas of tenderness on two occasions separated by an interval of several minutes, and compare the sites.

Between the two tests divert the patient's attention from his or her back by another examination.

Paradoxical straight leg raising test

Perform the usual straight leg raising test. The patient might manage a limited elevation, for example 30°. Keep the degree in mind. Ask the patient to sit up and swing the leg over the end of the couch. Distract attention with another test or some question, and then attempt to lift the straight leg to the same level achieved on the first occasion. If it is possible, then the patient's response is inconsistent.

Burn's 'kneeling on a stool' test

1. Ask the patient to kneel on a low stool, lean over and try to touch the floor.
2. The person with non-organic back pain will usually refuse on the grounds that it would cause great pain or that he or she might overbalance in the attempt.

Patients with even a severely herniated disc usually manage the task to some degree.

The axial loading test

1. Place your hands over the patient's head and press firmly downward (Fig. 33.13).
2. This will cause no discomfort to (most) patients with organic back pain.

Treatment options for back pain

General aspects of management

Relative rest

For acutely painful back problems 2 days strict rest lying on a firm surface is optimal treatment.[8] Resting for longer than 3 days does not produce any significant healing.

Patient education

Appropriate educational material leads to a clear insight into the causes and aggravation of the back disorder plus coping strategies.

Exercises

An early graduated exercise program as soon as the attack phase settles has been shown to promote healing and prevent relapses.[9] All forms of exercise (extension, flexion and isometric) appear to be equally effective with extension exercises being favoured for a discogenic problem and flexion exercises for most dysfunctional problems (see Figs 33.14a, b). Swimming is an excellent exercise for back disorders.

(a)

(b)

Fig. 33.14 *Examples of exercises for low back pain:* **(a)** *rotation exercise;* **(b)** *flexion exercise*

Pharmacological agents

Basic analgesics

Analgesics such as aspirin, paracetamol and codeine plus paracetomol (acetaminophen) should be used for pain relief.

NSAIDs

These are useful where there is clinical evidence of inflammation, especially with the spondyloarthropathies, severe spondylosis and in acute radicular pain, to counter the irritation on the nerve root. NSAIDs should not be used for mechanical dysfunction.

Antiepileptic drugs

These have been helpful in controlling acute radicular pain subject to repetitive bursts of lightning-like pains. Examples include carbamazepine and clonazepam.

Antidepressants

These have been used with success in the treatment of chronic back pain (especially without demonstrable pathology) and in patients with depression and associated back pain.

Fig. 33.13 *The axial loading test*

Injection techniques

Trigger point injection. This may be effective for relatively isolated points using 5–8 mL of local anaesthetic.

Chymopapain. This enzyme has been advocated for the treatment of acute nuclear herniation that

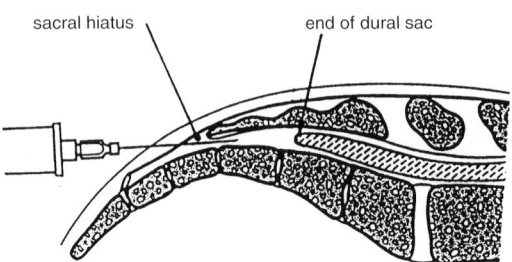

Fig. 33.15 *Caudal epidural injection: the needle should lie free in the space and be well clear of the dural sac*

is still intact. The indications are similar for surgical discectomy. However, its use is controversial.

Facet joint injection. Corticosteroid injection under radio image intensification is widely used in some clinics. The procedure is delicate and expertise is required. Some good results are obtained.

Epidural injections. Injections of local anaesthetic with or without corticosteroids are used, especially for nerve root pain. The author favours the caudal (trans-sacral) epidural injection for persistent sciatica using 15 mL of half-strength local anaesthetic only, e.g. 0.25% bupivacaine (Fig. 33.15).

Physical therapy

Active exercises are the best form of physical therapy (Fig. 33.14a, b).

Spinal mobilisation is a gentle, repetitive, rhythmic movement within the range of movement of the joint. It is safe and quite effective (Fig. 33.16).

Spinal manipulation is a high velocity thrust at the end range of the joint. It is generally more effective and produces a faster response but requires accurate diagnosis and greater skill. It is extremely effective for uncomplicated persistent dysfunctional low back pain (without radicular pain) and, together with exercises, is the treatment of choice (Fig. 33.17).[10, 11, 12]

Fig. 33.16 *Lumbar spinal mobilisation (for left-sided pain): illustration of the effective forces involved* REPRODUCED FROM C. KENNA AND J. MURTAGH, *BACK PAIN AND SPINAL MANIPULATION*, BUTTERWORTHS, SYDNEY, 1989, WITH PERMISSION

Fig. 33.17 *Lumbar spinal manipulation: illustration of the specific technique for the L4–L5 level with arrows indicating the direction of applied force* REPRODUCED FROM C. KENNA AND J. MURTAGH, *BACK PAIN AND SPINAL MANIPULATION*, BUTTERWORTHS, SYDNEY, 1989, WITH PERMISSION

Other treatments

The following treatments have a significant role in the management of back pain, although clear-cut evidence for the efficacy of these modalities is still lacking.

- hydrotherapy
- traction
- transcutaneous electrical nerve stimulation (TENS)
- facet joint injection
- posterior nerve root (medial branch) blocks with or without denervation (by cryotherapy or radiofrequency)
- deep friction massage (in conjunction with mobilisation and manipulation)
- acupuncture
- pain clinic (if unresponsive to initial treatments)
- biofeedback
- gravitational methods (home therapy)

Management guidelines for lumbosacral disorders (summary)

The management of 'mechanical' back pain depends on the cause. Since most of the problems are mechanical and there is a tendency to natural resolution, conservative management is quite appropriate. The rule is: 'if patients with uncomplicated back pain receive no treatment, one-third will get better within 1 week and by 3 weeks almost all the rest of the other two-thirds are better'.[13] Practitioners should have a clear-cut management plan with a firm, precise, reassuring and conservative clinical approach.

The problems can be categorised into general conditions for which the summarised treatment protocols are outlined.

- Acute pain   = pain less than 2 weeks.
- Subacute pain   = 2–12 weeks.
- Chronic pain   = greater than 3 months.

Acute low back pain—no spasm

The common problem of low back pain caused by facet joint dysfunction and/or limited disc disruption usually responds well to the following treatment. The typical patient is aged 20–55 years, is well and has no radiation of pain below the knee.[14]

- back education program
- encouragement of normal daily activities according to degree of comfort

- regular non-opioid analgesics, e.g. paracetamol
- exercise program (when exercises do not aggravate), swimming (if feasible)
- physical therapy: stretching of affected segment, muscle energy therapy, spinal mobilisation or manipulation (if no contraindication on first visit)[10,12,14]
- review in about 5 days (probably best time for physical therapy)
- no investigation needed initially

Most of these patients can expect to be relatively pain free in 14 days and can return to work early (some may not miss work and this should be encouraged). The evidence concerning spinal manipulation is that it reduces the period of disability.

Note: NSAIDs are not usually recommended. They can be used for 10–14 days if evidence of inflammation.

Acute low back pain (only) with spasm

- back education program
- strict rest lying on a firm surface for 2 days[8] (keep the spine as straight as possible)
- regular simple analgesics with review as the patient mobilises
- cold or hot compresses to the painful area
- simple mobilisation exercises as tolerated
- muscle energy therapy
- consider trigger point injection of local anaesthetic
- relaxant, e.g. diazepam (if appropriate) for 4–5 days
- review in 3–5 days

When the acute phase settles, treat as for uncomplicated low back pain.

Sciatica with or without low back pain

Sciatica is a more complex and protracted problem to treat, but most cases will gradually settle within 12 weeks.

Acute

- strict bed rest for 2–3 days (keep the spine straight—avoid sitting in soft chairs and for long periods)
- regular non-opioid analgesics with review as the patient mobilises
- NSAIDs for 10–14 days, then cease and review
- back education program
- resume normal activities as soon as possible

- exercises—straight leg raising exercises to pain tolerance
- swimming
- traction (a trial of intermittent traction is worthwhile)
- weekly or 2 weekly follow up

Chronic
- continue physiotherapy with possible traction
- reassurance that problem will subside (assuming no severe neurological defects)
- consider epidural anaesthesia (if slow response)

General guidelines for surgical intervention
- bladder/bowel disturbance
- progressive motor disturbance, e.g. significant foot drop, weakness in quadriceps
- severe prolonged pain
- failure of conservative treatment with persistent pain (problem of permanent nerve damage)

Note: An important controlled prospective study comparing surgical and conservative treatment in patients with sciatica over 10 years showed that there was significant relief of sciatica in the surgical group for 1 to 2 years but not beyond that time. At 10 years both groups had the same outcome including neurological deficits.[15]

Chronic back pain
The basic management of the patient with uncomplicated chronic back pain should follow the following guidelines:
- back education program and ongoing support
- encouragement of normal activity
- exercise program
- swimming
- analgesics, e.g. paracetamol
- NSAIDs for 10–14 days (only if inflammation, i.e. pain at rest—relieved by activity)
- trial of mobilisation or manipulation (at least 3 treatments)—if no contraindications[11,12]
- consider trigger point injection
- a multidisciplinary team approach is recommended

Prevention of further back pain
Patients should be informed that an ongoing back care program should give them an excellent outlook. Prevention includes:

- education about back care, including a good layperson's reference
- golden rules to live by: how to lift, sit, bend, play sport and so on
- an exercise program: a tailor-made program for the patient
- posture and movement training, e.g.
  — the Alexander technique[16]
  — the Feldenkrais technique[17]

When to refer
Urgent referral
- Myelopathy, especially acute cauda equina compression syndrome
- Severe radiculopathy with neurologic deficit
- Spinal fractures

Other referrals
- Neoplasia or infection
- Undiagnosed back pain
- Paget's disease
- Continuing pain of 3 months duration without a clearly definable cause

Practice tips
- Back pain that is related to posture, aggravated by movement and sitting, and relieved by lying down is due to vertebral dysfunction, especially a disc disruption.
- The pain from most disc lesions is generally relieved by rest.
- Plain X-rays are of limited use, especially in younger patients, and may appear normal in disc prolapse.
- Remember the possibility of depression as a cause of back pain; if suspected, consider a trial of antidepressants.
- If back pain persists, possibly worse during bed rest at night, consider malignant disease, depressive illness or other systemic diseases.
- Pain that is worse on standing and walking, but relieved by sitting, is probably caused by spondylolisthesis.
- If pain and stiffness is present on waking and lasts longer than 30 minutes upon activity, consider inflammation.
- Avoid using strong analgesics (especially opioids) in any chronic non-malignant pain state.
- Bilateral back pain is more typical of systemic diseases, while unilateral pain typifies mechanical causes.

- Back pain at rest and morning stiffness in a young person demand careful investigation: consider inflammation such as ankylosing spondylitis and Reiter's disease.
- A disc lesion of L5–S1 can involve both L5 and S1 roots. However, combined L5 and S1 root lesions should still be regarded with suspicion, e.g. consider malignancy.
- A large central disc protrusion can cause bladder symptoms, either incontinence or retention.
- Low back pain of very sudden onset with localised spasm and protective lateral deviation may indicate a facet joint syndrome.
- The T12–L1 and L1–L2 discs are the groin pain discs.
- The L4–L5 disc is the back pain disc.
- The L5–S1 disc is the leg pain disc.
- Severe limitation of SLR (especially to less than 30°) indicates lumbar disc prolapse.
- A preventive program for dysfunctional back pain based on back care awareness and exercises is mandatory advice.
- Remember that most back problems resolve within a few weeks, so avoid overtreatment.

References

1. Cormack J, Marinker M, Morrell D. *Practice: a handbook of primary health care.* London: Kluwer-Harrap Handbooks, 1980; 3(68):1–10.
2. Sloane P, Slatt M, Baker R. *Essentials of family medicine.* Baltimore: Williams and Wilkins, 1988, 228–235.
3. Maigne R. Manipulation of the spine. In: Basmajian JV ed, *Manipulation, traction and massage.* Paris: RML, 1986, 71–96.
4. Bogduk N. The sources of low back pain. In: Jaysom M ed. *The lumbar spine and back pain* (4th edn). Edinburgh: Churchill Livingstone, 1992: 61–88.
5. Deyo RA, Diehl AK. Lumbar spine films in primary care: Current use and effects of selective ordering criteria. J Gen Intern Med, 1986; 1:20–25.
6. Kenna C, Murtagh J. *Back pain and spinal manipulation* (2nd edn). Oxford: Butterworth Heinemann, 1997, 70–164.
7. Waddell G et al. Non-organic physical signs in low back pain. Spine, 1980; 5: 117–125.
8. Deyo RA, Diehl AK, Rosenthal M. How many days of bed rest for acute low back pain? A randomised clinical trial. N Eng J Med, 1986; 315:1064–1070.
9. Kendall PH, Jenkins SM. Exercises for backache: A double blind controlled study. Physiotherapy, 1968; 54:154–157.
10. Shekelle G et al. Spinal manipulation for low back pain. Ann Int Med, 1992; 117: 590–598.
11. Blomberg S, Svardsudd K, Mildenberger F. A controlled, multicentre trial of manual therapy in low back pain. Scand J Prim Health Care, 1992; 10:170–178.
12. Royal College of General Practitioners et al. *Clinical guidelines for the management of acute low back pain.* London: RCGP, 1996.
13. Kuritzky L. Low back pain. Audio-Digest Family Practice. California Medical Association, 1996; 44:14.
14. Deyo RA. Acute low back pain: A new paradigm for management. BMJ, 1996; 313:1343–1344.
15. Weber et al. A controlled prospective study with 10 years observation of patients with sciatica. Spine, 1983; 8: 131–140.
16. Hodgkinson L. *The Alexander technique.* London: Piatkus, 1988, 1–97.
17. Feldenkrais M. *Awareness through movement.* New York: Harper and Row, 1972.

34

Thoracic back pain

—

Since learning about the various causes of chest wall pain I am continually amazed about the number of pain syndromes that I am diagnosing as originating from the thoracic spine. I wonder what I was thinking beforehand.

Comments from LW
RACGP Back Pain Course participant, Brisbane 1986

Thoracic (dorsal) back pain is common in people of all ages including children and adolescents. Dysfunction of the joints of the thoracic spine, with its unique costovertebral joints (which are an important source of back pain), is very commonly encountered in medical practice, especially in people whose lifestyle creates stresses and strains through poor posture and heavy lifting. Muscular and ligamentous strains may be common, but they rarely come to light in practice because they are self-limiting and not severe.

This dysfunction can cause referred pain to various parts of the chest wall and can mimic the symptoms of various visceral diseases such as angina, biliary colic and oesophageal spasm. In similar fashion, heart and gall bladder pain can mimic spinal pain.

Key facts and checkpoints

- The commonest site of pain in the spine is the costovertebral articulations especially the costotransverse articulation (Fig. 34.1).
- Pain of thoracic spinal origin may be referred anywhere to the chest wall, but the commonest sites are the scapular region, the paravertebral region 2–5 cm from midline and, anteriorly, over the costochondral region.
- Thoracic (also known as dorsal) pain is more common in patients with abnormalities such as

kyphosis and Scheuermann's disorder.
- Trauma to the chest wall (including falls on the chest such as those experienced in body contact sport) commonly lead to disorders of the thoracic spine.
- Unlike the lumbar spine the joints are quite superficial and it is relatively easy to find the affected (painful) segment.
- The intervertebral disc prolapse is very uncommon in the thoracic spine.
- The older patient presenting with chest pain should be regarded as having a cardiac cause until proved otherwise.
- If the chest pain is non-cardiac, then the possibility of referral from the thoracic spine should be considered.
- The thoracic spine is the commonest site in the vertebral column for metastatic disease.

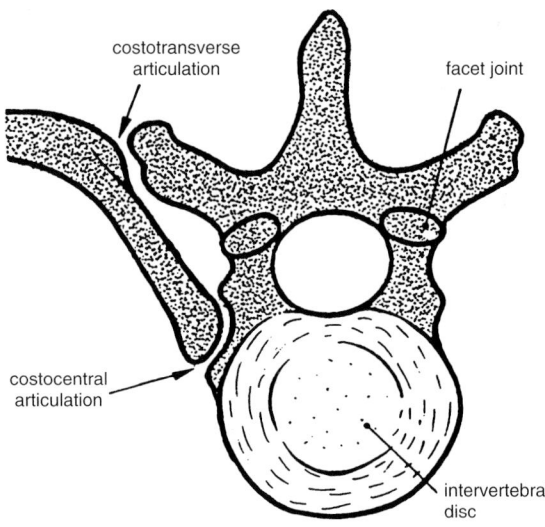

Fig. 34.1 *The functional unit of the thoracic spine*

- Scheuermann's disorder, which affects the lower thoracic spine in adolescents, is often associated with kyphosis and recurrent thoracic back pain. Always inspect the thoracic spine of the younger patient for kyphosis and scoliosis.
- Palpation is the most important component of the physical examination.

A diagnostic approach

A summary of the safety diagnostic model is presented in Table 34.1.

Table 34.1 *Thoracic back pain: diagnostic strategy model*

Q. *Probability diagnosis*
A. Musculoligamentous strains (mainly postural) vertebral dysfunction

Q. *Serious disorders not to be missed*
A. Cardiovascular
  - myocardial infarction
  - dissecting aneurysm
  - pulmonary infarction
  Neoplasia
  - myeloma
  - lung (with infiltration)
  - metastatic disease
  Severe infections
  - pleurisy
  - infectious endocarditis
  - osteomyelitis
  Pneumothorax
  Osteoporosis

Q. *Pitfalls (often missed)*
A. Angina
  Gastrointestinal disorders
  - oesophageal dysfunction
  - peptic ulcer (penetrating)
  - hepatobiliary
  - pancreatic
  Herpes zoster
  Spondyloarthropathies
  Fibromyalgia syndrome
  Polymyalgia rheumatica
  Chronic infection
  - tuberculosis
  - brucellosis

Q. *Seven masquerades checklist*
A. Depression   √
  Diabetes   —
  Drugs   —
  Anaemia   —
  Thyroid disease   —
  Spinal dysfunction   √√
  UTI   √

Q. *Is this patient trying to tell me something?*
A. Yes, quite possible with many cases of back pain.

Probability diagnosis

The commonest cause of thoracic back pain is musculoskeletal, due usually to musculoligamentous strains caused by poor posture. However, these pains are usually transitory and present rarely to the practitioner. The problems that commonly present are those caused by dysfunction of the lower cervical and thoracic spinal joints, especially those of the mid-thoracic (interscapular) area.

Arthritic conditions of the thoracic spine are not relatively common although degenerative osteoarthritis is encountered at times; the inflammatory spondyloarthropathies are uncommon.

The various systemic infectious diseases such as influenza and Epstein-Barr mononucleosis can certainly cause diffuse backache but should be assessed in context.

Not to be missed

A special problem with the thoracic spine is its relationship with the many thoracic and upper abdominal structures that can refer pain to the back. These structures are listed in Table 34.2 but, in particular, myocardial infarction and dissecting aneurysm must be considered.

Cardiopulmonary problems

The acute onset of pain can have sinister implications in the thoracic spine where various life-threatening cardiopulmonary and vascular

Table 34.2 *Non-musculoskeletal causes of thoracic back pain*

Heart	• myocardial infarction • angina • pericarditis
Great vessels	• dissecting aneurysm • pulmonary embolism (rare) • pulmonary infarction • pneumothorax • pneumonia/pleurisy
Oesophagus	• oesophageal rupture • oesophageal spasm • oesophagitis
Subdiaphragmatic disorders of	• gall bladder • stomach ⎫ including • duodenum ⎭ ulcers • pancreas • subphrenic collection
Miscellaneous infections	• herpes zoster • Boorholm disease • infective endocarditis
Psychogenic	

events have to be kept in mind. The pulmonary causes of acute pain include spontaneous pneumothorax, pleurisy and pulmonary infarction. Thoracic back pain may be associated with infective endocarditis due to embolic phenomena. The ubiquitous myocardial infarction or acute coronary occlusion may, uncommonly, cause interscapular back pain, while the very painful dissecting or ruptured aortic aneurysm may cause back pain with hypotension.

Osteoporosis

Osteoporosis, especially in elderly women, must always be considered in such people presenting with acute pain, which can be caused by a pathological fracture. The association with pain following inappropriate physical therapy such as spinal manipulation should also be considered.

Acute infections

Infective conditions that can involve the spine include osteomyelitis, tuberculosis, brucellosis, syphilis and salmonella infections. Such conditions should be suspected in young patients (osteomyelitis), farm workers (brucellosis) and migrants from South-East Asia and Third World countries (tuberculosis). The presence of poor general health and fever necessitates investigations for these infections.

Neoplasia

Fortunately, tumours of the spine are uncommon. Nevertheless, they occur frequently enough for the full-time practitioner in back disorders to encounter some each year, especially metastatic disease.

The three common primary malignancies that metastasise to the spine are those originating in the lung, breast and the prostate (all paired structures). The less common primaries to consider are the thyroid, the kidney and adrenals and malignant melanoma.

Reticuloses such as Hodgkin's disease can involve the spine. Primary malignancies that arise in the vertebrae include multiple myeloma and sarcoma.

Benign tumours to consider are often neurological in origin. An interesting tumour is the osteoid osteoma, which is aggravated by consuming alcohol and relieved by aspirin.

The tumours of the spine are summarised in Table 34.3.

Table 34.3 *Significant tumours affecting the thoracic and lumbar spine*

	Benign	Malignant
Of bone	• osteoid osteoma • haemangioma • osteoblastoma • aneurysmal bone cyst • eosinophilic granuloma	Primary • multiple myeloma • lymphomas, e.g. Hodgkin's • sarcoma
Spinal	Extradural • lipoma • neuroma • fibroma	Secondary • breast • lung • prostate • adrenals/kidney • thyroid • melanoma
	Intradural • neuroma • ependymoma • chordoma • meningioma	Direct spread • stomach • large bowel • pancreas • uterus/cervix/ovary

Source: After Kenna and Murtagh[1]

The symptoms and signs that should alert the clinician to malignant disease are:
• back pain occurring in an older person
• unrelenting back pain, unrelieved by rest (this includes night pain)
• rapidly increasing back pain
• constitutional symptoms, e.g. weight loss, fever, malaise
• a history of treatment for cancer, e.g. excision of skin melanoma

A common trap for the thoracic spine is carcinoma of the lung such as mesothelioma which can invade parietal pleura or structures adjacent to the vertebral column.

Pitfalls

Pitfalls include ischaemic heart disease presenting with interscapular pain, herpes zoster at the pre-eruption stage and the various gastrointestinal disorders. Two commonly misdiagnosed problems are a penetrating duodenal ulcer presenting with lower thoracic pain and oesophageal spasm which can cause thoracic back pain.

Inflammatory rheumatological problems are not common in the thoracic spine but occasionally a spondyloarthropathy such as ankylosing spondylitis manifests here, although it follows some time after the onset of sacroiliitis.

Seven masquerades checklist

Spinal dysfunction is the outstanding cause in this checklist, but urinary infection may occasionally cause lower thoracic pain. Depression always warrants consideration in any pain syndrome, especially back pain. It can certainly cause exaggeration of pre-existing pain from vertebral dysfunction or some other chronic problem.

Psychogenic considerations

Psychogenic or non-organic causes of back pain can present a complex dilemma in diagnosis and management. The causes may be apparent from the incongruous behaviour and personality of the patient, but often the diagnosis is reached by a process of exclusion. There is obviously some functional overlay to everyone with acute or chronic pain, hence the importance of appropriate reassurance to these patients that their problem invariably subsides with time and that they do not have cancer.

Anatomical and clinical features

The functional unit of the thoracic spine is illustrated in Figure 34.1. It appears that pain from the thoracic spine originates mainly from the apophyseal joints and rib articulations. Any one thoracic vertebra has ten separate articulations, so the potential for dysfunction and the difficulty in clinically pinpointing the precise joint at a particular level are apparent.

The costovertebral joints are synovial joints unique to the thoracic spine and have two articulations—costotransverse and costocentral. Together with the apophyseal joints, they are capable of presenting with well-localised pain close to the midline or as referred pain, often quite distal to the spine, with the major symptoms not appearing to have any relationship to the thoracic spine.

Generalised referral patterns are presented in Figure 34.2, while the dermatome pattern is outlined in Figure 34.3.

The pain pattern acts as a guide only because there is considerable dermatomal overlap within the individual and variation from one person to another. It has been demonstrated that up to five nerve roots may contribute to the innervation of any one point in the anterior segments of the trunk dermatomes, a fact emphasised by the clinical distribution of herpes zoster.

Upper thoracic pain[1]

Dysfunction of the joints of the upper thoracic spine usually gives rise to localised pain and stiffness posteriorly but also can cause distal symptoms, probably via the autonomic nervous system.

A specific syndrome called the T4 syndrome[2] has been shown to cause vague pain in the upper limbs and diffuse, vague head and posterior neck pain.

However, most of the pain, stiffness and discomfort arises from dysfunction of the upper and middle thoracic segments with patients presenting with the complaint of pain between 'my shoulder blades'.

Costovertebral joint dysfunction[1]

The unique feature of the thoracic spine is the costovertebral joint. Dysfunction of this joint commonly causes localised pain approximately 3–4 cm from the midline where the rib articulates with the transverse process and the vertebral body. In addition it is frequently responsible for referred pain ranging from the midline, posterior to the lateral chest wall, and even anterior chest pain. When the symptoms radiate laterally, the diagnosis is confirmed only when movement of the rib provokes pain at the costovertebral joint. This examination will simultaneously reproduce the referred pain.

Figure 34.4 presents the pattern of referred pain from these joints and highlights the capacity of the thoracic spine to refer pain centrally to the anterior chest and upper abdomen. Confusion arises for the clinician when the patient's history focuses on the anterior chest pain and fails to mention the presence of posterior pain, should it be present. The shaded areas on Figure 34.4 represent those areas where the patient experiences pain following the injection of hypertonic saline into the posterior elements of the spine.

The clinical approach
History

The history of a patient presenting with thoracic back pain should include a routine pain analysis, which usually provides important clues for the diagnosis. The age, sex and occupation of the patient are relevant. Pain in the thoracic area is very common in people who sit bent over for

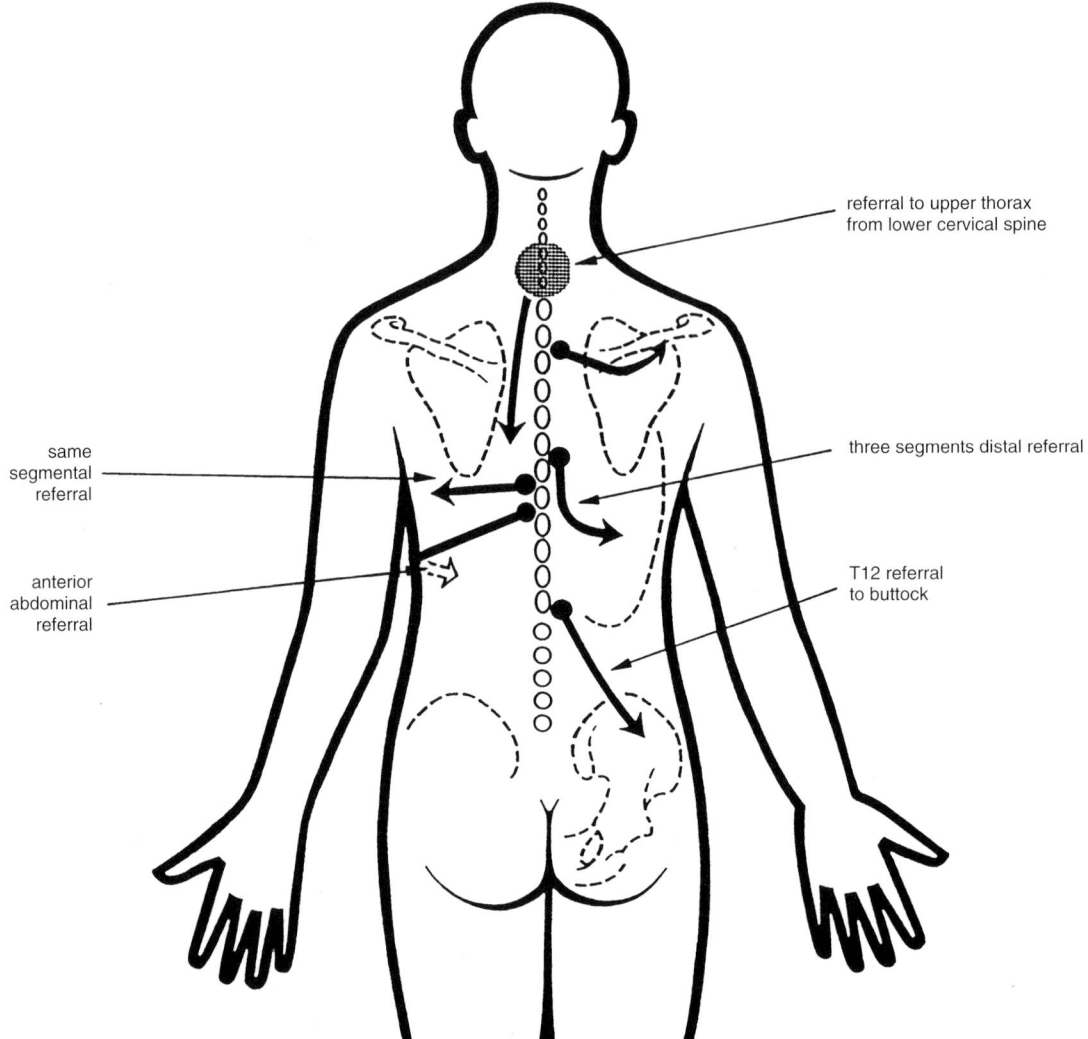

referral to upper thorax
from lower cervical spine

same
segmental
referral

three segments distal referral

anterior
abdominal
referral

T12 referral
to buttock

Fig. 34.2 *Examples of referral patterns for the thoracic spine*

long periods, especially working at desks. Students, secretaries and stenographers are therefore at risk, as are nursing mothers, who have to lift their babies.

People who are kyphotic or scoliotic or who have 'hunchbacks' secondary to disease such as tuberculosis and poliomyelitis also suffer from recurrent pain in this area.

Older people are more likely to present with a neoplastic problem in the thoracic spine and with osteoporosis. Senile osteoporosis is usually a trap because it is symptomless until the intervention of a compression fracture. Symptoms following such a fracture can persist for 3 months.

Pain that is present day and night indicates a sinister cause.

Features of the history that give an indication that the pain is arising from dysfunction of the thoracic spine include:

• *Aggravation and relief of pain on trunk rotation.* The patient's pain may be increased by rotating (twisting) towards the side of the pain but eased by rotating in the opposite direction.
• *Aggravation of pain by coughing, sneezing or deep inspiration.* This can produce a sharp catching pain which, if severe, tends to implicate the costovertebral joint.

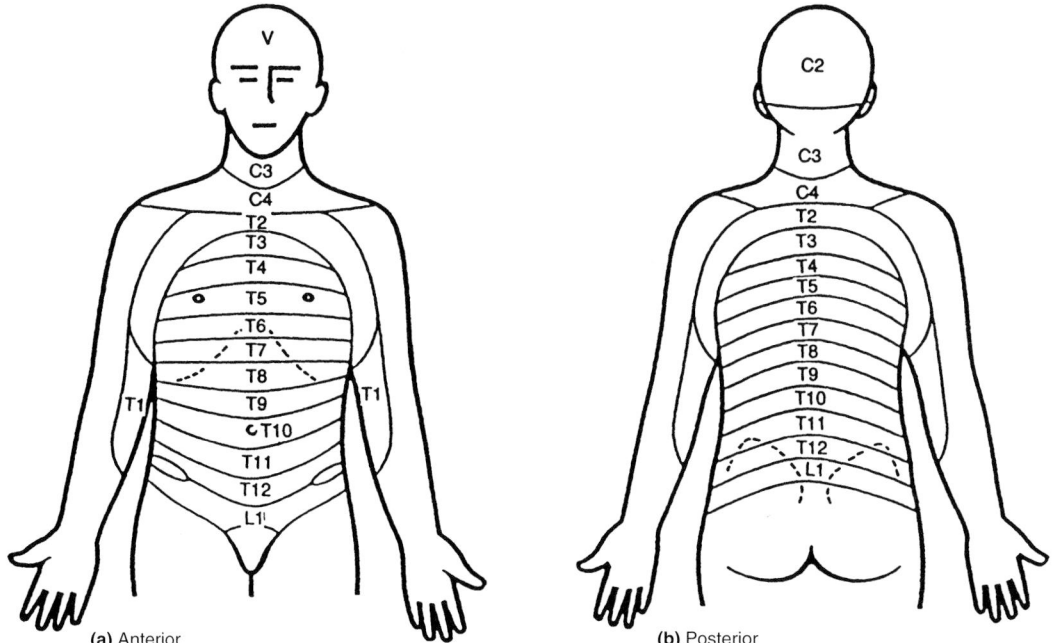

Fig. 34.3 *Dermatomes for the thoracic nerve roots, indicating possible referral areas* REPRODUCED FROM C. KENNA AND J. MURTAGH, *BACK PAIN AND SPINAL MANIPULATION (2ND EDN)*, BUTTERWORTH-HEINEMANN, OXFORD, 1997, WITH PERMISSION

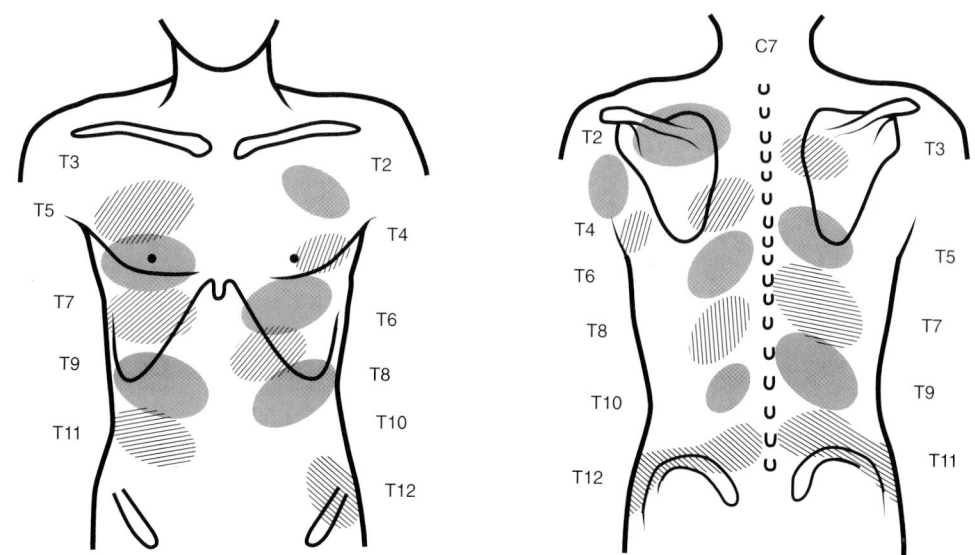

Fig 34.4 *Kellegren's (1939) pain referral patterns after stimulation of deep joints of the thoracic spine*

- *Relief of pain by firm pressure*: Patients may state that their back pain is eased by firm pressure such as leaning against the corner of a wall.

It is very important to be able to differentiate between chest pain due to vertebral dysfunction and that caused by myocardial ischaemia.

Key questions

- Can you recall injuring your back, such as by lifting something heavy?
- Did you have a fall onto your chest or back?
- Is the pain present during the night?
- Do you have low back pain or neck pain?

- Does the pain come on after walking or any strenuous effort?
- Does the pain come on after eating or soon after going to bed at night?
- Have you noticed a fever or sweating at any time, especially at night?
- Have you noticed a rash near where you have the pain?
- What drugs are you taking? Do you take drugs for arthritis or pain? Cortisone?
- What happens when you take a deep breath, cough or sneeze?

Physical examination

The examination of the thoracic spine is straight-forward with the emphasis on palpation of the spine—central and laterally. This achieves the basic objective of reproducing the patient's symptoms and finding the level of pain. The 'look, feel, move, X-ray' clinical approach is most appropriate for the thoracic spine.

Inspection

Careful inspection is important since it may be possible to observe at a glance why the patient has thoracic pain. Note the symmetry, any scars, skin creases and deformities, 'flat spots' in the spine, the nature of the scapulae or evidence of muscle spasm. Look for kyphosis and scoliosis.

Kyphosis may be generalised, with the back having a smooth uniform contour, or localised where it is due to a collapsed vertebra such as occurs in an older person with osteoporosis. Generalised kyphosis is common in the elderly, especially those with degenerative spinal disease. In the young it may reflect the important Scheuermann's disorder.

The younger person in particular should be screened for scoliosis, which becomes more prominent on forward flexion (Fig. 34.5). Look for any asymmetry of the chest wall, inequality of the scapulae and differences in the levels of the shoulders. A useful sign of scoliosis is unequal shoulder levels and apparent 'winging' of scapula. When viewed anteriorly a difference in the levels of the nipples indicates the presence of scoliosis, or other problems causing one shoulder to drop. Inspection should therefore take place with posterior, lateral (side) and anterior views.

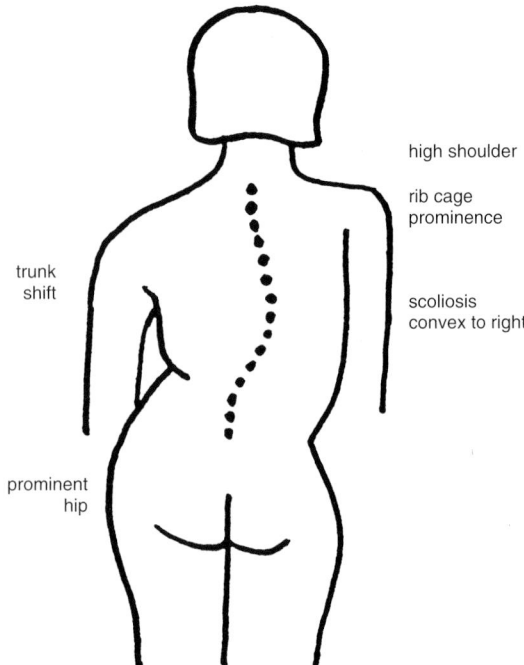

Fig. 34.5 *Screening for adolescent idiopathic scoliosis: configuration of the thoracic spine on forward flexion*

Palpation

The best position is to have the patient prone on the examination table with the thoracic spine preferably in slight flexion. This is achieved by lowering the top of the table.

Test passive extension of each joint with firm pressure from the pad of the thumbs or the bony hand (either the pisiform prominence or the lateral border of the fifth metacarpal). Spring up and down with a few firm oscillations, keeping the elbows straight, but being well above the patient. Ask the patient if the pressure reproduces the pain.

Apart from asking the patient 'Is that the pain?' note:

- the distribution of pain and its change with movement
- the range of movement
- the type of resistance in the joint
- any muscle spasm

Palpation must follow a set plan in order to reproduce the patient's pain. The sequence is as follows:

1. Central—over spinous processes
2. Unilateral—over apophyseal joints (2–3 cm from midline)

3. Transverse—on side of spinous processes
4. Unilateral—costotransverse junctions (4–5 cm from midline)
5. Unilateral—over ribs (spring over posterior rib curve with ulnar border of hand, along axis of rib)

Movements

There are four main movements of the thoracic spine to assess, the most important of which is rotation, as this is the movement that so frequently reproduces the patient's pain where it is facetal joint or costovertebral in origin.

The movements of the thoracic spine and their normal ranges are:

1. Extension   30°
2. Lateral flexion L and R   30°
3. Flexion   90°
4. Rotation L and R   60°

Ask the patient to sit on the table with hands placed behind the neck and then perform the movements. Check these four active movements noting any hypomobility, the range of movement, reproduction of symptoms and function and muscle spasm.

Passive movement, superimposed on active movements, is needed to stress the joints and reproduce pain if it has not been elicited by normal active movement. A passive 'overpressure' can be applied at the end range of each movement, especially with rotation. This is a sensitive method to stress the joint and reproduce the patient's pain. Record the patient's direction of movement, degree of restriction and presence of pain on the direction of movement diagram (Fig. 11.1).

Investigations

The main investigation is an X-ray, which may exclude the basic abnormalities and diseases such as osteoporosis and malignancy. If serious diseases such as malignancy or infection are suspected, and the plain X-ray is normal, a radionuclide bone scan may detect these disorders.

Other investigations to consider are:

• full blood examination and ESR
• serum alkaline phosphatase
• serum electrophoresis for multiple myeloma
• Bence-Jones protein analysis
• brucella agglutination test
• blood culture for pyogenic infection and bacterial endocarditis
• tuberculosis studies

• HLA-B$_{27}$ antigen for spondyloarthropathies
• ECG or ECG stress tests (suspected angina)
• gastroscopy or barium studies (peptic ulcer)

Thoracic back pain in children

The most common cause of thoracic back pain in children is 'postural backache', also known as 'TV backache', which is usually found in adolescent schoolgirls and is a diagnosis of exclusion.

Important, although rare, problems in children include infections (tuberculosis, discitis and osteomyelitis) and tumours such as osteoid osteoma and malignant osteogenic sarcoma.

Dysfunction of the joints of the thoracic spine in children and particularly in adolescents is very common and often related to trauma such as a heavy fall in sporting activities or falling from a height, e.g. off a horse. Fractures, of course, have to be excluded.

Inflammatory disorders to consider are juvenile ankylosing spondylitis and spinal osteochondritis (Scheuermann's disorder), which may affect adolescent males in the lower thoracic spine (around T9) and thoracolumbar spine. The latter condition may be asymptomatic, but can be associated with back pain, especially as the patient grows older. It is the commonest cause of kyphosis.

It is important to screen adolescent children for idiopathic scoliosis, which may be without associated backache.

Scheuermann's disorder

Typical features

• age 11–17
• males > females
• lower thoracic spine
• thoracic pain or asymptomatic
• increasing thoracic kyphosis over 1–2 months
• wedging of the vertebrae
• pain in the wedge, especially on bending
• short hamstrings
• cannot touch toes
• diagnosis confirmed by X-ray

Treatment

• explanation and support
• extension exercises, avoid forward flexion
• postural correction
• avoidance of sports involving lifting and bending
• consider bracing or surgery if serious deformity

Adolescent idiopathic scoliosis

A degree of scoliosis is detectable in 5% of the adolescent population.[3] The vast majority of curves, occurring equally in boys and girls, are mild and of no consequence. Eighty-five per cent of significant curves in adolescent scoliosis occur in girls.[4] Inheritance is a factor. The highest incidence is in first degree female relatives (12%). The scoliotic deformity develops at 10 years of age. Such curves appear during the peripubertal period usually coinciding with the growth spurt. The screening test (usually in 12–14 year olds) is to note the contour of the back on forward flexion (Fig. 34.6).

The test

The subject stands with the feet parallel and together, and bends forward as far as possible with outstretched hands, palms facing each other, pointed between the great toes.

Investigation

A single erect PA spinal X-ray is sufficient;[5] the Cobb angle (Fig. 34.7) is the usual measurement yardstick.

Management

Aims   • to preserve good appearance—level shoulders and no trunk shift
        • prevent increasing curve in adult life: less than 45°
        • *not* to produce a straight spine on X-ray

Methods • Braces: Milwaukee brace (rarely used)
            High density
            polyethylene
            underarm orthosis
        To be worn for 20–22 hours each day until skeletal maturity is reached.
        • Surgical correction: depends on curve and skeletal maturity

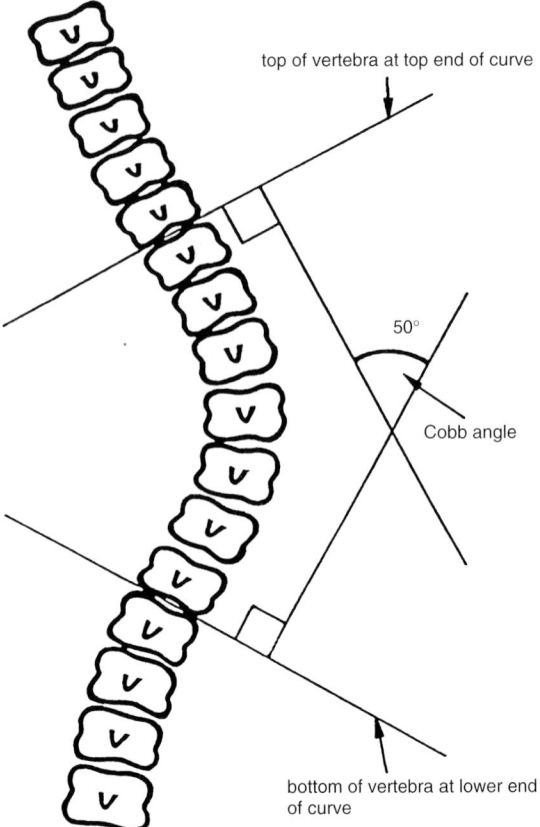

top of vertebra at top end of curve

50°

Cobb angle

bottom of vertebra at lower end of curve

Fig. 34.7 *Scoliosis: the Cobb method of curve measurement*

Guidelines for treatment

• Still growing: < 20°   observe (repeat examination + X-ray)
              20–30°   observe, brace if progressive
              30–45°   brace
              ≥45–50°   operate
• Growth complete:<45°   leave alone
                  >45°   operate
Referral to consultant: >20°

Thoracic back pain in the elderly

Thoracic back pain due to mechanical causes is not such a feature in the elderly although vertebral dysfunction still occurs quite regularly. However, when the elderly person presents with thoracic pain, a very careful search for organic

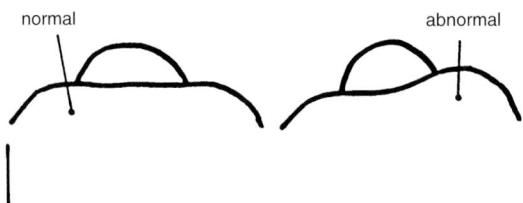

normal   abnormal

Fig. 34.6 *Screening for adolescent idiopathic scoliosis: testing asymmetry by forward flexion* disease is necessary. Special problems to consider are:

- malignant disease, e.g. multiple myeloma, lung, prostate
- osteoporosis
- vertebral pathological fractures
- polymyalgia rheumatica
- Paget's disease (may be asymptomatic)
- herpes zoster
- visceral disorders, e.g.
  - ischaemic heart disease
  - penetrating peptic ulcer
  - oesophageal disorders
  - biliary disorders

Dysfunction of the thoracic spine

This is the outstanding cause of pain presenting to the practitioner, is relatively easy to diagnose and usually responds dramatically to a simple spinal manipulation treatment.

Typical profile[1]

Age:	• Any age, especially between 20 and 40.
History of injury:	• Sometimes slow or sudden onset
Site and radiation:	• Spinal and paraspinal—e.g. interscapular, arms, lateral chest, anterior chest, substernal, iliac crest
Type of pain:	• Dull, aching, occasionally sharp; severity related to activity, site and posture
Aggravation:	• Deep inspiration, postural movement of thorax, slumping or bending, walking upstairs, activities (e.g. lifting children, making beds), beds too hard or soft, sleeping or sitting for long periods
Association:	• Chronic poor posture
Diagnosis confirmation:	• Examination of spine, therapeutic response to manipulation

Management

- explanation and reassurance
- analgesics for a painful episode
- spinal mobilisation or manipulation
- exercise program
- preventive program

Spinal mobilisation and manipulation

Spinal mobilisation is helpful but the more forceful manipulative therapy produces better and quicker results. There are many techniques that can be employed, the choice depending on which part of the back is affected.[1] The sternal thrust (Nelson hold) technique is widely used for upper thoracic segments and the crossed pisiform technique (patient prone) or posteroanterior indirect thrust (patient supine—Fig. 34.8), which is the most effective for mid-thoracic spine.

Preventive exercise program

A key to helping these patients who are prone to recurrences is to prescribe an exercise program for their thoracic spine.[1,6]

Thoracic disc protrusion

Fortunately, a disc protrusion in the thoracic spine is uncommon. This reduced incidence is related to the firm splintage action of the rib cage. Most disc protrusions occur below T9, with the commonest site, as expected, being T11–T12.

The common presentation is back pain and radicular pain that follows the appropriate dermatome.

However, disc lesions in the thoracic spine are prone to produce spinal cord compression, manifesting as sensory loss, bladder incontinence and signs of upper motor neurone lesion. The disc is relatively inaccessible to surgical intervention, but over the past decade there has been a significant improvement in the surgical

Fig. 34.8 *Manipulation of the mid-thoracic spine by the posteroanterior indirect thrust technique*
REPRODUCED FROM C. KENNA AND J. MURTAGH, *BACK PAIN AND SPINAL MANIPULATION (2ND EDN)*, BUTTERWORTH-HEINEMANN, 1997, WITH PERMISSION

treatment of thoracic disc protrusions, due to the transthoracic lateral approach.

Muscle injury

Muscular injuries such as tearing are uncommon in the chest wall. The strong paravertebral muscles do not appear to be a cause of chest pain, but strains of intercostal muscles, the serratus anterior and the musculotendinous origins of the abdominal muscles can cause pain. Injuries to these muscles can be provoked by attacks of violent sneezing or coughing or overstrain, for example lifting a heavy suitcase down from an overhead luggage rack.

Fibromyalgia, fibrositis and myofascial trigger points

Fibromyalgia is relatively uncommon but when encountered presents an enormous management problem. It is not to be confused with so-called fibrositis or tender trigger points.

Fibrositis is not a diagnosis but a symptom, indicating a localised area of tenderness or pain in the soft tissues, especially of the upper thoracic spine. It is probably almost always secondary to upper thoracic or lower cervical spinal dysfunction.

Myofascial trigger points

As described by Travell and Rinzler[7] a trigger point is characterised by:
• circumscribed local tenderness
• localised twitching with stimulation of juxtaposed muscle
• pain referred elsewhere when subjected to pressure

Trigger spots also tend to correspond to the acupuncture points for pain relief.

Treatment

Local injection is relatively easy and may give excellent results. Identify the maximal point of pain and inject 5–8 mL of local anaesthetic, e.g. lignocaine/lidocaine 1% into the painful point (Fig. 34.9). Post-injection massage or exercises should be performed.

Don't: use large volumes of LA; use corticosteroids; cause bleeding

Do: use a moderate amount of LA (only)

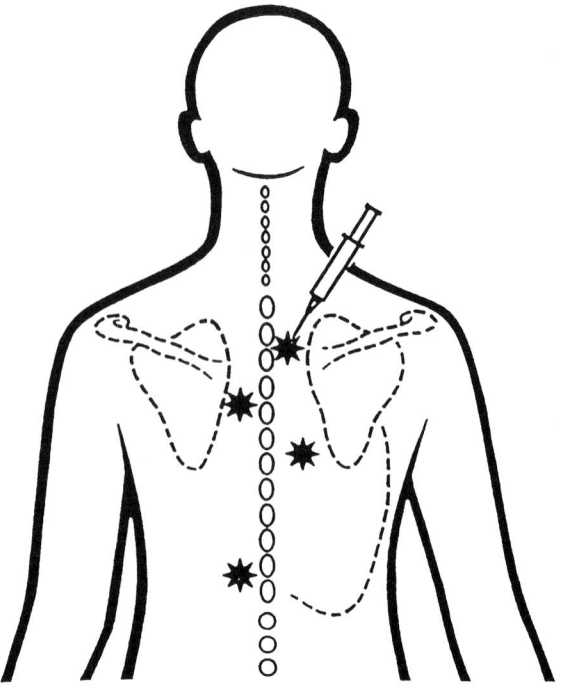

Fig 34.9 *Injection for myofascial trigger points*

Fibromyalgia syndrome[8]

The main diagnostic features are:

1. a history of widespread pain (neck to low back)
2. pain in 11 of 18 tender points on digital palpation

These points must be painful, not tender. Smythe and Moldofsky have recommended 14 of these points on a map as a guide for management[9] (see Fig. 34.10).

Other features

• female:male ratio 4:1
• usual age 29–37: diagnosis 44–53
• poor sleep pattern
• fatigue (similar to chronic fatigue syndrome)
• psychological disorders, e.g. anxiety, depression, tension headache, irritable digestive system.

This disorder is very difficult to treat and is usually unresponsive in the long term to passive physical therapy or injections.[10] Patients require considerable explanation, support and reassurance.

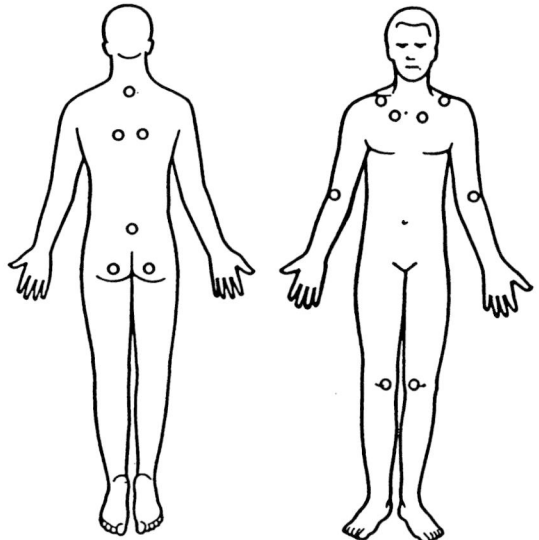

Fig. 34.10 *Fibromyalgia syndrome: typical tender points (the tender point map represents the 14 points recommended for use as a standard for diagnostic or therapeutic studies)*

Treatment

- explanation, reassurance and counselling
- attention to sleep disorders, stress factors and physical factors
- relaxation program
- rehabilitation exercise program, e.g. walking, swimming or cycling

Medication (often disappointing)

- antidepressants (of proven value) e.g. amitriptyline 10–75 mg (o) nocte or prothiaden 25–100 mg (o) nocte

or

- clonazepam (Rivotril) 0.5 mg bd

Serious pitfalls

The following points regarding serious vertebral organic disease are worth repeating in more detail.

Metastatic disease[11]

Secondary deposits in the thoracolumbar spine may be the first presenting symptoms of malignant disease. Any patient of any age presenting with progressive severe night pain of the back should be regarded as having a tumour and investigated with a technetium bone scan as part of the primary investigations.

Secondary deposits in the spine can lead to rapid onset paralysis due to spinal cord infarction. Many such metastases can be controlled in the early stages with radiotherapy.

Multiple myeloma

Osteoporotic vertebral body collapse should be diagnosed only when multiple myeloma has been excluded. Investigations should include an ESR, Bence-Jones protein analysis, and immunoglobulin electrophoresis.

Early treatment of multiple myeloma can hold this disease in remission for many years and prevent crippling vertebral fractures.

Infective discitis and vertebral osteomyelitis

Severe back pain in an unwell patient with fluctuating temperature (fever) should be considered as infective until proved otherwise. Investigations should include blood cultures, serial X-rays and nuclear bone scanning. Biphasic bone scans using technetium with either indium or gallium scanning for white cell collections usually clinch this diagnosis.

Strict bed rest with high-dose antibiotic therapy is usually curative. If left untreated, vertebral end plate and disc space collapse is common and extremely disabling.

When to refer

- Persistent pain or dysfunction—refer to a physical therapist.
- Evidence or suspicion of a sinister cause, e.g. neoplasia, infective discitis/osteomyelitis in a child.
- Suspicion of cardiac or gastrointestinal referred (persistent) pain.
- Significant idiopathic adolescent scoliosis or kyphosis, e.g. Scheuermann's disorder.

Practice tips

- Feelings of anaesthesia or paraesthesia associated with thoracic spinal dysfunction are rare.
- Thoracic back pain is frequently associated with cervical lesions.
- Upper thoracic pain and stiffness is common after 'whiplash'.
- The T4 syndrome of upper to mid-thoracic pain with radiation (and associated paraesthesia) to the arms is well documented.

- Symptoms due to a fractured vertebra usually last 3 months and to a fractured rib 6 weeks.
- The pain of myocardial ischaemia, from either angina or myocardial infarction, can cause referred pain to the interscapular region of the thoracic spine.
- Beware of the old trap of herpes zoster in the thoracic spine, especially in the older person.
- Consider multiple myeloma as a cause of an osteoporotic collapsed vertebra.
- Examine movements with the patient sitting on the couch and hands clasped behind the neck.
- Spinal disease of special significance in the thoracic spine includes osteoporosis and neoplasia, while disc lesions, inflammatory diseases and degenerative diseases (spondylosis) are encountered less frequently than with the cervical and lumbar spines.
- It is imperative to differentiate between spinal and cardiac causes of chest pain: either cause is likely to mimic the other. A working rule is to consider the cause as cardiac until the examination and investigations establish the true cause.
- Always X-ray the thoracic spine following trauma, especially after motor vehicle accidents, as wedge compression fractures (typically between T4 and T8) are often overlooked.

References

1. Kenna C, Murtagh J. *Back pain and spinal manipulation* (2nd edn). Oxford: Butterworth-Heinemann, 1997, 165–174.
2. McGuckin N. The T4 syndrome. In: Grieve GD ed, *Modern manual therapy of the vertebral column*. London: Churchill Livingstone, 1986, 370–6.
3. Stephens J. Idiopathic adolescent scoliosis. Aust Fam Physician, 1984, 13: 180–184.
4. Kane WJ, Moe JH. A scoliosis prevalence survey in Minnesota. Clin Orthop, 1970, 69:216–218.
5. Anonymous. *The Easter Seal Guide to Children's Orthopaedics*. Toronto: The Easter Seal Society, 1982, 64–67.
6. Murtagh J. *Patient education* (2nd edn). Sydney: McGraw-Hill, 1996.
7. Travell J, Rinzler SH. The myofascial genesis of pain. Postgrad Med, 1952; 11: 425–34.
8. Reilly P, Littlejohn G. Current thinking on fibromyalgia syndrome. Aust Fam Physician, 1990; 19:1505–1576.
9. Smythe HA, Moldofsky H. Two contributions to understanding of the 'fibrositis' syndrome. Bull Rheum Dis, 1977; 28:928–931.
10. McIndoe R, Littlejohn G. Management of fibromyalgia and regional pain syndromes. Mod Med Aust, 1995; 36(2): 56–69.
11. Young D, Murtagh J. Pitfalls in orthopaedics. Aust Fam Physician, 1989; 18:653–654.

35
Bruising and bleeding

—

My pa is one mask of brooses both blue and green.

Charles Dickens (1812–1870)
Nicholas Nickleby

Many patients present with the complaint that they bruise easily but only a minority turn out to have an underlying blood disorder. Purpura is bleeding into the skin or mucous membranes, appearing as multiple small haemorrhages that do not blanch on pressure. Smaller purpuric lesions that are 2 mm or less in diameter (pinhead size) are termed petechiae while larger purpuric lesions are called ecchymoses (Fig. 35.1).

Bruises are large areas of bleeding that are a result of subcutaneous bleeding. If bruising is abnormal and out of proportion to the offending trauma then a disturbance of coagulation is suggested.

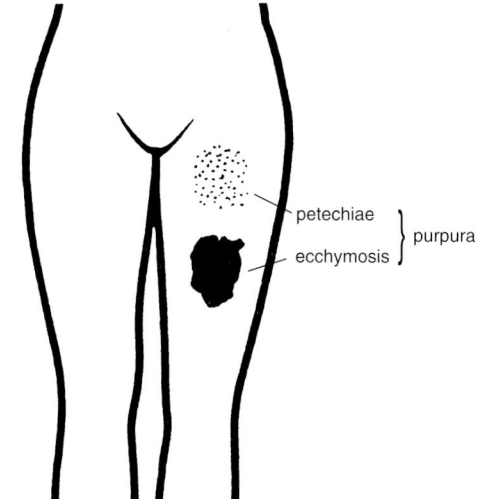

Fig. 35.1 *Purpuric rash (petechiae and ecchymoses)*

Differential diagnosis

'Palpable purpura' due to an underlying systemic vasculitis is an important differential problem. The petechiae are raised so finger palpation is important. The cause is an underlying vasculitis affecting small vessels, e.g. polyarteritis nodosa.

The decision to investigate is difficult because decisions have to be made about which patients warrant investigation and whether the haemostatic defect is due to local or systemic pathology.[1] The ability to identify a bleeding disorder is important because of implications for surgery, pregnancy, medication and genetic counselling.

Key facts and checkpoints
- Purpura = petechiae + ecchymoses.
- Abnormal bleeding is basically the result of disorders of (1) the platelet, (2) the coagulation mechanism, or (3) the blood vessel.
- There is no substitute for a good history in the assessment of patients with bleeding disorders.
- An assessment of the personal and family histories is the first step in the identification of a bleeding disorder.
- When a patient complains of 'bruising easily' it is important to exclude thrombocytopenia due to bone marrow disease and clotting factor deficiencies such as haemophilia.
- The commonest cause of an acquired bleeding disorder is drug therapy, e.g. aspirin, NSAIDs, cytotoxics and oral anticoagulants.
- In general, bleeding secondary to platelet defects is spontaneous, associated with a petechial rash and occurs immediately after trauma or a cut wound.[1]

- Laboratory assessment should be guided by the clinical impression.
- Bleeding caused by coagulation factor deficiency is usually traumatic and delayed, e.g. haemorrhage occurring 24 hours after a dental extraction in a haemophiliac.
- The routine screening tests for the investigation of patients with bleeding disorders can be normal despite the presence of a severe haemorrhagic state.

Causes of clinical disorders

The three major mechanisms of systemic bleeding disorders are:

1. coagulation deficiencies (reduction or inhibition of circulatory coagulation factors)
2. platelet abnormalities: of platelet number or function
3. vascular defects: of vascular endothelium

A list of differential diagnoses of systemic bleeding disorders is presented in Table 35.1.[1]

The clinical approach

Differentiation of coagulation factor deficiencies and platelet disorders as the cause of a bleeding problem can usually be determined by a careful evaluation of the history and physical examination.

History

Factors that suggest the presence of a systemic bleeding defect include:

- spontaneous haemorrhage
- severe or recurrent haemorrhagic episodes
- bleeding from multiple sites
- bleeding out of proportion to the degree of trauma

If a bleeding diathesis is suspected it is essential to determine whether local pathology is contributing to the blood loss, e.g. postoperative bleeding, postpartum bleeding, gastrointestinal haemorrhage.

Diagnostic tips

- Platelet abnormalities present as early bleeding following trauma.
- Coagulation factor deficiencies present with delayed bleeding after initial haemostasis is achieved by normal platelets.
- A normal response to previous coagulation stresses, e.g. dental extraction, circumcision or

Table 35.1 *Differential diagnoses of systemic bleeding disorders*

Vascular disorders
(a) Inherited
- hereditary haemorrhagic telangiectasia
- Marfan's syndrome

(b) Acquired
- purpura simplex
- senile purpura
- Henoch-Schönlein purpura
- steroid purpura
- scurvy

Coagulation factor deficiency or inhibitor
(a) Inherited
- haemophilia A
- haemophilia B
- von Willebrand's disease

(b) Acquired
- disseminated intravascular coagulation
- liver disease
- vitamin K deficiency
- oral anticoagulant therapy or overdosage

Thrombocytopenia
(a) Inherited
- Fanconi syndrome
- amegakaryocytic thrombocytopenia

(b) Acquired
- immune thrombocytopenic purpura
- drug-induced thrombocytopenia
- disseminated intravascular coagulation
- bone marrow replacement or failure
- thrombotic thrombocytopenic purpura
- post-transfusion purpura
- splenic pooling
- burns

Functional platelet disorders
(a) Inherited
- Glanzmann's thrombasthenia
- Bernard-Soulier syndrome
- storage pool deficiency

(b) Acquired
- drug-induced
- uraemia
- myeloproliferative disorders
- dysproteinaemias

Source: After Mitchell et al.[1] Adapted from Bleeding disorders, MIMS Disease Index 1996 with permission of MIMS Australia, a division of MediMedia Australia Pty Limited.

pregnancy, indicates an acquired problem.
- If acquired, look for evidence of drugs, malignancy and liver disease.
- A diagnostic strategy is outlined in Table 35.2.

Family history

A positive family history can be a positive pointer to the diagnosis:

- sex-linked recessive pattern
  — haemophilia A or B

Table 35.2 *Purpura: diagnostic strategy model*

Q. *Probability diagnosis*
A. Simple purpura (easy bruising syndrome)
   Senile purpura
   Corticosteroid-induced purpura
   Anaphylactoid purpura (Henoch-Schönlein)

Q. *Serious disorders not to be missed*
A. Malignant disease
   • leukaemia
   • myeloma
   Aplastic anaemia
   Myelofibrosis
   Severe infections
   • septicaemia
   • meningococcal infection
   • measles
   • typhoid
   Disseminated intravascular coagulation
   Thrombocytopenic purpura

Q. *Pitfalls (often missed)*
A. Haemophilia A,B
   von Willebrand's disease
   Connective tissue disorders, e.g. SLE, RA
   Post-transfusion purpura
   Trauma, e.g. domestic violence, child abuse
   Rare
   • hereditary telangiectasia
     (Osler-Weber-Rendu syndrome)
   • Ehlers-Danlos syndrome
   • scurvy
   • Fanconi syndrome

Q. *The masquerades*
A. Drugs
   • chloramphenicol
   • corticosteroids
   • sulphonamides
   • quinine/quinidine
   • thiazide diuretics
   • NSAIDs
   • cytotoxics
   • oral anticoagulants
   Anaemia
   • aplastic anaemia

Q. *Psychogenic factors*
A. Factitial purpura

Table 35.3 *Checklist for a bleeding history*

• Skin bruising	• Tonsillectomy
• Epistaxis	• Other operations
• Injury	• Childbirth
• Domestic violence	• Haematuria
• Menorrhagia	• Rectal bleeding
• Haemarthrosis	• Drugs
• Tooth extraction	• Family history

where possible and if none are present at the time of the consultation the patient should return if any bruises reappear.

Key questions

• How long has the problem been apparent to you?
• Do you remember any bumps or falls that might have caused the bruising?
• What sort of injuries cause you to bruise easily?
• Have you noticed bleeding from other areas such as your nose or gums?
• Has anyone in your family had a history of bruising or bleeding?
• What is your general health like?
• Do you have any tiredness, weight loss, fever or night sweats?
• Did you notice a viral illness or sore throat beforehand?
• How much alcohol do you drink?
• What happened in the past when you had a tooth extracted?
• Do you get widespread itchiness of your skin?
• Have you ever had painful swelling in your joints?

Medication record

It is mandatory to obtain a complete drug history. Examples of drugs and their responses are:
• vascular purpura
  — prednisolone
• thrombocytopenia
  — chloramphenicol
  — cytotoxic drugs
  — gold
  — heparin
  — phenylbutazone
  — sulphonamides
  — quinine, quinidine
  — thiazide diuretics

• autosomal dominant pattern
  — von Willebrand's disease
  — dysfibrinogenaemias
• autosomal recessive pattern
  — deficiency coagulation factors V, VII and X

Enquire whether the patient has noticed blood in the urine or stools and whether menorrhagia is present in women. A checklist for a bleeding history is presented in Table 35.3. The actual size and frequency of the bruises should be recorded

Table 35.6 *International nomenclature of clotting factors*

Factor	Common synonyms
I	Fibrinogen*
II	Prothrombin*
III	Thromboplastin*
IV	Calcium*
V*	Proaccelerin
VI	No longer used
VII*	Proconversion
VIII	Antihaemophilic factor
	Antihaemophilic globulin
IX*	Christmas factor, plasma thromboplastin component
X*	Stuart-Prower factor
XI*	Plasma thromboplastin antecedent
XII	Hageman factor, contact factor
XIII	Fibrin stabilising factor

Common terminology in use indicated by *

Management principles[1]

- Make the correct diagnosis.
- Stop or avoid drugs affecting the haemostatic system.
- Control bleeding episodes with appropriate drugs, blood products and local measures such as simple compression or topical haemostatic agents.
- Infuse appropriate blood components for the treatment of coagulation factor deficiencies and some platelet disorders, e.g. factor VIII for haemophilia A; fresh frozen plasma for multiple factor deficiency.
- Refer patients with identified defects to a consultant haematologist or haemophilia centre.
- Supervise advanced planning in patients seeking pregnancy, surgery or dental extraction.

When to refer[1]

- Management of haemorrhage is not amenable to simple measures such as local therapy with simple compression and other measures.
- Elective surgery or pregnancy is being planned.

Practice tips

- A careful history and physical examination will usually pinpoint the cause of the bleeding disorder.
- Drug therapy can lead to unmasking of pre-existing haemostatic disorders, e.g. platelet dysfunction induced by aspirin may cause spontaneous bleeding in patients with underlying von Willebrand's disease.
- Think of DIC in any acutely ill patient with abnormal bleeding from sites such as the mouth or nose, venepuncture or with widespread ecchymoses. The clinical situations are numerous, e.g. septicaemia, obstetric emergencies, disseminated malignant disease, falciparum malaria, snake bites.

References

1. Mitchell CA, Dear A, Salem H. Bleeding disorders. In: MIMS Disease Index (2nd edn). Sydney: IMS Publishing, 1996, 69–71.
2. McPherson J, Street A. Tests of haemostasis: Detection of the patient at risk of bleeding. Australian Prescriber 1995; 18(2):38–40.
3. Robinson MJ. *Practical paediatrics* (2nd edn). Melbourne: Churchill Livingstone, 1990, 349–356.
4. Kumer PJ, Clark ML. *Clinical medicine* (2nd edn). London: Bailliere Tindall, 1990, 335–344.

36

Chest pain

—

There is a disorder of the breast marked with strong and peculiar symptoms, considerable for the kind of danger belonging to it. The seat of it, and sense of strangling, and anxiety with which it is attended, may make it not improperly be called angina pectoris.

William Heberden (1710–1801)

The presenting problem of chest pain is common yet very threatening to both patient and doctor because the underlying cause in many instances is potentially lethal, especially with chest pain of sudden onset. The causes of acute chest pain are summarised and presented in Figure 36.1.

Checkpoints and golden rules

- Chest pain represents myocardial infarction until proved otherwise.
- Immediate life-threatening causes of spontaneous chest pain are:
  1. myocardial infarction/unstable angina
  2. pulmonary embolism
  3. dissecting aneurysm of the aorta
  4. tension pneumothorax
- The main differential diagnoses of myocardial infarction include angina, dissecting aneurysm, pericarditis, oesophageal reflux and spasm, and hyperventilation with anxiety.
- The history remains the most important clinical factor in the diagnosis of ischaemic heart disease. With angina a vital clue is the reproducibility of the symptom.

A diagnostic approach

The safety diagnostic model (Table 36.1) can be used to analyse chest pain according to the five self-posed questions.

Table 36.1 *Chest pain: diagnostic strategy model*

Q. *Probability diagnosis*
A. Musculoskeletal (chest wall)
   Psychogenic
   Angina

Q. *Serious disorders not to be missed*
A. Cardiovascular
   • myocardial infarction/unstable angina
   • dissecting aneurysm
   • pulmonary embolism
   Neoplasia
   • carcinoma lung
   • tumours of spinal cord and meningitis
   Severe infections
   • pneumonia-pleurisy
   • mediastinitis
   • pericarditis
   Pneumothorax

Q. *Pitfalls (often missed)*
A. Mitral valve prolapse
   Oesophageal spasm
   Gastro-oesophageal reflux
   Herpes zoster
   Fractured rib, e.g. cough fracture
   Spinal dysfunction

   Rarities
   • Bornholm disease (pleurodynia)
   • cocaine inhalation
   • hypertrophic cardiomyopathy

Q. *Seven masquerades checklist*
A. Depression   √ possible
   Diabetes   —
   Drugs   —
   Anaemia   √ indirect
   Thyroid disease —
   Spinal dysfunction √
   UTI   —

Q. *Is the patient trying to tell me something?*
A. Consider functional causes, especially anxiety with hyperventilation

Note: Chest pain is myocardial ischaemia until proved otherwise.

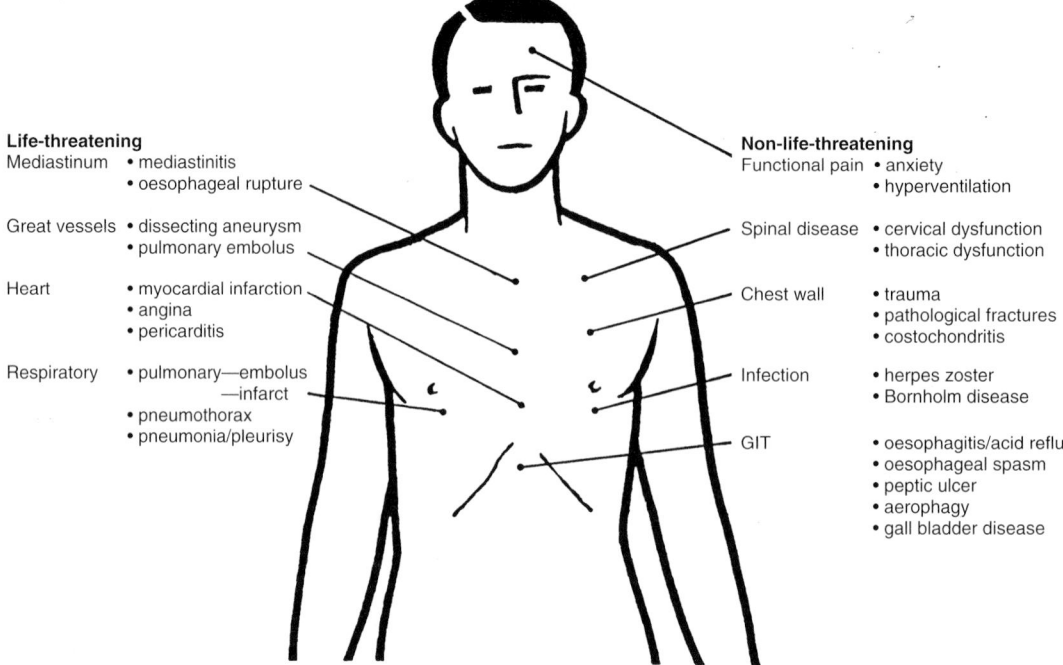

Life-threatening

Mediastinum • mediastinitis
• oesophageal rupture

Great vessels • dissecting aneurysm
• pulmonary embolus

Heart • myocardial infarction
• angina
• pericarditis

Respiratory • pulmonary—embolus
—infarct
• pneumothorax
• pneumonia/pleurisy

Non-life-threatening

Functional pain • anxiety
• hyperventilation

Spinal disease • cervical dysfunction
• thoracic dysfunction

Chest wall • trauma
• pathological fractures
• costochondritis

Infection • herpes zoster
• Bornholm disease

GIT • oesophagitis/acid reflux
• oesophageal spasm
• peptic ulcer
• aerophagy
• gall bladder disease

Fig. 36.1 *Causes of acute chest pain*

Probability diagnosis

The commonest causes encountered in general practice are musculoskeletal or chest wall pain and psychogenic disorders. The former is a very important yet often overlooked cause and sometimes inappropriately referred to as fibrositis or neuralgia. Causes include costochondritis, muscular strains, dysfunction of the sternocostal joints and dysfunction of the lower cervical spine or upper thoracic spine, which can cause referred pain to various areas of the chest wall. Angina is common and must always be considered. If angina-like pain lasts longer than 15 minutes myocardial infarction must be excluded.

Serious disorders not to be missed

The usual triad of malignancy, myocardial ischaemia and severe infections (Table 36.1) must be considered. In addition other cardiovascular catastrophes such as a dissecting aortic aneurysm and pulmonary embolus must be excluded, albeit uncommon, especially in those at risk. Spontaneous pneumothorax should also be considered especially in a young male of slight build. Malignancies of the lung are relatively common and may present as pain when the previously asymptomatic tumour invades nerves or the spine.

The severe infections that cause chest pain include pneumonia/pleurisy, pericarditis and mediastinitis.

Pitfalls

Unfortunately, myocardial infarction and angina are often missed. Referred pain from spinal dysfunction, especially if referred anteriorly, is commonly overlooked. Other pitfalls include a cough fracture of a rib, herpes zoster (prior to the eruption) and gastrointestinal disorders, including oesophageal spasm, reflux and cholecystitis. Oesophageal problems may be clinically indistinguishable from angina. Mitral valve prolapse can cause chest pain although the mechanism is unclear: think of it in an unwell female prone to palpitations and chest pain. The pain tends to be sharp, fleeting, non-exertional and located near the cardiac apex.

General pitfalls include:

• not being 'coronary aware' in patients presenting with chest pain
• referred pain from spinal disorders, especially of the lower cervical spine—one of the great pitfalls in medical practice

- labelling chest pain as psychological in an anxious patient presenting with acute chest pain
- assuming that pain radiating down the inside of the left arm is always cardiac in origin
- being unaware that up to 20% of myocardial infarctions are silent, especially in elderly patients, and that pulmonary embolism is often painless.

Seven masquerades checklist
Of this group spinal dysfunction is possible. Disc lesions from the lower cervical spine are unlikely to cause chest wall pain, but dysfunction of the facet joints of this area of the spine and the upper thoracic spine is a common cause of referred pain to the chest wall. Nerve root pain from spinal problems is rarely found in the chest wall. Pathological fractures secondary to osteoporosis or malignancy in the vertebrae cause posterior wall pain.

Psychogenic considerations
With psychogenic causes the pain can occur anywhere in the chest, and tends to be continuous and sharp or stabbing rather than constricting. Associated symptoms include palpitations, deep breathing, fatigue, tremor, agitation and anxiety. Abnormal stress, tension, anxiety or depression may precipitate the pain, which often lasts hours or days.

The clinical approach
History
A meticulous history of the behaviour of the pain is the key to diagnosis. The pain should be analysed into its usual characteristics: site and radiation, quality, intensity, duration, onset and offset, precipitating and relieving factors, and associated symptoms. Association with serious medical problems such as diabetes, Marfan's syndrome, anaemia and systemic lupus erythematosus should be kept in mind. The ability to take a detailed history will obviously be limited with severe acute pain.

Associated symptoms
- *Syncope.* Consider myocardial infarction, pulmonary embolus and dissecting aneurysm.
- *Pain on inspiration.* Consider pleurisy, pericarditis, pneumothorax and musculoskeletal (chest wall pain).

- *Thoracic back pain.* Consider spinal dysfunction, myocardial infarction, angina, dissecting aneurysm, pericarditis and gastrointestinal disorders such as a peptic ulcer, cholecystitis and oesophageal spasm.

Key questions
- Where exactly do you get the pain?
- Does the pain travel anywhere?
- Can you give me a careful description of the pain?
- How long did the pain last and could you do anything to relieve it?
- Is the pain brought on by exertion and relieved by rest?
- Do cold conditions bring it on?
- Do you have any other symptoms such as breathlessness, faintness, sweating or back pain?
- Is the pain made worse by breathing or coughing, or by movement or pressing on that area?
- Is there any blood in any sputum you bring up?
- Is your pain associated with what you eat and drink? Or with a bitter taste in your mouth?
- Do you get the pain on stooping over and after lying in bed at night?
- Do antacids relieve your pain?
- Have you noticed a rash where you get the pain?
- Have you had a blow to your chest or an injury to your back?

Physical examination
The examination should focus on the following areas:
- general appearance: evidence of atherosclerosis (senile arcus, thickened vessels), pale and sweating (myocardial infarction, dissecting aneurysm or pulmonary embolus), hemiparesis (? dissecting aneurysm)
- pulses—both radial and femoral: check for nature of pulse and absence of femoral pulses
- blood pressure
- temperature
- palpation of chest wall, lower cervical spine and thoracic spine: look for evidence of localised tenderness, pathological fracture, spinal dysfunction, herpes zoster
- palpation of legs: check for evidence of deep venous thrombosis
- examination of chest: check for evidence of pneumothorax
- auscultation of chest

— reduced breath sounds, hyper-resonant percussion note and vocal fremitus → pneumothorax
— friction rub → pericarditis or pleurisy
— basal crackles → cardiac failure
— apical systole murmur → mitral valve prolapse
— aortic diastolic murmur → proximal dissection (aortic regurgitation)

In the presence of a myocardial infarction, the examination may be normal but the patient, apart from being cold, clammy or shocked, may have muffled heart sounds, a gallop rhythm, a systolic murmur. With a dissecting aneurysm the patient may also appear cold, clammy and shocked, but may show absent femoral pulses, hemiparesis and a diastolic murmur of aortic regurgitation.

• upper abdominal palpation: check for tenderness suggestive of gall bladder disease or peptic ulceration

Possible findings on examination of a patient with chest pain are presented in Figure 36.2.[1]

Investigations

The following investigations to aid diagnosis are available, although the majority are sophisticated and confined to hospitals with high technology imaging departments. The fundamental

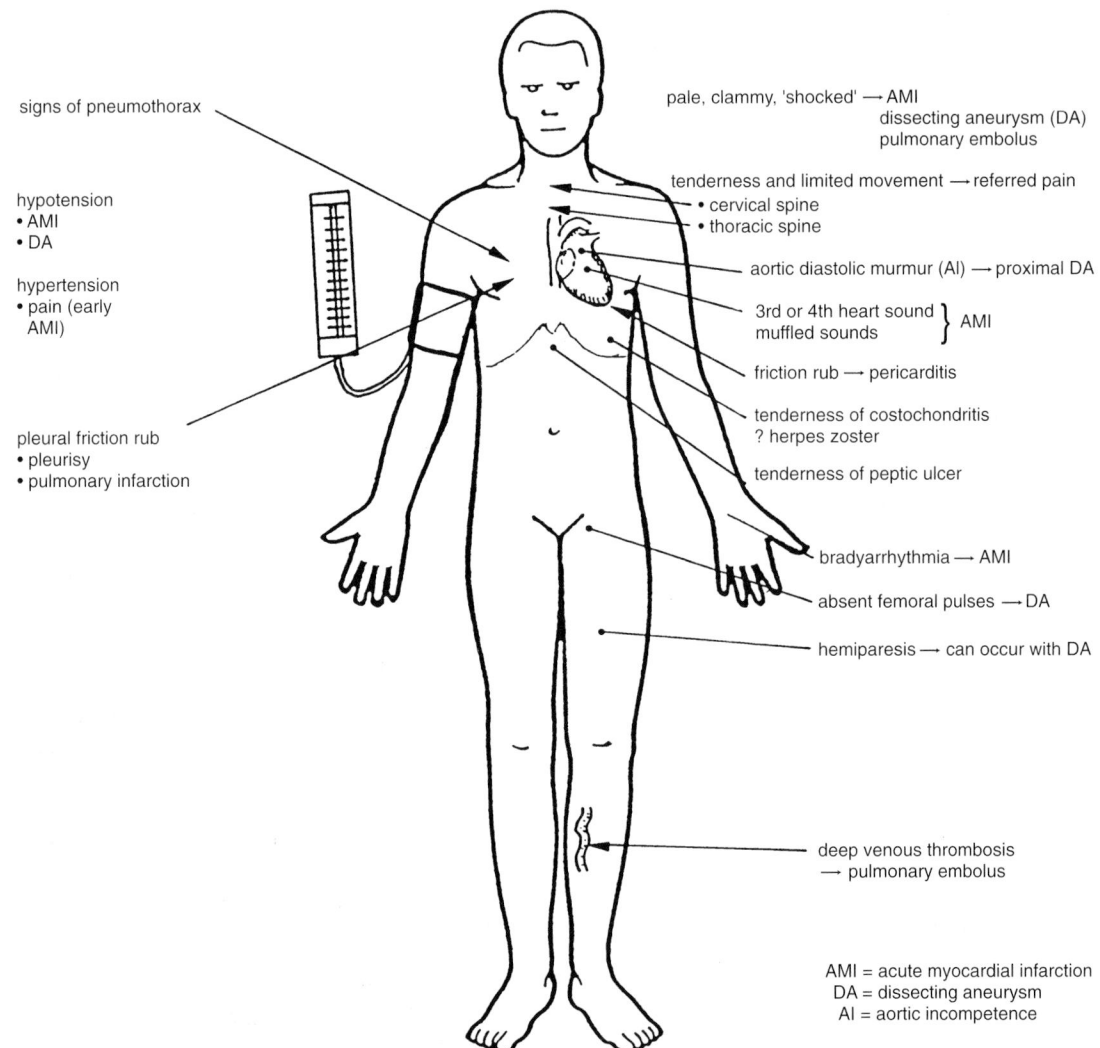

signs of pneumothorax

hypotension
• AMI
• DA

hypertension
• pain (early AMI)

pleural friction rub
• pleurisy
• pulmonary infarction

pale, clammy, 'shocked' → AMI
               dissecting aneurysm (DA)
               pulmonary embolus

tenderness and limited movement → referred pain
• cervical spine
• thoracic spine

aortic diastolic murmur (AI) → proximal DA

3rd or 4th heart sound ⎫
muffled sounds ⎭ AMI

friction rub → pericarditis

tenderness of costochondritis
? herpes zoster

tenderness of peptic ulcer

bradyarrhythmia → AMI

absent femoral pulses → DA

hemiparesis → can occur with DA

deep venous thrombosis
→ pulmonary embolus

AMI = acute myocardial infarction
DA = dissecting aneurysm
AI = aortic incompetence

Fig. 36.2 *Possible examination findings in a patient with chest pain* tests that are readily available to the GP—ECG, chest X-ray and cardiac enzymes—should help confirm the diagnosis in most instances.

Electrocardiogram (ECG)

This may be diagnostic for ischaemia and myocardial infarction although it is important to bear in mind that it may be normal with both, including the early minutes to hours of an acute infarction.

It can be helpful to differentiate between myocardial infarction, pulmonary embolism and pericarditis (Fig. 36.3). The ECG in pulmonary embolism may show right axis deviation. Pericarditis is characterised by low voltages and saddle-shaped ST segment elevation.

Exercise tolerance test

This is the key test for defining chest pain as cardiac in origin. Physical stress such as the motor-driven treadmill or a bicycle ergometer is used to elicit changes in the ECG to diagnose myocardial ischaemia.

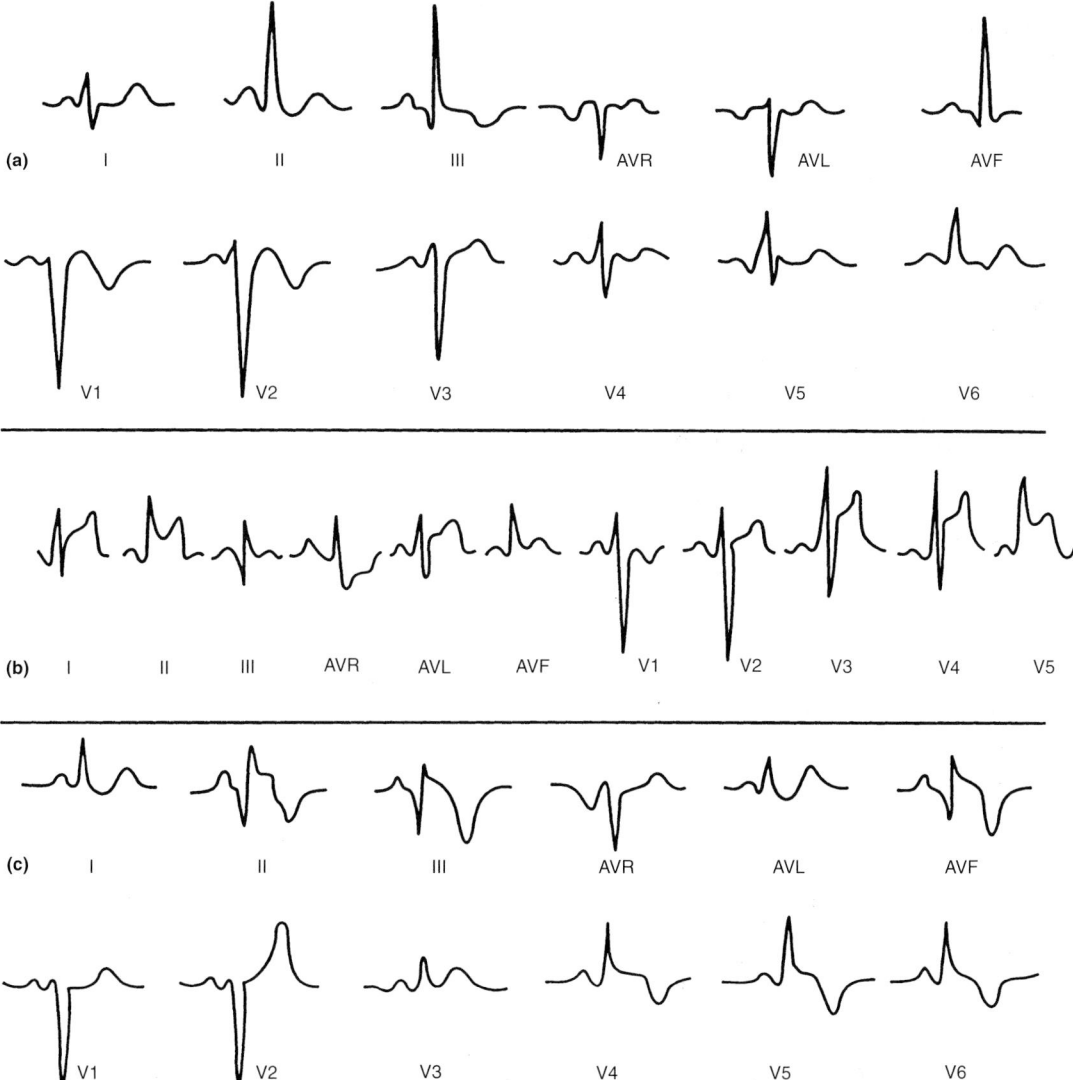

Fig. 36.3 *Typical ECG pattern for specific causes of acute chest pain:* **(a)** *acute pulmonary embolism;* **(b)** *acute pericarditis;* **(c)** *acute inferolateral myocardial infarction*

Exercise thallium scan

This radionuclide myocardial perfusion scan using thallium can complement the exercise ECG.

Ambulatory Holter monitor

This monitor is especially useful for silent ischaemia, variant angina and arrhythmias.

Chest X-ray

Blood glucose

Haemoglobin and blood film

Serum enzymes

Damaged necrosed myocardial tissue releases cellular enzymes, three of which are commonly assayed:

- creatinine kinase (CK) and creatinine kinase–myocardial bound fraction (CK–MB)
- aspartate aminotransferase (AST)
- lactic dehydrogenase (LDH)

Echocardiography

This can be used in the early stages of myocardial infarction to detect abnormalities in heart wall motion, when ECGs and enzymes are not diagnostic. Stress echocardiography is a new technique which is useful where standard exercise testing has been unhelpful.

Isotope scanning

1. Technetium 99 m pyrophosphate studies:
   A. myocardium: to diagnose posterolateral myocardial infarction in the presence of bundle branch block
   B. pulmonary: to diagnose pulmonary embolism
2. Gated blood pool nuclear scan (radionuclide ventriculography)—this scan tests left ventricular function at rest and exercise in patients with myocardial ischaemia.

Angiography (arteriography)

Angiography should be selective:

1. coronary—to evaluate coronary arteries
2. pulmonary—to diagnose pulmonary thromboembolism

Transoesophageal echocardiography (TOE)

This investigation is for dissecting aneurysm (immediate diagnosis).

Oesophageal studies

- endoscopy
- barium swallow
- oesophageal manometry
- radionuclide transit studies

Spine—X-ray

- cervical spine
- thoracic spine

Site, radiation and features of chest pain syndromes

Myocardial infarction and angina

The typical retrosternal distribution is shown in Figure 36.4. Retrosternal pain or pain situated across the chest anteriorly should be regarded as cardiac until proved otherwise.

The wide variation of sites of pain, umbilicus to jaw, including neck, inside of arms, epigastrium and interscapular, should always be kept in mind (Fig. 36.5). Pain is referred into the left arm twenty times more commonly than into the right arm.

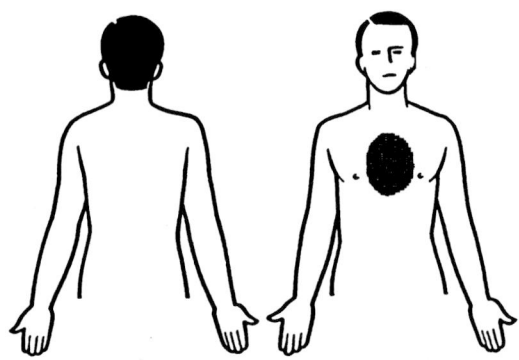

Fig. 36.4 *Pain of myocardial ischaemia: typical site*

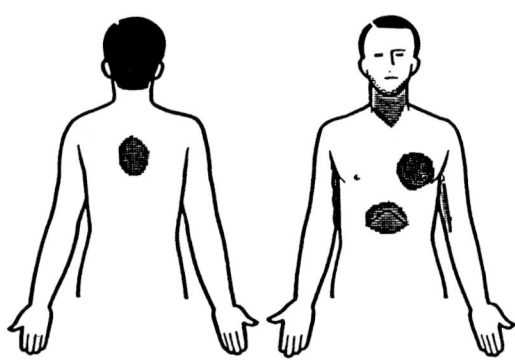

Fig. 36.5 *Pain of myocardial ischaemia: other sites*

The quality of the pain is usually typical. The patient often uses the clenched fist sign to illustrate a sense of constriction.

The radiation of pain will assist in differentiating ischaemic pain from that caused by pericarditis. Enquiry about precipitating and relieving factors will enable a differentiation to be made between ischaemic pain and the almost identical pain caused by reference from the spine.

If a retrosternal pain almost identical with that of myocardial ischaemia is precipitated not by exertion but by bending, lifting, straining or lying down, oesophageal reflux and spasm is a possible diagnosis. This is frequently confused with ischaemic heart disease and can cause radiation into the left arm.

The types of acute coronary syndromes are summarised in Table 36.2.

1. *Myocardial infarction.* Ischaemic pain lasting longer than 15 to 20 minutes is usually infarction. The pain is typically heavy and crushing, and can vary from mild to intense. Occasionally the attack is painless, typically in diabetics. Pallor, sweating and vomiting may accompany the attack.
2. *Stable Angina.* The pain tends to last a few minutes only (average 3–5 minutes) and is relieved by rest and glyceryl trinitrate (nitroglycerine). The pain may be precipitated by an arrhythmia.
3. *Unstable Angina.* This term includes rest angina, new onset effort angina, post infarct angina and post coronary procedure angina. Severe ischaemic chest pain can last 15–20 minutes or more. It is classified as low risk or high risk 'minor myocardial damage'.

Dissecting aneurysm

The pain, which is usually sudden, severe and midline, has a tearing sensation and is usually situated retrosternally and between the scapulae (Fig. 36.6). It radiates to the abdomen, flank and legs. An important diagnostic feature is the inequality in the pulses, e.g. carotid, radial and femoral. There may also be occlusion of the coronary or renal arteries with appropriate symptoms and signs. Hemiplegia, aortic incompetence or cardiac tamponade can occur.

Fig. 36.6 *Pain of dissecting aneurysm*

Pulmonary embolism

This has a dramatic onset following occlusion of the pulmonary artery or a major branch, especially if more than 50% of the cross-sectional area of the pulmonary trunk is occluded.

The diagnosis can present clinical difficulties, especially when dyspnoea is present without pain. Embolism usually presents with retrosternal chest pain (Fig. 36.7) and may be associated with syncope and breathlessness. In addition, hypotension, acute right heart failure or cardiac arrest occurs with a massive embolus. The physical examination can be deceptively

Table 36.2 *Types of acute coronary syndromes*

	Serum markers		
	Creatine Kinase	*Troponin*	*ECG at evaluation*
Unstable angina			
• low risk	normal	non–detectable	normal
• high risk	normal	detectable	ST depression
Myocardial infarction			
• non–ST elevation	elevated	detectable	ST depression, no Q wave
• ST elevation	elevated	detectable	± Q wave

Fig. 36.7 *Pain of pulmonary embolism*

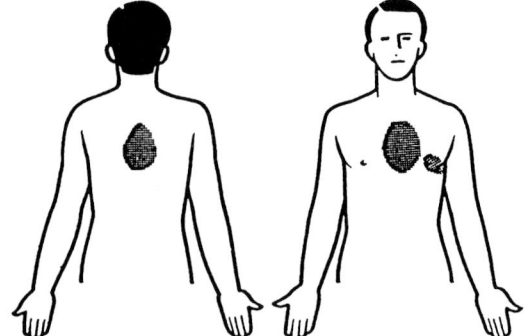

Fig. 36.8 *Pain of pericarditis*

normal. Pulmonary infarction is generally less dramatic than embolism and it is usually accompanied by pleuritic chest pain and haemoptysis. It complicates embolism in about 10% of patients.

Pleurisy
Inflammation of the pleura is due to underlying pneumonia (viral or bacterial), pulmonary infarction, tumour infiltration or connective tissue disease, e.g. SLE.

Features
- often sudden onset
- pain usually localised without radiation
- sharp knife-like pain
- continuous pain with sharp exacerbations
- aggravated by inspiration and coughing
- may be associated dyspnoea, cough, haemoptysis

Acute pericarditis
Pericarditis causes three distinct types of pain:
1. pleuritic (the commonest), aggravated by cough and deep inspiration, sometimes brought on by swallowing
2. steady, crushing, retrosternal pain that mimics myocardial infarction
3. pain synchronous with the heartbeat and felt over the praecordium and left shoulder

Occasionally two and rarely all three types of pain may be present simultaneously (Fig. 36.8).

Spontaneous pneumothorax
The acute onset of pleuritic pain and dyspnoea in a patient with a history of asthma or emphysema is the hallmark of a pneumothorax. It often occurs in young slender males without a history of lung disorders. The pain varies from

mild to severe and can be felt anywhere in the chest, sometimes being retrosternal. Typical pain distribution is shown in Figure 36.9.

If a tension pneumothorax becomes painful and dyspnoea becomes rapidly more intense, urgent decompression of air is essential. A comparison of the serious causes of acute chest pain is summarised in Table 36.3.

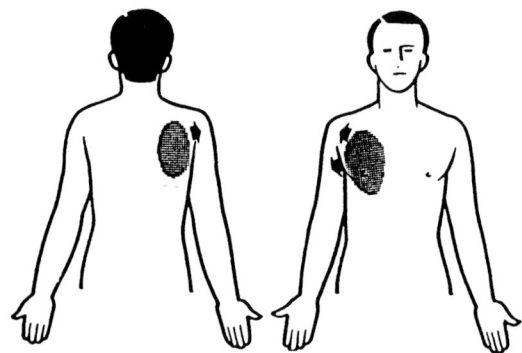

Fig. 36.9 *Pain of pneumothorax (right side)*

Oesophageal pain
Gastro-oesophageal reflux can cause oesophagitis characterised by a burning epigastric or retrosternal pain that may radiate to the jaw. The pain is aggravated or precipitated by lying flat or bending over, especially after meals, and is more frequent at night. The pain is worse if oesophageal spasm is present. Oesophageal motor disorders including spasm may occur in isolation. The pain may radiate uncommonly to the back (Fig. 36.10). It may be precipitated by eating, especially hot or cold food and drink, and may be relieved by eating or by glyceryl trinitrate (nitroglycerine) and other nitrates. Features differentiating angina-like oesophageal pain and cardiac pain are presented in Table

Table 36.3 *A comparison of the serious causes of acute chest pain*

	Myocardial infarction	Angina	Pulmonary embolus	Dissecting aneurysm	Pericarditis	Pneumothorax
Pain intensity	+ → ++++	+	+ → +++	+++++	+ → +++	+ → +++
Pain quality	Heavy Crushing Vice-like Burning	Heavy Aching Tightness Burning	Dull Heavy	Tearing Searing	Heavy Aching ± sharp	Tightness Sharp Stabbing
Pain site	Deep retrosternal	Deep retrosternal	Retrosternal	Anterior chest	Sternal surface	Lateral chest
Pain radiation	Throat/lower jaw Left arm (often) Right arm (uncommon) Back (uncommon)	As for infarction	Lateral chest (pleuritic)	Front to back of chest Down back to abdomen Arms	Left arm (uncommon) Right arm (rare) Throat (rare)	Lateral chest
History	Family, risk factors	Family, risk factors	Phlebitis Calf pain Immobility Surgery	Atherosclerosis Hypertension ? Marfan's	Viral infection M. infarction	Asthma COAD Old TB
Associated symptoms	Pallor, nausea, sweating, vomiting, dyspnoea, syncope	Strangling in throat	Dyspnoea, syncope, sweating, vomiting, cyanosis, agitation, ?haemoptysis	Syncope, pallor, cyanosis, Neurological • hemiparesis • paraplegia	Fever, malaise ± pleuritic pain	Dyspnoea, cough, ? cyanosis
Pulse	variable ? arrhythmias	variable ? arrhythmias	tachycardia	unequal some ?absent	weak if effusion	tachycardia
Cardiac auscultation	± gallop rhythm murmur of MI	S_3 during attack	↓ pulmonary S_2 S_3 or S_4	± murmur of AI	± pericardial friction rub	
Chest auscultation	basal crackles		± adventitious sounds			hyper-resonant ↓ breath sounds ↑ percussion
Chest X-ray			± localised oligaemia or infarction	widening of mediastinum	↑ cardiac silhouette if effusion	diagnostic— expiration film
ECG	Q waves ST elevation T inversion	normal or ST depression	normal or R heart strain S_1, Q_3, T_3	may show myocardial infarction	elevated S–T segments	
Special definitive diagnostic tests	• serum enzmes CK, CK–MB, AST, LDH • cardiac scanning	• stress ECG • coronary angiography	• lung scanning • pulmonary angiography	• TOE • ultrasound • aortic angiography • CT scan	• echocardio- graphy (if effusion)	

36.4.[2] Gastrointestinal causes of chest pain are summarised in Table 36.5.[1]

Spinal pain

The commonest cause of pain of spinal origin is vertebral dysfunction of the lower cervical or upper dorsal region. The spinal problem may be a disc prolapse (relatively common in the lower cervical spine, but rare in the upper thoracic spine) or dysfunction of the facet joints or costovertebral joints causing referred pain. This referred pain can be present anywhere in the chest wall including anterior chest, which causes confusion with cardiac pain (Fig. 36.11). The pain is dull and aching. It may be aggravated by exertion, certain body movements or deep

Fig. 36.10 *Oesophageal pain*

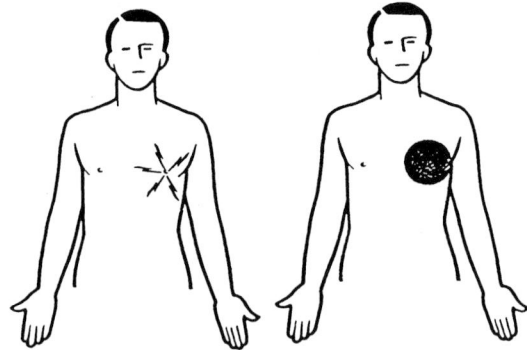

Fig. 36.12 *Typical sites of psychogenic pain*

Fig. 36.11 *Possible pain sites for thoracic spinal dysfunction (left side)*

inspiration. The old trap for unilateral nerve root pain is herpes zoster.

Psychogenic pain

Psychogenic chest pain can occur anywhere in the chest, but often it is located in the left submammary region, usually without radiation (Fig. 36.12). It tends to be continuous and sharp or stabbing. It may mimic angina but tends to last for hours or days. It is usually aggravated by tiredness or emotional tension and may be associated with shortness of breath, fatigue and palpitations.

Chest pain in children

Chest pain in children is rarely the result of serious pathology but is an important complaint especially in adolescents. A United States study has shown that the mean age for childhood chest pain is 11.9 years.[3,4] Most cases are of unknown aetiology (probably psychogenic), while common causes include musculoskeletal disorders, cough-induced pain, costochondritis, psychogenic disturbance (includes hyperventilation) and asthma. See Table 36.6.

Chest pain in children less than 12 years old is more likely to have a cardiorespiratory cause such as cough, asthma, pneumonia or heart disease, while chest pain in adolescents is more likely to be associated with a psychogenic disturbance.

Causes of musculoskeletal pain include strains to pectoral, shoulder or back muscles after excessive exercise, and minor trauma from sports such as football or wrestling.

Breast problems can present as chest pain.

Costochondritis

This causes mild to moderate anterior chest wall pain that may radiate to the chest, back or abdomen. It is usually unilateral, sharp in nature

Table 36.4 *Features differentiating angina-like, oesophageal pain and cardiac pain*[2]

	Favour oesophageal	*Favour cardiac*	*Non-discriminating*
Precipitating factors	Meals, posture	Consistently with exercise	Emotion
Relieving factors	Antacids		Rest, nitrates
Radiation	Epigastrium	Arm	Back
Associated symptoms	Heartburn, regurgitation, dysphagia	Dyspnoea	Sweating

Table 36.5   *A comparison of gastrointestinal causes of chest pain*

	Acid reflux	*Oesophageal spasm*	*Peptic ulcer*	*Gall bladder disease*
Site	• Epigastric	• Deep retrosternal	• Deep retrosternal	• Right hypochondrium
Radiation	• Retrosternal • Throat	• Back	• To back (DU)	• Below right scapula • Tip right shoulder
Quality	• Burning	• Constricting	• Gnawing	• Deep ache
Precipitation	• Heavy meals • Wine/coffee • Lying • Bending	• Eating hot/cold food and drinks	• Eating GU–30 mins DU–2 to 3 hrs	• Fatty food
Relief	• Standing • Antacids	• Antispasmodics • Nitroglycerine	• Antacids	
Associated symptoms	• Water brash	• Dysphagia	• Dyspepsia	• Flatulence • Dyspepsia

GU—gastric ulcer
DU—duodenal ulcer

Table 36.6   *Common causes of chest pain in children*

Cause	%
Idiopathic	21
Musculoskeletal	16
Cough	10
Costochondritis	9
Psychogenic	9
Asthma	7
Trauma	5
Pneumonia	4
GIT problems	4
Cardiovascular	4

Source: Adapted from Selbst[3]

and exaggerated by breathing, physical activity or a specific position. It may be preceded by exercise or an URTI and can persist for several months. It is diagnosed by eliciting tenderness at the chondrosternal junction of the affected ribs and needs to be differentiated from Tietze's syndrome where there is a tender, fusiform swelling at the chondrosternal junction.

Cardiac causes
Myocardial ischaemia is very rare in children but should be considered in any child with exercise-induced chest pain, adolescents with long-standing diabetes and children with sickle-cell anaemia.

Precordial catch (Texidor's twinge or stitch in the side)
This common complaint presents as a unilateral low chest pain that lasts a few seconds or minutes, typically with exercise such as long-distance running. The pain is relieved by straightening up and taking very slow deep breaths followed by shallow breaths.

Chest pain in the elderly
Chest pain is a very important symptom in the elderly as the life-threatening cardiovascular conditions—myocardial infarction and angina, dissecting aneurysm and ruptured aorta—are an increasing manifestation with age. In a community survey in Glasgow 20% of men and 12% of women over 65 were found to have ischaemic heart disease.[5] The elderly patient presenting with chest pain is most likely to have angina or myocardial infarction. Other important disorders to consider are herpes zoster, cough fracture of the rib, malignancy, pleurisy, pulmonary embolus and gastro-oesophageal reflux.

Angina pectoris
Main features
• There is a 2–3% incidence between 25 and 64 years.[6]
• The history is the basis of diagnosis.
• Angina is an oppressive discomfort rather than a pain.
• It is mainly retrosternal: radiates to arms, jaw, throat, back.
• It may be associated with shortness of breath.
• It occurs during exercise, emotion, after meals or in cold.
• It is relieved within a few minutes with rest.

- Physical examination is usually not helpful, except during an attack.
- Mitral valve prolapse, oesophageal spasm and dissecting aneurysm are important differential diagnoses.
- The causes of angina are summarised in Table 36.7.

Note: Ensure that the patient is not anaemic or thyrotoxic. Fever and tachycardia also have to be excluded.

Table 36.7 *Causes of angina*

Coronary artery atheroma
Valvular lesions, e.g. aortic stenosis
Rapid arrhythmias
Anaemia
Rarities
- trauma
- collagen disease

Variants of angina

1. *Stable angina.* Pain occurs with exertion and is usually predictable.
2. *Unstable angina* (also referred to as crescendo angina, pre-infarct angina and acute coronary insufficiency). It is increasing angina (severity and duration) over a short period of time, precipitated by less effort and may come on at rest, especially at night. It may eventually lead to complete infarction, often with relief of symptoms.
   Nocturnal angina. Pain occurs during the night. It is related to unstable angina.
   Decubitus angina. The pain occurs when lying flat and is relieved by sitting up.
   Variant angina or Prinzmetal angina or spasm angina.[7] The pain occurs at rest and without apparent cause. It is associated with typical transient ECG changes of ST elevation (as compared with the classical changes of ST depression during effort angina). It can lead to infarction and cause arrhythmias. It is caused by coronary artery spasm.

Aids to diagnosis

ECG. This may be normal or show ischaemia or evidence of earlier infarction. During an attack it may be normal or show well-marked depression of the ST segment, symmetrical T-wave inversion (Fig. 36.13) or tall upright T waves.

Exercise ECG. This is positive in about 75% of patients with severe coronary artery disease and

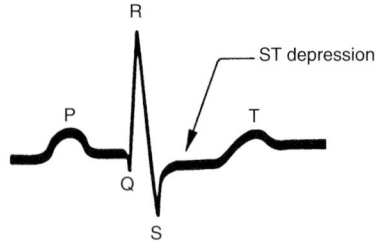

Fig. 36.13 *Typical ECG pattern for angina pectoris: this tracing is usually observed during an attack. Note: There is no specific ECG of angina; the most that can be said is that an ECG is consistent with angina*

should be performed if the diagnosis is in doubt, for prognostic reasons or to aid in the timing of additional investigations, e.g. coronary angiography. A normal stress test does not rule out coronary artery disease.

Exercise thallium 201 scan. This very expensive test is helpful in some difficult circumstances such as in the presence of LBBB, old infarction and WPW syndrome (when exercise test is of little use) and with mitral valve prolapse, which gives high false positive tests. It helps determine the presence and extent of reversible myocardial ischaemia since thallium is only taken up by perfused tissue.

Ambulatory Holter monitoring. This may be useful in some patients.

Gated blood pool nuclear scan. This test assesses the ejection fraction, which is a reliable index of ventricular function and thus aids assessment of patients for coronary artery bypass surgery.

Echocardiography. This assesses global and regional wall motion abnormalities and assesses valvular dysfunction and pericardium status.

Coronary angiography. This test accurately outlines the extent and severity of coronary artery disease. It is usually used to determine the precise coronary artery anatomy prior to surgery.

The relationship between the degree of angina and coronary artery disease is not clear cut. Some people with severe angina have normal coronary arteries.

Indications for coronary angiography are presented in Table 36.8.

'Ultrafast CT' may replace angiography.

Table 36.8 *Indications for coronary angiography*

- Strong positive exercise stress test
- Suspected left main CAD
- Unstable or variant angina
- Angina resistant to medical treatment
- Suspected but not otherwise proven angina
- Angina or myocardial infarction in young person < 50
- Angina after myocardial infarction
- Patients over 30 with aortic and mitral valve disease being considered for valve surgery

Management of angina

Prevention

This is especially important for those with a positive family history and an unsatisfactory lifestyle. Modification of risk factors:

- no smoking
- weight reduction
- optimal low-fat diet
- control of hypertension
- control of diabetes

General advice for the stable angina patient

- Reassure patient that angina has a reasonably good prognosis.
  - — 30% survive more than 10 years.[8]
  - — Spontaneous remission can occur.
- Attend to any risk factors.
- If inactive, take on an activity such as walking for 20 minutes a day.
- Take regular exercise to the threshold of angina.
- If tense and stressed, cultivate a more relaxed attitude to life—consider a stress management/relaxation course.
- Avoid precipitating factors.
- Don't excessively restrict lifestyle.

Medical treatment

The acute attack[9]

- glyceryl trinitrate (nitroglycerin) 600 µg tab or 300 µg (½ tab) sublingually (SL)

Alternatives

- isosorbide dinitrate 5 mg SL every 5 min (to maximum of 3)

or

- glyceryl trinitrate SL spray: 1–2 sprays to maximum of 3 in 15 minutes

or

- nifedipine 5 mg capsule (suck or chew) if intolerant of nitrates

Tips about glyceryl trinitrate tablets
- Warn patient about headache and other side effects.
- Sit down to take the tablet.
- Take ½ (initially) or 1 tablet every 5 minutes.
- Take a maximum of 3 tablets in 15 minutes.
- Tablets must be fresh.
- Discard the bottle opened for 3 months or after 2 days if carried on the person.
- Keep tablets out of light and heat.
- If pain relieved quickly, spit out residual tablet.
- Advise patient to get medical advice if no relief after 3 tablets.

Mild stable angina (angina that is predictable, precipitated by more stressful activities and relieved rapidly):
- aspirin 150 mg (o) daily
- gyceryl trinitrate (SL or spray) prn
- consider a beta-blocker or long-acting nitrate or nicorandil

Moderate stable angina (regular predictable attacks precipitated by moderate exertion):
add • beta-blocker, e.g. atenolol 25–100 mg (o) once daily

or

metoprolol 25–100 mg (o) once daily
- glyceryl trinitrate (transdermal: ointment or patches) daily (use for 12–16 hours only)

or

isosorbide mononitrate 60 mg (o) SR tablet mane
- consider calcium antagonist therapy as an alternative to a beta-blocker
  Note: Aim for a daily nitrate-free interval.

Persistent angina (not prevented by beta-blocker):
add a dihydropyridine Ca channel blocker (must have beta-blocker cover)
- nifedipine 10–20 mg (o) bd

or

nifedipine controlled release 30–60 mg (o) once daily

or

amlodipine or felodipine 2.5–10 mg (o) once daily
If beta-blocker contraindicated (use a non-dihydropyridine Ca channel blocker)

• diltiazem 60–90 mg (o) tds

or

verapamil (according to directions)

Consider potassium channel opener e.g. nicorandil

| Unstable angina | (includes onset of angina at rest, abrupt worsening of angina and angina following acute myocardial infarction):

Should be hospitalised for stabilisation and further evaluation. May need IV nitrate therapy.

The objectives are to optimise therapy and consider coronary angiography with a view to a corrective procedure.

Rules of practice

• For variant angina (spasm) use nitrates and calcium antagonist (avoid beta-blockers).
• As a rule avoid the combination of verapamil and a beta-blocker.
• Tolerance to nitrate use is a problem, so 24-hr coverage with long-acting preparations is not recommended.
• Consider using the newer vasodilator nicorandil 10–20 mg (o) bd.

Non-medical treatment

Coronary angioplasty

The current technique is dilating coronary atheromatous obstructions by inflating a balloon against the obstruction (Fig. 36.14). Other methods (which may supplant the balloon) include arthrectomy with laser devices or maintaining patency with intracoronary stent devices.

Two complications of the balloon inflation angioplasty are acute coronary occlusion (2–4%) and restenosis, which occurs in 30% in the first 6 months after angioplasty.[8]

Coronary artery surgery

The main surgical techniques in current use are coronary artery bypass grafting (CABG) using either a vein (usually the saphenous) (Fig. 36.15) or internal mammary arterial implantation (Fig. 36.16) or both and endarterectomy.

Symptomatic patients with significant left main coronary obstruction should undergo bypass surgery, and those with two or three

Fig. 36.14 *Percutaneous transluminal angioplasty with an inflatable balloon*

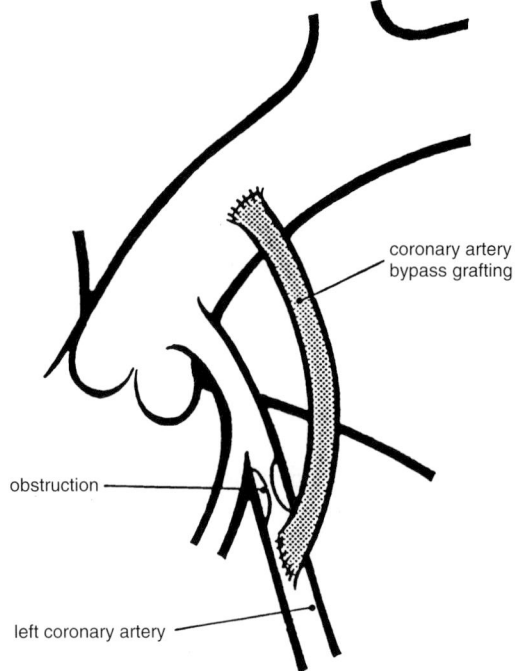

Fig. 36.15 *Coronary artery bypass grafting to relieve coronary obstruction*

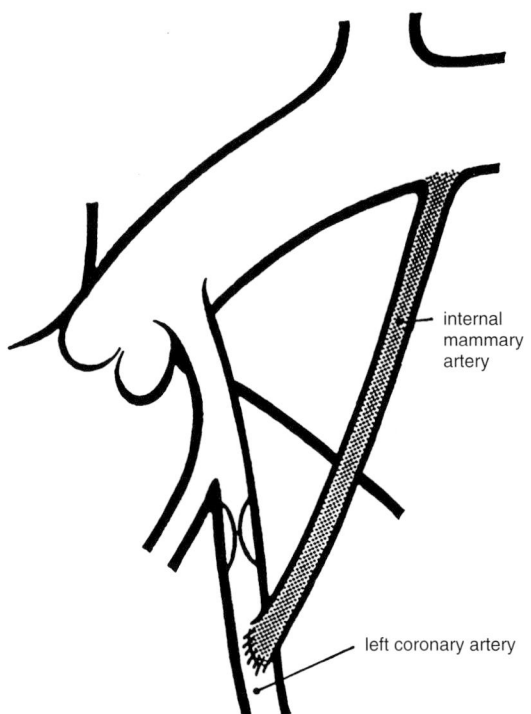

Fig. 36.16 *Internal mammary arterial transplantation to relieve coronary obstruction*

vessel obstruction and good ventricular function are often considered for angioplasty or surgery. A significant improvement in the quantity and quality of life can be expected.

Myocardial infarction
Clinical guidelines
- variable pain; may be mistaken for indigestion
- similar to angina but more oppressive
- so severe, patient may fear imminent death—*angor animi*
- about 20% have no pain
- 'silent infarcts' in diabetics, hypertensives and elderly
- 60% of those who die do so before reaching hospital, within 2 hours of the onset of symptoms
- hospital mortality is 8–10%[10]
- like CVA seems to peak at 6–10 am.
- diagnosis is based on 2 out of 3 criteria: history of prolonged ischaemic pain, typical ECG appearance, and rise and fall of cardiac enzymes

Aetiology
- thrombosis with occlusion
- haemorrhage under a plaque
- coronary artery spasm

Physical signs
These may be:

- no abnormal signs
- pale/grey, clammy, dyspnoeic
- restless and apprehensive
- variable BP ↑ with pain
            ↓ heart pump failure
- variable pulse: watch for bradyarrhythmias
- mild cardiac failure: 3rd or 4th heart sound, basal crackles

Investigations
1. *ECG.* The ECG is valuable with characteristic changes in a full thickness infarction. The features (Fig. 36.17) are:
   - The Q wave: broad (> 1 mm) and deep > 25% length R wave
     — occurs normally in leads AVR and V₁; III (sometimes)
     — abnormal if in other leads
     — occurs also with LBBB, WPW and VT
     — usually permanent feature after full thickness AMI

- T wave and ST segment
  — transient changes (inversion and elevation respectively).

The typical progression is shown in Figure 36.18.

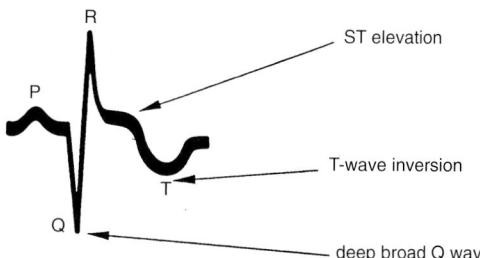

Fig 36.17 *Typical ECG features of myocardial infarction, illustrating a Q wave, ST elevation and T-wave inversion*

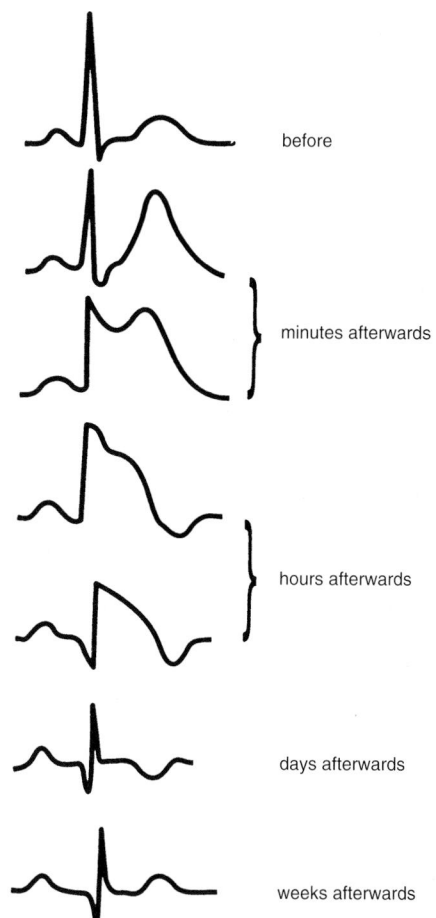

Fig. 36.18 *Typical evolution of ECG changes with myocardial infarction*

Note: • Q waves do not develop in subendocardial infarction.
  • A normal ECG, especially early, does not exclude AMI.

2. *Cardiac enzymes.* The typical enzyme patterns are presented in Figure 36.19. As a rule large infarcts tend to produce high serum enzyme levels. The elevated enzymes can help time the infarct:
   • Troponin I or T
     — Starts rising at 4–6 hours, peaks at 10 hours and persists for several days.
     — Now the preferred test.
     — Positive in unstable angina.
   • Creatinine kinase (CK)
     — After delay of 6–8 hours from the onset of pain it peaks at 20–24 hours and usually returns to normal by 48 hours.
     — CK–MB: myocardial necrosis is present if > 15% of total CK. Unlike CK, it is not affected by intramuscular injections.
   • Aspartate transferase (AST): formerly SGOT
     — It is slower to peak in the plasma (24–48 hours) and persists longer than CK.
     — It may fall to normal by 72 hours.
   • Lactic dehydrogenase (LD)
     — It peaks at 3–4 days and remains elevated for 7–14 days.

3. *Technetium pyrophosphate scanning*
   • It is performed from 24 hours to 14 days after onset.
   • It scans for 'hot spots', especially when a posterolateral AMI is suspected and ECG is unhelpful because of pre-existing LBBB.

4. *Echocardiography.* This is used to assist diagnosis when other tests are not diagnostic.

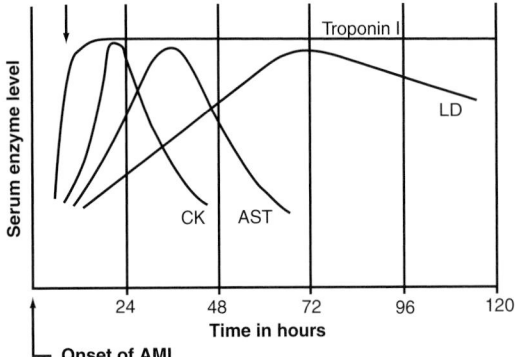

Fig. 36.19 *Typical cardiac enzyme patterns following myocardial infarction*

Note: The clinical diagnosis may be the most reliable, as the ECG and enzymes may be negative.

Management of myocardial infarction

General principles:[10]
• Aim for immediate attendance if suspected.
• Call a mobile coronary care unit, especially if severe.
• Optimal treatment is in a modern coronary care unit (if possible) with continuous ECG monitoring (first 48 hours), a peripheral IV line and intranasal oxygen.
• Pay careful attention to relief of pain and apprehension.
• Establish a caring empathy with the patient.
• Consider all patients for thrombolytic therapy, e.g. streptokinase (the sooner the better).
• Give aspirin as early as possible (if no contraindications).
• Prescribe a beta-blocker drug early (if no contraindications).
• Prevent possible sudden death in early stages from ventricular fibrillation by monitoring and availability of a defibrillator.

First-line management, e.g. outside hospital
• oxygen 4–6 L/min
• secure an IV line
• glyceryl trinitrate (nitroglycerin)
  300 μg (½ tab) SL (every 5 minutes as necessary to maximum of 3 doses)
  (beware of sildenafil (Viagra) use and bradycardia—correct with atropine)
• aspirin 300 mg
• morphine 5 mg IV statim bolus: 1 mg/min until pain relief (up to 15 mg)
  ± metoclopramide 10 mg IV (as antiemetic)
  (If feasible it is preferable to give IV morphine 1 mg/min until relief of pain; this titration is easier in hospital.)

Hospital management
• As for first-line management.
• Take blood for cardiac enzymes, urea and electrolytes.
• Consider urgent infarct embolectomy.
• Consider streptokinase:
  — 1 500 000 units IV infusion over 30–45 min (aim for 30 minutes and if problems such as hypotension occur slow down the infusion)

Rules for streptokinase infusion:

- must have ECG evidence of AMI
- ideal if evidence of transmural infarct
- need informed consent
- the earlier given, the lower the mortality
- give within 3–4 hours of onset AMI (max. 6 hrs)
- monitor for hypotension, allergy and arrhythmias
- local bleeding a problem but usually minor and controlled by local pressure
- contraindications
  - active bleeding
  - recent CVA/TIA (within 6 months)
  - poorly controlled hypertension
  - history of bleeding peptic ulcer
  - recent arterial (e.g. femoral) puncture
  - recent prolonged CPR
- do not use 3 days to 12 months after prior use; instead use recombinant tissue plasminogen activator (rt-PA)

  Note: Streptokinase and alteplase (rt-PA) are of similar efficiency but rt-PA is much more expensive (about 20 times).

- Full heparinisation for 24–36 hours (after rt-PA—not after streptokinase), especially for large anterior transmural infarction with risk of embolisation, supplemented by warfarin.
- Beta-blocker (if no thrombolytic therapy or contraindications) as soon as possible:

  atenolol 2–10 mg IV or 25 mg (o) statim → 25–50 mg (o) mane

  or

  metoprolol 5–10 mg IV or 25 mg (o) statim → 50 mg (o) bd

- Treat complications as necessary.
- Consider glyceryl trinitrate IV infusion if pain recurs.
- Consider early introduction of ACE inhibitors (after day 1) in those with significant left ventricular dysfunction.
- Treat hypokalaemia.
- Consider magnesium sulphate (after thrombolysis).
- Consider frusemide.

Ongoing management
- education and counselling
- bed rest 24–48 hours
- check serum potassium and magnesium
- early mobilisation to full activity over 7–12 days
- light diet

- sedation
- beta-blocker (o): atenolol or metoprolol
- warfarin where indicated (certainly if evidence of thrombus with echocardiography)
- consider ACE inhibitors for left ventricular failure and to prevent remodelling

On discharge
- rehabilitation program
- continued education and counselling
- no smoking
- reduce weight
- regular exercise, especially walking
- exercise test (to be considered)
- continue beta-blockers for 2 years
- consider ACE inhibitors
- aspirin 100–150 mg daily
- warfarin where indicated (at least 3 months)

Special management issues
Indications for coronary angiography
- development of angina
- strongly positive exercise test
- consider after use of streptokinase

Management of the extensive infarction
- ACE inhibitors (even if no CCF)
- radionuclide studies (to assess left ventricular function)
- beta-blockers (proven value in severe infarction) if no contraindications or LV dysfunction
- anticoagulation

> *Treating and recognising complications of AMI*

Acute left ventricular failure

Signs:
- basal crackles
- extra (3rd or 4th) heart sounds
- X-ray changes

Treatment: (according to severity)
- oxygen
- diuretic, e.g. frusemide
- glyceryl trinitrate: IV, SL, (o) or topical
- ACE inhibitors

Cardiogenic shock (a major hospital management procedure)

Dobutamine

Intra-aortic balloon pump

Urgent angiography ± angioplasty/surgery

Pericarditis. This occurs in first few days after AMI (usually anterior AMI), with onset of sharp pain.

Signs:
- pericardial friction rub

Treatment:
- anti-inflammatory medication
  e.g. aspirin 600 mg (o) 4 hourly
  or
  indomethacin 25 mg (o)
  4 hourly (or by suppository)
  or
  corticosteroids (keep in
  reserve)

Note: Avoid anticoagulants.

Post-AMI syndrome (Dressler's syndrome). This occurs weeks or months later, usually around 6 weeks.

Features:
- pericarditis
- fever
- pericardial effusion (an auto-immune response)

Treatment:
- as for pericarditis

Left ventricular aneurysm. This is a late complication.

Clinical:
Features:
- cardiac failure
- arrhythmias
- embolisation

Signs:
- double ventricular impulse
- 4th heart sound
- visible bulge on X-ray

Diagnosis:
- 2D electrocardiography

Treatment:
- antiarrhythmic drugs
- anticoagulants
- medication for cardiac failure
- possible aneurysmectomy

Ventricular septal rupture and mitral valve papillary rupture. This presents with severe cardiac failure and a loud pansystolic murmur. Both have a poor prognosis and early surgical intervention may be appropriate.

Management of other serious causes of chest pain

Dissecting aneurysm
- Early definitive diagnosis is necessary: best achieved by transoesophageal echocardiography.
- 50% of patients are hypertensive; so need pharmacological control of hypertension with IV nitroprusside beta-blockers.
- Emergency surgery needed for many, especially for type A (ascending aorta involved).

  Note: There is an increased risk during pregnancy.

Pulmonary embolus
Needs supportive medical care and anti-coagulation:
- Heparin IV: 5000 U as immediate bolus
  continuous infusion 30 000 U over 24 hours
  or
  heparin 12 500 U (sc) bd

  Note: The dose of heparin should then be adjusted daily to maintain the APTT between 1.5 and 2 times control.
- Continue heparin 5–10 days.
- Warfarin (o) after 3 to 4 days; then continue heparin for 3 days after INR at desired level.

  Note: Thrombolytic therapy either IV or into the pulmonary artery can be used for major embolism. Surgical embolectomy is rarely necessary but needed if very extensive.

Ruptured oesophagus
Refer for early thoracotomy and repair of the defect, usually a longitudinal repair in the supra-diaphragmatic lower oesophagus—with mediastinal and pleural drainage.[12]

Pneumothorax
- Most episodes resolve spontaneously without drainage (at least 20% lung collapse).
- Drainage of the pleural space indicated for a large pneumothorax > 30% pleural area, with persistent dyspnoea.
- For recurrent attacks, excision of cysts or pleurodesis may be necessary.

Methods
1. *Simple aspiration without underwater drainage.* Under strict sepsis insert a 16-gauge polyethylene IV catheter into the second intercostal space in the mid-clavicular line on the affected side (under local anaesthetic). Then aspirate air into a 20 mL syringe to confirm entry into the pleural space, remove the stilette, connect the catheter via a flexible extension tube to a three-way tap and a 50 mL syringe. Aspirate and expel air via the three-way tap until resistance indicates lung re-expansion. Obtain a follow-up X-ray. Repeat aspiration may be necessary, but most patients do not require inpatient admission.

2. *Standard intercostal catheter insertion with connection to an underwater seal drainage*

| Acute tension pneumothorax |

For urgent cases insert a 12–16 gauge needle into the pleural space through the second intercostal space on the affected side. Replace with a formal intercostal catheter connected to underwater seal drainage.

Treatment of oesophageal disorders

Gastro-oesophageal reflux

- Achieve normal weight if overweight.
- Avoid coffee, alcohol and spicy foods.
- Avoid large meals and overeating (keep to small meals).
- Use antacids or alginate compounds, e.g. Gaviscon, Mylanta Plus.
  If persistent:
    acid suppression
      H$_2$ blockers, e.g. cimetidine, ranitidine
              or
      proton-pump inhibitors, e.g. omeprazole

Oesophageal spasm

      long-acting nitrates, e.g. isosorbide dinitrate 10 mg tds
                  or
      calcium channel blockers, e.g. nifedipine 10 mg tds
Note: Attend to lifestyle and dietary factors, as for reflux.

Oral anticoagulation

Many patients with cardiovascular problems are now being discharged from hospital on oral anticoagulants (warfarin) or aspirin (150–300 mg daily). A greater responsibility rests with the patient's GP for careful monitoring of this anticoagulation lest bleeding, including intracerebral haemorrhage, occurs. For all practical purposes the only orally active anticoagulant is warfarin. Indications and contraindications are presented in Table 36.9.

Warfarin

Actions[11]

- antagonises vitamin K
- depresses factors VII, IX and X (half-life of 30–40 hours)

Table 36.9   *Warfarin anticoagulation*

Indications

- Prosthetic cardiac valves
- Deep venous thrombosis
- Deep venous thrombosis, pulmonary thromboembolism
- Atrial fibrillation (selected cases)
- Transient ischaemic attacks
- Severe peripheral vascular disease
- Perioperatively in lower limb orthopaedic surgery (low dose)
- Postcoronary bypass surgery (selected cases)

Contraindications

- Active bleeding
- Recent surgery
- History of intracranial haemorrhage
- Uncontrolled hypertension
- Liver disease with impaired synthetic function— based on international normalised ratio (INR)
- Pregnancy

- achieves full anticoagulation effect after 3–4 days
- prothrombin time (INR ratio) of 2 times normal control indicates therapeutic effect
- duration of effect is 2–3 days
- antidote is vitamin K

Initiation of warfarin treatment

An estimate of the patient's final steady dose is made. The patient is commenced on this dose and the INR monitored daily and the dose altered accordingly.

- Measure INR first to establish baseline.
- Generally warfarin is commenced on same day or day after heparin is commenced.
- Heparin can be ceased when INR > 2 for two consecutive days.
- Typical loading dose is 5–10 mg (o) daily for 2 days (avoid dose > 30 mg over 3 days without INR).
- Adjust the dosage according to the INR table (Table 36.10) from the third day.
- Establish the INR in the therapeutic range, usually 2–3.
- Maintenance dose is usually reached by day 5.
- The INR reflects the warfarin dose given 48 hours earlier.

Table 36.10 *Warfarin dosages adjustment**

Day	INR	Dose
1	—	5 to 10 mg**
2	—	5 to 10 mg**
3	<2	10 mg
	2.0 to 2.4	5 mg
	2.5 to 2.9	3 mg
	3.0 to 3.4	2 mg
	3.5 to 4.0	1 mg
	> 4.0	nil
4, and until stabilised	< 1.4	10 mg
	1.4 to 1.9	7 mg
	2.0 to 2.4	5 mg
	2.5 to 2.9	4 mg
	3.0 to 3.9	3 mg
	4.0 to 4.5	miss 1 day, then 2 mg
	> 4.5	miss 2 days, then 1 mg

* This table should be used only if the pretreatment INR is normal.

** 5 mg of warfarin should be given to patients who are more likely to be sensitive to warfarin. This includes the elderly, the very ill, the malnourished and patients with abnormal liver function or significant chronic renal failure.

INR measurement schedule

before treatment
on third day
↓
daily for 1 week
↓
2 times daily for 2 weeks
↓
weekly for 4 weeks
↓
monthly

Note: • Warfarin should be continued for 3 to 6 months and longer if major risk factors are present.
• Watch for potential drug interactions.

Recommended target values
• prophylaxis atrial fibrillation   1.5–2.7
• treatment DVT   2–3
• tissue heart valve replacement   2–3
• mechanical heart replacement   2.5–3.5

Overdosage of warfarin

Signs of warfarin overdosage include:

• unexpected bleeding after minor trauma
• epistaxis
• spontaneous bruising
• unusually heavy menstrual bleeding
• gastrointestinal bleeding

Management of overdosage

1. Urgent measurement of INR is required.
2. If the only evidence of overdosage is a small increase of the INR above the therapeutic range, cessation of warfarin for 1 to 2 days followed by a continuation at a lower dose is appropriate.
3. If bleeding is minor, transient action as in point 2 is still appropriate.
4. If bleeding is persistent, or severe, or involves closed body cavities (such as pericardium, intracranial, fascial compartment), urgent admission to hospital is essential. The anticoagulation may need to be reversed by administering oral or parenteral vitamin K. Infusion of fresh frozen plasma may also be necessary.

Drug interactions

There are so many potential interactions between warfarin and other drugs that the following general principles should be applied:

1. Maintain the simplest possible drug regimens. Avoid polypharmacy.
2. Aspirin is contraindicated while the patient is on warfarin because of the combined antiplatelet and anticoagulation effects. The risk of gastrointestinal bleeding is also increased. Other non-steroidal anti-inflammatory drugs should also be avoided (Table 36.11).
3. If the patient's drug regimen must be altered during warfarin therapy then the INR should be followed closely until stable.

Practice tips

• The INR result reflects the warfarin dose administered 48–72 hours earlier.
• Advise and encourage patients to keep a record in an 'anticoagulant diary' of drug dosage and INR results.

Advice to the patient

• Keep to a consistent diet.
• Do not take aspirin or liquid paraffin.
• Always mention that you take warfarin to any doctor, dentist or chemist you are consulting.
• Remember to take tablets strictly as directed and have your blood tests.
• Report signs of bleeding, e.g. black motions, blood in urine, easy bruising, unusual nose bleeds, heavy periods.

Table 36.11 *Some important drug interactions with warfarin*

Effects on warfarin activity	Drug
↑ Increased	allopurinol
	amiodarone
	anabolic steroids
	antibiotics (broad spectrum)
	aspirin—salicylates (high doses)
	chloral hydrate
	cimetidine
	clofibrate
	gemfibrozil
	metronidazole
	miconazole
	NSAIDs
	phenytoin
	proton-pump blockers
	quinidine/quinine
	ranitidine
	sulphonamides
	tamoxifen
	thyroxine
↓ Decreased	antacids
	antihistamines
	barbiturates
	carbamazepine
	cholestyramine (reduced absorption)
	haloperidol
	oestrogen/oral contraceptives
	rifampicin
	vitamin C
Increased or decreased	alcohol
	chloral hydrate
	diuretics
	ranitidine

Table 36.12 *Causes/origins of chest wall pain (front and back)*

Musculoskeletal causes
Injury to thoracic spine → dysfunction
Vertebral fracture
- trauma
- pathological
  - osteoporosis
  - metastatic disease
  - multiple myeloma

Intercostal muscle strains/tears
Rib disorders
- fractures
- slipping rib

Costochondritis
Tietze's syndrome
Fibromyalgia

Non-musculoskeletal causes

Heart	• myocardial infarction
	• angina
	• pericarditis
Great vessels	• dissecting aneurysm
	• pulmonary embolism
Pulmonary	• pulmonary embolus/infarction
	• pneumothorax
	• pneumonia/pleurisy
Oesophagus	• oesophageal rupture
	• oesophageal spasm/reflux
	• oesophagitis
	• aerophagy
Subdiaphragmatic disorder of	• gall bladder
	• stomach } including
	• duodenum } ulcers
	• pancreas
	• subphrenic collection
Miscellaneous infections	• herpes zoster
	• Bornholm disease
	• infective endocarditis

Musculoskeletal causes of chest wall pain

There are many musculoskeletal causes, most of which can be eliminated by the history and physical examination. Some of the causes listed in Table 36.12 are very uncommon and often part of a general disorder such as ankylosing spondylitis. Muscular tears or strains of the chest wall are quite common. A differential diagnosis is a fractured rib including a cough fracture.

Musculoskeletal chest pain is typically aggravated or provoked by movements such as stretching, deep inspiration, sneezing and coughing. The pain tends to be sharp and stabbing in quality but can have a constant aching quality.

Costochondritis is a common cause of anterior pain, which is generally well localised to the costochondral junction and may also be a component of an inflammatory disorder such as one of the spondyloarthropathies.

Management is generally conservative with analgesics, gentle massage with analgesic creams and NSAIDs if there is an inflammatory component. Other measures that can help for very painful chest wall problems are localised injections of local anaesthetic with or without corticosteroids (with care not to penetrate the parietal pleura) and a modified support (especially for rib injuries) in the form of a special elasticised rib belt (called a universal rib belt) that gives excellent support and symptom relief while permitting adequate lung expansion.

Posterior chest (thoracic back) pain

Disorders of the musculoskeletal system represent the most common cause of thoracic (dorsal) back pain, especially dysfunction of the joints of the thoracic spine. Refer to Chapter 34 for more detail. Probably the commonest cause is costovertebral dysfunction caused by overstress of rib articulations with vertebrae (the costovertebral joints). This fact is clearly demonstrated with the midline thoracic back pain following cardiac surgery when these joints are compressed during sternotomy and splaying of the chest walls.

The back pain may be associated with simultaneous referred anterior chest pain or abdominal pain (Fig. 34.4).

Acute thoracic back pain

Although posterior pain is invariably caused by vertebral dysfunction, there are several other important causes including serious bone disease (leading to compression fractures) and life-threatening visceral and vascular causes. Refer to Tables 34.2 and 34.3.

Note: • Intervertebral disc protrusions are rare in the thoracic spine.
• Rarely, a penetrating peptic ulcer can present with mid to lower thoracic back pain.

Management
Management has to be according to the cause. The most appropriate treatment for thoracic spine dysfunction (in the absence of organic disease such as osteoporosis and inflammation, and if the patient is not on anticoagulants) is physical therapy: mobilisation or manipulation, as described in Chapter 34.

When to refer

• Obvious or suspected myocardial infarction, especially with extensive infarction
• Transfer to major centre with complications of AMI
— rupture of septum or papillary muscle
— aneurysm
— refractory arrhythmias
— cardiogenic shock

• Patients with persistent postinfarction angina
• Angina
— patient with angina not responding to drug treatment
— patient with unstable angina
— angina lasting for longer than 15 minutes (unresponsive to sublingual nitrate) needs urgent hospital admission
• Suspected or proven pulmonary embolus or dissecting aneurysm or other serious life-threatening problem (after initial first-line measures, e.g. decompression of tension pneumothorax)
• Suspected oesophageal or other gastrointestinal disorder, e.g. duodenal ulcer, for endoscopy or appropriate gastroenterological evaluation.

Practice tips

• All sudden acute chest pain is cardiac (and potentially fatal) until proven otherwise.
• A careful history is the basis of the diagnosis.
• Mitral valve prolapse is often an undiagnosed cause of chest pain: keep it in mind, especially if pain is recurrent and intermittent (proved by echocardiography).
• Calcium antagonists can cause peripheral oedema so be careful not to attribute this to heart failure.
• The pain of oesophageal spasm can be very severe and mimic myocardial infarction.
• Oesophageal spasm responds to glyceryl trinitrate: do not confuse with angina.
• Intervertebral disc protrusions are a very rare cause of severe sudden thoracic pain (T2–T9).
• Infective endocarditis can cause pleuritic posterior chest pain.
• Family doctors need to monitor carefully patients who are on anticoagulants. The INR ratio, which needs to be kept between 2 and 3, should be tested at least monthly.
• The sudden onset of dyspnoea without chest pain can occur frequently with (painless) myocardial infarction and pulmonary embolism.
• If a patient recovering from an AMI suddenly develops shortness of breath, consider ventricular septal rupture, mitral valve papillary rupture (with mitral regurgitation), pulmonary embolus and other serious complications.

References

1. Sandler G, Fry J. *Early clinical diagnosis*. Lancaster: MTP Press, 1986; 5–24.

2. Lambert J. Chest pain. From *Oesophageal disorders* in Proceedings of Monash University Faculty of Medicine 4th Annual Postgraduate Medical Refresher Course, 1991.

3. Selbst S. Chest pain in children. Amer Fam Physician, January 1990; 179–186.

4. Selbst S, Ruddy R, Clark B et al. Paediatric chest pain: A prospective study. Paediatrics, 1988; 82:319–23.

5. Kennedy RD, Andrews GR, Mitchell JRA. Ischaemic heart disease in the elderly. Br Heart J, 1977; 39:1121–1127.

6. Caspari P. Angina pectoris. In: MIMS Disease Index (2nd edn). Sydney: IMS Publishing, 1996, 35–38.

7. Kincaid-Smith P, Larkins R, Whelan G. *Problems in clinical medicine*. Sydney: MacLennan and Petty, 1990; 10–11.

8. Kumar P, Clark M. *Clinical medicine*. London: Bailliere Tindall, 1990; 569–582.

9. Mashford ML (Chairman). *Cardiovascular drug guidelines* (2nd edn). Victorian Medical Postgraduate Melbourne Foundation, 1996; 87–112.

10. Thompson P. Myocardial infarction. In: MIMS Disease Index (2nd edn). Sydney: IMS Publishing, 1996, 327–330.

11. Coughlin PB, Salem H. Management and prevention of venous thromboembolism. Aust Fam Physician, 1990; 19:1249–1256.

12. Hunt P, Marshall V. *Clinical problems in general surgery*. Sydney: Butterworths, 1991; 87–88.

37

Constipation

—

I have finally kum to the konklusion, that a good reliable set of bowels iz wurth more tu a man, than enny quantity of brains.

Henry Shaw (1818–85)
'Josh Billings'

Definition

Constipation is the difficult passage of small hard stools. It has also been defined as infrequent bowel actions or a feeling of unsatisfied emptying of the bowel. However, the emphasis is on the consistency of the stool rather than on the frequency of defecation; for example, a person passing a hard stool with difficulty once or twice a day is regarded as constipated, but the person who passes a soft stool comfortably every two or three days is not constipated. Various causes of chronic constipation are summarised in Figure 37.1.

Key facts and checkpoints

- A UK study[1] showed that the diagnostic range is 12 per 1000 patients per year.
- The survey showed 10% of adults and 6% of children reported constipation in the preceding 2 weeks.
- Up to 20% of British adults take regular laxatives.[2]
- Constipation from infancy may be due to Hirschsprung's disease.
- Diet is the single most important factor in preventing constipation.
- Beware of the recent onset of constipation in the middle aged and the elderly.
- Bleeding suggests carcinoma, haemorrhoids, diverticular disease and inflammatory bowel disease.

- Unusually shaped stools (small pellets or ribbon-like) suggest the irritable bowel syndrome.
- Always examine the abdomen and rectum.
- Plain abdominal X-rays are generally not useful in the diagnosis of chronic constipation.
- The flexible sigmoidoscope is far superior to the rigid sigmoidoscope in investigation of the lower bowel.

A diagnostic approach

Using the safe diagnostic strategy model (Table 37.1) the five self-posed questions can be answered as follows.

Probability diagnosis

The commonest is 'idiopathic' constipation where there is no structural or systemic disease. This is also referred to as 'functional' constipation.

Probably the most frequent single factor causing constipation in Western society is deficiency in dietary fibre including fruit, green leafy vegetables and wholemeal products. The amount of fibre in our diet is directly related to stool weight and to colonic transit time. The average colonic transit time in the large bowel for Westerners is 60 hours; for a rural African on a very high fibre diet it is 30 hours. Constipation is also a common problem in pregnancy.

Serious disorders not to be missed

Neoplasia

It is obvious that colonic or anorectal neoplasms must not be missed in a patient, especially middle-aged or elderly, presenting with constipation or other change in bowel habit. Most

360

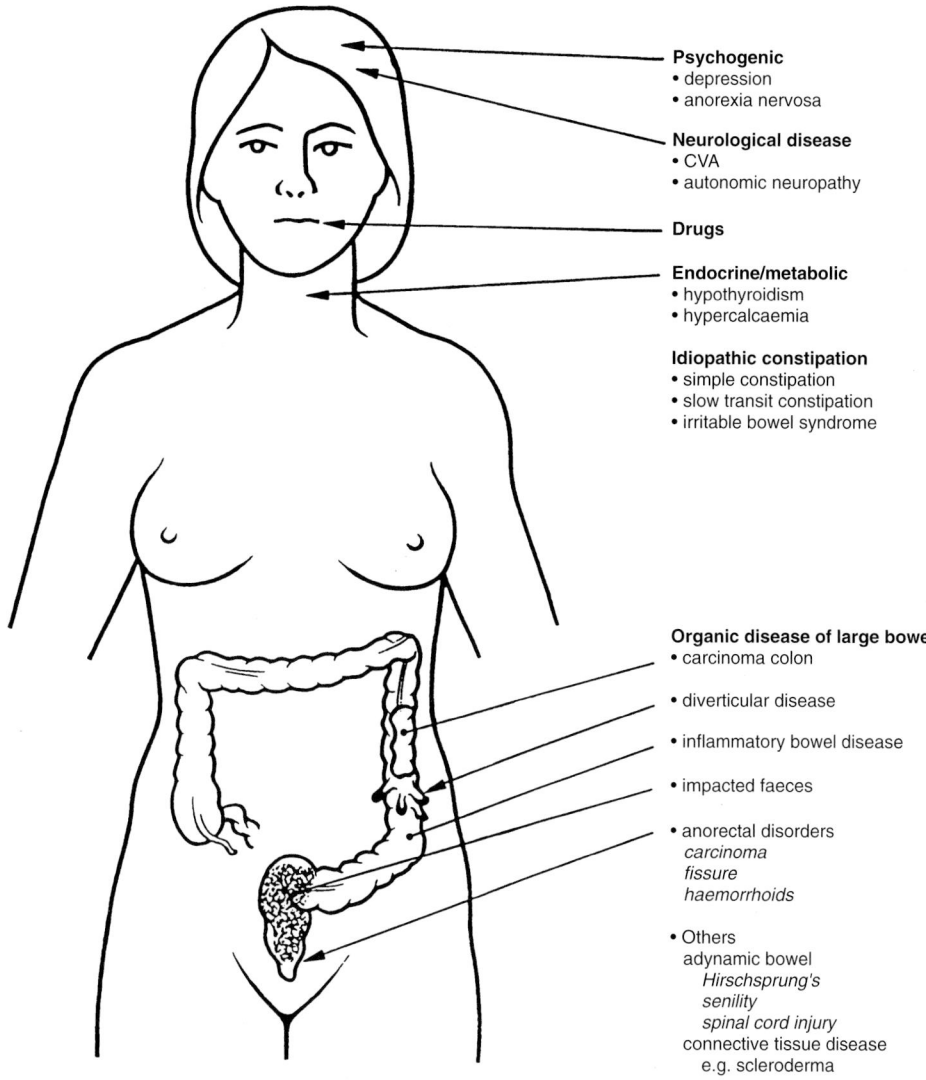

Fig. 37.1 *Causes of chronic constipation*

Within the figure:

Psychogenic
• depression
• anorexia nervosa

Neurological disease
• CVA
• autonomic neuropathy

Drugs

Endocrine/metabolic
• hypothyroidism
• hypercalcaemia

Idiopathic constipation
• simple constipation
• slow transit constipation
• irritable bowel syndrome

Organic disease of large bowel
• carcinoma colon
• diverticular disease
• inflammatory bowel disease
• impacted faeces
• anorectal disorders
  carcinoma
  fissure
  haemorrhoids
• Others
  adynamic bowel
    Hirschsprung's
    senility
    spinal cord injury
  connective tissue disease
    e.g. scleroderma

cases present with either complete or incomplete bowel obstruction.

Extrinsic malignancy such as lymphoma or carcinoma of the ovary, compressing or invading the rectum, also have to be considered. Carcinoma of the large bowel is most prevalent in our society and appropriate screening examinations, including rectal examination, sigmoidoscopy and colonoscopy, must be considered where appropriate.

Megacolon
In children it is important to detect the presence of megacolon, for example megacolon secondary to Hirschsprung's disease. Symptoms dating from birth suggest Hirschsprung's disease, which occasionally may present for the first time in adult life.[3]

Neurological disorders
Constipation, often with faecal impaction, is a common accompaniment to paraplegia, multiple sclerosis, cerebral palsy and autonomic neuropathy.

Alarm symptoms
• recent constipation in > 40-year-old
• rectal bleeding
• family history of cancer

Table 37.1 *Chronic constipation: diagnostic strategy model*

Q. Probability diagnosis
A. Simple constipation:
   low-fibre diet and bad habit

Q. Serious disorders not to be missed
A. Intrinsic neoplasia: colon, rectum or anus,
   especially carcinoma of colon
   Extrinsic malignancy, e.g. lymphoma, ovary
   Hirschsprung's (children)

Q. Pitfalls (often missed)
A. Impacted faeces
   Local anal lesions
   Drug/purgative abuse
   Hypokalaemia
   Depressive illness
   Acquired megacolon
   Diverticular disease

   Rarities
   • Lead poisoning
   • Hypercalcaemia
   • Hyperparathyroidism
   • Dolichocolon (large colon)
   • Chagas' disease
   • Systemic sclerosis

Q. Seven masquerades checklist
A. Depression   √
   Diabetes   rarely
   Drugs   √
   Anaemia   –
   Thyroid   √ hypo
   Spinal dysfunction   severe only
   UTI   –

Q. Is the patient trying to tell me something?
A. May be functional, e.g. depression, anorexia
   nervosa.

Pitfalls

The pitfalls can be summarised as follows:

• impacted faeces
• depressive illness
• purgative abuse
• local anal lesions
• drugs

Although patients with impacted faeces usually present with spurious diarrhoea, it is a form of idiopathic constipation and is very commonly encountered in general practice, especially in bedridden elderly people.

Anal pain or stenosis, such as fissure-in-ano, thrombosed haemorrhoids, perianal haematoma, or ischiorectal abscess, leads to constipation when the patient is hesitant to defecate.

General pitfalls and tips

• Ensure the patient is truly constipated, and not having unreal expectations of regularity.

• Ensure that the anthraquinone group of laxatives, including 'Ford pills', is never used long-term because they cause melanosis coli and associated megacolon.
• Be very wary of alternating constipation and diarrhoea, e.g. carcinoma of colon.
• In a busy practice be careful not to let 'familiarity breed contempt', e.g. onset of hyperparathyroidism, carcinoma.
• Avoid relying solely on the rectal examination to exclude carcinoma.

Seven masquerades checklist

Three of the primary masquerades (Table 37.1) are important causes of constipation, namely drugs, depression and hypothyroidism. Many drugs (Table 37.2) may be associated with constipation, especially codeine and its derivatives, antidepressants, aluminium and calcium antacids. A careful drug history is thus mandatory. Fortunately the constipation is usually relieved once the drug is withdrawn. Constipation can be a significant symptom in all types of depressive illness and may be aggravated by treatment with antidepressants.

The metabolic causes of constipation include hypothyroidism, hypercalcaemia and porphyria. We occasionally encounter the patient with hypercalcaemia, for example hyperparathyroidism, but thyroid dysfunction is relatively common in general practice.

Diabetes rarely can be associated with constipation when an autonomic neuropathy can lead to alternating bouts of constipation and diarrhoea.

Psychogenic considerations

Constipation may be a manifestation of an underlying functional problem and psychiatric disorder such as depression, anorexia nervosa, schizophrenia or drug abuse. Drug abuse must always be considered, keeping in mind that narcotics and laxatives present with rebound constipation. More commonly, it may reflect the inactive lifestyle of the patient and provide a good opportunity for appropriate counselling.

The clinical approach
History

It is important to ask patients to define exactly what they mean by constipation. Some people believe that just as the earth rotates on its axis once a day, so should their bowels open daily

Table 37.2 *Drugs associated with constipation*

Analgesics (inhibitors of prostaglandin synthesis)

Antacids (containing calcium carbonate or aluminium hydroxide)

Anticholinergic agents

Antidiarrhoeal agents

Antihistamines (H₁ blockers)*

Antiparkinsonian drugs*

Barbiturates

Barium sulphate

Benzodiazepines

Clonidine

Cough mixtures

Cytotoxic drugs

Diuretics that cause hypokalaemia

Ganglionic blocking agents

Heavy metal (especially lead)

Iron supplements

Laxatives (chronic use)

Monoamine oxidase inhibitors

Muscle relaxants

Opiate analgesics (e.g. codeine)

Phenothiazines*

Polystyrene resins

Tricyclic antidepressants*

Calcium channel blockers (verapamil)

* denotes anticholinergic effect

to ensure good health. As always, a careful history is appropriate, including stool consistency, frequency, ease of evacuation, pain on defecation and the presence of blood or mucus. A dietary history is very relevant in the context of constipation.

Key questions
• How often do you go to the toilet?
• What are your bowel motions like?
• Are they bulky, hard, like rabbit pellets or soft?
• Is there pain on opening your bowels?
• Have you noticed any blood?
• Have you noticed any lumps?
• Do you have any soiling on your underwear?
• How do you feel in yourself?
• What medications are you taking?

Diary
Ask the patient to keep a 10-day diary recording frequency and nature of stools, and whether any difficulty was experienced when passing stool.

Physical examination

The important aspects are abdominal palpation and rectal examination. Palpation may reveal the craggy mass of a neoplasm, faecal retention (especially in the thin patient) or a tender spastic colon. The perianal region should be examined for localised disease. The patient should be asked to bear down to demonstrate perianal descent, haemorrhoids or mucosal prolapse.[3] Perianal sensation and the anal reflex should be tested. Digital rectal examination is mandatory, and may reveal a rectal tumour and faecal impaction, as well as testing for rectal size and tone. If there is a history from infancy, a normal or narrow rectum suggests congenital megacolon (Hirschsprung's disease) but, if dilated, acquired megacolon.

General signs that may be significant in the diagnosis of constipation are summarised in Figure 37.2.

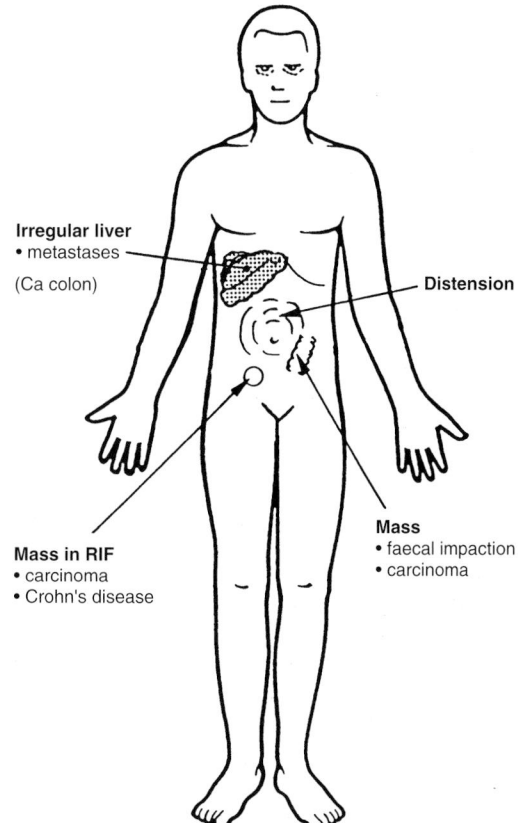

Fig. 37.2 *Possible significant abdominal signs in the patient with constipation*

The rectal examination

The most important first step is to *do* the examination.

| Method |

- Explain to the patient what will happen.
- After inspection with the patient in the left lateral position and with knees drawn up, a lubricated gloved index finger is placed over the anus.
- Ask the patient to concentrate on slow deep breathing.
- With gentle backwards pressure the finger is then inserted slowly into the anal canal and then into the rectum (it helps patient comfort if they push down or squeeze to accommodate the finger).
- Rotate the finger anteriorly to feel the prostate in males and the cervix in females.
- The finger will reach to about 7–8 cm with gentle thrusting into the perineum.
- Gently withdraw the finger and examine the whole circumference of the rectum by sweeping the finger from posterior on both sides.

Points to note

- any pain, e.g. fissure, proctitis, excoriation from diarrhoea (a rectal examination will not be possible in the presence of a fissure)
- induration from a chronic fissure or fistula in the anal canal
- the sphincter tone
- the nature of the faeces (? impaction)
- the rectal wall
  — carcinoma is usually indurated, elevated and ulcerated
  — a villous adenoma has a soft velvety feel
- posteriorly—the sacrum and coccyx
- laterally—the side walls of the pelvis
- anteriorly — cervix and pouch of Douglas in the female
  — prostate and rectovesical pouch in the male (Fig. 37.3)

| The prostate |

- It feels larger if the patient has a full bladder.
- The normal prostate is a firm smooth rubbery bilobed structure (with a central sulcus) about 3 cm in diameter.
- A craggy hard mass suggests carcinoma.

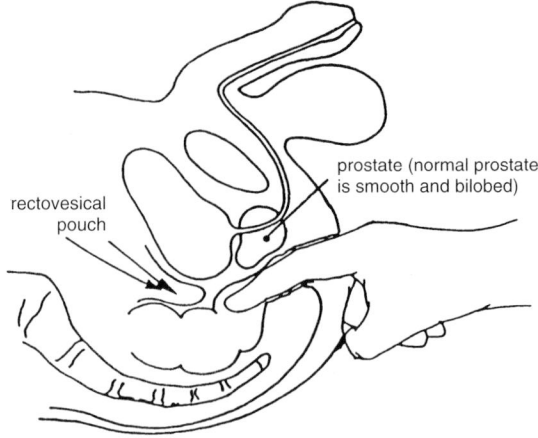

Fig. 37.3 *Rectal examination in the male: the normal prostate is bilobed with a central sulcus*

- An enlarged smooth mass suggests benign hypertrophy.
- A tender, nodular or boggy mass suggests prostatitis.

A common pitfall. In the female the cervix or a vaginal tampon can be mistaken for a mobile extrarectal tumour (Fig. 37.4).

Endoscopy

Sigmoidoscopy—in particular, flexible sigmoidoscopy with examination of the rectosigmoid—is important in excluding local disease; search for abnormalities such as blood, mucus or neoplasia. The insufflation of air sometimes reproduces the pain of the irritable bowel syndrome.

It is worth noting that 60% of polyps and cancers will occur in the first[5] 60 cm of the bowel and diverticular disease should be

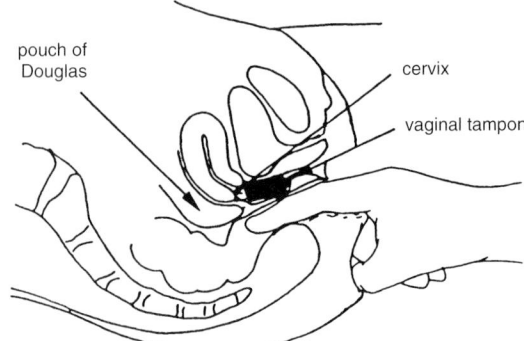

Fig. 37.4 *Rectal examination in the female: the cervix or vaginal tampon may be mistaken for a rectal mass*

evident with the flexible sigmoidoscope.

The presence of melanosis coli is an important sign—it may give a pointer to the duration of the constipation and the consequent chronic intake (perhaps denied) of anthraquinone laxatives.

Investigations
These can be summarised as follows.

Haematological
• haemoglobin
• erythrocyte sedimentation rate

Stools for occult blood

Biochemistry (where suspected)
• thyroid function tests
• serum calcium
• serum potassium
• carcinoembrogenic antigen (a tumour marker)

Radiological
• double contrast barium enema (especially for primary colonic disease, e.g. megacoln)
• bowel transit studies, using radio-opaque shapes taken orally and checking progresses by abdominal X-ray or stool collection

Physiological tests
• anal manometry—test anal tone
• rectal sensation and compliance, using an inflatable rectal balloon
• dynamic proctography, to determine disorders of defecation
• rectal biopsy, to determine aganglionia

Endoscopy

Constipation in children
Constipation is quite common in children and often related to diet. Most children develop normal bowel control by 4 years of age (excluding any physical abnormality). It is important to differentiate between encopresis and constipation.
• *Encopresis* is the inappropriate passage of normal stool, which usually indicates a psychological disorder or stress.
• *Constipation* is difficulty or delay in passing the stool with incomplete emptying of the rectum. This can present as

soiling, due to faecal retention with overflow of liquid faeces.

Other important conditions
Hirschsprung's disease
• Consider if delay in passing first meconium stool and subsequent constipation.

Anal fissure in infants
• Consider if stool hard and associated with pain or bleeding.

Principles of treatment of functional constipation
• Encourage relaxed child–parent interaction with toilet training, e.g. appropriate encouragement; 'after breakfast habit' training.
• Introduce psychotherapy or behaviour modification program, especially where 'fear of the toilet' exists.
• Establish an empty bowel: remove any impacted faeces with microenemas, e.g. Microlax, and even disimpaction under anaesthesia if necessary.
• Advice for parents of children over 18 months:
  — Drink ample fluids each day, e.g. several glasses of water, unsweetened fruit juice or milk.
  — Get regular exercise, e.g. walking, running, outside games or sport.
  — Provide high-fibre foods, e.g. high-fibre cereals, wholegrain bread, brown rice, wholemeal pasta, fresh fruit with skins left on where possible, dried fruits such as sultanas, apricots or prunes, fresh vegetables.
• Use a pharmaceutical preparation as a last resort to achieve regularity:
• *First line*: bulk-producing agent, e.g. psyllium granules, 1 teaspoonful, once or twice daily
• *Second line*: osmotic laxative, e.g. lactulose:
  1–5 years: 5 mL bd
  6–12 years: 10 mL bd
  > 12 years: 15 mL bd

Constipation in the elderly
Constipation is a common problem in the elderly with a tendency for idiopathic constipation to increase with age. In addition the chances of organic disease increase with age, especially colorectal carcinoma; so this problem requires attention in the older patient. Faecal impaction is a special problem in the aged confined largely

to bed. Constipation is often associated with Parkinson's disease. In the elderly an osmotic laxative such as sorbitol or lactulose may be required for long-standing refractory constipation but stimulant and other non-osmotic laxatives should be avoided.

Practice tip on treatment

A suitable method of doing a rectal examination on a home visit (in the absence of gloves in the doctor's bag) is to apply moist soap around the finger and caked under the nail (in case of breakage), then plastic wrap and finally petroleum jelly (e.g. Vaseline).

Before resorting to a good old-fashioned '3H' enema (hot water, high and a hell of a lot), use a sorbitol compound, e.g. Microlax 5 mL enema. It can be carried in the doctor's bag, is very easy to insert and is most effective.

Manual disimpaction

However, if manual disimpaction should be necessary, the unpleasant procedure can be rendered virtually odourless if the products are 'milked' or scooped directly into a container of water. A large plastic cover helps restrict the permeation of the smell.

Discomfort and embarrassment are reduced by this method and by adequate premedication (e.g. IV midazolam and IV fentanyl) if large faecaliths are present.

Idiopathic constipation

It is best to classify idiopathic constipation into three subgroups:[3]

1. simple constipation
2. slow transit constipation
3. normal transit constipation (irritable bowel syndrome)

Of these, the commonest is simple constipation, which is essentially related to a faulty diet and bad habit. Avery-Jones,[4] who defined the disorder, describes it as being due to one or more of the following causes:

- faulty diet
- neglect of the call to stool
- unfavourable living and working conditions
- lack of exercise
- travel

Dyschezia, or lazy bowel, is the term used to describe a rectum that has become unresponsive

to faecal content, and this usually follows repeated ignoring of calls to defecate.

Slow transit constipation occurs primarily in women with an apparently normal colon, despite a high-fibre intake and lack of the other causes described by Avery-Jones. Many are young, with a history dating from early childhood or, more commonly, adolescence. Constipation may follow childbirth, uncomplicated abdominal surgery or a period of severe dieting. However, in the majority no precipitating cause is evident.

Management

Most patients have simple constipation and require reassurance and education once an organic cause has been excluded.

Basic advice to the patient

- Adequate exercise, especially walking, is important.
- Develop good habit: answer the call to defecate as soon as possible. Develop the 'after breakfast habit'. Allow time for a good relaxed breakfast and then sit on the toilet.
- Avoid laxatives and codeine compounds (tablets or mixture).
- Take plenty of fluids, especially water and fruit juices.
- Eat an optimal bulk diet. Eat foods that provide bulk and roughage such as vegetables and salads, cereals (especially wheat fibre), fresh and dried fruits, and wholemeal bread. Enough fibre should be taken to convert stools that sink to stools that float.[3]

Examples of food with good bulk properties are presented in Table 37.3.[6] Fruit has good fibre, especially in the skin, and some have natural laxatives (e.g. prunes, figs, rhubarb, apricots).

Table 37.3 *Foods with bulk-forming properties (from least to most)*

• Potato
• Banana
• Cauliflower
• Peas
• Cabbage
• Lettuce
• Apple
• Carrot
• Bran

Pharmaceutical preparations

Some patients may not tolerate unprocessed bran but tolerate pharmaceutical preparations better (Table 37.4). An appropriate choice would be one of the hydrophilic bulk-forming agents such as ispaghula or psyllium. Avoid stimulant laxatives except for short sharp treatments.

First-line therapy[7]

Use a general bulking agent
e.g. psyllium or ispaghula granules
    1–2 teaspoonsful (o) once or twice daily

Second-line therapy

Use an osmotic laxative or a fibre-based stimulant preparation
e.g. sorbitol 70% liquid, 10 mL (o) bd increasing
    as required
        or
    lactulose syrup, 15–30 mL (o) daily until response, then 10–20 mL daily
        or
    dried fruits with senna leaf (Nu-Lax) 10 g nocte

Third-line therapy

(Recheck cause.)
    magnesium sulphate, 1–2 teaspoons in water once or twice daily (if normal renal function)
        or
    a stimulating agent, e.g. bisacodyl 10–20 mg (o) nocte
        or
    glycerin suppository
        or
    citrate or phosphate enema

Colorectal cancer
Clinical features
- commonest GIT malignancy
- second most common cause of death from cancer in Western society
- generally men over 50 years
- mortality rate about 60%
- good prognosis if diagnosed early
- two-thirds in descending colon and rectum

Predisposing factors
- ulcerative colitis (long-standing)
- familial polyposis coli
- colonic adenomata
- decreased dietary fibre

Lifetime risk
- general population   1 in 25
- family history (first-degree relative)   1 in 3
- familial polyposis coli   100% by age 40–50

Symptoms
- blood in the stools
- mucus
- recent change in bowel habits (constipation more common than diarrhoea)
- bowel leakage when flatus passed
- unsatisfactory defecation (the mass is interpreted as faeces)
- abdominal pain (colicky) or discomfort (if obstructing)
- rectal discomfort
- symptoms of anaemia

Various forms of presentation of large bowel cancers are shown in Figure 37.5.

Table 37.4 *Therapeutic agents to treat constipation (with examples)*

Hydrophilic bulk-forming agents
  psyllium mucilloid (Agiofibe, Metamucil)
  sterculia (Granocol, Normacol)
  ispaghula (Agiolax, Fybogel)
  methylcellulose (Cellulone)
  wheat bran
  crude fibre (Fibyrax Extra)

Stimulant (irritant) laxatives
  phenolphthalein (Laxettes, Figsen, Ford pills)
  senna (Senokot)
  cascara
  castor oil
  bisacodyl (Durolax)

Osmotic laxatives
  magnesium sulphate (Epsom salts)
  magnesium hydroxide (Milk of Magnesia)
  lactulose (Duphalac)
  mannitol
  sorbitol (Sorbilax)

Stool-softening agents
  liquid paraffin (Agarol)
  dioctyl sodium sulphosuccinate (Coloxyl)
  glycerin suppositories
  sorbital/sodium compounds (Microlax)

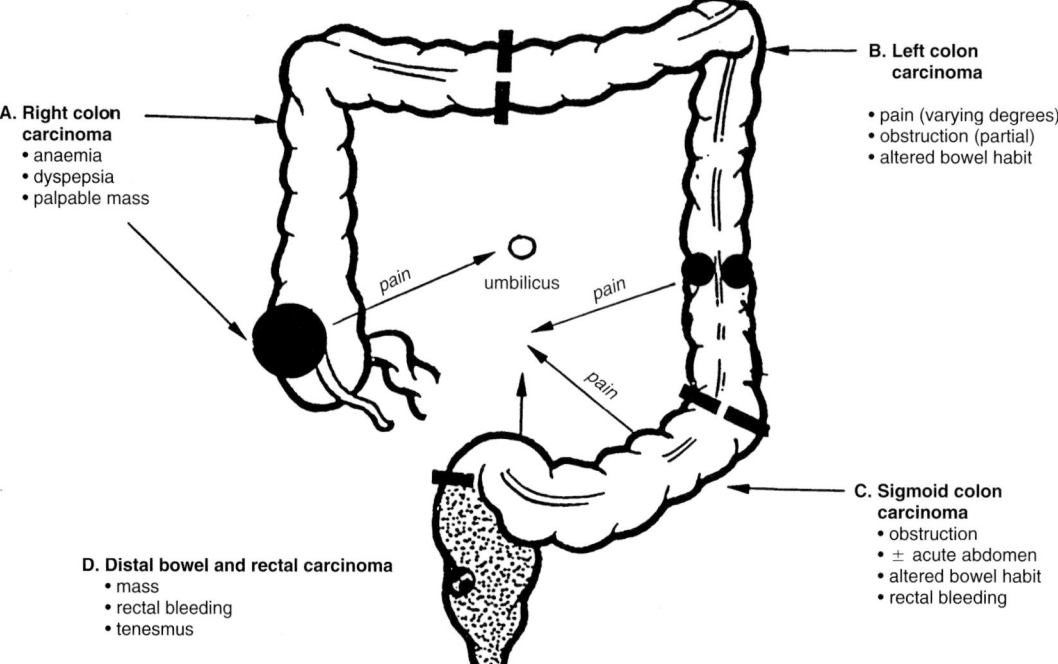

A. Right colon carcinoma
• anaemia
• dyspepsia
• palpable mass

B. Left colon carcinoma
• pain (varying degrees)
• obstruction (partial)
• altered bowel habit

C. Sigmoid colon carcinoma
• obstruction
• ± acute abdomen
• altered bowel habit
• rectal bleeding

D. Distal bowel and rectal carcinoma
• mass
• rectal bleeding
• tenesmus

Fig. 37.5 *Various forms of presentation of large bowel carcinoma*

Investigations
• faecal occult blood (FOBT)
• sigmoidoscopy, especially flexible sigmoidoscopy
• barium enema (accurate as a double contrast study) but may miss tumours
• colonoscopy: essential if suspicion on clinical grounds remains and barium enema normal (more useful if rectal bleeding)
• ultrasonograph and CT scanning not useful in primary diagnosis; valuable in detecting spread especially hepatic metastases

If FOBT is positive—investigate by colonoscopsy or by flexible sigmoidoscopy.

Screening
Faecal occult blood testing is now recommended (see guidelines p. 73). Colonoscopy is recommended for those at risk and, in addition, flexible sigmoidoscopy and rectal biopsy for those with ulcerative colitis.

Management
Early surgical excision is the treatment, with the method depending on the site and extent of the carcinoma. Duke's classification gives a guide to prognosis (Table 37.5).

Table 37.5 *Modified Duke's classification of colorectal cancer[8]*

Stage	Pathologic description	Approx. 5 year survival %
A	Cancer limited to mucosa and submucosa	> 90
B	Cancer extends into muscularis or serosa	70–80
C	Cancer involves regional lymph nodes	30
D	Distant metastases, e.g. liver	5

Megacolon
Hirschsprung's disease (aganglionosis)

Features
• congenital
• constipation from infancy
• abdominal distension from infancy
• possible anorexia and vomiting
• male:female 8:1
• rectal examination—narrow or normal rectum
• abdominal X-ray/barium enema—distended colon full of faeces to narrow rectum

- diagnosis, confirmed by full thickness biopsy, shows absence of ganglion cells
- absent rectoanal reflex on anal manometry

Treatment
Resect narrow segment after preliminary colostomy.

Acquired megacolon
Features
- in older children and adults
- mainly due to bad habit
- can be caused by
  — chronic laxative abuse
  — milder form of Hirschsprung's disease
  — Chagas' disease (Latin America)[2]
  — hypothyroidism (cretinism)
  — systemic sclerosis
- marked abdominal distension
- rectal examination—dilate loaded rectum, lax sphincter
- abdominal X-ray/barium enema—distended colon full of faeces but no narrowed segment

Treatment
Re-education of bowel habit is required.

When to refer[5]

Patients with constipation or change in bowel habit of recent onset without obvious cause need further investigation.
- Patients with chronic symptoms that do not respond to simple measures should be referred.

Practice tips
- The objectives of treatment should be to exclude organic disease and then reassure and re-educate the patient about normal bowel function.
- Discourage long-term use of laxatives, suppositories and microenemas.
- The laxatives to discourage should include anthraquinone derivatives, bisacodyl, phenolphthalein, magnesium salts, castor oil and mineral oils.

- First-line treatment of functional constipation (unresponsive to simple measures) is a bulking agent. An osmotic laxative is good second-line therapy.
- Bleeding with constipation indicates associated organic illness—exclude carcinoma of the bowel. Bright red blood usually means haemorrhoids.
- Beware of hypokalaemia causing constipation in the elderly patient on diuretic treatment.
- If carcinoma can be felt on rectal examination an abdominal perineal procedure with colostomy usually follows; if not, an anterior resection is generally the rule.

An appropriate management plan for the patient presenting with constipation is that given by Barnes[3] as in Table 37.6 on page 370.

References
1. Cormack JJC. *Practice: A handbook of primary medical care.* London: Kluwer-Harrap, 1980; 3(47):1–2.
2. Sandler G, Fry J. *Early clinical diagnosis.* Lancaster: MTP Press, 1986, 209.
3. Barnes PRH. Assessment and management of constipation. What's new in gastroenterology? Gastroenterological Society of Australia 1989; 34:1–4.
4. Avery-Jones F, Godding FW. *Management of constipation.* Oxford: Blackwell Scientific Publications, 1972, 16.
5. Bolin T. Constipation. In: MIMS Disease Index (2nd edn). Sydney: IMS Publishing, 1996, 127–129.
6. Sali A. Preventive initiatives in medicine and surgery. Aust Fam Physician, 1985; 14:1314.
7. Moulds RFW (chairman). *Gastrointestinal guidelines.* Victorian Medical Postgraduate Foundation, 1994, 60–62.
8. Wilson JD et al. *Harrison's principles of internal medicine* (12th edn). New York: McGraw-Hill, 1991, 1292.

Table 37.6 *Management plan for constipation*[3]

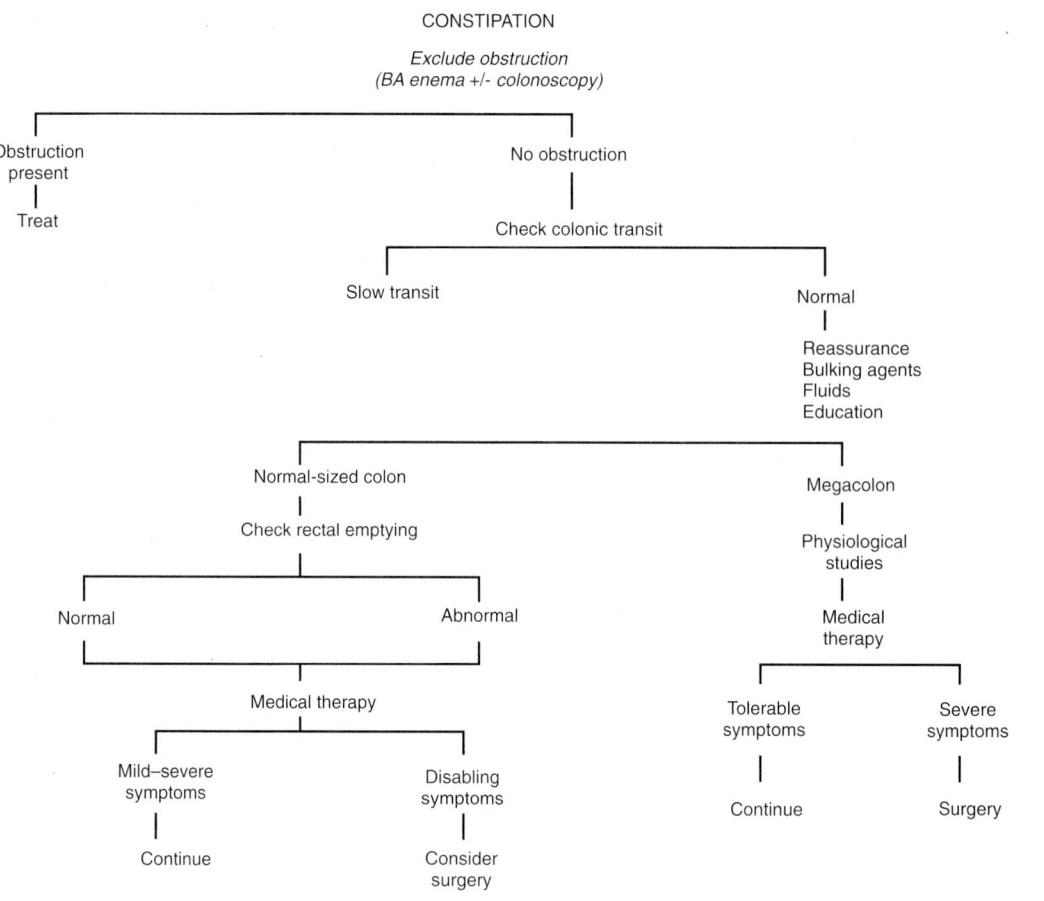

Source: After Barnes[3]

38
Cough

I bounded into bed. The bound made me cough—I
spat—it tasted strange—it was bright red blood—I
don't want to find this is real consumption—I shan't
have my work written. That's what matters. How
unbearable it would be to die—nothing real finished.

Katherine Mansfield (1888–1923)
Diary entry 1918

Cough is one of the five most common symptoms
presenting in family practice. There is a wide range
of causes (Table 38.1) with the great majority
being minor and self-limiting, although the possibility of serious causes such as bronchogenic carcinoma should always be kept in mind.

It is a feature of smokers, who often have a
morning cough with little sputum. Coughing can
also be initiated by pleural irritation. It is a reflex
that provides an essential protective service. It
serves to remove substances that may have been
accidentally inhaled and removes excess secretions or exudates that may accumulate in the
airway.

Key facts and checkpoints

- Cough is the commonest manifestation of
  lower respiratory tract disease.
- Cough is the cardinal feature of chronic
  bronchitis.
- Cough is a feature of asthma with sputum production, especially at night.
- Cough can have a psychogenic basis.
- Cough may persist for many weeks following
  an acute URTI as a result of persisting bronchial inflammation and increased airway
  responsiveness.[1]
- Postnasal drip is the commonest cause of a
  persistent or chronic cough, especially causing
  nocturnal cough due to secretions (mainly

Table 38.1 *Significant causes of cough*

Non-productive (dry cough)
- Upper respiratory tract infection
- Lower respiratory tract infection
  — viral
  — mycoplasma
- Inhaled irritants
  — smoke
  — dust
  — fumes
- Inhaled foreign body
- Bronchial neoplasm
- Pleurisy
- Interstitial lung disorders
  — fibrosing alveolitis
  — extrinsic allergic alveolitis
  — pneumoconiosis
  — sarcoidosis
- Tuberculosis
- Left ventricular failure
- Whooping cough (pertussis)
- GORD and hiatus hernia
- post nasal drip

Productive cough
- Chronic bronchitis
- Bronchiectasis
- Pneumonia
- Asthma
- Foreign body (later response)
- Bronchial carcinoma (dry or loose)
- Lung abcess
- Tuberculosis (when cavitating)

from chronic sinusitis) tracking down the
larynx and trachea during sleep.
- The commonest causes of haemoptysis are
  URTI (24%), acute or chronic bronchitis (17%),
  bronchiectasis (13%), TB (10%). Unknown

causes totalled 22% and carcinoma 4% (figures from a UK study).[2]

A diagnostic approach

A summary of the safety diagnostic model is presented in Table 38.2.

Probability diagnosis

The most common cause of cough is an acute respiratory infection, whether an upper respiratory infection (URTI) or acute bronchitis.[3] Persistent coughing with an URTI is usually due to the development of sinusitis with a postnasal drip.

Chronic bronchitis is also a common cause of cough.

Table 38.2 *Cough: diagnostic strategy model*

Q. *Probability diagnosis*
A. Upper respiratory infection
   Postnasal drip
   Smoking
   Acute bronchitis
   Chronic bronchitis

Q. *Serious disorders not to be missed*
A. Cardiovascular
   • left ventricular failure
   Neoplasia
   • carcinoma of lung
   Severe infections
   • tuberculosis
   • pneumonia
   • influenza
   • lung abscess
   • HIV infection
   Asthma
   Cystic fibrosis
   Foreign body
   Pneumothorax

Q. *Pitfalls (often missed)*
A. Atypical pneumonias
   Gastro-oesophageal reflux (nocturnal)
   Smoking (children/adolescents)
   Bronchiectasis
   Whooping cough (pertussis)
   Interstitial lung disorders
   Sarcoidosis

Q. *Seven masquerades checklist*
A. Depression   —
   Diabetes   —
   Drugs   √
   Anaemia   —
   Thyroid disease   —
   Spinal dysfunction —
   UTI   —

Q. *Is the patient trying to tell me something?*
A. Anxiety and habit

Serious disorders not to be missed

Bronchial carcinoma must not be overlooked. A worsening cough is the commonest presenting problem. A bovine cough is suggestive of carcinoma: the explosive nature of a normal cough is lost when laryngeal paralysis is present, usually resulting from bronchial carcinoma infiltrating the left recurrent laryngeal nerve.

Chronic cough may be the first presentation of *Pneumocystis carinii* pneumonia in an HIV-infected patient. Careful but tactful questioning of the patient in relation to IV drug use, sexual practice and previous blood transfusions is important. Important causes of a chronic cough are summarised in Table 38.3.

The possibility of a foreign body should always be kept in mind, especially in children, and severe infections such as tuberculosis and pulmonary abscess must not be misdiagnosed.

It is also important not to overlook asthma in which a nocturnal cough, without wheezing, is a feature in children.

Pitfalls

Causes that tend to be overlooked, especially in the presence of a normal X-ray, are gastro-oesophageal reflux, postnasal drip and asthma. Gastro-oesophageal reflux is more common as a

Table 38.3 *Some causes of chronic cough*[2,4,5]

Normal chest X-ray (includes most causes)
• Chronic postnasal drip
• Asthma
• Asthma + postnasal drip
• Postinfective bronchial hyper-responsiveness
• Gastro-oesophageal reflux
  — symptomatic
  — asymptomatic
• Chronic bronchitis
• Drugs, e.g. ACE inhibitors, inhaled steroids
• Snoring and obstructive sleep apnoea
• Irritants: occupational and household
• Whooping cough (pertussis)
• Habit
• Functional
• Idiopathic

Abnormal chest X-ray
• Bronchiectasis
• Carcinoma: bronchogenic, larynx
• Cardiac failure
• COAD
• cystic fibrosis
• inhaled foreign body
• interstitial lung disorders, e.g. sarcoidosis
• tuberculosis

cause of reflex coughing, especially at night, than appreciated. Whooping cough, especially immunisation-modified, can be difficult to diagnose particularly if the characteristic whoop is absent.

General pitfalls

- Attributing cough due to bronchial carcinoma in a smoker to 'smoker's cough'
- Overlooking TB, especially in the elderly, by equating symptoms to old age, bronchitis or even smoking
- Overlooking the fact that bronchial carcinoma can develop in a patient with other pulmonary conditions such as chronic bronchitis
- Being slow to order a chest X-ray
- Failing to recognise that pertussis presents in adults

Seven masquerades checklist

The applicable masquerade is drugs, many of which can produce a wide variety of disorders of the respiratory tract that cause a cough. Pulmonary infiltration with fibrosis may result from some cytotoxic drugs, especially bleomycin. Over 20 different drugs are known to produce an SLE-like syndrome, sometimes complicated by pulmonary infiltrates and fibrosis. Cough can be a feature of some of the ACE inhibitors and beta-blockers, inhaled steroids and salazopyrin.

Psychogenic considerations

A cough can occur for psychosocial reasons. Coughing is under cerebral control and a slight cough before commencing a speech is normal and presumably assists in clearing mucus from around the vocal cords.[6] This can readily become a nervous habit or mannerism. A typical 'psychogenic' cough is barking in quality, the 'Cape Barren goose' cough. It does not occur during sleep.

The clinical approach

History

The nature of the cough may provide important diagnostic clues but it is the associated symptoms, such as the nature of the sputum, breathlessness, wheezing and constitutional symptoms, that provide the most helpful diagnostic value. A history of smoking habits, past and present, is essential and an occupational and hobby history requires investigation. Significant occupations

(past or present) include mining (pneumoconiosis), aircraft manufacturing (asbestosis and mesothelioma), farming ('farmer's lung'— allergic pneumonitis from mouldy hay) and bird handling ('bird fancier's lung'—allergic alveolitis or psittacosis from pigeons or budgerigars). A past history of recurrent lung infections from childhood is suggestive of cystic fibrosis and bronchiectasis; a history of hay fever and eczema suggests asthma, while a family history involves asthma, cystic fibrosis, emphysema (α_1– antitrypsin deficiency) and tuberculosis.

Key questions[7]

- How would you describe the cough?
- How long has the cough been present?
- Do you cough up sputum?
- Describe the sputum, especially its colour.
- Is there any blood in the sputum?
- How much sputum do you produce—a teaspoonful, an eggcupful or more?
- Is there a burning sensation in your throat or chest when you cough?
- Have you noticed any other symptoms?
- What about chest pain or fever, shivers or sweats?
- Do you have a wheeze?
- Have you had previous attacks of wheezing or hay fever?
- Is there a history of asthma in your family?
- Have you lost weight?
- Has anyone in the family had tuberculosis or a persistent cough?
- How much do you smoke?
- Are you exposed to any smoke or fumes?
- What kind of work do you do?
- Where have you worked in the past?
- Is there a chance you have been exposed to asbestos?
- Do you keep birds at home?
- Do you have any birds nesting outside your bedroom?
- Is there a possibility of a foreign body such as a peanut 'having gone down the wrong way'?
- Have you had an operation recently or been confined to bed?
- Have you noticed any swelling of your legs?
- Have you been exposed to birds such as pigeons?

Physical examination

Physical examination includes a general examination with a search for features such as enlarged cervical or axillary glands which may indicate bronchial carcinoma, as would Horner's syndrome (constricted pupil, ptosis). A careful examination of the lungs and cardiovascular system is also appropriate. Careful inspection of the sputum forms an important part of the physical examination of the lungs. This should include its colour and consistency, presence of particulate matter and a 24 hour sputum watch.

Investigations

This applies particularly to patients with haemoptysis. Investigations include:

- haemoglobin, blood film and white cell count
- sputum cytology and culture
- ESR (elevated with bacterial infection, bronchiectasis, TB, lung abscess and bronchial carcinoma)
- respiratory function tests
- radiology
  — plain chest X-ray (shows many problems)
  — tomography
    • helps more precise localisation of lesion
    • may show cavitation
  — bronchography
    • shows bronchiectasis (a very unpleasant procedure)
  — CT scanning (more sensitive than plain X-ray)
  — ventilation/perfusion isotope scan
    • for pulmonary infarction
- skin tests
- lung biopsy
- bronchoscopy (best at time of haemoptysis)

A schema for the investigation of chronic cough is presented in Figure 38.1.[8]

However, all that is needed initially is a plain chest X-ray.

Diagnostic characteristics

There are important characteristics of cough that may point to the causation. Table 38.1 compares typical causes of dry and productive cough.

Character of the cough

- brassy → • tracheitis and bronchitis (major bronchi)
  • extrinsic pressure on trachea
- barking → laryngeal disorders, e.g. laryngitis
- croupy (with stridor) → laryngeal disorders, e.g. laryngitis, croup
- bovine (no power) → vocal cord paralysis (left recurrent laryngeal nerve)
- weak cough → indicates bronchial carcinoma
- paroxysmal with whoops → whooping cough
- painful → • tracheitis
    • left ventricular failure

Timing

- nocturnal cough → • asthma
    • left ventricular failure
    • postnasal drip
    • chronic bronchitis
    • whooping cough
- waking cough → • bronchiectasis
    • chronic bronchitis
    • gastro-oesophageal reflux

Associations

- changing posture → • bronchiectasis
    • lung abscess
- meals → • hiatus hernia (possible)
    • oesophageal diverticulum
    • tracheo-oesophageal fistula
- wheezing → • asthma
- breathlessness → • asthma
    • left ventricular failure
    • chronic obstructive airways disease

Sputum

A healthy non-smoking individual produces approximately 100–150 mL of mucus a day. This normal bronchial secretion is swept up the airways towards the trachea by the mucociliary clearance mechanism and is usually swallowed. The removal from the trachea is assisted also by occasional coughing although this is carried out almost subconsciously.[6]

Excess mucus is expectorated as sputum. The commonest cause of excess mucus production is cigarette smoking. Mucoid sputum is clear and white.

Character of sputum

- clear white (mucoid) → normal or uninfected bronchitis
- yellow or green (purulent) → due to cellular material (neutrophils or eosinophil granulocytes)

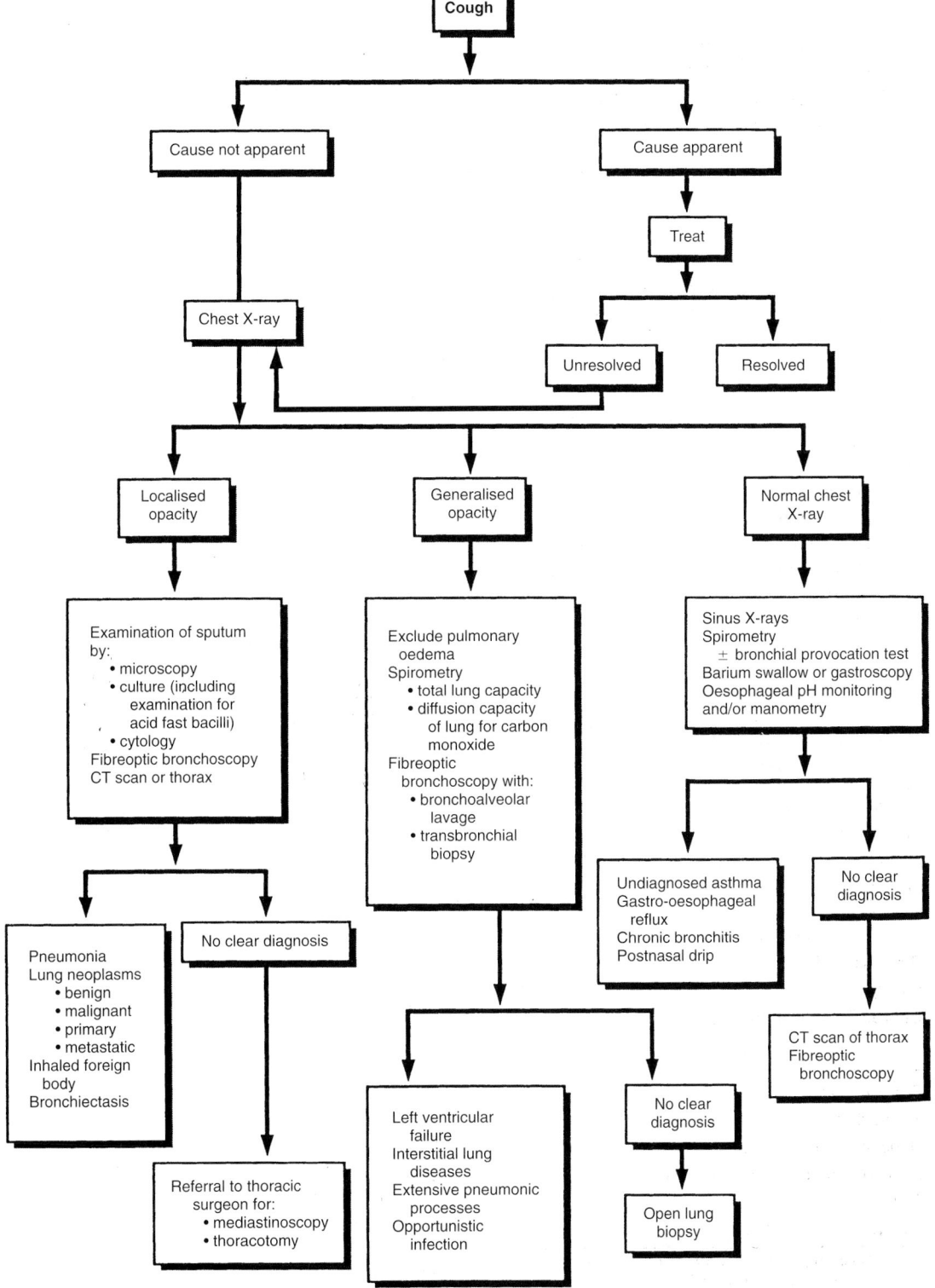

Fig. 38.1 *A recommended schematica for investigation of chronic cough* REPRODUCED FROM T.J. WILLIAMS AND G. BOWES, *MOD MED AUST*, JUNE 1992, WITH PERMISSION

- ± infection (not necessarily bacterial infection)
- asthma due to eosinophils
- bronchiectasis (copious quantities)
- rusty → lobar pneumonia (*Strep. pneumoniae*): due to blood
- thick and sticky → asthma
- profuse, watery → alveolar cell carcinoma
- thin, clear mucoid → viral infection
- redcurrant jelly → bronchial carcinoma
- profuse and offensive → • bronchiectasis
  - lung abscess
- thick plugs (cast-like) → • allergic bronchopulmonary aspergillus
  - bronchial carcinoma
- pink frothy sputum → • pulmonary oedema

Haemoptysis

Blood-stained sputum (haemoptysis), which varies from small flecks of blood to massive bleeding, requires thorough investigation. Often the diagnosis can be made by chest X-ray. Causes are presented in Table 38.4. Haemoptysis must be distinguished from blood-stained saliva

Table 38.4   *Causes of haemoptysis (blood-stained sputum)*

Acute infection • URTI
• acute bronchitis } commonest cause[1]
Chronic bronchitis
Bronchiectasis
Lobar pneumonia (rusty sputum)
Tuberculosis
Neoplasic • bronchogenic carcinoma
• metastatic carcinoma
Pulmonary infarction
Foreign body
Cardiac • left ventricular failure
• mitral stenosis
Unknown
Rarer causes
Idiopathic pulmonary haemosiderosis
Goodpasture's syndrome
Blood disorders including anticoagulants
Trauma
Iatrogenic, e.g. endotracheal tubes

Note: Haemoptysis must be distinguished from blood-stained saliva caused by nasopharyngeal bleeding or sinusitis.[6] Copious haemoptysis is due to bronchiectasis or tuberculosis.

caused by nasopharyngeal bleeding or sinusitis and also from haematemesis.[6]

Productive cough

- chronic bronchitis — mucoid or purulent
  — rarely exceeds 250 mL per day[6]
- bronchiectasis — purulent sputum
  — up to 500 mL/day
- asthma — mucoid or purulent
  — tenacious sputum
- lung abscess — purulent and foul-smelling
- foreign body — can follow impaction

Cough in children

Cough in children is a very common symptom, but troublesome persistent cough is a great cause of anxiety among parents and probably the commonest symptom for which the family doctor is consulted. Age-related causes of chronic cough (present at least 4 weeks) are presented in Table 38.5. Most children with chronic cough do NOT have asthma.

Common causes are:

- asthma
- recurrent viral bronchitis
- acute URTIs
- allergic rhinitis

Disorders not to be missed are:

- asthma

Table 38.5   *Chronic cough in children: age-related causes to consider*

Early months of life
• milk inhalation/reflux
• asthma
Toddler/preschool child
• asthma
• bronchitis
• whooping cough
• cystic fibrosis
• croup
• foreign body inhalation
• tuberculosis
• bronchiectasis
Early school years
• asthma
• bronchitis
• mycoplasma pneumonia
Adolescence
• asthma
• psychogenic
• smoking

Source: After Selecki and Helman[10]

- cystic fibrosis
- inhaled foreign body
- tracheo-oesophageal fistula

Several clinicians describe the catarrhal child syndrome as the commonest cause of cough.[3] This refers to children who develop a postnasal drip following acute respiratory infection and allergic rhinitis.

Psychogenic causes

Habit cough can occur in children, especially those with a history of school phobia. The cough does not occur during sleep and remains unchanged with exertion or infection.

Croup (laryngotracheobronchitis)

Clinical features:

- characteristic barking cough with stridor
- children 9 months to 3 years
- usually 11 p.m. to 2 a.m.
- occurs in small local epidemics

Management—refer Chapter 77.

Cough in the elderly

Important causes of cough to consider in the elderly include chronic bronchitis, carcinoma of the lung, bronchiectasis and left ventricular failure in addition to the acute upper and lower respiratory infections to which they are prone. It is important to be surveillant for bronchial carcinoma in an older person presenting with cough, bearing in mind that the incidence rises with age.

Common respiratory infections

Respiratory infections, especially those of the upper respiratory tract, are usually regarded as trivial, but they account for an estimated one-fifth of all time lost from work and three-fifths of time lost from school, and are thus of great importance to the community. The majority of respiratory infections are viral in origin and antibiotics are therefore not indicated.

Upper respiratory tract infections (URTIs) are those involving the nasal airways to the larynx, while lower respiratory tract infections (LRTIs) affect the trachea downwards.

Combined URTI and LRTI include influenza, measles, whooping cough and laryngotracheo-bronchitis.

The common cold (acute coryza)

This highly infectious URTI, which is often mistakenly referred to as 'the flu', produces a mild systemic upset and prominent nasal symptoms (Fig. 38.2).

Typical clinical features

- malaise and tiredness
- sore, runny nose
- sneezing
- sore throat
- slight fever

Other possible symptoms:

- headache
- hoarseness
- cough

The watery nasal discharge becomes thick and purulent in about 24 hours and persists for up to a week. Secondary bacterial infection is uncommon.

Management

Advice to the patient includes:

- rest: adequate sleep and rest
- analgesics: paracetamol (acetaminophen) or aspirin (maximum 8 tablets a day in adults)

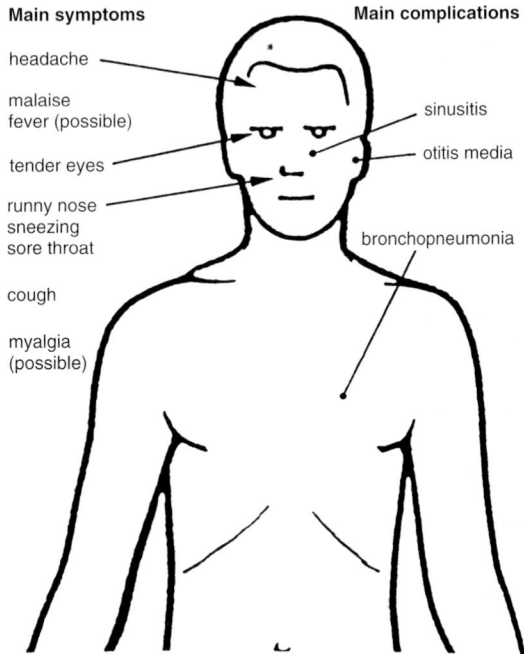

Fig. 38.2 *The main symptoms and complications of the common cold*

- steam inhalations (as per Fig. 48.3) for a blocked nose
- cough mixture for a dry cough
- gargling aspirin in water or lemon juice for a sore throat
- vitamin C powder or tablets, e.g. 2 g daily, may aid recovery

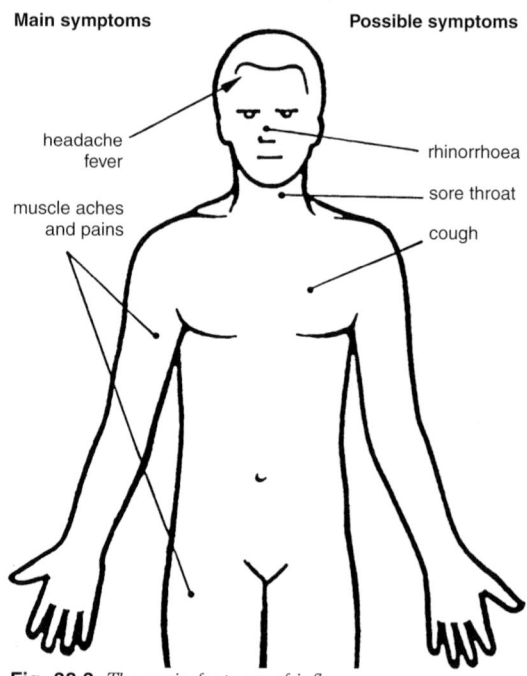

Influenza

Influenza causes a relatively debilitating illness and should not be confused with the common cold. The differences are presented in Table 38.6. The incubation period is usually 1–3 days and the illness commences abruptly with a fever, headache, shivering and generalised muscle aching (Fig. 38.3).

Typical clinical features
Initial:
- fever, shivering
- headache
- generalised muscle aching, especially limbs

Followed by:
- sore throat
- dry cough (can last several weeks)
- rhinorrhoea
- depression (a common sequela)

Fig. 38.3 *The main features of influenza*

Complications
- secondary bacterial infection
- pneumonia due to *Staphylococcus aureus* (mortality up to 20%)[1]
- encephalomyelitis (rare)

Management
Advice to the patient includes:
- rest in bed until the fever subsides
- analgesics: aspirin is effective or codeine and aspirin (or paracetamol), especially if a dry cough
- fluids: maintain high fluid intake

Consider a neuraminidase inhibitor e.g. zanamivir 10 mg by inhalation, 12 hrly for 5 days (commence with 36 hours onset)

Table 38.6 *Comparison of common cold and influenza*

	Common cold	Influenza
Incubation period	12 hours to 5 days	1–3 days
Fever	±	+ +
Cough	(later)	+
Sore throat	+ +	±

Rhinitis
  sneezing
  rhinorrhoea
	+	−

Muscle aches	−	+
Toxaemia	−	±
Causes	rhinoviruses parainfluenza influenza B, C corona virus respiratory syncytial virus	influenza A influenza B

Prophylaxis
Influenza vaccination offers some protection for up to 70% of the population for about 12 months.[1]

Bronchitis

Acute bronchitis
This is acute inflammation of the tracheobronchial tree that usually follows an upper respiratory infection. Although generally mild and self-limiting it may be serious in debilitated patients.

Features
Features of acute infectious bronchitis are:
• cough and sputum (main symptoms)
• wheeze and dyspnoea
• usually viral infection
• can complicate chronic bronchitis—often due to *Haemophilus influenzae* and *Streptococcus pneumoniae*
• scattered wheeze on auscultation
• fever or haemoptysis (uncommon)

Outcome
• It improves spontaneously in 4–8 days in healthy patients.

Treatment[11]
• symptomatic treatment
• inhaled bronchodilators for airflow limitation
• antibiotics usually not needed in previously healthy adult or child
• use antibiotics if severe infection with fever
  e.g. amoxycillin/clavulanate tds for 5 days
     doxycycline or erythromycin if mycoplasma suspected

Chronic bronchitis
This is a chronic productive cough for at least 3 successive months in 2 successive years.

• wheeze, progressive dyspnoea
• recurrent exacerbations with acute bronchitis
• occurs mainly in smokers

Refer to COAD (pp. 457–459).

Pneumonia

This is inflammation of lung tissue. It usually presents as an acute illness with cough, fever and purulent sputum plus physical signs and X-ray changes if consolidation.

However, the initial presentation of pneumonia can be misleading, especially when the patient presents with constitutional symptoms (fever, malaise and headache) rather than respiratory symptoms. A cough, although usually present, can be relatively insignificant in the total clinical picture. This diagnostic problem applies particularly to atypical pneumonia but can occur with bacterial pneumonia especially lobar pneumonia.

Typical pneumonia
The commonest community-acquired infection is with *Streptococcus pneumoniae* (majority) or *Haemophilus influenzae*.[11]

Clinical features
• often history of viral respiratory infection
• rapidly ill with high temperature, dry cough, pleuritic pain
• 1–2 days later maybe rusty-coloured sputum
• rapid and shallow breathing follows
• X-ray and examination: consolidation

The atypical pneumonias
Clinical features
• fever, malaise
• headache
• minimal respiratory symptoms, non-productive cough
• signs of consolidation absent
• chest X-ray (diffuse infiltration) incompatible with chest signs

Causes
Mycoplasma pneumoniae—the commonest:
• adolescents and young adults
• treat with doxycycline 100 mg bd for 10–14 days

Legionella pneumophila (legionnaires' disease):
• related to cooling systems in large buildings
• incubation 2–10 days

Diagnostic criteria include:
• prodromal influenza-like illness
• a dry cough, confusion or diarrhoea
• very high fever (may be relative bradycardia)
• lymphopenia with moderate leucocytosis
• hyponatraemia

Patients can become very prostrate with complications—treat with erythromycin.

Chlamydia pneumoniae
• similar to mycoplasma

Chlamydia psittaci (psittacosis)
• treat with doxycycline (as above)
Coxiella burnetii (Q fever)
• treat with doxycycline (as above)

Antibiotic treatment according to severity[11,12]

Mild pneumonia

This does not require hospitalisation.
• roxithromycin 150 mg 12 hourly
  — covers most likely pathogens including mycoplasma and chlamydia
     or
• amoxycillin/clavulanate 500/125 mg 8 hourly
  — especially if *S. pneumoniae* isolated or suspected
     or
• doxycycline 200 mg loading dose, then 100 mg daily
  — if atypical pneumonia suspected

Moderately severe pneumonia

This requires hospitalisation—see Table 38.7.
• benzylpenicillin 600 mg IV 4–6 hourly for 5–10 days
  (drug of choice for *S. pneumoniae*)
     or
• cephalothin 1 g IV 4–6 hourly for 5–10 days
  (in penicillin-allergic patient)
• If not so severe and oral medication tolerated can use amoxycillin/clavulanate or cefaclor or doxycycline
• If atypical pneumonia use doxycycline, erythromycin or roxithromycin

Table 38.7   *Pneumonia: Guidelines for hospitalisation*[11]

• Age over 65 years
• Coexisting illness
• High temperature: > 38°C
• Clinical features of severe pneumonia
• Involvement of more than one lobe
• Inability to tolerate oral therapy

Severe pneumonia

The criteria for severity are presented in Table 38.8.
• erythromycin 500 mg IV slowly 6 hourly
  (covers mycoplasma, chlamydia and legionella)
     plus

• cefotaxime 1 g IV 8 hourly
     or
ceftriaxone 1 g IV daily

Table 38.8   *Guidelines for severe pneumonia*[11]

• Altered mental state
• Rapidly deteriorating course
• Respiratory rate > 30 per minute
• BP < 90/60 mmHg
• Hypoxia P_aO_2 < 60 mmHg
• Leucocytes < 4 × 10⁹/L or > 20 × 10⁹/L

Pneumonia in children

Features
• tachypnoea, expiratory grunt
• possible focal chest signs
• diagnosis often only made by chest X-ray

Pathogens
• Viruses are the most common cause in infants.
• Mycoplasma are common in children over 5 years.
• *S. pneumoniae* is a cause in all age groups.
• Pathogens are difficult to isolate—may need blood culture.

Treatment
Almost all those under 48 months should be admitted to hospital
• Minimal handling
• Careful observations including pulse oximetry
• Attend to hydration
• Antibiotics indicated in all cases. Refer to guidelines.[12]
  Mild to moderate (general guidelines only):[13]
  < 24 months—penicillin IV or IM initially
  > 24 months—penicillin or erythromycin
  Severe:[11]
  flucloxacillin IV + cefotaxime IV

Chronic persistent cough

A cough associated with a viral respiratory infection should last no more than 2 weeks. If it does it is termed *persistent*. A cough lasting 2 months or more is defined as a chronic cough. A cough that lasts longer than 3 to 4 weeks requires scrutiny. Table 38.3 includes some causes of chronic cough.

A chronic cough can be divided into productive and non-productive. If productive, the presence of pus is significant, as purulent sputum usually means bacterial infection in the bronchi and/or sinuses.[4] The main organisms are *Haemophilus influenzae* (the most common), *Streptococcus pneumoniae* and *Moraxella*. Such infections are most susceptible to amoxycillin or amoxycillin/clavulanate or parenteral cephalosporins.

Non-productive cough

Some of the many causes of a non-productive cough are included in Table 38.1 and more than one may be operative in a patient simultaneously; for example, an allergic snorer with oesophageal reflux taking an ACE inhibitor for hypertension may have a viral respiratory infection.[4] It has been shown that a non-productive or irritating cough is usually caused by persistent stimulation of irritant receptors in the trachea and major bronchi, and may result in the production of small amounts of mucoid sputum.

Investigations to be considered in intractable chronic cough include a chest X-ray, spirometry, CT scan of the thorax (searching in particular for a tumour) and ambulatory oesophageal pH monitoring.

If bronchial hyper-responsiveness is proven a trial of inhaled or oral corticosteroids can be used in these patients.[5]

Gastro-oesophageal reflux

This common condition is the most likely cause of a persistent, non-productive cough in an apparently well patient with a history of reflux. Recent studies utilising 24 hour ambulatory oesophageal pH monitoring have demonstrated that in patients with persistent unexplained cough the predominant cause is asymptomatic gastro-oesophageal reflux.[4,5] In the absence of evidence of aspiration the cough is considered to be due to stimulation of a distal oesophageal-tracheobronchial reflex. Other studies have established a relationship between bronchial asthma and reflux or swallowing disorders whereby micro-aspiration can initiate an inflammatory response in the airways.

Indication for 24 hour ambulatory oesophageal pH monitoring in chronic cough include:

- unexplained chronic cough after clinical assessment
- symptomatic gastro-oesophageal reflux
- chronic cough with known aetiology unresponsive to therapy

If reflux is proven or suspected, treat with routine conservative antireflux measures and at least a 4 week trial of histamine H_2-receptor antagonists. If cough persists, refer for further evaluation.[5]

If all investigations and treatment trials (including antireflux and corticosteroids) prove unrewarding, a trial of ipratropium bromide both nebulised (500 µg, qid) and to a lesser degree metered dose inhaler (4 × 20 µg puffs qid) has been found to be effective.[5,14]

However, for patients with idiopathic chronic cough it is important to provide ongoing interest and support, and not eventually to dismiss them as 'just a cough'.

Bronchial carcinoma

Lung cancer accounts for 33% of cancer deaths in men and 24% of cancer deaths in women (rapidly rising) in the United States, with cigarette smoking being the most common cause of lung cancer in both sexes.[9] It is also the most common lethal cancer in both sexes in Australia.

Clinical features

- most present between 50 and 70 years
- only 10–25% asymptomatic at time of diagnosis[9]
- if symptomatic—usually advanced and not resectable

Local symptoms

- cough (42%)
- chest pain (22%)
- wheezing (15%)
- haemoptysis (7%)
- dyspnoea (5%)

General

- anorexia, malaise
- weight loss

Others

- hoarseness
- symptoms from metastases

The possible physical findings are summarised in Figure 38.4.

Investigations

- chest X-ray
- computerised tomography
- fibreoptic bronchoscopy
- PET scanning

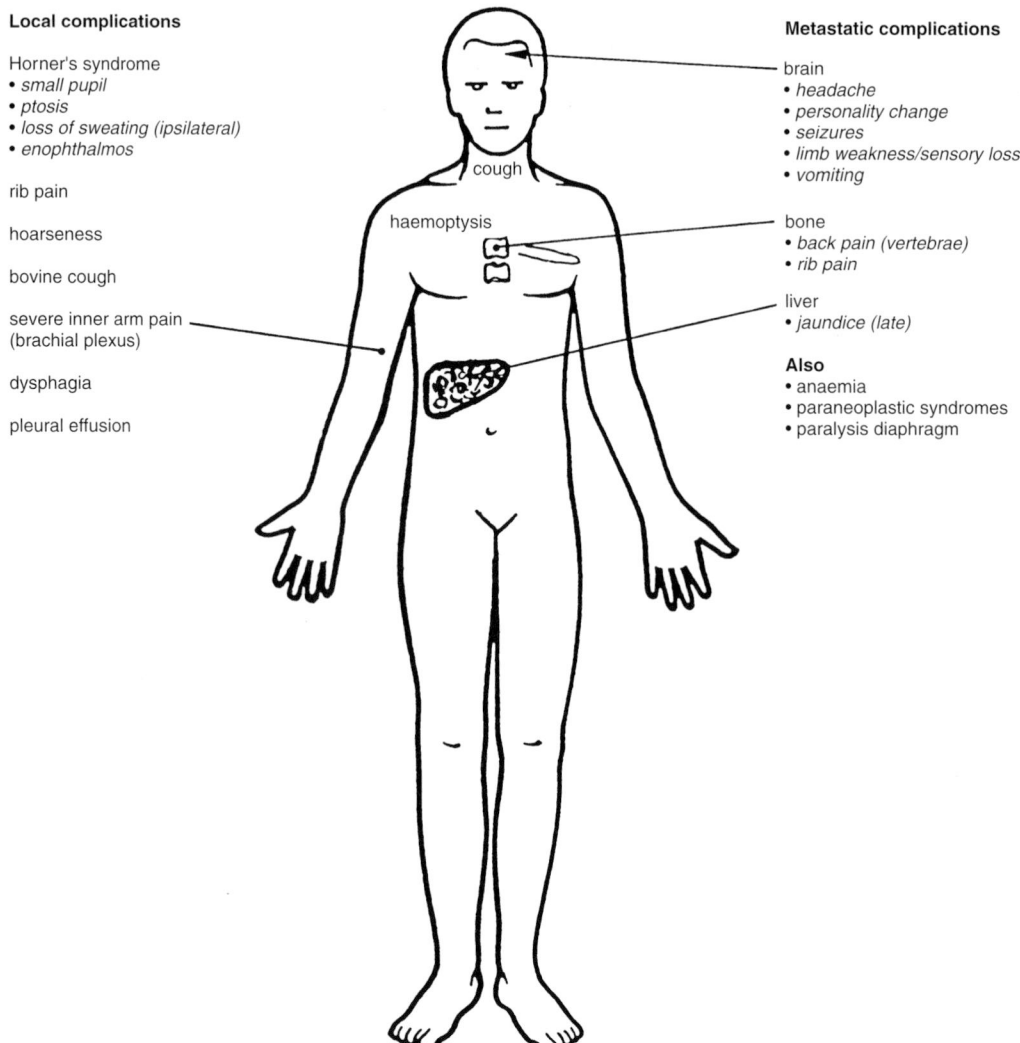

Local complications

Horner's syndrome
• *small pupil*
• *ptosis*
• *loss of sweating (ipsilateral)*
• *enophthalmos*

rib pain

hoarseness

bovine cough

severe inner arm pain
(brachial plexus)

dysphagia

pleural effusion

cough

haemoptysis

Metastatic complications

brain
• *headache*
• *personality change*
• *seizures*
• *limb weakness/sensory loss*
• *vomiting*

bone
• *back pain (vertebrae)*
• *rib pain*

liver
• *jaundice (late)*

Also
• anaemia
• paraneoplastic syndromes
• paralysis diaphragm

Fig. 38.4 *Possible physical findings of bronchial carcinoma*

Management

Refer to a respiratory physician to determine the type of carcinoma. They are usually classified as small cell lung cancer (SCLC) and non-small cell lung cancer (NSCLC). The main aim of management is a curative resection of NSCLC in those who can benefit from it. Chemotherapy is suitable for the deadly SCLC but currently only extends life expectancy from 3 to 18 months (at best). It has little place in treating NSCLC. The main role of radiotherapy is palliative.

Bronchiectasis

Bronchiectasis is dilatation of the bronchi when their walls become inflamed, thickened and irreversibly damaged, usually following obstruction followed by infection. Predisposing causes include whooping cough, measles, tuberculosis, inhaled foreign body (e.g. peanuts in children), bronchial carcinoma, cystic fibrosis and congenital ciliary dysfunction (Kartagener's syndrome). The left lower lobe and lingula are the commonest sites for localised disease.

Clinical features

• chronic cough—worse on waking
• mild cases: yellow or green sputum only after infection
• advanced — profuse purulent offensive sputum

— persistent halitosis
— recurrent febrile episodes
— malaise, weight loss
• episodes of pneumonia
• sputum production related to posture
• haemoptysis (blood-stained sputum or massive) possible

Physical examination
• clubbing
• coarse crackles over infected areas (usually lung base)
• other respiratory signs in Table 45.5

Investigations
• chest X-ray (normal or bronchial changes)
• sputum examination — for resistant pathogens
                      — to exclude TB
• main pathogens: *Staphylococcus aureus, Pseudomonas aeruginosa, Haemophilus influenzae*
• CT scan: can show bronchial wall thickening
• bronchograms: very unpleasant and used only if diagnosis in doubt or possible localised disease amenable to surgery (rare)

Management
• explanation and preventive advice
• postural drainage, e.g. lie over side of bed with head and thorax down for 10–20 minutes 3 times a day
• antibiotics according to organism—it is important to eradicate infection to halt the progress of the disease
• bronchodilators if evidence of bronchospasm

Tuberculosis
Pulmonary tuberculosis may be symptomless and detected by mass X-ray screening.[8]

Typical clinical features
Respiratory symptoms
• cough
• sputum: initially mucoid, later purulent
• haemoptysis
• dyspnoea (especially with complications)
• pleuritic pain

General (usually insidious)
• anorexia
• fatigue
• weight loss
• fever (low grade)
• night sweats

Physical examination
• may be no respiratory signs or signs of fibrosis, consolidation or cavitation (amphoric breathing)
• finger clubbing

Investigations
• chest X-ray
• micro and culture sputum (for tubercle bacilli)
• ESR
• tuberculin test (misleading if previous BCG vaccination)

Management
Tuberculosis is a notifiable disease and must be reported to state (and local) health departments. Hospitalisation for the initial therapy of pulmonary TB is not necessary in most patients. Monthly follow-up is recommended including sputum smear and culture. Multiple drug therapy is initiated primarily to guard against the existence and/or emergence of resistant organisms. Standard initial therapy consists of rifampicin + ethambutol + isoniazid + pyrazinamide daily for at least 2 months, followed by rifampicin + isoniazid for 4 months if the organism is susceptible to these drugs.[12] If isoniazid resistance is suspected, streptomycin (with care) is added.

Symptomatic treatment of cough
Symptomatic treatment of cough should be reserved for patients who have acute self-limiting causes of cough, especially an acute viral infection. There are many cough mixtures available and the major constituents of these mixtures are shown in Table 38.9.[8] The recommended mixture should be tailored to the patient's individual requirements. These mixtures should be used only in the short term.

When to refer
• Patients in whom bronchoscopy is necessary to exclude bronchial carcinoma
• Persistent hoarseness in a patient who requires expert laryngeal examination
• Evidence of pulmonary tuberculosis

Table 38.9 *Cough mixtures: major constituents*

Cough suppressants	Decongestants
Opiate	*Sympathomimetic*
Codeine	Ephedrine
Dihydrocodeine	Pseudoephedrine
Hydrocodone	Phenylephrine
Pholcodine	Phenylpropanolamine
Ethylmorphine	Methoxyphenamine
Normethadone	
	Antihistamine
Other	Promethazine
Carbetapentane	Pheniramine
Dextromethorphan	Chlorpheniramine
Expectorants/mucolytics	Diphenhydramine
Senega	Dexchlorpheniramine
Ammonia	Brompheniramine
Guaiphenesin	Triprolidine
Bromhexine	
	Anticholinergic
Analgesics/antipyretics	Atropine
Paracetamol (acetaminophen)	Isopropamide
Salicylates (e.g. aspirin)	

Source: After William and Bowes[8]

Practice tips

- Unexplained cough over the age of 50 is bronchial carcinoma until proved otherwise (especially if there is a history of smoking).
- Bronchoscopy is essential to exclude adequately a suspicion of bronchial carcinoma when the chest X-ray is normal.
- Bright red haemoptysis in a young person may be the initial symptom of pulmonary tuberculosis.
- Avoid settling for a diagnosis of bronchitis as an explanation of haemoptysis until bronchial carcinoma has been excluded.
- Coughing may be so severe that it terminates in vomiting or loss of consciousness (posttussive syncope).
- Large haemoptyses are usually due to bronchiectasis or tuberculosis.
- The presence of white cells in the sputum renders it yellow or green (purulent) but does not necessarily imply infection.

References

1. Kumar PJ, Clarke ML. *Clinical medicine* (2nd edn). London: Bailliere Tindall, 1990, 637–638.
2. Walsh TD. *Symptom control.* Oxford: Blackwell Scientific Publications, 1989; 81:81–88 and 235–239.
3. Sandler G, Fry J. *Early clinical diagnosis.* Lancaster: MTP Press, 1986, 233–257.
4. Burns M. Chronic cough. Aust Fam Physician, 1996; 25:161–167.
5. Ing A. Intractable cough. In: MIMS Disease Index (2nd edn). Sydney: IMS Publishing, 1996, 130–133.
6. Kincaid-Smith P, Larkins R, Whelan G. *Problems in clinical medicine.* Sydney: MacLennan & Petty, 1990, 105–108.
7. Davis A, Bolin T, Ham J. *Symptom analysis and physical diagnosis* (2nd edn). Sydney: Pergamon Press, 1990, 56–60.
8. Williams TJ, Bowes G. Cough as a symptom in adult life. Mod Med Aust, June 1992, 84–92.
9. Tierney LM et al. *Current medical diagnosis and treatment.* Stamford: Appleton and Lange, 1996, 179–180.
10. Selecki Y, Helman A. Chronic cough in children. Australian Dr Weekly, 18 Sept. 1989.
11. Christiansen K. Antibiotics for common respiratory infections. Aust Fam Physician, 1995; 24:49–56.
12. Mashford ML (Chairman). *Antibiotic guidelines* (9th edn). Melbourne: Victorian Medical Postgraduate Foundation, 1996–97, 108–118.
13. Efron D. *Paediatric handbook* (5th edn). Melbourne: Blackwell Science, 1996, 70–72.
14. Holmes PW, Barter CE, Pierce RJ. Chronic persistent cough: Use of ipratropium bromide in undiagnosed cases following URTI. Respiratory Medicine, 1992; 86:425–429.

39

Deafness and hearing loss

—

There are two kinds of deafness. One is due to wax and is curable; the other is not due to wax and is not curable.

Sir William Wilde (1815–1876)

Deafness is defined as impairment of hearing, regardless of its severity.[1] It is a major community health problem requiring a high index of suspicion for diagnosis, especially in children. Deafness may be conductive, sensorineural or a combination of both (mixed).

Fig. 39.1 *Prevalence of hearing problems with increasing age*

Key facts and checkpoints

- Deafness occurs at all ages but is more common in the elderly (Fig. 39.1).
- The threshold of normal hearing is from 0 to 20 decibels (dB), about the loudness of a soft whisper.
- One in seven of the adult population suffers from some degree of significant hearing impairment (over 20 dB in the better hearing ear).[2]
- One child in every 1000 is born with a significant hearing loss.
- Degrees of hearing impairment:[2,3]
  - mild = loss of 20–40 dB (20 dB is soft-spoken voice)
  - moderate = loss of 40–70 dB (40 dB is normal-spoken voice)
  - severe = loss of 70–90 dB (shout)
  - profound = loss of over 90 dB
- More women than men have a hearing loss.
- People who have worked in high-noise levels (> 85 dB) are more than twice as likely to be deaf.
- There is a related incidence of tinnitus with deafness.

A diagnostic approach

It is useful to consider the causes of deafness in terms of pathophysiology (conductive or sensorineural hearing loss) and anatomical sites (Fig. 39.2).

Conductive hearing loss is caused by an abnormality in the pathway conducting sound waves from the outer ear to the inner ear,[1] as far as the footplate of the stapes.

Sensorineural hearing loss is a defect central to the oval window involving the cochlear (sensor), cochlear nerve (neural) or, more rarely, in central neural pathways.[1]

Congenital deafness is an important consideration in children, while presbyacusis is very common in the aged. The commonest acquired causes of deafness are impacted cerumen (wax), serous otitis media and otitis externa. Noise-induced deafness is also a common problem.

It is important not to misdiagnose an acoustic neuroma which can present as acute deafness, although slow progressive loss is more typical. A

Fig. 39.2 *Causes of deafness according to anatomical site*

summary of the diagnostic strategy, which includes several important causes of deafness, is presented in Table 39.1 and a checklist of oto-toxic drugs in Table 39.2.

Symptoms

The symptoms vary so that some barely notice a problem while others are severely disabled.

Common symptoms include inability:

- to hear speech and other sounds loudly enough
- to hear speech and music clearly, even when loud enough
- to understand speech even when loud enough—a problem of language reception

People with mild hearing loss notice only subtle differences and may have trouble hearing certain high-frequency sounds such as 's', 'f' or 'th'. They may also have trouble hearing in certain situations such as at a party or in a crowd where there is a lot of background noise. Those with moderate hearing loss have trouble hearing in many situations.

The clinical approach

History

The history should include an account of the onset and progression of any deafness; noise exposure; drug history; a history of swimming or diving, air travel and head injury; and family history. A recent or past episode of a generalised infection would be relevant and the presence of associated aural symptoms such as ear pain, discharge, tinnitus and vertigo. Vertigo may be a symptom of Ménière's disease, multiple sclerosis, acoustic neuroma or syphilis.

Several important clues can be obtained from the history. The often sudden onset of hearing loss in an ear following swimming or showering is suggestive of wax, which swells to block the ear canal completely.

Patients with conductive loss may hear better in noisy conditions (paracusis) because we raise our voices when there is background noise. Conversely, people with sensorineural deafness (SND) usually have more difficulty hearing in noise as voices become unintelligible.

Table 39.1 *Deafness and hearing loss: diagnostic strategy model*

Q. Probability diagnosis
A. Impacted cerumen
   Serous otitis media
   Otitis externa
   Congenital (children)
   Presbyacusis

Q. Serious disorders not to be missed
A. Neoplasia
   • acoustic neuroma
   • temporal lobe tumours (bilateral)
   • otic tumours
   Severe infections
   • generalised infections, e.g. mumps
   • syphilis
   Perforated tympanic membrane
   Cholesteatoma
   Perilymphatic fistula (post-stapedectomy)

Q. Pitfalls (often missed)
A. Foreign body
   Temporal bone fracture
   Otosclerosis
   Barotrauma
   Noise-induced deafness

   Rarities
   • Paget's disease of bone
   • Multiple sclerosis
   • Osteogenesis imperfecta

Q. Seven masquerades checklist
A. Depression   —
   Diabetes   √
   Drugs   √
   Anaemia   —
   Thyroid disease   √ hypo
   Spinal dysfunction —
   UTI   —

Q. Is this patient trying to tell me something?
A. Unlikely.

Table 39.2 *Known ototoxic drugs*

Alcohol

Aminoglycosides
• amikacin
• gentamicin
• kanamycin
• neomycin
• streptomycin
• tobramycin

Diuretics
• ethacrynic acid
• frusemide

Chemotherapeutic agents

Quinine and related drugs

Salicylates

Examination

Inspect the facial structures, skull and ears. The ears are inspected with an otoscope to visualise the external meatus and the tympanic membrane (TM) and the presence of obstructions such as wax, inflammation or osteomata. The examination requires a clean external auditory canal. Gentle suction is useful for cleaning pus debris. Syringing is reserved for wax in people with an intact TM and a known healthy middle ear.

It is an advantage to have a pneumatic attachment to test drum mobility. Reduction of TM mobility is an important sign in secretory otitis media.

There are several simple hearing tests. The distance at which a ticking watch can be heard can be used but the advent of the digital watch has affected this traditional method.

The hair-rubbing method

In children and in adults with a reasonable amount of hair grab several hairs close to the external auditory canal between the thumb and index finger. Rub the hairs lightly together to produce a relatively high-pitched 'crackling' sound (Fig. 39.3). If this sound cannot be heard, a moderate hearing loss is likely (usually about 40 dB or greater). Like the whisper test, this test is a rough guide only.

Tuning fork tests

If deafness is present, its type (conduction or sensorineural) should be determined by tuning fork testing. The most suitable tuning fork for preliminary testing is the C_2 (512 cps) fork. The

Fig. 39.3 *The simple hair-rubbing method of testing possible deafness*

fork is best activated by striking it firmly on the bent elbow.

1. *Weber test*

The vibrating tuning fork is applied firmly to the midpoint of the skull or to the central forehead or to the teeth.

This test is of value only if the deafness is unilateral or bilateral and unequal (Fig. 39.4). Normally the sound is heard equally in both ears in the centre of the forehead. With sensorineural deafness the sound is transmitted to the normal ear, while with conduction deafness it is heard better in the abnormal ear.

Fig. 39.4 *Weber test*

2. *Rinne's test*

The tuning fork is held:

• outside the ear (tests air conduction) and
• firmly against the mastoid bone (tests bone conduction).

It therefore compares air and bone conduction in the same ear (Fig. 39.5). A variation of the test includes placing the tuning fork on the mastoid

Fig. 39.5 *Rinne's test*

process and the patient indicates when it can no longer be heard. The fork is then placed at the external auditory meatus and the patient indicates whether the sound is now audible. Normally air conduction is better than bone conduction and the sound will again be heard.

A comparison of the interpretation of these tests is summarised in Table 39.3.

Audiometric assessment

Audiometric assessment has two basic parts:

1. puretone audiometry
2. impedance tympanometry

Puretone audiometry[4]

Puretone audiometry is a graph of frequency expressed in Hertz versus loudness expressed in decibels. The tone is presented either through the ear canal (a test of the conduction and the cochlear function of the ear) or through the bone (a test of cochlear function).

Figures 39.6 and 39.7 are typical examples of puretone audiograms.

The difference between the two is a measure of conductance. If the two ears have different thresholds, a white noise masking sound is applied to the better ear to prevent it hearing sound presented to the test ear. The normal speech range occurs between 0 and 20 decibels across the frequency spectrum.

Tympanometry

Tympanometry measures the mobility of the tympanic membrane, the dynamics of the ossicular chain and the middle ear air cushion. The test consists of a sound applied at the external auditory meatus, otherwise sealed by the soft probe tip.

Deafness in children

Deafness in childhood is relatively common and often goes unrecognised. One to two of every 1000 newborn infants suffer from sensorineural deafness.[1] Congenital deafness may be due to inherited defects, to prenatal factors such as maternal intrauterine infection or drug ingestion during pregnancy, or to perinatal factors such as birth trauma, and haemolytic disease of the newborn.

Deafness may be associated with Down syndrome and Waardenburg's syndrome. Waardenburg's syndrome, which is dominantly inherited, is diagnosed in a patient with a white

Table 39.3 *A comparison of the Rinne and Weber tests*

State of the hearing	Rinne test	Weber test
Normal	Positive: A.C.>B.C.	Equal in both ears
Conduction deafness	Negative: B.C.>A.C.	Louder in the deaf ear
Very severe conduction deafness	Negative: B.C.>A.C. May hear B.C. only	Louder in the deaf ear
Sensorineural deafness	Positive: A.C.>B.C.	Louder in the better ear
Very severe sensorineural deafness	'False' negative (without masking)	Louder in the better ear

A.C. = air conduction; B.C. = bone conduction

forelock of hair and different coloured eyes.

Acquired deafness accounts for approximately half of all childhood cases. Purulent otitis media and secretory otitis media are common causes of temporary conductive deafness. However, 1 in 10 children will have persistent middle ear effusions and mild to moderate hearing loss in the 15–40 decibel range.[5] Permanent deafness in the first few years of life may be due to virus infections such as mumps, meningitis, ototoxic antibiotics and several other causes.

Screening[1]

The aim of screening should be to recognise every deaf child by the age of 8 months to 1 year—before the vital time for learning speech is wasted. High-risk groups should be identified and screened, for example a family history of deafness, maternal problems of pregnancy, perinatal problems, cerebral palsy and those with delayed or faulty speech. The guidelines for early signs of normal hearing are presented in Table 39.4.

Optimal screening times:

• 8 to 9 months
• school entry

Fig. 39.6 *Puretone audiogram for severe conductive deafness in right ear* AFTER B. BLACK[4]

R. air conduction ○—○—○
L. air conduction ✕—✕—✕
R. bone conduction]---]---]
L. bone conduction :---[---[

Fig. 39.7 *Puretone audiogram for unilateral (right) sensorineural deafness. Suspect a viral or congenital origin in children; check adults for acoustic neuroma*

Table 39.4 *Early signs of normal hearing*

Age	Typical response
1 month	Should notice sudden constant sounds (e.g. car motor, vacuum cleaner) by pausing and listening.
3 months	Should respond to loud noise, e.g. will stop crying when hands are clapped.
4 months	Should turn head to look for source of sound such as mother speaking behind the child.
7 months	Should turn instantly to voices or even to quiet noises made across the room.
10 months	Should listen out for familiar everyday sounds.
12 months	Should show some response to familiar words and commands, including his or her name.

Early signs of hearing loss

A high index of suspicion is essential in detecting hearing loss in children and any parental concern should be taken seriously. The presentation of hearing loss will depend on whether it is bilateral or unilateral, its severity and age of onset.

Typical presentations include:

- malformation of skull, ears or face
- failure to respond in an expected way to sounds, especially one's voice
- preference for, or response only to, loud sounds
- no response to normal conversation or to television
- speech abnormality or delay
- absence of 'babbling' by 12 months
- no single words or comprehension of simple words by 18 months
- learning problems at school
- disobedience
- other behavioural problems
- inability to detect sound direction (unilateral loss)
- inability to follow simple commands or less than 20 spoken words by 2 years

Screening methods

Hearing can be tested at any age. No child is too young to be tested and this includes the newborn. Informal office assessments, such as whispering in the child's ear or rattling car keys, are totally inadequate for excluding deafness and may be potentially harmful if they lead to false reassurance.

Pneumatic otoscopy is essential to exclude middle ear effusions.

Puretone audiometry is unreliable in children under 4 years of age; so special techniques such as tympanometry are required. Tympanometry assesses TM compliance, and is highly sensitive and specific for detecting middle-ear pathology in children beyond early infancy.

Auditory brain stem response testing is used to evaluate children (particularly young infants) for whom information on behavioural hearing tests is either unobtainable or unreliable.[5]

Management

Children with middle ear pathology and hearing loss should be referred to a specialist. All children with SNHL (even those with profound deafness), as well as children with conductive losses

not correctable by surgery, benefit from amplification. All children need referral to a specialist centre skilled in educational and language remediation.

Deafness in the elderly

The prevalence of hearing loss increases exponentially with age. The commonest reason for bilateral progressive SND is presbyacusis, which is the high-frequency hearing loss of advancing age (Fig. 39.8). There appears to be a genetic predisposition to presbyacusis.

Some features include:

- loss of high-frequency sounds
- usually associated with tinnitus
- intolerance to very loud sounds
- difficulty picking up high-frequency consonants, e.g. 'f', 's'—these sounds are often distorted or unheard, and there is confusion with words such as 'fit' and 'sit', 'fun' and 'sun'

Deafness is associated with various types of mental illness in the aged including anxiety, depression, paranoid delusions, agitation and confusion because of sensory deprivation. The possibility of deafness should be kept in mind when assessing these problems.

Signs indicating referral for hearing test

Possible indications for referring the older person:

- speaking too loudly
- difficulty understanding speech
- social withdrawal
- lack of interest in attending parties and other functions

Fig. 39.8 *Presbyacusis: bilateral high-frequency sensorineural deafness*

- complaints about people mumbling
- requests to have speech repeated
- complaints of tinnitus
- setting television and radio on high volume

Sudden deafness

Sudden deafness refers to sudden sensorineural hearing loss of greater than 30–35 dB with an onset period of between 12 hours and 3 days.[6] It specially excludes gradual progressive causes of sensorineural deafness such as cumulative noise trauma or presbyacusis and also excludes causes of sudden deafness that may be related to pathology in the external auditory canal, TM or middle ear.

The main causes are given in Table 39.5.

In several instances, despite a careful clinical examination and investigation, an explanation for sudden SND cannot be found. The cause of deafness in these cases is thought to be either vascular obstruction of the end artery system or viral cochleitis.[5,6] Fortunately spontaneous recovery usually results.

Patients with sudden SND require immediate referral. It is a difficult problem both in diagnosis and management. Early diagnosis and a high index of suspicion are fundamental.[6] Two important conditions that deserve special reference are perilymphatic fistula, which occurs after stapedectomy, and an acoustic neuroma presumably causing compression of the internal auditory artery by the tumour in the internal auditory meatus.

Otosclerosis

Otosclerosis is a disease of the bone surrounding the inner ear and is the most common cause of conductive hearing loss in the adult with a normal tympanic membrane.

Features[3]
- a progressive disease
- develops in the 20s and 30s
- family history (autosomal dominant)
- female preponderance
- affects the footplate of the stapes
- conductive hearing loss
- SND may be present
- impedance audiometry shows characteristic features (Fig. 39.9).
- maybe associated with Meniere's syndrome

Management
- stapedectomy (approximately 90% effective)
- hearing aid (less effective alternative)

Noise-induced hearing loss
Features
- onset of tinnitus after work in excessive noise
- speech seems muffled soon after work
- temporary loss initially but becomes permanent if noise exposure continues
- high-frequency loss on audiogram

Sounds exceeding 85 dB are potentially injurious to the cochlea, especially with prolonged exposures. Common sources of injurious noise are industrial machinery, weapons and loud music.

Table 39.5 *Causes of sudden deafness*

Trauma
- head injury
- diving
- flying
- acoustic blast

Postoperative
- previous stapedectomy

Viral infections, e.g. mumps, measles, herpes zoster

Ototoxic drugs, e.g. aminoglycosides

Cerebellopontine angle tumours, e.g. acoustic neuroma

Vascular disease
- polycythaemia
- diabetes

Ménière's syndrome

Cochlear otosclerosis

Fig. 39.9 *Otosclerosis: the conductive loss is commonly associated with a mild sensorineural loss at 2000 cycles per second (Carhardt's notch)*

Hearing aids

Hearing aids are most useful in conductive deafness. This is due to the relative lack of distortion, making amplification simple. In SND the dual problem of recruitment and the hearing loss for higher frequencies may make hearing aids less satisfactory. Modern aids selectively amplify higher frequencies and 'cut out' excessive volume peaks that would cause discomfort. A trial of such aids should be made by a reliable hearing-aid consultant following full medical assessment.

Advice for families

Relatives and close friends need considerable advice about coping with deaf members. They should be told that the deaf person may hear in a quiet room but not in a crowd, and advised of the range of aids and services available and the importance of proper maintenance of any hearing aids (especially with aged people).

Do

- Face the light when speaking to them.
- Speak directly to them.
- Speak clearly and naturally.
- Speak at a uniform pitch: avoid lowering your voice during or at the end of a sentence.
- Speak within 2 metres.
- Be tolerant and relaxed.
- Be patient with mistakes.
- Write key words on a paper pad when necessary.

Don't

- Speak with your back to them.
- Mumble your words.
- Use exaggerated lip movements.
- Shout.
- Put your hand or fingers over your mouth when talking.
- Repeat one word over and over.

When to refer

- Sudden deafness.
- Any child with suspected deafness, including poor speech and learning problems, should be referred to an audiology centre.
- Any child with middle ear pathology and hearing loss should be referred to a specialist.
- Unexplained deafness.

Practice tips

- A mother who believes her child may be deaf is rarely wrong in this suspicion.
- Suspect deafness in an infant with delayed development and in children with speech defects or behavioural problems.
- Audiological assessment should be performed on children born to mothers with evidence of intrauterine infection by any of the TORCH organisms (toxoplasmosis, rubella, cytomegalovirus and herpes virus).
- No child is too young for audiological assessment. Informal office tests are inadequate for excluding hearing loss.
- Sounds tend to be softer in a conductive hearing loss and distorted with sensorineural loss.
- People with conductive deafness tend to speak softly, hear better in a noisy environment, hear well on the telephone and have good speech discrimination.
- People with SND tend to speak loudly, hear poorly in a noisy environment, have poor speech discrimination and hear poorly on the telephone.

References

1. Ludman H. *ABC of otolaryngology (3rd edn)*. London: British Medical Association, 1993, 10–22.
2. Stephens S. Hearing problems. Medical Observer, 14 September, 1990, 51–52.
3. Tierney LM et al. *Current medical diagnosis and treatment (35th edn)*. Stamford: Appleton & Lange, 1996, 181–183.
4. Black B. Pure tone audiograms. Aust Fam Physician, 1988; 17:906–907.
5. Jarman R. Hearing impairment. In: *Australian Paediatric Review*, 1991, 4:2.
6. Pohl DV. Sudden deafness. Mod Med Aust, June 1990, 72–78.

40
Diarrhoea

—

Diarrhoea is defined as the frequent passage of loose or watery stools.

Essential features are:

- an increase in frequency of bowel action
- an increase in softness, fluidity or volume of stools

Acute self-limiting diarrhoea, which is very common and frequently not seen by the medical practitioner, is usually infective and mild, and resolves within days. In Australia most infective cases are viral. The causes of diarrhoea are numerous, thus making a detailed history and examination very important in leading to the diagnosis. Important causes are presented in Figure 40.1.

The terminology for acute infective diarrhoea can be confusing. A simple classification is:

- vomiting and diarrhoea = gastroenteritis
- diarrhoea (only) = enteritis

Key facts and checkpoints

- The characteristics of the stool provide a useful guide to the site of the bowel disorder.
- Disease of the upper GIT tends to produce diarrhoea stools that are copious, watery or fatty, pale yellow or green.
- Colonic disease tends to produce stools that are small, of variable consistency, brown and may contain blood or mucus.
- Acute gastroenteritis should be regarded as a diagnosis of exclusion.

- Chronic diarrhoea is more likely to be due to protozoal infection (amoebiasis, giardiasis or cryptosporidium) than bacillary dysentery.
- A history of travel, especially to countries at risk of endemic bowel infections, is essential.
- Certain antibiotics can cause an overgrowth of *Clostridium difficile*, which produces pseudo-membranous colitis.
- Coeliac disease, although a cause of failure to thrive in children, can present at any age.
- In disorders of the colon the patient experiences frequency and urgency but passes only small amounts of faeces.

A diagnostic approach

A summary of the safety diagnostic model is presented in Table 40.1.

Probability diagnosis

Acute diarrhoea

Common causes are:

- gastroenteritis/enteritis
  - bacterial
    - salmonella sp
    - *Campylobacter jejuni*
    - *Shigella* sp
    - enteropathic *Escherichia coli*
    - *Staphylococcus aureus* (food poisoning)
  - viral
    - rotavirus (50% of children hospital admissions[1])
- dietary indiscretions, e.g. binge eating
- antibiotic reactions

Chronic diarrhoea

Irritable bowel syndrome was the commonest cause of chronic diarrhoea in a UK study.[2]

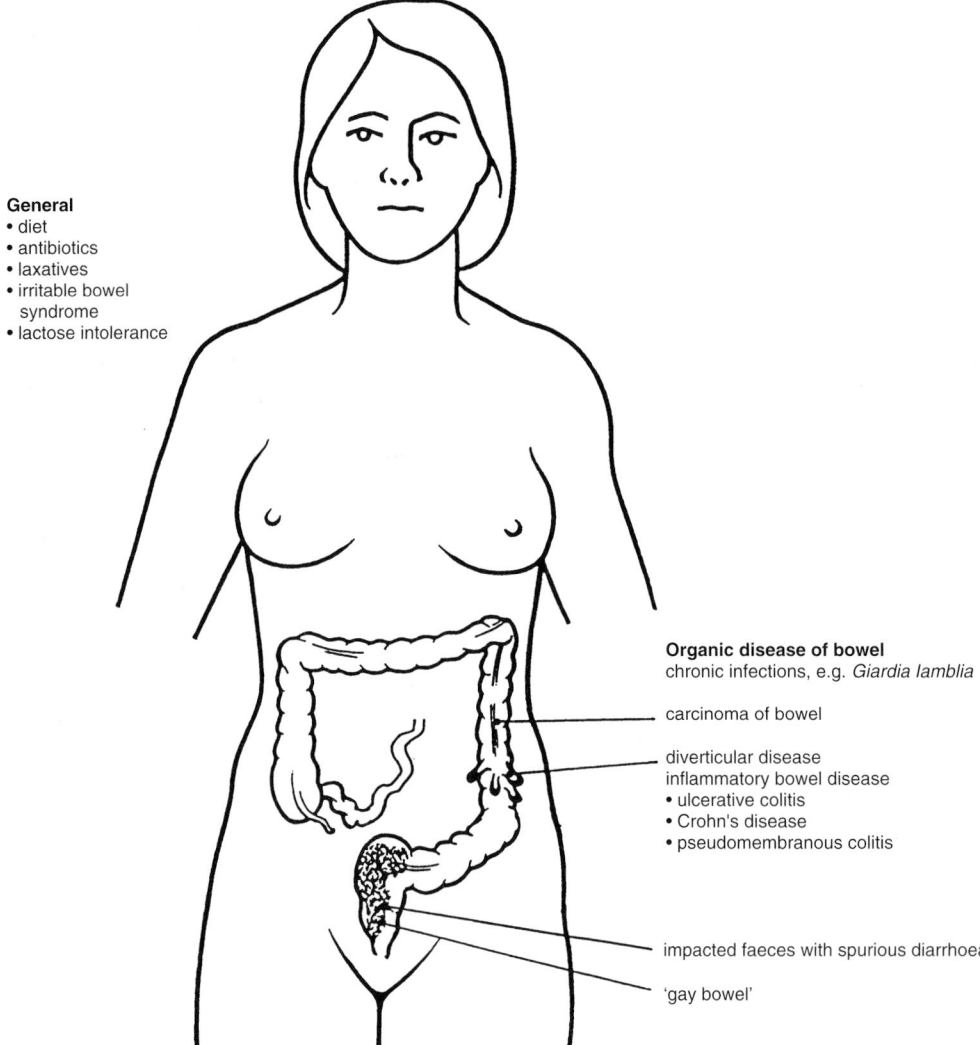

General
• diet
• antibiotics
• laxatives
• irritable bowel
  syndrome
• lactose intolerance

Organic disease of bowel
chronic infections, e.g. *Giardia lamblia*

carcinoma of bowel

diverticular disease
inflammatory bowel disease
• ulcerative colitis
• Crohn's disease
• pseudomembranous colitis

impacted faeces with spurious diarrhoea

'gay bowel'

Fig. 40.1 *Important causes of chronic diarrhoea*

Drug reactions are also important. These include ingestion of laxatives, osmotic agents such as lactose and sorbitol in chewing gum, alcohol, antibiotics, thyroxine and others.

Acute gastroenteritis that persists into a chronic phase is relatively common, especially in travellers returning from overseas. Important considerations are *Giardia lamblia*, *Clostridium difficile*, *Yersinia*, *Entamoeba histolytica*, *Cryptosporidium* and HIV infection.

Serious disorders not to be missed

Colorectal carcinoma must be considered with persistent diarrhoea, especially if of insidious onset.

AIDS due to symptomatic HIV infection needs consideration, especially in those at risk. The serious infectious disorders that can affect international travellers such as cholera, typhoid, paratyphoid and amoebiasis should also be kept in mind.

In children coeliac disease and fibrocystic disease can present as chronic diarrhoea while intussusception, although not causing true diarrhoea, can present as loose redcurrant jelly-like stools and should not be misdiagnosed (as gastroenteritis). Appendicitis must also be considered in the onset of acute diarrhoea and vomiting.

Infection with enterohaemorrhagic strains of

Table 40.1   *Diarrhoea: diagnostic strategy model*

Q   Probability diagnosis
A.   *Acute*
   • Gastroenteritis/infective enteritis
   • Dietary indiscretion
   • Antibiotic reaction
   Chronic
   • Irritable bowel syndrome
   • Drug reactions, e.g. laxatives
   • Chronic infections
Q.   Serious disorders not to be missed
A.   Neoplasia
   • Carcinoma of bowel
   HIV infection (AIDS)
   Infections
   • Cholera
   • Typhoid/paratyphoid
   • Amoebiasis
   • Malaria
   • Enterohaemorrhagic *E. coli* enteritis
   Inflammatory bowel disease
   • Crohn's/ulcerative colitis
   • Pseudomembranous colitis
   Intussusception
   Pelvic appendicitis/pelvic abscess
Q.   The pitfalls
A.   Faecal impaction with spurious diarrhoea
   Lactase deficiency
   Giardia lamblia infection
   Cryptosporidium infection
   Malabsorption states, e.g coeliac disease
   Vitamin C and other oral drugs
   Radiotherapy
   Diverticulitis
   Post GIT surgery
   'Gay bowel'
   Ischaemic colitis (elderly)
   Rarities
   • Addison's disease
   • Carcinoid tumours
   • Short bowel syndrome
   • Amyloidosis
   • Toxic shock
   • Zollinger–Ellison syndrome
Q.   Seven masquerades checklist
A.   Depression   —
   Diabetes   √
   Drugs   √
   Anaemia   —
   Thyroid disease   √ hyper
   Spinal dysfunction   —
   UTI   —
Q.   Is the patient trying to tell me something?
A.   Yes, diarrhoea may be a manifestation of anxiety state or irritable bowel syndrome.

Escherichia coli, e.g. O157:H7, O111:H8, may lead to the haemolytic uraemic syndrome or thrombotic thrombocytopenic purpura, particularly in children. What appears to be simple enteritis can eventuate to be fatal.

Pitfalls

There are many traps in evaluating the patient with diarrhoea including drug ingestion, especially vitamin C (sodium ascorbate powder) which causes diarrhoea. Faecal impaction with spurious diarrhoea is an age-old pitfall, as is lactase deficiency, which may go undiagnosed for many years. In recent times infection with *Giardia lamblia* may smoulder on for months with watery offensive stools before diagnosis.

General pitfalls

• Not considering acute appendicitis in acute diarrhoea—can be retrocaecal or pelvic appendicitis
• Missing faecal impaction with spurious diarrhoea
• Failing to perform a rectal examination
• Failing to consider acute ischaemic colitis in an elderly patient with the acute onset of bloody diarrhoea stools (following sudden abdominal pain in preceding 24 hours)

Seven masquerades checklist

The significant masquerades include diabetes, when an autonomic neuropathy may cause alternating bouts of constipation and diarrhoea, thyrotoxicosis and drugs. Drugs that can cause diarrhoea are summarised in Table 40.2.

Table 40.2   *Drugs that can cause diarrhoea*

Alcohol, esp. chronic abuse (often overlooked!)

Antibiotics, esp. penicillin derivatives

Antihypertensives, selected, e.g. methyldopa

Cardiac agents, e.g. digoxin, quinidine

Chenodeoxycholic acid

Cisapride

Colchicine

Cytotoxic agents, e.g. methotrexate

Heavy metals

H_2-antagonists

Iron-containing compounds

Laxatives

Magnesium-containing antacids

Metformin

Misoprostol

Prostaglandins

Salicylates

Theophylline

Thyroxine

Pseudomembranous colitis (antibiotic-associated diarrhoea)

This colitis can be caused by the use of any antibiotic, especially clindamycin, lincomycin, ampicillin and the cephalosporins (an exception is vancomycin). It is usually due to an overgrowth of *Clostridium difficile*, which produces a toxin that causes specific inflammatory lesions, sometimes with a pseudomembrane. It may occur, uncommonly, without antibiotic usage.

Features

- profuse watery diarrhoea
- abdominal cramping and tenesmus, maybe fever
- within 2 days of taking antibiotic (can start up to 4 to 6 weeks after usage)
- persists 2 weeks (up to 6) after ceasing antibiotic

Diagnosed by characteristic lesions on sigmoidoscopy and a tissue culture assay for *C. difficile* toxin.

Treatment[7]

- cease antibiotic
- choice 1: metronidazole 400 mg (o) tds for 7–10 days

  or
- choice 2: vancomycin 125 mg (o) qid for 10 days

Psychogenic considerations

Anxiety and stress can cause looseness of the bowel. The irritable bowel syndrome, which is a very common condition, may reflect underlying psychological factors and most patients find that the symptoms are exacerbated by stress. Look for evidence of depression.

In children chronic diarrhoea can occur with the so-called 'maternal deprivation syndrome', characterised by growth and developmental retardation due to adverse psychosocial factors.

The clinical approach

History

As always, the history is the key to the diagnosis. First establish what the patient means by the term 'diarrhoea', his or her normal pattern and how the presenting problem varies from normal.

It is important to analyse the nature of the stools, the frequency of diarrhoea, associated symptoms including abdominal pain and constitutional symptoms such as fever. Food intake in the past 72 hours and recent travel abroad may give a clue to acute gastroenteritis or food poisoning (an acute self-limiting illness of diarrhoea and vomiting). The difference between food poisoning and infective gastroenteritis is presented in Table 40.3. However, there can be an overlap

Table 40.3 *Comparison of acute diarrhoea due to bacterial food poisoning and infective gastroenteritis*

	Food poisoning	Infective gastroenteritis

Responsible organisms	Toxins from:
	Staphylococcus aureus
	Clostidrium perfringens
	Vibrio parahaemolyticus
	Aeromonas hydrophilia
	Bacillus cereus
		viral
		bacterial
		e.g. *Campylobacter jejuni*
		  Escherichia coli
		  Shigella sp
		  Salmonella sp

Incubation period (onset from contact)	short—within 24 hours average—12 hours *S. aureus*—2–4 hours	3–5 days
Diarrhoea	watery	diarrhoea ± blood
Other features	abdominal cramps (milder) dehydration headache vomiting	abdominal cramps
Typical foods	chicken meat seafood rice custards and cream (*S. aureus*)	milk water chicken

Table 40.4 *Non-microbial food poisoning*

Food (specific types)	Toxin	Onset	Features (symptoms)
Mushrooms Toadstools	Muscarine	Minutes to hours	• N,V,D,P • multiple CNS symptoms
Immature or sprouting potatoes	Solanine	Within hours	• N,V,D,P • throat constriction
Fish	Ichthysarcotoxin Various	10–60 minutes (occasionally longer)	• N,V,D,P • circumoral tingling • CNS symptoms • collapse
Mussels	Mytilotoxism	5–30 minutes	• N,V,P • CNS: paralysis
Grain, esp. rye	Ergot fungus	Minutes to 24 hours	• N,V,P • circulatory and CNS
Fava beans (favism)	Enzyme deficiency	Rapid	• V,D • acute haemolysis

N = nausea; V = vomiting; D = diarrhoea; P = abdominal pain

of features from a specific organism and the exercise may be semantic, but it may provide a clue to food-borne causation. A summary of non-microbial food poisoning is presented in Table 40.4.

A drug history is relevant and a family history of diarrhoea, which may be significant for coeliac disease, Crohn's disease and cystic fibrosis.

Patients at risk from HIV infection should be discretely evaluated.

Key questions

| Acute diarrhoea |

• Where did you eat in the 24 hours before the diarrhoea started?
• What food did you eat during this time?
• Did you have chicken or seafood recently? (Chicken may be contaminated with *Salmonella* or *Campylobacter* and seafood with *Vibrio parahaemolyticus*.)
• Did any other people get the same problem?
• Have you travelled overseas recently? Where?
• Have you noticed any blood or mucus in your motions?
• Have you had any previous attacks?
• Have you noticed fever, weakness or other symptoms?

| Chronic diarrhoea |

• Have you noticed any blood or mucus in the motion?
• Have you travelled overseas recently? Where?

• Do you have pain and is it relieved by opening your bowels or passing wind?
• Does anyone else in your family have diarrhoea?
• Have you had any operations on your abdomen recently?
• What medications are you taking?
• Are you taking antibiotics?
• Do you take vitamin C for your health?
• Do you take laxatives?
• How much alcohol do you drink?
• How much milk do you drink?
• What about thick shakes, ice-cream and yoghurt?
• Do you get clammy or shaky, or have you lost weight?
• Have you had trouble with pain in your joints, back pain, eye trouble or mouth ulceration?
• Do you have trouble flushing your motions down the toilet?
• Do you get diarrhoea during the night?
• Are you under a lot of stress?

Significance of symptoms

| Abdominal pain |

Central colicky abdominal pain indicates involvement of the small bowel, while lower abdominal pain points to the large bowel.

| Nature of stools |

If small volume consider inflammation or carcinoma of colon, and if large volume consider laxative abuse and malabsorption.

If there is profuse bright red bleeding consider diverticulitis or carcinoma of colon, and if small amounts with mucus or mucopus consider inflammatory bowel disease. The presence of blood in the stools excludes functional bowel disease. Diarrhoea at night suggests organic disease. In steatorrhoea the stools are distinctively pale, greasy, offensive, floating and difficult to flush. It is exacerbated by fatty foods.

The consistency of the stool as an aid to diagnosis[2,3] is summarised in Table 40.5, and the characteristics that distinguish between small and large bowel diarrhoea[1] are presented in Table 40.6.

Table 40.5 *Stool consistency as an aid to diagnosis*

Consistency	Probable cause
Liquid and uniform	Small bowel disease, e.g. gastroenteritis
Loose with bits of faeces	Colonic disease
Watery, offensive, bubbly	*Giardia lamblia* infection
Liquid or semiformed, mucous ± blood	*Entamoeba histolytica*
Bulky, pale, offensive	Malabsorption
Pellets or ribbons	Irritable bowel syndrome

Table 40.6 *Distinction between small and large bowel diarrhoea*

	Small bowel	Large bowel
Volume	Large	Small
Pain	Central	Lower/LIF
Borborygmi	++	–
Undigested food	+	–
Steatorrhoea	+/–	–
Blood	–	+
Mucus	–	+
Urgency	–	+
Tenesmus	–	+

Physical examination

The extent of the examination depends on the nature of the presenting problem. If it is acute, profuse and associated with vomiting, especially in a child, the examination needs to be general to assess the effects of fluid, electrolyte and nutritional loss. An infant's life is in danger from severe gastroenteritis and this assessment is a priority. The general nutritional and electrolyte assessment is also relevant in chronic diarrhoea with malabsorption, and this includes looking for evidence of muscle weakness (e.g. hypokalaemia, hypomagnesaemia, tetany [hypocalcaemia], bruising [vitamin K loss]).

The examination should also focus on the abdomen (systematic palpation), the rectum and the skin. Possible helpful signs are included in Figure 40.2.

The stool

In all cases the stool should be examined. Note the presence of blood or mucus or steatorrhoea.

Investigations

The following list includes a range of tests that may be required. Appropriate tests should be judiciously selected and in some instances, such as acute self-limiting diarrhoea, no investigations are necessary.

- Stool tests
  — microscopy for parasites and red and white cells (warm specimen for amoebiasis)
  — cultures: may need special requests for Campylobacter sp, *Clostridium difficile* and toxin, *Yersinia* sp, *Cryptosporidium* sp, *Aeromonas* sp (stools must be collected fresh on three occasions)
- Blood tests
  — haemoglobin; MCV; WCC; ESR; iron; ferritin; folate; vitamin B_{12}; calcium; electrolytes; thyroid function; HIV tests
- Haemagglutination tests for amoebiasis
- *Clostridium difficile* tissue culture assay
- Malabsorption studies
- Endoscopy
  — proctosigmoidoscopy
  — flexible sigmoidoscopy/colonoscopy (with biopsy)
  — small bowel biopsy (coelic disease)
- Radiology
  — plain X-ray abdomen—of limited value
  — small bowel enema
  — barium enema, especially double contrast

Note: HIV patients should be investigated in specialist centres.

Principles of treatment[4]

When an underlying cause of diarrhoea can be identified, apart from some common infections, management should be directed at that cause. There are a few situations in which the causative bacterial or parasitic pathogen requires specific treatment, for example giardiasis. The management is determined by the nature of the pathogen and the severity of the illness.

Fig. 40.2 *Possible significant signs in the patient with diarrhoea*

However, in Australia most infective cases are viral. The basic principle therefore is to achieve and maintain adequate hydration until the illness resolves. In adults and children oral rehydration is indicated unless there is evidence of impending circulatory 'shock' demanding intravenous therapy. Oral rehydration solution containing sodium, potassium and glucose should be considered for patients with mild to moderate dehydration. Adults should drink 2 to 3 litres of the solution in 24 hours.

In general, treatment should not be directed specifically at altering the frequency and consistency of the stools. The antimotility drugs (loperamide, diphenoxylate and codeine) have a role restricted to short-term control of symptoms in adults during periods of significant social inconvenience such as travel. It must be emphasised that antimotility drugs are never indicated for management of acute diarrhoea in infants and children.[4]

The traditional absorbent agents such as kaolin/pectin mixtures, activated charcoal and other mineral clays have not been shown to be of value and may interfere with absorption of other drugs. They should not be used.

Specific antibiotics are reserved for the treatment of giardiasis, amoebiasis, antibiotic-associated diarrhoea, cholera and typhoid. Although antibiotics are usually unnecessary in most cases they may be indicated for severe cases of campylobacter enteritis, salmonella, enteritis, shigellosis and traveller's diarrhoea.

Malabsorption

It is important to distinguish the steatorrhoea of various malabsorption syndromes from diarrhoea. Important causes are presented in Table 40.7.

The common causes are coeliac disease, chronic pancreatitis and postgastrectomy.

Clinical features
- bulky, pale, offensive, frothy, greasy stools
- stools difficult to flush down toilet
- weight loss
- failure to thrive (in infants)
- increased faecal fat
- signs of multiple vitamin deficiencies, e.g. A,D,E,K
- sore tongue (glossitis)
- hypochromic or megaloblastic anaemia (possible)

Refer for specific investigations, e.g. FBE, barium studies, small bowel biopsy, faecal fat (>21 g/3 days).

Coeliac disease
Synonyms: coeliac sprue, gluten-sensitive enteropathy
Note: It can appear at *any* age; refer to coeliac disease in children (pp. 403–404).

Table 40.7 *Important causes of malabsorption*

Primary mucosal disease
- gluten-sensitive enteropathy (coeliac disease)
- tropical sprue
- lactose intolerance (lactase deficiency)
- Crohn's disease (regional enteritis)
- parasite infections, e.g. *Giardia lamblia*
- lymphoma

Maldigestion states
Lumenal abnormalities
- postsurgery, e.g. gastrectomy, ileal resection
- systemic sclerosis

Pancreatic disease
- chronic pancreatitis
- cystic fibrosis
- pancreatic tumours, e.g. Zollinger-Ellison

Diagnosis
- classic triad: diarrhoea, weight loss, iron/folate deficiency
- elevated faecal fat
- characterisic small bowel biopsy (key test)
- antigliadin antibodies (screening—limited)

Management
- diet control: high complex carbohydrate and protein, low fat, gluten-free (no wheat, barley, rye and oats)
- treat specific vitamin deficiencies

Gluten-free diet
Avoid foods containing gluten either as obvious component, e.g. flour, bread, oatmeal, or as a hidden ingredient, e.g. dessert mix, stock cube.
Forbidden foods include:
- standard bread, pasta, crispbreads, flour
- standard biscuits and cakes
- breakfast cereals made with wheat or oats
- oatmeal, wheat bran, barley/barley water
- 'battered' or bread-crumbed fish, etc.
- meat and fruit pies
- most stock cubes and gravy mixes

Diarrhoea in the elderly

The older the patient the more likely a late onset of symptoms that reflect serious underlying organic disease, especially malignancy. Colorectal cancer needs special consideration. The older the patient, especially the bedridden elderly patient, the more likely the presentation of faecal impaction with spurious diarrhoea. The possibility of drug interactions, including digoxin, should also be considered. Ischaemic colitis must be considered in an elderly patient.

Ischaemic colitis
This is due to atheromatous occlusion of mesenteric vessels.

Clinical features
Clinical features include:
- sharp abdominal pain in an elderly patient with bloody diarrhoea
  or
- periumbilical pain and diarrhoea about 15–30 minutes after eating
- maybe loud bruits over central abdomen
- other evidence of generalised atherosclerosis
- barium enema shows 'thumb printing' sign due to submucosal oedema

- the definitive test is aortography and selective angiography of mesenteric vessels
- most episodes resolve—may be followed by a stricture

Diarrhoea in children

The commonest cause of diarrhoea in children is acute infective gastroenteritis, but there are certain conditions that develop in childhood and infancy and require special attention. The presentation of small amounts of redcurrant jelly stool with intussusception should also be kept in mind. Of the many causes only a few are commonly seen. The two commonest causes are infective gastroenteritis and antibiotic-induced diarrhoea.

Important causes of diarrhoea in children are:
- infective gastroenteritis
- antibiotics
- overfeeding (loose stools in newborn)
- dietary indiscretions
- sugar (carbohydrate) intolerance
- food allergies, e.g. milk, soya bean, wheat, eggs
- maternal deprivation
- malabsorption states
  — cystic fibrosis
  — coeliac disease

Note: Exclude surgical emergencies, e.g. acute appendicitis, infections, e.g. pneumonia, septicaemia, otitis media < 5 years.

Acute gastroenteritis

Note: Dehydration from gastroenteritis is an important cause of death, particularly in obese infants (especially if vomiting accompanies the diarrhoea).

Definition

It is an illness of acute onset, of less than 10 days duration associated with fever, diarrhoea and/or vomiting, where there is no other evident cause for the symptoms.[5]

Features

Causes
- mainly rotavirus (developed countries) and adenovirus: viruses account for about 80%
- bacterial: *Campylobacter jejuni* and *Salmonella* sp (two commonest), *Escherichia coli* and *Shigella* sp
- protozoal: *Giardia lamblia, Entamoeba histolytica, Cryptosporidium*

- food poisoning—staphylococcal toxin

Differential diagnoses. These include septicaemia, urinary tract infection, intussusception, appendicitis, pelvic abscess, partial bowel obstruction, diabetes mellitus and antibiotic reaction[3] (see Table 40.8).
Note: Exclude acute appendicitis and intussusception in the very young.

Symptoms

- anorexia, nausea, poor feeding, vomiting, fever, diarrhoea (fever and vomiting may be absent)
- fluid stools (often watery) 10–20 per day
- crying—due to pain, hunger, thirst or nausea
- bleeding—uncommon (usually bacterial)
- anal soreness

Viral indication: large volume, watery, typically lasts 2–3 days, systemic symptoms uncommon

Bacterial indication: small motions, blood, mucus, abdominal pain and tenesmus

Dehydration must be assessed (see Table 40.9).

Complications
- febrile convulsions
- sugar (lactose) intolerance (common)
- septicaemia esp. *Salmonella*

Management

Management is based on the assessment and correction of fluid and electrolyte loss.[5,6] Since dehydration is usually isotonic with equivalent loss of fluid and electrolytes, serum electrolytes will be normal.

Table 40.8 *Differential diagnosis of acute diarrhoea and vomiting in children*

Bowel infection
- viruses
- bacteria
- protozoal
- food poisoning—staphylococcal toxin

Systemic infection

Abdominal disorders
- appendicitis
- pelvic abscess
- intussusception
- malrotation

Urinary tract infection

Antibiotic reaction

Diabetes mellitus

Table 40.9 *Assessment of hydration*

	Mild	*Moderate*	*Severe*
Body weight loss	• 5%	• 6–9%	• $\geq$ 10%
Symptoms/general observations	• thirsty • alert • restless	• thirsty • restless • lethargic • irritable	• *Infants*: drowsy, limp, cold, sweaty, cyanotic limbs, comatose • *Older*: apprehensive, cold and sweaty, cyanotic limbs
Signs	• normal	• dry mucous membranes, absent tears	• rapid feeble pulse • hypotensive • sunken eyes and fontanelles • very dry mucous membranes
Pinched skin test	• normal	• retracts slowly (1–2 seconds)	• retracts very slowly > 2 seconds
Urine output	• normal	• decreased	• nil

Treatment	• *Oral rehydration*
	  — small amounts of fluids often
	  — continue breast-feeding
	  — solids after 24 hours
	  — provide maintenance fluid and loss
		• *Oral rehydration*
		  — consider nasogastric tube for steady fluid infusion
		    or
		  — IV infusion
			• urgent IV infusion: isotonic fluid

Note: The most accurate way to monitor dehydration is to weigh the child, preferably without clothes, on the same scale each time. However the easiest is clinical assessment (e.g. vomiting, no urine, lethargy and thirst).

Avoid

• Drugs: antidiarrhoeals, antiemetics and antibiotics
• Lemonade: osmotic load too high: can use if diluted 1 part to 4 parts water but sugar may be poorly tolerated

To treat or not to treat at home

• Treat at home—if family can cope, vomiting is not a problem and no dehydration.
• Admit to hospital—if dehydration or persisting vomiting or family cannot cope; also infants < 6 months and high-risk patients.

Advice to parents (for mild to moderate diarrhoea)

General rules

• Give small amounts of fluids often.
• Start solids after 24 hours.

• Continue breast-feeding
  or
  start bottle feeding after 24 hours.

Day 1

Give fluids, a little at a time and often (e.g. 50 mL every 15 minutes if vomiting a lot). A good method is to give 200 mL (about 1 cup) of fluid every time a watery stool is passed or a big vomit occurs.

The ideal fluid is Gastrolyte or New Repalyte. Other suitable oral rehydration preparations are WHO recommended solutions 'Electrolade' and 'Glucolyte'.

Alternatives are:

• lemonade (not low-calorie)	1 part to 6 parts water
• sucrose (table sugar)	1 teaspoon to 120 mL water
• glucose	1 teaspoon to 120 mL water
• cordials (not low-calorie)	1 part to 16 parts water
• fruit juice	1 part to 4 parts water

Warning: Do *not* use straight lemonade or mix up Gastrolyte with lemonade or fluids other than water.

Method of assessing fluid requirements[4]

Fluid loss (mL) = % dehydration × body weight (kg) × 10

Maintenance (mL/kg/24 hr): 1–3 mo: 120 mL; 4–12 mo: 100 mL; > 12 mo: 80 mL

Allow for continuing loss,

e.g. 8 month 10 kg child with 5% dehydration

Fluid loss = 5 × 10 × 10 = 500 mL

Maintenance = 100 × 10 = 1000 mL

Total 24 hour requirement (minimum) = 1500 mL

Approx. average hourly requirement = 60 mL

> - Aim to give more (replace fluid loss) in the first 6 hours.
> - Rule of thumb: 100 mL/kg (infants) and 50 mL/kg (older children) in first 6 hours.

Days 2 and 3

Reintroduce your baby's milk or formula diluted to half strength (i.e. mix equal quantities of milk or formula and water).

Do not worry that your child is not eating food. Solids can be commenced after 24 hours. Start with bread, plain biscuits, jelly, stewed apple, rice, porridge or non-fat potato chips. Avoid fatty foods, fried foods, raw vegetables and fruit, and wholegrain bread.

Day 4

Increase milk to normal strength and gradually reintroduce the usual diet.

Breast-feeding. If your baby is not vomiting, continue breast-feeding but offer extra fluids (preferably Gastrolyte) between feeds. If vomiting is a problem, express breast milk for the time being while you follow the oral fluid program.

NB: Watch for lactose intolerance as a sequela— explosive diarrhoea after introducing formula. Replace with a lactose-free formula.

Chronic diarrhoea in children

Sugar intolerance

Synonyms: carbohydrate intolerance, lactose intolerance.

The commonest offending sugar is lactose.

Diarrhoea often follows acute gastroenteritis when milk is reintroduced into the diet. Stools may be watery, frothy, smell like vinegar and tend to excoriate the buttocks. They contain sugar.

A simple test

- Line the napkin with thin plastic and collect fluid stool.
- Mix 5 drops of liquid stool with 10 drops of water and add a Clinitest tablet (detects lactose and glucose but not sucrose).
- A positive result indicates sugar intolerance.

Treatment

- Remove the offending sugar from the diet.
- Use milk preparations in which the lactose has been split to glucose and galactose by enzymes, or use soya protein.

Milk allergy

This is not as common as lactose intolerance. Diarrhoea is related to taking a cows milk formula and relieved when it is withdrawn.

Inflammatory bowel disorder

These disorders, which include Crohn's disease and ulcerative colitis, can occur in childhood. A high index of suspicion is necessary to make an early diagnosis. Approximately 5% of cases of chronic ulcerative colitis have their onset in childhood.[5]

Chronic enteric infection

Responsible organisms include *Salmonella* sp, *Campylobacter, Yersinia, Giardia lamblia* and *Entamoeba histolytica*. With persistent diarrhoea it is important to obtain microscopy of faeces and aerobic and anaerobic stool cultures. *Giardia lamblia* infestation is not an uncommon finding and may be associated with malabsorption, especially of carbohydrate and fat. Giardiasis can mimic coeliac disease.

Coeliac disease

Clinical features in childhood:

- usually presents at 9–18 months, but any age
- previously thriving infant
- anorexia, lethargy, irritability
- failure to thrive
- malabsorption: abdominal distension
- offensive frequent stools

Diagnosis: duodenal biopsy

Treatment: remove gluten from diet

Cystic fibrosis

Cystic fibrosis is the commonest of all inherited disorders (1 per 2500 live births). Clinical features include:

- family history
- presents in infancy
- meconium ileus in the neonate
- recurrent chest infections (cough and wheeze)
- failure to thrive
- malabsorption

Diagnosis: can be diagnosed antenatally (in utero)

neonatal screening—immunoreactive trypsin

Treatment: • pancreatic enzyme replacement for malabsorption

• attention to respiratory problems

Acute gastroenteritis in adults

Features

- invariably a self-limiting problem (1–3 days)
- abdominal cramps
- possible constitutional symptoms, e.g. fever, malaise, nausea, vomiting
- other meal sharers affected → food poisoning
- consider dehydration, especially in the elderly
- consider possibility of enteric fever

Traveller's diarrhoea

The symptoms are usually as above but very severe diarrhoea, especially if associated with blood or mucus, may be a feature of a more serious bowel infection such as amoebiasis. Possible causes of diarrhoeal illness are presented in Table 12.1. Most traveller's diarrhoea is caused by an *Escherichia coli*, which produces a watery diarrhoea within 14 days of arrival in a foreign country. For specific treatment refer to pages 92–93.

Persistent traveller's diarrhoea

Any traveller with persistent diarrhoea after visiting less developed countries, especially India and China, may have a protozoal infection such as amoebiasis or giardiasis.

If there is a fever and blood or mucus in the stools, suspect amoebiasis. Giardiasis is characterised by abdominal cramps, flatulence and bubbly foul-smelling diarrhoea.

Principles of treatment

Acute diarrhoea

- maintenance of hydration
- antiemetic injection (for severe vomiting)
  prochlorperazine IM, statim
  or
  metoclopramide IV, statim
- antidiarrhoeal preparations
  (avoid if possible: loperamide preferred)
  loperamide 2 mg caps (Imodium) 2 caps statim then 1 after each unformed stool (max: 8 caps/day)
  or
  diphenoxylate with atropine (Lomotil) 2 tabs statim then 1–2 (o) 8 hourly

General advice to patient

Rest

Your bowel needs a rest and so do you. It is best to reduce your normal activities until the diarrhoea has stopped.

Diet

It is vital that you starve but drink small amounts of clear fluids such as water, tea, lemonade and yeast extract (e.g. Marmite) until the diarrhoea settles. Then eat low-fat foods such as stewed apples, rice (boiled in water), soups, poultry, boiled potatoes, mashed vegetables, dry toast or bread, biscuits, most canned fruits, jam, honey, jelly, dried skim milk or condensed milk (reconstituted with water).

Avoid alcohol, coffee, strong tea, fatty foods, fried foods, spicy foods, raw vegetables, raw fruit (especially with hard skins), Chinese food, wholegrain cereals and cigarette smoking.

On the third day introduce dairy produce such as a small amount of milk in tea or coffee and a little butter or margarine on toast. Add also lean meat and fish (either grilled or steamed).

Antimicrobial drugs[7]

It is advisable not to use these except where the following specific organisms are identified. The drugs should be selected initially from the list below or modified according to the results of culture and sensitivity tests.[7] Adult doses are shown.

Pseudomembranous colitis. See page 396.

Shigella dysentery (moderate to severe)
- co-trimoxazole (double strength) 1 tab (o) 12 hourly for 7–10 days
  or
- norfloxacin 400 mg (o) 12 hourly for 7–10 days
  or
- ampicillin 1 g (o) 6 hourly for 7–10 days

Campylobacter jejuni (if prolonged)
- norfloxacin 400 mg (o) 12 hourly for 7 days
  or
- erythromycin 500 mg (o) qid for 7 days (preferable)

Giardiasis
- tinidazole 2 g (o), single dose
  or
- metronidazole 400 mg (o) tds for 7 days
(in children: 30 mg/kg/day (to max 1.2 g/day) as single daily dose for 3 days)

Salmonella enteritis
Antibiotics are not generally advisable but if severe or prolonged use
- ciprofloxacin 500 mg (o) bd for 2 weeks

Amoebiasis (intestinal)
- metronidazole 600–800 mg (o) tds for 6–10 days
  plus
- diloxanide furoate 500 mg (o) tds for 10 days

Specialist advice should be sought.

Special enteric infections
Typhoid/paratyphoid fever
- ciprofloxacin 500 mg (o) 12 hourly for 14 days (use IV if oral therapy not tolerated)
  If ciprofloxacin is contraindicated (e.g. in children) or not tolerated, then use:
- ceftriaxone 3 g IV daily until culture and sensitivities available, then choose oral regimens

Alternative oral regimens (based on sensitivity)
- chloramphenicol 500–750 mg (o) 6 hourly for 14 days
  or
- co-trimoxazole (DS) 1 tablet (o) 12 hourly for 14 days
  or
- amoxycillin 1 g (o) 6 hourly for 14 days

If severe: administer same drug and dosage IV for first 4–5 days.

Cholera
Antibiotic therapy reduces the volume and duration of diarrhoea.
- doxycycline 100 mg (o) 12 hourly for 4 days
  or
- co-trimoxazole (DS) 1 tablet (o) 12 hourly for 4 days
  or
- norfloxacin 400 mg (o) 12 hourly for 4 days

Inflammatory bowel disease
Inflammatory bowel disease should be considered when a young person presents with:
- bloody diarrhoea and mucus
- colonic pain and fever
- extra-abdominal manifestations such as arthralgia, low back pain (spondyloarthropathy), eye problems (iridocyclitis), liver disease and skin lesions (pyoderma granulosum, erythema nodosum)

Two important diseases are ulcerative colitis and Crohn's disease which have equal sex incidence and can occur at any age, but onset peaks between 20 and 40 years.

Ulcerative colitis
Features
- mainly a disease of Western societies
- mainly in young adults (15–40) years
- high-risk factors—family history, previous attacks, low-fibre diet
- recurrent attacks of loose stools
- blood, or blood or pus, or mucus in stools
- abdominal pain slight or absent
- fever, malaise and weight loss uncommon
- begins in rectum (continues proximally)—affects only the colon
- an increased risk of carcinoma after 7–10 years

Main symptom
- bloody diarrhoea

Diagnosis
- proctosigmoidoscopy: a granular red proctitis with contact bleeding
- barium enema: characteristic changes

Prognosis
- 5% mortality in an acute attack
- recurrent attacks common
- 75% ten year survival rate

Crohn's disease
Synonyms: regional enteritis, granulomatous colitis

Features
- recurrent diarrhoea in a young person (20–40 years)
- blood and mucus in stools (less than ulcerative colitis)
- colicky abdominal pain (small bowel colic)
- right iliac fossa pain (confused with appendicitis)
- constitutional symptoms, e.g. fever, weight loss, malaise
- signs include perianal disorders, e.g. anal fissure, fistula, ischiorectal abscess
- skip areas in bowel: ½ ileocolic, ¼ confined to small bowel, ¼ confined to colon

Main symptom
- colicky abdominal pain

Diagnosis
- sigmoidoscopy: 'cobblestone' appearance (patchy mucosal oedema)
- colonoscopy: useful to differentiate from ulcerative colitis (UC)

Prognosis
Less favourable than UC with both medical and surgical treatment.

Management principles for both diseases
- Treat under consultant supervision.
- Treatment of acute attacks depends on severity of the attack and the extent of the disease:
  - mild attacks: manage out of hospital
  - severe attacks: hospital, to attend to fluid and electrolyte balance.
- Role of diet controversial: consider a high-fibre diet but maintain adequate nutrition.
- Pharmaceutical agents (the following can be considered):
  - 5-aminosalicylic acid derivatives (mainly UC)
    - sulfasalazine (mainstay)
    - olsalazine; mesalazine

  - corticosteroids (mainly for acute flares)
    - oral
    - parenteral
    - topical (rectal foam, suppositories or enemas)
  - immunomodifying drugs, e.g. azathioprine, cyclosporin, methotrexate
- Surgical treatment: reserve for complications.

Alternating diarrhoea and constipation
Alternating diarrhoea and constipation are well-known symptoms of incomplete bowel obstruction (carcinoma of colon and diverticular disease) and irritable bowel syndrome.

Irritable bowel syndrome (IBS)

Clinical features

- typically in younger women (21–40)
- any age or sex can be affected
- may follow attack of gastroenteritis/traveller's diarrhoea
- cramping abdominal pain (central or iliac fossa)—Fig. 40.3
- pain usually relieved by passing flatus or by defecation
- variable bowel habit (constipation more common)
- diarrhoea usually worse in morning—several loose, explosive bowel actions with urgency
- often precipitated by eating

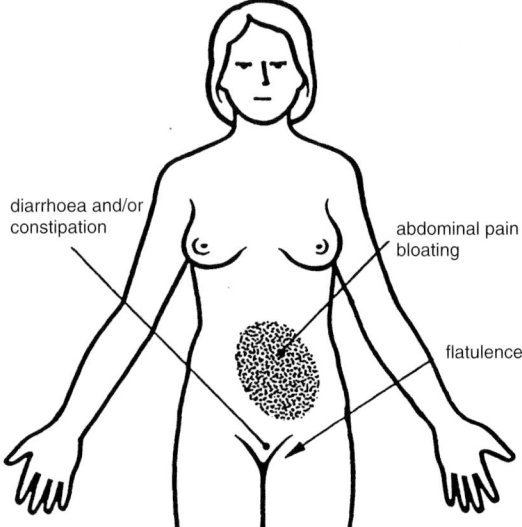

diarrhoea and/or constipation

abdominal pain bloating

flatulence

Fig. 40.3 *Classic symptoms of irritable bowel syndrome*

- faeces sometimes like small, hard pellets or ribbon-like
- anorexia and nausea (sometimes)
- bloating, abdominal distension, ↑ borborygmi
- tiredness common

IBS is a diagnosis of exclusion. A thorough physical examination, investigations (FBE, ESR and stool microscopy or culture) and sigmoidoscopy are necessary. Insufflation of air at sigmoidoscopy may reproduce the abdominal pain of IBS.

Possible related causes
Bowel infection, food irritation (e.g. spicy foods), lactose (milk) intolerance, low-fibre diet, high fatty foods, laxative overusage, use of antibiotics and codeine-containing analgesics, psychological factors.

Management
The patient must be reassured and educated with advice that the problem will not cause malignancy or inflammatory bowel disease and will not shorten life expectancy. The basis of initial treatment is simple dietary modification and non-drug therapy. Drugs that have been used with mixed success include mebeverine, dicyclomine and peppermint oil.

Self-help advice to the patient
Anyone with irritable bowel should try to work on the things that make the symptoms worse. If you recognise stresses and strains in your life, try to develop a more relaxed lifestyle. You may have to be less of a perfectionist in your approach to life.

Try to avoid any foods that you can identify as causing the problem. You may have to cut out smoking and alcohol and avoid laxatives and codeine (in painkillers). A high-fibre diet may be the answer to your problem.

Diverticular disease
Diverticular disease is a problem of the colon (90% in descending colon) and is related to lack of fibre in the diet. It is usually symptomless.

| Clinical features |

- typical in middle aged or elderly—over 40 years
- increases with age
- present in 1 in 3 people over 60 years (Western world)

- diverticulosis—symptomless
- diverticulitis—infected diverticula and symptomatic
- constipation or alternating constipation/diarrhoea
- intermittent cramping lower abdominal pain in LIF
- tenderness in LIF
- rectal bleeding—may be profuse (± faeces)
- may present as acute abdomen or subacute obstruction
- usually settles in 2–3 days

Complications (of diverticulitis)
- abscess
- perforation
- peritonitis
- obstruction
- fistula—bladder, vagina

Investigations
- WBC and ESR—to determine inflammation
- sigmoidoscopy
- barium enema

Management
It usually responds to a high-fibre diet.

Advice to the patient
The gradual introduction of fibre with plenty of fluids (especially water) will improve any symptoms you may have and reduce the risk of complications. Your diet should include:
1. cereals, such as bran, shredded wheat, muesli or porridge
2. wholemeal and multigrain breads
3. fresh or stewed fruits and vegetables

Bran can be added to your cereal or stewed fruit, starting with 1 tablespoon and gradually increasing to 3 tablespoons a day. Fibre can make you feel uncomfortable for the first few weeks, but the bowel soon settles to your improved diet.

When to refer
Children with diarrhoea
- infant under 3 months
- moderate to severe dehydration
- diagnosis of diarrhoea and vomiting in doubt, e.g. blood in vomitus or stool, bile-stained vomiting, high fever or toxaemia, abdominal signs suggestive of appendicitis or obstruction

- failure to improve or deterioration
- a pre-existing chronic illness

Adults

- patient with chronic or bloody diarrhoea
- any problem requiring colonoscopic investigation
- patients with anaemia
- patients with weight loss, abdominal mass or suspicion of neoplasia
- patients with anal fistulae
- patients not responding to treatment for giardiasis
- infection with *Entamoeba histolytica*
- long-term asymptomatic carrier of typhoid or paratyphoid fever
- patient with persistent undiagnosed nocturnal diarrhoea
- patients with 'irritable bowel syndrome' with a significant change in symptoms
- patients with inflammatory bowel disorders with severe exacerbations, possibly requiring immunosuppressive therapy and with complications
- patients with ulcerative colitis of more than 7 years duration (screening by colonoscopy for carcinoma)

Practice tips

- Oral antidiarrhoeal drugs are contraindicated in children; besides being ineffective they may prolong intestinal recovery.
- Antiemetics can readily provoke dystonic reactions in children, especially if young and dehydrated.
- Acute diarrhoea is invariably self-limiting (lasts 2–5 days). If it lasts longer than 7 days investigate with culture and microscopy of the stools.
- If diarrhoea is associated with episodes of facial flushing or wheezing, consider carcinoid syndrome.
- Recurrent pain in the right hypochondrium is

usually a feature of the irritable bowel syndrome (not gall bladder disease).
- Recurrent pain in the right iliac fossa is more likely to be irritable bowel syndrome than appendicitis.
- Beware of false correlations or premature conclusions, e.g. attributing the finding of diverticular disease on barium meal to the cause of the symptoms.
- Undercooked chicken is a common source of enteropathic bacterial infection.
- Consider alcohol abuse if a patient's diarrhoea resolves spontaneously on hospital admission.

References

1. Selby W. Diarrhoea—Differential diagnosis. Aust Fam Physician, 1990; 19: 1683–1689.
2. Sandler G, Fry J. *Early clinical diagnosis.* Lancaster: MTP Press, 1986, 25–30.
3. Borody TJ. Diarrhoea (acute and chronic). In: MIMS Disease Index (2nd edn). Sydney: IMS Publishing, 1996, 153–154.
4. Moulds RFW (Chairman). *Gastrointestinal drug guidelines.* Melbourne: Victorian Medical Postgraduate foundation, 1994–95, 69–96.
5. Barnes G. The child with diarrhoea. In: Robinson MJ ed, *Practical paediatrics.* Melbourne: Churchill Livingstone, 1990, 505–508.
6. Oberklaid F. Management of gastroenteritis in children. In: *The Australian paediatric review.* Melbourne: Royal Children's Hospital, 1990, 1–2.
7. Mashford ML. *Antibiotic guidelines* (9th edn). Melbourne: Victorian Medical Postgraduate Foundation, 1996, 54–56.
8. Schmidt G. Irritable bowel syndrome. In: MIMS Disease Index (2nd edn). Sydney: IMS Publishing, 1996, 279–280.

41
The disturbed patient

—

There is not a sight in nature so mortifying as that of a Distracted Person, when his imagination is troubled, and his whole soul is disordered and confused.

Joseph Addison (1672–1719)

The disturbed and confused patient is a complex management problem in general practice. The cause may be a single one or a combination of several abnormal mental states (see Table 41.1)[1]. The cause may be an organic mental disorder which may be a long-term insidious problem such as dementia, or an acute disorder (delirium), often dramatic in onset. On the other hand the cause of the disturbance may be a psychiatric disorder such as panic disorder, mania, major depression or schizophrenia.

The manifestations of the disturbance are many and include perceptual changes and hallucinations, disorientation, changes in consciousness, changes in mood from abnormally elevated to gross depression, agitation and disturbed thinking including delusions.

Table 41.1 *A general classification of psychiatric disorders*[1]

Organic mental disorders
Acute organic brain syndrome (delirium)
Chronic organic brain syndrome (dementia)

Psychoactive and substance use disorders
Toxic states
Drug dependency
Withdrawal states

Schizophrenic disorders

Mood disorders
Major depression
Bipolar (manic depressive) disorder
Adjustment disorders with depressed mood
Dysthymia

Anxiety disorders
Generalised anxiety disorder
Panic disorder
Obsessive-compulsive disorder
Phobic disorders
Post-traumatic stress disorder

Disorders specific to children

Other disorders
Postpartum psychiatric illness
Eating disorders
Personality disorders

Key facts and checkpoints

- Depression affects 15% of people over 65 and can mimic or complicate any other illness including delirium and dementia.[1]
- Elderly patients with depression are at a high risk of suicide.
- Always search vigorously for the cause or causes of delirium.
- Seeing patients in their home is the best way to evaluate their problem and support systems: it allows opportunities for a history from close contacts and for checking medication, alcohol intake and other factors.

- The diagnosis of dementia can be overlooked: a Scottish study showed that 80% of demented patients were not diagnosed by their GP.[2]
- Patients with a chronic brain syndrome (dementia) are at special risk of an acute brain syndrome (delirium) in the presence of infections and many prescribed drugs.[1]
- Consider prescribed and illicit substances, including the severe anticholinergic delirium syndrome.
- The key feature of dementia is impaired memory.

• The two key features of delirium are disorganised thought and attention.

Definitions

• *Delirium* (also termed 'toxic confusional state') is a relatively acute disorder in which impaired consciousness is associated with abnormalities of perception or mood.
• *Confusion* is disorientation in time, place and person. It may be accompanied by a disturbed conscious state (Table 67.1).
• *Dementia* is an acquired, chronic and gradually progressive deterioration of memory, intellect and personality. Presenile dementia or early onset dementia is dementia under 65 years of age. Senile dementia refers to older patients (usually over 80 years).
• *Alzheimer's disease* is a term used for both senile and presenile dementia which has characteristic pathological degenerative changes in the brain.
• *Cognition* refers to the mental functions of perception, thinking and memory. It is the process of 'knowing'.
• *Hallucinations* are disorders of perception quite divorced from reality. Features:
   — mostly auditory or visual
   — a false perception—not a distortion
   — perceived as normal perceptions
   — independent of the person's will
• *Illusions* are false interpretations of sensory stimuli such as mistaking people or familiar things.
• *Delusions* are abnormal, illogical or false beliefs that are held with absolute conviction despite evidence to the contrary.
• *Obsessions* are recurrent or persistent thoughts, images or impulses that enter the mind despite efforts to exclude them.
• *Compulsions* are repeated, stereotyped and seemingly purposeful actions that the person feels compelled to carry out but resists, realising they are irrational (most are associated with obsessions).

A diagnostic approach

A summary of the diagnostic strategy model for the disturbed or confused patient is presented in Table 41.2.

Table 41.2 *The disturbed mind: diagnostic strategy model*

Q.	*Probability diagnosis*
A.	The 4 D's
	• dementia
	• delirium (look for cause)
	• depression
	• drugs — toxicity
	— withdrawal
Q.	*Serious disorders not to be missed*
A.	Cardiovascular
	• CVAs
	• cardiac failure
	• arrhythmia
	• myocardial ischaemia/AMI
	Neoplasia
	• cerebral
	• carcinoma, e.g. lung
	Severe infections
	• septicaemia
	• HIV infection
	• infective endocarditis
	Hypoglycaemia
	Bipolar disorder/mania
	Schizophrenia states
	Anxiety/panic
	Subdural haematoma
Q.	*Pitfalls (often missed)*
A.	Illicit drug withdrawal
	Fluid and electrolyte disturbances
	Faecal impaction (elderly)
	Urinary retention (elderly)
	Hypoxia
	Pain syndromes (elderly)
	Rarities
	• Hypocalcaemia
	• Renal failure
	• Hepatic failure
	• Prion diseases e.g. Creutzfeldt–Jakob disease
Q.	*Seven masquerades checklist*
A.	Depression √√
	Diabetes √
	Drugs √√
	Anaemia √
	Thyroid disease √
	Spinal dysfunction √ (severe pain in elderly)
	UTI √
Q.	*Is the patient trying to tell me something?*
A.	Consider anxiety, depression, emotional deprivation or upset, change in environment, serious personal loss.

Probability diagnosis

The diagnosis depends on the age and presentation of the patient. In a teenager the probable causes of acute confusion or irrational behaviour include drug toxicity or withdrawal, schizophrenia, severe depression or a behavioural disorder.

It is the elderly who commonly present with confusion. The questions that must be asked are:

- Is the problem one of the 4D's—dementia, delirium, depression, drugs or something else?
- If delirium is the problem, what is the cause?

Depression affects 15% of people over 65, and can mimic other causes of confusion and behavioural disturbance.

Significant prescribed drugs include hypnotics, sedatives, oral hypoglycaemics, antihypertensives, digoxin, antihistamines, anticholinergic drugs and antipsychotics.

Serious disorders not to be missed

There are many serious underlying disorders that must be considered, especially with delirium (Table 41.3). Cerebral organic lesions including space-occupying lesions (e.g. cerebral tumour,

subdural haematoma), severe infection (systemic or intracerebral) and carcinoma at any site, especially lung, breast, lymphoma or bowel, must be ruled out.

The sudden onset of delirium may suggest angina, myocardial infarction or a cerebrovascular accident. Twenty per cent of patients with delirium also have underlying heart failure.[3]

Pitfalls

There are many pitfalls, especially with drug toxicity or withdrawal from the so-called illicit drugs. In the elderly in particular, fluid and electrolyte disturbances such as dehydration, hypokalaemia, hyponatraemia and hypocalcaemia can cause delirium. Bowel disturbances such as

Table 41.3 *Important causes of delirium (typical examples of each group)*

Drug intoxication and drug sensitivity	• anticholinergics • antidepressants • sedatives • alcohol, opiates, etc.
Withdrawal from substances of abuse and prescribed drugs	• alcohol • opiates • amphetamines • cannabis • sedatives and anxiolytics
Infections specific	• urinary tract • lower respiratory, e.g. pneumonia • otitis media • cellulitis
intracranial	• meningitis • encephalitis
systematic	• infective endocarditis • septicaemia • HIV virus • other viral infections • malaria
Metabolic disturbances	• uraemia, hepatic failure • electrolyte disturbances • dehydration
Endocrine disturbances	• diabetes ketosis, hypoglycaemia • hypothyroidism
Nutritional and vitamin deficits	• Wernicke's encephalopathy
Hypoxia	• respiratory failure, cardiac failure, anaemia
Vascular	• CVA
Head injury and other intracranial problems	
Seizures	• complex partial seizures
'Subtle' causes	• pain, e.g. herpes zoster • emotional upset • environmental change • perioperative • faecal impaction • urinary retention

faecal impaction or constipation can cause delirium and incontinence of both faeces and urine.

Seven masquerades checklist

All the following disorders can cause disturbed or confused behaviour, particularly in the elderly:

- depression: a very important cause of 'pseudodementia'
- drugs: toxicity or withdrawal (see Table 41.4)
- diabetes: especially hypoglycaemia, which can occur with NIDDM
- anaemia: often from self-neglect or chronic blood loss
- thyroid disorders: both hyperthyroidism and hypothyroidism can present with disturbed behaviour; 'myxoedemic madness' may be precipitated by atropine compounds
- urinary tract infection: causes or contributes to 20% of cases of hallucinations or illusions[2]
- spinal dysfunction: with its many severe pain syndromes, such as sciatica, it can be a significant factor.

Table 41.4 *Prescribed drugs that can cause delirium*

Anticholinergic
- antiparkinsonian, e.g. benztropine
- tricyclic antidepressants

Tranquillisers and hypnotics
- major tranquillisers
  e.g. chlorpromazine
- minor tranquillisers
  e.g. diazepam
- hypnotics
- lithium

Antiepileptics

Antihistamines 1 and 2

Antihypertensives

Corticosteroids

Cardiac drugs
- digoxin
- diuretics
- beta-blockers
Opioids
Sympathomimetics

Psychogenic factors

Apart from the primary psychiatric disorders of anxiety, depression, mania and schizophrenia, relatively simple and subtle social problems such as loneliness, boredom, a domestic upset, financial problem or similar issue can trigger a confusional state.

The clinical approach
History

Developing rapport with the disturbed or confused patient is essential and can be helped by a warm handshake or a reassuring pat on the shoulder. The basis of the history is a careful account from relatives or witnesses about the patient's behaviour.

When communicating with the patient, speak slowly and simply (avoid shouting), face the patient and maintain eye contact. Important features are the past history, recent psychosocial history including recent bereavement, family upsets and changes in environment. Search for evidence of depression and note any organic symptoms such as cough, constipation and so on.

Mental status examination

The most practical bedside screening test of mental function is the Mental Status Questionnaire of Kahn[4] which includes ten simple questions.

1. What is the name of this place?
2. What city are you in now?
3. What year is it?
4. What month is it?
5. What is the date today?
6. What year were you born?
7. When is your birthday?
8. How old are you?
9. Who is the prime minister/president?
10. Who was the prime minister/president before him?

(Interpretation: normal 9–10; mildly impaired 8–9; confused/demented 7 or less.)

If the patient has appropriate mental function ask questions related to possible depressive illness, e.g.

- Do you feel hopeful about your future?
- Do you have good things to look forward to?
- Do you think life is worth living?
- Have you ever thought of taking your life?

Physical examination

The patient's general demeanour, dress and physical characteristics should be noted at all times. Assess the patient's ability to hear, see, speak, reason, obey commands, stand and walk. Any problems related to the special senses can cause confusion.

Look for features of alcohol abuse, Parkinson's disease and hypothyroidism.

Examine the neurological system and keep in mind the possibility of a subdural haematoma which may have followed a forgotten fall.

Don't omit the rectal examination to exclude faecal impaction, melaena, cancer and prostatomegaly (in males) and also check the bladder for evidence of chronic retention.

Investigations

Investigations to consider for delirious or demented patients (unknown cause):

- urinalysis and microscopy
- cultures of blood and urine
- total and differential blood count; ESR
- blood glucose
- urea and creatinine and electrolytes
- calcium and phosphate
- thyroid function tests
- liver function tests
- serum B_{12} and folate levels
- ECG
- chest X-ray
- cerebral CT scan
- syphilis serology

Management of the acutely disturbed patient

Delirious or psychotic patients can be paranoid and respond defensively to the world around them. This behaviour can include aggressive and violent behaviour resulting in danger to themselves, their friends and family and to their medical attendants.

Dangerousness should be assessed from features such as the patient's past history (especially previous dangerous behaviour), age and sex, recent stress, victim behaviour, muscle bulk, presence of weapons, degree of overactivity and the manner of handling of the present distress by others. The patient may be in a state of acute panic and trying to flee a situation or in an agitated psychotic state prepared to confront the

situation. It should be emphasised that most violent individuals are not mentally ill.

Most cases require an injection (the ideal intravenous administration can be extremely difficult and hazardous) which is often interpreted as a physical attack. It may not be possible to diagnose the cause of the problem before giving the injection.

Approach to management

- Assess the environment and don't move into the patient's space until in a position of control.
- React calmly. Communicate calmly and simply.
- State your task firmly and simply.
- Try to control the disturbed patient gently.
- Ensure the safety of all staff and make certain that heroics are not attempted in dangerous circumstances.
- An adequate number of staff to accompany the doctor is essential—six is ideal (one for immobilisation of each limb, one for the head and one to assist with drugs).[1]
- Patients should be placed on the floor in the prone position.

Principles of sedative administration[1]

- Use the safest possible route of administration whenever possible, i.e. oral in preference to parenteral. Intravenous administration has the lowest margin of safety.
- Parenteral administration should be restricted to severely disturbed patients.
- Closely monitor vital signs during and after sedative administration.
- Avoid intramuscular diazepam because of poor absorption.
- Avoid intravenous midazolam (Hypnovel) in such patients because of the risk of respiratory depression.
- Avoid benzodiazepines in patients with respiratory insufficiency. Haloperidol is an alternative.
- Patients have died from cardiopulmonary arrest after repeated sedative administration (especially benzodiazepines); so intensive monitoring is essential.

Monitor the following adverse effects:
- respiratory depression
- hypotension
- dystonic reactions, including choking
- neuroleptic malignant syndrome

Treatment options[1]

- diazepam 10–20 mg (o) as single dose (if patient co-operates); repeat every 2–6 hours (up to 120 mg daily) depending on response
- if intramuscular benzodiazepines required— midazolam (Hypnovel) 2.5–5 mg IM as single dose
- if intravenous benzodiazepines required
  — diazepam 5–20 mg IV (slow injection over several minutes) as single dose

Alternatives

- droperidol (Droleptan) 5–10 mg IM
  or
- haloperidol 5–10 mg IM

(These injections can be repeated in 15–30 minutes if required. Droperidol is similar to haloperidol but more sedating. Keep in mind the rare but potentially fatal laryngeal dystonia with high doses—cover with benztropine 2 mg IM.)
  or (orally)
- chlorpromazine 100 mg (o) by tablet or syrup; repeat in 60 minutes if required. IV use is dangerous.

(Syrup may be preferred as it is less likely to be hidden in the mouth.)
  or
- haloperidol 5–10 mg (o), repeat every 2–6 hours
  or
- combination of diazepam and haloperidol

Postdisturbance evaluation

Determine the likely cause, such as:

- acute organic brain syndrome
  e.g. toxic causes
    infection
- alcohol or drugs (illicit or prescribed)
  — intoxication
  — withdrawal
- manic illness
- severe depression
- schizophrenic syndrome
- severe panic

Acute organic brain syndrome (delirium)

The many labels of acute organic brain syndrome include:

- delirium
- acute confusional state
- toxic confusional state
- confusional episode
- acute brain syndrome

Main features

- clouding of conscious state
- disorientation
- impaired attention
- impaired memory

Refer to Table 41.5.

Table 41.5   *DSM-III (R) criteria for delirium*

Diagnosis of delirium requires evidence of:
A.   Clouding of consciousness
B.   Two or more of
     1. perceptual disturbance
     2. incoherent speech
     3. disturbance of sleep
     4. increased or decreased psychomotor activity
C.   Disorientation or memory impairment
D.   Clinical features appearing over a short period
E.   Evidence of a cause

Other clinical features[1]

- The patients are usually elderly.
- Anxiety and agitation can be severe but in hypoactive deliria (usually due to metabolic disturbance) the conscious state can vary from drowsiness to coma.
- Psychotic symptoms can occur.
- Delusions are usually fleeting.
- The disturbance is usually worse at night and may be aggravated by sedation.
- Visual hallucinations are a feature of alcohol withdrawal.
- Attacks on bystanders may result (uncommon).

Always seek a cause.[1] A list of causes is presented in Table 41.3. The most important causes are:

- infections (usually in urinary tract, lungs or ear, or systemic in young or elderly)
- prescribed drugs.

Anticholinergic delirium

Consider this cause (from drugs with anticholinergic properties or illicit substances). Features include hyperactiviy, marked thought disorder, vivid visual hallucinations and very disturbed behaviour.

Differential diagnosis of delirium

In the earlier stages it may mimic the various psychiatric disorders including anxiety, depression, various hallucinatory states, particularly agitated schizophrenia (rarely), extreme manic states and complex partial seizures.

Investigations

Investigations are those listed under clinical approach (p. 413).

Treatment

Principles:

- Acute delirium is a medical emergency.
- Establish normal hydration, electrolyte, balance and nutrition.
- Attend to helpful environmental factors, e.g. calm atmosphere, a night-light, orientation clues, presence of friends and relatives.

Medication

Medication[1] may not be needed but will be in the presence of anxiety, aggression or psychotic symptoms.

For anxiety and agitation

- diazepam 5–10 mg (o) as a single dose
  or
- midazolam 1.25–5 mg IM
  or
- diazepam 2–20 mg IV (over several minutes)

For psychotic behaviour, add

- haloperidol 1.5–10 mg (o) according to response

For severe symptoms, when parenteral medication required (cover with benztropine 2 mg (o) or IM)

- haloperidol 5–10 mg (IM) as single dose
  or
- droperidol 5–10 mg (IM) as single dose
  (more sedating)

For anticholinergic delirium

- tacrine hydrochloride 15–30 mg with caution by slow IV injection (an antidote)

Note: • Benzodiazepines should be avoided in children and in patients with respiratory insufficiency.
- Consider necessity for pain relief.
- Use lower doses of parenteral medications in the very old and frail.

Dementia (chronic organic brain syndrome)

Dementia is an important diagnosis to consider in the elderly patient. The DSM-III (R) criteria for dementia are presented in Table 8.2 and elaborated in more detail in Chapter 8.

The main feature of dementia is impairment of memory, especially recent memory, when the person cannot remember what has happened a few hours (or even moments) earlier but may clearly remember the events of the past.

The more serious behavioural changes encountered with dementia tend to occur in the advanced stages. However, these disturbances may be precipitated by illness such as infections, emotional upset and drugs. These serious disturbances include:

- uninhibited behaviour
- hallucinations (generally uncommon)
- paranoid delusions

If a stable patient becomes acutely disturbed, delirium should be suspected.

Presenile dementia—Alzheimer's type

The main features are:

- onset in late 50s and early 60s
- insidious onset
- early loss of short-term memory
- progressive decline in intellect
- death in 5–10 years
- more common in Down syndrome

Differential diagnosis of dementia

There are two approaches to the differential diagnosis, including consideration of the classic causes of disturbed behaviour as summarised in the mnemonic in Table 41.6[5] and those more everyday subtle causes presented in Table 8.2, in the chapter on the elderly patient.

However, the foremost differential diagnosis should be 'pseudodementia' caused by severe depression.

A simple comparison between schizophrenia and dementia is shown in Table 41.7.

A vigorous search for a possible cause of dementia is warranted since there are a significant number of reversible causes. In particular it is important to exclude the psychiatric conditions that may mimic dementia.

Table 41.6 *Differential diagnosis of dementias*

D	delirium
	drugs (*see* toxic)
E	emotional disorder = depression
	endocrine = thyroid
M	memory = benign forgetfulness
E	elective = anxiety disorders/neuroses
N	neurological—CVA
	—head trauma
T	toxic—drugs/medication
	—metabolic disease
I	intellect—low or retarded
A	amnesic disorders—Korsakov's
S	schizophrenia (chronic)

Source: After McLean[5]

Treatment

See page 62.
- To control psychotic symptoms or disturbed behaviour
  - risperidone 0.5–2 mg (o) daily
- To control symptoms of anxiety and agitation—oxazepam 15 mg (o) 1 to 4 times daily. Avoid benzodiazepines for longer than 2 weeks.

Schizophrenia and associated disorders

The term schizophrenia (Bleuler 1911) refers to a group of severe psychiatric illnesses characterised by severe disturbances of emotion, language, perception, thought processes, volition and motor activity. The causes of schizophrenia disorders are unknown.

Main abnormal clinical features include:[6]
- disorders of thinking
  - poverty of thinking
  - disordered form of thought: 'woolly'
  - impaired planning ability
  - disordered content, e.g. delusional
  - impaired communication
- disorders of emotion
  - blunted affect (lack of emotion)
  - inappropriate affect
- disorders of perception
  - auditory hallucinations
  - visual and somatic hallucinations may occur
- disorders of volition
  - apathy
  - lack of motivation
  - social withdrawal
  - social and personality deterioration
- disorders of motor activity
  - slow or unusual movements
- reduced speech output

Other features include:
- bizarre behaviour
- subject to tension, anxiety or depression
- deterioration in work and study performance
- peak incidence 15–25 years[6]—smaller peak at 40 years
- lifetime prevalence 1 in 100
- equal sex incidence
- high risk of suicide

Differential diagnosis

Organic factors need to be excluded, especially drugs:
- amphetamines
- hallucinogens, e.g. LSD
- marijuana

A comparison of delirium, dementia and functional psychosis is presented in Table 41.8.[7]

Management

Drug treatment is only a part of the total management. Explanation and appropriate reassurance to the family with patient and family supportive care is obviously essential. A team approach is necessary to cope with the disorder, which usually has a devastating effect on the family.

Table 41.7 *Comparison of schizophrenia and dementia*

	Dementia	Schizophrenia
Onset	Middle-aged or elderly	Young
Memory	Always impaired	Usually unaffected
Delusions	Rare	Frequent
Hallucinations	Uncommon	Frequent
Thought broadcasting	Never	Frequent

Table 41.8   *Comparison of the clinical features of delirium, dementia and acute functional psychoses*[7]

Feature	Delirium	Dementia	Acute psychosis
Onset	Rapid	Slow—insidious	Rapid
Duration	Hours to weeks	Months to years	Depends on response to treatment
Course over 24 hours	Fluctuates—worse at night	Minimal variation	Minimal variation
Consciousness	Reduced	Alert	Alert
Perception	Misperceptions common, especially visual	Misperceptions rare	May be misperceptions
Hallucinations	Common, visual (usually) or auditory	Uncommon	Common, mainly auditory
Attention	Distractable	Normal to impaired	Variable—may be impaired
Speech	Variable, may be incoherent	Difficulty finding correct words	Variable: normal, rapid or slow
Organic illness or drug toxicity	One or both present	Often absent	Usually absent

Acute phase
- hospitalisation usually necessary
- drug treatment for the psychosis[1]
1. When oral medication possible, first line treatment is
   - olanzapine 2.5–10 mg (o) nocte

   or

   - risperidone 1 mg (o) at night increasing to 1 mg bd and then titrated in 1 mg steps over several days to 2–4 mg (o) bd (beware of hypotension)

   or

   - quetiapine 25 mg (o) bd (day 1) increasing gradually as tolerated to 300–450 mg day in divided doses
2. When parenteral medication required
   - haloperidol 5–10 mg IV or IM, initially, up to 20 mg in 24 hours, depending on the response

   add

   - benztropine 1–2 mg (o) bd (to avoid dystonic reaction)
   If dystonic reaction
   - benztropine 1–2 mg IV or IM
   If very agitated, use
   - diazepam 10–20 mg (o) or 5–10 mg IV

Chronic phase of schizophrenia
Long-term antipsychotic medication recommended to prevent relapse.[1]

- Examples of oral medication regimens:[1]
— olanzapine 10–20 mg (o) nocte

   or

— risperidone 1–2 mg (o) bd

   or

— quetiapine 150 mg (o) bd
- Aim for lowest possible dose to maintain control.
- Chlorpromazine is not recommended for long-term use because of photosensitivity reactions.
- Use depot preparations if compliance is a problem:
— fluphenazine decanoate 12.5–75 mg IM, every 2–4 weeks (12.5 mg statim test dose)

   or

— haloperidol decanoate 50–300 mg IM, every 4 weeks (50 mg statim)

   or

— flupenthixol decanoate 20–80 mg IM, every 2–4 weeks (10 mg statim)

Tips with depot preparations:
- Start with IM test doses and then titrate to recommended controlling levels.
- May take 2–4 months to produce a stable

response; so oral supplements may be necessary.
• Not as effective as oral therapy.
• Give as deep IM injection with 21 gauge needle in buttock.
• Use lowest possible dose to avoid tardive dyskinesia.
• Reassess at least every 3 months.
• Closely monitor patient for movement disorders.

Drug-resistant schizophrenia
Consider other causes, e.g. substances abuse. ECT may help the agitated patient, especially if catatonic. Consider a trial of clozapine (300–600 mg daily) with strict monitoring for blood dyscrasias or olanzapine (5–20 mg daily).

Movement disorders from antipsychotic medication[1]
Acute dystonias
• usually bizarre muscle spasms affect face, neck, tongue and trunk
• oculogyric crises, opisthotonos and laryngeal spasm

Rx: benztropine 1–2 mg IV or IM

Akathisia
• subjective motor restlessness of feet and legs
• generally later onset in course of treatment

Rx: — reduce dosage until akathisia less troublesome or substitute thioridazine
— can use oral propranolol, diazepam or benztropine as short-term measure

Parkinsonian
• seen relatively early in treatment
• the akinesia can be confused with drug-induced depression

Rx: — use lower dose or substitute a phenothiazine in low dosage
— alternatively, use benztropine or benzhexol

Tardive dyskinesia
Tardive dyskinesia is a syndrome of abnormal involuntary movements of the face, mouth, tongue, trunk and limbs. This is a major problem with use of long-term antipsychotic drugs and may occur months or years (usually) after starting treatment.
Differential diagnosis:
• spontaneous orofacial dyskinesia
• senile dyskinesia

• ill-fitting dentures
• neurological disorders causing tremor and chorea

There is no specific treatment for tardive dyskinesia. The risks and benefits of continuing therapy have to be weighed.

Note: Because of the inability to manage tardive dyskinesia, prevention in the form of using the lowest possible dosage of antipsychotic medication is essential. This involves regular review and adjustment if necessary.

Neuroleptic (antipsychotic) malignant syndrome
This is a potentially fatal adverse effect that can develop at any time. It develops in hours to days.
  Syndrome: high temperature, muscle rigidity, altered consciousness. Milder variants can occur.
  Treatment:
• discontinue medication
• ensure adequate hydration with IV fluids
• if life-threatening
— bromocriptine 2.5 mg (o) bd, gradually increasing to 5 mg (o) tds
      and
— dantrolene 50 mg (IV) every 12 hours for up to 7 doses
• consultant referral

Bipolar disorder
The mood disorders are divided into depressive disorders and bipolar disorders. The swing in moods in bipolar disorders (manic depressive disorders) is illustrated in Figure 41.1. The symptoms of mania may appear abruptly.

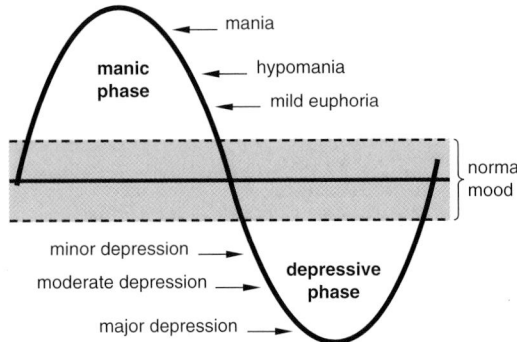

Fig. 41.1 *Bipolar disorder (manic depression): possible mood swings*

The main clinical features of mania are:
- elevated, expansive or irritable mood
- accelerated speech
- agitation
- racing thoughts or flights of ideas
- increased activity
- reduced sleep

Other features include:
- grandiose ideas, sometimes paranoid
- reckless behaviour, overspending
- impaired judgment
- increased sexual drive and activity
- poor insight into the problem

Note: The peak onset is in early adult life. There is a strong hereditary basis.

Hypomania is the term used to describe the symptoms of mania that are less severe and of shorter duration.

Management of acute mania

Hospitalisation
- for protection of patient and family
- usually involuntary admission necessary

Drugs of choice[1]
1. *Co-operative patient*
   lithium carbonate 750–1000 mg (o) daily[1]
   - this is the initial dose
   - give in 2 to 3 divided doses
   - can increase by increments of 250–500 mg per day
   - monitor by plasma levels
   - therapeutic plasma level 0.8–1.4 mmol/L
   - required daily dosage usually 1000–2500 mg
   - elderly patients may require reduced dosage   or
   (if not tolerated or for rapid cycling disorder)
   sodium valproate 400–800 mg (o) daily
   - give in 2 divided doses
   - introduce stepwise every 2–3 days
   - check plasma levels after 7 days
   - therapeutic level 350–700 μmol/L
                or
   carbamazepine 200–400 mg (o) daily
   - give as above
   - therapeutic plasma level 20–50 μmol/L
2. *Unco-operative patients and manic behaviour problematic*
   haloperidol 10–20 mg (o) as single dose
   - can be repeated up to 40 mg daily, depending on response

- use minimum possible dose to achieve control
- there is a risk of tardive dyskinesia
If parenteral antipsychotic drug required
             haloperidol 5–10 mg IM or IV
                        or
             droperidol 5–10 mg IM (more sedating)
- repeat in 15–30 minutes if necessary
- change to oral medication as soon as possible
Note: Benzodiazepines, e.g. diazepam, can be used with lithium and also the anti-epileptics.

If not responding to medication consider ECT.

Maintenance
- Lithium carbonate—continue for 6 months; if not tolerated or ineffective use antiepileptics, carbamazepine or sodium valproate.
  Give at minimum dose and for minimum time to gain control.
- Antiepileptics are claimed to be more effective in patients with rapid cycling illness (4 or more episodes per year).

Prophylaxis for recurrent bipolar disorder
(Over 90% will have a recurrence at some time: consider medication if two or more episodes of either mania or depression in the previous 4 years.)
- Use long-term lithium, e.g. 3–5 years. Target plasma level for maintenance is usually 0.6–0.8 mmol/L.
- If poor response use carbamazepine or sodium valproate.
- Unwanted side effects of lithium include
  — a fine tremor
  — muscle weakness
  — weight gain
  — gastrointestinal symptoms
- With antiepileptics adjust dosage according to clinical response and toxicity.

Depression

Depression is very common and presents in a great range of severity. In the context of 'the disturbed patient' depression can be confused with dementia or a psychosis, particularly if the following are present:
- psychomotor agitation
- psychomotor retardation
- delusions
- hallucinations

Assessment[1]

The following questions need to be addressed:

- Is the depression primary (i.e. not secondary to another psychiatric condition such as schizophrenia or anxiety disorder)?
- Is it part of a bipolar disorder? Has there been a previous manic or hypomanic episode? If so, a different approach to treatment is required.
- Is the depression caused by another illness or physical factor (e.g. hypothyroidism, cerebrovascular disease or medication)?
- Is the patient psychotic?
- Is the patient a suicide risk?

The treatment of depression is presented in Chapter 16.

Psychoactive substance use disorders

It is important for the general practitioner to be aware of the effects of self-administration of psychoactive substances, especially their toxic or withdrawal effects. They form significant consideration for the differential diagnosis of disturbed patient behaviour.

Alcohol

Toxic and withdrawal effects, including delirium tremens, are outlined in Chapter 106. Abrupt withdrawal can cause symptoms ranging from tremors, agitation and dysphoria (feeling thoroughly miserable) to fully developed delirium tremens. Epileptic seizures may also occur.

Barbiturate dependence

Tolerance and symptoms on withdrawal are the main features. Barbiturate withdrawal is a very serious life-threatening problem and may be encountered in elderly people undergoing long-standing hypnotic withdrawal. Symptoms include anxiety, tremor, extreme irritability, twitching, seizures and delirium.

Management[1]

Undertake withdrawal with medical supervision as an inpatient.

Transfer the patient to phenobarbitone or diazepam.

- phenobarbitone 120 mg (o) hourly until sedation

or

- phenobarbitone 30 mg for each 100 mg of shorter-acting barbiturate
  reduce the dose gradually over 10 to 14 days

or

- diazepam 20–40 mg orally, daily,
  reduce the dose gradually over 10 to 14 days

Benzodiazepine dependence

Withdrawal symptoms in the dependent patient include anxiety, restlessness, irritability, palpitation and muscle aches and pains, but delirium and seizures are uncommon except with very high doses. The shorter the half-life the greater the dependence.

Withdrawal is best achieved by supervising a gradual reduction in dosage aided by relaxation techniques and behavioural strategies to help patients cope with insomnia and anxiety.

Opioid dependence[1]

Withdrawal symptoms include anxiety and panic, sweating, musculoskeletal pain ('aching bones'), gooseflesh, diarrhoea and abdominal colic. These peak at 36–72 hours and tend to subside after 10 days.

Management includes methadone withdrawal (short-term withdrawal) or methadone maintenance. The new oral opioid antagonist, naltrexone, appears to have an important role. It also shows promise in alcoholic detoxification.

- Starting dose:
  methadone 30–40 mg (o) daily (do not exceed 50 mg daily if patient unwell—beware of doses >40 mg)
- Maintenance (if necessary):
  methadone 30–80 mg (o) daily
  Note: Methadone used appropriately can save lives, but it can be fatal if used inappropriately.
  If autonomic signs use clonidine
  If anxiety and depression use diazepam

Stimulant substance abuse

The stimulants include amphetamines and their analogues, ephedrine, cocaine and certain appetite suppressants.

Stimulant-induced syndrome[1]

- aggressive behaviour
- paranoid behaviour
- irritability
- transient toxic psychosis
- delirium
- schizophrenic-like syndrome

Treatment:
- withdrawal of drugs
- chlorpromazine 200–600 mg (o) daily for short term

Stimulant-withdrawal syndrome[1]
This syndrome should be suspected in people whose occupation involves shift work, interstate transport driving or multiple jobs presenting with the following symptoms:
- drowsiness
- hypersomnia then insomnia
- irritability
- aggressive behaviour
- dysphoria
- urge to resume drugs

Treatment:
- psychological support and encouragement
- desipramine (or similar tricyclic antidepressant)
  75 mg (o) nocte (increasing as necessary)
  - bromocriptine 1.25 mg (o) bd has also been used for cocaine withdrawal

Hallucinogen abuse
Hallucinogens in use include lysergic acid (LSD), phencyclidine (Angel dust), diethylamide and many synthetics. Symptoms include psychotic behaviour including severe hallucinations. Withdrawal from these drugs is not usually a problem but 'flashbacks' can occur.

Medication to counter symptoms[1]
- haloperidol 2.5–10 mg (o) daily
        or
- diazepam 10–40 mg (o) daily

Cannabis use and dependence
Users of cannabis are typically detached and apathetic in nature (Chapter 18).

Psychosis may occur, especially in chronic users, and it is believed that the drug appears to unmask an underlying schizophrenia-type psychosis. No specific treatment is used for use or withdrawal.

Psychiatric disorders of childhood and adolescence[1]

The following disturbance problems do occur and must be taken seriously, especially the potential for suicide in the second decade. Many of these disorders are presented in more detail in Chapter 75.

Attention deficit hyperactivity disorder
Clinical features:
- short attention span
- distractability
- overactivity
- impulsiveness
- antisocial behaviour

Depression
Major depression follows the same criteria as for adults. Suicidal ideation has to be considered and taken very seriously if present. Imipramine is probably the drug of choice.

Bipolar disorders
Mania is seldom diagnosed before puberty. Adolescents may present (uncommonly) with symptoms of mania or hypomania.

Schizophrenia and related disorders
Schizophrenia is rare before puberty. The criteria for diagnosis are similar to adults:
- delusion
- thought disorder
- hallucinations
- six months or more of deterioration in functioning

Autism
Aggression and irritability can be a feature, especially during adolescence.

Tourette's syndrome
Behavioural problems can be part of this syndrome, which requires the attention of an experienced consultant.

Obsessive-compulsive disorders
In about one-third of cases the onset is between 5 and 15 years of age.

Violence and dangerousness

Dangerousness has been defined as a 'propensity to cause serious physical injury or lasting psychological harm to others' and, in the context of the mentally abnormal, 'the relative probability of their committing a violent crime'.[8]

Dangerousness is not related only to mental illness and, interestingly, most offenders have no psychiatric diagnosis. It is not an inherited, immutable characteristic of an individual but tends to surface on impulse in a particular context given a whole range of situational factors. Prediction of the risk of violence is not straightforward.

Various groups have been identified as contributing risk factors for violent conduct.[8]

- schizophrenic psychoses, including
  - older male paranoid schizophrenics
  - younger males prone to act violently and impulsively, presumably due to hallucinatory commands
- morbid jealousy
  - associated with delusions of infidelity
- antisocial personality disorder
- mood disorder
  - violence, usually associated with depression (rarely mania)
  - married women with severe depression (violence against young children)
  - history of suicide attempts in depression
- episodic discontrol syndrome (similar to intermittent explosive disorder)
- mental retardation combined with personality disorder and behavioural disturbances
- alcohol abuse or dependency
- amphetamine or benzodiazepine abuse or dependency

From a management viewpoint, homicidal threats must be taken very seriously.

Suicide and parasuicide

The haunting issue of suicide and parasuicide is presented in Chapter 16. The disturbed patient is always a suicide risk rather than a homicide risk. The importance of recognising depression with an associated suicide risk in the elderly patient has been emphasised heavily in this chapter.

Facts and figures[9]

- More than 90% of suicides occur without underlying chronic conditions but most people are significantly depressed at the time.
- In Australia suicide is the second most common cause of death between the ages of 11 and 25 years. Children as young as 5 years of age have committed suicide.
- Those who talk about suicide may attempt it later.
- About half those committing suicide have seen a doctor within their last month of life.

- Around 80–90% of suicides have given clear or subtle warnings to family, friends or doctors.
- There is no evidence that asking patients about suicidal ideation provokes suicidal acts.
- Doctors in Australia and other Western countries have a high suicide rate.

Suicide risk

Blumenthal's[10] overlapping model lists five groups of risk factors (Fig. 41.2):

1. Psychiatric disorders, e.g.
   - affective disorder and alcohol abuse in adults
   - schizophrenia
   - depression and conduct disorder in young people
2. Personality traits, e.g.
   - impulsiveness and aggression
3. Environmental and psychosocial factors, e.g.
   - poor social supports
   - chronic medical illness, e.g. AIDS
   - significant loss
4. Family history and genetics (both nature and nurture) e.g.
   - emulation of relatives
   - specific ethnic groups in custody
5. Biological factors, e.g.
   - possible serotonin deficiency

Parasuicide

Parasuicide is attempted suicide; in many cases patients are drawing attention to themselves as a 'plea for help'. It is important for the GP to take an active role in the support of the patient and family after discharge from hospital, but preferably in conjunction with a psychiatric or counselling service. Arrange frequent consultations at first and ensure adequate follow-up, especially for missed appointments.

Personality disorders

People with personality disorders may become very distressed and acutely disturbed under stress or provocation, and this may involve dramatic scenes including public suicide threats. It is important to recognise personality disorders because they usually cause considerable distress to the patients, their family, society and GPs.

In practice the personality disorders of most concern are those that present with hostility, either verbal or physical, particularly if a suicide or homicide threat is involved. It is a mistake to assume that those patients who manifest violent

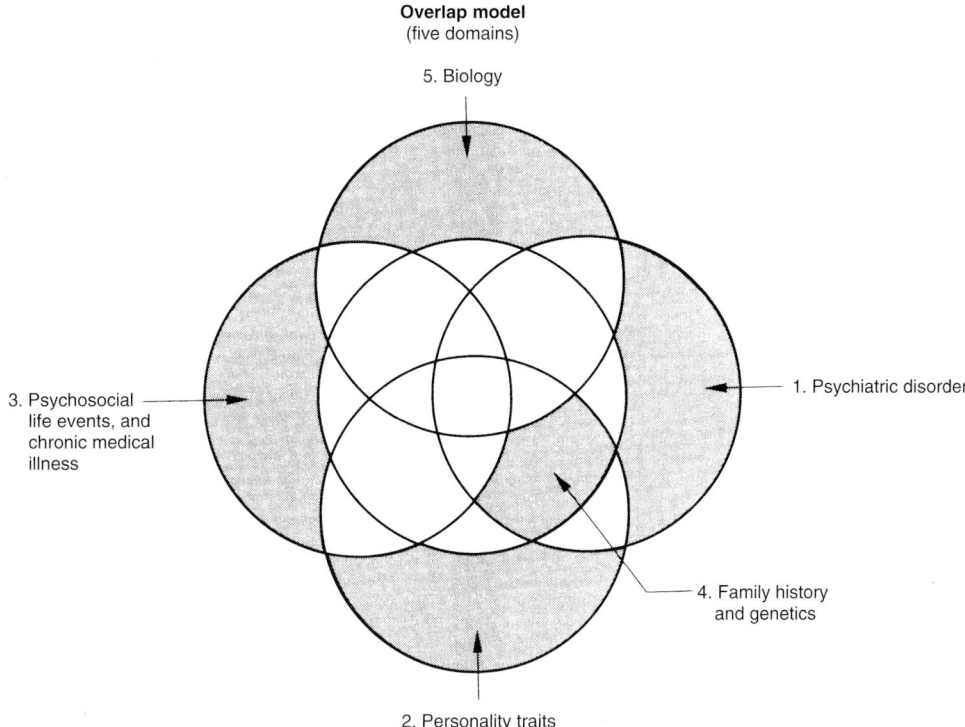

Overlap model
(five domains)

5. Biology

3. Psychosocial
life events, and
chronic medical
illness

1. Psychiatric disorder

4. Family history
and genetics

2. Personality traits

Fig. 41.2 *Overlap model for understanding suicidal behaviour* AFTER BLUMENTHAL AND KUPFER

or psychopathic behaviour have a personality disorder or, conversely, the meek and mild are free from personality disorder.

The diagnosis of personality disorder can be difficult. As practitioners we tend to have a 'gut feeling' about the diagnosis but often find it difficult to classify the personality of the patient and then to manage it appropriately.

The main characteristics of a personality disorder are:[11]
- lack of confidence and low self-esteem
- long history from childhood
- difficulties with interpersonal relationships and society
- recurrent maladaptive behaviour
- relatively fixed, inflexible and stylised reaction to stress
- minimal insight
- perception of difficulties as external to themselves

The medical/psychiatric significance:
- maladaptive relationships with GPs and society
- problem of sexually dysfunctional lives
- risk of substance abuse and self-destructive behaviour

- prone to depression and anxiety (usually low grade)
- susceptible to 'breakdown' under stress

Personality is the result of a genetic template and the continuing interaction of the person with outside influences (peer pressures, family interactions, influential events) and personal drives in seeking an identity. The outcome is a unique behaviour pattern manifest as a personality trait or character reflective of the individual's self-image and fundamental to his or her sense of personal identity.[11]

Although personality is unique it is possible to make a hypothesis that one is normal or abnormal. If abnormal it is possible to stereotype it according to the predominant symptoms or behaviours.

Using the International Classification of Disease (ICD-10) and the DSM IV classification[12] various subtypes are readily identifiable (Table 41.9),[12] which can be considered in four main groups. There is a considerable overlap between the subtypes within the group.[13]

The antisocial group tend to come to the attention of GPs more frequently with some

Table 41.9 *Summary of main personality disorders*

Main cluster group	Subtypes	Main features of disorder
A. Withdrawn *synonyms* odd eccentric	• Paranoid	• Suspicious, oversensitive, argumentative, defensive, hyperalert, cold and humourless
	• Schizoid	• Shy, emotionally cold, introverted, detached, avoids close relationships
	• Schizotypal	• Odd and eccentric, sensitive, suspicious and superstitious, socially isolated, odd speech, thinking and behaviour. Falls short of criteria for schizophrenia
B. Antisocial *synonyms* dramatic emotional sociopathic flamboyant erratic	• Antisocial (sociopathic, psychopathic)	• Impulsive, insensitive, selfish, callous, superficial charm, lack of guilt, low frustration level, doesn't learn from experience, relationship problems e.g. promiscuous
	• Histrionic (hysterical)	• Self-dramatic, egocentric, immature, vain, dependent, manipulative, easily bored, emotional scenes, inconsiderate, seductive
	• Narcissistic ('prima-donna')	• Morbid self-admiration, exhibitionist, insensitive, craves and demands attention, exploits others, preoccupied with power, lacks interest in others
	• Impulsive ('mad dog')	• Mood swings, impulsiveness, prone to violence and threats (esp. if criticised) but doesn't lack guilt
	• Borderline ('hell-raiser')	• Confused self-image, impulsive, reckless, 'all or nothing' relationships—unstable and intense, damaging reckless behaviour, full of anger and guilt, lacks self-control ± uncontrolled gambling, spending etc. *Note:* High incidence suicide and parasuicide; drug abuse
C. Dependent *synonyms* anxious fearful inhibited	• Avoidant (anxious)	• Anxious, self-conscious, fears rejection, timid and cautious, low self-esteem, overreacts to rejection and failure
	• Dependent	• Passive, weak willed, lacks vigour, lacks self-reliance and confidence, overaccepting, avoids responsibility, seeks support
	• Obsessional (obsessive-compulsive)	• Rigid, perfectionist, pedantic, indecisive, egocentric
	• Passive-aggressive	• Procrastinates, childishly stubborn, dawdles, sulks, argumentative, clings, deliberately inefficient and hypercritical of authority figures
D. Other	• Hypochondrial	• Health-conscious, disease fearing, symptom preoccupation
	• Depressive (dysthymic, cyclothymic)	• Pessimistic, anergic, low self-esteem, gloomy, chronic mild depression

individuals representing 'heart-sink' patients because of demanding, angry or aggressive behaviour. The withdrawn group are typically withdrawn, suspicious and socially isolated but fall short of a true psychotic syndrome. GPs have problems communicating with them because they are often suspicious, which can make proper physical examination and management difficult.

In the dependent and inhibited groups, which may overlap with an anxiety state, the main features are nervousness, timidity, emotional dependence and fear of criticism and rejection. They are frequent attenders (the 'fat file' syndrome) and are often accompanied by friends and relatives because of their insecurity.

Management

The best treatment is a supportive 'therapeutic' community and an understanding and supportive GP. It is vital to understand that people with personality disorders perceive the world from a fundamentally different perspective. Problematic patients, if agreeable, may respond well to psychological intervention and behavioural techniques, especially operant conditioning (reinforcing acceptable behaviour) and averse conditioning (correcting inappropriate behaviour).[11]

The borderline and narcissistic disorders in particular respond well to specific types of psychotherapeutic intervention. Patients' self-esteem needs careful support while maladaptive modes of behaviour are confronted. Hospitalisation is rarely required except for those at risk of suicide, e.g. antisocial patients.

Medication has limitations but may be useful to treat those individuals who temporarily decompensate into a psychosis, an anxiety state or depression. One study has shown that antipsychotic medication in low dosage (e.g. haloperidol 5 mg daily) is effective in treating the problematic behaviours in paranoid and some antisocial personality disorders.[14]

When to refer[9]

Indications for referral to a psychiatrist:

- Severe depression
- High suicide risk
- Actual suicide attempt: recent or in the past
- Suspected psychiatric disorders in the elderly
  ? depression or schizophrenia
  ? depression or dementia
- Failure to improve with treatment
- Poor family and social supports.

References

1. Bochner F. et al. *Psychotropic drug guidelines* (4th edn). Melbourne: Therapeutic Guidelines Ltd, 2000, 88–145.
2. Biro G. Dementia. Australian Dr Weekly, 16 February 1990, I–VIII.
3. Biro G. Delirium in the elderly. Australian Dr Weekly, 1 December 1989, I–VIII.
4. Kahn RL et al. Brief objective measures of the determination of mental status in the aged. American Journal of Psychiatry, 1960; 117: 326–329.
5. McLean S. Is it dementia? Aust Fam Physician, 1992; 21:1762–1776.
6. Norman T, Judd F. Schizophrenia. In: MIMS Disease Index (2nd edn). Sydney: IMS Publishing, 1996, 455–457.
7. Kumar PJ, Clark ML. *Clinical medicine* (2nd edn). London: Bailliere Tindall, 1990.
8. Beaumont PJV, Hampshire RB. *Textbook of psychiatry*. Melbourne: Blackwell Scientific Publications, 1989, 283–284.
9. Biro G. Suicide. Australian Dr Weekly, 26 April 1991, I–VIII.
10. Blumenthal S. Suicide—a guide to risk factors, assessment and treatment of suicidal patients. Medical Clinics of North America, 1988; 72:937–963.
11. Tierney LM. *Current medical diagnosis and treatment*. Stamford. Appleton & Lange, 1996, 930–931.
12. American Psychiatric Association: *Diagnostic and statistical manual of mental disorders* (4th edn). Washington DC; American Psychiatric Association, 1994.
13. Pullen I, Wilkinson G et al. *Psychiatry and general practice today*. London: RC Psych and RCGP, 1994, 180–183.
14. Soloff PH et al. Progress in pharmacotherapy of borderline disorders: A double blind study of amitriptyline, haloperidol and placebo. Archives of General Psychiatry, 1986; 43: 691–697.

42
Dizziness

—

When patients complain of 'dizziness', they can be using this term to describe many different phenomena, and hence a careful history is required to unravel the problem. Other patients may use different terms to explain the same sensation, for example, 'giddiness', 'swimming in the head', 'my brain spinning', 'whirling' and 'swinging'.

'Dizzy' comes from an old English word, *dysig*, meaning foolish or stupid. Strictly speaking, it means unsteadiness or lightheadedness—without movement or motion or spatial disorientation.

'Vertigo', on the other hand, comes from the Latin word for turning. The modern medical definition of vertigo is 'a sudden sense of movement'.[1] It should describe a hallucination of rotation of self or the surroundings in a horizontal or vertical direction.

The term 'dizziness', however, is generally used collectively to describe all types of equilibrium disorders and, for convenience, can be classified as shown in Figure 42.1.

Key facts and checkpoints

- Approximately one-third of the population will have suffered from significant dizziness by age 65 and about a half by age 80.[2]

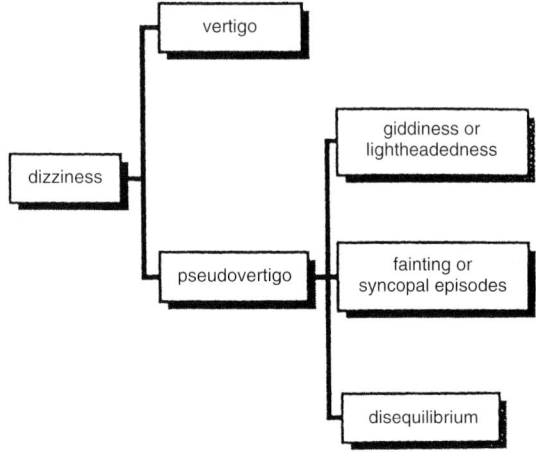

Fig. 42.1 *Classification of dizziness*

- The commonest causes in family practice are postural hypotension and hyperventilation.
- The ability to examine and interpret the sign of nystagmus accurately is important in the diagnostic process.
- A drug history is very important, including prescribed drugs and others such as alcohol, cocaine, marijuana and illicit drugs.
- Ménière's syndrome is overdiagnosed. It has the classical triad: vertigo–tinnitus–deafness (sensorineural).
- Vertebrobasilar insufficiency is also overdiagnosed as a cause of vertigo. It often causes dizziness and sometimes vertigo but rarely in isolation.

Defined terminology
Vertigo
Vertigo is an episodic sudden sensation of circular motion of the body or of its surroundings.

Other terms used by the patient to describe this symptom include 'everything spins', 'my head spins', 'the room spins', 'whirling', 'reeling', 'swaying', 'pitching' and 'rocking'.

Vertigo is characteristically precipitated by standing or turning the head or by movement. Patients have to walk carefully and may become nervous about descending stairs or crossing the road and usually seek support. Therefore the vertiginous patient is usually very frightened and tends to remain immobile during an attack.

Patients may feel as though they are being impelled by some outside force that tends to pull them to one side, especially while walking.

True vertigo is a symptom of disturbed function involving the vestibular system or its central connections. It invariably has an organic cause. Important causes are presented in Table 42.1, while Figure 42.2 illustrates central neurological centres that can cause vertigo.

Nystagmus is often seen with vertigo and, since 80–85% of causes are due to an ear problem, tinnitus and hearing disorders are also associated. In acute cases there is usually a reflex autonomic discharge producing sweating, pallor, nausea and vomiting.

Table 42.1 *Causes of vertigo*

1. Peripheral disorders

Labyrinth
- labyrinthitis: viral or suppurative
- Ménière's syndrome
- benign paraxysmal positional vertigo (BPPV)
- drugs
- trauma
- chronic suppurative otitis media

8th nerve
- vestibular neuronitis
- acoustic neuroma
- drugs

Cervical vertigo

2. Central disorders

Brain stem
- vertebrobasilar insufficiency
- infarction

Cerebellum
- degeneration
- tumours

Migraine

Multiple sclerosis

Giddiness

Giddiness is a sensation of uncertainty or ill-defined lightheadedness. Other terms used by

Fig. 42.2 *Diagrammatic illustration of central centres that can cause vertigo*

patients include 'a swimming sensation', 'walking on air' and 'ground going beneath me'. It usually contains no elements of rotation, impulsion, tinnitus, deafness, nausea or vomiting.

The patient with giddiness, although fearful of falling or swooning, can nonetheless walk without difficulty if forced to do so.

Giddiness is a typical psychoneurotic symptom.

Syncopal episodes

Syncope may present as a variety of dizziness or lightheadedness in which there is a sensation of impending fainting or loss of consciousness. Common causes are cardiogenic disorders and postural hypotension, which are usually drug-induced.

Disequilibrium

Disequilibrium implies a condition in which there is a loss of balance or instability while walking, without any associated sensations of spinning. Other terms used to describe this include 'unsteadiness on feet', 'the staggers', 'swaying feeling' and 'dizzy in the feet'.

Disequilibrium is usually of neurogenic origin.

A diagnostic approach

A summary of the safety diagnostic model is presented in Table 42.2.

Probability diagnosis

In medical school we gain the wrong impression that the common causes of dizziness or vertigo are the relatively uncommon causes such as Ménière's syndrome, aortic stenosis, Stokes-Adams attacks, cerebellar disorders, vertebrobasilar disease and hypertension. In the real world of medicine one is impressed by how often dizziness is caused by relatively common benign conditions such as hyperventilation associated with anxiety, simple syncope, postural hypotension due to drugs and old age, inner ear infections, wax in the ears, post head injury, motion sickness and alcohol intoxication. In most instances making the correct diagnosis (which, as ever, is based on a careful history) is straightforward, but finding the underlying cause of true vertigo can be very difficult.

The common causes of vertigo seen in general practice are benign positional vertigo (so often

Table 42.2 *Dizziness/vertigo: diagnostic strategy model*

Q.	*Probability diagnosis*
A.	Anxiety-hyperventilation (G)
	Postural hypotension (G/S)
	Simple faint—vasovagal (S)
	Ear infection—acute labyrinthitis (V)
	Vestibular neuronitis (V)
	Benign paroxysmal positional vertigo (V)
	Motion sickness (V)
	Post head injury (V/G)
	Cervical dysfunction/spondylosis

Q.	*Serious disorders not to be missed*
A.	Neoplasia
	• acoustic neuroma
	• posterior fossa tumour
	• other brain tumours 1° or 2°
	Intracerebral infection, e.g. abscess
	Cardiovascular
	• arrhythmias
	• myocardial infarction
	• aortic stenosis
	Cerebrovascular
	• vertebrobasilar insufficiency
	• brain stem infarct
	Multiple sclerosis

Q.	*Pitfalls (often missed)*
A.	Ear wax—otosclerosis
	Arrhythmias
	Hyperventilation
	Alcohol and other drugs
	Cough or micturition syncope
	Vertiginous migraine
	Parkinson's disease
	Ménière's syndrome (overdiagnosed)
	Rarities
	• Addison's disease
	• Neurosyphilis
	• Autonomic neuropathy
	• Hypertension
	• Subclavian steal
	• Perilymphatic fistula
	• Shy-Dragar syndrome

Q.	*Seven masquerades checklist*	
A.	Depression	✓
	Diabetes	possible
	Drugs	✓
	Anaemia	✓
	Thyroid disease	possible
	Spinal dysfunction	✓
	UTI	possible

Q.	*Is the patient trying to tell me something?*
A.	Very likely. Consider anxiety and/or depression.

G = giddiness; S = syncope; V = vertigo

related to cervical vertebral dysfunction), vestibular neuronitis and acute viral labyrinthitis.

Viral labyrinthitis is basically the same as vestibular neuronitis, except that the whole of the inner ear is involved so that deafness and tinnitus arise simultaneously with severe vertigo.

Serious disorders not to be missed

Neoplasia

The important serious disorders to keep in mind are space-occupying tumours, such as acoustic neuroma; medulloblastoma and other tumours (especially posterior fossa tumours) capable of causing vertigo; intracerebral infections and cardiovascular abnormalities.

It is important to bear in mind that the commonest brain tumour is a metastatic deposit from carcinoma of the lung.[3]

Cardiac disorders

Cardiac disorders that must be excluded for giddiness or syncope are the various arrhythmias, such as Stokes-Adams attacks caused by complete heart block, aortic stenosis and myocardial infarction.

Cerebrovascular

The outstanding cerebrovascular causes of severe vertigo are vertebrobasilar insufficiency and brain stem infarction. Vertigo is the commonest symptom of transient cerebral ischaemic attacks in the vertebrobasilar distribution.[1]

Severe vertigo, often in association with hiccoughs and dysphagia, is a feature of the variety of brain stem infarctions known as the lateral medullary syndrome.

Neurological causes

Important neurological causes of dizziness are multiple sclerosis and complex partial seizures.

The lesions of multiple sclerosis may occur in the brain stem or cerebellum. Young patients who present with a sudden onset of vertigo with 'jiggly' vision but without auditory symptoms should be considered as having multiple sclerosis. Five per cent of cases of multiple sclerosis present with vertigo.

Pitfalls

A list of conditions causing dizziness that may be misdiagnosed is presented in Table 42.2. Wax in the ear certainly causes dizziness, though its mechanism of action is controversial. Cough and micturition syncope do occur, although they are uncommon.

Ménière's syndrome is a pitfall in the sense that it tends to be overdiagnosed.

Seven masquerades checklist

Of these conditions drugs and vertebral dysfunction (of the cervical spine) stand out as important causes. Depression demands attention because of the possible association of anxiety and hyperventilation.

Diabetes mellitus has an association through the possible mechanisms of hypoglycaemia from therapy or from an autonomic neuropathy.

Drugs

Drugs usually affect the vestibular nerve rather than the labyrinth. Drugs that cause dizziness are presented in Table 42.3.

Table 42.3 *Drugs that can cause dizziness*

Alcohol
Aspirin and salicylates
Antibiotics: streptomycin, gentamicin, kanamycin, tetracyclines especially minocycline
Antiepileptics: phenytoin
Antidepressants
Antihypertensives
Antihistamines
Cocaine
Quinine-quinidine
Tranquillisers: phenothiazines, phenobarbitone, benzodiazepines
Diuretics in large doses: intravenous frusemide, ethacrynic acid
Glyceryl trinitrate

Cervical spine dysfunction

It is not uncommon to observe vertigo in patients with cervical spondylosis or post cervical spinal injury. It has been postulated[4] that this may be caused by the generation of abnormal impulses from proprioceptors in the upper cervical spine, or by osteophytes compressing the vertebral arteries in the vertebral canal. Some instances of benign positional vertigo are associated with disorders of the cervical spine.

Psychogenic considerations

This may be an important aspect to consider in the patient presenting with dizziness, especially if the complaint is giddiness or lightheadedness. An underlying anxiety may be the commonest cause of this symptom in family practice and clinical investigation of hyperventilation may confirm the diagnosis. The possibility of depression must also be kept in mind.[5] Many of these patients harbour the fear that they may be suffering from a serious disorder, such as a brain tumour or multiple sclerosis, or face an impending stroke or insanity. Appropriate reassurance to the contrary is often positively therapeutic for that patient.

The clinical approach

The essentials of the diagnostic approach include careful attention to the history and physical examination, and judicious selection of specific office tests and special investigations.

History

It is important to get patients to explain the precise nature of the symptoms, even `asking their opinion as to the cause of their dizziness.

The following questions should be addressed:

- Is it vertigo or pseudovertigo?
- Symptom pattern:
  — paroxysmal or continuous?
  — effect of position and change of posture?
- Any aural symptoms?
  — tinnitus?
  — deafness?
- Any visual symptoms?
- Any neurological symptoms?
- Any nausea or vomiting?
- Any symptoms of psychoneurosis?
- Any recent colds?
- Any recent head injury (even trivial)?
- Any drugs being taken?
  — alcohol?
  — marijuana?
  — hypotensives?
  — psychotropics?
  — other drugs?

Physical examination

A full general examination is appropriate with particular attention being paid to the cardiovascular and central nervous systems and the auditory and vestibular mechanisms.

Examination guidelines are:

1. ear disease
   - auroscopic examination: wax? drum?
   - hearing tests
   - Weber and Rinne's tests
2. the eyes
   - visual acuity
   - test movements for nystagmus

3. cardiovascular system
   - evidence of atherosclerosis
   - blood pressure: supine, standing, sitting
   - cardiac arrhythmias
4. cranial nerves
   - 2nd, 3rd, 4th, 6th and 7th
   - corneal response for 5th
   - 8th—auditory nerve
5. the cerebellum or its connections
   - gait
   - co-ordination
   - reflexes
   - Romberg test
   - finger nose test: ? past pointing
6. the neck, including cervical spine
7. general search for evidence of:
   - anaemia
   - polycythaemia
   - alcohol dependence

Special office tests for dizziness

- Ask the patient to perform any manoeuvre that may provoke the symptom.
- Carry out head positional testing to induce vertigo and nystagmus (Fig. 42.3).
- Take blood pressure measurements in three positions.
- Perform forced hyperventilation (20 to 25 breaths per minute) for 2 minutes.

Fig. 42.3 *Positional testing for benign positional vertigo (head taken rapidly from sitting position to hanging position with head turned to right: one of the three positions)*

- Carry out palpation of carotid arteries and carotid sinus (with care).

Investigations

Appropriate laboratory tests should be selected from Table 42.4.

Table 42.4 *Investigations*

Haemoglobin
Blood glucose
ECG: ? Holter monitor
Audiometry
Brain-stem evoked audiometry
Caloric test
Visual evoked potentials (MS)
Electrocochleography
Electro-oculography (electronystagmography)
Rotational tests
Radiology
- chest X-ray (? bronchial carcinoma)
- cervical spine X-ray
- CT scan
- MRI (the choice to locate acoustic neuroma or other tumour—may detect MS)

Diagnostic guidelines

- A sudden attack of vertigo in a young person following a recent URTI is suggestive of vestibular neuronitis.
- Dizziness is a common symptom in menopausal women and is often associated with other features of vasomotor instability.
- Phenytoin therapy can cause cerebellar dysfunction.
- Postural and exercise hypotension are relatively common in the older atherosclerotic patient.
- Acute otitis media does not cause vertigo but chronic otitis media can, particularly if the patient develops a cholesteatoma which then erodes into the internal ear causing a perilymph fistula.

Dizziness in children

Dizziness is not a common symptom in children. Vertigo can have sinister causes and requires referral because of the possibility of tumours such as a medulloblastoma. A study by Eviatar and Eviatar[6] of vertigo in children found that the commonest cause was a seizure focus particularly affecting the temporal lobe. Other causes included psychosomatic vertigo, migraine and vestibular neuronitis.

Apart from the above causes it is important to consider:
- infection, e.g. meningitis, meningoencephalitis, cerebral abscess
- trauma, especially to the temporal area
- middle ear infection
- labyrinthitis, e.g. mumps, measles, influenza
- benign paroxysmal vertigo (short-lived attacks of vertigo in young children between 1 and 4 years of age: tends to precede adulthood migraine)[7]
- hyperventilation
- drugs—prescribed
- illicit drugs, e.g. cocaine, marijuana
- cardiac arrhythmias
- alcohol toxicity

A common trap is the acute effect of alcohol in curious children who can present with the sudden onset of dizziness.

Dizzy turns in girls in late teens

- These are commonly due to blood pressure fluctuations.
- Give advice related to reducing stress, lack of sleep and excessive exercise.
- Reassure that it settles with age (rare after 25 years).

Dizziness in the elderly

Dizziness is a relatively common complaint of the elderly. Common causes include postural hypotension related mainly to drugs prescribed for hypertension or other cardiovascular problems. Cerebrovascular disease, especially in the areas of the brain stem, is also relevant in this age group. True vertigo can be produced simply by an accumulation of wax in the external auditory meatus, being more frequent than generally appreciated.

Middle ear disease is also sometimes the cause of vertigo in an older person but disease of the auditory nerve, inner ear, cerebellum, brain stem and cervical spine are common underlying factors.

Malignancy, primary and secondary, is a possibility in the elderly. The possibility of cardiac arrhythmias as a cause of syncopal symptoms increases with age.

Dizzy turns in elderly women

If no cause such as hypertension is found, advise them to get up slowly from sitting or lying, and to wear firm elastic stockings.

Vestibular neuronitis and labyrinthitis

These are considered to be a viral infection of the vestibular nerve and labyrinth respectively, causing a prolonged attack of vertigo that can last for several days and be severe enough to require admission to hospital.

- acute vertigo with nausea and vomiting = vestibular neuronitis
- same symptoms + hearing loss ± tinnitus = acute labyrinthitis

It is analogous to a viral infection of the 7th nerve causing Bell's palsy. The attack is similar to Ménière's syndrome except that there is no hearing disturbance. Characteristic features are:

- single attack of vertigo without tinnitus or deafness
- usually preceding upper respiratory tract infection
- mainly in young adults
- abrupt onset with vertigo, nausea and vomiting
- may take 6 weeks or so to subside
- examination shows nystagmus—rapid component away from side of lesion (no hearing loss)
- caloric stimulation confirms impaired vestibular function

Note: Acute labyrinthitis has a similar pattern. It is the diagnosis if hearing loss is present.

Treatment

The following drugs can be used:
- dimenhydrinate (Dramamine) 50 mg 4–6 hourly

or

- prochlorperazine (Stemetil) 12.5 mg IM (if severe)

or (recommended as best)

- diazepam (which decreases brain-stem response to vestibular stimuli),[2] 5–10 mg IM for the acute attack, then 5 mg (o) tds and possibly droperidol.

Outcome

Both are self-limiting disorders and usually settle over 5–7 days or several weeks. Labyrinthitis usually lasts longer and during recovery rapid head movements may bring on transient vertigo.

Benign paroxysmal positional vertigo

BPPV is a common type of acute vertigo that is induced by changing head position—particularly tilting the head backwards, changing from a recumbent to a sitting position or turning to the affected side. Characteristic features:

- It affects all ages especially the elderly.
- The female to male ratio is 2:1.
- It recurs periodically for several days.
- Each attack is brief, usually lasts 10–60 seconds, and subsides rapidly.
- Attacks are not accompanied by vomiting, tinnitus or deafness (nausea may occur).
- In one large series 17% were associated with trauma, 15% with viral labyrinthitis while about 50% had no clear predisposing factor other than age. One accepted theory of causation is that fine pieces of debris that are loose in the labyrinth settle on the bottom of the ear and generate endolymphatic movement.[8] It may also be a variation of cervical dysfunction.
- Diagnosis is confirmed by head position testing. (From a sitting position the patient's head is rapidly taken to a head-hanging position 30° below the level of the couch—do three times, with the head (1) straight, (2) rotated to the right, (3) rotated to the left. Hold on for 30 seconds and observe the patient carefully for vertigo and nystagmus. There is a latent period of a few seconds before the onset of the symptoms—see Fig. 42.3.)
- Tests of hearing and vestibular function are normal.
- There is usually spontaneous recovery in weeks (most return to regular activity after 1 week).
- Recurrences are common: attacks occur in clusters.

Management

- Give appropriate explanation and reassurance.
- Drugs are not recommended.

Positional vestibular exercises

Most patients appear to benefit from exercise such as the Brandt and Daroff procedure[9] or the Cawthorne Cooksie exercises that consist essentially of repeatedly inducing the symptoms of vertigo. Rather than resorting to avoidance measures the patient is instructed to perform positional exercises to induce vertigo, hold this position until it subsides, and repeat this many times until the manoeuvre does not precipitate vertigo. The attacks then usually subside in a few days.

Surgical treatment
Rarely surgical treatment is required; it involves occlusion of the posterior semicircular canal rather than selective neurectomy.

Ménière's syndrome
- It is commonest in 30–50 age group.
- It is characterised by paroxysmal attacks of:
  — vertigo
  — tinnitus
  — nausea and vomiting
  — sweating and pallor
  — deafness (progressive)
- Onset is abrupt—patient may fall and then be bed-ridden for 1–2 hours.
- Attacks last 30 minutes to several hours.
- There is a variable interval between attacks (twice a month to twice a year).
- Nystagmus is observed only during an attack (often to side opposite affected inner ear).
- Examination:
  — sensorineural deafness (low tones)
  — caloric test: impaired vestibular function
  — audiometry
    • sensorineural deafness
    • loudness recruitment
  — special tests
- There are characteristic changes in electro-cochleography

Treatment

Acute attack[10]
Anticipation of attack (fullness, tinnitus)
- prochlorperazine 25 mg suppository
- 30 g urea crystals in orange juice (preferably 30 minutes before)

Treatment
- diazepam 5 mg IV ± prochlorperazine 12.5 mg IM
- consider betahistine 8 mg (o) tds if persistent or episodic

Long term
- reassurance with a careful explanation of this condition to the patient who often associates it with malignant disease
- excess intake of salt, tobacco and coffee to be avoided
- a low-salt diet is the mainstay of treatment

- alleviate abnormal anxiety by using stress management, meditation or possibly long-term sedation
- referral for neurological assessment
- diuretic, e.g. hydrochlorothiazide/amiloride daily

Surgery may be an option for intractable cases.

Vestibular migraine
Migraine is a relatively common cause of vertigo and often unrecognised because of its many guises. It should be strongly suspected if there is a past and/or family history of migraine and also where there is a history of vertigo or ataxia that persists for hours or days in the absence of aural symptoms.[11] Vertigo, which is usually not violent, may take the place of the aura that precedes the headache or may be a migraine equivalent whereby the vertigo replaces the symptoms of headache. Pizotifen or propranolol are recommended for prophylaxis.

When to refer
- Vertigo of uncertain diagnosis, especially in children
- Possibility of tumour, or bacterial infection
- Vertigo in presence of suppurative otitis media despite antibiotic therapy
- Presumed viral labyrinthitis not abating after 3 months
- Vertigo following trauma
- Presumed Ménière's syndrome, not responding to conservative medical management
- Evidence of vertebrobasilar insufficiency
- BPPV persisting for more than 12 months despite treatment with particle repositioning exercises

Practice tips
A careful drug history often pinpoints the diagnosis.
- Always consider cardiac arrhythmias as a cause of acute dizziness.
- Consider phenytoin therapy as a cause of dizziness in an epileptic patient.
- If an intracerebral metastatic lesion is suspected, consider the possibility of carcinoma of the lung as the primary source.
- Three important office investigations to perform in the evaluation are blood pressure measurement (lying, sitting and standing),

hyperventilation and head positional testing.

- Cervical vertigo is very common and appropriate cervical mobilisation methods should be considered.
- BPPV is also common and prescribing a set of exercises to desensitise the labyrinth is recommended. Use either the Brandt and Daroff procedure or the Cawthorne-Cooksey program.[12]

References

1. Kincaid-Smith P, Larkins R, Whelan G. *Problems in clinical medicine*. Sydney: MacLennan and Petty, 1989, 165.

2. Sloane PD, Slatt LM, Baker RM. *Essentials of family medicine*. Baltimore: Williams and Wilkins, 1988.

3. Sandler G, Fry J. *Early clinical diagnosis*. Lancaster: MTP Press, 1986, 361–382.

4. Lance JW. *A physiological approach to clinical neurology*. London: Butterworths, 1970, 162–179.

5. Ell J. The dizzy patient. Mod Med, 1991; 34:26–32.

6. Eviatar L, Eviatar A. Vertigo in children. Differential diagnosis and treatment. Paediatrics, 1977; 59:833–837.

7. Tunnessen WW Jr. *Signs and symptoms in paediatrics*. Philadelphia: Lippincott, 1988, 591–594.

8. Horne M. Neurology quiz. Aust Fam Physician, 1994; 23:1563–1564.

9. Brandt T, Daroff DB. Physical therapy for BPPV. Arch Otolaryngol, 1980; 106: 484–485.

10. Tonkin JP. Ménière's disease. Current Therapeutics, 1995; 36:39–43.

11. Pohl D. Vertigo: In MIMS Disease Index (2nd edn). Sydney: IMS Publishing, 1996, 568–571.

12. Moulds RFW. *Therapeutic guidelines: Neurology*. Melbourne: Therapeutic Guidelines Limited, 1997–98, 60–63.

43
Dyspepsia (indigestion)

—

Half the patients who get you up in the middle of the night and think they are dying are suffering from wind!

Francis Young (1884–1954)
Advice to a younger doctor

Dyspepsia or indigestion is a difficult, sometimes vague, symptom to define or evaluate and requires very careful questioning to clarify the exact nature of the complaint.

Definitions

Dyspepsia. This is pain or discomfort centred at the upper abdomen that is chronic or recurrent in nature. It embraces the following:

- nausea
- heartburn/regurgitation
- upper abdominal discomfort
- lower chest discomfort
- acidity
- epigastric fullness or unease
- abdominal distension

The discomfort can sometimes amount to pain. Diagnoses to consider in dyspeptic patients are summarised in Table 43.1.[1]

Heartburn. This is a central retrosternal or epigastric burning sensation that spreads upwards to the throat.

Flatulence. This is excessive wind. It includes belching, abdominal bloating or passing excessive flatus.[2]

Table 43.1 *Diagnoses to consider in dyspeptic patients*

Gastrointestinal disorders
- Gastro-oesophageal reflux including hiatus hernia
- Functional (non-ulcer) dyspepsia
- Oesophageal motility disorders (dysmotility)
- Peptic ulcer
- Upper GIT malignancies
  e.g. oesophagus, stomach, pancreas
- Hepatobiliary disease
  e.g. hepatitis, biliary dyskinesia, cholelithiasis
- Pancreatitis
- Upper GIT inflammation
  — gastritis
  — giardiasis
  — Crohn's disease
- Irritable bowel syndrome

Non-gastrointestinal disorders
- Myocardial ischaemia
- Drug reaction
- Alcohol effect
- Anxiety/stress
- Depression

Excessive belching
- usually functional
- organic disease uncommon
- due to air swallowing (aerophagy)
- common in anxious people who gulp food and drink
- associated hypersalivation

Key facts and checkpoints
- Dyspepsia or indigestion is a common complaint; 80% of the population[1] will have experienced it at some time.
- Consider heartburn as ischaemic heart disease until proved otherwise.

- The presence of oesophagitis is suggested by pain on swallowing hot or cold liquids (odynophagia).
- All reflux is not due to hiatus hernia.
- Many patients with hiatus hernia do not experience heartburn.
- All patients with dysphagia must be investigated to rule out malignancy.
- 10% of people in the community develop peptic ulcer disease.
- The major feature of peptic ulcer disease is epigastric pain.
- The pain of duodenal ulcer classically occurs at night.
- At any time 10–20% of chronic NSAIDs users have peptic ulceration (greater than non-users).[3]
- NSAIDs mainly cause gastric ulcers (gastric antrum and prepyloric region) with duodenum affected to a lesser extent.
- Dyspeptic symptoms correlate poorly with NSAID-associated ulcer.

A diagnostic approach

A summary of the safety diagnostic model is presented in Table 43.2.

It is best to consider dyspepsia as:

- ulcer-like—localised pain
- dysmotility-like—diffuse discomfort, feeling full after meals (early satiety), nausea, bloating
- acid-reflux-like—indigestion or heartburn with acid reflux or regurgitation.

The ulcer-like category may be due to an ulcer and if not is termed functional (non-ulcer) dyspepsia.

Pitfalls

Perhaps the commonest mistake is to attribute the discomfort of myocardial ischaemia to a disorder of the GIT. A sense of fullness or pressure in the epigastrium can certainly accompany ischaemia.

General pitfalls

- Reflux oesophagitis and peptic ulcer can mimic ischaemic heart disease.
- Overlooking gastric carcinoma as a cause of dyspepsia.

Table 43.2   *Dyspepsia: diagnostic strategy model*

Q. *Probability diagnosis*
A. Irritable upper GIT (functional dyspepsia)
Gastro-oesophageal reflux
Oesophageal motility disorder (dysmotility)

Q. *Serious disorders not to be missed*
A. Neoplasia
• carcinoma: stomach, pancreas, oesophagus
Cardiovascular
• ischaemic heart disease
• congestive cardiac failure
Pancreatitis
Peptic ulcer

Q. *Pitfalls (often missed)*
A. Myocardial ischaemia
Food allergy, e.g. lactose intolerance
Pregnancy (early)
Biliary motility disorder
Other gall bladder disease
Post vagotomy
Duodenitis
Rarities
• Hyperparathyroidism
• Mesenteric ischaemia
• Zollinger-Ellison syndrome
• Renal failure

Q. *Seven masquerades checklist*
A. Depression   √
Diabetes   rarely
Drugs   √
Anaemia   –
Thyroid disease   –
Spinal dysfunction   –
UTI   –

Q. *Is this patient trying to tell me something?*
A. Anxiety and stress are common associations of which patients are often unaware. Consider irritable bowel syndrome.

- Failing to stress that weight reduction to ideal level will generally alleviate gastro-oesophageal reflux.
- Overlooking drugs as a cause (Table 43.3).

The clinical approach
History

It is worthwhile spending some time clarifying the exact nature of the presenting complaint: what the patient means by 'indigestion' or 'heartburn'.[4] The relationship of the symptom to eating is very important, and whether it occurs after each meal or after specific meals.

In particular, care should be taken to consider and perhaps exclude ischaemic heart disease.

Table 43.3 *Drugs that may cause dyspepsia*

Alcohol
Anticholinergics
Aspirin
Calcium channel blockers
Corticosteroids
Digitalis
Lipid-lowering agents
Narcotics
Nicotine
NSAIDs
Potassium supplements (slow release)
Theophylline
Tricyclic antidepressants
Tetracycline

Key questions

- How would you describe the discomfort?
- Can you show me exactly where it is and where it radiates?
- What makes your discomfort worse?
- What relieves your discomfort?
- What effect do food, milk and antacids have?
- What effect do coffee, onions or garlic have?
- What effect does a big meal have?
- What about drinking alcohol? Wine?
- What effect does exercise have?
- Do fried or fatty foods make it worse?
- Do hot spicy foods affect it?
- Does the problem come on at night soon after you go to bed?
- Does it wake you up at night?
- Does bending over, e.g. gardening, make it worse?
- Do you have periods of freedom from the problem?
- Are you under a lot of stress or have a lot of worry?
- Do you go flat out all day?
- Do you rush your meals?
- Do you chew your food properly?
- What drugs or medicines do you take?
- How much alcohol do you have? Do you smoke?
- Have you noticed anything else when you have the problem?
- Do you get constipated or have diarrhoea?
- Have you lost weight recently?
- Do you feel the discomfort between your shoulder blades, or in your shoulders or throat?

Symptoms analysis

Site and radiation

The site and radiation of pain or discomfort can provide a lead to the diagnosis.[5] Refer to Figure 36.10. If it is felt in the interscapular area consider oesophageal spasm, gall bladder disease or a duodenal ulcer. Retrosternal discomfort indicates oesophageal disorders or angina, while epigastric discomfort suggests disorders of the biliary system, stomach and duodenum.

Character of the pain

There tends to be considerable overlap in the character of the pain from the various disorders but some general characteristics apply.

- burning pain → gastro-oesophageal (G-O) reflux
- constricting pain → ischaemic heart disease or oesophageal spasm
- deep gnawing pain → peptic ulcer
- heavy ache or 'killing' pain → psychogenic pain

Aggravating and relieving factors

Examples of these factors include:

- Eating food may aggravate a gastric ulcer but relieve a duodenal ulcer.
- Eating fried or fatty foods will aggravate biliary disease, functional dyspepsia and oesophageal disorders.
- Bending will aggravate G-O reflux.
- Alcohol may aggravate G-O reflux, oesophagitis, gastritis, peptic ulcer, pancreatitis.

Associated symptoms

Relevant examples:

- difficulty in swallowing → oesophageal disorders
- lump or constricting in throat → psychogenic
- acid regurgitation → G-O reflux; oesophagitis
- anorexia, weight loss → carcinoma of the stomach
- waterbrash → G-O, hiatus hernia, peptic ulcer
- symptoms of anaemia → chronic oesophagitis or gastritis, peptic ulcer, carcinoma (stomach, colon)
- flatulence, belching, abnormal bowel habits → irritable bowel syndrome
- diarrhoea 30 minutes after meal → mesenteric ischaemia

Physical examination

The physical examination does not often provide the key to the diagnosis but it is important to perform very careful palpation and inspection. Look for evidence of clinical anaemia and jaundice. Diffuse mild abdominal tenderness and a pulsatable abdominal aorta are common findings but do not necessarily discriminate between organic and functional problems. Specific epigastric tenderness suggests peptic ulceration while tenderness over the gall bladder area (Murphy's sign) indicates gall bladder disease. An epigastric mass indicates carcinoma of the stomach.

Investigations

Do not overinvestigate. Investigations tend to be unrewarding in most instances of dyspepsia and could be postponed if the history is suggestive of a functional cause and the symptoms are not severe.[1] A trial of treatment such as changing adverse lifestyle factors, dietary modification and antacids could be the initial approach. Age is important in determining the extent of investigations, which are more relevant in those over 40 years.

The investigation of choice is endoscopy, which is superior to barium studies in investigation of the upper GIT. Gastroscopy is indicated for the *alarm* symptoms.

- abnormal symptoms of reflux/dyspepsia
- change of symptoms
- dysphagia
- unexplained weight loss
- GIT bleeding
- pain radiating to back
- pain waking at night
- abnormal signs on examination

Dyspepsia in the elderly

An organic disorder is more likely in the older patient in whom it is important to consider carcinoma of the stomach. Symptoms such as anorexia, vomiting and weight loss point to such a problem.

Other conditions causing dyspepsia that are more prevalent in this age group are:

- constipation
- mesenteric artery ischaemia
- congestive cardiac failure

Dyspepsia in children

Dyspepsia is an uncommon problem in children but can be caused by drugs, oesophageal disorders and gastro-oesophageal reflux in particular.[6] Reflux can be considered to be physiological or pathological.

Gastro-oesophageal reflux

Regurgitation of feeds because of gastro-oesophageal reflux is a common physiological event in newborn infants. A mild degree of reflux is normal in babies, especially after they burp; this condition is called *posseting*.

Symptoms

Milk will flow freely from the mouth soon after feeding, even after the baby has been put down for a sleep. Sometimes the flow will be forceful and may even be out of the nose.

Despite this vomiting or regurgitation, the babies are usually comfortable and thrive. Some infants will cry, presumably because of heartburn.[6]

In a small number the reflux may be severe enough (pathological) to cause serious problems such as oesophagitis with haematemesis or anaemia, stricture formation, failure to thrive, apnoea and aspiration.

Prognosis

Reflux gradually improves with time and usually ceases soon after solids are introduced into the diet. Most cases clear up completely by the age of 9 or 10 months, when the baby is sitting. Severe cases tend to persist until 18 months of age.

Investigations

These are not necessary in most cases but in those with persistent problems or complications referral to a paediatrician is recommended. The specialist investigations include barium meal with cine scanning, oesophageal pH monitoring or endoscopy and biopsy.

Management

Appropriate reassurance with parental education is important. It should be pointed out that changes in feeding practice and positioning will control most reflux.

The infant should be placed on the left side for sleeping with the head of the cot elevated about 10–20 degrees. The old bucket method, in which the child is placed in a bucket, is not necessary. Suspending the child in one of the new suspended swings for periods of 30–60 minutes after feeds will help.

Smaller, more frequent feeds and thickening agents are appropriate.

Thickening of feeds

Giving the baby thicker feeds usually helps those with more severe reflux. The old-fashioned remedy of using cornflour blended in bottles is still useful.

Bottle-fed babies (powdered milk formula)

Carobel: Add slightly less than 1 full scoop per bottle.

Gaviscon: Mix slightly less than ½ teaspoon of Infant Gaviscon Powder with 120 mL of formula in the bottle.

Cornflour: Mix 1 teaspoon with each 120 mL of formula. Check with your doctor or nurse for the proper method.

Karicare: This is very simple to use but more expensive.

Breast-fed babies

Carobel: Add slightly less than 1 full scoop to 20 mL cool boiled water or 20 mL expressed breast milk and give just before the feed.

Gaviscon: Mix slightly less than ½ teaspoon of Infant Gaviscon Powder with 20 mL cool boiled water or expressed breast milk and give just after the feed.

For persistent or complicated reflux, including oesophagitis, specialist-monitored treatment will include the use of antacids, H_2-receptor blocking agents or prokinetic agents, e.g. cisapride.

Dyspepsia in adults

Gastro-oesophageal reflux disease (GORD)

Features
- heartburn
- acid regurgitation, especially lying down at night
- waterbrash
- diagnosis usually made on history
- investigation usually not needed

(reserve for danger signs and non-responsive treatment)

Complications
- oesophagitis
- iron-deficiency anaemia
- stricture
- respiratory: chronic cough, asthma, hoarseness
- Barrett's oesophagus (from prolonged reflux)

Barrett's oesophagus
- a premalignant condition
- lower oesophagus lined with gastric mucosa (at least 3 cm)
- prone to ulceration
- needs careful management
- consider 2 yearly endoscopies with biopsies

Management[7]

Stage 1

- Patient education/appropriate reassurance
- Consider acid suppression or neutralisation
- Attend to lifestyle:
  — weight reduction if overweight (this alone may abolish symptoms)
  — reduction or cessation of smoking
  — reduction or cessation of alcohol (especially with dinner)
  — avoid fatty foods, e.g. pastries
  — reduction or cessation of coffee, tea and chocolate
  — avoid coffee and alcohol late at night
  — avoid gaseous drinks
  — leave at least 3 hours between the evening meal and retiring
  — have main meal at midday with light evening meal
  — avoid spicy foods and tomato products
- Drugs to avoid
  — anticholinergics, theophylline, calcium channel blocks, doxycycline. Pill-induced oesophagitis occurs especially with tetracyclines, slow release K, iron sulphate, corticosteroids, NSAIDs—avoid taking dry; use ample fluids
- Antacids (see Table 43.4)
  — best is liquid alginate/antacid mixture
  — e.g. Gaviscon/Mylanta plus
      20 mL on demand or 1½–2 hours before meals and bedtime
- Elevation of head of bed
  — if GORD occurs in bed, sleep with head of bed elevated 10–20 cm on wooden blocks

Table 43.4 *Antacids in common use*

Antacids

Water soluble	Calcium carbonate
	Sodium — bicarbonate
	— citrotartrate

Note: Excess is prone to cause alkalosis—apathy, mental changes, stupor, renal dysfunction, tetany

Water insoluble	Aluminium — hydroxide
	— glycinate
	— phosphate
	Magnesium — alginate
	— carbonate
	— hydroxide
	— trisilicate

Combination antacids

Antacid +	alginic acid
+	oxethazaine
+	simethicone

Table 43.5 *Side effects of common antacids*

Aluminium hydroxide	— constipation
Magnesium trisilicate	— diarrhoea
Sodium bicarbonate	— alkalosis
	— milk alkali syndrome
Calcium carbonate	— alkalosis
	— constipation
	— milk alkali syndrome
	— hypercalcaemia

Stage 2[8]

If no relief after several weeks, the following guidelines may be appropriate.

Step 1 Reduce acid secretion (select from)
- H$_2$-receptor antagonists (oral use for 8 weeks)
  — cimetidine 400 mg bd pc or 800 mg nocte
      or
  — famotidine 40 mg nocte
      or
  — nizatadine 150 mg bd or 300 mg nocte
      or
  — ranitidine 150 mg bd pc or 300 mg nocte
- Proton-pump inhibitor (PPI) (if no response to above) for 4–8 weeks
  — lansoprazole 30 mg mane
      or
  — omeprazole 20–40 mg mane
      or
  — pantoprazole 40 mg mane
    (all very effective for ulcerative oesophagitis and reflux)

If step 1 is not fully effective:

Step 2 Prokinetic agents (select from)
- to facilitate gastric emptying
- very useful in reflux and dysmotility
  — domperidone 10 mg tds or qid ac
      or
  — metoclopramide 10 mg tds
      or
  — cisapride 5–10 mg tds

Note: Long-term use of metoclopramide may cause agitation, confusion or extrapyramidal side effects, e.g. dystonia

Resistant reflux: Combined PPI and cisapride very effective. May be advised to eradicate *H. pylori* if present.

Surgery. This is usually for young patients with severe reflux. The gold standard is a short loose 360° fundoplication.

Functional (non-ulcer) dyspepsia[8]

There is discomfort on eating in the absence of demonstrable organic disease. This can be considered in two categories:
- ulcer-like dyspepsia
      or
- dysmotility-like dyspepsia

Ulcer-like dyspepsia
Treat as for GORD.

Dysmotility-like dyspepsia
Features of dysmotility
- discomfort with early sense of fullness on eating
- nausea
- overweight

- emotional stress
- poor diet, e.g. fatty foods
- similar lifestyle guidelines to GORD

Management
- Treat as for GORD (stage 1).
- Include antacids.
- If not responsive:
  — *Step 1:* H$_2$-antagonists
  — *Step 2:* Prokinetic agents

Peptic ulcer disease
General features
- common: 10–20% incidence over a lifetime
- point prevalence of ulcer disease: 3–5%
- DU:GU = 4:1
- DUs common in men 3:1
- cumulative mortality of 10%
- risk factors
  — male sex
  — family history
  — smoking (cause and delayed healing)
  — stress
  — common in blood group O
  — NSAIDs 2–4 times increase in GU and ulcer complications
  — *Helicobacter pylori*: if absent, no ulcer; now proved to cause DUs.
- unproven risk factors
  — corticosteroids
  — alcohol
  — diet (does reduce recurrence of PU)
- types of ulcers
  — lower oesophageal
  — gastric
  — stomal (post gastric surgery)
  — duodenal

Clinical features
- episodic burning epigastric pain related to meals (1–2 hours after)
- relieved by food or antacids (generally)
- dyspepsia common
- may be 'silent' in elderly on NSAIDs
- physical examination often unhelpful

Investigations
- endoscopy (investigation of choice)[9]
    92% predictive value
- barium studies
    54% predictive value
- serum gastrin (consider if multiple ulcers)

- *H. pylori* test: serology or urea breath test; diagnosis usually based on urease test performed at endoscopy

Complications
- perforation
- bleeding → haematemesis and melaena
- obstruction—pyloric stenosis
- (blood loss) anaemia
- carcinoma (in gastric ulcer)
- oesophageal stenosis

Management
Aims of treatment:
- relieve symptoms
- accelerate ulcer healing
- prevent complications
- minimise risk of relapse

The treatment of a gastric ulcer is similar to that for a DU except that GUs take about 2 weeks longer to heal and the increased risk of malignancy has to be considered.

Stage 1: Treatment
General measures
- same principles as for GORD
- stop smoking
- avoid irritant drugs
  —NSAIDs
  —aspirin
- normal diet but avoid foods that upset
- antacids

H$_2$-receptor antagonists (first-line agent)
    8 week oral course of
- cimetidine 400 mg bd pc
      or 800 mg nocte
                or
- famotidine 40 mg nocte
                or
- nizatadine 300 mg nocte
                or
- ranitidine 150 mg bd pc

Use with caution in:
- the elderly
- those on drugs, especially warfarin, anticonvulsants, beta-blockers
- liver disease

Outcome[9,10]
- DU: 80% healing rate
  — prone to spontaneous remissions and relapse

— once healed:
- 60% relapse within 1 year
- 20% persist but asymptomatic
- GU: 50% do not recur
  other 50% recurrence within 2 years

Note: Use maintenance or continuous treatment for two or more exacerbations in 12 months.

Stage 2: Pharmacological agents

The following can be used for ulcers not responding to an H_2-receptor antagonist, for frequent relapses or complicated ulcers.

Proton-pump blocker
- omeprazole 20 mg cap (o) mane for 4–8 weeks
  or
- lansoprazole 30 mg (o) mane
  — used for resistant ulcers
  — 100% inhibition of acid
  — high healing rates

Other possible agents

Cytoprotective agents
- sucralfate 1 g tab (o) qid, 1 hour ac and nocte

Prostaglandin analogue
- misoprostol 800 μg daily (divided doses)

Colloidal bismuth subcitrate (CBS)
- bismuth subcitrate (De-Nol)
  2 tabs (chewed) bd for 6–8 weeks
  — effective for relapsing ulcers
  — appears to be effective against *H. pylori*

Therapy to eradicate *Helicobacter pylori*

This organism has a proven link with peptic ulcer disease (both DU and benign non-drug induced GU) gastric carcinoma and maltoma (a gastric lymphoma) because of mucosal infection. This hypothesis is supported by a very low relapse of DU in subjects eradicated of *H. pylori*.

Treatment regimens

(use for 7–14 days)[11]
1. CBS 1 tab qid
     +
   2 antibiotics: tetracycline or amoxycillin
     + metronidazole (14 days)

or
2. proton-pump blocker + amoxycillin
     + metronidazole (14 days)
   or
3. proton-pump blocker + clarithromycin + either amoxycillin or metronidazole (7 days)
   or
other combinations

Surgical treatment

Indications include:
- failed medical treatment after 1 year
- complications
  — uncontrollable bleeding
  — perforation
  — pyloric stenosis
- suspicion of malignancy in gastric ulcer
- recurrent ulcer after previous surgery

NSAIDs and peptic ulcers

1. *Ulcer identified in NSAID user*
   - stop NSAID (if possible)
   - check smoking and alcohol use
   - try alternative anti-inflammatory analgesic e.g. paracetamol
         enteric-coated, slow-release aspirin
         corticosteroids intra-articular or oral
   - H_2-receptor antagonist (full dose)
       or
   misoprostol 800 μg a day (used for GU)

   Note: Healing time is doubled if NSAID continued.[3] About 90% heal within 12 weeks. Check healing by endoscopy at 12 weeks.

2. *Prevention of ulcers in NSAID user*
   Try alternatives (as above). Prophylactic drugs are rarely justified but reasonable in those over 75 years and in those with a past history of peptic ulcer.
   - misoprostol (prevents GU recurrence)
   - H_2-receptor antagonist (prevents DU, not GU)
   Increased dietary fibre assists DU healing and prevention.

Carcinoma of stomach
Clinical features
- male:female 3:1
- usually asymptomatic early
- consider if upper GIT symptoms in patients > 40, especially weight loss

- recent onset dyspepsia in middle age
- dyspepsia unresponsive to treatment
- vague fullness or epigastric distension
- anorexia, nausea, ± vomiting
- dysphagia—a late sign
- onset of anaemia
- changing dyspepsia in gastric ulcer
- changing symptoms in pernicious anaemia
- *H. pylori* now implemented as a cause

Limited physical findings
- palpable abdominal mass (20%)
- signs (Fig. 43.1) in advanced cases

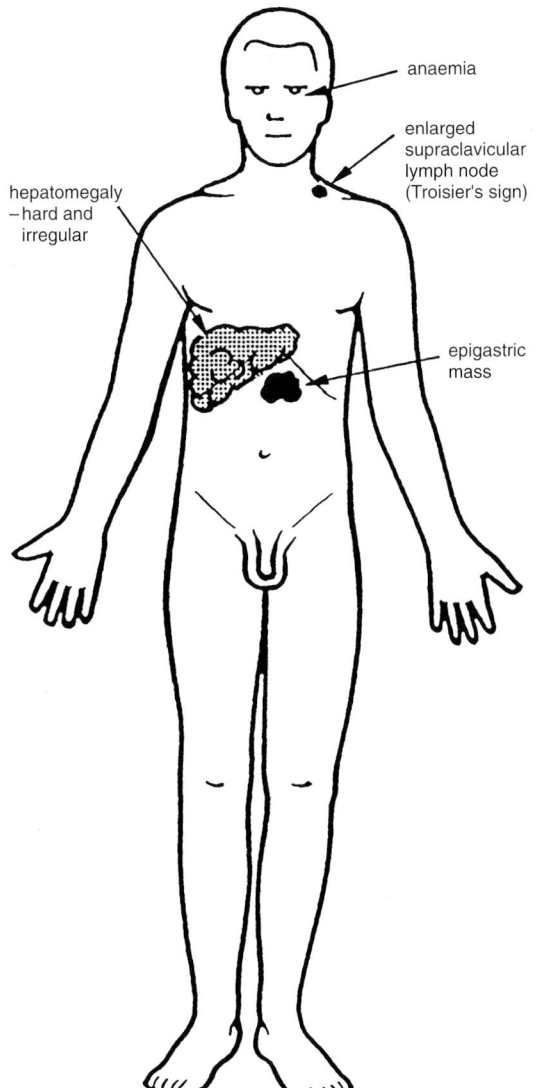

Fig. 43.1 *Late signs of carcinoma of the stomach*

anaemia

enlarged
supraclavicular
lymph node
(Troisier's sign)

hepatomegaly
–hard and
irregular

epigastric
mass

Investigations
- endoscopy and biopsy is optimal test
- barium meal—false negatives

Treatment
- surgical excision

Overall survival is poor.

When to refer

- Infants with persistent gastro-oesophageal reflux not responding to simple measures
- Failure to respond to stage 1 therapy for heartburn, when endoscopy is required
- Patients with persistent or recurrent ulcers
- Any patient with a peptic ulcer complication such as haemorrhage, obstruction or perforation

Practice tips

- Scleroderma is a rare but important cause of oesophagitis.
- Advise patients never to 'dry swallow' medications.
- Dysphagia always warrants investigation, not observation.
- Beware of attributing anaemia to oesophagitis.
- Epigastric pain aggravated by any food, relieved by acids = chronic gastric ulcer.
- Epigastric pain before meals, relieved by food = chronic duodenal ulcer
- Keep in mind the malignant potential of a gastric ulcer.
- A change in the nature of symptoms with a gastric ulcer suggests the possibility of malignant change.
- Avoid the long-term use of water-soluble antacids.
- Investigate the alarm symptoms—dysphagia, bleeding, anaemia, weight loss, waking at night, pain radiating to the back.

References

1. Smallwood R. Dyspepsia. Medical Observer, 27 September, 1991:33–34.

2. Holvey DN. *The Merck manual* (12th edn). Rahway: Merck Sharp & Dohme, 1975, 679–682.

3. Pritchard P. The management of upper gastrointestinal problems in patients taking NSAIDs. Aust Fam Physician, 1991; 20:1739–1741.

4. Kincaid-Smith P, Larkins R, Whelan G. *Problems in clinical medicine*. Sydney: MacLennan and Petty, 1989, 207–212.

5. Sandler G, Fry J. *Early clinical diagnosis*. Lancaster: MTP Press, 1986, 99–135.

6. Sewell J. Gastro-oesophageal reflux. Aust Paed Review, 1991; 3:2.

7. Hansky J. Gastro-oesophageal reflux. In: MIMS Disease Index (2nd edn). Sydney: IMS Publishing, 1996, 189–191.

8. Moulds RFW (Chairman). *Gastrointestinal drug guidelines*. Melbourne: Victorian Medical Postgraduate Foundation, 1994, 29–38.

9. Korman M, Sievert W. Peptic ulcers. In: MIMS Disease Index (2nd edn). Sydney: IMS Publishing, 1996, 400–402.

10. Sandler G. *Common medical problems*. London: ADIS, 1984, 139–176.

11. Lambert J. *Helicobacter pylori* and acid-pepsin disease. In: MIMS Disease Index (2nd edn). Sydney: IMS Publishing, 1996, 223–225.

44

Dysphagia

—

We swallow approximately 1200 times daily, largely subconsciously. While we take the fundamental function for granted, disordered swallowing can be a devastating condition, with substantial morbidity for those affected.

Ian Cook 1996

Dysphagia is difficulty in swallowing. It is usually associated with a sensation of hold-up of the swallowed bolus and is sometimes accompanied by pain.

Its origin is considered as either oropharyngeal or oesophageal. Oropharyngeal dysphagia is usually related to neuromuscular dysfunction and is commonly caused by stroke. Oesophageal dysphagia is usually due to motor disorders such as achalasia or diffuse oesophageal spasm and to peptic oesophageal strictures often secondary to reflux. In this type of dysphagia there is a sensation of a hold-up, which may be experienced in either the cervical or retrosternal region.[1] Causes are usually classified as functional, mechanical and neurological (Table 44.1)

Dysphagia must not be confused with globus hystericus, which is the sensation of the constant 'lump in the throat' although there is no actual difficulty swallowing food.

Table 44.1 *Causes of dysphagia*

• Functional	e.g. muscle tension, 'express swallowing'
• Neurological	e.g. stroke, myasthenia
• Mechanical	
Luminal	e.g. foreign body
Mural	e.g. stricture, tumour
Extramural	e.g. extrinsic compression, i.e. goitre

There are only a few common causes of dysphagia and these are usually readily diagnosed on the history and two or three investigations.

Diagnostic guidelines

- Any disease or abnormality affecting the tongue, pharynx or oesophagus can cause dysphagia.
- Patients experience a sensation of obstruction at a definite level with swallowing food or water; hence, it is convenient to subdivide dysphagia into oropharyngeal and oesophageal.
- Pain from the oropharynx is localised to the neck.
- Pain from the oesophagus is usually felt over the T2–T6 area of the chest.
- Oropharyngeal causes: difficulty initiating swallowing; food sticks at the supersternal notch level; regurgitation; aspiration.
- Oesophageal causes: food sticks to mid to lower sternal level; pain on swallowing solid foods, especially meat, potatoes and bread, and then eventually liquids.
- A pharyngeal pouch usually causes regurgitation of undigested food and gurgling may be audible over the side of the neck.
- Neurological disorders typically result in difficulty swallowing or coughing or choking due to food spillover, especially with liquids.
- Dysphagia for solids only indicates a structural lesion such as a stricture or tumour.
- Dysphagia for liquids and solids is typical of an oesophageal motility disorder.
- Gastroenterologists claim that the big three common causes referred to them are benign peptic stricture, carcinoma and achalasia.[2]
- Malignant oesophageal obstruction is usually evident when there is a short history of rapidly

progressive dysphagia and significant weight loss.[3]

A summary of the safety diagnostic model is presented in Table 44.2

Examination

It is worthwhile focusing on the following features:

- general examination including hands and skin
- mouth, pharynx, larynx (look for paralysis)
- neck, especially for lymph nodes and thyroid
- neurological, especially cranial nerve function and muscle weakness disorders
- special oesophageal obstruction test:
  — hand the patient a glass of water and place a stethoscope over the left upper quadrant of abdomen

Table 44.2 *Dysphagia: diagnostic strategy model (excluding oropharyngeal infections and strokes)*

Q. *Probability diagnosis*
A. Functional, e.g. 'express' swallowing, psychogenic
   Tablet-induced irritation
   Reflux oesophagitis

Q. *Serious disorders not to be missed*
A. Neoplasia
   • carcinoma pharynx, oesophagus, stomach
   • extrinsic tumour
   AIDS (opportunistic oesophageal infection)
   Stricture, usually benign peptic stricture
   Scleroderma
   Neurological causes
   • pseudobulbar palsy
   • multiple sclerosis
   • amyotrophic sclerosis
   • Parkinson's disease

Q. *Pitfalls (often missed)*
A. Foreign body
   Drugs, e.g. phenothiazines
   Subacute thyroiditis
   Extrinsic lesions, e.g. lymph nodes, goitre
   Upper oesophageal web, e.g. Plummer-Vinson syndrome
   Radiotherapy
   Achalasia
   Upper oesophageal spasm (mimics angina)
   Rarities (some)
   • Sjögren's syndrome
   • Aortic aneurysm
   • Aberrant right subclavian artery
   • Lead poisoning
   • Cervical osteoarthritis (large osteophytes)
   • Other neurological causes
   • Other mechanical causes

— measure time between swallowing and murmur produced by bolus passing the cardia (normal: 7–10 seconds)

Investigations

- full blood examination: ? anaemia
- neurological cause: oesophageal motility study (manometry)
- mechanical:
  — extrinsic compression, e.g. barium swallow, CT scan
  — intrinsic, e.g. endoscopy ± barium swallow

The primary investigation in suspected pharyngeal dysphagia is a video barium swallow[3] while endoscopy is generally the first investigation in cases of suspected oesophageal dysphagia. Barium swallow should precede endoscopy in the latter when there is a suspected oesophageal 'ring' and suspected oesophageal dysmotility. If endoscopy and radiology are negative, consider oesophageal motility studies to look specifically for achalasia or other less common motility disorders.

Specific conditions
Benign peptic stricture

- fibrous stricture of lower third oesophagus (can be higher)
- follows years of reflux oesophagitis
- usually older patients
- dysphagia with solid food
- diagnosis confirmed by endoscopy and barium swallow

Treatment

- Dilate the stricture.
- Treat reflux vigorously.

Carcinoma of oesophagus

- dysphagia at beginning of meal
- dysphagia for solid food steadily progressive over weeks
- can remain silent and tend to be invasive when diagnosed
- weight loss can be striking
- diagnosis confirmed by barium swallow and endoscopy
- both SCC (commonest) and adenocarcinoma
- adenocarcinoma associated with Barrett's mucosa
- treatment is usually palliative surgery

Achalasia

- a disorder of oesophageal motility
- widely dilated oesophagus
- empties poorly through a smoothly tapered lower end
- gradual onset of dysphagia for both liquids and solids
- fluctuating symptoms
- diagnosis confirmed by barium swallow or manometry
- manometry is the only way to diagnose with certainty[1]

Treatment

- conservative in the elderly, e.g. nifedipine
- pneumatic dilatation of lower oesophageal sphincter or surgical myotomy

Drug-induced oesophageal ulceration[2]

- Tetracycline, especially doxycycline, can cause painful ulceration in all age groups.
- Delayed passage of some drugs (due to pre-existing disorders) can cause local ulceration, even perforation (especially in elderly), e.g. iron tablets, slow-release potassium, aspirin, NSAIDs.
- The elderly are prone to the problem if they ingest drugs upon retiring to bed with insufficient liquid washdown.

Practice tips

- Although dysphagia is a common psychogenic symptom it must always be taken seriously and investigated.

- Mechanical dysphagia represents carcinoma until proved otherwise.
- Carcinoma of the oesophagus usually causes pain (odynophagia), wasting and regurgitation.
- Globus hystericus, an anxiety disorder, should not be confused with dysphagia. It is the subjective sensation of a lump or mass in the throat.
- Carcinoma-induced achalasia occurs with tumours at the gastro-oesophageal junction usually due to adenocarcinoma of the stomach.
- Severe oesophageal reflux predisposes to adenocarcinoma.
- Oesophageal strictures can be benign, usually secondary to chronic reflux oesophagitis, or due to malignancy.

References

1. Tally NJ, Martin CJ. *Clinical gastroenterology: A practical problem-based approach.* Sydney: MacLennan & Petty, 1996, 31–32.

2. Breen K. A practical approach to patients with dysphagia or pain on swallowing. Mod Med Aust, 1992; 3:50–56.

3. Cook I. Swallowing disorders. Current Therapeutics, 1996; 37:81–85.

45

Dyspnoea

In the year 1775 my opinion was asked concerning a family recipe for the cure of the dropsy. I was told that it had long been kept a secret by an old woman in Shropshire who had sometimes made cures after the more regular practitioners had failed—this medicine was composed of twenty or more different herbs and the active herb could be no other than the Foxglove.

William Withering (1741–99)
On the use of Foxglove (digitalis) in the
treatment of heart disease

Dyspnoea is the subjective sensation of breathlessness that is excessive for any given level of physical activity. It is a cardinal symptom affecting the cardiopulmonary system and can be very difficult to evaluate. Appropriate breathlessness following activities such as running to catch a bus or climbing several flights of stairs is not abnormal but may be excessive due to obesity or lack of fitness.

Key facts and checkpoints

- Determination of the underlying cause of dyspnoea in a given patient is absolutely essential for effective management.
- The main causes of dyspnoea are lung disease, heart disease, obesity and functional hyperventilation.[1]
- The most common cause of dyspnoea encountered in family practice is airflow obstruction, which is the basic abnormality seen in chronic asthma and chronic obstructive airways disease (COAD).[2]
- Wheezing, which is a continuous musical or whistling noise, is an indication of airflow obstruction.
- Some patients with asthma do not wheeze and some patients who wheeze do not have asthma.

- Other important pulmonary causes include restrictive disease such as fibrosis, collapse and pleural effusion.
- Dyspnoea is not inevitable in lung cancer but occurs in about 60% of cases.[3]
- Normal respiratory rate is 12–16 breaths/minute.

Terminology

It is important to emphasise that dyspnoea or breathlessness is a subjective sensation of the desire for increased respiratory effort and must be considered in relation to the patient's lifestyle and individual tolerance of discomfort. It also depends on the age, physical fitness and physical expectations of the person. Patients may complain of tightness in the chest and this must be differentiated from angina.

The New York Heart Association functional and therapeutic classification applied to dyspnoea:

Grade 1	No breathlessness
Grade 2	Breathlessness on severe exertion
Grade 3	Breathlessness on mild exertion
Grade 4	Breathlessness at rest

Orthopnoea. This is breathlessness lying down flat.

Paroxysmal nocturnal dyspnoea. This is inappropriate breathlessness causing waking from sleep.

Tachypnoea. This is an increased rate of breathing.

Hyperpnoea. This is an increased level of ventilation, e.g. during exertion.

Hyperventilation. This is overbreathing.

448

Table 45.1 *Comparison of distinguishing features between dyspnoea due to heart disease and to lung disease*

Lung disease	Heart disease
History of respiratory disease	History of hypertension, cardiac ischaemia or valvular heart disease
Slow development	Rapid development
Present at rest	Mainly on exertion
Productive cough common	Cough uncommon, and then 'dry'
Aggravated by respiratory infection	Usually unaffected by respiratory infection

Source: After Sandler[1]

Difference between heart and lung causes

The distinguishing features between dyspnoea due to heart disease and to lung disease are presented in Table 45.1. The history is a good indication, and a useful guideline is that dyspnoea at rest is typical of lung disease, especially asthma, while it tends to be present on effort with heart disease as well as with COAD.

Wheezing

Wheezing is any continuous musical expiratory noise heard with the stethoscope or otherwise. Wheeze includes stridor, which is an inspiratory wheeze.

Common causes of wheezing
Localised:
• partial bronchial obstruction
  — impacted foreign body
  — impacted mucus plugs
  — extrinsic compression

Generalised:
• asthma
• obstructive bronchitis

'Cardiac asthma' and bronchial asthma

The term 'cardiac asthma' is used to describe a wheezing sensation such as that experienced with paroxysmal nocturnal dyspnoea. Differentiating features are presented in Table 45.2.

A diagnostic approach

A summary of the diagnostic strategy model is presented in Table 45.3.

Probability diagnosis
The common causes of dyspnoea are lung disease, heart disease, obesity, anaemia (tissue hypoxia) and functional hyperventilation. More specifically, bronchial asthma, COAD, acute pulmonary infections and left heart failure (often insidious) are common individual causes.

Serious disorders not to be missed
Severe cardiovascular events such as acute heart failure which may be precipitated by myocardial infarction (may be silent especially in diabetics), a life-threatening arrhythmia, pulmonary embolism, dissecting aneurysm or a cardiomyopathy (such as viral myocarditis) require early diagnosis and corrective action. Recurrent pulmonary embolism may present a diagnostic problem. There may be a history of deep venous thrombosis, pregnancy, malignancy or taking the contraceptive pill.[4]

Table 45.2 *Comparison of distinguishing features between 'cardiac asthma' and bronchial asthma*

	Cardiac	Bronchial
Dyspnoea	Mainly inspiratory	Mainly expiratory
Cough	Follows dyspnoea	Precedes dyspnoea
Sputum	Pink and frothy	Thick and gelatinous
Relief	Standing up (by an open window) Intravenous diuretic/morphine	Coughing up sputum Bronchodilator
Lung signs	Mainly crackles	Mainly wheezes

Source: After Sandler[1]

Table 45.3 *Dyspnoea: diagnostic strategy model*

Q. *Probability diagnosis*
A. Bronchial asthma
    Bronchiolitis (children)
    Left heart failure
    COAD
    Obesity
    Lack of fitness

Q. *Serious disorders not to be missed*
A. Cardiovascular
    • acute heart failure, e.g. AMI
    • pulmonary embolism
    • pulmonary hypertension
    • dissecting aneurysm
    • cardiomyopathy
    • pericardial tamponade
    • anaphylaxis
    Neoplasia
    • bronchial carcinoma
    Severe infections
    • pneumonia
    • acute epiglottitis (children)
    Respiratory disorders
    • inhaled foreign body
    • upper airways obstruction
    • pneumothorax
    • atelectasis
    • pleural effusion
    • tuberculosis
    Neuromuscular disease
    • infective polyneuritis
    • poliomyelitis

Q. *Pitfalls (often missed)*
A. Interstitial lung disorder
    • fibrosing alveolitis
    • extrinsic allergic alveolitis
    Chemical pneumonitis
    Metabolic acidosis
    Radiotherapy
    Renal failure (uraemia)
    Multiple small pulmonary emboli

Q. *Seven masquerades checklist*
A. Depression   ✓
    Diabetes   ✓
    Drugs   ✓
    Anaemia   ✓
    Thyroid disease   ✓
    Spinal dysfunction   (ankylosing spondylitis)
    UTI   –

Q. *Is the patient trying to tell me something?*
A. Consider functional hyperventilation (anxiety and panic attacks).

Severe infections such as lobar pneumonia, tuberculosis and myocarditis must be considered. In children acute epiglottitis, croup, bronchiolitis, pneumonia and bronchitis are serious infections responsible for respiratory distress.

Primary carcinoma is an important consideration especially in dyspnoea of gradual onset.

Other malignant conditions to consider are metastases, lymphangitis carcinomatosis, lymphomas and pleural mesothelioma. Pleural effusion may be the mode of presentation of some of these serious disorders.

Pitfalls

Interstitial pulmonary disease can be a diagnostic dilemma because the physical signs and X-ray appearances can be minimal in the early stages despite the presence of significant dyspnoea. Allergic alveolitis, such as that caused by birds (e.g. hypersensitivity to their droppings), can be a pitfall. The diagnosis is easier if a known disease associated with pulmonary infiltration, such as sarcoidosis, is present. Measuring the diffusing capacity will help with diagnosis.

Pericardial tamponade may cause difficulty in diagnosis either with an acute onset, such as malignancy involving pericardium, or insidiously. The patient usually has a weak pulse with pulsus paradoxus, hypotension and a raised jugular venous pressure.

It is important to be careful not to attribute dyspnoea simply to obesity or lack of fitness when it could have a true organic disorder such as heart failure.

Seven masquerades checklist

Most of the masquerades have to be considered as underlying causes. Depression can be associated with dyspnoea, anaemia is an important cause of dyspnoea, thyrotoxicosis can present with dyspnoea, and diabetic ketoacidosis can cause rapid deep breathing.

Drugs must also be considered, especially as a cause of interstitial pulmonary fibrosis that presents with dyspnoea, cough and fever. Drugs that cause this disorder include several cytotoxic agents (especially bleomycin, cyclophosphamide, methotrexate), amiodarone, sulfasalazine, penicillamine, nitrofurantoin, gold salts and adrenergic nasal sprays.[3] Poisons that may cause hyperventilation are salicylate, methyl alcohol, theophylline overdosage and ethylene glycol. Anaemia must be considered especially in those at risk. Dyspnoea is unlikely to be caused solely by chronic anaemia unless the haemoglobin is less than 8 g/dL.[4] It is more likely to occur if another predisposing cause such as ischaemic heart disease is present.

Psychogenic considerations

Functional dyspnoea or hyperventilation is common. However, it is important to exclude organic causation such as asthma, drugs and thyrotoxicosis before settling with the psychogenic label and to reassure the patient strongly if there is no organic cause. Any uncomfortable sensation in the chest may be interpreted as dyspnoea by anxious patients. Depression, anxiety and panic attacks may be underlying the problem. Characteristic associated features of hyperventilation with anxiety include dizziness, faintness, palpitations, yawning, paraesthesia of the hands and legs, inability to take a deep breath or a sensation of smothering. These patients may exhibit sighing and irregular breathing on examination. In true psychogenic dyspnoea, chest X-rays and pulmonary function tests are normal but symptoms are often reproduced after 15–30 seconds of voluntary hyperventilation. It is important to remember that it may be present in a patient who has organic disease of a mild degree such as asthma.

The clinical approach
History

Special attention should be paid to evaluating exactly what the patient means by breathlessness or restriction of breathing. The analysis should then include provoking factors and associated symptoms with a view to differentiating between pulmonary causes such as asthma and COAD. Wheeze is often (but not always) present in asthma and chronic airflow obstruction. Most respiratory causes of dyspnoea also produce cough. The rate of development of dyspnoea gives an indication of the possible cause (Table 45.4).[5] The sudden onset of dyspnoea at rest is suggestive of pulmonary embolism or pneumothorax. Severe dyspnoea developing over one or two hours is most likely due to left heart failure or bronchial asthma. Bronchial asthma is usually easily distinguished from left heart failure by the history of previous attacks, by the absence of chest pain and the absence of cardiac murmurs. 'My breathing feels tight' indicates asthma. A complaint of 'suffocation or feeling smothered' or 'just not getting enough air' may be a pointer to functional dyspnoea.

The dyspnoea of asthma tends to occur at rest and at night, while that with chronic airflow obstruction occurs with exertion.

Table 45.4 *Typical causes of dyspnoea related to time of onset*

Sudden
- lung collapse
- inhaled foreign body
- spontaneous pneumothorax
- pulmonary embolism

Rapid (over a few hours)
- asthma
- diabetic ketoacidosis
- extrinsic allergic alveolitis
- high altitude
- left heart failure (acute pulmonary oedema)
- pericardial tamponade
- poisons

Over days or weeks
- congestive heart failure
- pleural effusion
- carcinoma of the bronchus/trachea

Over months or years
- COAD
- tuberculosis
- fibrosing alveolitis
- pneumoconiosis

Non-respiratory causes
- anaemia
- hyperthyroidism
- obesity

Examination

The routine findings from inspection, percussion and auscultation will determine whether the underlying lung disease is localised or generalised. The generalised findings for various disorders of the lungs are summarised in Table 45.5. Careful inspection is mandatory. The patient should be stripped to the waist and observed for factors such as cyanosis, clubbing, mental alertness, dyspnoea at rest, use of accessory muscles, rib retraction and any other abnormalities of the chest wall. A coarse tremor or flap of the outstretched hands indicates CO_2 intoxication.[5] To obtain maximum value from auscultation request the patient to open his or her mouth and take deep breaths. Adventitious sounds that are not audible during tidal breathing may then be heard. Wheezes are high-pitched continuous sounds heard either in expiration or inspiration, being more pronounced in expiration.

Crackles are short interrupted sounds heard mainly at the end of inspiration, resembling the crackling sound of hair being rubbed between the fingers near the ear. Fine crackles, previously referred to as crepitations, occur typically in

Table 45.5 *Comparison of examination findings for various lung disorders*

	Trachea	Chest wall movement	Percussion note	Breath sounds	Vocal fremitus	Adventitious sounds
Normal	Midline	Equal expansion	Resonant	Vesicular	Normal	Nil: ± few transient inspiratory basal crackles
Asthma	Midline	Decreased (bilateral)	Resonant	Vesicular— prolonged expiration	Normal or decreased	Expiratory wheezes
Emphysema	Midline	Decreased (bilateral)	Resonant to hyper-resonant	Vesicular— decreased	Decreased	Nil or the crackles and wheezes of chronic bronchitis
Consolidation, e.g. lobar pneumonia	Midline	Decreased on affected side	Dull	Bronchial	Increased	Fine late inspiratory crackles
Collapse: major bronchus	Towards affected side	Decreased (unilateral)	Dull	Absent or decreased	Absent or decreased	Nil
Collapse: peripheral bronchus	Towards affected side	Decreased (unilateral)	Dull	Bronchial	Increased	Coarse crackles
Pleural effusion > 500 mL	Towards opposite side (if massive)	Decreased (unilateral)	Stony dull	Absent or decreased	Absent or decreased	None
Pneumothorax (large)	Towards opposite side (if tension)	Decreased (unilateral)	Hyper-resonant	Absent or decreased	Absent or decreased	None
Fibrosis (generalised)	Midline	Decreased (bilateral)	Normal	Vesicular	Increased	Fine crackles
Bronchiectasis	Midline	Slight decrease	Resonant to dull	Bronchial	Normal or decreased	Coarse crackles ± localised wheeze

lobar pneumonia and diffuse interstitial fibrosis, and are not cleared by coughing. Medium crackles are typical of congestive cardiac failure, and coarse crackles indicate airway mucus and usually clear on coughing.

Investigations
The two most important initial investigations for respiratory disease are chest X-ray and respiratory function tests.

| Respiratory function tests |

These relatively simple tests provide considerable information.

Peak expiratory flow rate
The most practical instrument for office use to detect chronic airway obstruction due to asthma or chronic bronchitis is the mini peak flow meter, which measures peak expiratory flow rate (PEFR).

The interpretation of the tests, which vary according to sex, age and height, requires charts of predicted normal values. A chart for PEFR in normal adult subjects is presented in Appendix V. The value for a particular patient should be the best of three results.

Spirometry
The measurement of the forced vital capacity (FVC) and the forced expiratory volume in one second (FEV_1) will provide a very useful guide to the type of ventilatory deficit. Both the FVC and the FEV_1 are related to sex, age and height.

The FEV_1 expressed as a percentage of the FVC is an excellent measure of airflow limitation. In normal subjects it is approximately 70%.

Figure 45.1 summarises the relative values for these conditions.

Lung volume

Tidal volume and vital capacity can be measured by a simple spirometer but the total lung capacity and the residual volume are measured by the helium dilution method in a respiratory laboratory.

Gas transfer factor

This test measures the carbon monoxide uptake by a single breath analysis for whole lungs. In normal lungs the transfer factor is a true measure of the diffusing capacity of the lungs for oxygen and depends on the thickness of the alveolar-capillary membrane.[5] Gas transfer is usually reduced in patients with severe degrees of emphysema and fibrosis, anaemia and congestive cardiac failure.

Histamine challenge test

This test indicates the presence of airway or bronchial hyper-reactivity, which is a fundamental feature with asthma. The test should not be performed on those with poor lung function and only performed by a respiratory technician under medical supervision. The test is potentially dangerous.

Other investigations (to select from)

- haemoglobin, red cell indices and PCV
- white blood cell count, e.g. eosinophilia of asthma
- ESR
- arterial blood gas analysis
- oximetry: pulse oximeters monitor oxygen saturation
- cardiological investigations
  — ECG including exercise
  — echocardiography (technically difficult in emphysema)
  — nuclear gated blood pool scan to assess heart function
  — cardiac enzymes
- other medical imaging
  — high resolution computerised tomography
  — magnetic resonance imaging
  — ventilation and perfusion radionuclide scan (pulmonary embolism)
- bronchoscopy, especially fiberoptic bronchoscopy
- thoracocentesis and pleural biopsy
- open lung biopsy
- alpha$_1$-antitrypsin measurement

Dyspnoea in children

There are numerous causes of dyspnoea in children but the common causes are asthma, bronchiolitis and pulmonary infections. The important infections that can be fatal—croup, epiglottitis and myocarditis—must be kept in mind and intensively managed.

Sudden breathlessness or stridor may be due to an inhaled foreign body. Signs of lobar collapse may be present but physical examination may be of little help and a chest X-ray is essential.

Cardiovascular disorders including congenital heart disease can cause dyspnoea. Extra respiratory causes include anaemia, acidosis, aspiration, poisoning and hyperventilation.

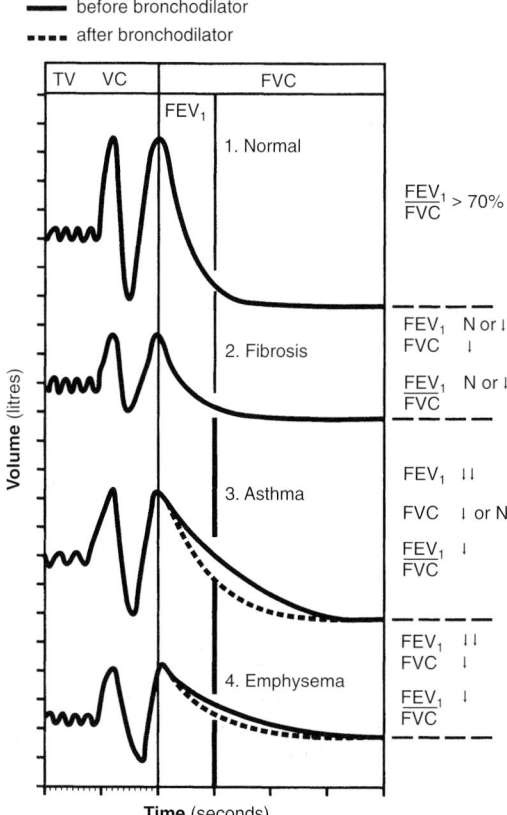

Fig. 45.1 *Spirometry patterns for respiratory disorders*

Dyspnoea in the elderly

Dyspnoea in the elderly is common and is caused usually by heart failure and COAD. The other associations with ageing such as carcinoma of the lungs, pulmonary fibrosis and drugs are relevant. The classic problem of the aged is acute heart failure that develops typically in the early morning hours. The acute brain syndrome is a common presentation of all these disorders.

Respiratory disease in the elderly

The respiratory system, like most other bodily systems, matures until about the age of 25 years and subsequently slowly loses efficiency due to a variety of factors such as disease, smoking, pollution and ageing. There is a decline in lung function and gas exchange and decreased ventilatory responses to hypoxia and hypercapnia.

Heart failure

Heart failure occurs when the heart is unable to maintain sufficient cardiac output to meet the demands of the body. Dyspnoea is a common early symptom as pulmonary congestion causes hypoxia (increased ventilation) and decreased compliance (increased work). The incidence of congestive cardiac failure (CCF) has been increasing steeply, partly due to the ageing population.

Symptoms

- increasing dyspnoea
  progressing to (in order)
- fatigue, especially exertional fatigue
- paroxysmal nocturnal dyspnoea
- weight change: gain or loss

It is convenient to divide heart failure into left and right heart failure but they rarely occur in isolation and often occur simultaneously. Right failure is invariably secondary to left failure. Furthermore some cardiologists stress the importance of differentiating between systolic and diastolic dysfunction. Both present in the same way clinically, and hence referral for cardiac studies to obtain measurement of the left ventricular function is required. This permits an accurate diagnosis and guide to treatment, and an accurate prognosis.

Signs

It is helpful clinically to differentiate between the signs of right and left heart failure.

Left heart failure

- tachycardia
- low volume pulse
- tachypnoea
- bilateral basal crackles
- gallop rhythm
- pleural effusion
- poor peripheral perfusion

Right heart failure

- elevated venous pressure
- peripheral/ankle oedema
- hepatomegaly
- ascites

Heart failure may cause pleural effusions, which are usually bilateral. The common causes of left heart failure are ischaemic heart disease (there is often a history of at least one AMI), hypertension, cardiomyopathy and valvular disease. Many acute cases are precipitated by an arrhythmia. Right heart failure is usually secondary to left ventricular failure but can occur in isolation when due to primary respiratory conditions (cor pulmonale).

Systolic versus diastolic heart failure

The classic heart failure is systolic failure due to an inadequate pumping action of the heart. However, diastolic heart failure, which is being recognised more widely, is due to impairment of left ventricular filling. It should be suspected in the elderly with hypertension and a normal heart size on chest X-ray who present with dyspnoea or pulmonary oedema.[5]

The oedema of heart failure

Peripheral oedema appears initially on the lower legs and is 'pitting'. To assess the presence of pitting, which is usually graded on a 4-point scale, press firmly yet gently with the thumb for 5–10 seconds over the dorsum of the feet, behind each medial malleolus and over the shins. With increasing severity of failure the oedema extends proximally to involve the abdomen. In the recumbent position it may only be apparent over the sacrum.[7]

Investigations

Investigations for heart failure include:

- renal function tests
- serum electrolytes
- full blood count
- chest X-ray
- ECG
- serum digoxin (if appropriate)
- echocardiogram
- nuclear gated blood pool scan

Left ventricular function should be measured by echocardiography or nuclear gated blood pool scanning to determine the ejection fraction, which is usually very low in heart failure.[6] Echocardiography also provides objective information on the size and function of the cardiac chambers. It helps to differentiate between systolic and diastolic failure.

Determining severity of heart failure

The severity of heart failure can be considered from three different perspectives: the severity of the symptoms, the degree of impairment of cardiac function and the severity of the congestive state. The severity of the symptoms or the degree of functional disability is usually described according to the New York Heart Association criteria (Table 45.6). The left ventricular ejection fraction provides an indication of cardiac function.

Table 45.6 *New York Heart Association classification of functional disability in heart failure*

Class I (asymptomatic)	No limitation; cardiac disease present, but ordinary physical activity; causes no symptoms such as fatigue, breathlessness or palpitation, or rapid forceful breathing.
Class II (mild)	Slight limitation; ordinary activity causes symptoms but patients comfortable at rest.
Class III (moderate)	Marked limitation; symptoms with less than ordinary physical activity although patients still comfortable at rest.
Class IV (severe)	Unable to carry on any activity without symptoms; may have symptoms at rest.

Treatment of heart failure

The treatment of heart failure includes appropriate patient education, determination and treatment of the cause, removal of any precipitating factors, general non-pharmaceutical measures and drug treatment.

Prevention of heart failure

The emphasis on prevention is very important since the onset of heart failure is generally associated with a very poor prognosis. Approximately 50% of patients with severe heart failure die within 2 years of diagnosis.[8]

The scope for prevention includes the following measures.[9]

- dietary advice, e.g. achievement of ideal weight
- emphasising the dangers of smoking and excessive alcohol
- control of hypertension
- control of other risk factors such as hypercholesterolaemia
- early detection and control of diabetes mellitus
- early intervention in myocardial infarction to preserve myocardial function, e.g. thrombolytic therapy
- secondary prevention after the occurrence of myocardial infarction, e.g. beta-blockers and aspirin
- appropriate timing of surgery or angioplasty for ischaemic or valvular heart disease

Treatment of causes and precipitating factors

Determination and treatment of the causes has been largely covered in the section on prevention. Precipitating factors that should be treated include:

- arrhythmias, e.g. atrial fibrillation
- electrolyte imbalance, especially hypokalaemia
- anaemia
- myocardial ischaemia, especially myocardial infarction
- dietary factors, e.g. malnutrition, excessive salt or alcohol
- adverse drug reactions, e.g. fluid retention with NSAIDs
- infection, e.g. bronchopneumonia, endocarditis
- thyrotoxicosis
- lack of compliance with therapy

General non-pharmacological management

- reduction in physical activity: rest if symptoms severe; moderate activity when symptoms are absent or mild
- weight reduction, if patient obese
- avoid smoking and alcohol
- salt restriction: advise no-added-salt diet (60–100 mmol/day)
- water restriction: water intake should be limited to 1.5L/day or less in patients with advanced heart failure, especially when the serum sodium falls below 130 mmol/day[8]
- fluid aspiration if a pleural effusion or pericardial effusion is present

Drug therapy of systolic heart failure

Any identified underlying factor should be treated. Initial drug therapy should consist of a diuretic. Loop diuretics such as frusemide are preferred for acute episodes although other diuretics may be used for long-term maintenance therapy.

Atrial fibrillation should be treated with digoxin. Vasodilators are widely used for heart failure and ACE inhibitors are currently the most favoured vasodilator.

Note: Monitor and maintain potassium level in all patients.

Initial therapy of heart failure

1. ACE inhibitor (start low, aim high)
   Dosage of ACE inhibitor: Commence with ¼ to ½ lowest recommended therapeutic dose and then adjust it for the individual patient by gradually increasing it to the maintenance dose (Table 45.7).
2. Add a Diuretic[9]
   - frusemide 20–40 mg (o) once or twice daily
     or
   - spironolactone 12.5–25 mg (o) daily (monitor K+)
     or
   - hydrochlorothiazide 25 mg (o) daily

Table 45.7 *Some ACE inhibitors in common usage*

	Initial daily dose	Usual maintenance daily dose
Captopril	6.25 mg (o) nocte	25 mg (o) tds
Enalapril	2.5 mg (o) nocte	10 mg (o) bd
Lisinopril	2.5 mg (o) nocte	5–20 mg (o) nocte
Perindopril	2 mg (o) nocte	4 mg (o) nocte
Ramipril	1.25 mg (o) nocte	5 mg (o) nocte

ACE inhibitors

- Many authorities now promote ACE inhibitors as the drugs of first choice because they correct neuroendocrine abnormalities and reduce cardiac load by their vasodilator action.
- In practice the usual initial treatment of heart failure is a diuretic plus an ACE inhibitor. This optimises response and improves diuretic safety.
- The first dose should be given at bedtime to prevent orthostatic hypotension.
- Potassium-sparing diuretics or supplements should be given with care with ACE inhibitors because of the danger of hyperkalaemia.
- Renal function and potassium levels should be monitored in all patients.

Some authorities are concerned about the over-reliance on diuretics and also about compliance as well as side effects. Once the diuretic effect has been achieved, diuretics may be withdrawn and fluid restriction advised. The ACE inhibitor is then used alone.

Heart failure (unresponsive to first-line therapy)

- frusemide 40–80 (o) bd
  +
- ACE inhibitor
  +
- carvedilol (a selective β blocker)
  +
- digoxin (if not already taking it)[9]
  - 0.5–0.75 mg (o) statim (depending on renal function)
  - then 0.5 mg (o) 4 hours later
  - then 0.5 mg the following day
  - then individualise maintenance

Severe heart failure[9]

Hospitalise with bed rest.

- ACE inhibitor
  +
- frusemide to max. 500 mg/day
  If poorly controlled,
- consider metolazone 2.5–5 mg (o) statim, repeated in 2–7 days according to diuretic response
  +
- digoxin
  +
- heparin (if confined to bed)
  If still uncontrolled consider other vasodilators:
  - isosorbide dinitrate and hydralazine
    or
  - spironolactone

Consider cardiac transplantation for appropriate patients with end-stage heart failure, e.g. patients under 50 with no other major disease.

A flow chart for the basic management of heart failure is presented in Figure 45.2.

Pitfalls in management

- The most common treatment error—excessive use of diuretics[5]
- Giving an excessive loading dose of ACE inhibitor
- Failure to correct remedial causes or precipitating factors
- Failure to measure left ventricular function
- Failure to monitor electrolytes and renal function

Acute severe heart failure

For the treatment of acute pulmonary oedema refer to page 1113 under emergency care.

Diastolic heart failure

The basic treatment is with inotropic agents such as calcium antagonists (verapamil or diltiazem) and beta-blockers. If possible avoid diuretics, digoxin, nitrates, nifedipine.

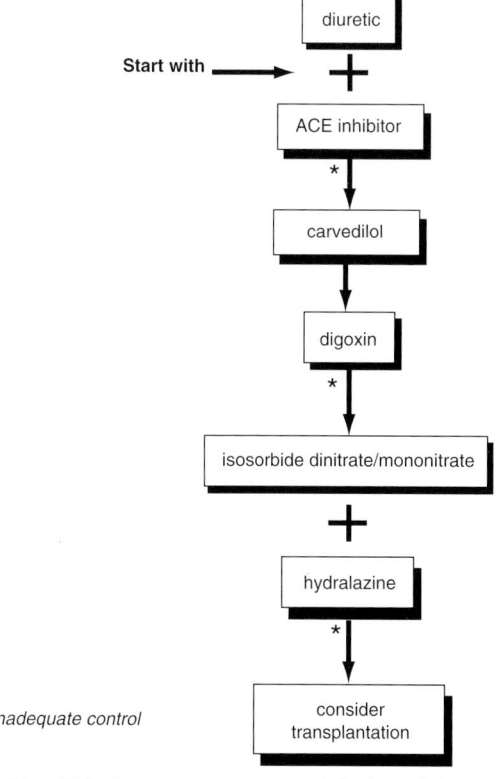

*Inadequate control

Fig. 45.2 *A management approach for heart failure*

Chronic obstructive airways disease

Chronic bronchitis and emphysema should be considered together as both these conditions usually coexist to some degree in each patient. An alternative, and preferable, term—chronic obstructive airway or pulmonary disease (COAD)—is used to cover chronic bronchitis and emphysema with chronic airflow limitation.

Chronic bronchitis. This is a clinical condition characterised by a productive cough on most days for at least 3 months of the year for at least 2 consecutive years in the absence of any other respiratory disease that could be responsible for such excessive sputum production (such as tuberculosis or bronchiectasis).

Emphysema. This is defined in pathological rather than clinical terms, as permanent dilatation and destruction of lung tissue distal to the terminal bronchioles.

Chronic airflow limitation. This is a physiological process measured as impairment of forced expiratory flow and is the major cause of dyspnoea in these patients.

Cigarette smoking is undoubtedly the major cause of both chronic bronchitis and emphysema although only 10–15% of smokers develop the diseases.[11]

Factors in causation

- cigarette smoking
- air pollution
- airway infection
- familial factors
- alpha$_1$-antitrypsin deficiency (emphysema)

Clinical features

Symptoms

- onset in 5th or 6th decade
- excessive cough
- sputum production (chronic bronchitis)
- dyspnoea (chronic airflow limitation)
- wheeze (chronic bronchitis)
- susceptibility to colds

Signs

The signs vary according to the nature of the disease and the presence of infection. Signs may be completely absent in the early stages of emphysema and there may be wheezing only with chronic bronchitis and dyspnoea with chronic airflow limitation.

Signs may include:

• tachypnoea
• reduced chest expansion
• hyperinflated lungs
• hyper-resonant percussion
• diminished breath sounds
• 'pink puffer'—always breathless
• 'blue bloater'—oedematous and central cyanosis
• signs of respiratory failure
• signs of cor pulmonale

The diagnosis is usually clinical with a history of increasing dyspnoea and sputum production in a lifetime smoker. It is unwise to make a diagnosis of chronic bronchitis and emphysema in the absence of cigarette smoking unless there is a family history suggestive of alpha$_1$-antitrypsin deficiency.[6]

Investigations

Chest X-ray. This can be normal (even with advanced disease) but characteristic changes occur late in disease.

Pulmonary function tests

• peak expiratory flow rate—low with minimal response to bronchodilator
• ratio FEV$_1$/FVC—reduced with minimal response to bronchodilator
• gas transfer coefficient of CO is low if significant emphysema

Blood gases

• may be normal
• PaCO$_2$ ↑; PaO$_2$ ↓ (advanced disease)

ECG. This may show evidence of cor pulmonale. Haemoglobin and PCV may be raised.

Management

Advice to the patient

• If you smoke, you must stop (persuading the patient to stop smoking is the key to management). Nicotine replacement therapy should be considered.
• Avoid places with polluted air and other irritants, such as smoke, paint fumes and fine dust.
• Go for walks in clean, fresh air.
• A warm dry climate is preferable to a cold damp place (if prone to infections).
• Get adequate rest.
• Avoid contact with people who have colds or flu.

Physiotherapy

Refer to a physiotherapist for chest physiotherapy, breathing exercises and an aerobic physical exercise program.

Drug therapy

Consider the use of bronchodilators, e.g. inhaled β$_2$ agonists and ipratropium bromide and corticosteroids, because of associated (often unsuspected) asthma. A carefully monitored trial of these drugs with a peak flow meter is recommended.

Bronchodilators.[12,13] A bronchodilator, either a β$_2$-adrenoreceptor agonist or ipratropium bromide, should be used in patients who have a proven response to bronchodilator therapy (by respiratory function tests). These drugs can be trialled for efficacy in individual patients commenced with metered dose inhalers (MDI). For patients unable to use an MDI or a spacer, a nebuliser should be used with ipratropium bromide, salbutamol or terbutaline. In those who have failed to respond adequately to inhaled agents, oral theophylline may help, starting with sustained release 200–250 mg (o) bd and then increasing to 300–400 mg (o) bd as tolerated. Plasma concentration should be assayed at higher doses and maintained at 50–110 µmol/L.

Corticosteroids. Approximately one-third of patients with COAD improve with either inhaled or oral corticosteroids.[13] It is recommended that patients with COAD be given a trial of inhaled corticosteroids, e.g. 1500 µg beclomethasone daily, and closely monitored with daily peak flow and 2 weekly FEV$_1$ measurements. After 6 weeks of evaluation, only those who clearly benefit should continue.[12]

Antibiotics. The prompt use of antibiotics for acute episodes of infection is important to help prevent further lung damage. Patients should be instructed to commence antibiotics (a supply should be kept at home) as soon as they develop an infection and notice their increased sputum turn yellow or green together with increased cough and dyspnoea.

The antibiotics of choice are:[13]

• amoxycillin 500 mg (o) tds
    or
• cefaclor 500 mg (o) tds   } for 5–12 days
    or
• doxycycline 100 mg (o) daily

A sputum micro and culture may help to identify those patients with organisms resistant to antibiotics.

Other treatment

- Annual influenza vaccine should be considered.
- Consider home oxygen therapy for advanced cases with persistent hypoxia at rest.
- Surgery for appropriate patients: lung volume reduction[16] or lung transplantation.

Acute exacerbation[13]

Treat patients with acute exacerbation with nebulised salbutamol or terbutaline together with ipratropium bromide. Administer oxygen (4–6 L/min) if the patient is hypoxic. If the patient is seriously ill and unable to tolerate oral medication (prednisolone 50 mg daily) use intravenous corticosteroids (dexamethasone 4 mg IV 6 hourly or hydrocortisone 100 mg IV 6 hourly).

A decision about giving antibiotics will have to be made on clinical judgment including past experience.

Interstitial lung diseases

Interstitial lung diseases comprise a group of disorders that have the common features of inflammation and fibrosis of the interalveolar septum, representing a non-specific reaction of the lung to injury of various causes.[11]

Causes of pulmonary infiltration include:

- sarcoidosis
- cryptogenic fibrosing alveolitis (interstitial pulmonary fibrosis)
- extrinsic allergic alveolitis (hypersensitivity pneumonitis)
- drug-induced
- lymphangitis carcinomatosis
- acute pulmonary oedema

Common clinical features
- dyspnoea and dry cough (insidious onset)
- fine inspiratory crackles at lung base
- finger clubbing
- RFTs: restrictive ventilatory deficit
        decrease in gas transfer factor
- characteristic X-ray changes

High resolution CT scanning has been a major advance in diagnosis.

Sarcoidosis

Sarcoidosis is a multisystemic disorder of unknown aetiology which is characterised by non-caseating granulomatous inflammation that involves the lung in about 90% of affected patients. A characteristic feature is bilateral hilar lymphadenopathy, which is often symptomless and detected on routine CXR. Radiological lung involvement can be associated with or occur independently of hilar lymphadenopathy.

Clinical features:
- may be asymptomatic (one-third)
- onset usually 3rd or 4th decade (but any age)
- bilateral hilar lymphadenopathy (on CXR)
- cough
- fever, malaise, arthralgia
- erythema nodosum
- ocular lesions, e.g. anterior uveitis
- other multiple organ lesions (uncommon)
- overall mortality 2–5%

Erythema nodosum with acute fever, malaise and arthralgia in a young adult female is diagnostic of sarcoidosis.

Diagnosis

Histological evidence from biopsy specimen, usually transbronchial biopsy (essential if an alternative diagnosis, e.g. lymphoma, cannot be excluded) or skin biopsy in cases of erythema nodosum.

Supporting evidence:
- elevated serum ACE (non-specific)
- PFTs: restrictive pattern; impaired gas transfusion in advanced cases.
- ±ve Kveim test (not recommended these days)

Treatment

Sarcoidosis may resolve spontaneously (hilar lymphadenopathy without lung involvement does not require treatment).

Indications for treatment with corticosteroids:
- no spontaneous improvement after 6 months
- symptomatic pulmonary lesions
- eye, CNS and other systems involvement
- hypercalcaemia, hypercalcuria
- erythema nodosum with arthralgia
- persistent cough

Corticosteroid treatment
- Prednisolone 30 mg daily for 4–6 weeks, then reduce to lowest dose that maintains

improvement.[6] If there is no response, taper the dose to zero. If there is a response, taper the dose to 10–15 mg (o) daily as a maintenance dose for 6–12 months.[14]

- Prednisolone 20–30 mg for 2 weeks for erythema nodosum of sarcoidosis.

Fibrosing alveolitis

Cryptogenic fibrosing alveolitis (idiopathic pulmonary fibrosis) is the most common diagnosis among patients presenting with interstitial lung disease.

Patients usually present in the 5th to 7th decade with the clinical features as outlined under interstitial lung diseases. CXR abnormalities are variable but include bilateral diffuse nodular or reticulonodular shadowing favouring the lung bases. Open lung biopsy may be needed for diagnosis and staging. The usual treatment is high doses of oral corticosteroids with or without cyclophosphamide.[14]

Extrinsic allergic alveolitis

This disease is characterised by a widespread diffuse inflammatory reaction in both the small airways of the lung and alveoli, due to the inhalation of allergens, which are usually spores of micro-organisms such as *Thermophilic actinomycetes* in 'farmer's lung' or (more commonly) avian proteins from droppings or feathers in 'bird fancier's lung'. Occupational causes of extrinsic alveolitis have been described by Molina[15] (Table 45.8). Illness may present as acute or subacute episodes of pyrexia, chills and malaise with dyspnoea and a peripheral neutrophilia several hours after exposure.[14] Management is based on prevention, namely avoiding exposure to allergens or wearing protective fine-mesh masks. Prednisolone can be used (with caution) to control acute symptoms. It should be pointed out that this allergic disease is different from the infection psittacosis.

Drug-induced interstitial lung disease[14]

Drugs are an important cause of this disorder and have three main effects:

- *Alveolitis with or without pulmonary fibrosis.* This is mainly due to cytotoxic drugs, nitrofurantoin and amiodarone. The drug should be removed and consideration given to prescribing prednisolone 50–100 mg (o) daily.
- *Eosinophilic reactions.* This is presumably an immunological reaction, which may present as

Table 45.8 *Various causes of extrinsic allergic alveolitis*

Occupation/disease	Source of antigen
Farmer's lung	Mouldy hay, grain and straw
Bagassosis	Mouldy sugar cane fibre (bagasse)
Bird fancier's lung	Dropping dust, e.g. pigeons, budgerigars 'bloom' on feathers
Mushroom workers	Mushroom compost
Cheese washer's lung	Moulds or mites on cheese
Wheat weevil lung	Infested wheat flour (insect)
Ventilator pneumonitis	Humidified hot air system Air-conditioning system
Wood pulp worker's disease	Contaminated wood dust
Detergent worker's disease	Proteolytic enzymes
Suberosis	Mouldy cork bark
Rat handler's lung	Rat urine and serum
Malt worker's lung	Mouldy barley
Coffee worker's lung	Coffee dust
Sisal worker's lung	Sisal dust
Sericultural workers	Silkworms
Furrier's lung	Fur dust
Sausage workers	Dust
Prawn workers	Prawn fumes

wheezing, dyspnoea, a maculopapular rash and pyrexia. The many implicated drugs include various antibiotics, NSAIDs, cytotoxic agents, major tranquillisers and antidepressants, and antiepileptics. Treatment is drug removal and a short course of prednisolone 20–40 mg (o) daily for 2 weeks.

- *Acute pulmonary oedema.* This is rare and has been reported to occur with opioids, aspirin, hydrochlorothiazide, β_2-adrenoceptor agonists (given IV to suppress premature labour) and cytotoxics.

Occupational pulmonary disease

Various types of acute and chronic pulmonary diseases are related to exposure to noxious substances such as dusts, gases and vapours in the workplace. GPs have a crucial role in the identification of the possible work-relatedness of lung disease.

Disorders due to chemical agents include:
- obstructive airways disorders, e.g. occupational asthma, acute bronchitis, (chronic) industrial bronchitis, byssinosis (asthma-like condition due to cotton dust)
- extrinsic allergic alveolitis
- pulmonary fibrosis (pneumoconiosis) due to mineral dust
- lung cancer due to industrial agents such as asbestos, various hydrocarbons
- pleural diseases, usually associated with asbestosis

Pneumoconiosis

The term *pneumoconiosis* refers to the accumulation of dust in the lungs and the reaction of tissue to its presence, namely chronic fibrosis. The main cause worldwide is inhalation of coal dust, a specific severe variety being progressive massive fibrosis (complicated coal worker's pneumoconiosis) in which the patient suffers severe dyspnoea of effort and cough often productive of black sputum. Table 45.9 summarises the important causes.

Of particular concern are diseases caused by inhalation of fibres of asbestos, which is a mixture of silicates of iron, magnesium, cadmium, nickel and aluminium. The diseases include asbestosis, diffuse pleural thickening, pleural plaques, mesothelioma and increased bronchial carcinoma in smokers. It usually takes 20 to 40 years from exposure for mesothelioma

Table 45.9 *Selected pneumoconioses*

Fibrotic lung disease	Agent	Typical occupations
Coal dust		
Coal worker's pneumoconiosis	Coal dust	• Coal mining
Metal dust		
Siderosis	Metallic iron or iron oxide	• Mining • Welding • Foundry work
Inorganic dusts		
Silicosis	Silica (silicon dioxide)	• Quarrying • Rock mining • Stone cutting • Sandblasting
Silicate dusts		
Asbestosis	Asbestos	• Mining • Shipbuilding • Insulation • Power stations • Wharf labouring

to develop, while bronchial carcinoma is caused by the synergistic effects of asbestosis and cigarette smoking.

Bronchial carcinoma

Dyspnoea is associated with about 60% of cases of lung cancer.[3] It is not a common early symptom unless bronchial occlusion causes extrinsic collapse. In advanced cancer, whether primary or secondary, direct spread or metastases may cause dyspnoea. Other factors include pleural effusion, lobar collapse, metastatic infiltration, upper airway obstruction due to SVC obstruction and lymphangitis carcinomatosis. A special problem arises with coexisting chronic bronchitis and emphysema.

When to refer

- Patients with acute onset of severe dyspnoea
- All patients with heart failure resistant to initial therapy or where the diagnosis is in doubt
- Patients with pulmonary disease of uncertain aetiology, especially those requiring respiratory function tests
- Those in whom carcinoma of the lung is suspected

Practice tips

- Remember to order a chest X-ray and pulmonary function tests in all doubtful cases of dyspnoea.
- All heart diseases have dyspnoea as a common early symptom.
- Increasing dyspnoea on exertion may be the earliest symptom of incipient heart failure.
- Several drugs can produce a wide variety of respiratory disorders, particularly pulmonary fibrosis and pulmonary eosinophilia. Amiodarone and cytotoxic drugs, especially bleomycin, are the main causes.
- Dyspnoea in the presence of lung cancer may be caused by many factors such as pleural effusion, lobar collapse, upper airway obstruction and lymphangitis carcinomatosis.
- The abrupt onset of severe dyspnoea suggests pneumothorax or pulmonary embolism.
- If a patient develops a relapse of dyspnoea while on digoxin therapy, consider the real possibility of digoxin toxicity and/or electrolyte abnormalities leading to left heart failure.

- Recurrent attacks of sudden dyspnoea, especially waking the patient at night, are suggestive of asthma or left heart failure.
- Causes of hyperventilation include drugs, asthma, thyrotoxicosis and panic attacks/anxiety.

References

1. Sandler G. *Common medical problems*. London: ADIS Press, 1984, 31–56.

2. Cormack J, Marinker M, Morrell D. *Practice: A handbook of primary health care*. London: Kluwer-Harrap Handbooks, 1980; 3:29:3.

3. Walsh TD. *Symptom control*. Boston: Blackwell Scientific Publications, 1989, 157–164.

4. Beck ER, Francis JL, Souhami RL. *Tutorials in differential diagnosis* (3rd edn). Edinburgh: Churchill Livingstone, 1993, 37.

5. Kelly DT. Cardiac failure. In: MIMS Disease Index (2nd edn). Sydney: IMS Publishing, 1996, 97–99.

6. Kumer PJ, Clark ML. *Clinical medicine* (2nd edn). London: Bailliere Tindall, 1990, 637–690.

7. Davis A, Bolin T, Ham J. *Symptom analysis and physical diagnosis* (2nd edn). Sydney: Pergamon Press, 1990, 173.

8. Kumer PJ, Clark ML. *Clinical medicine* (2nd edn). London: Bailliere Tindall, 1990, 562.

9. Mashford ML. *Cardiovascular drug guidelines* (2nd edn). Melbourne: Victorian Medical Postgraduate Foundation, 1995–96, 129–139.

10. DiBianco R. A practical approach to the management of heart failure. Aust Fam Physician, 1993; 22:764–781.

11. Tierney LM et al. *Current medical diagnosis and treatment* (35th edn). Stamford: Appleton and Lange, 1996, 228–268.

12. Seale JP. Chronic obstructive pulmonary disease. In: MIMS Disease Index (2nd edn). Sydney: IMS Publishing, 1996, 109–111.

13. Naismith NW (Chairman). *Respiratory drug guidelines*. Melbourne: Victorian Medical Postgraduate Foundation, 1994–95, 72–77.

14. Naismith NW (Chairman). *Respiratory drug guidelines*. Melbourne: Victorian Medical Postgraduate Foundation, 1994–95, 109–114.

15. Molina C. Occupational extrinsic allergic alveolitis. In: Pepys J, ed. *Clinics in immunology and allergy*. London: WB Saunders, 1984, 173–190.

16. Snell GI, Solin P, Chin W. Lung volume reduction surgery for emphysema. Med J Aust, 1997; 167:529–532.

46
The painful ear

—

Pain in the ear (otalgia) is a common symptom in general practice. It affects all ages, but is most prevalent in children, where otitis media is the commonest cause. Ear pain may be caused by disorders of the ear or may arise from other structures, and in many instances the precise diagnosis is difficult to make. Important causes of ear pain are summarised in Table 46.1.[1]

A patient with a painful ear often requests urgent attention, and calls in the middle of the night from anxious parents of a screaming child are commonplace. Infants may present with nothing except malaise, vomiting or screaming attacks.

Key facts and checkpoints

- Of patients presenting with earache, 77% can be expected to have acute otitis media and 12% otitis externa.[2]
- Approximately 1 of every 25 patients in general practice will present with an earache.
- Two-thirds of children will sustain at least one episode of otitis media by their second birthday; 1 in 7 children will have had more than six episodes by this age.[3]
- Otitis media is unlikely to be present if the tympanic membrane is mobile. Pneumatic otoscopy greatly assists diagnosis since the most valuable sign of otitis media is absent or diminished motility of the tympanic membrane (TM).

Table 46.1 *Causes of ear pain*

1. **Ear**
   External ear
   Perichondritis
   Otitis externa:
   - *Candida albicans*
   - *Aspergillus nigra*
   - *Pseudomonas pyocyaneus*
   - *Staphylococcus aureus*
   Furunculosis
   Trauma
   Neoplasia
   Herpes zoster (Ramsay Hunt syndrome)
   Viral myringitis
   Wax-impacted

   Middle ear
   Acute eustachian insufficiency
   Barotrauma
   Acute otitis media
   Chronic otitis media and cholesteatoma
   Acute mastoiditis

2. **Periotic cause**
   Dental disorders
   Upper cervical spinal dysfunction
   Temporomandibular joint arthralgia
   Parotitis
   Temporal arteritis
   Lymph node inflammation

   Other referred causes
   Pharyngeal disorders
   Tonsillitis
   Glossopharyngeal neuralgia

- Bullous myringitis, which causes haemorrhagic blistering of the eardrum or external ear canal, is an uncommon cause of severe pain. It is caused by a virus, probably influenza.[4]
- The antibiotic of first choice for acute otitis media (children and adults) is amoxycillin.
- Otitis externa can be distinguished from otitis media by pain on movement of the pinna.

463

A diagnostic approach

Using the safe diagnostic approach model (Table 46.2) the five self-posed questions can be answered as follows.

Table 46.2 *The painful ear: diagnostic strategy model*

Q. *Probability diagnosis*
A. Otitis media (viral or bacterial)
   Otitis externa
   TMJ arthralgia
   Eustachian dysfunction

Q. *Serious disorders not to be missed*
A. Neoplasia of external ear
   Carcinoma of other sites, e.g. tongue, throat
   Herpes zoster (Ramsay Hunt syndrome)
   Acute mastoiditis
   Cholesteatoma

Q. *Pitfalls (often missed)*
A. Foreign bodies in ear
   Hard ear wax
   Barotrauma
   Dental causes
   Referred pain: neck, throat
   Unerupted wisdom tooth and other dental causes
   TMJ arthralgia
   Facial neuralgias, esp. glossopharyngeal
   Post tonsillectomy
   • from the wound
   • from TMJ due to mouth gag

Q. *Seven masquerades checklist*
A. Depression   √
   Diabetes   –
   Drugs   –
   Anaemia   –
   Thyroid disease   –
   Urinary infection   –
   Spinal dysfunction   √

Q. *Is the patient trying to tell me something?*
A. Unlikely, but always possible with pain.
   More likely in children. Consider factitious pain.

Probability diagnosis

The commonest cause of ear pain is acute otitis media. Chronic otitis media and otitis externa are also common. In the tropics, 'tropical ear' due to acute bacterial otitis is a particular problem. TMJ arthralgia, which may be acute or chronic, is also common and must be considered, especially when otitis media and otitis externa are excluded.

Serious disorders not to be missed

As always, it is important not to overlook malignant diseases, especially the obscure ones such as carcinoma of the tongue, palate or tonsils that cause referred pain.

Locally destructive cholesteatoma associated with chronic otitis media must be searched for. It signifies the 'unsafe' ear (Fig. 46.1) that must be distinguished from the so-called 'safe' ear (Fig. 46.2).

Herpes zoster should be considered, especially if it does not erupt on the pinna and is confined to the ear canal (usually the posterior wall), and especially in the older person.

Pitfalls

The medical aphorism 'more things are missed by not looking than by not knowing' applies particularly to the painful ear—good illumination and focusing the auroscope are mandatory. Particular attention should be paid to the external canal—look for hard wax, otitis externa, furuncles and foreign objects such as insects.

It may not be possible to visualise the tympanic membrane; so it is important to clean the canal to permit this (if possible, on the first visit). Otitis media may coexist with otitis externa. Barotrauma should be considered, especially if pain follows air travel or diving.

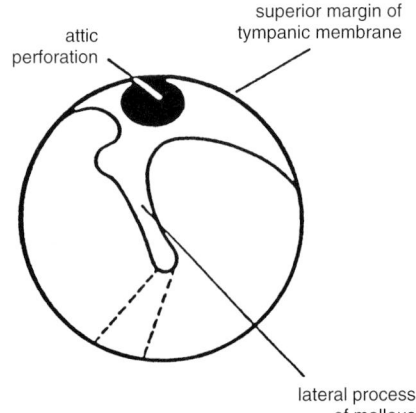

Fig. 46.1 *Infected ear: unsafe perforation*

Fig. 46.2 *Infected ear: safe perforation*

General pitfalls
- Failing to visualise the tympanic membrane before diagnosis and treatment
- Not checking out possible referral sites such as the oropharynx and teeth
- Overlooking common musculoskeletal causes such as TMJ arthralgia and cervical spondylosis
- Failing to recognise the unsafe ear

Seven masquerades checklist
Of the conditions in the checklist, depression and dysfunction of the upper cervical spine have to be considered. Depressive illnesses should be considered in any patient complaining of chronic pain.

Disorders of the upper cervical spine are a commonly overlooked cause of periotic pain. Pain from the C2 and C3 levels are referred to the posterior region of the ear.

Psychogenic considerations
Such factors are unlikely, unless the pain causes discomfort in the periotic region, which is likely to be magnified by a depressive state.

The clinical approach
History
In assessing the painful ear the relevant features are:
- site of pain and radiation
- details of the onset of pain
- nature of the pain
- aggravating or relieving factors, especially swimming
- associated features such as deafness, discharge, vertigo, tinnitus and irritation of the external ear, sore throat

Agonising pain may be caused by perichondritis or furunculosis of the external ear and by the rare problem of herpes zoster (Ramsay Hunt syndrome). Movement of the pinna markedly increases the pain of acute otitis externa and perichondritis, and movement of the jaw usually causes an exacerbation of temporomandibular joint (TMJ) arthralgia or severe otitis externa.

Key questions (especially children)
- Where is the pain?
- Is it in the ear, behind or below it?
- Is it in one ear or both ears?
- Have you noticed any other symptoms such as sore throat, fever or vomiting?
- Has anyone hit you over the ear?
- Has there been a discharge from the ear?
- Have you noticed any deafness?
- Are you allergic to penicillin?
- Have you been swimming in a spa, and where?
- Have you been in an aeroplane?

Physical examination
The patient's general state and behaviour is observed during the history taking. Sudden, jabbing pain may indicate neuralgia, particularly glossopharyngeal neuralgia or a severe infection. The external ear is carefully inspected and the pinna manipulated to determine any tenderness.

Palpate the face and neck and include the parotid glands, regional lymph nodes and the skin. Inspect the TMJs—tenderness from dysfunction typically lies immediately in front of the external auditory meatus. Palpate the TMJ over the lateral aspect at the joint disc. Ask the patient to open the mouth fully when tenderness is maximal. The TMJ can be palpated posteriorly by inserting the little finger into the external canal.

Inspect both ear canals and tympanic membranes with the auroscope, using the largest earpiece that comfortably fits into the canal. Better visualisation of the tympanic membrane (TM) can be achieved by pulling the pinna back in young children and up and back in older children. Impacted wax may not explain the otalgia. If herpes zoster involves the facial nerve, vesicles may be noted in and around the external auditory meatus (notably the posterior wall).

If the diagnosis is still doubtful look for causes of referred pain; inspect the cervical spine, the nose and postnasal space and the mouth, including the teeth, pharynx and larynx.

Pharyngeal and mandibular causes of periotic pain are summarised in Figures 46.3 and 46.4.

Inspect sites supplied by the nerves V2, IX, X, XI, C1, C2 and C3 to exclude other causes of referred pain.

Investigations
Investigations are seldom necessary. Hearing tests are essential, especially for children. Simple tests such as speech discrimination, hair rubbing and tuning fork tests can be used. Otherwise audiometry can be used. Audiometry combined with tympanometry and physical measurement of the volume of the ear canal can be performed in children, irrespective of age.

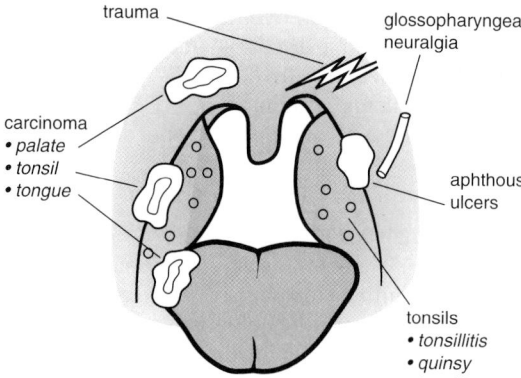

Fig 46.3 *Pharangeal causes of otalgia*
COURTESY OF B. BLACK

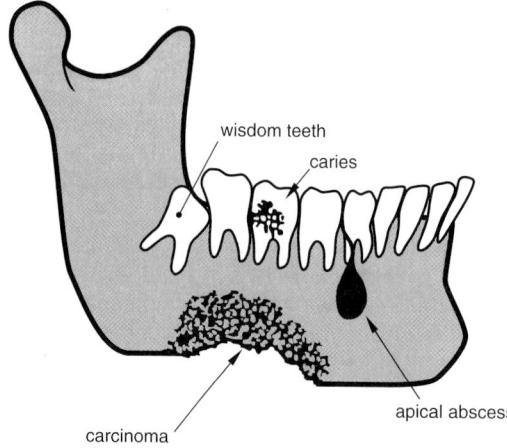

Fig 46.4 *Mandibular causes of otalgia*
COURTESY OF B. BLACK

Swabs from discharge, especially to determine bacterial causes such as *Staphylococcus aureus* or *Pseudomonas pyocyaneus* infection, may be necessary. However swabs are of no value if the TM is intact.

Radiology and computerised tomography may be indicated for special conditions such as a suspected extraotic malignancy.

Ear pain in children

Important causes of primary otalgia in children include otitis media, otitis externa, external canal furuncle or abscess, chronic eczema with fissuring of the auricle, impacted wax, foreign body, barotrauma, perichondritis, mastoiditis and bullous myringitis. Secondary otalgia includes pharyngeal lesions, dental problems, gingivostomatitis, mumps and postauricular lymphadenopathy. Peritonsillar abscess (quinsy) may cause ear pain.

Foreign bodies

Foreign bodies are frequently inserted into the ear canal. They can usually be syringed out or lifted with thin forceps. Various improvised methods can be used to remove foreign bodies (FB) in co-operative children. These include a probe to roll out FB or a rubber catheter used as a form of suction or otherwise a fine sucker.[6]

Probe method

This requires good vision using a head mirror or head light and a thin probe. The probe is inserted under and just beyond the FB. Lever it in such a way that the tip of the probe 'rolls' the foreign body out of the obstructed passage (Figs 46.5a,b).

Rubber catheter suction method

The only equipment required for this relatively simple and painless method is a straight rubber catheter (large type) and perhaps a suction pump. The end of the catheter is cut at right

(a)

(b)

Figs. 46.5 *Probe method of removing a foreign body:* **(a)** *the tip of the probe is lifted by depressing the outer end of the probe;* **(b)** *continued gentle levering 'rolls' the foreign body out*

angles, a thin smear of petroleum jelly is applied to the rim and this end is applied to the FB (Figs 46.6a,b). Suction is applied either orally or by a pump. Gentle pump suction is preferred but it is advisable to pinch closed the suction catheter until close to the FB as the hissing noise may frighten the child.

Insects in the ear

Live insects should be immobilised by first instilling Aquaear drops or olive oil, and then syringing the ear with warm water (Figs 46.7a,b). Dead flies that have originally been attracted to pus are best removed by suction.

Note: If simple methods such as syringing fail to dislodge the FB it is important to refer for examination and removal under microscopic vision. Syringing should not be performed if there is a possibility of the FB perforating the tympanic membrane (TM).

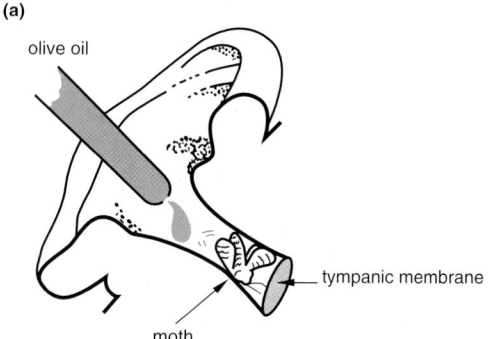

Figs. 46.6 *Extracting the foreign body using a rubber catheter:* **(a)** *catheter cut straight across near its extremity;* **(b)** *application of suction (orally or by pump)*

Otitis media in children

Otitis media is very common in children and is the most common reason a child is brought in for medical attention. Persistent middle ear effusions may follow and affect the language and cognitive development of young children.

Features

- Two peaks of incidence: 6–12 months of age and school entry.
- Seasonal incidence coincides with URTIs.
- Bacteria cause two-thirds of cases.[6]
- The two commonest organisms are *Streptococcus pneumoniae* and *Haemophilus influenzae.*
- Fever, irritability, otalgia and otorrhoea may be present.
- The main symptoms in older children are increasing earache and hearing loss.
- Pulling at the ears is a common sign in infants.
- Removal of wax is necessary in about 30% to visualise the TM.

Visualisation of the tympanic membrane

Use the largest ear speculum that will comfortably fit in the child's ear. A good technique to enable the examination of the ears (also nose and throat) in a reluctant child is where the child is held against the parent's chest while the parent's arm embraces the child's arm and trunk.

Note the following features of the TM: translucency, colour, position and motility.

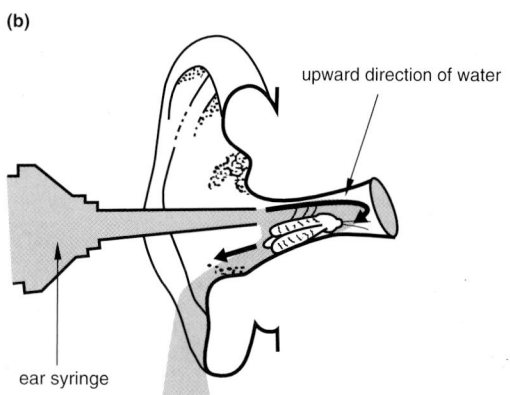

Figs. 46.7 *Insect in the ear:* **(a)** *first aid;* **(b)** *office procedure*

Treatment

Many children with viral URTIs have mild reddening or dullness of the eardrum and antibiotics are not warranted.[7] In contrast, where the eardrum is red or yellow and bulging, with loss of anatomical landmarks, antibiotic therapy is indicated.

The antibiotic of choice is amoxycillin 40 mg/kg/day (maximum 1.5 g/day) orally in three divided doses for 10 days.

If β-lactamase producing bacteria are suspected or documented, or initial treatment fails, use:

- cefaclor 10 mg/kg/day (maximum 750 mg/day) orally in three divided doses for 10 days (cefaclor is second choice irrespective of cause)

or

- (if resistance to amoxycillin is suspected or proven) amoxycillin/potassium clavulanate

With appropriate treatment most children with acute otitis media are significantly improved within 48 hours. Parents should be encouraged to contact their doctor if no improvement occurs within 72 hours. This problem is usually due to a resistant organism or suppuration. The patient should be re-evaluated at 10 days.

It is of interest that some practitioners refer to the 'Pollyanna' phenomenon when treating otitis media; that is, all antibiotics seem to work!

Symptomatic treatment

Rest the patient in a warm room with adequate humidity. Use analgesics such as paracetamol (acetaminophen) in high dosage. Although the use of antihistamines and decongestants has not been verified scientifically, the author has found nasal decongestants (as oxymetazoline nasal drops or sprays) effective in distressed children with an associated URTI. Otherwise, avoid antihistamines and decongestants.

Follow-up: adequate follow-up with hearing assessment is mandatory.

Complications

- *Middle ear effusion.* 70% of children will have an effusion present 2 weeks from the time of diagnosis, 40% at 4 weeks, with 10% having persistent effusions for 3 months or more. If the effusion is still present at 6–8 weeks, a second course of antibiotics should be prescribed.[2] If the effusion persists beyond 3 months refer for an ENT opinion.

- *Acute mastoiditis.* This is a major complication that presents with pain, swelling and tenderness developing behind the ear associated with a general deterioration in the condition of the child. Such a complication requires immediate referral.[8]
- *Chronic otitis media*
- *Rare complications.* These include labyrinthitis, petrositis, facial paresis and intracranial abscess.
- *Serous otitis media (glue ear).* This represents incomplete resolution of suppurative otitis media. Signs include loss of drum mobility, hearing loss and abnormal impedance. Most resolve spontaneously but any necessary treatment includes medications such as bromhexine elixir and Demazin syrup, auto-inflations and 'Oto-vent' assisted nasal inflation.

Recurrent acute otitis media

Prevention of acute otitis media (AOM) is indicated if it occurs more often than every other month or for three or more episodes in 6 months.

- Chemoprophylaxis (for about 4 months)
  — amoxycillin twice daily (first choice)

or

  — cefaclor twice daily

Consider pneumococcus vaccine in children over 18 months of age in combination with the antibiotic.

Viral infections

Most children with viral URTIs have mild reddening or dullness of the eardrum and antibiotics are not warranted. If painful bullous otitis media is present, either prick the bulla with a sterile needle for pain relief, or instil dehydrating ear drops such as anhydrous glycerol.

Ear pain in the elderly

Causes of otalgia that mainly afflict the elderly include herpes zoster (Ramsay Hunt syndrome), temporomandibular joint arthralgia, temporal arteritis and neoplasia. It is especially important to search for evidence of malignancy.

Acute otitis media

Acute otitis media causes deep-seated ear pain, deafness and often systemic illness. The sequence of symptoms is a blocked ear feeling, pain and fever. Discharge may follow if the TM perforates, with relief of pain and fever.

The commonest organisms are viruses (adenovirus and enterovirus), and the bacteria *Haemophilus influenzae*, *Streptococcus pneumoniae*, *Branhamella* (previously *Neisseria*) *catarrhalis* and β-*haemolytic streptococci*.

The two cardinal features of diagnosis are inflammation and middle ear effusion.

Appearance of the tympanic membrane (all ages)

Translucency. If the middle ear structures are clearly visible through the drum, otitis media is unlikely.

Colour. The normal TM is a shiny pale-grey to brown: a yellow colour is suggestive of an effusion.

Diagnosis

The main diagnostic feature is the redness of the TM. The inflammatory process usually begins in the upper posterior quadrant and spreads peripherally and down the handle of the malleus (Fig. 46.8). The TM will be seen to be reddened and inflamed with engorgement of the vessels particularly along the handle of the malleus. The loss of light reflex follows and anatomical features then become difficult to recognise as the TM becomes oedematous. Bulging of the drum is a late sign. Blisters are often seen on the TM and this is thought to be due to a viral infection in the epidermal layers of the drum.

Treatment of acute otitis media (adults)

- analgesics to relieve pain
- adequate rest in a warm room
- nasal decongestants for nasal congestion
- antibiotics until resolution of all signs of infection
- treat associated conditions, e.g. adenoid hypertrophy
- follow-up: review and test hearing audiometrically

Antibiotic treatment

First choice:

- amoxycillin 750 mg (o) bd for 5 days[7]

    or

    500 mg (o) tds for 5 days

A longer course (up to 10 days) may be required depending on severity and response to 5-day course.

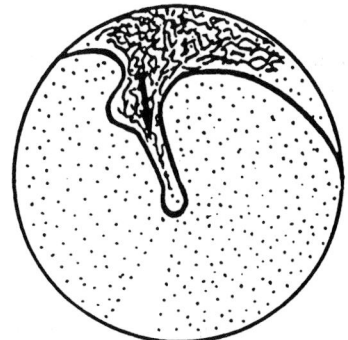

- erythema of prominent blood vessels progressing down handle of malleolus
- normal drum

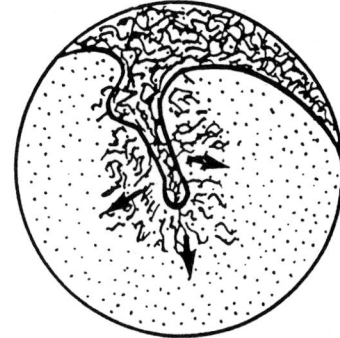

- progressive erythema

- loss of light reflex

- bulging pars flaccida

- red pars tensa
- anatomical structures unidentifiable

Fig. 46.8 *The appearances of the left tympanic membrane in the progressive development of acute otitis media*

Alternatives:

- doxycycline 100 mg (o) bd for 5 days (daily for milder infections)

or

- cefaclor 250 mg (o) tds for 5 days

or

(if resistance to amoxicillin is suspected or proven) amoxicillin/potassium clavulanate 500/125 mg (o) tds for 5 days (the most effective antibiotic).

Consider surgical intervention for failed therapy.

Chronic otitis media

There are two types of chronic suppurative otitis media and they both present with deafness and discharge without pain. The discharge occurs through a perforation in the TM: one is safe, the other unsafe.

Recognising the unsafe ear

Examination of an infected ear should include inspection of the attic region, the small area of drum between the lateral process of the malleus, and the roof of the external auditory canal immediately above it. A perforation here renders the ear 'unsafe' (Fig. 46.1); other perforations, not involving the drum margin (Fig. 46.2), are regarded as 'safe'.

The status of a perforation depends on the presence of accumulated squamous epithelium (termed cholesteatoma) in the middle ear, because this erodes bone. An attic perforation contains such material; safe perforations do not.

Cholesteatoma is visible through the hole as white flakes, unless it is obscured by discharge or a persistent overlying scab. Either type of perforation can lead to chronic infective discharge, the nature of which varies with its origin. Mucus admixture is recognised by its stretch and recoil when this discharge is being cleaned from the external auditory canal. The types of discharge are compared in Table 46.3.

Management

If an attic perforation is recognised or suspected, specialist referral is essential. Cholesteatoma cannot be eradicated by medical means: surgical removal is necessary to prevent a serious infratemporal or intracranial complication.

Table 46.3 *Comparison of types of discharge*

	Unsafe	*Safe*
Source	Cholesteatoma	Mucosa
Odour	Foul	Inoffensive
Amount	Usually scant, never profuse	Can be profuse
Nature	Purulent	Mucopurulent

Otitis externa

Otitis externa (Fig. 46.9), also known as 'swimmer's ear', 'surfer's ear' and 'tropical ear', is common in a country whose climate and coastal living leads to extensive water sport. It is more prevalent in hot humid conditions and therefore in the tropics.

Predisposing factors are allergic skin conditions, ear canal trauma, water penetration (swimming, humidity, showering), water and debris retention (wax, dermatitis, exostoses), foreign bodies, contamination from swimming water including spas, and use of Q tips and hearing aids.

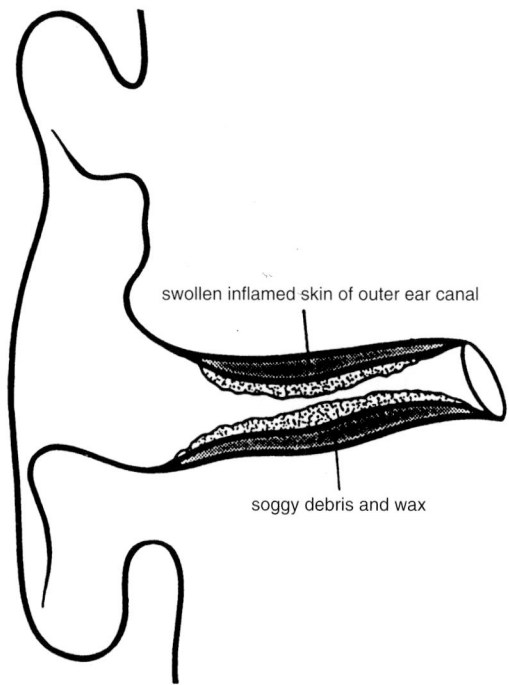

swollen inflamed skin of outer ear canal

soggy debris and wax

Fig. 46.9 *Otitis externa*

Common responsible organisms

- Bacteria: — *Pseudomonas* sp.
  — *Escherichia coli*
  — *Staphylococcus aureus*
  — *Proteus* sp.
  — *Klebsiella* sp.
- Fungi: — *Candida albicans*
  — *Aspergillus* sp.

Clinical features

- itching at first
- pain (mild to intense)
- fullness in ear canal
- scant discharge
- hearing loss

Signs

- oedema (mild to extensive)
- tenderness on moving auricle or jaw
- erythema
- discharge (offensive if coliform)
- pale cream 'wet blotting paper' debris— *Candida albicans*
- black spores of *Aspergillus nigra*
- TM granular or dull red

Obtain culture, especially if resistant *Pseudomonas* sp. suspected, by using small ear swab.

Note: 'Malignant' otitis externa occurs in diabetics due to *Pseudomonas* infection at base of skull.

Management

Aural toilet

Meticulous aural toilet by gentle suction and dry mopping with a wisp of cotton wool on a fine broach under good lighting is the keystone of management. This enables topical medication to be applied directly to the skin.

Syringing

This is appropriate in some cases but the canal must be dried meticulously afterwards. For most cases it is not recommended.

Dressings

Dressings are essential in all but the mildest forms. After cleaning and drying, insert 10–20 cm of 4 mm Nufold gauze impregnated with a steroid and antibiotic cream.

For severe otitis externa a wick is important and will reduce the oedema and pain in 12 to 24 hours (Fig. 46.10). The wick can be soaked

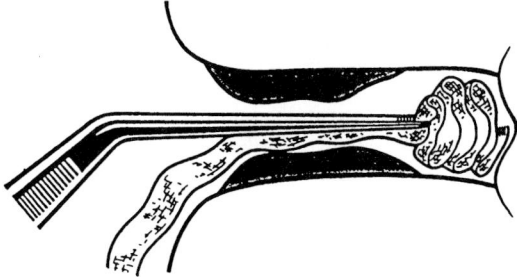

Fig. 46.10 *Insertion of a wick; it is packed gradually by short back-and-forth movements of the forceps* COURTESY OF B. BLACK

in an astringent, e.g. aluminium acetate 4% solution or glycerin and 10% ichthammol. The wick needs replacement daily until the swelling has subsided.

Topical antimicrobials

The most effective, especially when the canal is open, is an antibacterial, antifungal and corticosteroid preparation, e.g. Kenacomb or Sofradex drops (2–3 drops tds) or Locacorten-Vioform drops (2–3 drops bd).

Other measures

- Strong analgesics are essential.
- Antibiotics have little place in treatment unless a spreading cellulitis has developed.
- Prevent scratching and entry of water.

Practice tip for severe 'tropical ear'

- prednisolone (o) 15 mg statim then 10 mg 8 hourly for 6 doses
  followed by
- Merocel ear wick
- topical Kenacomb or Sofradex drops

Prevention

- Keep the ear dry, especially those involved in water sports.
- Protect the ear with various water-proofing methods, e.g.:
  — cotton wool coated with petroleum jelly
  — tailor-made ear plugs, e.g. EAR foam plugs
  — silicone putty or Blu-tack
  — a bathing cap pulled well forward allows these plugs to stay *in situ*.
- Avoid poking objects such as hairpins and cotton buds in the ear to clean the canal.
- If water enters, shake it out or use Aquaear drops (spirit drops help dry the canal).

Furunculosis

Furunculosis is a staphylococcal infection of the hair follicle in the outer cartilaginous part of the ear canal. It is usually intensely painful. Fever occurs only when the infection spreads in front of the ear as cellulitis. The pinna is tender on movement—a sign that is not a feature of acute otitis media. The furuncle (boil) may be seen in the external auditory meatus (Fig. 46.11).

Management

- If pointing, it can be incised after a local anaesthetic or freezing spray.
- Warmth, e.g. use hot face washer, hot water bottle.
- If fever with cellulitis—dicloxacillin.

Perichondritis

Perichondritis is infection of the cartilage of the ear characterised by severe pain of the pinna which is red, swollen and exquisitely tender. It is rare and follows trauma or surgery to the ear. As the organism is frequently *Pseudomonas pyocyaneus* the appropriate antibiotics must be carefully chosen (e.g. ciprofloxacin).

Infected ear lobe

The cause is most likely a contact allergy to nickel in an earring, complicated by a *Staphylococcus aureus* infection.

Management

- Discard the earrings.
- Clean the site to eliminate residual traces of nickel.
- Swab the site and then commence antibiotics, e.g. flucloxacillin or erythromycin.
- Instruct the patient to clean the site daily, and then apply the appropriate ointment.
- Use a 'noble metal' stud to keep the tract patent.
- Advise the use of only gold, silver or platinum studs in future.

Otic barotrauma

Barotrauma is damage caused by undergoing rapid changes in atmospheric pressure in the presence of an occluded eustachian tube (Fig. 46.12). It affects scuba divers and aircraft travellers. The symptoms include temporary or persisting pain, deafness, vertigo, tinnitus and perhaps discharge.

Inspection of the TM may reveal (in order of seriousness): retraction; erythema; haemorrage (due to extravasation of blood into the layers of the TM); fluid or blood in the middle ear; perforation. Perform conductive hearing loss tests with tuning fork.

Fig. 46.11 *Furuncle (boil) in hair-bearing area at opening of the ear canal*

Fig. 46.12 *Mechanism of barotrauma, with blocking of the eustachian tube due to increased pressure at the sites indicated* COURTESY OF B. BLACK

Treatment

Most cases are mild and resolve spontaneously in a few days; so treat with analgesics and reassurance. Menthol inhalations are soothing and effective. Refer if any persistent problems for consideration of the Politzer bag inflation or myringotomy.

Prevention

Flying. Perform repeated Valsalva manoeuvres during descent. Use decongestant drops or sprays before boarding the aircraft, and then 2 hours before descent.

Diving. Those with nasal problems, otitis media or chronic tubal dysfunction should not dive.

Penetrating injury to tympanic membrane

A penetrating injury to the TM can occur in children and adults from various causes such as pencils and slivers of wood or glass. Bleeding invariably follows and infection is the danger.

Management

- Remove blood clot by suction toilet or gentle dry mopping.
- Ensure no foreign body is present.
- Check hearing.
- Prescribe a course of broad spectrum antibiotics, e.g. co-trimoxazole.
- Prescribe analgesics.
- Instruct patient not to let water enter ear.
- Review in 2 days and then regularly.
- At review in 1 month the drum should be virtually healed.
- Check hearing 2 months after injury.

Complete healing can be expected within eight weeks in 90–95% of such cases.[9]

Temporomandibular joint arthralgia

If rheumatoid arthritis is excluded, a set of special exercises, which may include 'chewing' a piece of soft wood over the molars, invariably solves this problem (Chapter 48). If an obvious dental malocclusion is present, referral is necessary.

When to refer
Otitis media

- Incomplete resolution of acute otitis media
- Persistent middle ear effusion for 3 months after an attack of acute otitis media
- Persistent apparent or proved deafness
- Evidence or suspicion of acute mastoiditis or other severe complications
- Frequent recurrences, e.g. four attacks a year
- Presence of craniofacial abnormalities

Other ear problems

- attic perforation/cholesteatoma
- foreign bodies in ear not removed by simple measures such as syringing
- no response to treatment after 2 weeks for otitis externa
- suspicion of carcinoma of the ear canal
- acute tympanic membrane perforation that has not healed in 6 weeks
- chronic tympanic membrane perforation (involving lower two-thirds of TM)

Practice tips

- The pain of acute otitis media may be masked by fever in babies and young children.
- A red tympanic membrane is not always caused by otitis media. The blood vessels of the drum head may be engorged from crying, sneezing or nose blowing. In crying babies the TM as well as the face may be red.
- In otitis externa, most cases will resolve rapidly if the ear canal is expanded and then cleaned meticulously.
- If an adult presents with ear pain but normal auroscopy, examine possible referral sites, namely TMJ, mouth, throat, teeth and cervical spine.
- Antibiotics have no place in the treatment of otic barotrauma.
- It is good medicine to make relief of distressing ear pain a priority. Adequate analgesics must be given. There is a tendency to give too low a dose of paracetamol in children. The installation of nasal drops in infants with a snuffy nose and acute otitis media can indirectly provide amazing relief of pain.
- Spirit ear drops APF are a cheap and simple agent to use for recurrent otitis externa where wetness of the ear canal is a persistent problem.

References

1. Black B. Otalgia. Aust Fam Physician, 1987; 16:292–296.

2. Shires DB, Hennen BK, Rice DI. *Family medicine* (2nd edn). New York: McGraw-Hill, 1987: 86–93.

3. Jarman R. Otitis media. Aust Paed Review, 1991; 4:1–2.

4. Ludman H. *ABC of otolaryngology* (3rd end). London: BMJ, 1993.

5. Sandler G, Fry J. *Early clinical diagnosis*. Lancaster: MTP Press, 1986, 285–287.

6. Murtagh J. *Practice tips* (2nd edn). Sydney: McGraw-Hill, 1995, 109–113.

7. Mashford L (Chairman). *Antibiotic guidelines* (9th edn). Melbourne: Victorian Medical Postgraduate Foundation, 1996.

8. Robinson MJ. *Practical paediatrics*. Melbourne: Churchill Livingstone, 1990, 607.

9. Kruger R, Black B. Penetrating injury eardrum. Aust Fam Physician, 1986; 15: 735.

47

The red and tender eye

—

Those with sore eyes . . . find the light painful, while the darkness, which permits them to see nothing, is restful and agreeable.

Dio Chryostom (40–115)

A red eye accounts for at least 80% of patients with eye problems encountered in general practice.[1] An accurate history combined with a thorough examination will permit the diagnosis to be made in most cases without recourse to specialist ophthalmic equipment. A summary of the diagnostic strategy model is presented in Table 47.1.

Key facts and checkpoints

- Acute conjunctivitis accounts for over 25% of all eye complaints seen in general practice.[2]
- A purulent discharge indicates bacterial conjunctivitis.[3]
- A clear or mucous discharge indicates viral or allergic conjunctivitis.
- Viral conjunctivitis can be slow to resolve and may last for weeks.
- Pain and visual loss suggest a serious condition such as glaucoma, uveitis (including acute iritis) or corneal ulceration.
- Beware of the unilateral red eye—think beyond bacterial or allergic conjunctivitis. It is rarely conjunctivitis and may be a corneal ulcer, keratitis, foreign body, trauma, uveitis or acute glaucoma.[4]
- Keratitis (inflammation of the cornea) is one of the most common causes of an uncomfortable red eye. Apart from the well-known viral causes (herpes simplex, herpes zoster, adenovirus and measles), it can be caused by fungal

Table 47.1 *The red and tender eye: diagnostic strategy model*

Q. *Probability diagnosis*
A. Conjunctivitis
- bacterial
- adenovirus
- allergic

Q. *Serious disorders not to be missed*
A. Acute glaucoma
Uveitis
- acute iritis
- choroiditis
Corneal ulcer
Herpes simplex keratitis
Fungal keratitis
Herpes zoster ophthalmicus
Penetrating injury
Orbital cellulitis

Q. *Pitfalls (often missed)*
A. Scleritis/episcleritis
Foreign body
Trauma
Ultraviolet light 'keratitis'
Blepharitis
Cavernous sinus arteriovenous fistula

Q. *Seven masquerades checklist*
A. Depression —
Diabetes —
Drugs √ hypersensitivity
Anaemia —
Thyroid disease √ hyperthyroidism
Spinal dysfunction —
UTI —

Q. *Is the patient trying to tell me something?*
A. Unlikely.

infection (usually on a damaged cornea), bacterial infection or inflammatory disease such as ankylosing spondylitis.[5]
- Herpes simplex keratitis (dendritic ulcer) often presents painlessly as the neurotrophic effect grossly diminishes sensation.

The clinical approach

The five essentials of the history are:

- history of trauma (especially as indicator of IOFB)
- vision
- the degree and type of discomfort
- presence of discharge
- presence of photophobia

The social and occupational history is also very important. This includes a history of exposure to a 'red eye' at school, work or home; incidents at work such as injury, welding, foreign bodies or chemicals; and genitourinary symptoms.

When examining the unilateral red eye keep the following diagnoses in mind:

- trauma
- foreign body including IOFB
- corneal ulcer
- iritis (uveitis)
- viral conjunctivitis (commonest type)
- acute glaucoma

The manner of onset of the irritation often gives an indication of the cause. Conjunctivitis or uveitis generally has a gradual onset of redness, while a small foreign body will produce a very rapid hyperaemia. Photophobia occurs usually with uveitis and keratitis. It is vital to elicit careful information about visual acuity. The wearing of contact lenses is very important as these are prone to cause infection or the 'overwear syndrome', which resembles an acute ultraviolet burn.

Key questions

- Have you noticed blurring of your vision?
- Have you been in close contact with others with the same condition?
- Have you had a cold or running nose recently?
- Do you wear contact lenses?
- Can you recall scratching or injuring your eye?
- What were you doing at the time you noticed trouble?
- Have you been putting any drops, ointments or cosmetics in or around your eye?
- Do you suffer from hay fever?
- Do you have any problems with your eyelids?
- Had your eyes been watering for some time beforehand?
- Have you had any other problems?
- Have you been exposed to arc welding?

Physical examination

The basic equipment:

- eye testing charts at 45 cm (18 in) and 300 cm (10 ft)
- multiple pinholes
- torch, e.g. Cobalt blue
- magnifying aid, e.g. binocular loupe
- glass rod or cotton bud to aid eyelid eversion
- fluorescein sterile paper strips
- anaesthetic drops
- Schiotz tonometer
- ophthalmoscope
- Ishihara's colour vision test

The four essentials of the examination are:

- testing and recording vision
- meticulous inspection under magnification
- testing the pupils
- testing ocular tension[4]

Also

- local anaesthetic test
- fluorescein staining
- subtarsal examination

Inspection

A thorough inspection is essential, noting the nature of the inflammatory injection, whether it is localised (episcleritis) or diffuse, viewing the iris for any irregularity, observing the cornea, and searching for foreign bodies, especially under the eyelids, and for any evidence of penetrating injury. No ocular examination is complete until the eyelid is everted and closely inspected. Both eyes must be examined since many patients presenting with conjunctivitis in one eye will have early signs of conjunctivitis in the other. Use fluorescein to help identify corneal ulceration. Local anaesthetic drops instilled prior to the examination of a painful lesion is recommended. The local anaesthetic test is a sensitive measure of a surface problem—if the pain is unrelieved a deeper problem must be suspected.

Palpate for enlarged preauricular lymph nodes, which are characteristic of viral conjunctivitis.

The nature of the injection is important. In conjunctivitis the vessels are clearly delineated and branch from the corners of the eye towards the cornea, since it involves mainly the tarsal plate. Episcleral and scleral vessels are larger than conjunctival vessels and are concentrated towards the cornea (Fig. 47.1). Ciliary injection

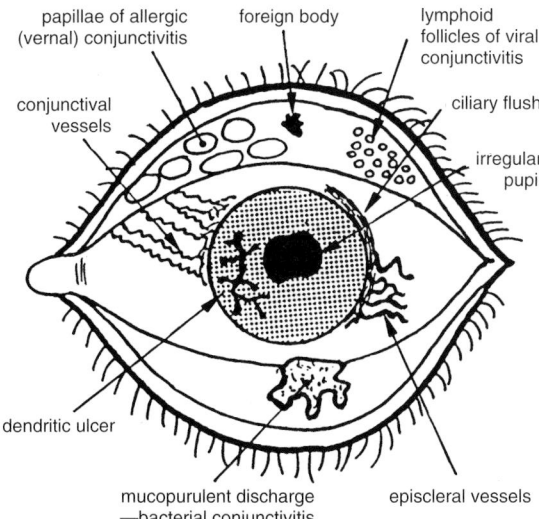

papillae of allergic (vernal) conjunctivitis

foreign body

lymphoid follicles of viral conjunctivitis

conjunctival vessels

ciliary flush

irregular pupil

dendritic ulcer

mucopurulent discharge —bacterial conjunctivitis

episcleral vessels

Fig. 47.1 *Physical signs to search for in a patient with a red eye (eyelids everted)*

appears as a red ring around the limbus of the cornea (the ciliary flush), and the individual vessels, which form a parallel arrangement, are not clearly visible. Ciliary injection may indicate a more serious deep-seated inflammatory condition such as anterior uveitis or a deep corneal infection. The presence of fine follicles on the tarsal conjuctivae indicates viral infection while a cobblestone appearance indicates allergic conjunctivitis.

Note: Slit lamp examination is ideal for the examination of the eye.

Red eye in children

Children can suffer from the various types of conjunctivitis (commonly), uveitis and trauma. Of particular concern is orbital cellulitis, which may present as a unilateral swollen lid and can rapidly lead to blindness if untreated. Bacterial, viral and allergic conjunctivitis are common in all children. Conjunctivitis in infants is a serious disorder because of the immaturity of tissues and defence mechanisms. Serious corneal damage and blindness can result.

Neonatal conjunctivitis (ophthalmia neonatorum)

This is conjunctivitis in an infant less than 1 month old and is a notifiable disease. Chlamydial and gonococcal infections are uncommon but must be considered if a purulent discharge

is found in the first few days of life.[6] In both conditions the parents must be investigated for associated venereal disease and treated accordingly. *Chlamydia trachomatis* accounts for 50% or more of cases. Its presentation in neonates is acute, usually 1–2 weeks after delivery, with moderate mucopurulent discharge. It is a systemic disease and may be associated with pneumonia. The diagnosis is confirmed by serological tests on the conjunctival secretions.

Treatment is with oral erythromycin and local sulfacetamide eye drops.

Neisseria gonorrhoeae conjunctivitis, which usually occurs within 1–2 days of delivery, requires vigorous treatment with intravenous cephalosporins or penicillin and local sulfacetamide drops. The discharge is highly infectious and the organism has the potential for severe corneal infection or septicaemia.[6]

Other common bacterial organisms can cause neonatal conjunctivitis, and herpes simplex virus type II can cause conjunctivitis and/or eyelid vesicles or keratitis.[2]

Trachoma

Trachoma is a chlamydial conjunctivitis that is prevalent in outback areas and in the Aboriginal population. *Chlamydia trachomatis* is transmitted by human contact and by flies, especially where hygiene is inadequate. It is the most common cause of blindness in the world. Recurrent and untreated disease leads to lid scarring and inturned lashes with corneal ulceration and visual loss. It is important to commence control of the infection in childhood.

Blocked nasolacrimal duct

Delayed development of the nasolacrimal duct occurs in about 6% of infants,[6] resulting in blocked lacrimal drainage; the lacrimal sac becomes infected, causing a persistent discharge from one or both eyes. In the majority of infants spontaneous resolution of the problem occurs by the age of 6 months.

Management

- local antibiotics for infective episodes
- bathing with normal saline
- frequent massage over the lacrimal sac
- referral for probing of the lacrimal passage before 6 months if the discharge is profuse and irritating or between 6 and 12 months if the problem has not self-corrected.

Red eye in the elderly

In an elderly patient there is an increased possibility of acute glaucoma, uveitis and herpes zoster. Acute angle closure glaucoma should be considered in any patient over the age of 50 presenting with an acutely painful red eye.

Eyelid conditions such as blepharitis, trichiasis, entropion and ectropion are more common in the elderly.

Acute conjunctivitis

Acute conjunctivitis is defined as an episode of conjunctival inflammation lasting less than 3 weeks.[2] The two major causes are infection (either bacterial or viral) and acute allergic or toxic reactions of the conjunctiva (see Table 47.2).

Clinical features

- diffuse hyperaemia of both tarsal or bulbar conjunctivae
- absence of ocular pain; good vision; clear cornea
- infectious conjunctivitis is bilateral (usually) or unilateral (depending on the cause), with a discharge, and a gritty or sandy sensation

Bacterial conjunctivitis

Bacterial infection may be primary, secondary to a viral infection or secondary to blepharitis.

History

Purulent discharge with sticking together of eyelashes in the morning is typical. It usually starts in one eye and spreads to the other. There may be a history of contact with a person with similar symptoms. The organisms are usually picked up from contaminated fingers, face cloths or towels.

Examination

There is usually a bilateral mucopurulent discharge with uniform engorgement of all the conjunctival blood vessels and a non-specific papillary response. Fluorescein staining is negative.

Causative organisms

These include:

- *Streptococcus pneumoniae*
- *Haemophilus influenzae*
- *Staphylococcus aureus*
- *Streptococcus pyogenes*
- *Neisseria gonorrhoeae* (a hyperacute onset)
- *Pseudomonas aeruginosa*

Diagnosis is usually clinical but a swab should be taken for smear and culture with:[2]

- hyperacute or severe purulent conjunctivitis
- prolonged infection
- neonates

Management

Limit the spread by avoiding close contact with others, use of separate towels and good ocular hygiene.

Mild cases

Mild cases may resolve with saline irrigation of the eyelids and conjunctiva but may last up to 14 days if untreated.[7] An antiseptic eye drop such as propamidine isethionate 0.1% (Brolene) 1–2 drops 6–8 hourly for 5–7 days can be used.

More severe cases

- chloramphenicol 0.5% eye drops, 1–2 hourly for 2 days,[1] decrease to 4 times a day for another 7 days (maximum 10 days—cases of aplastic anaemia have been reported with long-term use)
  Use also chloramphenicol 1% eye ointment each night

  or preferably[7]
- polymyxin B sulphate 5000 units/mL + gramicidin 25 mcg/mL + neomycin 2.5 mg/mL, 1–2 drops hourly, decreasing to 6 hourly as the infection improves.

Specific organisms

Pseudomonas and other coliforms: use topical gentamicin and tobramycin.

Neisseria gonorrhoeae. Use appropriate systemic antibiotics.

Viral conjunctivitis

The most common cause of this very contagious condition is adenovirus.

History

It is commonly associated with upper respiratory tract infections and is the type of conjunctivitis that occurs in epidemics (pink eye).[1] The conjunctivitis usually has a 2–3 week course; it is initially one-sided but with cross-infection occurring days later in the other eye.

Table 47.2 Major causes of a red eye

	Site of inflammation	Pain	Discharge	Vision	Photophobia	Pupil	Cornea	Ocular tension
Bacterial conjunctivitis	Conjunctiva, including lining of lids (usually bilateral)	Irritation—gritty	Purulent, lids stuck in morning	Normal	No	Normal	Normal	Normal
Viral conjunctivitis	Conjunctiva, lining of lids often follicular (uni or bilateral)	Gritty	Watery	Normal	No	Normal	Normal	Normal
Allergic (vernal) conjunctivitis	Conjunctiva, papillary swellings on lid linings (bilateral)	Gritty—itching	Watery	Normal	No	Normal	Normal	Normal
Contact hypersensitivity (dermato-conjunctivitis)	Conjunctiva and eyelids. Oedema	Itching	Watery	Normal—may be blurred	No	Normal	Normal	Normal
Subconjunctival haemorrhage	Beefy red area fading at edge (unilateral)	No	No	Normal	No	Normal	Normal	Normal
Herpes simplex keratitis	Unilateral—circumcorneal. Dendritic ulcer	Yes—gritty	No, reflex lacrimation	Blurred, but variable, depends on site	Yes	Normal	Abnormal	Normal
Corneal ulcer	Unilateral—circumcorneal (exclude foreign body)	Yes	No, reflex lacrimation	Blurred but variable, depends on site	Yes	Normal	Abnormal	Normal
Scleritis/episcleritis	Localised deep redness. Tender area	Yes	No	Normal	No	Normal	Normal	Normal
Acute iritis	Maximum around cornea	Yes—radiates to brow, temple, nose	No, reflex lacrimation	Blurred	Yes	Constricted, may be irregular	Normal	Normal or low
Acute glaucoma	Diffuse but maximum circumcorneal	Yes, severe with nausea and vomiting	No, reflex lacrimation	Haloes around lights	Yes	Dilated. Absent light reflex	Hazy	Hard, elevated

Examination

It is usually bilateral with diffuse conjunctival infection and productive of a scant watery discharge. Viral infections typically but not always produce a follicular response in the conjunctivae (tiny, pale lymphoid follicles) and an associated preauricular lymph node. Subconjunctival haemorrhages may occur with adenovirus infection. High magnification, ideally a slit lamp, may be necessary to visualise some of the changes, such as small corneal opacities, follicles and keratitis.

Diagnosis is based on clinical grounds and a history of infected contacts. Viral culture and serology can be performed to identify epidemics.

Treatment

- Limit cross-infection by appropriate rules of hygiene and patient education.
- Treatment is symptomatic, e.g. cool compress and topical lubricants (artificial tear preparations), naphazoline e.g. Albalon, vasoconstrictors e.g. phenylephrine
- Do not pad.
- Watch for secondary bacterial infection.

Primary herpes simplex infection

This viral infection produces a follicular conjunctivitis. About 50% of patients have associated lid or corneal ulcers/vesicles which are diagnostic.[2] Only a minority (less than 15%) develop corneal involvement with the primary infection.

Dendritic ulceration highlighted by fluorescein staining is diagnostic. Antigen detection or culture may allow confirmation.

Treatment of herpes simplex keratitis

- aciclovir 3% ointment, 5 times a day for 14 days or for at least 3 days after healing[7]
- atropine 1% 1 drop, 12 hourly, for the duration of treatment will prevent reflex spasm of the pupil (specialist supervision)
- debridement by a consultant

Allergic conjunctivitis

Allergic conjunctivitis results from a local response to an allergen. It includes:
- vernal (hay fever) conjunctivitis, and
- contact hypersensitivity reactions

Vernal (hay fever) conjunctivitis

This is usually seasonal and related to pollen exposure. There is usually associated rhinitis.

Treatment

Tailor treatment to the degree of symptoms. Antihistamines may be required but symptomatic measures usually suffice.

- Use sodium cromoglycate 2% drops, 1–2 drops per eye 4 times daily.
- Artificial tear preparations may give adequate symptomatic relief.

Contact hypersensitivity

Common topical allergens and toxins include topical ophthalmic medications, especially antibiotics, contact lens solutions (often the contained preservative) and a wide range of cosmetics, soaps, detergents and chemicals. Clinical features include burning, itching and watering with hyperaemia and oedema of the conjunctiva and eyelids. A skin reaction of the lids usually occurs.

Treatment

- Withdraw the causative agent.
- Apply normal saline compresses.
- Treat with naphazoline or phenylephrine.
- If not responding, refer for possible corticosteroid therapy.

Chlamydial conjunctivitis

Chlamydial conjunctivitis is encountered in three common situations:

- neonatal infection (first 1–2 weeks)
- young patient with associated venereal disease
- isolated Aboriginal people with trachoma

Systemic antibiotic treatment:[7]

- Neonates: erythromycin for 3 weeks
- Children over 6 kg and adults: azithromycin 1 g (o) as single dose.

Subconjunctival haemorrhage

Subconjunctival haemorrhage, which appears spontaneously, is a beefy red localised haemorrhage with a definite posterior margin. If it follows trauma and extends backwards it may indicate an orbital fracture. It is usually caused by a sudden increase in intrathoracic pressure such as coughing and sneezing. It is not related to hypertension but it is worthwhile measuring the blood pressure to help reassure the patient.

Management

No local therapy is necessary. The haemorrhage absorbs over 2 weeks. Patient explanation and reassurance is necessary. If haemorrhages are recurrent a bleeding tendency should be excluded.

Episcleritis and scleritis

Episcleritis and scleritis present as a localised area of inflammation (Figs 47.1 and 47.2). The episclera lies just beneath the conjunctiva and adjacent to the sclera. Both may become inflamed but episcleritis (which is more localised) is essentially self-limiting while scleritis (which is rare) is more serious as the eye may perforate.[3] Either conditions may be confused with inflammation associated with a foreign body, pterygium or pinguecula.

History

A red and sore eye is the presenting complaint. There is usually no discharge but there may be reflex lacrimation. Scleritis is much more painful than episcleritis.[3]

Examination

With scleritis there is a localised area of inflammation that is tender to touch, and more extensive than with episcleritis. The inflamed vessels are larger than the conjunctival vessels.

Management

An underlying cause such as an autoimmune condition should be identified. Refer the patient, especially for scleritis. Corticosteroids or NSAIDs may be prescribed.

Uveitis

The iris, ciliary body and the choroid form the uveal tract, which is the vascular coat of the eyeball.[6]

Anterior uveitis (acute iritis or iridocyclitis) is inflammation of the iris and ciliary body and this is usually referred to as acute iritis (Fig. 47.2). The pupil may become small because of adhesions, and the vision is blurred.

Causes include the seronegative arthropathies, e.g. ankylosing spondylitis, sarcoidosis and some infections, e.g. toxoplasmosis and syphilis. The examination findings are summarised in Table 47.2. The affected eye is red with the injection being particularly pronounced over the area covering the inflamed ciliary body (cilary flush). However, the whole bulbar conjunctivae can be injected. The patient should be referred to a consultant. Slit lamp examination aids diagnosis.

Management involves finding the underlying cause. Treatment includes pupil dilatation with atropine drops and topical steroids to suppress inflammation. Systemic corticosteroids may be necessary. The prognosis of anterior uveitis is good if treatment and follow-up are maintained, but recurrence is likely.

Posterior uveitis (choroiditis) may involve the retina and vitreous. Blurred vision and floating opacities in the visual field may be the only symptoms. Pain is not a feature. Referral to detect the causation and for treatment is essential.

Acute glaucoma

Acute glaucoma should always be considered in a patient over 50 years presenting with an acutely painful red eye. Permanent damage will result from misdiagnosis. The attack characteristically strikes in the evening when the pupil becomes semidilated.[3]

Features

- patient > 50 years
- pain in one eye
- ± nausea and vomiting
- impaired vision

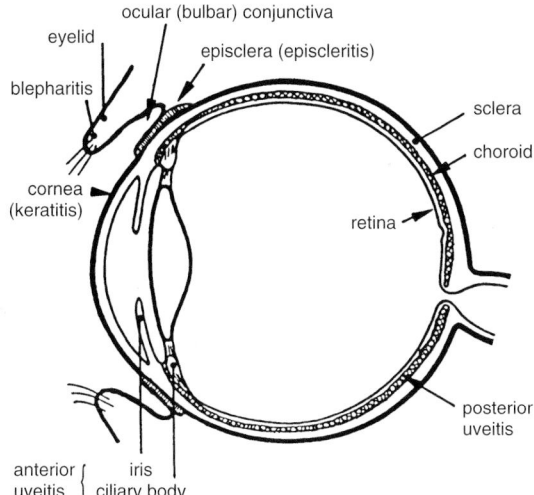

Fig. 47.2 *Diagrammatic representation of eye structures involved in inflammatory disorders*

- haloes around lights
- hazy cornea
- fixed semidilated pupil
- eye feels hard

Management
Urgent ophthalmic referral is essential since emergency treatment is necessary to preserve eyesight. If immediate specialist attention is unavailable, treatment can be initiated with acetazolamide (Diamox) 500 mg IV and pilocarpine 4% drops to constrict the pupil.

Keratoconjunctivitis sicca
Dry eyes are a common problem, especially in elderly women. Lack of lacrimal secretion can be functional (e.g. ageing), or due to systemic disease e.g. rheumatoid arthritis, SLE, Sjögren's syndrome, drugs or other factors.

Features
- dryness, grittiness and redness
- photophobia if severe
- slit light examination diagnostic

Treatment
- Treat the cause.
- Use artificial tears: hypromellose e.g. Tears Naturale; polyvinyl alcohol e.g. Tears Plus.
- Be cautious of adverse topical reactions.

Eyelid and lacrimal disorders
There are several inflammatory disorders of the eyelid and lacrimal system that present as a 'red and tender' eye without involving the conjunctiva. Any suspicious lesion should be referred.

Stye
A stye is an acute abscess of a lash follicle or associated glands of the anterior lid margin, caused usually by *Staphylococcus aureus*. The patient complains of a red tender swelling of the lid margin, usually on the medial side. A stye may be confused with a chalazion, orbital cellulitis or dacryocystitis.

Management
- Use heat to help it discharge by using direct steam from a thermos (Fig. 47.3) onto the enclosed eye or by hot compresses.

Fig. 47.3 *Steaming the painful eye: allow steam to rise from a thermos onto the closed eye for 10–15 minutes*

- Perform lash epilation to allow drainage of pus (incise with a D_{11} blade if epilation does not work).
- Use chloramphenicol ointment if the infection is spreading locally.[3]

Chalazion (meibomian cyst)
This granuloma of the meibomian gland in the eyelid may become inflamed and present as a tender irritating lump in the lid. Look for evidence of blepharitis.

Management
Conservative treatment may result in resolution. This involves heat either as steam from a thermos or a hot compress (a hand towel soaked in hot water) and the application of chloramphenicol ointment for 5 days. If the chalazion is very large, persistent or uncomfortable, or is affecting vision, it can be incised and curetted under local anaesthesia. This is best performed through the inner conjunctival surface using a chalazion clamp (blepharostat) (Fig. 47.4).

Blepharitis
This common chronic condition is characterised by inflammation of the lid margins and is commonly associated with secondary ocular effects such as styes, chalazia and conjunctival or corneal ulceration. Blepharitis is frequently associated with seborrhoeic dermatitis (especially) and atopic dermatitis, and less so with rosacea.[8] There is a tendency to colonisation of the lid

Fig. 47.4 *Excision of a meibomian cyst, using a chalazion clamp and curette*

margin with *Staphylococcus aureus*, which causes an ulcerative infection.

The two main types are:
- seborrhoeic blepharitis
- staphylococcal blepharitis

Features[8]
- persistent sore eyes or eyelids
- irritation, grittiness, burning, dryness and 'something in the eye' sensation
- lid or conjunctival swelling and redness
- crusts or scales around the base of the eyelids
- discharge or stickiness, especially in morning
- inflammation and crusting of the lid margins

Management
- Eyelid hygiene is the mainstay of therapy. The crusts and other debris should be gently cleaned with a cotton wool bud dipped in a 1:10 dilution of baby shampoo or a solution of sodium bicarbonate, once or twice daily.
- For chronic blepharitis short-term use of a corticosteroid ointment, eg. hydrocortisone 0.5%, can be very effective.
- Ocular lubricants such as artificial tear preparations may greatly relieve symptoms of keratoconjunctivitis sicca (dry eyes).
- Control scalp seborrhoea with regular medicated shampoos.
- Treat infection with an antibiotic ointment smeared on the lid margin (this may be necessary for several months) e.g. tetracycline

hydrochloride 1% or chloramphenicol 1% ointment to lid margins 3–6 hourly.[7]
- Systemic antibiotics such as flucloxacillin may be required for lid abscess.

Dacryocystitis
Acute dacryocystitis is infection of the lacrimal sac secondary to obstruction of the nasolacrimal duct at the junction of the lacrimal sac. Inflammation is localised over the medial canthus. There is usually a history of a watery eye for months beforehand. The problem may vary from being mild (as in infants) to severe with abscess formation.

Management
- Use local heat: steam or a hot moist compress.
- Use analgesics.
- In mild cases, massage the sac and duct, and instil astringent drops e.g. zinc sulfate.
- For acute cases systemic antibiotics are best guided by results of Gram's stain and culture.
- Measures to establish drainage are required eventually. Recurrent attacks or symptomatic watering of the eye are indications for surgery such as dacryocystorhinostomy.

Orbital cellulitis
Orbital cellulitis includes two basic types—periorbital (or preseptal) and orbital (or postseptal) cellulitis. The latter is a potentially blinding and life-threatening condition. It is especially important in children in whom blindness may develop in hours. The patient, often a child, presents with unilateral swollen eyelids that may be red.

Features to look for in orbital cellulitis include:[3]
- an unwell patient
- tenderness over the sinuses
- restricted and painful eye movements (Fig. 47.5)

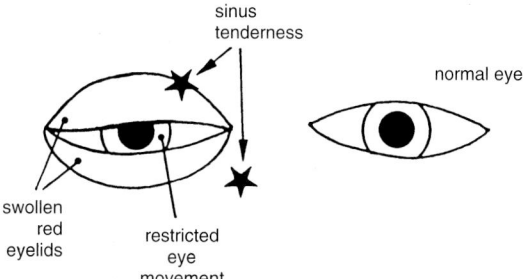

Fig. 47.5 *Important signs in the patient presenting with orbital cellulitis*

In periorbital cellulitis, which usually follows an abrasion, there is no pain or restriction of eye movement.

Immediate referral to hospital for specialist treatment is essential for both types. Treatment is with IV cefotaxime until afebrile, then amoxycillin/clavulanate for 7–10 days.

Herpes zoster ophthalmicus

Herpes zoster ophthalmicus (shingles) affects the skin supplied by the ophthalmic division of the trigeminal nerve. The eye may be affected if the nasociliary branch is involved. Ocular problems include conjunctivitis, uveitis, keratitis and glaucoma.

Immediate referral is necessary if the eye is red, vision is blurred or the cornea cannot be examined. Apart from general eye hygiene, treatment usually includes one of the oral anti-herpes virus agents, e.g. oral aciclovir 800 mg, five times daily for 10 days or (if sight is threatened) aciclovir 10 mg/kg IV slowly 8 hourly for 10 days (provided this is commenced within 3 days of the rash appearing),[5,7] and topical aciclovir ointment 4 hourly.

Pinguecula and pterygium

Pinguecula is a yellowish elevated nodular growth on either side of the cornea in the area of the palpebral fissure. It is common in people over 35 years. The growth tends to remain static but can become inflamed—pingueculitis. Usually no treatment is necessary unless they are large, craggy and uncomfortable, when excision is indicated. If irritating, topical astringent drops such as naphazoline compound drops, e.g. Albalon, can give relief.

Pterygium is a fleshy overgrowth of the conjunctiva onto the nasal side of the cornea and usually occurs in adults living in dry, dusty, windy areas. Excision of a pterygium by a specialist is indicated if it is likely to interfere with vision by encroaching on the visual axis, or if it becomes red and uncomfortable or disfiguring.

Problems with contact lenses

Because a contact lens is a foreign body, various complications can develop and a history of the use of contact lenses is important in the management of the red eye.

Infection

Infection is more likely to occur with soft rather than hard lenses. They should not be worn for sleeping since this increases the risk of infection tenfold.[10] One cause is *Acanthamoeba* keratitis acquired from contaminated water that may be used for cleaning the lenses.

Hard lens trauma

This may cause corneal abrasions with irreversible endothelial changes or ptosis, especially with the older polymethyl methacrylate based lenses. Patients should change to modern gas permeable hard lenses.

Lost lenses

Patients should be reassured that lenses cannot go behind the eye. The edge of the lens can usually be seen by everting the upper lid.

Preventive measures[11]

• Wash hands before handling lenses.
• Do not use tap water or saline.
• Clean lenses with disinfecting solution.
• Store overnight in a clean airtight case with fresh disinfectant.
• Change the lens container solution daily.
• Discard disposable lenses after 2 weeks.
• Do not wear lenses while sleeping.
• Do not wear lenses while swimming in lakes, rivers or swimming pools.

Refer to an ophthalmologist if a painful red eye develops.

Flash burns

A common problem usually presenting at night is bilateral painful eyes caused by ultraviolet 'flash burns' to both corneas some 5–10 hours previously. The mechanism of injury is ultraviolet rays from a welding machine causing superficial punctate keratitis. Other sources of UV light such as sunlamps and snow reflection can cause a reaction.

Management

• Local anaesthetic (long-acting) drops: once only application (do not allow the patient to take home more drops).
• Instil homatropine 2% drops statim or other short-acting ocular dilating agent (be careful of glaucoma).
• Use analgesics, e.g. codeine plus paracetamol, for 24 hours.

- Use broad spectrum antibiotic eye ointment in lower fornix (to prevent infection).
- Use firm eye padding for 24 hours, when eyes reviewed (avoid light).

The eye usually heals completely in 48 hours. If not, check for a foreign body.

Note: Contact lens 'overwear syndrome' gives the same symptoms.

Cavernous sinus arteriovenous fistula

Such a fistula produces conjunctival hyperaemia but no inflammation or discharge. The lesion causes raised orbital venous pressure. The fistula may be secondary to head injuries or may arise spontaneously, particularly in postmenopausal women. They need radiological investigation.

The classic symptom is a 'whooshing' sound synchronous with the pulse behind the eye, and the sign is a bruit audible with the stethoscope placed over the orbit.

Penetrating eye injuries

These require urgent referral to an ophthalmologist. If significant delay is involved give one dose (in adults) of:[7]

- gentamicin 1.5 mg/kg IV plus
- cefotaxime 1 g or ceftriaxone 1 g IV
  (can give ceftriaxone IM but with lignocaine 1%)

When to refer

- Uncertainty about the diagnosis
- Patients with uveitis, acute glaucoma, episcleritis/scleritis or corneal ulceration
- Deep central corneal and intraocular foreign bodies
- Prolonged infections, with a poor or absent response to treatment or where therapy may be complicating management
- Infections or severe allergies with possible ocular complications
- Sudden swelling of an eyelid in a child with evidence of infection suggestive of orbital cellulitis—this is an emergency
- Emergency referral is also necessary for hyphaema, hypopyon, penetrating eye injury, acute glaucoma, severe chemical burn
- Herpes zoster ophthalmicus: if the external

nose is involved then the internal eye may be involved
- Summary for urgent referral:
  — trauma (significant)
  — corneal ulcer
  — severe conjunctivitis
  — uveitis/acute iritis
  — acute glaucoma
  — orbital cellulitis
  — acute dacryocystitis
  — episcleritis/scleritis
  — herpes zoster ophthalmicus

Note: As a general rule never use corticosteroids or atropine in the eye before referral to an ophthalmologist.

Practice tips

- Avoid long-term use of any medication, especially antibiotics, e.g. chloramphenicol: course for a maximum of 10 days.[2]
- *Note*: Beware of allergy or toxicity to topical medications, especially antibiotics, as a cause of persistent symptoms.
- As a general rule avoid using topical corticosteroids or combined corticosteroid/antibiotic preparations.
- Never use corticosteroids in the presence of a dendritic ulcer.
- To achieve effective results from eye ointment or drops, remove debris such as mucopurulent exudate with bacterial conjunctivitis or blepharitis by using a warm solution of saline (dissolve a teaspoon of kitchen salt in 500 mL of boiled water) to bathe away any discharge from conjunctiva, eyelashes and lids.
- A gritty sensation is common in conjunctivitis but the presence of a foreign body must be excluded.[3]
- Beware of the contact lens 'overwear syndrome', which is treated in a similar way to flash burns.

References

1. McDonnell P. Red eye: An illustrated guide to eight common causes. Mod Med Aust, October 1989, 37–39.

2. Della NG. Acute conjunctivitis. In: MIMS Disease Index. Sydney: IMS Publishing, 1991–92, 113–115.

3. Elkington AR, Khaw PT. *ABC of eyes*. London: British Medical Association, 1990, 6–10.

4. Colvin J. Systematic examination of the red eye. Aust Fam Physician, 1976; 5: 153–165.

5. Maclean H. Keratitis (viral and fungal). In: MIMS Disease Index. Sydney: IMS Publishing, 1991–92, 301–303.

6. Robinson MJ. *Practical paediatrics* (2nd edn). Melbourne: Churchill Livingstone, 1990, 595–597.

7. Mashford ML. *Antibiotic guidelines* (9th edn). Melbourne: Victorian Medical Postgraduate Foundation, 1996/97.

8. Barras CW. Blepharitis. In: MIMS Disease Index. Sydney: IMS Publishing, 1991–92, 80–82.

9. Colvin J. Painful eye: An emergency call. Aust Fam Physician, 1985; 14:1258

10. Schein OD, Poggio EC. Ulcerative keratitis in contact lens wearers. Cornea, 1990; 9(1):55–58.

11. Lazarus MG. Complications of contact lenses. In: MIMS Disease Index (2nd edn). Sydney: IMS Publishing, 1996, 121–123.

48
Pain in the face

—

It's as though the devil suddenly thrust red hot electric needles through my right cheek towards my ear.

Patient (anonymous)
Describing 'tic douloureux'

When a patient complains of pain in the face rather than the head, the physician has to consider foremost the possibilities of dental disorders, sinus disease, especially of the maxillary sinuses, temporomandibular joint dysfunction, eye disorders, lesions of the oropharynx or posterior third of the tongue, trigeminal neuralgia and chronic paroxysmal hemicrania.

The key to the diagnosis is the clinical examination because even the most sophisticated investigation may provide no additional information.

A basic list of causes of facial pain is presented in Table 48.1.[1] The causes can vary from the simple, such as aphthous ulcers, herpes simplex and dental caries, to serious causes such as carcinoma of the tongue, sinuses and nasopharynx or osteomyelitis of the mandible or maxilla.

Table 48.1 *Diagnoses to consider in orofacial pain*

Positive physical signs
Cervical spinal dysfunction
Dental pathology
Erysipelas
Eye disorders
Herpes zoster
Nasopharyngeal carcinoma
Oropharyngeal disorders
• ulceration (aphthous, infective, traumatic, others)
• carcinoma
• gingivitis/stomatitis
• tonsillitis
• erosive lichen planus
Paranasal sinus disorders
Parotid gland
• mumps
• sialectasis
• carcinoma
• pleomorphic adenoma
Temporomandibular joint dysfunction
Temporal arteritis

Absent physical signs
Atypical facial pain
Chronic paroxysmal hemicrania
Depression-associated facial pain
Facial migraine (lower half headache)
Glossopharyngeal neuralgia
Migrainous neuralgia (cluster headache)
Trigeminal neuralgia (tic douloureux)

Key facts and checkpoints

• Dental disorders are the commonest cause of facial pain, accounting for up to 90% of pain in and about the face.[2]
• The most common dental disorders are dental caries and periodontal diseases.
• Trigeminal neuralgia is relatively uncommon with a prevalence of 155 persons per million of the population.[3]

• The mean age of onset of trigeminal neuralgia is 50–52 years.
• There is a similarity in the 'occult' causes of pain in the ear and in the face (refer to Figs 46.3 and 46.4).
• Sinusitis occurs mainly as part of a generalised upper respiratory infection. Swimming is another common predisposing factor.
• Dental root infection must be sought in all cases of maxillary sinusitis.

A diagnostic approach

A summary of the safety diagnostic model is presented in Table 48.2.

Probability diagnosis

The commonest cause of facial pain is dental disorders, especially dental caries. Another common cause is sinusitis, particularly maxillary sinusitis.

Temporomandibular joint (TMJ) dysfunction causing TMJ arthralgia is a very common problem encountered in general practice and it

Table 48.2 *Pain in the face: diagnostic strategy model*

Q. *Probability diagnosis*
A. Dental pain   — caries
                    — periapical abscess
    Maxillary sinusitis
Q. *Serious disorders not to be missed*
A. Cardiovascular
    • aneurysm of cavernous sinus
    • internal carotid aneurysm
    • ischaemia of posterior inferior cerebellar artery
    Neoplasia
    • carcinoma   — mouth
                     — sinuses
                     — nasopharynx
                     — tonsils
                     — tongue
                     — larynx
    • metastases   — orbital
                     — base of brain
                     — bone
    Severe infections
    • erysipelas
    • periapical abscess → osteomyelitis
    • acute sinusitis → spreading infection
    Temporal arteritis
Q. *Pitfalls*
A. Temporomandibular joint dysfunction
    Migraine variants
    • facial migraine
    • chronic paroxysmal hemicrania
    Eye disorders—glaucoma, iritis, optic neuritis
    Chronic dental neuralgia
    Parotid gland—mumps, carcinoma, sialectasis
    Acute glaucoma (upper face)
    Cranial nerve neuralgias
    • trigeminal neuralgia
    • glossopharyngeal neuralgia
Q. *Seven masquerades checklist*
A. Depression   √
    Diabetes   —
    Drugs   —
    Anaemia   —
    Thyroid disease   —
    Spinal dysfunction   √
    UTI   —
Q. *Is the patient trying to tell me something?*
A. Quite probably. Atypical facial pain has underlying psychogenic elements.

is important to have some simple basic strategies to give the patient.

Serious disorders not to be missed

It is important not to overlook carcinoma of various structures such as the mouth, sinuses, nasopharynx, tonsils, tongue, larynx and parotid gland.

It is important therefore to inspect these areas, especially in the elderly, but lesions in the relatively inaccessible nasopharynx can be easily missed. Nasopharynx carcinoma spreads upwards to the base of the skull early and patients can present with multiple cranial nerve palsies before either pain or bloody nasal discharge.[1]

Tumours may arise in the bones of the orbit, for example lymphoma or secondary carcinoma, and may cause facial pain and proptosis. Similarly, any space-occupying lesion or malignancy arising from the region of the orbit or base of the brain can cause facial pain by involvement (often destruction) of trigeminal sensory fibres. This will lead to a depressed ipsilateral corneal reflex.

Also, aneurysms developing in the cavernous sinus[1] can cause pain via pressure on any of the divisions of the trigeminal nerve, while aneurysms from the internal carotid arising from the origin of the posterior communicating artery can cause pressure on the oculomotor nerve.

Temporal arteritis typically causes pain over the temporal area but can cause ischaemic pain in the jaws when chewing.

Pitfalls

Commonly overlooked causes of facial pain include TMJ arthralgia and dental disorders, especially of the teeth, which are tender to percussion, and oral ulceration. Diagnosing the uncommon migraine variants, particularly facial migraine and chronic paroxysmal hemicrania, often presents difficulties including differentiating between the neuralgias. Glossopharyngeal neuralgia, which is rare, causes pain in the back of the throat, around the tonsils and adjacent fauces. The lightning quality of the pain of neuralgia gives the clue to diagnosis.

Common pitfalls

- failing to refer unusual or undiagnosed causes of facial pain
- overlooking infective dental causes which can cause complications
- failing to consider the possibility of malignant disease of 'hidden' structures in the older patient

Seven masquerades checklist

Of these, depression and cervical spinal dysfunction must be considered. The upper cervical spine can cause facial pain from lesions of C2 or C3 via the lesser occipital or greater auricular (Fig. 48.1) nerves, which may give pain around the ear. It is important to remember that C2 and C3 share a common pathway with the trigeminal nerve (Chap. 56).

Depressive illness can present with a variety of painful syndromes and facial pain is no exception. The features of depression may be apparent and thus antidepressants should be prescribed. Usually the facial pain and the depression subside concomitantly.

Psychogenic considerations

Psychogenic factors have to be considered in every painful condition. They are considered to be high in patients with atypical facial pain.

The clinical approach

History

Diagnosis of nearly all types of facial pain must be based almost entirely on the history. It is often difficult to delineate the exact nature and distribution of the pain. The history should include the typical analysis of pain, especially noting the site and radiation of the pain.

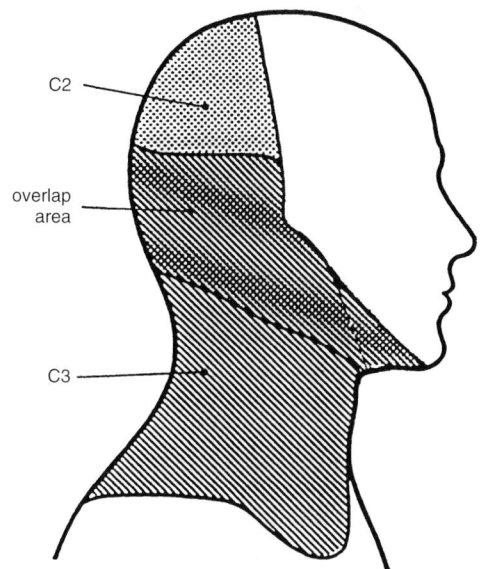

C2

overlap area

C3

Fig.48.1 *Dermatomes of C2 and C3, with the overlap area indicated*

Examination

The patient's general state and behaviour should be noted. Any sudden jabbing pain in the face causing the characteristic 'tic' may indicate neuralgia.

Palpate the face and neck to include the parotid glands, eyes, regional lymph nodes and the skin. Inspect the TMJs and cervical spine. Carefully inspect the nose, mouth, pharynx and postnasal space. In particular inspect the teeth, percussing each tooth if dental disorder is suspected. Bimanual palpation of the floor of the mouth is performed to detect induration or submandibular and submental lymph node enlargement.

The sinuses, especially the maxillary sinuses, should be inspected and a torch light should be placed inside the mouth to test transillumination of the maxillary sinuses. It works best when one symptomatic side can be compared with an asymptomatic side.

Perform a neurological examination on the cranial nerves with special emphasis on the trigeminal, oculomotor and glossopharyngeal nerves.

Investigations

If investigations are being contemplated referral may be appropriate. The association of multiple sclerosis and tumours with neuralgias may have to be investigated. Radiological investigations include plain X-rays such as the paranasal sinuses, CT scans, MRI and orthopantomograms.

Facial pain in children

Apart from trauma, facial pain in children is invariably due to dental problems, rarely migraine variants and occasionally childhood infections such as mumps and gingivostomatitis. A serious problem sometimes seen in children is orbital cellulitis secondary to ethmoiditis.

Sinusitis occurs in children, especially older children, and it should be suspected with persistent bilateral mucopurulent rhinorrhoea (beyond 10 days).

Facial pain in the elderly

Many of the causes of facial pain have an increased incidence with age, in particular trigeminal neuralgia, herpes zoster, carcinoma, glaucoma, TMJ dysfunction and cervical spondylosis. Glossopharyngeal neuralgia does not seem to have a particular predilection for the elderly. Xerostomia due to decreased secretions of salivary glands may cause abrasion with minor trauma. It may aggravate the pain of glossitis, which is common in the elderly.

Dental disorders

Dental caries, impacted teeth, infected tooth sockets and dental roots can cause pain in the maxillary and mandibular regions. Caries with periapical and apical abscess formation produces pain from infection extending around the apex of the tooth into the alveolar bone. Retention of a fractured root may cause unilateral paroxysmal pain. Impacted third molars (wisdom teeth) may be associated with surrounding soft tissue inflammation (pericoronitis), causing pain that may be localised to the mandible or radiate via the auriculotemporal nerve to the ear. *Candida albicans*, which are oral commensals, may colonise dentures causing hyperaemia and painful superficial ulceration of the denture-bearing mucosa.

Features of dental caries
- Pain is usually confined to the affected tooth but it may be diffuse.
- Pain is almost always aggravated by thermal changes in the mouth:
  cold — if dental pulp vital
  hot — if dental pulp is necrotic.
- Pain may be felt in more than one tooth.
- Dental pain will not cross the midline.

Treatment of dental pain
- Arrange urgent dental consultation.
- Pain relief[4]
  - aspirin 600 mg (o) 4–6 hourly
                 or
  - paracetamol 0.5–1 g (o) 4–6 hourly
- If pain severe add:
  - codeine 30 mg (o) 4–6 hourly

Tooth abscess, inflamed wisdom tooth (pericoronitis) or root canal infection[7]
Dental treatment will usually alleviate the problem; however, if severe:
- metronidazole 400 mg (o), 12 hourly for 3 days
if unresponsive, add:
- phenoxymethylpenicillin 500 mg (o), 6 hourly for 3 days

for patients hypersensitive to penicillin:
- clindamycin 300 mg (o), 8 hourly for 3 days

Pain from paranasal sinuses

Infection of the paranasal sinuses may cause localised pain. Localised tenderness and pain may be apparent with frontal or maxillary sinusitis. Sphenoidal or ethmoidal sinusitis causes a constant pain behind the eye or behind the nose, often accompanied by nasal blockage. Chronic infection of the sinuses may be extremely difficult to detect. The commonest organisms are *Streptococcus pneumoniae*, *Haemophilus influenzae* and *Moraxella catarrhalis*.

Expanding lesions of the sinuses, such as mucocoeles and tumours, cause local swelling and displace the contents of the orbit—upwards for maxillary, laterally for the ethmoids and downwards for the frontal.

Maxillary sinusitis
The maxillary sinus is the one most commonly infected.[5] It is important to determine whether the sinusitis is caused by stasis following an URTI or acute rhinitis, or due to dental root infection.

Clinical features of acute sinusitis
- facial pain and tenderness (over sinuses)
- toothache
- headache
- purulent postnasal drip
- nasal discharge
- nasal obstruction
- rhinorrhoea
- cough (worse at night)
- prolonged fever
- epistaxis
Suspect bacterial cause if high fever and purulent nasal discharge

Clinical features of chronic sinusitis
- vague facial pain
- offensive postnasal drip
- nasal obstruction
- toothache
- malaise
- halitosis

Some simple office tests
Diagnosing sinus tenderness[6]
To differentiate sinus tenderness from non-sinus bone tenderness palpation is useful. This is best

done by palpating a non-sinus area first and last (Fig. 48.2), systematically exerting pressure over the temporal bones (T), then the frontal (F), ethmoid (E) and maxillary (M) sinuses, and finally zygomas (Z), or vice versa.

Differential tenderness both identifies and localises the main sites of infection (Fig. 48.2).

Diagnosis of unilateral sinusitis

A simple way to assess the presence or absence of fluid in the frontal sinus, and in the maxillary sinus (in particular), is the use of transillumination. It works best when one symptomatic side can be compared with an asymptomatic side.

It is necessary to have the patient in a darkened room and to use a small, narrow-beam torch. For the maxillary sinuses remove dentures (if any). Shine the light inside the mouth, on either side of the hard palate, pointed at the base of the orbit. A dull glow seen below the orbit indicates that the antrum is air-filled. Diminished illumination on the symptomatic side indicates sinusitis.

Management of acute bacterial sinusitis

Principles

- Exclude dental root infection.
- Control predisposing factors.
- Use appropriate antibiotic therapy.

(F = frontal sinuses; E = ethmoid sinuses; M = maxillary sinuses)

Fig. 48.2 *Diagnosing sinus tenderness: T (temporal) and Z (zygoma) represent no sinus bony tenderness, for purposes of comparison*

- Establish drainage by stimulation of mucociliary flow and relief of obstruction.

Measures

- analgesics
- antibiotics[7,9]
  - amoxycillin tds for 7–10 days

    or

    (if sensitive to penicillin)
  - doxycycline 100 mg (o) bd for 10 days

    or
  - cefaclor 500 mg (o) tds for 10 days

    or
- in complicated or severe disease use intravenous cephalosporins or flucloxacillin
- nasal decongestants (ephedrine-containing nasal drops or sprays)[5] only if congestion
- inhalations (a very important adjunct).

Invasive methods

Surgical drainage may be necessary by atrial lavage or frontal sinus trephine.

Inhalations for sinusitis

The old method of towel over the head and inhalation bowl can be used, but it is better to direct the vapour at the nose. Equipment needed is a container, which can be an old disposable bowl, a wide-mouthed bottle or tin, or a plastic container.

For the inhalant, several household over-the-counter preparations are suitable, e.g. friar's balsam (5 mL), Vicks Vapo-rub (1 teaspoon), or menthol (5 mL).

The cover can be made from a paper bag (with its base cut out), a cone of paper (Fig. 48.3) or a small cardboard carton (with the corner cut away).

Method

1. Add 5 mL or 1 teaspoon of the inhalant to 0.5 L (or 1 pint) of boiled water in the container.
2. Place the paper or carton over the container.
3. Get the patient to apply nose and mouth to the opening and breathe in the vapour deeply and slowly through the nose, and then out slowly through the mouth.
4. This should be performed for 5–10 minutes, three times a day, especially before retiring.

After inhalation, upper airway congestion can be relieved by autoinsufflation.

cone of paper

vapour

inhalant

Fig. 48.3 *Method of inhalation for sinusitis*

Temporomandibular joint

This condition is due to abnormal movement of the mandible, especially during chewing. The basic cause is dental malocclusion. The pain is felt over the joint and tends to be localised to the region of the ear and mandibular condyle but may radiate forwards to the cheek and even the neck.

Examination of the TMJ

- Check for pain and limitation of mandibular movements, especially on opening the mouth.
- Palpate about the joint bilaterally for tenderness, which typically lies immediately in front of the external auditory meatus; palpate the temporalis and masseter muscles.
- Palpate the TMJ over the lateral aspect of the joint disc.
- Ask the patient to open the mouth fully when tenderness is maximal. The TMJ can be palpated posteriorly by inserting the little finger into the external canal.
- Check for crepitus in mandibular movement.

Treatment of TMJ dysfunction

If organic disease such as rheumatoid arthritis and obvious dental malocclusion is excluded, a special set of instructions or exercises can alleviate the annoying problem of TMJ arthralgia in about 3 weeks.

| Method 1 | *'Chewing' the piece of soft wood*

- Obtain a rod of soft wood approximately 15 cm long and 1.5 cm wide. An ideal object is a large carpenter's pencil.
- Instruct the patient to position this at the back of the mouth so that the molars grasp the object with the mandible thrust forward.
- The patient then rhythmically bites on the object with a grinding movement for 2–3 minutes at least 3 times a day.

| Method 2 | *The 'six by six' program*

This is a specific program recommended by some dental surgeons. The six exercises should be carried out six times on each occasion, six times a day, taking about 1–2 minutes.
Instruct the patient as follows:

1. Hold the front one-third of your tongue to the roof of your mouth and take six deep breaths.
2. Hold the tongue to the roof of your mouth and open your mouth six times. Your jaw should not click.
3. Hold your chin with both hands keeping the chin still. Without letting your chin move, push up, down and to each side. Remember, do not let your chin move.
4. Hold both hands behind your neck and pull chin in.
5. Push on upper lip so as to push head straight back.
6. Pull shoulders back as if to touch shoulder blades together.

These exercises should be pain-free. If they hurt, do not push them to the limit until pain eases.

| Method 3 | *The TMJ 'rest' program*

This program is reserved for an acutely painful TMJ condition.

- For eating avoid opening your mouth wider than the thickness of your thumb and cut all food into small pieces.
- Do not bite any food with your front teeth—use small bite-size pieces.
- Avoid eating food requiring prolonged chewing, e.g. hard crusts of bread, tough meat, raw vegetables.
- Avoid chewing gum.
- Always try to open your jaw in a hinge or arc motion. Do not protrude your jaw.

- Avoid protruding your jaw, e.g. talking, applying lipstick.
- Avoid clenching your teeth together—keep your lips together and your teeth apart.
- Try to breathe through your nose at all times.
- Do not sleep on your jaw: try to sleep on your back.
- Practise a relaxed lifestyle so that your jaws and face muscles feel relaxed.

Injection into the TMJ

Indications: painful rheumatoid arthritis, osteoarthritis or TMJ dysfunction not responding to conservative measures.

> Method

- The patient sits on a chair, facing away from the therapist. The mouth is opened to at least 4 cm.
- The joint line is palpated anterior to the tragus of the ear: this is confirmed by the opening and closing of the jaw. A 25-gauge needle is inserted into the depression above the condyle of the mandible, below the zygomatic arch and one finger-breadth (2 cm) anterior to the tragus. The needle is directed inwards and slightly upwards to lie free within the joint cavity. The 1 mL solution containing 0.5 mL of local anaesthetic and 0.5 mL of corticosteroid should flow quite freely.[8]

Other treatments

- Dental management that may be required for malfunction of the bite includes dental occlusal splinting.
- NSAIDs: A trial of NSAIDs for TMJ inflammation may need consideration.

Inflammatory or ulcerative oropharyngeal lesions

A variety of ulcerative conditions and infections of structures such as gingivae, tongue, tonsils, larynx and pharynx can cause facial pain. Gingivostomatitis, herpes labialis (cold sores) and aphthous ulceration are common examples. Lesions of the posterior third of the tongue, the oropharynx, tonsils and larynx may radiate to the region of the ear via the tympanic branch of the ninth nerve or the auricular branch of the tenth nerve.

Trigeminal neuralgia

Trigeminal neuralgia (tic douloureux) is a condition of often unknown cause that typically occurs in patients over the age of 50, affecting the second and third divisions of the trigeminal nerve and on the same side of the face.[3] Brief paroxysms of pain, often with associated trigger points, are a feature.

Typical clinical features

- Site: sensory branches of the trigeminal nerve (Fig. 48.4) almost always unilateral (often right side)

- Radiation: tends to commence in the mandibular division and spreads to the maxillary division and (rarely) to the ophthalmic division

- Quality: excruciating, searing jabs of pain like a burning knife or electric shock

- Frequency: variable and no regular pattern
- Duration: 1–2 minutes (up to 15 minutes)
- Onset: spontaneous or trigger point stimulus

- Offset: spontaneous

Fig. 48.4 *Typical cutaneous sensory distribution of the trigeminal nerve and its branches*

- Precipitating factors: talking; chewing; touching trigger areas on face, e.g. washing, shaving, eating; cold weather or wind; turning onto pillow
- Aggravating factors: trigger points usually in the upper and lower lip, nasolabial fold or upper eyelid (Fig. 48.5)
- Relieving factors: nil
- Associated features: — rarely occurs at night — spontaneous remissions for months or years
- Signs: there are no signs, normal corneal reflex
- Causes: — unknown — local pressure on the nerve root entry zone by tortuous pulsatile dilated small vessels (probably up to 75%) — multiple sclerosis — neurosyphilis — tumours of the posterior fossa

Note: Precise diagnosis is essential.

Treatment

- Patient education, reassurance and empathic support is very important in these patients.
- Medical therapy:

Fig. 48.5 *Trigeminal neuralgia: typical trigger points*

— carbamazepine (from onset of the attack to resolution)[4] 100 mg (o) bd initially, gradually increase the dose to avoid drowsiness by 200 mg every four days to 300–400 mg bd (maintenance); testing serum levels is unnecessary
— alternative drugs if carbamazepine not tolerated or ineffective (but question the diagnosis if lack of response)
  · phenytoin 300–500 mg daily
  · clonazepam
  · sodium valproate
  · baclofen
- Surgery:
— refer to a neurosurgeon if medication ineffective
— possible procedures include:
  · decompression of the trigeminal nerve root, e.g. gel foam packing between the nerve and blood vessels
  · thermocoagulation/radiofrequency neurolysis
  · surgical division of peripheral branches

Glossopharyngeal neuralgia[9]

This is a rare condition of the 9th cranial nerve with similar clinical features of severe lancinating pains.

- Sites: back of throat around tonsillar fossa and adjacent fauces deep in ear
- Radiation: ear canal, neck
- Triggers: swallowing, coughing, talking
- Treatment: as for trigeminal neuralgia.

Migrainous neuralgia (cluster headache)

As described in Chapter 52 the pain is unilateral and centred around the eye with associated lacrimation and stuffiness of the nose.

Facial migraine (lower half headache)[9]

Migraine may rarely affect the face below the level of the eyes, causing pain in the area of the cheek and upper jaw. It may spread over the nostril and lower jaw. The pain is dull and throbbing, and nausea and vomiting are commonly present. The treatment is as for other varieties of migraine with simple analgesics or ergotamine for infrequent attacks.

Chronic paroxysmal hemicrania

In the rare condition of chronic or episodic paroxysmal hemicrania there is a unilateral facial pain that can resemble chronic cluster headache but the duration is briefer, about 15 minutes, and it may recur many times a day even for years. It responds dramatically to indomethacin.[10]

Herpes zoster and postherpetic neuralgia

Herpes zoster may present as hyperaesthesia or a burning sensation in any division of the fifth nerve, especially the ophthalmic division.

Atypical facial pain

This is mainly a diagnosis of exclusion whereby patients, usually middle-aged women, complain of diffuse pain in the cheek (unilateral or bilateral) without demonstrable organic disease. The pain does not usually conform to a specific nerve distribution (although in the maxillary area), varies in intensity and duration and is not lancinating as in trigeminal neuralgia. It is usually described as deep-seated and 'boring', severe, continuous and throbbing in nature. It is a very confusing and difficult problem to treat. These patients tend to show psychoneurotic tendencies but caution is needed in labelling them as functional.

Treatment
Trial of an antidepressant[4] e.g.
- dothiepin 25–150 mg nocte
  or
- amitriptyline 50–150 mg nocte

When to refer

- Severe trigeminal neuralgia
- Unusual facial pain, especially with a suspicion of malignancy
- Positive neurological signs, e.g. impaired corneal reflex, impaired sensation in a trigeminal dermatome, slight facial weakness, hearing loss on the side of the neuralgia
- Possible need for surgical drainage of sinusitis—indications for surgery include failure of

appropriate medical treatment, anatomical deformity, polyps, uncontrolled sinus pain[5]
- Dental root infection causing maxillary sinusitis
- Other dental disorders

Practice tips

- Malignancy must be excluded in the elderly with facial pain.
- Problems from the molar teeth, especially the third (wisdom), commonly present with periauricular pain without aural disease and pain in the posterior cheek.
- Facial pain never crosses the midline; bilateral pain means bilateral lesions.

References

1. Beck ER, Francis JL, Souhami RL. *Tutorials in differential diagnosis.* Edinburgh: Longman Cheshire, 1987: 161–164.
2. Gerschman JA, Reade PC. Orofacial pain. Aust Fam Physician, 1984;13: 14–24.
3. Selby G. Trigeminal neuralgia. In: MIMS Disease Index (2nd edn). Sydney: IMS Publishing, 1996, 531–533.
4. Moulds RFW. *Analgesic guidelines* (3rd edn) Melbourne: Victorian Medical Postgraduate Foundation, 1997–98, 211–217.
5. Stevens M. The diagnosis and management of acute and chronic sinusitis. Mod Med Aust, April 1991: 16–26.
6. Bridges-Webb C. Diagnosing sinus tenderness. Practice tip. Aust Fam Physician, 1981; 10:742.
7. Mashford ML (Chairman). *Antibiotic guidelines* (9th edn). Melbourne: Victorian Medical Postgraduate Foundation, 1996, 49–50 and 101–102.
8. Corrigan B, Maitland G. *Practical orthopaedic medicine.* Sydney: Butterworths, 1986: 220.
9. Moulds RFW (Chairman). *Therapeutic guidelines: Neurology.* Melbourne: Therapeutic Guidelines Limited, 1997, 52–58.
10. Burns R. Pitfalls in headache management. Aust Fam Physician, 1990; 19:1825.

49
Fever and chills

—

Why! the fever itself is nature's instrument.

Thomas Sydenham (1624–89)
Medical observations

Although fever is a sign of disease and usually occurs in response to infection (mainly viral), its presence is recognised to play an important role in the individual's defence against infection. The infecting pathogen triggers hypothalmic receptors, causing the thermostatic mechanisms to be reset to maintain core temperature at a higher level. The elevation in body temperature activates T-cell production, increases the effectiveness of interferons and limits the replication of some common viruses.[1]

Facts and figures

- Fever plays an important physiological role in the defence against infection.
- Normal body temperature (measured orally) is 36–37.3°C (average 36.8°C).
- Normal average values: mouth   36.8°C
                            axilla   36.4°C
                            rectum   37.3°C
- Fever (pyrexia):   mouth   > 37.3°C
                            rectum   > 37.7°C
- There can be a normal diurnal variation of 1°C (lowest in early morning and highest in late afternoon).
- Fevers due to infections have an upper limit of 40.5–41.1°C (105–106°F).
- Hyperthermia (temperature above 41.1°C) and hyperpyrexia appear to have no upper limit.
- Infection remains the most important cause of acute fever.[2]
- Symptoms associated with fever include sweats, chills, rigors and headache.

- General causes of fever include infections; malignant disease; mechanical trauma, e.g. crush injury; vascular accidents, e.g. infarction, cerebral haemorrhage; immunogenic diseases, e.g. drug reactions, SLE; acute metabolic disorders, e.g. gout; and haemopoietic disorders, e.g. acute haemolytic anaemia.[2]
- Drugs can cause fever, presumably because of hypersensitivity.[2] Important examples are allopurinol, antihistamines, barbiturates, cephalosporins, cimetidine, methyldopa, penicillins, isoniazid, quinidine, phenolphthalein (including laxatives), phenytoin, procainamide, salicylates, sulphonamides.
- Infectious diseases at the extremes of age (very young and aged)[2] often present with atypical symptoms and signs. Their condition may deteriorate rapidly.
- Overseas travellers or visitors may have special, even exotic, infections and require special evaluation (refer Chap. 12).
- Immunologically compromised patients, e.g. AIDS patients, pose a special risk for infections including opportunistic infections.
- A febrile illness is characteristic of the acute infection of HIV: at least 50% have an illness like glandular fever. Think of it!

Chills

The abrupt onset of fever with a chill or rigor is a feature of some diseases. Examples include:

- pneumococcal pneumonia
- pyogenic infection with bacteraemia
- lymphoma
- pyelonephritis

Features of a true chill are teeth chattering and bed shaking, which is quite different from the chilly sensations that occur in almost all fevers, particularly those in viral infections.

Hyperthermia

Hyperthermia or hyperpyrexia is a temperature greater than 41.1°C (106°F). A more accurate definition is a state when the body's metabolic heat production or environmental heat load exceeds normal heat loss capacity. Hyperthermia may be observed particularly in the tropics, in malaria and heatstroke. It can occur with CNS tumours, infections or haemorrhages because of its effect on the hypothalamus.

Malignant hyperthermia

This is a rare hereditary disorder characterised by rapidly developing hyperpyrexia, muscular rigidity and acidosis in patients undergoing major surgery.

Sweats

Sweating is a heat loss mechanism, and diffuse sweating that may soak clothing and bedclothing permits rapid release of heat by evaporation. In febrile patients the skin is usually hot and dry—sweating occurs in most when the temperature falls. It is characteristic of only some fevers, e.g. septic infections and rheumatic fever.

Factitious fever

Factitious fever is usually encountered in hospitalised patients attempting to malinger. The situation is usually suspected when:

- a series of high temperatures is recorded to form an atypical pattern of fluctuation
- there is excessively high temperature (41.1°C) and above
- a recorded high temperature is unaccompanied by warm skin, tachycardia and other signs of fever such as a flushed face and sweating

The patient may have surreptitiously dipped the thermometer in warm water, placed it in contact with a heat source or heated the bulb by friction with bedclothes or even mucous membranes of the mouth.

Neuroleptic malignant syndrome

This is often confused with 'malignant' hyperthermia and heat stroke. The syndrome includes high temperature, muscle rigidity, autonomic dysfunction and altered consciousness. It is a rare and potentially lethal reaction in patients taking antipsychotic drugs, particularly occurring with haloperidol alone or with other drugs especially lithium carbonate.

Measurement of temperature

Temperature can be measured by several methods, including the mercury thermometer, the liquid crystal thermometer and the electronic probe thermometer. The mercury thermometer, however, is probably still the most widely used and effective temperature-measuring instrument.

Basic rules of usage

1. Before use, shake down to 35–36°C.
2. After use:
   — shake down and store in antiseptic
   — do not run under hot water
   — wipe rectal thermometer with alcohol and store separately
3. Recording time is 3 minutes orally and 1–2 minutes rectally.

Oral use

1. Place under the tongue at the junction of the base of the tongue and the floor of the mouth to one side of the frenulum—the 'heat' pocket.
2. Ensure that the mouth is kept shut.
3. Remove dentures.

Note: This is unsuitable for children 4 years and under, especially if irritable.

Rectal use

This is an excellent and recommended route for babies and young children under the age of 4 years.

Method
1. Lubricate the stub with petroleum or KY jelly.
2. Insert for 3 cm (1 in) past anal verge.
3. Keep the thermometer between the flexed fingers with the hand resting on the buttocks (Fig. 49.1).

Don't:
- dig thermometer in too hard
- hold it too rigidly
- allow the child to move around

Axillary use

This is very unreliable, and should be avoided.

Fig. 49.1 *Rectal temperature measurement in infants*

Groin use
This route is not ideal but is more reliable than the axilla. It closely approximates oral temperature. In infants, the thigh should be flexed against the abdomen.

Vaginal use
This is mainly used as an adjunct to the assessment of ovulation during the menstrual cycle. It should be placed deeply in the vagina for 5 minutes before leaving bed in the morning.

Accidental breakage in the mouth
If children bite off the end of a mercury thermometer there is no need for alarm, as the small amount of mercury is non-toxic and the piece of glass will usually pass in the stool.

The clinical approach
The initial approach is to evaluate the severity of the problem and the nature of the illness. Some infections, particularly bacterial infections, are life-threatening and this requires urgent diagnosis and hospital admission.

According to Yung and Stanley[2] it is helpful to consider fever in three categories: less than 3 days duration; between 4 and 14 days duration and protracted fever (more than 14 days).

Fever of less than 3 days duration
This is very commonly encountered in family practice, often due to a self-limiting viral infection of the respiratory tract. It is important, however, to be vigilant for other infections; so

evidence of an infectious disease, urinary tract infection, pneumonia or other infection should be sought. A routine urine examination, especially in females, is an important screening investigation. The majority of patients can be managed conservatively.

Fever present for 4 to 14 days
If fever persists beyond 4–5 days a less common infection should be suspected since most common viral infections will have resolved by about four days.[2] A checklist of causes is presented in Table 49.1. The careful history is mandatory as outlined for FUO. The basic examination and investigations are along similar lines.

Temperature chart
Charting the patterns of fever may be a diagnostic help because some febrile conditions follow a predictable temperature pattern.[4] Examples are presented in Figure 49.2.

Intermittent fever
This is a fever in which the temperature rises for a few hours and then returns to normal (Fig. 49.2a). Malaria is the classic example: in quartan fever, caused by *Plasmodium malariae*, the attacks occur every 72 hours (the term *quartan* means every 4th day by inclusive counting). This compares with tertian fever from *Plasmodium*

Table 49.1 *Common causes of fever of 4–14 days duration*

- Influenza
- Sinusitis
- Epstein-Barr mononucleosis
- Enteroviral infection
- Infective endocarditis
- Dental infections
- Hepatobiliary infections: hepatitis, cholecystitis, empyema of gall bladder
- Abscess
- Pelvic inflammatory disease
- Cytomegalovirus infection
- Lyme disease
- Travel-acquired infection: typhoid, dengue, hepatitis, malaria, amoebiasis
- Zoonosis: brucellosis, Q fever, leptospirosis, psittacosis
- Drug fever

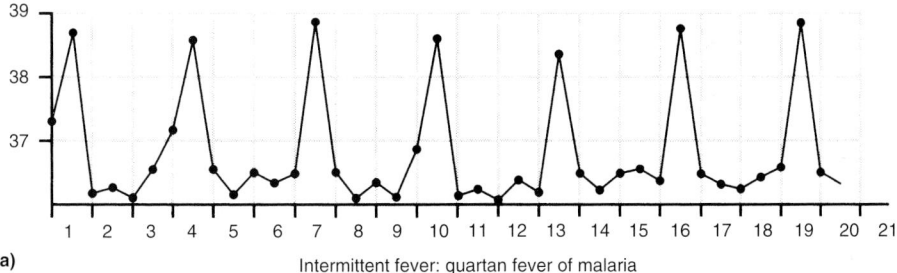

(a) Intermittent fever: quartan fever of malaria

(b) Undulant fever: due to lymphoma

(c) Continuous pattern

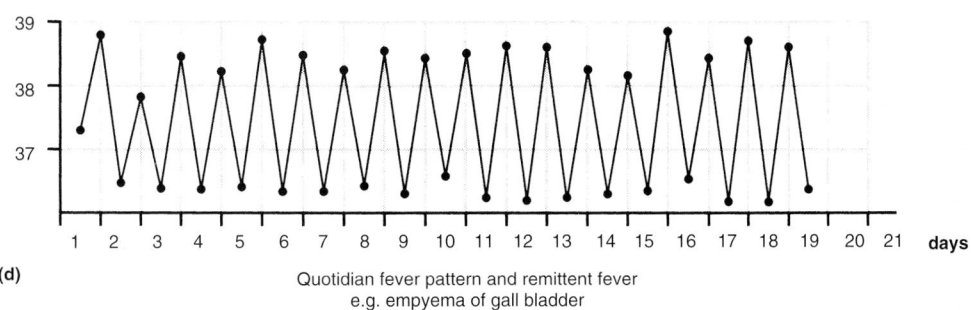

(d) Quotidian fever pattern and remittent fever
e.g. empyema of gall bladder

Fig. 49.2 *Examples of fever patterns from temperature charts* *vivax* in which paroxysms of malaria occur every 48 hours. Other examples are cytomegalovirus, Epstein-Barr mononucleosis and various pyogenic infections, e.g. ascending cholangitis.

Remittent fever
This is a fever in which the temperature returns towards normal for a variable period but is always elevated (Fig. 49.2d). Common examples are collections of pus, e.g. pelvic abscess, wound infection, empyema and carcinoma. It is a common feature of empyema.

Undulant fever
Undulant fever is characterised by bouts of continuous or remittent fever for several days, followed by afebrile remissions lasting a variable number of days. It is commonly a feature of brucellosis infection but is also seen in the lymphomas, especially Hodgkin's lymphoma (Fig. 49.2b).

Continuous fever pattern
This is common with viral infections such as influenza (Fig. 49.2c).

Quotidian fever
In this pattern the fever recurs daily (Fig. 49.2d). Daily fever spikes in the morning are characteristic of pseudomonas infection, e.g. pulmonary superinfection; afternoon spikes are indicative of cytomegalovirus infection; and evening spikes suggest localised collection of pus, e.g. empyema of the gall bladder.

Double quotidian fever (two fever spikes in a day) is caused by adult Still's disease, gonococcal endocarditis and visceral leishmaniasis.

If risk factors are present, especially if on antibiotics, consider the investigations outlined in Table 77.1.

Fever in children
The fever is usually a response to a viral infection. Fever itself is not harmful until it reaches a level of 41.5°.[1] Hyperthermia is uncommon in children. Temperatures above 41°C are usually due to CNS infection or the result of human error, e.g.
• shutting a child in a car on a hot day
• overwrapping a febrile child

Complications include dehydration (usually mild) and febrile convulsions, which occur in 5%

of febrile children between 6 months and 5 years. Febrile convulsions are triggered by a rapid rise in temperature rather than its absolute level.

Approach to the febrile infant
It is important to decide whether the child looks well or seriously ill. Identification of the very ill child is presented in Chapter 77.

If the child is well and has no risk factors (e.g. unreliable caregiver, poor access to treatment, medical risk factors, on antibiotics) treat expectantly. The only test required is urine microscopy and culture. Educate the caregiver about review if serious signs develop. Treat the fever as outlined in Table 77.1.

Management
• Treatment of low-grade fevers should be discouraged.
• Treatment of high-grade fevers includes:
  — treatment of the causes of the fever (if appropriate)
  — adequate fluid intake
  — paracetamol (acetaminophen) is the preferred antipyretic since aspirin is potentially dangerous in young children (use if temperature > 38.5°C). The usual dose of 10–15 mg/kg every 4–6 hours may represent undertreatment. Use 20 mg/kg as a loading dose and then 15 mg/kg maintenance.

Advice to parents
• Dress the child in light clothing (stripping off is unnecessary).
• Do not overheat with too many clothes, rugs or blankets.
• Give frequent small drinks of light fluids, especially water.
• Sponging with cool water and using fans is not effective.

Febrile convulsions
Refer to page 787.

Fever in the elderly
The elderly tend to have a problem with impaired thermoregulation and so they may not develop a fever in response to suppurative infection compared with younger people. This can be misleading in the diagnostic process.

Important facts

- Any fever in the elderly is significant.
- Viral infection is a less common cause of fever in the elderly.
- Fever in the elderly is sepsis until proven otherwise (common sites are the lungs and urinary tract).

The elderly are more vulnerable to hyperthermia and hypothermia. Heatstroke classically occurs in epidemic form during a heatwave. The syndrome consists of hyperpyrexia, decreased sweating, delirium and coma. The core temperature is usually over 41°C.

'Alarm bell' signs

In many patients the existence of a life-threatening infective illness is obvious and prompt action is essential. In others the diagnosis is not clear cut but there are certain warning signs:

- high fever
- repeated rigors
- drenching night sweats
- severe myalgia
- severe pain anywhere   } ? sepsis
- severe sore throat or dysphagia (? *Haemophilus influenzae* epiglottitis)
- altered mental state
- incessant vomiting
- unexplained rash
- jaundice
- marked pallor
- tachycardia
- tachypnoea

These symptoms and signs are obviously super 'sensitive'. Patients with some of these features may have potentially life-threatening diseases, but this list would include many with viral infections.

Fever of undetermined origin (FUO)

FUO, also referred to as pyrexia of unknown origin (PUO), has the following criteria:

- illness for at least 3 weeks
- fevers > 38°C (100.4°C)
- undiagnosed after 1 week of intensive study

Most cases represent unusual manifestations of common diseases and not rare or exotic diseases. Examples are tuberculosis, bacterial endocarditis, hepatobiliary disease and carcinoma of the lung.[5]

Patients with FUO in definite need of further investigation are:

- babies < 3 months of age
- children with fever > 40°C
- adults > 50 years
- diabetics
- the immunocompromised
- travellers

A diagnostic approach

A knowledge of the more common causes of FUO is helpful in planning a diagnostic approach (refer Table 49.2).

History

The history should include consideration of past history, occupation, travel history, sexual history, animal contact, and other relevant factors. Symptoms such as pruritus, a skin rash and fever patterns may provide clues for the diagnosis. The average patient with a difficult FUO needs to have a careful history taken on at least three separate occasions.[3]

Physical examination

A common mistake is the tendency to examine the patient only once and not re-examine. The patient should be examined regularly (as for history taking) as physical signs can develop eventually. Special attention should be paid to the following (Fig. 49.3):

- skin: look for rashes, vesicles and nodules
- the eyes and ocular fundi
- temporal arteries
- sinuses
- teeth and oral cavity: ? dental abscess, other signs
- heart: murmurs, pericardial rubs
- lungs: abnormalities including consolidation, pleuritic rub
- abdomen: enlarged/tender liver, spleen or kidney
- rectal and pelvic examination (note genitalia)
- lymph nodes, especially cervical (supraclavicular)
- blood vessels, especially of the legs ? thrombosis
- urine (analysis)

Investigations

Basic investigations include:

- haemoglobin, red cell indices and blood film
- white cell count

Table 49.2 *Common causes of FUO*

Common examples of each group selected

Infection (40%)

Bacteria
- pyogenic abscess, e.g. liver, pelvic
- urinary infection
- biliary infection, e.g. cholangitis
- chronic septicaemia
- infective endocarditis
- Lyme disease
- tuberculosis
- brucellosis
- osteomyelitis
- typhoid/paratyphoid fever

Viral, rickettsial, chlamydia
- Epstein-Barr mononucleosis
- cytomegalovirus
- HIV virus infection (AIDS, ARC)
- Q fever
- psittacosis

Parasitic
- malaria
- toxoplasmosis
- amoebiasis

Malignancy (30%)

Reticuloendothelial
- leukaemia
- lymphomas

Solid (localised) tumours
- kidney
- liver
- pancreas
- stomach
- lung

Disseminated

Immunogenic (20%)

Drugs

Connective tissue diseases/vasculitides
- rheumatic fever
- rheumatoid arthritis
- systemic lupus erythematosus
- polyarteritis nodosa
- giant cell arteritis/polymyalgia

Sarcoidosis

Crohn's disease

Factitious (1–5%)

Remain unknown (5–9%)

Source: After Kumar and Clark[6]

- ESR/C-reactive protein
- chest X-ray and sinus films
- urine examination (analysis and culture)
- routine blood chemistry
- blood cultures

Further possible investigations:

- stool microscopy and culture
- culture of sputum (if any)

- specific tests for typhoid, E-BM, Q fever, brucellosis, psittacosis, cytomegalovirus, toxoplasmosis, syphilis
- HIV screening
- tests for rheumatic fever
- tuberculin test
- tests for connective tissue disorders, e.g. DNA antibodies, C-reactive protein
- upper GIT series with small bowel follow-through
- CT and ultrasound scanning for 1° and 2° neoplasia
  — gall bladder functioning
  — occult abscesses
- isotope scanning for specific causes
- aspiration or needle biopsy
- laparoscopy for suspected pelvic infection
- tissue biopsies, e.g. lymph nodes, skin, liver, bone marrow (as indicated)

FUO in children

Fever in children is usually a transient phenomenon and subsides within 4–5 days. At least 70% of all infections are viral. Occasionally a child will present with FUO which may be masked from antibiotic administration. Common causes of prolonged fever in children differ from those in adults. Most cases are not due to unusual or esoteric disorders,[7] the majority representing atypical manifestation of common diseases.

A summary of the common causes (with the most common ranked first) is as follows.[7]

Infectious causes (40%)

- viral syndrome
- urinary tract infection
- pneumonia
- pharyngitis
- sinusitis
- meningitis

Collagen-vascular disorders (15%)

- rheumatic arthritis
- systemic lupus erythematosus
- rheumatic fever
- Henoch-Schönlein syndrome

Neoplastic disorders (7%)

- leukaemia
- reticulum cell sarcoma
- lymphoma

Inflammatory diseases of the bowel (4%)

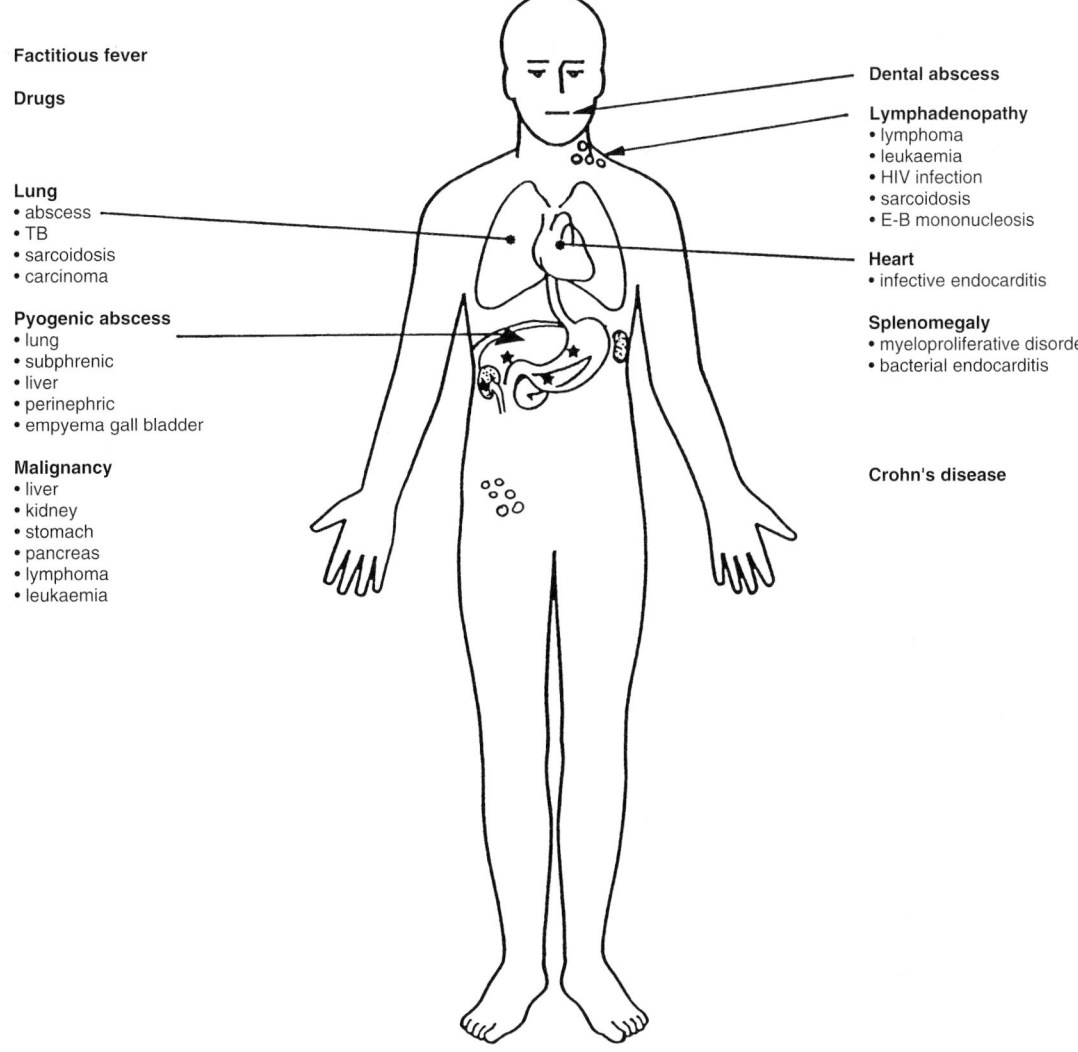

Factitious fever

Drugs

Lung
• abscess
• TB
• sarcoidosis
• carcinoma

Pyogenic abscess
• lung
• subphrenic
• liver
• perinephric
• empyema gall bladder

Malignancy
• liver
• kidney
• stomach
• pancreas
• lymphoma
• leukaemia

Dental abscess

Lymphadenopathy
• lymphoma
• leukaemia
• HIV infection
• sarcoidosis
• E-B mononucleosis

Heart
• infective endocarditis

Splenomegaly
• myeloproliferative disorder
• bacterial endocarditis

Crohn's disease

Fig. 49.3 *Sites to consider in FUO (malignancy is indicated by a star)*

Septicaemia
Definitions
Bacteraemia. This refers to the transient presence of bacteria in the blood (usually asymptomatic) caused by local infection or trauma.

Septicaemia. This refers to the multiplication of bacteria or fungi in the blood, usually causing severe systemic symptoms such as fever and hypotension. Septicaemia has a very high mortality and demands urgent attention.

Pyaemia. This is a serious manifestation of septicaemia whereby organisms and neutrophils undergo embolisation to many sites, causing abscesses especially in the lungs, liver and brain.

Primary septicaemia. This refers to septicaemia where the focus of infection is not apparent, while in *secondary septicaemia* a primary focus can be identified. Examples of secondary septicaemia in adults are:

• urinary tract, e.g. *Escherichia coli* (*E.coli*)
• respiratory tract, e.g. *Streptococcus pneumoniae*
• pelvic organs, e.g. *Neisseria gonorrhoea*
• skin, e.g. *Staphylococcus aureus*
• gall bladder, e.g. *E.coli*, *Streptococcus faecalis*

Patients with septicaemia require urgent referral.

References

1. Sewell J. Fever in childhood. Problems in clinical medicine. Aust Paed Review, 1990; 2:2.

2. Yung A, Stanley P. Problems in infectious diseases. In: Kincaid Smith et al. *Problems in clinical medicine*. Sydney: MacLennan and Petty, 1990, 326–335.

3. Wilson J et al. *Harrison's principles of internal medicine* (12th edn). New York: McGraw-Hill, 1991, 129–131.

4. Beck ER, Francis JL, Souhami RL. *Tutorials in differential diagnosis* (3rd edn). Edinburgh: Churchill Livingstone, 1995, 209–213.

5. Tierney LM et al. *Current medical diagnosis and treatment* (35th edn). Stamford: Appleton & Lange, 1996, 1111–1112.

6. Kumer PJ, Clark ML. *Clinical medicine* (2nd edn). London: Bailliere Tindall, 1990, 9.

7. Tunnessen WW Jr. *Signs and symptoms in paediatrics* (2nd edn). Philadelphia: JB Lippincott, 1988, 3–6.

50
Faints, fits and funny turns

—

Persons who have had frequent and severe attacks of swooning, without any manifest cause, die suddenly.

Hippocrates (?460–377 BC)
Aphorisms, 11, 41

When patients present with the complaint of a 'funny turn' it is usually possible to determine that they have one of the more recognisable presenting problems such as fainting, 'blackouts', lightheadedness, weakness, palpitations, vertigo or migraine. However, there are patients who do present with confusing problems that warrant the label of 'funny turn'. The most common problem with funny turns is that of misdiagnosis; so a proper and adequate history taking is of great importance.

It is important to remember that seemingly 'funny turns' may be the subjective interpretation of cultural and linguistic communication barriers, especially in an emotional and frustrated patient.[1] Various causes of faints, fits and funny turns are presented in Table 50.1. A useful simple classification is to consider them as:

- syncope
- seizures
- sleep disorders—sleep apnoea/narcolepsy/cataplexy
- labyrinthine

Key facts and checkpoints

- The commonest cause of 'funny turns' presenting in general practice is lightheadedness, often related to psychogenic factors such as anxiety, panic and hyperventilation.[2] Patients usually call this 'dizziness'.

- Absence attacks occur with minor forms of epilepsy and with partial seizures such as complex partial seizures.
- The psychomotor attack of complex partial seizure presents as a diagnostic difficulty. The most commonly misdiagnosed seizure disorder

Table 50.1 *Faints, fits and funny turns: checklist of causes (excluding tonic-clonic seizure and stroke)*

Psychogenic/communication problems
Conversion reactions (hysteria)
Culture/language conflicts
Fugue states
Hyperventilation
Malingering
Personality disorders
Phobia/anxiety states
Psychoses/severe depression

Other conditions
Transient ischaemic attacks
Complex partial seizure (temporal lobe epilepsy)
Tonic, clonic or atonic seizures
Primary absence seizure
Migraine variants or equivalents
Cardiovascular disorders
- arrhythmias
- postural hypotension
- aortic stenosis
Vertigo
Drug reaction
Alcohol and other substance abuse
Hypoglycaemia
Anaemia
Amnesic episodes
Metabolic/electrolyte disturbances
Vasovagal/syncope
Carotid sinus sensitivity
Cervical spondylosis
Sleep disorders
- sleep apnoea
- narcolepsy/cataplexy
Autonomic failure

is that of complex partial seizures or variants of generalised tonic clonic seizures (tonic or clonic or atonic).

- The diagnosis of epilepsy is made on the history (or video EEG), rather than on the standard EEG, although a sleep-deprived EEG is more effective.
- The triad—angina/dyspnoea/blackout or light-headedness—indicates aortic stenosis.
- Severe cervical spondylosis can cause vertebrobasilar ischaemia by causing pressure on the vertebral arteries that pass through the intervertebral foramina, especially with head turning or looking up.

The diagnostic approach

A summary of the diagnostic strategy model is presented in Table 50.2.

Table 50.2 *Faints, fits and funny turns: diagnostic strategy model*

Q. *Probability diagnosis*
A. Anxiety related/hyperventilation
Vasovagal syncope
Postural hypotension
Q. *Serious disorders not to be missed*
A. Cardiovascular
- arrhythmias
- aortic stenosis
Cerebrovascular
- TIAs
Neoplasia
- space-occupying lesions
Severe infections
- infective endocarditis
Hypoglycaemia
Q. *Pitfalls (often missed)*
A. Atypical migraine
Cardiac arrhythmias
Simple partial seizures
Complex partial seizures
Atypical tonic clonic seizures
Drugs/alcohol/marijuana
Electrolyte disturbances, e.g. hypokalaemia
Sleep disorders
  Rarities
  - Atrial myxoma
Q. *Seven masquerades checklist*
A. Depression   ✓
Diabetes   ✓ hypoglycaemia
Drugs   ✓
Anaemia   ✓
Thyroid disease   –
Spinal dysfunction   ✓ cervical spondylosis
UTI   –
Q. *Is this patient trying to tell me something?*
A. Highly likely. Psychogenic and 'communication' disorders quite significant.

History

The clinical history is of paramount importance in unravelling the problem. A reliable eye witness account of the 'turn' is invaluable, as is the setting or circumstances in which the 'episode' occurred.

It is essential at first to determine exactly what the patient means by 'funny turn'. In the process of questioning it is appropriate to evaluate the mental state and personal and social factors of the patient. It may be appropriate to confront the patient about feelings of depression, anxiety or detachment from reality.

It is important to break up the history into three components. The first is the lead-up to the episode, the second is adequate description of what took place during the episode and, thirdly, the events that took place after the episode.

Apart from the events note the patient's feelings, symptoms, circumstances and provocative factors. Search for possible secondary gain.

Onset

A sudden onset may be due to cardiovascular causes, especially arrhythmias, which may include the more common supraventricular tachycardias in addition to the less common but more dramatic arrhythmias that may cause unconsciousness. Other causes of a sudden onset include the various epilepsies, vasovagal attacks and TIAs.

Precipitating factors[2]

Enquire about precipitating factors such as emotion, stress, pain, heat, fright, exertion, suddenly standing up, coughing, head movement or hypersomnolence.

- emotion and stress suggest hyperventilation
- fright, pain → vasovagal attack
- standing up → postural hypotension
- exertion → aortic stenosis
- head movement → cervical spondylosis with vertebrobasilar insufficiency
- hypersomnolence → narcolepsy

Associated symptoms[2]

Certain associated symptoms give an indication of the underlying disorder:

- breathing problems and hyperventilation suggest an anxiety state
- tingling in extremities or tightening of the hand → anxiety/hyperventilation
- visual problems → migraine, TIA
- fear or panic → anxiety or complex partial seizure

- hallucinations (taste/smell/visual) → complex partial seizure
- speech problems → TIA/anxiety
- sweating, hunger feelings → hypoglycaemia
- related to food → migraine
- first thing in morning → consider 'hangover'

Drug history

This requires careful analysis and includes alcohol intake and illicit drugs such as marijuana, cocaine and amphetamines. Prescribed drugs that can cause lightheadedness or unconsciousness are listed in Table 50.3.

Sudden cessation of certain drugs such as phenothiazines can also be responsible for 'funny turns'.

Past history

The past history may give an indication of the cause of the 'turn'. Such conditions include hypertension, migraine, epilepsy, rheumatic heart disease, atherosclerosis, e.g. angina, vascular claudication, alcohol or other substance abuse and psychiatric disorders.

Diary of events

If the diagnosis is elusive it may help to get the patient to keep a diary of circumstances in which events take place, keeping in mind the importance of the time period prior, during and post episode.

The examination

Important focal points of the physical examination include:

- evaluation of the mental state, especially for anxiety

Table 50.3 *Typical drugs that may cause lightheadedness or blackouts*

Alcohol
Peripheral vasodilators
- ACE inhibitors
- glyceryl trinitrate
- hydralazine
- prazosin
Antiepileptics
Antihypertensives
Barbiturates
Benzodiazepines
Phenothiazines
Phenoxybenzamine
Tricyclic antidepressants
OTC anticholinergic compounds

- looking for evidence of anaemia, alcohol abuse and infection
- cerebrovascular examination: carotid arteries, ocular fundi, bruits
- cardiovascular examination: pulses, BP, heart (the BP should be taken lying, sitting and standing)
- the cervical spine

Various manoeuvres

Subject the patient to a number of manoeuvres to try to induce various sensations in order to try to identify the one that affects them. These should include sudden assumption of the erect posture from a squat, spinning the patient and then a sudden stop, head positioning with either ear down (Fig. 42.3), Valsalva manoeuvre, and hyperventilation for 60 seconds. Children can spin a showbag 'windmill' while hyperventilating (blowing). Ask 'Which one mimics your complaint?'

Investigations

Depending on the clinical findings, investigations can be selected from the following tests:

- Full blood count ? anaemia ? polycythaemia
- Blood sugar ? diabetes ? hypoglycaemia
- Urea and electrolytes
- ECG ? ischaemia ? arrhythmia
- 24 hour ambulatory cardiac (Holter) monitor ? arrhythmia
- Radiology/imaging
  - cervical X-ray
  - chest X-ray
  - carotid duplex Doppler scan: ? carotid artery stenosis
  - CT scan
  - MRI scan
- Electroencephalogram (EEG) or video EEG; EEGs include those recorded with sleep deprivation, hyperventilation or photic stimulation.
- Positron emission tomography (PET) or single photon emission computerised tomography (SPECT) may show localised brain dysfunction when others are negative.

Children

The various forms of seizures are also encountered in childhood when most patients with epilepsy are diagnosed.

Epilepsy syndromes

The following are special age-related epilepsy syndromes seen in children.[3,9]

Febrile seizures

Tonic-clonic seizures occur in 2–5% of children usually aged 6 months to 5 years who have a high fever generally caused by a viral infection. The long-term prognosis is good.

Infantile spasms (hypsarrhythmia)

These are generalised tonic seizures with sudden flexion of the arms, forward flexion of the trunk and extension of the legs, lasting only a few seconds, with usual age onset between 3 and 7 months. They are usually restricted to the first 3 years of life and are replaced by other forms of attacks. Prognosis for cognitive development is also unfavourable. The most effective therapy is corticotrophin (ACTH) IM injection. Otherwise, oral prednisolone or valproate can be used.

Lennox-Gastaut syndrome (myoclonic epilepsy of infancy)

This uncommon syndrome refers to a triad of severe difficult-to-control seizures (usually tonic with drop attack), mental retardation and characteristic EEG. The seizures usually begin between ages 1 and 6 years with a peak onset at 3 to 5 years. Prognosis is also poor. Sodium valproate is the therapy of choice.

Benign rolandic epilepsy

This disorder usually begins in children aged 2–13 years with a peak age of 5 to 8 years. There is a strong family history of epilepsy. The feature is a simple partial motor or somatosensory seizure involving the face and mouth during sleep, producing a typical 'glugging' sound. The child usually wakes from sleep, goes to the parents and is unable to speak and has hemifacial contortions. It may progress to a tonic–clonic seizure. There is a characteristic EEG pattern. The prognosis is excellent as remission usually occurs around puberty. Carbamazepine is the therapy of choice.

Childhood absence syndrome

These children present with frequent absence seizures, often over a hundred daily. Peak age of onset is 6 to 7 years. The absence seizures can be very subtle. Signs include alteration of awareness (usually in the classroom), sudden onset, facial and other automatisms.

Juvenile myoclonic epilepsy (myoclonic epilepsy of Janz)

There is a triad of seizures: myoclonic jerks, tonic–clonic seizures and absences. Onset is around puberty but may occur earlier. The myoclonic jerks and tonic–clonic seizures usually occur in the early morning after waking. Mental development is usually normal but the disorder is usually lifelong and is well controlled with sodium valproate.

Medial temporal lobe epilepsy

This syndrome of complex partial seizures, which usually last 1 to 3 minutes, is seen in childhood. Transient post-ictal confusion and speech dysfunction is common. Those with medically intractable seizures respond well to surgery.

Non-epileptic events resembling epileptic seizures[3]

Many normal and abnormal behaviours seen in children resemble seizures but are unrelated to epilepsy. A careful history is very important. The following are examples:

- *Postures of spasticity and movement disorders.* These occur in neurologically handicapped children such as those with cerebral palsy.
- *Syncope.* The child may describe a 'sinking feeling', or 'everything getting louder' prior to the loss of consciousness.
- *Breath-holding.* This often occurs after a crying spell and clonic movements may be seen at the end of the event.
- *Masturbation.* This behaviour leads to a tonic-like posture of the legs and preoccupation, especially in young girls.[4]
- *Münchausen-by-proxy.*[5] This syndrome of fictitious epilepsy described by a parent is becoming more recognised.
- *Psychogenic seizures (pseudo seizures).* A diagnostic dilemma exists when these co-exist with genuine seizures. These should be suspected when they occur in particular circumstances and the description of the 'seizure' is bizarre.
- *Shuddering.* Shuddering or shivering spells can resemble myoclonic jerks.
- *Night terrors.*[6] These episodes, which usually affect 2–4 year olds and 6–9 year olds, generally develop within 2 hours of sleep onset and last 1 to 2 minutes (sometimes longer). They are alarming and the child usually cannot be reassured or settled. A 6 week trial of phenytoin or imipramine can be used for severe problems.
- *Tics.* Motor tics can be quite complex but are usually brief involuntary movements involving the face and upper limbs.

Blackouts

The important causes of blackout include the various syncopes that are listed in Table 67.3 and the various forms of epilepsy. The classic tonic–clonic seizure is described in Chapter 67 (The unconscious patient) while descriptions of other seizures producing blackouts or funny turns now follow.

Important causes of convulsions (tonic–clonic seizures) are listed in Table 50.4.

Complex partial seizures

In complex partial seizures (known also as temporal lobe epilepsy) the symptomatology varies considerably from patient to patient and is often a diagnostic problem. It is the commonest type of focal epilepsy and the attacks vary in time from momentary to several minutes (usually 1 to 3 minutes).

Possible manifestations[2]

- Commonest: slight disturbance of perception and consciousness
- Hallucinations   — visual
       — taste
       — smell
       — sounds

Table 50.4 *Important causes of convulsive seizures*

- Epilepsy
  — first presentation
  — known patient with recurrence
- Cerebral hypoxia
- Hypoglycaemia
- Poor cerebral perfusion, e.g.
  — oedema of eclampsia
- Neurotrauma
- Cerebrovascular accident
- CNS infections, e.g.
  — meningitis
  — encephalitis
  — septicaemia
  — septic emboli
  — cerebral abscess
- Toxins
- Hyperthermia
- Metabolic disorders
- Drugs, e.g.
  — antidepressants
  — theophylline
  — amphetamine
  — cocaine
  — local anaesthetics
- Anaphylaxis
- Expanding brain lesion, e.g.
  — neoplasm
  — haematoma

- Absence attacks or vertigo
- Illusions—objects/people shrink or expand
- Affective feelings—fear, anxiety, anger
- Dyscognitive effects   — *déjà vu* (familiarity)
       — *jamais vu* (unreality)
       — waves emanating from epigastrium
- Objective signs   — lip-smacking
       — swallowing/chewing/ sucking
       — unresponsive to commands or questions
       — pacing around a room

Unreal or detached feelings are common in complex partial seizures. There can be permanent short-term memory loss. The sensation of strange smells or tastes is more common than auditory or visual hallucinations.[1] They can progress to tonic–clonic seizures.

Diagnosis

- EEG   — diagnostic in 50–60% of cases
       — a repeat EEG will increase rate to 60–80%
- EEG/video telemetry helpful with frequent attacks
- CT or MRI scan—to exclude tumour when diagnosis confirmed

Medication

- carbamazepine (1st choice)[7]
       or
- phenytoin (2nd choice)
       or (others)
- vigabatrin, sodium valproate, phenobarbitone

Tonic–clonic seizures

Variants of tonic–clonic seizures are more common than realised. Some patients may simply stiffen or drop to the ground while others may have one or two jerks or shakes only.

- stiffen and fall = tonic
- floppy and fall = atonic
- shaking only = clonic

Simple partial seizures

In simple partial seizures (Jacksonian epilepsy) there is no loss of consciousness. These include focal seizures, which may proceed to a generalised tonic–clonic seizure or to motor seizures.

Jacksonian (motor seizure)

Typically, jerking movements begin at the angle of the mouth or in the thumb and index finger and 'march' to involve the rest of the body, e.g. thumb → hand → limb → face ± leg on one side and then on to the contralateral side. A tonic–clonic or complex partial seizure may follow.

Medication

• carbamazepine (1st choice)[7]
             or
• phenytoin (2nd choice)
             or (others)
• sodium valproate, vigabatrin, gabapentin

Absence seizure (previously called petit mal)

This type of generalised epilepsy typically affects children from 4 years up to puberty.[2]

• child ceases activity and stares suddenly
• child is motionless (may blink or nod)
• no warning
• sometimes clonic (jerky) movement of eyelids, face, fingers
• may be lip-smacking or chewing (called complex absence)
• only lasts a few seconds—usually 5–10 seconds
• child then carries on as though nothing happened
• usually several per day (not just one or two)
• may lead to generalised seizures in adulthood

Diagnosis

Best evoked in the consulting room by hyperventilation and 'windmill'.
EEG • classic 3-H$_z$ wave and spike
     • may be normal
     • always include hyperventilation
     • easier with sleep deprivation

Medication

• ethosuximide (1st choice)[8]
             or
• sodium valproate (2nd choice)
             or (others)
• clonazepam, gabapentin

Note: Beware of hepatoxicity with sodium valproate, especially in those under 2 years.

Narcolepsy

Narcolepsy is characterised by brief spells of irresistible sleep during daytime hours, usually at times when the average person simply feels sleepy. Although patients are usually aware of their disorder some may have no insight into the problem and present with the complaint of unusual turns. Narcolepsy can present as 'attacks' in which the patient may crumple and fall without losing consciousness. It can be part of a tetrad syndrome (narcolepsy, cataplexy, hypnogogic hallucinations, sleep paralysis).

Other features:

• onset in teens or twenties
• can have several attacks per day

Diagnosis

• a clinical diagnosis

If doubtful

• EEG monitoring
• sleep laboratory studies (sleep latency test)—rapid eye movement is a hallmark

Medication

• amphetamines (in slowly increasing doses)
             or
          methylphenidate (Ritalin)
• tricyclic antidepressants, e.g. clomipramine, for associated cataplexy

Amnesic episodes

Amnesic episodes in which people cannot recall events or their own identity can be psychogenic (commonly) or related to an organic problem such as epilepsy, sleep apnoea or a cerebrovascular disorder. In the latter an unusual disorder—transient global amnesia—can occur.

Cerebrovascular disorders

Cerebrovascular disease is one of the major causes of mortality and morbidity in developed countries and can cause recurrent attacks of ischaemia in the carotid and vertebrobasilar systems (particularly vertebrobasilar insufficiency) which may present as 'funny turns'. In particular, brain stem ischaemia causes 'funny turns' such as impaired consciousness including transient global amnesia, drop attacks and the 'locked in' syndrome.

Psychogenic or communication disorders

Psychogenic causes have to be considered. 'Hysterical fugue' is one such manifestation. The problem can be a communication disorder, such as an emotional person trying to communicate a problem in a language foreign to them.

Patients with psychiatric disorders such as schizophrenia or depression may experience feelings of depersonalisation or unreality, which can be interpreted as a 'turn' or even temporal lobe epilepsy.

Patients who complain of vague and bizarre symptoms such as 'queer feelings in the head', 'swimming sensation', 'unreal feelings' and 'walking on air' are likely to have an anxiety state.

Severe anxiety or panic attacks typically cause lightheadedness that presents as a 'funny turn'. Other somatic symptoms include palpitations, sweating, inability to swallow, headache, breathlessness and manifestations of hyperventilation.

When to refer

- Transient ischaemic attacks, especially if the diagnosis is in doubt
- Clinical suspicion of or proven cardiac arrhythmias
- Evidence of aortic stenosis
- Seizures
- General uncertainty of the diagnosis

Pitfalls in management[2]

- The main pitfall associated with seizure disorders and epilepsy is misdiagnosis (not all seizures are generalised tonic–clonic in nature).
- Failing to place appropriate emphasis on the history in making the diagnosis.
- Misdiagnosing syncope with some involuntary movements for epilepsy.
- Overlooking cardiac arrhythmias as a cause of funny turns including recurrent dizziness.
- Failing to consider the possibility of aortic stenosis with syncopal attacks.
- Misdiagnosing vertigo and syncope for TIA.
- Mistaking visual or sensory migraine equivalents in young adults for TIA.
- Overlooking drugs (including self-administered drugs) as a cause of lightheadedness.

Practice tips

- A detailed clinical analysis is more important in the first instance than laboratory tests. The key to accurate diagnosis is a very careful history, taking the patient second by second through the attack and events preceding the turn.
- Talk to as many eye witnesses as possible in unravelling the cause.
- For 'undiagnosed turns' ask the patient to keep a diary with an accurate record of the attack including preceding events.
- Remember that migraine is a great mimic and can cause confusion in diagnosis.
- Remember that the EEG can be normal in the confirmed epileptic.
- The more bizarre the description of a 'funny turn', the more likely a functional problem is the cause.

References

1. Kincaid-Smith P, Larkins R, Whelan G. *Problems in clinical medicine*. Sydney: MacLennan & Petty, 1990, 159–164.
2. Sandler G, Fry J. *Early clinical diagnosis*. Lancaster: MTP Press, 1986, 411–430.
3. Stewart I, Bye A. The diagnosis of childhood fits and funny turns. Mod Med Aust, 1994; 37(8):65–72.
4. Fleisher DR, Morrison A. Masturbation mimicking abdominal pain or seizures in young girls. J Paediatr, 1990; 116: 810–814.
5. Meadow R. Fictitious epilepsy. Lancet, 1984; 2:25–28.
6. Rothner AD. Not everything that shakes is epilepsy: The differential diagnosis of paroxysmal nonepileptiform disorders. Cleve Clin J Med, 1989; 56 Suppl part 2: 206S–213S.
7. Scott AK. Management of epilepsy. In: *Central nervous system*. London: British Medical Association, 1995, 1–2.
8. Levine M et al. *Drugs of choice: A formulary for general practice*. Ottawa: Canadian Medical Association, 1995, 98–99.
9. Moulds RFW (Chairman). *Therapeutic Guidelines: Neurology*. Melbourne: Therapeutic Guidelines Limited, 1997, 87–102.

51

Haematemesis and melaena

—

*The 'once smelt never forgotten' sickly smell of
melaena can be diagnosed from a distance of 20
metres without trying.*

Emergency room supervisor
Brisbane 1985

Acute severe upper gastrointestinal (GI) haemorrhage is an important medical emergency. The
dramatic symptom of haematemesis follows
bleeding from the oesophagus, stomach and
duodenum. Over half the patients are over 60
years of age.[1]

Haematemesis is the vomiting of blood.
Melaena is the passage of black tarry stools, with
50 mL or more of blood required to produce
melaena stool. Melaena occurs in most patients
with upper GI haemorrhage and haematemesis
occurs in over 50%.[1]

Key facts and checkpoints

- Chronic peptic ulceration accounts for most
  cases of upper GI haemorrhage.
- Haematemesis is almost always associated
  with some degree of blood in the stools,
  although melaena may not necessarily accompany it, especially if bleeding occurs from the
  oesophagus.
- Black stool caused by oral iron therapy or
  bismuth-containing antacid tablets can cause
  confusion.
- Always check for a history of drug intake, especially aspirin and NSAIDs.
- Corticosteroids in conventional therapeutic
  doses are thought to have no influence on GI
  haemorrhage.
- The volume of the bleeding is best assessed by
  its haemodynamic effects rather than relying
  on the patient's estimation, which tends to be
  excessive.

- Melaena is generally less life-threatening than
  haematemesis.
- Resuscitation of the patient is the first task.
- A sudden loss of 20% or more circulatory blood
  volume usually produces signs of shock such as
  tachycardia, hypotension, faintness and sweating. Younger patients can compensate better
  and tolerate a larger loss prior to the development of shock.[1] A useful guide is that shock in a
  previously well 70 kg man indicates an acute
  blood loss of at least 1000–1500 mL.

Causes of upper GI bleeding

The major cause of bleeding is chronic peptic
ulceration of the duodenum and stomach, which
accounts for approximately half of all cases.[2] The
other major cause is acute gastric ulcers and erosions, which account for at least 20% of cases.
Aspirin and NSAIDs are responsible for many of
these bleeds. Causes are summarised in Table
51.1 and illustrated in Figure 51.1.

Table 51.1 *Causes of upper gastrointestinal
bleeding*[3,4]

Common causes
1. Duodenal ulcer
2. Gastric erosion
3. Gastric ulcer
4. Reflux oesophagitis
5. Oesophageal varices
6. Mallory-Weiss syndrome

Others
- Gastric or oesophageal carcinoma
- Stomal ulcer
- Blood dyscrasias
- Anticoagulant therapy
- Vascular malformations
- Hereditary haemorrhagic telangiectasia
  (Rendu-Osler-Weber syndrome)

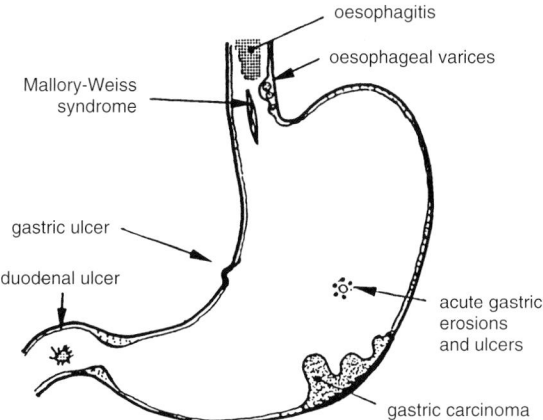

Fig. 51.1 *Important causes of haematemesis and melaena*

Mallory-Weiss syndrome

In this condition a tear occurs at the lower end of the oesophageal mucosa (at the oesophago-gastric junction) because of an episode of severe or protracted vomiting or coughing. Blood appears in the vomitus after a bout of heavy vomiting or dry retching. It is usually seen in alcoholic patients. It is usually a self-limiting lesion. A definite diagnosis can only be made by oesophagoscopy.

Gastro-oesophageal varices

Such varices are caused by portal hypertension, which in turn is usually due to cirrhosis of the liver. There is a raised incidence of peptic ulcer in those with liver cirrhosis, especially in biliary and alcohol-induced cirrhosis; so this should be kept in mind as a possible source of bleeding. Mortality is about 30%, despite advances.[4]

Management includes injection sclerotherapy, and then intravenous octreotide if it fails. Passage of a Sengstaken-Blakemore or Minnesota tube into the oesophagus and stomach to provide tamponade and the radiological procedure of using a transjugular intrahepatic porto-systemic stent are possible options.

The clinical approach
History

It is important to establish the nature of the vomitus and the possibility of bleeding arising from the mouth, nose or pharynx. A coffee grounds vomitus indicates that the blood has been in contact with gastric acid. Oesophageal bleeding tends to lead to vomiting of fresh blood. Questions to help pinpoint the possible aetiology should be asked.

Key questions

- What drugs have you been taking?
- Have you been taking aspirin or tablets for arthritis or back pain?
- How much have you vomited?
- What did the vomit look like?
- Do you notice black dots like coffee grounds or any blood clots?
- Have you had any indigestion, heartburn or stomach pains recently?
- Have you opened your bowels and if so what was the colour?
- Have you noticed whether your bowel motions were black or unusual in any way?
- How much alcohol do you drink?
- Have you had any previous operations on your stomach for a peptic ulcer?
- Were you vomiting normal vomit before the blood appeared?

Physical examination

The patient's general state, particularly the circulation, should be assessed immediately on presentation. A careful abdominal examination should be performed including a digital rectal examination. As a rule abdominal findings are not remarkable except when a mass, hepatomegaly or splenomegaly is found. Other evidence of liver disease should be sought.

Investigations

Investigations to determine the source of the bleeding should be carried out in a specialist unit. Upper gastrointestinal endoscopy is the single most useful test and will detect the cause of the bleeding in at least 80% of cases.[2]

The haemoglobin level will not be an appropriate guide to blood loss or the need for transfusion during the early stages, because haemodilution occurs gradually over the 24 hours following a severe bleed. However, a level below 90 g/L during this period is usually regarded as an indication for transfusion.

Management

The immediate objectives are:

1. restore an effective blood volume (if necessary)
2. establish a diagnosis to allow definitive treatment

A diagnostic approach

A summary of the safety diagnostic model is presented in Table 52.1.

Probability diagnosis

The commonest cause of headache presenting in general practice is respiratory infection.[1] For chronic recurrent headache the author has found that tension and combination headaches

Table 52.1 *Headache: diagnostic strategy model*

Q.	*Probability diagnosis*
A.	Acute: respiratory infection
	Chronic: • tension-type headache
	• combination headache
	• migraine
Q.	*Serious disorders not to be missed*
A.	Cardiovascular
	• subarachnoid haemorrhage
	• intracerebral haemorrhage
	• temporal arteritis
	Neoplasia
	• cerebral tumour
	• pituitary tumour
	Severe infections
	• meningitis, esp. fungal
	Haematoma: extradural/subdural
	Glaucoma
	Benign intracranial hypertension
Q.	*Pitfalls (often missed)*
A.	Cervical spondylosis/dysfunction
	Dental disorders
	Refractive errors of eye
	Sinusitis
	Ophthalmic herpes zoster (pre-eruption)
	Exertional headache
	Hypoglycaemia
	Post-traumatic headache
	Post-spinal procedure, e.g. epidural
	Sleep apnoea
	Rarities
	• Paget's disease
	• Post-sexual intercourse
	• Cushing's syndrome
	• Conn's syndrome
	• Addison's disease
	• Dysautonomic cephalgia
Q.	*Seven masquerades checklist*
A.	Depression ✓✓
	Diabetes ✓
	Drugs ✓✓
	Anaemia ✓
	Thyroid disease ✓
	Spinal dysfunction ✓
	UTI ✓
Q.	*Is the patient trying to tell me something?*
A.	Quite likely if there is an underlying psychogenic disorder.

are the commonest, with combination (mixed) headache responsible for 21% of these presentations. Combination headaches, typified by relatively constant pain lasting for many days, have a mix of components such as tension, depression, cervical dysfunction, vascular headache and drug dependence. Migraine is not as common in general practice as it is in consultant practice. Tension headache too is far less common than previously promulgated.[3]

Serious disorders not to be missed

For the acute onset of headache it is vital not to miss subarachnoid haemorrhage or meningitis. Intracranial haemorrhage, especially involving cerebellar, intraventricular and frontal lobe areas, needs to be considered. It is worth keeping in mind the special problem of people taking monoamine (MAO) inhibitors who imbibe foodstuffs containing tyramine and other catechol derivatives, for example, cheese, yeast extracts, broad beans, cream, chocolate and alcohol. For chronic headache, space-occupying lesions including subdural haematomas must be considered. Since headaches tend to decrease with age, headaches developing in the elderly should be viewed with suspicion and this includes considering temporal arteritis. Benign intracranial hypertension should be considered, especially in young obese women. The dangerous cryptococcal meningitis can be difficult, as the CT scan may be normal.

Pitfalls

The list (Table 52.1) contains some controversial causes of headache, although some should be obvious if a careful history is elucidated. These include post-traumatic headache; postprocedural headache, for example lumbar puncture and spinal anaesthesia; and exertional headache. Sinusitis can be overlooked in the absence of respiratory signs. Refractive errors of the eye, although an uncommon cause of headache, do warrant consideration.

General pitfalls

- Overinvestigating the patient with headache, especially as a substitute for a careful history and examination
- Failing to appreciate that a combination of factors and cervical dysfunction are common causes of headache

- Omitting to measure the blood pressure in the patient complaining of headache
- Rushing in with antibiotics for a patient (especially children) with fever and headache—bacterial meningitis may be masked
- Attributing the early headache of a space-occupying lesion to tension or hypertension

Seven masquerades checklist

Of the masquerades, depression and drugs are important causes of headache. Cervical dysfunction is certainly an important cause and tends to be ignored by some doctors. Australian figures are misleading because many of these patients gravitate to alternative health professionals.

A United Kingdom study placed headache from cervical spondylosis on almost equal terms with migraine.[1]

The explanation for referral of pain from disorders of the upper cervical spine to the head and eye is that some afferent fibres from the upper three cervical nerve roots converge on cells in the posterior horn of the spinal cord (which can also be excited by trigeminal afferent fibres), thus conveying to the patient the impression of head pain through this shared pathway (Fig. 52.1).

Significant drug causes are listed in Table 52.2. Anaemia can cause headache, usually if the haemoglobin level falls below 10 g/dL.[1] Hypo- and hyper-thyroidism may also cause headache, and in diabetics hypoglycaemia is often responsible.

Table 52.2 *Drugs that can cause headache*

Alcohol
Analgesics (rebound), e.g. aspirin
                                     codeine
Antibiotics and antifungals
Antihypertensives, e.g. methyldopa
                          beta-blockers, e.g. atenolol
                          hydralazine
                          reserpine
                          calcium channel blockers, e.g.
                          nifedipine
Caffeine
Corticosteroids
Cyclosporin
Dipyridamole
Ergotamine (rebound)
H_2-antagonists, e.g. cimetidine
                          ranitidine
MAO inhibitors
Nicotine
Nitrazepam
Nitrous oxide
NSAIDs, e.g. indomethacin
Oral contraceptives
Retinoids
Sympathomimetics
Theophylline
Vasodilators, e.g. calcium channel blockers, nitrates

Psychogenic considerations

Headache, like tiredness, is one of those symptoms that may reflect a 'hidden agenda'. Of course the patient may be depressed (overt or masked) or may have a true anxiety state. The most characteristic feature of psychogenic headache is that the headache is present virtually every minute of the day for weeks or months on end. However, it is common for patients to deny that they are anxious, depressed or unduly stressed. For this reason a detailed history is important to identify lifestyle factors and historical events that can be associated with headache.

Some patients are fearful of their headache lest it represent a cerebral tumour, stroke or hypertension and need appropriate reassurance.

Conversion reactions and other aspects of compensation rewards, especially following an accident, e.g. rear-end collision, may make the symptom of headache difficult to manage. Headache, like backache, is one of the prime symptoms perpetuated or exaggerated for secondary gain.

Severe headaches, especially simulated migraine, are common 'tickets of entry' for drug

Fig. 52.1 *Typical headache referral patterns for dysfunction of the upper cervical spinal segments*

addicts seeking narcotics from empathic practitioners. Such patients require very skilled management.

Diurnal patterns of pain

Plotting the fluctuation of headache during the day provides vital clues to the diagnosis (Fig. 52.2). The patient who wakes up with headache could have vascular headache (migraine), cervical spondylosis, depressive illness, hypertension or a space-occupying lesion. It is usual for migraine to last hours, not days, which is more characteristic of tension headache. The pain of frontal sinusitis follows a typical pattern, namely onset around 9 a.m., building to a maximum by about 1 p.m., and then subsiding over the next few hours. In the absence of respiratory symptoms it is likely to be misdiagnosed as tension headache. The pain from combination headache tends to follow a most constant pattern throughout the day and does not usually interrupt sleep.

Fig. 52.2 *Typical diurnal patterns of various causes of headache; the relative intensity of pain is plotted on the vertical axis*

The clinical approach
History
A full description of the pain including a pain analysis should be obtained. This includes:

• site
• radiation
• quality
• frequency
• duration
• onset and offset
• precipitating factors
• aggravating and relieving factors
• associated symptoms

It is useful to get the patient to plot on a prepared grid the relative intensity of the pain and the times of day (and night) that the pain is present.

Key questions[5]
• Can you describe your headaches?
• How often do you get them?
• Can you point to exactly where in the head you get them?
• Do you have any pain in the back of your head or neck?
• What time of the day do you get the pain?
• Do you notice any other symptoms when you have the headache?
• Do you feel nauseated and do you vomit?
• Do you experience any unusual sensations in your eyes, such as flashing lights?
• Do you get dizzy, weak or have any strange sensations?
• Does light hurt your eyes?
• Do you get any blurred vision?
• Do you notice watering or redness of one or both of your eyes?
• Do you get pain or tenderness on combing your hair?
• Are you under a lot of stress or tension?
• Does your nose run when you get the headache?
• What tablets do you take?
• Do you get a high temperature, sweats or shivers?
• Have you had a heavy cold recently?
• Have you ever had trouble with your sinuses?
• Have you had a knock on your head recently?
• What do you think causes the headaches?

Differences between the clinical features of migraine and tension headache are presented in Table 52.3.

Table 52.3 *A comparison of typical clinical features of migraine and tension headache*

	Migraine	Tension headache
Family history	✓	
Onset before 20	✓	
Prodromata	✓	
Bilateral		✓
Unilateral	✓	
Throbbing	✓	
Constant		✓
Less than 1 per week	✓	
Continuous daily		✓
Lasts less than 24 hrs	✓	
Vomiting	✓	
Aggravated by the pill	✓	
Aggravated by alcohol	✓	
Relieved by alcohol		✓

Physical examination

For the physical examination it is appropriate to use the basic tools of trade, namely the thermometer, sphygmomanometer, pen torch, and diagnostic set, including the ophthalmoscope and the stethoscope. Inspect the head, temporal arteries and eyes. Areas to palpate include the temporal arteries, the facial and neck muscles, the cervical spine and sinuses, the teeth and temporomandibular joints. Search especially for signs of meningeal irritation and papilloedema.

A mental state examination is mandatory and includes looking for altered consciousness or cognition and assessment of mood, anxiety–tension–depression, and any mental changes. Neurological examination includes assessment of visual fields and acuity, reactions of the pupils and eye movements in addition to sensation and motor power in the face and limbs.

Special signs

Upper cervical pain sign: Palpate over the C2 and C3 areas of the cervical spine, especially two finger-breadths out from the spinous process of C2. If this is very tender and even provokes the headache it indicates headache of cervical origin.

Ewing's sign for frontal sinusitis. Press your finger gently upwards and inwards against the orbital roof medial to the supraorbital nerve. Pain on pressure is a positive finding and indicates frontal sinusitis.

The invisible pillow sign. The patient lies on the examination table with head on a pillow. The examiner then supports the head with his or her hands as the pillow is removed. The patient is instructed to relax the neck muscles and the examiner removes the supporting hands. A positive test indicating tension from contracting neck muscles is when the patient's head does not readily change position. This is uncommon.

Investigations

Investigations can be selected from:

- Haemoglobin: ? anaemia
- WCC: leucocytosis with bacterial infection
- ESR: ? temporal arteritis
- Radiography
  - chest X-ray, if suspected intracerebral malignancy
  - cervical spine
  - skull X-ray, if suspected brain tumour, Paget's disease, deposits in skull
  - sinus X-ray, if suspected sinusitis
  - CT scan • detection of brain tumour (most effective)
    - cerebrovascular accidents (valuable)
    - subarachnoid haemorrhage
  - radioisotope scan (technetium-99) to localise specific tumours and haematoma
  - magnetic resonance imaging: very effective for intracerebral pathology but expensive; produces better definition of intracerebral structures than CT scanning but not as sensitive for detecting bleeding
  - lumbar puncture
    - diagnosis of meningitis
    - suspected SAH (only if CT scan normal)
  - *Note:* Dangerous if raised intracranial pressure.

Headache in children

Respiratory infections and febrile illnesses are a common cause of headache in children but there are other causes that reflect the common causes in adults. Many childhood headaches are isolated but are chronic in a significant number. Migraine is relatively common before adolescence, while tension or muscle contraction headache is more common after adolescence.

Young children rarely experience sinus headache and this should not really be considered until the sinuses develop, around 5 years for the frontal sinuses.

From 1% of 7-year-olds to 5% or more of 15-year-old children suffer from migraine, with girls developing it at a higher rate[2] with increasing age. There is a strong family history. As a rule the prognosis is good as the majority will have no migraines in the long term. The type is mainly common migraine with symptoms such as malaise or nausea: classic migraine with the typical aura is not a feature of childhood migraine. The rather dramatic migraine, such as vertebrobasilar migraine, is frequent in adolescent girls and hemiplegia occurs in infants and children, especially with their first migraine attack .[7] Vomiting is not necessarily an associated symptom in children.

The possibility of cerebral space-occupying lesions requires due consideration, especially if the headaches are progressive. These are present typically in the morning and are associated with symptoms such as vomiting, dizziness, diplopia, ataxia, personality changes and deterioration of school performance. Symptoms that indicate a cerebral tumour or other serious problem are outlined in Table 52.4.

Table 52.4 *Pointers to serious causes of headache in children*

Headache features

Persistent

Present first thing in morning

Wakes child at night

No past history

No family history

Associated poor health

Associated neurological symptoms

Unilateral localisation

Source: After Wright[2]

Neonates and children aged 6–12 months are at the greatest risk from meningitis and it is important to keep this in mind.

Management of the non-serious causes of headache includes reassurance (especially of parents), discouragement of excessive emphasis on the symptom and simple medications such as paracetamol for the younger child and aspirin for the adolescent.

Headaches in the elderly

The recent onset of headache in the elderly has to be treated with caution because it could herald a serious problem such as a space-occupying lesion (e.g. neoplasm, subdural haematoma), temporal arteritis, trigeminal neuralgia or vertebrobasilar insufficiency. Cervical spondylosis is age-related and may be an important factor in the ageing patient. Age-related headaches are summarised in Table 52.5.

Late-life migraine can be mistaken for cerebrovascular disease, especially in the presence of preceding neurological symptoms. It is the sequence of the visual and sensory symptoms with the spread from face to tongue to hand over some minutes, with clearing in one area as it appears, that helps distinguish migraine from transient ischaemic attacks (TIAs). Although some patients experience headache with TIAs it is not a distinguishing feature. Vomiting is suggestive of migraine rather than cerebrovascular disease.[7]

Table 52.5 *Age-related causes of headache*

Children	• Intercurrent infections
	• Psychogenic
	• Migraine
	• Meningitis
	• Post-traumatic
Adults including middle age	• Migraine
	• Cluster headache
	• Tension
	• Cervical dysfunction
	• Subarachnoid haemorrhage
	• Combination
Elderly	• Cervical dysfunction
	• Cerebral tumour
	• Temporal arteritis
	• Neuralgias
	• Paget's disease
	• Glaucoma
	• Cervical spondylosis
	• Subdural haemorrhage

Tension-type headache

Tension or muscle contraction headaches are typically a symmetrical tightness. They tend to last for hours and recur each day. They are often associated with cervical dysfunction and stress or tension, although the patient usually does not realise the headaches are associated with tension until it is pointed out. Seventy-five per cent of patients are female.[3]

Typical clinical features

• Site: frontal, over forehead and temples (Fig. 52.3)

• Radiation: occiput

Fig. 52.3 *Typical distribution of pain in tension-type headache*

- Quality: dull ache, like a 'tight pressure feeling', 'heavy weight on top of head', 'tight band around head'; may be tightness or vice-like feeling rather than pain.
- Frequency: almost daily
- Duration: hours (can last days)
- Onset: after rising, gets worse during day
- Aggravating factors: stress, overwork with skipping meals
- Relieving factors: alcohol
- Associated features: lightheadedness, fatigue; neck ache or stiffness (occiput to shoulders); perfectionist personality; anxiety/depression
- Physical examination: muscle tension, e.g. frowning; scalp often tender to touch; 'invisible pillow' sign may be positive

IHS criteria for tension-type headache

The International Headache Society (IHS) criteria for episodic tension-type headaches involve the following:

1. The patient should have had at least ten of these headaches.
2. The headaches last from 30 minutes to 7 days.
3. The headaches must have at least two of the following four:
   (a) non-pulsating quality
   (b) mild or moderate intensity
   (c) bilateral location
   (d) no aggravation with routine physical activity

4. The headaches must have both of the following:
   (a) no nausea or vomiting
   (b) photophobia and phonophobia are absent, or one but not the other is present
5. There should be less than 15 days of headache per month and less than 180 days per year.
6. Secondary causes are excluded.

Management

- Careful patient education: explain that the scalp muscles get tight like the calf muscles when climbing up stairs.
- Counselling and relevant advice, e.g.
  — Learn to relax your mind and body.
  — During an attack, relax by lying down in a hot bath and practise meditation.
  — Be less of a perfectionist: do not be a slave to the clock.
  — Don't bottle things up, stop feeling guilty, approve of yourself, express yourself and your anger.
- Advise and demonstrate massage of the affected area with a soothing analgesic rub.
- Advise stress reduction, relaxation therapy and yoga or meditation classes.
- Medication—use mild analgesics such as aspirin or paracetamol. Discourage stronger analgesics. Avoid tranquillisers and antidepressants if possible, but consider these drugs if symptoms warrant medication, e.g. amitriptyline 10–75 mg (o) nocte increasing to 150 mg if necessary. Diazepam (short-term use) appears to be very effective in middle-aged men; it is prone to cause depression in women.

Special notes
- The general aim is to direct patients to modify their lifestyle and avoid tranquillisers and analgesics.
- It is unusual to be awoken from sleep.
- Beware of depression.
- Consider muscle energy therapy and/or mobilisation of the neck followed by exercises if there is evidence of cervical dysfunction.
- Recommend a meditation program.

Migraine

Migraine, or the 'sick headache', is derived from the Greek word meaing 'pain involving half the head'. It affects at least 1 person in 10, is more common in females and peaks between 20 and 50 years. There are various types of migraine

Table 52.6 *Types of vascular headache*

Common migraine (aura is vague or absent)

Classic migraine

Complicated migraine

Unusual forms of migraine
• hemiplegic
• basilar
• retinal
• migrainous stupor
• ophthalmoplegic
• migraine equivalents
• status migrainosus

Cluster headache

Chronic paroxysmal hemicrania

Menstrual migraine

Lower half headache

Benign exertional-sex headache (beware of SAH)

Miscellaneous, e.g. icepick pains, ice-cream headache

Source: After Day[8]

(Table 52.6) with classic migraine (headache, vomiting and aura) and common migraine (without the aura) being the best known.

The most common trigger factor is stress.[3]

Typical clinical features of classic migraine

• Site: temporofrontal region
                       (unilateral) (Fig. 52.4);
                       can be bilateral
• Radiation: retro-orbital and occipital
• Quality: intense and throbbing
• Frequency: 1 to 2 per month
• Duration: 4 to 72 hours (average
                       6–8 hours)
• Onset: paroxysmal, often wakes
                       with it
• Offset: spontaneous (often after
                       sleep)

• Precipitating   tension and stress
  factors: (commonest); others in
                       Table 52.7
• Aggravating factors: tension, activity
• Relieving factors: sleep, vomiting
• Associated factors: nausea, vomiting (90%)
                       irritability
                       aura —visual 25%
                            (scintillation,
                            scotoma,
                            hemianopia,
                            fortification)
                       —sensory (unilateral
                            paraesthesia)
• Other pointers: abdominal pain in child-
                       hood; family history of
                       migraine, asthma and
                       eczema

IHS criteria for common migraine
The IHS criteria for migraine without aura involves this checklist.

Table 52.7 *Migrainous trigger factors*

Exogenous

• Foodstuffs—chocolate, oranges, tomatoes, citrus fruits, cheeses
• Alcohol—especially red wine
• Drugs—vasodilators, oestrogens, monosodium glutamate, nitrites ('hot dog' headache), indomethacin, OCP
• Glare or bright light
• Emotional stress
• Head trauma (often minor) e.g. jarring—'footballer's migraine'
• Allergens
• Climatic change
• Excessive noise
• Strong perfume

Endogenous

• Tiredness, physical exhaustion, oversleeping
• Stress, relaxation after stress: 'weekend migraine'
• Exercise
• Hormonal changes
    — puberty
    — menstruation
    — climacteric
    — pregnancy
• Hunger
• Familial tendency
• ? Personality factors

Fig. 52.4 *Typical distribution of pain in migraine (right side)*

1. The patient should have had at least five of these headaches.
2. The headaches last 4–72 hours.
3. The headache must have at least two of the following:
   (a) unilateral location
   (b) pulsing quality
   (c) moderate or severe intensity, inhibiting or prohibiting daily activities
   (d) headache worsened by routine physical activity
4. The headache must have at least two of the following:
   (a) nausea and/or vomiting
   (b) photophobia and phonophobia
5. Secondary causes of headache are excluded (e.g. normal exam and/or imaging study)

IHS criteria for migraine with typical aura (classic)
There should be at least two attacks, including at least three of the following:
1. reversible brain symptoms (cortical or brain stem)
2. gradual development over 4 minutes
3. aura duration less than 60 minutes
4. headache follows aura in less than 1 hour
Note: If the aura lasts longer than 1 hour, it is migraine with prolonged aura. If it lasts longer than 24 hours, it is a migrainous infarction (stroke).

Management
Patient education—provide explanation and reassurance, especially if bizarre visual and neurological symptoms are present. Patients should be reassured about the benign nature of their migraine.

Counselling and advice
- Tailor the advice to the individual patient.
- Avoid known trigger factors, especially tension, fatigue, hunger and constant physical and mental stress.
- Advise keeping a diary of foodstuffs or drinks that can be identified as trigger factors. Consider a low amine diet: eliminate chocolate, cheese, red wine, walnuts, tuna, vegemite, spinach and liver.
- Practise a healthy lifestyle, relaxation programs, meditation techniques and biofeedback training.
- Be open to non-drug therapies, e.g. trial of acupuncture, hypnotherapy.

Treatment of the acute attack
- Commence treatment at earliest impending sign.
- Mild headaches may require no more than conventional treatment with '2 aspirin (or paracetamol), and a good lie down in a quiet dark room'.[8]
- Rest in a quiet, darkened, cool room.
- Place cold packs on the forehead or neck.
- Avoid drinking coffee, tea or orange juice.
- Avoid moving around too much.
- Do not read or watch television.
- For patients who find relief from simply 'sleeping off' an attack, consider prescribing temazepam 10 mg or diazepam 10 mg in addition to the following measures.[3]
- For moderate attacks use oral ergotamine or sumatriptan and for severe attacks use injection therapy.

Medication (if necessary)

| First-line medication |
- Aspirin or paracetamol + antiemetic:
  e.g. soluble aspirin 600–900 mg (o)
                    and
  metoclopramide 10 mg (o)
- Paracetamol (for children)
- Consider NSAIDs, e.g. ibuprofen

| Alternatives |

Choose an ergotamine preparation or sumatriptan.
- Ergotamine (helps about 80% of patients)
  — oral: e.g. ergotamine 1 mg + caffeine
            100 mg (Cafergot)
            2 tabs at 1st warning then 60 minutes
            if necessary (maximum 6 per day)
     May need metoclopramide (o), IM or IV
                    or
  — suppository: e.g. ergotamine 2 mg + caffeine 100 mg (Cafergot S)
            1 suppository at 1st warning
            then ½ every 60 minutes
            (maximum 3 per day)
                    or
  — medihaler: e.g. 1 inhalation statim then
            every 5 minutes (maximum 6
            per day)
                    or
  — IM injection: e.g. dihydroergotamine 0.5–1
            mg, preceded by metoclopramide 10 mg
            IM, 20 minutes beforehand.

- Sumatriptan (a serotonin receptor agonist)[9]
  — 50–100 mg (o) at the time of prodrome, repeat in 2 hours if necessary to maximum dose 300 mg/24 hours
    or
  — nasal spray 10–20 mg per nostril
    or
  — 6 mg, SC injection, repeat in 1 or more hours to maximum dose 12 mg/24 hours
  Avoid sumatriptan in patients with coronary artery disease, Prinzmetal angina, uncontrolled hypertension or during pregnancy. Do not use it with ergotamine simultaneously and cease if chest pain develops, albeit transient in a young patient.
- zolmitriptan 2.5 mg (o), repeat in 2 hours if necessary
    or
- naratriptan 2.5 mg (o), repeat in 4 hours

| *The severe attack* | (if other preparations ineffective)

Caution: Consider the possibility of underlying cerebral vascular malformation, subarachnoid haemorrhage or pethidine addiction.
- If at home:[10]
  — dihydroergotamine 0.5–1 mg (IM) + metoclopramide 10 mg (IM)
    or
  — sumatriptan 6 mg (SC)
- If in surgery or emergency room:
  — metoclopramide 10 mg (IV) slowly over 2 minutes + oral analgesics
    or
  — metoclopramide 10 mg (IV) + dihydroergotamine 0.5 mg IV slowly
    or
  — sumatriptan 6 mg (SC)

Caution: Do not use ergotamine preparations if sumatriptan used in previous 6 hours, and do not use sumatriptan if ergotamine preparations used in previous 24 hours.
- Consider lignocaine 1% IV infusion of 1 mg/kg slowly over 90 seconds, e.g. 7 mL in a 70 kg adult.

Note: Lignocaine is reportedly successful but awaiting trials. Contraindications include known hypersensitivity to local anaesthetics, bradycardia, patients with pacemakers or those on antiarrhythmic medication.

Status migrainosis: IV dihydroergotamine (may have to be given over 3–7 days in hospital).

Consider corticosteroids, e.g. dexamethasone 10–20 mg IV statim and then taper.

Prophylaxis

Consider prohylactic therapy for frequent attacks that cause disruption to the patient's lifestyle and well-being, a rule of thumb being two or more migraine attacks per month; certainly consider it for weekly attacks and a poor response to therapy for the acute attack. Do not give ergotamine.

The most commonly used drugs include:
- beta-blockers: propranolol, metoprolol, atenolol
- pizotifen 1.5–2.0 mg at night
- cyproheptadine (ideal for children)
- tricyclic antidepressants—amitriptyline
- clonidine
- methysergide (reserve for unresponsive severe migraine) 1 mg tds after food—up to 4 months only
- calcium channel blockers: nifedipine, verapamil
- NSAIDs: naproxen, indomethacin, ibuprofen
- MAO inhibitors: phenelzine, moclobemide
- sumatriptan
- sodium valproate[11]

Guidelines[9,10]

Select the initial drug according to the patient's medical profile.
- if low or normal weight—pizotifen
- if hypertensive—a beta-blocker
- if depressed or anxious—amitriptyline
- if tension—a beta-blocker
- if cervical spondylosis—naproxen
- food-sensitive migraine—pizotifen
- menstrual migraine—naproxen or ibuprofen

Commonly prescribed first-line drugs are propranolol or pizotifen[9]
- propranolol 40 mg (o) bd or tds (at first) increasing to 240 mg daily (if necessary)
- pizotifen 0.5–1 mg (o) nocte (at first) increasing to 3 mg a day (if necessary)

Each drug should be tried for 2 months before it is judged to be ineffective. Amitriptyline 50 mg nocte can be added to propranolol, pizotifen (beware of weight gain) or methysergide and may convert a relatively poor response to very good control.[3]

Cluster headache

Cluster headache is also known as migrainous neuralgia. It occurs in paroxysmal clusters of unilateral headache that typically occur nightly, usually in the small hours of the morning, although patients may have headaches that occur at other times. A hallmark is the pronounced cyclical nature of the attacks. It occurs typically in males (6:1 ratio) and is rare in childhood. There are no visual disturbances or vomiting.

Typical clinical features

- Site: over or about one eye (Fig. 52.5); always same side
- Radiation: frontal and temporal regions
- Quality: severe
- Frequency: 1–3 times a day, at regular times like clockwork
- Duration: 15 minutes to 2–3 hours (average 30 minutes); the clusters last 4–6 weeks (can last months)

- Onset: suddenly during night (usually), same time about 2–3 hours after falling asleep. The 'alarm clock' headache e.g. 2–4 a.m.
- Offset: spontaneous
- Aggravating factors: alcohol (during cluster)
- Relieving factors: drugs
- Associated features: family history; rhinorrhoea, ipsilateral nose; lacrimation; flushing of forehead and cheek; redness of ipsilateral eye; Horner's syndrome (uncommon) (Fig. 52.6)

Fig. 52.5 *Typical distribution of pain in cluster headache*

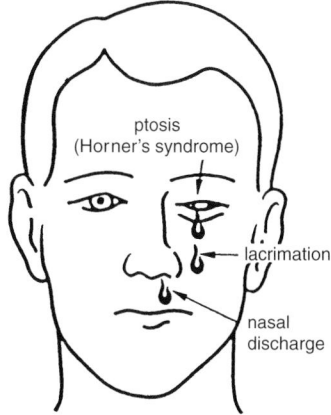

ptosis
(Horner's syndrome)

lacrimation

nasal
discharge

Fig. 52.6 *Features of an attack of cluster headache: ptosis, lacrimation and a discharge from the nostril on the side of pain*

Management

Acute attack (brief treatment seldom effective):

- avoid alcohol during cluster
- consider 100% oxygen 6 L/min for 15 min (usually good response)
- sumatriptan 6 mg SC injection
  or
- ergotamine, e.g. medihaler or rectally
- metoclopramide 10 mg IV + dihydroergotamine 0.5 mg IV slowly
- consider local anaesthetic—greater occipital nerve block

Prophylaxis (once a cluster starts)
Consider the following:

- ergotamine (the drug of choice: take at night during a cluster): oral or dihydroergotamine IM (preferably given 1 hour prior to predicted times)
- methysergide 2 mg/tds
- prednisolone 50 mg/day for 3 days then reduce
- lithium carbonate
- verapamil
- pizotifen
- indomethacin (helps confirm diagnosis)
- sodium valproate

Note: Some of the above can be used long term for frequent clusters.

Cervical dysfunction/spondylosis

Headache from neck disorders, often referred to as occipital neuralgia, is far more common than realised and is very rewarding to treat by physical therapy, including mobilisation and manipulation and exercises in particular.

Headache can be caused by abnormalities in any structure innervated by the upper two cervical nerves C2, C3 (usually the C1–2, C2–3 facet joints). Pain from cervical structures can be referred retro-orbitally and over one-half of the head. The headache is often incorrectly diagnosed as migraine.[12]

Typical clinical features
- Site: occipital region (Fig. 52.7)
- Radiation: parietal region (unilateral), vertex of skull, behind an eye
- Quality: nagging dull aching pain of mild to moderate intensity
- Frequency: usually daily
- Duration: 1 to 6 hours
- Onset: usually on waking in morning
- Offset: usually settles towards midday
- Precipitating factors: often an accident—MVA or striking head
- Aggravating factors: neck movement, especially reversing car
- Relieving factors: heat or cold compress to neck
- Associated features: paraesthesia posterior half of scalp (uncommon); stiffness and grating in neck
- Other pointers: head can feel very heavy (like a metal ball)
- Examination: tenderness to palpation over C1, C2 or C3 levels of cervical spine, especially on side of headache (if unilateral)

Fig. 52.7 *Typical distribution of pain in cervical dysfunction (right side)*

Treatment
- physiotherapy modalities: hydrotherapy, muscle energy therapy, mobilisation, manipulation (from experts) and neck exercises (very important)
- supportive neck pillow
- NSAIDs for cervical spondylosis
- for intractable cases consider manipulation under general anaesthesia, injections of corticosteroids around, or surgical section of, the greater occipital nerve.[12]

Combination headache

Combined (also known as mixed) headaches are common and often diagnosed as psychogenic headache or atypical migraine. They have a combination of various degrees of:

- tension and/or depression
- cervical dysfunction
- vasospasm (migraine)
- drugs, e.g.
  — analgesics (rebound)
  — alcohol
  — nicotine
  — caffeine
  — NSAIDs

The headache, which has many of the features of tension headache, is usually described as a heavy deep ache 'as though my head is ready to burst'. It tends to be constant, being present throughout every waking moment. It tends to last for days (average 3–7) but can last for weeks or months. It is often related to stress and adverse working conditions, and sometimes follows an accident.

Management
An important strategy is to evaluate each possible component of the headache as a stepwise trial by an elimination process:

- drug evaluation and modification
- cervical dysfunction—physical therapy if present
- depression
- tension and stress
- other psychogenic factors, e.g. conversion reaction
- vasospasm

Treatment includes insight therapy, reassurance that the patient does not have a cerebral tumour, and lifestyle modification. The most effective medication is amitriptyline or other antidepressant.

Temporal arteritis

Temporal arteritis (TA) is also known as giant cell arteritis or cranial arteritis. There is usually a persistent unilateral throbbing headache in the temporal region and scalp sensitivity with localised thickening, with or without loss of pulsation of the temporal artery. It is related to polymyalgia rheumatica—20% of sufferers will develop TA.

Fig. 52.8 *Typical distribution of pain in temporal arteritis (right side)*

Typical clinical features

- Age: over 50 years (mean age 70 years)
- Site: forehead and temporal region (unilateral) (Fig. 52.8)
- Radiation: down side of head towards occiput
- Quality: severe burning pain
- Frequency: daily, a constant ache
- Duration: usually constant (getting worse)
- Onset: non-specific, tends to be worse in morning
- Offset: nil
- Aggravating factors: stress and anxiety
- Relieving factors: nil
- Associated features: malaise, vague aches and pains in muscles (especially of neck), weight loss
- Other pointers: — intermittent blurred vision
  - — tenderness on brushing hair
  - — jaw claudication on eating
  - — polymyalgia rheumatica
  - — hypertension
  - — abnormal emotional behaviour

Description

Temporal arteritis is a type of collagen disease causing inflammation of extracranial vessels, especially the superficial temporal artery. It usually presents as a unilateral intermittent headache in a person over 50 years.

TA may also involve the intracranial vessels, especially the ophthalmic artery or posterior ciliary arteries, causing optic atrophy and blindness. Vision is impaired in about one-half of patients at some stage. Once the patient goes blind it is usually irreversible.

Diagnosis

Diagnosis is by biopsy and histological examination of the superficial temporal artery. The ESR is usually markedly elevated but may be normal. The biopsy may be normal as TA has a focal nature.

Note: Consider it with any 'new' headache.

Treatment

TA is very responsive to corticosteroids; start treatment immediately to prevent permanent blindness. Initial medication is prednisolone 60–100 mg orally daily. Dose reduction and progress is monitored by the clinical state and ESR levels.[9] Concomitant use of H_2-receptor antagonists may be appropriate initially. Temporal arteritis may take 1–2 years to resolve.

Frontal sinusitis

The headache of frontal sinusitis can be a diagnostic problem especially in the absence of, or a lapse in time since, an obvious upper respiratory infection or vasomotor rhinitis. Some patients do not have a history of a preceding respiratory infection nor have signs of nasal obstruction or fever. Contrary to popular belief, sinusitis is a relatively uncommon source of headache.

Typical clinical features

- Site: frontal and retro-orbital (unilateral > bilateral) (Fig. 52.9)
- Radiation: vertex

Fig. 52.9 *Typical distribution of pain of frontal sinusitis (right side)*

- Quality: dull and throbbing, moderate severity
- Frequency: daily
- Duration: about 6 to 9 hours
- Onset: develops in morning around 9 a.m.
- Offset: late afternoon around 6 p.m.
- Precipitating factors: URTI
- Aggravating factors: bending forward
- Relieving factors: drainage from nose
- Associated features: malaise ± fever

Examination
There is tenderness over frontal sinus, and pain on percussion over the sinus. Ewing's sign may be elicited. Fever and oedema of the upper eyelid may be present.

Management
Principles of treatment:
- drain the sinus conservatively using steam inhalations
- antibiotics: amoxycillin/clavulanate or cefaclor or doxycycline
- analgesics

Referral
If resolution cannot be accomplished by conservative means then referral to an ENT specialist is advisable. Acute purulent sinusitis can be treacherous if it persists and spreads, causing collections of pus in the extradural or subdural space, cerebral abscess or blood-borne spread of infection.

Complications
- orbital cellulitis
- subdural abscess
- osteomyelitis
- cavernous sinus thrombosis

Symptoms indicating spread of infection:
- increase in fever and chills
- vomiting
- oedema of the eyelids and forehead
- visual disturbances
- dulling of the sensorium
- convulsions

Raised intracranial pressure
Important causes of a space-occupying lesion include a cerebral tumour and subdural haematoma. Sometimes it is not possible to differentiate between a subdural and an extradural haematoma although the latter classically follows an acute injury. Typical features are generalised headache, usually worse in the morning, aggravated by abrupt changes in intracranial pressure and later associated with vomiting and drowsiness. Headache is an uncommon presenting symptom of a cerebral tumour.

Typical clinical features of the headache
- Site: generalised, often occipital
- Radiation: retro-orbital
- Quality: dull, deep steady ache
- Frequency: daily
- Duration: may be hours in morning
- Onset: worse in mornings, usually intermittent, can awaken from sleep
- Offset: later in day (if at all)
- Aggravating factors: coughing, sneezing, straining at toilet
- Relieving factors: analgesics, e.g. aspirin, sitting, standing
- Associated features: vomiting (without preceding nausea); vertigo/dizziness; drowsiness; confusion (later); neurological signs (depending on side)

Examination
- focal CNS signs
- papilloedema (but may be absent)

Intracerebral tumours
- Incidence is 5–10 per 100 000 population
- Two peaks of incidence: children < 10 years[3]   35–60 years

- Main types of tumour:
  - children
    - medulloblastoma
    - astrocytoma (posterior fossa)
    - ependymoma
    - glioma (brain stem)
  - adults
    - cerebral glioma
    - meningioma
    - pituitary adenoma
    - cerebral metastases, e.g. lung

Investigations
CT scan and MRI

Subarachnoid haemorrhage (SAH)

SAH is a life-threatening event that should not be overlooked at the primary care level. The incidence is 12 per 100 000 population per annum. About 40% of patients die before treatment, while about one-third have a good response to treatment.
   Clinical features:

- sudden onset headache (moderate to intense severity)
- occipital location
- localised at first, then generalised
- pain and stiffness of the neck follows
- vomiting and loss of consciousness often follow
- Kernig's sign positive
- neurological deficit may include
  - hemiplegia (if intracerebral bleed)
  - third nerve palsy (partial or complete) (Fig. 52.10)

About one-third of patients experience a 'senital' headache.

Diagnosis
CT scanning is the investigation of choice and should be performed in the first few hours. Lumbar puncture is not necessary if the diagnosis can be made by CT, but is used if the CT scan is negative (usually 10–20% of cases). Even

blood staining of CSF and xanthochromia is a positive feature on lumbar puncture.

Special notes
- Less severe headaches can cause diagnostic difficulties.
- Consider an angioma rather than an aneurysm as the cause of SAH if previous episodes.

Management
Immediate referral is required. If there is lingering doubt review the patient within 12–24 hours.

Meningitis

The headache of meningitis is usually generalised and radiates to the neck. It is constant and severe, and occasionally may begin abruptly. It is aggravated by flexion of the neck. Kernig's sign is positive. Fever and neck stiffness is usually present. Urgent referral to hospital is necessary. If meningitis is suspected or if a child or adult has headache with fever and neck stiffness, antibiotics must not be given until a lumbar puncture has been performed.

Drug rebound headache

Rebound headaches are usually associated with analgesic and ergotamine dependence. A long list of over-the-counter and prescription medications can cause rebound, for example aspirin, paracetamol, ibuprofen, opioids and caffeine. The headache is present on waking and typically persists throughout the day but fluctuates in intensity. It is a mild to moderate, dull, bilateral ache with a distribution similar to tension headache. Drug rebound headaches should be suspected in any patient who complains of headache 'all day, every day'. A careful drug history should be taken. Treatment includes gradual withdrawal of the drugs and the substitution of antiemetics and sedatives or beta-blockers over about 14 days.

Chronic paroxysmal hemicrania

This is a rare headache syndrome which overlaps with cluster headache and facial pain. The unilateral pain, which can be excruciating, is located in the area of the temple, forehead, eye and upper face. It can radiate to the ear, neck and shoulder. It differs from cluster headaches

ptosis

eye turned down and outwards

dilated pupil

Fig. 52.10 *Third nerve palsy (right side)*

in that the patients are invariably female, the paroxysms are short (average 20–30 minutes) and more frequent, with attacks occurring up to 14 times a day. The disorder resembles cluster headaches in nature and distribution and associated autonomic features such as ipsilateral nasal stuffiness or rhinorrhoea, lacrimation, conjunctival injection and ptosis. The aetiology is unknown but the headache often responds dramatically to indomethacin (25 mg (o) tds).[9]

Trigeminal neuralgia

The pain of trigeminal neuralgia comes in excruciating paroxysms, which last for seconds to minutes only and usually affect the face rather than the head (see pp. 493–494). The lightning-like jabs of searing or burning pain usually last 1 to 2 minutes but can last as long as 15 minutes.

Icepick headache

Icepick headaches are similar sudden stabbing pains usually at the temple and are more common in migraine sufferers. Treatment is with indomethacin 25 mg tds.

Hypertension headache

It tends to occur only in severe hypertension such as malignant hypertension or hypertensive encephalopathy. The headache is typically occipital, throbbing and worse on waking in the morning.

The headache may be psychogenic in origin, developing after the diagnosis of hypertension is disclosed to the patient. However, the occasional patient has genuine headache related to milder hypertension and this serves as an accurate indicator of their blood pressure level.

Benign intracranial hypertension (pseudotumour cerebri)

This is a rare but important sinister headache condition that typically occurs in young obese women. Key features are headache, visual blurring and obscurations, nausea, papilloedema. The CT and MRI scans are normal but lumbar puncture reveals increased CSF pressure and normal CSF analysis.

It is sometimes linked to drugs including tetracyclines (most common), nitrofurantoin, oral contraceptive pill and vitamin A preparations. The main concern is visual deficits from the high intracranial pressure. Medical treatment includes weight reduction, corticosteroids and diuretics. The treatment of choice to alleviate symptoms is repeated lumbar puncture. Surgery, which involves decompression of the optic nerves or lumboperitoneal shunting, is sometimes required for failed medical therapy.

Headaches related to specific activities

Sex headache

This can manifest as a dull or explosive headache, provoked by sexual arousal and activity especially with orgasm. Some are clearly a form of exertional headache. Sometimes sex headache is mistaken for SAH but if the severe headache coincided with orgasm, was not associated with vomiting or neck stiffness, or settled within hours, SAH is unlikely. Treatment is with prophylactic beta-blockers.

Cough and exertional headache

Some people experience a severe transient pain with factors such as coughing, sneezing, stooping, straining, lifting and various sporting activities. It is usually benign and examination is normal. A CT scan is indicated if there are focal signs or if the symptoms do not settle.

Gravitational headache

Occipital headache, coming on when standing upright and relieved by lying down, is characteristic of a postlumbar puncture, an epidural block or low pressure headache. It can last for several weeks after the procedure.

'Ice-cream' headache

Frontal or global headache can be provoked by the rapid ingestion of very cold food and drink. It is a form of vascular headache.

When to refer

- Evidence or suspicion of subarachnoid haemorrhage or intracerebral haematoma
- Complicated migraine
- Uncertain diagnosis
- Positive neurological signs despite typical headaches
- Headaches increasing in frequency, despite prophylaxis
- Danger signals with headache:
  — sudden onset without previous history
  — recent onset for first time in an older person

— recurrent in children
— progressive
— wakes the patient at night
— localised pain in definite area or structure, e.g. ear, eye
— precipitated by raised intracranial pressure, e.g. coughing
— associated neurological symptoms or signs:
  • convulsions
  • fever
  • confusion
  • impaired consciousness
  • neck stiffness
  • dizziness/vertigo
  • personality change

Practice tips

• A middle-aged or elderly patient presenting with unaccustomed headache has an organic disorder such as temporal arteritis, intracerebral tumour or subdural haematoma until proved otherwise.
• The ESR is an excellent screening test to diagnose temporal arteritis but occasionally can be normal in the presence of active TA.
• If a patient presents twice within 24 hours to the same practice or hospital with headache and vomiting, consider other causes apart from migraine before discharging the patient.[7]
• Treat an unusual or unaccustomed headache with a lot of respect.
• If migraine attacks are severe and unusual (e.g. always on the same side) consider the possibility of cerebral vascular malformation.
• CT scans and MRI have superseded other investigations in the diagnosis of cerebral tumours and intracranial haemorrhage but should be ordered sparingly and judiciously.
• If a headache is occipital in origin or accompanied by neck pain, consider the likely possibility of cervical dysfunction and refer to the appropriate therapist once the diagnosis is established.
• For recurrent migraine sufferers emphasise the importance of trigger factor avoidance and of taking aspirin and metoclopramide medication at the earliest warning of an attack.
• A severe headache of sudden onset is subarachnoid haemorrhage until proved otherwise.
• SAH is overlooked sometimes, mainly because it is not considered in the differential diagnosis. Suspect with very severe and protracted headache, drowsiness and neck stiffness.

• A 'stranger' presenting with a severe migraine attack may well be a pethidine addict. Your regular migraine patient may also be a narcotic addict. Avoid giving narcotic analgesics to your migraine patients—establish a conservative drug regimen backed by patient education and empathy.
• Prophylactic ergotamine medication commonly causes a dull, constant, steady headache.
• If women with migraine demand the oral contraceptive, use a low-dose oestrogen preparation and monitor progress.
• The use of narcotics for migraine treatment (such as pethidine and codeine) is to be avoided whenever possible—the frequent use of ergotamine, analgesics or narcotics can transform episodic migraine into chronic daily headache.

References

1. Cormack J, Marinker M, Morrell D. The patient complaining of headache. In: *Practice*. London: Kluwer Medical, 3.12.
2. Wright M. Recurrent headaches in children. The Aust Paed Review, 1991; 1(6):1–2.
3. Anthony M. Migraine and tension headache. In: MIMS Disease Index (2nd edn). Sydney: IMS Publishing, 1996, 313–316.
4. Sandler G, Fry J. *Early clinical diagnosis*. Lancaster: MTP Press, 1986, 297–325.
5. Davis A, Bolin T, Ham J. *Symptom analysis and physical diagnosis*. Sydney: Pergamon, 1990.
6. Lance JW. *Mechanism and management of headache* (3rd edn). London: Butterworths, 1978, 109–112.
7. Burns R. Pitfalls in headache management. Aust Fam Physician, 1990; 19:1821–1826.
8. Day TJ. Migraine and other vascular headaches. Aust Fam Physician, 1990; 19:1797–1804.
9. Moulds RFW (Chairman). *Therapeutic guidelines: Neurology*. Melbourne: Therapeutic Guidelines Limited, 1997, 39–49.
10. Heywood J, Zagami A. Treating acute migraine attack. Current Therapeutics, 1997; 37(12): 33–37.
11. Silberstein, S, Wilmore J. Divalproex sodium: Migraine treatment and monitoring. Headache, 1996; 36:239–242.
12. Anthony M. The treatment of migraine—old methods, new ideas. Aust Fam Physician, 1993; 22:1401–1405.

53

Jaundice

—

How is jaundice diagnosed? In natural sunlight is the answer. When I was an army doctor I recall how many sick troops confined below deck were found to be jaundiced when they came onto the deck.

Experienced physician to students

Jaundice is a yellow discolouration of the skin and mucosal surfaces caused by the accumulation of excessive bilirubin.[1] It is a cardinal symptom of hepatobiliary disease and haemolysis. Important common causes include gallstones, hepatitis A, hepatitis B, hepatitis C, drugs, alcohol and Gilbert's disease. The commonest clinical encounter with jaundice, especially physiological jaundice, is in the newborn. As for all patients, the history and examination are paramount, but investigations are essential to clinch the diagnosis of jaundice.

The three major categories of jaundice are (Fig. 53.1):

- obstructive
  — extrahepatic
  — intrahepatic
- hepatocellular
- haemolysis

Key facts and checkpoints

- Jaundice is defined as a serum bilirubin exceeding 17 µmol/L.[2]
- Clinical jaundice manifests only when the bilirubin exceeds 50 µmol/L.[1]
- However, jaundice is difficult to detect visually below 85 µmol/L if lighting is poor.
- It can be distinguished from yellow skin due to hypercarotenaemia (due to dietary excess of carrots, pumpkin, mangoes or pawpaw) and hypothyroidism by involving the sclera.

Table 53.1 *Abbreviations used in this chapter*

Hepatitis A virus	HAV
Hepatitis A antibody	anti-HAV
Immunoglobulin M	IgM
Immunoglobulin G	IgG
Hepatitis B virus	HBV
Hepatitis B surface antigen	HBsAg
Hepatitis surface antibody	anti-HBs
Hepatitis B core antibody	anti-HBc
Hepatitis Be antigen	HBeAg
Hepatitis C virus	HCV
Hepatitis C virus antibody	anti-HCV
Hepatitis D (Delta) virus	HDV
Hepatitis E virus	HEV
Hepatitis F virus	HFV
Hepatitis G virus	HGV

- The most common causes of jaundice recorded in a general practice population are (in order) viral hepatitis, gallstones, carcinoma of pancreas, cirrhosis, pancreatitis and drugs.[3]
- Always take a full travel, drug and hepatitis contact history in any patient presenting with jaundice.
- A fatty liver (steatosis) can occur not only with alcohol excess but also with obesity, diabetes and starvation. There is no liver damage and thus no jaundice.

A diagnostic approach

A summary of the diagnostic safety model is presented in Table 53.2.

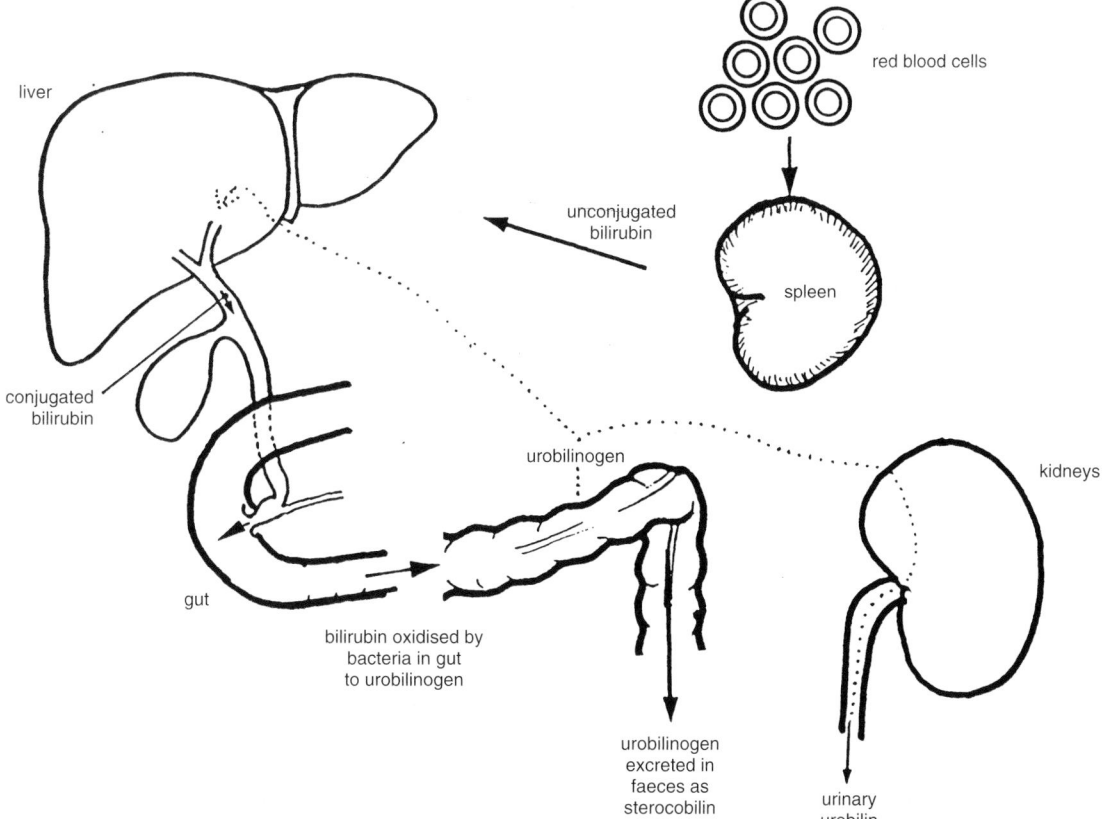

Fig. 53.1 *The jaundice pathway*

Probability diagnosis

The answer depends on the age and social grouping of the patient, especially if the patient indulges in risk-taking behaviour or has travelled overseas.

Viral hepatitis A, B or C accounts for the majority of cases of jaundice.

In the middle-aged and elderly group, a common cause is obstruction from gallstones or cancer. It is common for older people to have painless obstructive jaundice; bear in mind that the chances of malignancy increase with age.

Alcoholic liver disease is common and may present as chronic alcoholic cirrhosis with liver failure or as acute alcoholic hepatitis. It is worth emphasising that such patients can make a dramatic recovery when they cease drinking alcohol.

In family practice we encounter many cases of drug-induced jaundice, especially in the elderly. These drugs are outlined later in the chapter, under the 'seven masquerades'.

Serious disorders not to be missed

Malignancy must always be suspected, especially in the elderly patient and those with a history of chronic active hepatitis, e.g. post hepatitis B infection. The former is more likely to have carcinoma of the head of the pancreas and the latter, hepatocellular carcinoma (hepatoma).

Metastatic carcinoma must be kept in mind, especially in those with a history of surgery, such as large bowel cancer, melanoma and stomach cancer.

Hepatic failure can be associated with severe systemic infection, e.g. septicaemia and pneumonia, and after surgery in critically ill patients. A patient who has the classic Charcot's triad of upper abdominal pain, fever (and chills) and jaundice should be regarded as having ascending cholangitis until proved otherwise. Wilson's disease, although rare, must be considered in all young patients with acute hepatitis. A history of neurological symptoms, such as a tremor or a clumsy gait, and a family history is important. If

Table 53.2 *Jaundice (adults): diagnostic strategy model*

Q. *Probability diagnosis*
A. Hepatitis A,B,C (mainly B, C)
   Gallstones
   Alcoholic hepatitis/cirrhosis

Q. *Serious disorders not to be missed*
A. Malignancy
   • pancreas
   • biliary tract
   • hepatocellular (hepatoma)
   • metastases
   Severe infections
   • septicaemia
   • ascending cholangitis
   • fulminant hepatitis
   • HIV/AIDS
   Rarities
   • Wilson's disease
   • Reye's disease
   • Acute fatty liver of pregnancy

Q. *Pitfalls (often missed)*
A. Gallstones
   Gilbert's disease
   Cardiac failure
   Primary biliary cirrhosis
   Autoimmune chronic active hepatitis
   Chronic viral hepatitis
   Haemochromatosis
   Viral infections

Q. *Seven masquerades checklist*
A. Depression   –
   Diabetes   –
   Drugs   √
   Anaemia   √
   Thyroid disease   –
   Spinal dysfunction   –
   UTI   –

Q. *Is this patient trying to tell me something?*
A. Not usually applicable.

Wilson's disease is suspected the patient should have an ocular slit lamp examination, serum ceruloplasmin levels (low in 95% of patients) and a liver biopsy. Early diagnosis and treatment mean a better prognosis.

Reye's syndrome is a rare and severe complication of influenza and some other viral diseases, especially in children when given aspirin. There is rapid development of hepatic failure and encephalopathy.

Pitfalls

Gallstones, especially in the absence of upper abdominal pain, can be overlooked; so this possibility should be kept in mind in the elderly.

Gilbert's disease is worth considering, especially as it is the commonest form of unconju-

gated hyperbilirubinaemia. It affects at least 3% of the population. Like the more severe but rarer Crigler-Najjar syndrome there is a deficiency of glucuronyl transferase. In Gilbert's disease the serum bilirubin, which may rise to 50 μmol/L but seldom higher,[2] tends to fluctuate and to rise during intercurrent infections, such as influenza and in episodes of fasting. All other liver function tests are normal, as is liver serology, but a history of intermittent mild jaundice, a family history or vague right upper quadrant pain may be useful pointers. Patients diagnosed by the author appeared to have a consistently coloured skin resembling a 'suntan' despite living in a cool climate. Gilbert's disease is benign with an excellent prognosis and no treatment is required.

Cardiac failure can present as jaundice with widespread tenderness under the right costal margin. It can be insidious in onset or manifest with gross acute failure. It can be confused with acute cholecystitis. The biochemical abnormalities seen are very variable. Usually there is a moderate rise in bilirubin and alkaline phosphatase and sometimes, in acute failure, a marked elevation of transaminase may occur, suggesting some hepatocellular necrosis.

There are many other pitfalls for a family doctor, who may encounter the conditions very rarely, if at all. Such disorders include:

• inherited conjugated hyperbilirubinaemias (Dubin-Johnson and Rotor syndromes) caused by faulty excretion by liver cells
• haemochromatosis (associated pigmentation and diabetes)
• chronic active hepatitis
• primary biliary cirrhosis
• sclerosing cholangitis (associated with ulcerative colitis)

General pitfalls

• Excluding jaundice by examining the sclera in artificial light
• Not realising that the sclera in elderly patients often have an icteric appearance (without jaundice)
• Omitting to take a careful history including illicit drugs
• A liver biopsy is essential in all patients with chronic hepatitis

Seven masquerades checklist

Of this group the haemolytic anaemias and drugs have to be considered.

Drug-related jaundice

Drug-induced jaundice is common and many drugs are implicated. The patterns of drug-related liver damage include cholestasis, necrosis ('hepatitis'), granulomas, chronic active hepatitis, cirrhosis, hepatocellular tumours and veno-occlusive disease.[4] Some drugs, such as methyldopa, can initiate haemolysis.

The important drugs to consider are presented in Table 53.3. Antibiotics, especially flucloxacillin and erythromycin, are commonly implicated.

Haemolysis

The patient may present with the symptoms of underlying anaemia and jaundice with no noticeable change in the appearance of the urine and stool. The degree of haemolysis may vary from the lemon yellow tinge of pernicious

Table 53.3 *Drugs that can cause jaundice*

Haemolysis
• methyldopa

Hepatocellular damage
dose-dependent
• paracetamol (can cause acute hepatic necrosis)
• salicylates
• tetracycline
dose-independent

• anaesthetics	e.g. halothane
• antidepressants	e.g. MAO inhibitors
• antiepileptics	e.g. phenytoin
	sodium valproate
	carbamazepine
• antibiotics	e.g. penicillins
	sulphonamides
• antimalarials	e.g. Fansidar
• antituberculosis	e.g. isoniazid
• anti-inflammatories	e.g. NSAIDs (various)
• carbon tetrachloride	
• cardiovascular	e.g. amiodarone
	methyldopa
	perhexilene

Cholestasis
• antithyroid drugs
• chlorpromazine
• erythromycin estolate
• penicillins
• gold salts
• oral contraceptives/oestrogens
• synthetic anabolic steroids, e.g. methyltestosterone
• hypoglycaemic drugs, e.g. chlorpropamide

Others
• allopurinol
• cimetidine (aggravated by alcohol)
• cytotoxics, e.g. methotrexate
• etretinate
• hydralazine
• nitrofurantoin
• vitamin A (mega dosage)

anaemia in an elderly patient to a severe haemolytic crisis precipitated by drugs or broad beans (favism) in a patient with an inherited red cell deficiency of glucose-6-phosphate dehydrogenase. More common causes include the hereditary haemolytic anaemias, such as congenital spherocytosis and thalassaemia major. Acquired causes include incompatible blood transfusions, malignancies, such as lymphoma, severe sepsis and some drugs.

Splenomegaly occurs in most patients with haemolytic anaemia, and decreased red cell survival can be measured.

Psychogenic considerations

This is not really applicable for an organic problem such as jaundice. Nevertheless, the cause may be related to factors in the patient's lifestyle such as homosexuality, sexual promiscuity or intravenous drug abuse, and the patient may be reluctant to offer this information. Discreet, concerned probing will be necessary.

The clinical approach

History

The history should include questioning about the following:

• any episodes of jaundice
• change in colour of faeces and urine
• anorexia, sore throat, weight loss, pruritus
• abdominal pain
• residence and members of household
• contact with patients with hepatitis or jaundice
• recent overseas travel
• exposure to blood or blood products
• needle-stick injuries or exposure to needles, such as acupuncture, tattooing and intravenous drugs
• dietary history: shellfish, drinking water
• sexual history: evidence of promiscuity
• drug history, including alcohol
• recent medical history, including surgery
• family history: family contacts who have had jaundice, haemolytic disease and other genetic liver diseases
• ethnic history: liable to haemolytic disease, contact with hepatitis B
• occupational history: exposure to hazards

Significance of various symptoms

• pain in the right hypochondrium
— gallstones

— acute hepatitis (a constant ache)
— cholecystitis
- anorexia, dark urine, fever
  — viral hepatitis probable
  — alcoholic liver disease possible
  — drug-induced hepatitis possible
- pruritus
  — cholestasis probable
  — possible with all liver diseases
- arthralgia, rash
  — viral hepatitis
  — autoimmune hepatitis

The examination

The abdominal examination is very important. The liver should be palpated carefully for enlargement, consistency and tenderness under the right costal margin. Search for enlargement of the gall bladder and the spleen. The gall bladder lies in the transypyloric line. A palpable gall bladder indicates extrahepatic biliary obstruction, and splenomegaly may indicate haemolytic anaemia, portal hypertension or viral hepatitis. Test for ascites.

Skin excoriation may indicate pruritus, which is associated with cholestatic jaundice. Look for evidence of chronic liver disease, such as palmar erythema, easy bruising, spider naevi and muscle wasting, and testicular atrophy and gynaecomastia. Test for hepatic flap (asterixis) and fetor, which indicate liver failure. Search for lymphadenopathy which may be indicative of malignancy.

A summary of the possible findings is presented in Figure 53.2.

Investigations

The main investigations are the standard liver function tests and viral serology for the infective causes, particularly hepatitis B virus.

A summary of the general findings for liver function tests is shown in Table 53.4. Consideration should be given to ordering fractionalisation of bilirubin to determine whether it is conjugated or unconjugated (important in diagnosis of Gilbert's disease).

Markers for hepatitis

Serology includes the test for hepatitis B virus (HBV) surface antigen (HBsAg), which is diagnostic of infection. Other markers of HBV are HBeAg antigen and the antibodies (anti-HBs and anti-HBc).

Hepatitis A virus is diagnosed by the presence of IgM antibody for recent infection and IgG antibody which indicates past infection and lifelong immunity.

Specific serological tests for the previously designated non-A, non-B hepatitis are more complex, but tests to identify two of these causative agents (C and D) are now available.

Hepatobiliary imaging

Tests to identify causes such as malignancy or gallstones are now sophisticated and should be chosen with care.
- X-ray: a plain abdominal X-ray shows up to 10% of gallstones
- Ultrasound: the most useful investigation for detecting gallstones and dilatation of the common bile duct; also detects liver metastases and other diffuse liver diseases
- HIDA scintiscan: useful in diagnosis of acute cholecystitis
- CT scan: for diagnosis of enlargement of the head of the pancreas and other pathology; indicated if US unsatisfactory
- PTC: percutaneous transhepatic cholangiography
- ERCP: endoscopic retrograde cholangiopancreatography; PTC and ERCP (best) determine the cause of the obstruction
- Liver isotopic scan: useful for liver cirrhosis, especially of the left lobe

Specific tests

Some specific tests include:
- autoantibodies for autoimmune chronic active hepatitis and primary biliary cirrhosis
- carcinoembryonic antigen to detect liver secondaries, especially colorectal
- serum iron and ferritin—elevated in haemochromatosis
- alpha-fetoprotein—elevated in hepatocellular carcinoma; mild elevation with acute or chronic liver disease e.g. cirrhosis
- serum ceruloplasmin—low in Wilson's disease
- liver biopsy
- E-B virus/cytomegalovirus serology (consider if hepatitis serology negative)

Jaundice in children
Jaundice in the infant
Jaundice in the newborn is clinically apparent in 50% of term babies and more than 80% of

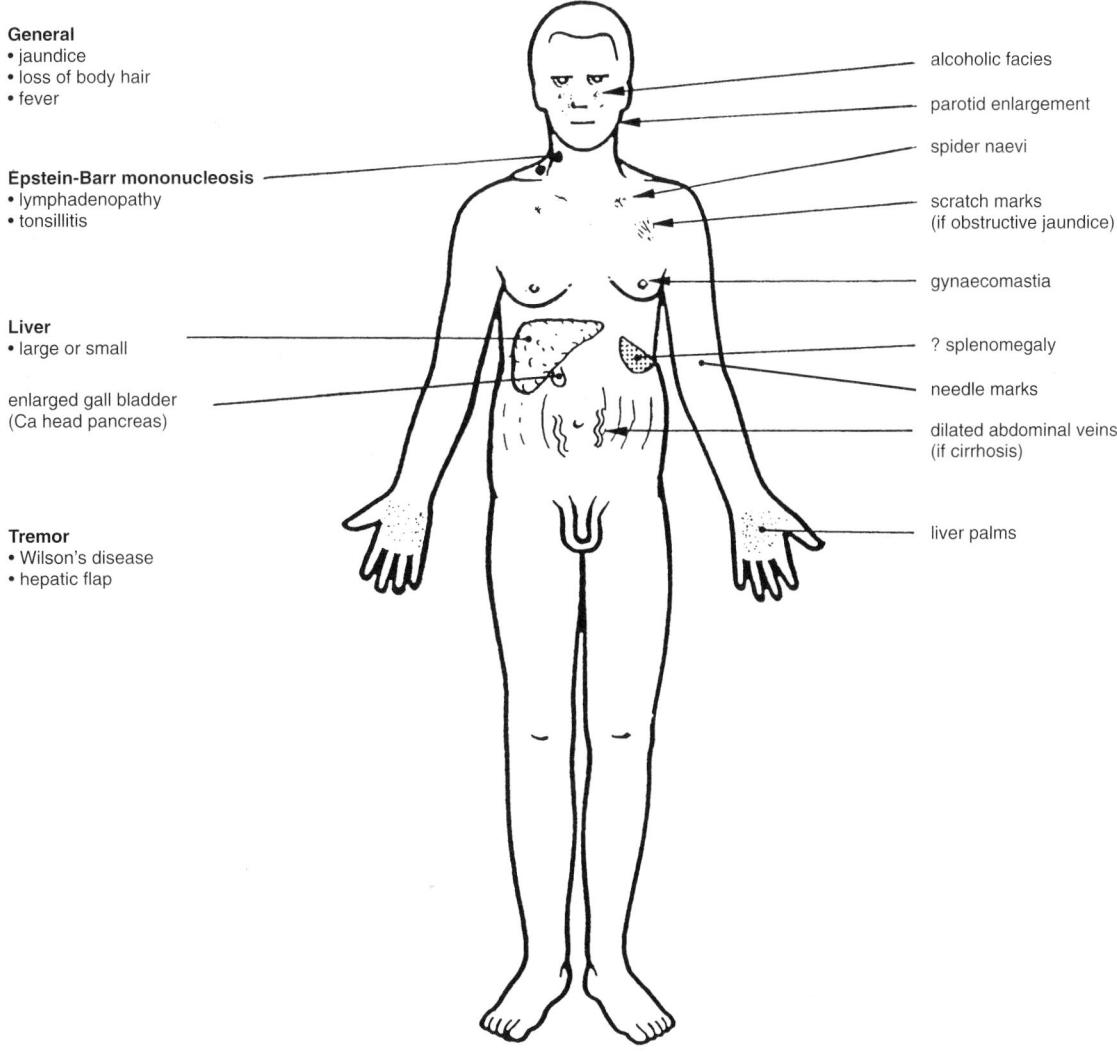

General
• jaundice
• loss of body hair
• fever

Epstein-Barr mononucleosis
• lymphadenopathy
• tonsillitis

Liver
• large or small

enlarged gall bladder
(Ca head pancreas)

Tremor
• Wilson's disease
• hepatic flap

alcoholic facies

parotid enlargement

spider naevi

scratch marks
(if obstructive jaundice)

gynaecomastia

? splenomegaly

needle marks

dilated abdominal veins
(if cirrhosis)

liver palms

Fig. 53.2 *Possible findings on examining the jaundiced patient*

Table 53.4 *Characteristic liver function tests for selected types of liver disease*

Liver function tests (serological)	Hepatocellular (viral) hepatitis	Haemolytic jaundice	Obstruction	Gilbert's disease	Liver metastases/ abscess	Alcoholic liver disease
Bilirubin	↑ to ↑↑↑	↑ unconjugated	↑ to ↑↑↑	↑ up to 50 unconjugated	↑ to N	↑ to N
Alkaline phosphatase	↑ < 2N	N	↑↑↑ > 2N	N	↑↑ to ↑↑↑	↑
Aspartate transferase	↑↑↑ > 5N	N	N or ↑	N	↑	↑
Gamma glutamyl transferase	N or ↑	N	↑↑	N	↑	↑↑↑
Albumin	N or ↓	N	N	N	N to ↓	N to ↓↓
Globulin	N or ↑	N	N	N	N	N to ↑

N: is within normal limits

preterm.[5] Icterus is therefore common and invariably physiologically benign. However, there are many other causes and investigation is needed to determine whether the bilirubin is conjugated or unconjugated.

Bilirubin encephalopathy

Unconjugated bilirubin can be regarded as a neurological poison. With increasing serum levels an encephalopathy (which may be transient) can develop, but if persistent can lead to the irreversible brain damage known as kernicterus. The level of bilirubin causing kernicterus is totally unpredictable, but a guideline as a cause for concern in babies with Rh disease is a serum unconjugated bilirubin of 340 μmol/L (20 mg/dL).

Physiological jaundice

This mild form of jaundice, which is very common in infants, is really a diagnosis of exclusion. In a term infant the serum bilirubin rises quickly after birth to reach a maximum by day 3–5, then declines rapidly over the next 2–3 days before fading more slowly for the next 1–2 weeks. Management includes phototherapy.

Pathological jaundice

There are many causes of pathological jaundice, including:

- haemolysis, e.g. blood grouping incompatibilities
- polycythaemia, e.g. intrauterine growth retardation
- inherited conjugation defects, e.g. uridyl diphoshate glucuronyl transferase deficiency
- breast milk jaundice
- drugs
- sepsis
- hypothyroidism
- biliary atresia

Such cases require referral for evaluation and management.

Jaundice in older children

Viral infection is the commonest cause of jaundice in the older child, especially hepatitis A and hepatitis B. It is uncommon for viral hepatitis to become chronic in childhood.

Jaundice in the elderly

If an elderly person presents with jaundice the usual causes and investigations have to be considered. Obstructive jaundice is the commonest form of jaundice in the elderly and may be caused by gallstones blocking the common bile duct (may be painless) and carcinoma of the head of the pancreas, the biliary tract itself, the stomach or multiple secondaries for other sites. While it is not uncommon for a gallstone to produce marked obstructive jaundice and yet be painless, it is appropriate to adhere to the old adage that painless obstructive jaundice is due to neoplasm—particularly if the gall bladder is palpable (Courvoisier's law).

Alcoholic liver disease, although most frequently affecting patients between 40 and 60 years, can present for the first time over age 60 years. The commonest cause of hepatocellular jaundice in the elderly is probably alcoholic cirrhosis; hepatitis A is still relatively uncommon in old persons.

Drugs do not cause jaundice in the elderly as frequently as they once did, particularly as phenothiazines, especially chlorpromazine, are not prescribed as often as previously. However, drugs should be considered as a potential cause and a careful check of the drug history is important.

Infective causes of jaundice

A generation ago hepatitis A (infectious hepatitis or yellow jaundice) was the commonest recognised form of viral hepatitis, presenting usually with an abrupt onset of fever, anorexia, nausea and vomiting. It usually occurred in epidemics and hence was common in overcrowded institutions and camps. Now hepatitis B and C are the most commonly reported types of viral hepatitis with an onset that is more insidious and with a longer incubation period.[6,7] Symptoms include malaise, anorexia, nausea and polyarthritis.

The various forms of hepatitis are summarised in Table 53.5. All forms of hepatitis are common in developing countries and travellers are at risk of contracting these diseases: hepatitis A and E from faeco-oral transmission; and hepatitis B,C,D and G from intravenous drugs and bodily fluids (from sexual transmission, in particular, for hepatitis B).

Table 53.5 *Characteristic profiles of viral hepatitis A–E*

Characteristic	Hepatitis A	Hepatitis B	Hepatitis C	Hepatitis D	Hepatitis E
Pseudonyms	Infectious hepatitis	Serum hepatitis	Parenterally transmitted non A, non B	Delta hepatitis	Enterically transmitted non A, non B
Agent (virus)	27nm RNA	42nm DNA	50nm RNA	35nm RNA	30 nm RNA
Transmission	Faecal-oral	Blood and other body fluids	Blood ? other body fluids	Blood and other body fluids	Faecal-oral
Incubation period	15–45 days	40–180 days	14–180 days	30–50 days	15–45 days
Severity of acute illness	Mild to moderate; often subclinical —no jaundice	Mild to severe; Jaundice common; arthralgia and rash common	Mild to moderate; often subclinical	Moderate to severe; high mortality; usually jaundice	Mild to moderate; often subclinical
Chronic liver disease	No	Yes 5–10%	Yes 20–50%	Yes Potentially worst	No
Mortality	0.1–0.2%	1–3%	1–2%	Variable	Variable; high (10–20%) in pregnant women
Carrier state	No	Yes	Yes	Yes	Uncertain
Risk in travellers	Yes, applies to all A–E: East and South-East Asia, Asian subcontinent (e.g. India), South Pacific Islands (e.g. Fiji), sub-Saharan Africa, Mexico, CIS, other developing countries. A and E with poor sanitation; B, C, D also with IV drug use; B, D, sexual contact.				
Antigens	HA Ag	HBsAg, HBcAg, HBeAg	HC Ag	HD Ag	?
Serology	IgM anti-HAV diagnosis	HBsAg diagnosis anti-HBs ⎫ exposure ⎬ immunity ⎭	anti-HCV (antibody)	HBsAg + ve HDsAg + ve anti-HDV (antibody)	Being developed
Immuno-prophylaxis	Normal Ig	HB Ig	? Ig effective	None	None
Vaccine	Hepatitis A vaccine	Hepatitis B vaccine	None	Hepatitis B vaccine	None

Evidence points to more viruses causing non-ABC hepatitis.[8] Hepatitis F virus has been claimed to be transmitted enterically while the newly designated hepatitis G virus (HGV) is transmitted parenterally. It does not appear to cause a severe illness in recipients. It can be predicted that the hepatitis alphabet will continue to expand.

In hepatitis A liver damage is directly due to the virus, but in hepatitis B and C it is due to an immunologic reaction to the virus.

Other infections that can present with jaundice as part of a systemic disease are malaria, Epstein-Barr mononucleosis, cytomegalovirus, Q fever, toxoplasmosis, leptospirosis and, rarely, measles, varicella, yellow fever, rubella, herpes simplex, dengue fever, Lassa fever and Marburg and Ebola virus.

Hepatitis A

Hepatitis A is becoming relatively less prevalent in First World countries. It is enterically transmitted and arises from the ingestion of contaminated food such as shellfish or water. There is no carrier state and it does not cause chronic liver disease. Hepatitis A most often causes a subclinical or self-limited clinical illness.

Clinical features

Preicteric (prodromal) phase:
• anorexia, nausea, ± vomiting
• malaise
• headache
• distaste for cigarettes in smokers
• mild fever
• ± diarrhoea
• ± upper abdominal discomfort

Icteric phase (many patients do not develop jaundice):

• dark urine
• pale stools
• hepatomegaly
• splenomegaly (palpable in 10%)

Recovery usually in 3–6 weeks.

Fulminant hepatitis with liver coma and death may occur but is rare.

Investigations

Liver function tests and viral markers confrm the diagnosis. The antibodies to HAV are IgM, which indicates active infection, and IgG antibodies, which means immunity and which is common in the general population. Ultrasound is useful to exclude bile duct obstruction, especially in an older patient.

Outcome and treatment

Hepatitis A has an excellent prognosis with most patients making a complete recovery, and patients should be reassured. The mortality is less than 0.5%. Admission to hospital is not usually necessary. There is no specific treatment; so management is as follows.

• Provide appropriate reassurance and patient education.
• Rest as appropriate.
• Follow a fat-free diet.
• Avoid alcohol, smoking and hepatotoxic drugs (until recovery).
• Advise on hygiene at home to prevent spread to close contacts and family members.
• Wash hands carefully after using the toilet and disinfect them with antiseptic.
• Do not handle food for others with your fingers.
• Do not share cutlery and crockery during meals.
• Do not use tea towels to dry dishes.

Prevention

Simple health measures such as good sanitation, effective garbage disposal and hand washing are probably responsible for the major decrease in the disease. Immune serum globulin (0.03–0.06 mL/kg IM) confers satisfactory passive immunity for close contacts (within 2 weeks of contact) and for travellers to endemic areas for up to 3 months. An active vaccine consisting of a 2-dose primary course is the best means of prevention.

Hepatitis B

Hepatitis B has protean clinical manifestations. Transmission is by blood-spread, sexual transmission, perinatal spread or by close prolonged family contact. Infection may be subclinical or self-limited acute hepatitis. Fulminant hepatitis is rare. Five per cent of subjects go on to become chronic carriers of the virus. Most are 'healthy carriers' but some may develop chronic active hepatitis, cirrhosis and hepatoma. The serology of hepatitis B involves antibody responses to the four main antigens of the virus (core, DNA polymerase, protein X and surface antigens). Passive and active vaccines are available, and should be used freely in groups at risk including babies of infected mothers. High-risk groups are presented in Table 53.6. The clinical features are the same as those found in hepatitis A infection but may be less abrupt in onset but more severe in the long term.[6] A serum sickness-like immunological syndrome may be seen with transient rashes, e.g. urticaria or a maculopapular rash, and polyarthritis affecting small joints in up to 25% of cases in the prodromal period.

Investigations

The main viral investigation for HBV is HBsAg (surface antigen), which is searched for routinely. If detected, a full viral profile is then formed.

HBsAg may disappear or persist. Its presence indicates a current or chronic infection as well as a carrier state (Fig. 53.3). Hepatitis B carriage is the presence of HBsAg for at least 6 months.

Table 53.6 *Higher risk groups for contracting hepatitis B (vaccination advisable)*[6]

Babies born to hepatitis B positive (carrier) mothers

Sexual partners of hepatitis B carriers (especially acute HBV)

Household contacts of hepatitis B carriers

Intravenous drug users

Recipients of blood or blood products (prior to testing)

Male homosexuals

Renal dialysis patients

Sex industry workers

Health care workers

Garbage collectors

Institutionalised mentally retarded patients

Prisoners

Travellers to endemic areas

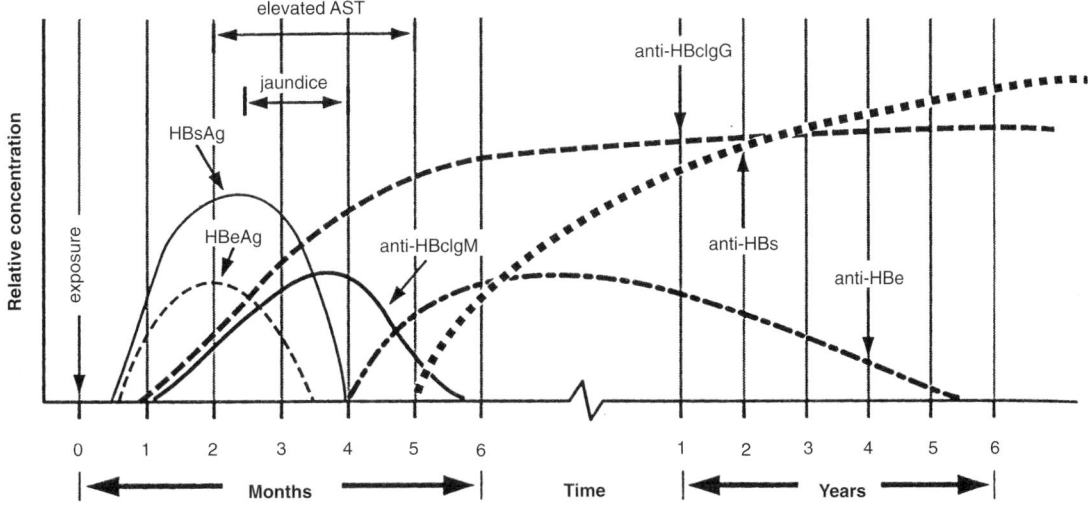

Fig. 53.3 *Time course of clinical events and serological changes following infection with hepatitis B*

Outcome and treatment

The possible course of events is shown in Figure 53.4. The majority of patients recover completely with the outcome depending on several factors including the virulence of the virus and the immune state and age of the patient. Some will develop chronic hepatitis, some will develop a fulminant course, and others will become asymptomatic carriers and present a health risk to others.

There is no specific treatment, and appropriate reassurance and patient education is necessary. Treatment of chronic hepatitis B infection is with the immunomodulatory and antiviral agents interferon and lamivudine. This is expensive but it achieves permanent remission in 25% of patients, and temporary remission in a further 25%.[6] Liver transplantation has been performed, but is often followed by recurrence of hepatitis B in the grafted liver. Follow up with regular LFTs and $\propto$ fetoprotein.

Prevention

Active immunisation through hepatitis B vaccination has been a major breakthrough in the management of this serious illness. There is a course of three injections. If there is a negative antibody response after 3 months, revaccinate with a double dose. If the response is positive, consider a test in 5 years with a view to a booster injection.

For non-immune patients at risk, e.g. after a needle-stick injury, hepatitis B immunoglobin (HBIg), which contains a high level of HBV surface antibody, is appropriate.

Prenatal screening of pregnant women and appropriate use of HBIg and HB vaccine is useful in preventing perinatal vertical transmission of HBV.

Hepatitis C

Hepatitis C virus is responsible for most cases of viral hepatitis in Australia. It is primarily contracted from intravenous drug use or tattooing. It does not seem to be spread very readily by sexual contact although there is a small risk during heterosexual and homosexual intercourse. It is also not readily spread perinatally.

Hepatitis C infection may be self-limiting, but more commonly (in 50% of cases) causes a slow, relentless progression to chronic hepatitis, cirrhosis (20%) and also hepatoma.[7]

Diagnosis

This is by the presence of HCV antibody.

There is no vaccine yet available. Treatment of chronic hepatitis C infection is also with interferon alpha and ribaviran.

Those at increased risk of having hepatitis B and C

- blood transfusion recipients (prior to HCV testing)
- intravenous drug users (past or present)
- male homosexuals who have practised unsafe sex
- renal dialysis patients
- sex industry workers

Fig. 53.4 *Natural history of hepatitis B infection*

- those with abnormal LFTs with no obvious cause
- tattooed people

Prevention of transmission of hepatitis B and C viruses
Advice to those who are positive for HCV:
- Do not donate blood or any body organs.
- Do not share needles.
- Advise health care workers, including your dentist.
- Do not share intimate equipment such as toothbrushes, razors, nail files and nail scissors.
- Wipe up blood spills in the home with household bleach.
- Cover up cuts or wounds with an adequate dressing.
- Dispose of bloodstained tissues, sanitary napkins and other dressings safely.
- Use safe sex practices such as condoms.

Hepatitis D
Hepatitis D is a small defective virus that lacks a surface coat. This is provided by hepatitis B virus, and so hepatitis D infection occurs only in patients with concomitant hepatitis B.

It is usually spread parenterally and if chronic is usually associated with progressive disease with a poor prognosis. Treatment with interferon has a poor success rate. Antibodies to the delta virus, both anti-HDV and anti-HDV IgM (indicating a recent infection) as well as HDV Ag can be measured.[9]

Hepatitis E
Hepatitis E is an enterically transmitted virus that occurs in outbreaks in certain countries with a poor water supply such as some Asian sub-continent countries. Epidemiologically, HEV behaves like HAV with well-documented waterborne epidemics in areas of poor sanitation. There is a high case fatality rate (up to 20%) in pregnant females.

Hepatitis F
Researchers claim to have identified HGF virus that is spread enterically.[10]

Hepatitis G

HGV has been identified as a transfusion spread virus. It has subsequently been found to be prevalent among Queensland blood donors.[8,11]

Cholestatic jaundice

Cholestasis refers to the syndrome of biliary obstructive jaundice whereby there is obstruction to the flow of bile from the hepatocyte to the duodenum, thus causing bilirubin to accumulate in the blood. It is classified into two main groups:

- intrahepatic cholestasis—at the hepatocyte or intrahepatic biliary tree level
- extrahepatic cholestasis—obstruction in the large bile ducts

The significant causes are listed in Table 53.7.

Symptoms

- jaundice (greenish tinge)
- dark urine and pale stools
- pruritus—worse on palms and soles
- pain varies from nil to severe

Gallstones and jaundice

Gallstones can be found in the following (Fig. 53.5):

- gall bladder (asymptomatic up to 75%)—the majority remain here
- neck of gall bladder ⎱ biliary 'colic'
  ⎰ or
- cystic duct ⎰ acute cholecystitis
- common bile duct: may cause severe biliary 'colic', cholestatic jaundice or cholangitis

Table 53.7 *Significant causes of cholestasis in adults*

Intrahepatic
- viral hepatitis
- alcoholic hepatitis/cirrhosis
- drugs
- primary biliary cirrhosis

Extrahepatic
- common bile duct gallstones
- cancer of pancreas
- cancer of bile ducts
- other cancer: primary or secondary spread
- cholangitis
- primary sclerosing cholangitis (? autoimmune)
- pancreatitis
- postsurgical biliary stricture or oedema

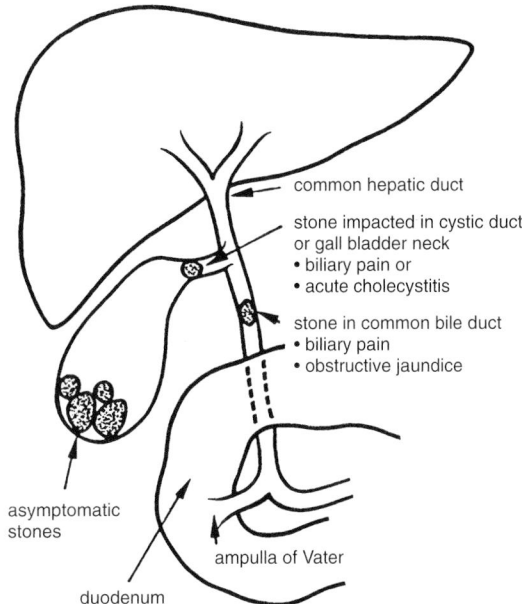

Fig. 53.5 *Clinical presentation of gallstones*

common hepatic duct

stone impacted in cystic duct or gall bladder neck
- biliary pain or
- acute cholecystitis

stone in common bile duct
- biliary pain
- obstructive jaundice

asymptomatic stones

ampulla of Vater

duodenum

Acute cholecystitis is accompanied by mild jaundice in 20% of cases, due to accompanying common duct stones.[9]

Common bile duct stones may be asymptomatic or may present with any one or all of the triad of abdominal pain, jaundice and fever. The jaundice varies, depending on the amount of obstruction. The liver is moderately enlarged if the obstruction lasts for more than a few hours.

The investigations of choice for cholestatic jaundice are ultrasound and ERCP.

Acute cholangitis

This is due to bacterial infection of the bile ducts secondary to abnormalities of the bile duct, especially gallstones in the common duct. Other causes are neoplasms and biliary strictures.

Charcot's triad (present in 70%) for acute cholangitis is:

Fever (often with rigor) + *upper abdominal pain* + *jaundice*

Older patients can present with circulatory collapse and Gram-negative septicaemia. Urgent referral is necessary.

Carcinoma of head of the pancreas

Pancreatic carcinoma is the fourth commonest cause of cancer death in the UK and USA.[9]

Typical clinical features
- M > F
- mainly > 60 years of age
- obstructive jaundice
- pain (over 75%)—epigastric and back
- enlarged gall bladder (50–75%)

Possible features
- weight loss, malaise, diarrhoea
- migratory thrombophlebitis
- palpable hard, fixed mass
- metastases, e.g. left supraclavicular gland of Virchow
- occult blood in stool
- glycosuria

Diagnosis
- scanning by ultrasound or CT scan may show mass
- ERCP

Prognosis
Very poor: 5 year survival 1–2%.

Cirrhosis of the liver

Cirrhosis is accompanied by jaundice as a late and serious manifestation with the exception of primary biliary cirrhosis where jaundice appears before advanced liver failure. The development of jaundice usually indicates that there is minimal hepatic reserve and is therefore found in conjunction with other signs of liver failure (Fig. 53.6).

Causes
Common:
- alcohol excess
- chronic viral hepatitis (esp. HBV, HCV)

Others:
- autoimmune chronic active hepatitis
- primary biliary cirrhosis (autoimmune)
- haemochromatosis
- Wilson's disease
- drugs, e.g. methotrexate
- cryptogenic (no cause found)

Clinical features
- anorexia, nausea, ± vomiting
- swelling of legs
- abdominal distension
- bleeding tendency
- drowsiness, confusion or coma (if liver failure)

Signs
- spider naevi (distribution of superior vena cava)
- palmar erythema of hands
- peripheral oedema and ascites
- jaundice (obstructive or hepatocellular)
- enlarged tender liver (small liver in long-term cirrhosis)
- ascites
- gynaecomastia
- ± splenomegaly (portal hypertension)

Complications
- ascites
- portal hypertension and GIT haemorrhage
- portosystemic encephalopathy
- hepatoma
- renal failure

Autoimmune chronic active hepatitis

Also termed idiopathic ACAH, it usually affects young females (10–40 years) who present insidiously with progressive fatigue, anorexia and jaundice. Diagnosis is made by abnormal LFTs, positive smooth muscle antibodies, a variety of other autoantibodies and a typical liver biopsy. If untreated most patients die within 3–5 years. Treatment is with prednisolone orally, monitored according to serum alanine aminotransferase levels, and supplemented with azathioprine.

Alcoholic liver disease

The main effects of alcohol excess on the liver are:
- fatty liver
- alcoholic hepatitis (progresses to cirrhosis if alcohol consumption continues)
- alcoholic cirrhosis

If diagnosed, patients are advised to stop drinking alcohol for life except for fatty liver when small amounts can be drunk later.

Special patient groups
The returned overseas traveller

The overseas traveller presenting with jaundice may have been infected by any one of the viruses—hepatitis A, B, C, D or E. All are prevalent in developing countries, especially in south-eastern and eastern Asia, some Pacific islands and Africa.

Other causes to consider are malaria, ascending cholangitis and drug-induced hepatic

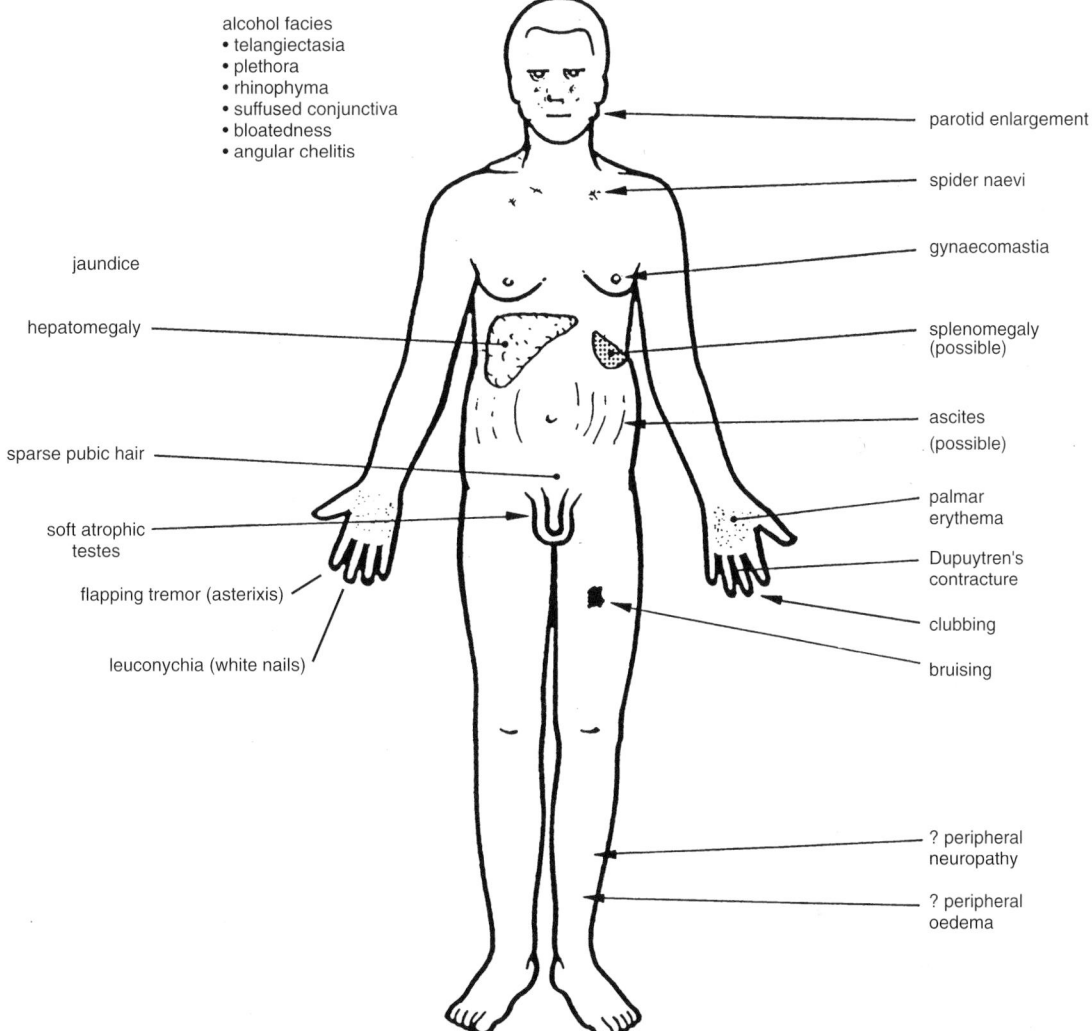

alcohol facies
• telangiectasia
• plethora
• rhinophyma
• suffused conjunctiva
• bloatedness
• angular chelitis

parotid enlargement

spider naevi

gynaecomastia

jaundice

hepatomegaly

splenomegaly
(possible)

ascites
(possible)

sparse pubic hair

palmar
erythema

soft atrophic
testes

Dupuytren's
contracture

flapping tremor (asterixis)

clubbing

leuconychia (white nails)

bruising

? peripheral
neuropathy

? peripheral
oedema

Fig. 53.6 *Possible features of chronic alcoholic liver disease*

damage due to, for example, the antimalarials, including mefloquine (Lariam) and Fansidar.

The pregnant patient

Specific types of jaundice related to pregnancy are rare. Viral hepatitis accounts for 40% of all cases of jaundice during pregnancy. Cholestasis of pregnancy is due to an oestrogen sensitivity. The symptoms are mild and the condition clears up rapidly after delivery, but it often recurs if the patient is prescribed oral contraceptives.[12]

Severe pre-eclampsia, eclampsia and hyperemesis gravidarum may cause hepatic damage and failure but the most dramatic condition is acute fatty liver of pregnancy, which is now very

rare. It is a serious condition of unknown aetiology and may follow the administration of hepatotoxic agents, especially in the more debilitated patient, usually in the third trimester. Acute fatty liver presents in the last trimester with symptoms of fulminant hepatitis, namely jaundice, vomiting, abdominal pain, possibly coma.[9] It has a high mortality (about 75%) and necessitates urgent termination of pregnancy, which may save both mother and baby.

Postoperative jaundice

There are many possible causes of postoperative jaundice either in the immediate or the long-term postoperative phase. Hypoxia associated with shock in a severely ill patient or in a patient with cardiopulmonary disease may lead to transient abnormalities in liver function. Other causes include:

- post-transfusion hepatitis
- coincident viral hepatitis
- drugs, including anaesthetics
- transfusion overload (haemolysis)
- sepsis
- unmasked chronic liver disease and biliary tact disease
- cholestasis: post major abdominal surgery

Neonates of HBeAg positive mothers

The neonates should have the following:

- hepatitis B immunoglobulin IM within 24 hours of birth
- hepatitis B vaccine at birth, 1 month and 6 months

This is not 100% effective because some infants can be infected *in utero*.

When to refer

- All patients with fulminant hepatitis
- All patients with chronic liver disease
- Painless obstructive jaundice
- Evidence of malignancy
- Symptomatic gallstones
- Patients with cirrhosis
- Acute fatty liver of pregnancy (very urgent)
- Suspected rare conditions, e.g. Wilson's disease

Practice tips

- All drugs should be suspected as potential hepatotoxins.
- With hepatitis A the presence of IgM antibodies reflects recent infection, and IgG antibody indicates past infection and lifelong immunity.
- There is no chronic carrier state of hepatitis A and E.
- All patients with jaundice should be tested for hepatitis B surface antigen (HBsAg).
- Hepatitis B infection is usually benign and short-lived, but it can be fatal if chronic hepatitis develops, which may lead later to cirrhosis and hepatocellular carcinoma.
- Up to 5–10% of patients with hepatitis B will become chronic carriers (especially drug addicts and homosexuals).

- Such carriers are identified by persistent titres of HBsAg and possibly HBeAg, the latter indicating the presence of the whole virus, and active replication and high infectivity.
- A raised gamma glutamyl transferase accompanied by a raised MCV is a good screening test for alcohol abuse.
- A systolic murmer may be heard over the liver in alcoholic hepatitis and hepatoma.
- A distaste for smoking (with jaundice) suggests acute viral hepatitis.

References

1. Kincaid-Smith R, Larkins R, Whelan G. *Problems in clinical medicine*. Sydney: McLennan & Petty, 1989, 251.
2. Coffman D, Chalstrey J, Smith-Laing G. *Gastrointestinal disorders*. Edinburgh: Churchill Livingstone, 1986, 106.
3. Sandler G. Fry J. *Early clinical diagnosis*. Lancaster: MTP Press, 1986, 468–490.
4. Taggart G. Viral hepatitis. Sigma Clinical Review, 1988, no 17:15.
5. Robinson MJ. *Practical paediatrics*. Melbourne: Churchill Livingstone, 1990, 192.
6. Smith BC, Watson KR. Management of the chronic hepatitis B carrier. Aust Fam Physician, 1995; 24:331–339.
7. Ruff TA, Gust I. Hepatitis, viral (acute and chronic). In: MIMS disease index (2nd edn). Sydney: IMS Publishing, 1996, 226–230.
8. Bowden DS, Moaven LD. Locarnini SA. New hepatitis viruses: Are there enough letters in the alphabet? Med J Aust, 1996; 164:87–89.
9. Kumer PJ, Clarke ML. *Clinical medicine* (2nd edn). London: Bailliere Tindall, 1990, 237–292.
10. Deka N, Sharma MD, Mukerjee R. Isolation of the novel agent from human stool that is associated with sporadic human hepatitis. J Virol, 1994; 68: 7810–7815.
11. Moaven LD et al. Prevalence of hepatitis G virus in Queensland blood donors. Med J Aust, 1996; 165:369–371.
12. Beischer NA, MacKay EV. *Obstetrics and the newborn*. Sydney: Saunders, 1986, 307–308.

54
Nausea and vomiting

—

Nausea, retching and hypersalivation frequently precede the act of vomiting, which is a highly integrated sequence of involuntary visceral and somatic motor events.

Harrison's Principles of Internal Medicine 1994

Vomiting or emesis is a rather dramatic event with a diverse number of causes. It is usually preceded by nausea.

Definitions

Nausea. This is the unpleasant sickly sensation that can herald the onset of vomiting or can be present without vomiting.

Vomiting. This is the forceful expulsion of gastric contents through the mouth.

Regurgitation. This is the expulsion of food in the absence of nausea and without diaphragmatic muscular contractions.

Retching. This is an involuntary act with all the movements of vomiting without the expulsion of gastric contents because the cardiac orifice remains closed.

Haematemesis. This is vomiting of blood. It is presented on pages 512–514.

Key checkpoints

- Nausea and vomiting have a wide range of potential causes emanating from every body system.
- The common cause of acute nausea and vomiting in most age groups is gastroenteritis.
- The most common causes of vomiting in children are infections—viral (especially) and

bacterial—including otitis media and urinary infection.
- Drug ingestion is a common cause of nausea and vomiting; thus a drug history is vital in assessment.
- Vomiting is commonly associated with migraine and may be the only symptom of a variety of migraine.
- The nature of the vomitus provides a clue:
    faecalent = intestinal obstruction
    blood = bleeding from oesophagus, stomach or duodenum (mostly)
    coffee-grounds = bleeding from stomach or duodenum

The clinical approach
History
A careful history is essential with an emphasis on drug intake, possible psychogenic factors including self-induced emesis, weight loss, other GIT symptoms or symptoms suggestive of systemic disease.

Diagnostic guidelines

- Surgical GIT causes are unlikely in the absence of abdominal pain.
- Vomiting without bile-stained vomitus = pyloric obstruction.
- Vomiting of bile = obstruction below duodenal ampulla.
- Vomiting of ingested food = oesophageal obstruction.
- Vomiting without nausea and possibly projectile = ↑ intracranial pressure.

A summary of the diagnostic strategy model is presented in Table 54.1

Table 54.1 *Vomiting: diagnostic strategy model*

Q. *Probability diagnosis*
A. All ages: acute gastroenteritis
                                motion sickness
                                drugs
                                various infections
    Neonates: feeding problems
    Children: viral infections/fever
                                otitis media
                                urinary tract infection
    Adults: gastritis
                                alcohol intoxication
                                pregnancy
                                migraine

Q. *Serious disorders not to be missed*
A. Bowel obstruction
   • oesophageal atresia (neonates)
   • pyloric obstruction < 3 months
   • intestinal malrotation
   • intussusception
   • malignancy, e.g. oesophagus
   Severe infection
   • septicaemia
   • meningitis/encephalitis
   • infective endocarditis
   • others, e.g. acute viral hepatitis
   Malignancy
   Intracranial disorders
   • malignancy
   • cerebellar haemorrhage
   Acute appendicitis
   Acute pancreatitis
   Acute myocardial infarction, e.g. painless

Q. *Pitfalls (mainly adults)*
A. Pregnancy (early)
   Organic failure
   • liver, renal, heart, respiratory
   Labyrinthine disorders
   • Ménière's syndrome
   • labyrinthitis
   Poisoning
   • food
   • chemicals
   Gut motility disorders
   • achalasia
   Substance abuse
   Radiation therapy
   Hypercalcaemia
   Functional obstruction
   • diabetic gastroparesis
   • idiopathic gastroparesis

Q. *Seven masquerades checklist*
A. Depression   possible
   Diabetes   √ ketoacidosis
   Drugs   √ √
   Anaemia   —
   Thyroid and other   √
     endocrine
   Spinal dysfunction   —
   UTI   √ √

Q. *Is this patient trying to tell me something?*
A. Possible: extreme stress, e.g. panic attacks
   Consider bulimia (self-induced vomiting)

Examination

If fever is present possible sources of infection, e.g. middle ear, meninges and urinary tract, should be checked.

A careful abdominal examination is appropriate in most instances and this includes urinalysis. Look particularly for scars indicating previous surgery. Look for a succussion splash—this indicates pyloric obstruction.

A neurological examination needs to be considered including ophthalmoloscopy. Consider raised intracranial pressure.

No examination is complete without assessment of the patient's physical fitness including the level of hydration, especially in infants.

Investigations

These should consider the underlying cause and also biochemical abnormalities resulting from fluid and electrolyte loss.

The following need to be considered:
• pregnancy test
• microscopy and culture of stools
• radiology of GIT
• oesophageal motility studies
• neurological investigation for suspected intracranial pressure
• drug toxicity studies
• biochemistry

Vomiting in infancy

First question: Is the vomiting bile-stained?

• Green vomiting = urgent surgical referral for possible intestinal malrotation (6 hours leeway before gangrene of bowel)[1]
• Non bile-stained vomitus
  Consider pyloric stenosis, gastro-oesophageal reflux (GOR), feeding problems, concealed infection, e.g. UTI, meningitis. Both pyloric stenosis and GOR cause projectile vomiting.

Important warning signs in neonates

• excessive drooling of frothy secretions from mouth
• bile-stained vomitus—always abnormal
• delayed passage of meconium (beyond 24 hours)
• inguinal hernias

Specific conditions

Oesophageal atresia

- Vomiting occurs with the first feeding.
- There is excessive drooling of frothy secretions from the mouth.
- Pass a 10 French gauge catheter through the mouth to aid diagnosis.

Congenital hypertrophic pyloric stenosis

- usually sudden onset 3rd–6th week
- projectile vomitus
- failure to thrive
- male:female = 5:1
- gastric peristalsis during test feeding (L→R)
  - feel for pyloric tumour either during test feeding or immediately after vomiting (deep in right epigastrium)—Figure 54.1. Once felt, further investigation is not necessary.
- biochemistry
  - metabolic alkalosis: sodium usually < 130 mmol/L, chloride < 100 mmol/L
- special investigations (if necessary)
  - barium meal (string sign)
  - abdominal ultrasound
- treatment
  - correct fluid and electrolyte deficiency (hypochloraemic alkalosis)
  - surgical management (longitudinal pyloromyotomy)

Acute gastroenteritis

See pages 401 and 404.

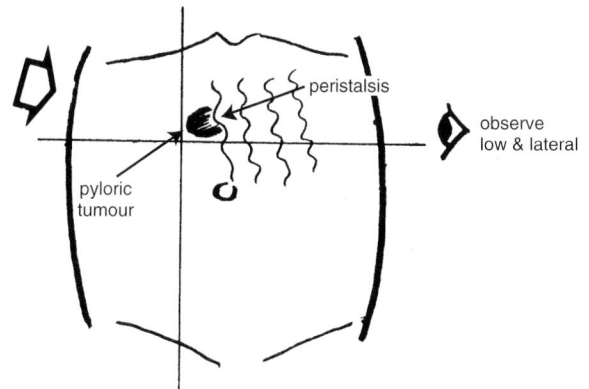

Fig. 54.1 *Signs of pyloric stenosis*

Symptomatic relief of vomiting

The first-line management is to ensure that any fluid and electrolyte imbalance is corrected and that any underlying cause is identified and treated. Various antiemetics can give symptomatic relief.

Drug-induced nausea and vomiting[2]

- metoclopramide 10 mg (o) or IM 8 hourly prn

For cytotoxic drugs, e.g. cisplatin and radiotherapy:

- metoclopramide 10 mg (o) or IM 1 to 2 hours prior to therapy then 8 hourly (if mild)

For severe cases:

- ondansetron 8 mg (o) or IV prior to therapy then 2 doses 6 hourly
  plus
- dexamethasone 8 mg IV 30 minutes prior to therapy, then 2 doses 6 hourly

Note: Restrict ondansetron to 8 mg daily for those with hepatic dysfunction

Motion sickness

- promethazine theoclate 25 mg (o) 60 minutes prior to travel
  or
- dimenhydrinate 50 mg (o) 60 minutes prior to travel
  or
- hyoscine 300–600 μg (o) 30 minutes prior to travel
  or
- hyoscine 1.5 mg dermal disc: applied to dry hairless skin behind the ear 5–6 hours before travel (effective for 72 hours)[2]

For treatment: repeat oral presentations 4–6 hourly during trip (maximum 4 doses in 24 hours)

Vestibular disturbances[2]

The phenothiazine derivatives are the most effective, while the dopamine D_2-receptor antagonists are ineffective.

- prochlorperazine 5–10 mg (o) or 10 mg rectally, SC or IM 4 times daily prn
  or
- promethazine theoclate 25 mg (o) or IM 4 hourly prn (maximum 100–150 mg per 24 hours)

Note: Beware of tardive dyskinesia with prolonged use.

Gastroenteritis

For severe cases in adults:

• metoclopramide 10 mg (o) or IM 8 hourly prn

Gastroparesis[2]

• metoclopramide 5–10 mg (o) 30 minutes before meals

or

• cisapride 5–20 mg (o) qid 15 minutes before meals

Pregnancy

• pyridoxine hydrochloride 25–50 mg tds

if still ineffective add

• metoclopramide 10 mg (o) tds or IM (if oral intolerance)

Postoperative vomiting[2]

• metoclopramide 10 mg IM or IV (slowly), 8 hourly prn

or

• prochlorperazine 12.5 mg IM, 8 hourly prn

Note: A list of some drugs that can cause nausea and vomiting is presented in Table 54.2.

Practice tips

• Consider the possibility of anorexia nervosa and bulimia in adolescent females with a history of vomiting immediately after meals, especially after binge eating.
• If weight loss accompanies nausea and vomiting consider GIT malignancy and obstruction as well as the above psychogenic conditions.
• Early morning nausea and vomiting can be caused typically by alcohol, pregnancy, renal failure and raised intracranial pressure.

Table 54.2 *Some drugs that can cause nausea and vomiting*

• Alcohol (including binge drinking)
• Antibiotics (various) esp. erythromycin
• Antidepressants, e.g. serotonin reuptake inhibitors
• Antihypertensives
• Bromocriptine
• Codeine
• Corticosteroids
• Cytotoxic agents
• Digoxin
• Levodopa
• Iron preparations
• Nicotine and nicotine gum
• NSAIDS, e.g. indomethacin
• Opiates, e.g. morphine, codeine
• Oral contraceptives
• Salicylates
• Theophylline

• Intracranial space-occupying lesions can cause vomiting without associated anorexia or nausea.
• Gastroparesis commonly occurs in long-standing diabetes or may be idiopathic. Intense nausea and anorexia are a feature.
• Antiemetic drug therapy should not be used in infants and children with gastroenteritis.
• Antiemetic treatment must be tailored to the specific cause of the problem.
• The major complications of severe vomiting include trauma of the distal oesophagus such as a Mallory-Weiss tear and severe fluid and electrolyte disturbances.

References

1. Efron D. *Paediatric handbook* (5th edn). Melbourne: Blackwell Science, 1996, 232–233.

2. Moulds RFW et al. *Gastrointestinal drug guidelines*. Melbourne: Victorian Medical Postgraduate Foundation, 1994–95, 21–27.

55
Neck lumps

—

There are approximately 800 lymph nodes in the body; no fewer than 300 of them lie in the neck and inflammation of these is exceedingly common.

McNeill Love (Editor of Bailey & Love) 1965

In the management of lumps in the neck it is important to distinguish between the various midline and lateral causes, especially cervical lymphadenopathy, which may be caused by occult malignancy such as in the aerodigestive tract. With increasing ageing in the population

the number of patients presenting with a malignant neck lump is also increasing. The neck is divided into anterior and posterior triangles by the sternomastoid muscle and the anatomical areas are helpful in identifying the origin of the primary lesion (Fig. 55.1).

Key points

- Lymph nodes are normally palpable in children between 3 and 8 years of age; soft

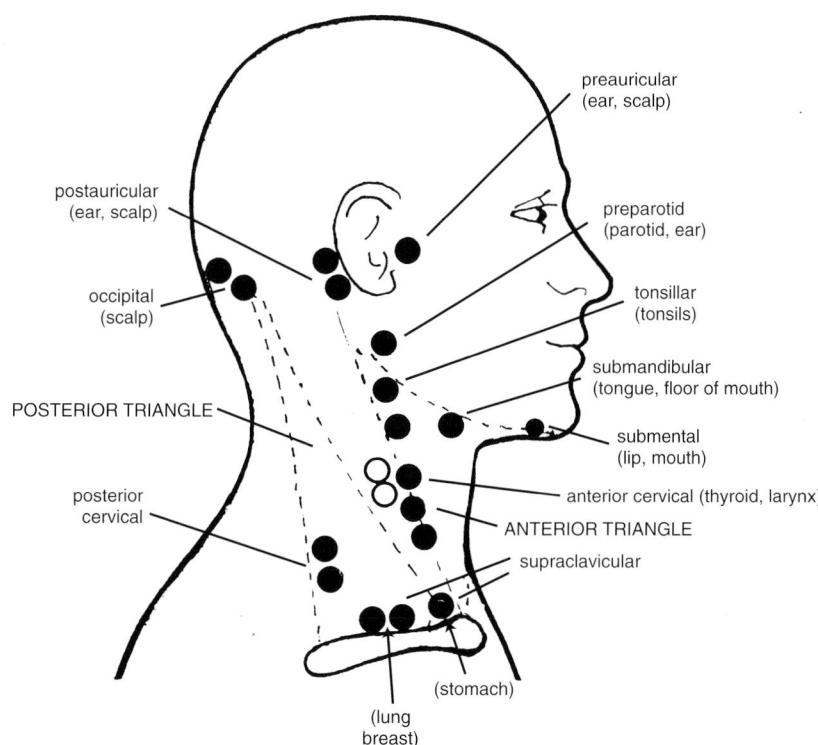

Fig. 55.1 *Lymph glands of the neck including common sources of adenopathy (excluding lymphomas)*

mobile nodes up to 1 cm in diameter are commonly felt in the anterior and posterior triangle. A node > 2 cm is considered to be enlarged. Some cervical glands are very prominent, especially tonsillar nodes.

- These prominent nodes often enlarge during intercurrent viral infection.
- Causes of neck swellings are lymph nodes 85%, goitres 8%, others 7%.[1]
- Solitary nodules in the thyroid move on swallowing.
- Consider the possibility of tuberculosis.
- A knowledge of the areas drained by lymph nodes is important (Fig. 55.1).
- Examination must extend beyond the neck for lymphadenopathy.
- To examine cervical glands slightly rotate head and palpate with palmar aspect of fingers.
- Palpate submental area with head slightly flexed.
- Biopsy of a complete lymph node is necessary to establish diagnosis for unknown or suspicious causes but do not consider it as the first step in diagnosis.[2]
- Other investigations are chest X-ray and FBE. Bone marrow biopsy or fine-needle aspiration of thyroid nodule or other masses may be considered. Fine-needle aspiration, which is a relatively simple procedure, is the single most helpful investigation for diagnosing the cause.[3]
- Imaging techniques that may assist diagnosis include axial CT scan (especially in fat necks), MRI scan (distinguishes a malignant swelling from scar tissue or oedema), tomogram of larynx (laryngocele or malignancy), barium swallow (pharyngeal pouch), sialogram and carotid angiogram.

The 20:40 and 80:20 rules[3]

The age of the patient is a helpful guide, as causes of neck lumps can be roughly categorised by the '20:40 rule':

- 0–20 years: congenital, inflammatory, lymphoma
- 20–40 years: inflammatory, salivary, thyroid, lymphoma
- > 40 years: lymphoma, metastases

Most neck lumps (80%) are benign in children while the reverse applies to adults.

Cervical lymphadenopathy

- There are many causes varying from local infections to lymphoproliferative disorders.
- Most malignant nodes in the supraclavicular area have their primary tumour below the clavicle.
- Eighty-five per cent of malignant nodes in the anterior triangle have their primary tumour in the head and neck.[2]
- Always search for:
  — other nodes at distant sites
  — possible primary source of infections or neoplasia
  — hepatosplenomegaly
- Hodgkin's disease usually presents with rubbery, painless nodes in the neck.
- Most swellings are lateral.

Consistency of enlarged nodes

Rules of thumb are:[4]
- hard: secondary carcinoma
- rubbery: lymphoma
- soft: sarcoidosis or infection
- tender and
  multiple: infection

Causes of cervical lymph node enlargement (lateral cervical swelling)

Acute cervical lymphadenitis
- acute viral lymphadenitis
- acute bacterial lymphadenitis—coccal infection

Chronic lymph node infection
- MAIS lymphadenitis (atypical tuberculosis)
- viral infection, e.g. E-B mononucleosis, rubella, cytomegalovirus, HIV
- *Toxoplasma gondii* infection

Neoplastic lymphadenopathy
- lymphomas, esp. Hodgkin's disease
- leukaemia

Metastatic
- Check mouth, pharynx, sinuses, larynx, scalp, oesophagus, stomach, breast, lungs, thyroid, skin. A working rule is upper neck (from skin to upper aerodigestive tract); lower neck (from below clavicles, e.g. lung, stomach, breast, colon).

- Examples:
  — occipital or preauricular—check scalp
  — submental—check mouth, tongue, teeth
  — submandibular—check floor of mouth
  — left supraclavicular (under sternomas-toid)—consider stomach (Troisier's sign)
  — deep anterior cervical—consider larynx, thyroid, oesophagus, lungs

Non lymph node swellings

Widespread
- sebaceous cysts
- lipomas

Midline
- thyroid nodule (moves upon swallowing)
- thyroglossal cysts (move up on tongue protrusion)
- dermoid cyst (beneath chin)
- midline cervical lymph node swelling

Anterior triangle
- branchial cyst (in upper part)
  — usually adulthood (20–25 years)
- carotid body tumour
  — opposite thyroid cartilage
  — smooth and pulsatile
  — can be moved laterally but not vertically
  — usually 40–60 years
  — requires excision (with care)
- carotid aneurysm
- lateral thyroid tumours

Posterior triangle
- developmental remnants
  — cystic hygroma
  — bronchial sinuses and cysts
- Pancoast's tumour (from apex lung)
- cervical rib

Submandibular swellings
- submandibular salivary gland
- cervicofacial actinomycosis (lumpy jaw syndrome)
  — infection follows dental extraction or poor dental hygiene
  — treat with high dose penicillin G, 4 months

Sternomastoid tumour

Pharyngeal pouch
- a soft, squelchy indefinite mass
- base of left neck
- history of difficulty in swallowing

Neck lumps in children

Eighty per cent of neck lumps are benign while 20% are malignant. Benign lumps usually occur in the anterior triangle, while malignant lumps are more likely in the posterior triangle. The common midline lump in children is the thyroglossal cyst.[3]

Lymphadenopathy
- Most enlarged lymph nodes are either 'normal' or local infections (mainly viral), especially if < 2 cm diameter, and not hard or fixed.
- Inflammatory nodes may be caused by infection in the tonsils, the teeth or other oral or nasopharyngeal cavities.
- They are of concern if supraclavicular node enlargement and fever < 1 week.
- Suspicious nodes are > 2.5 cm, with firmer consistency than normal and less mobility (investigate especially with biopsy).

MAIS lymphadenitis[5]
- child usually 2–3 years of age
- caused by *Mycobacterium avium intracellulare* or *M. scrofulaceum*
- a relatively common infection of cervical nodes yet often unrecognised
- painless swelling due to development of a cold abscess in healthy child
- common sites are submandibular, tonsillar and preauricular nodes
- invariably unilateral, confined to one lymph node group
- no pulmonary involvement
- unresponsive to antimicrobials: treatment is by surgical excision

Acute bacterial lymphadenitis
- usually coccal infections—staphylococcus, streptococcus
- can progress to abscess formation (fluctuant): requires drainage

When to refer
- A persisting lump, depending on its location and size
- A lymph node or group of nodes that are abnormally enlarged and fail to respond to antibiotics

References

1. Fry J, Berry H. *Surgical problems in clinical practice*. London: Edward Arnold, 1987, 38.

2. Coman WB. Neck lumps in adults. In: MIMS disease index (2nd edn). Sydney: IMS Publishing, 1996, 340–341.

3. Cole IE, Turner J. Neck lumps: Clues to the diagnosis and management. Mod Med Aust, 1997; 37–55.

4. Larkins R, Smallwood R. *Clinical skills*. Melbourne: Melbourne University Press, 1993, 133–134.

5. Stokes K. *Lumps in the neck in children*. Proceedings notes. Box Hill Hospital Seminar, 1995: 1–2.

56

Neck pain

—

Neck pain is a very common symptom in both sexes at all ages and although most pain is experienced in the posterior aspect of the neck, anterior neck pain can occur from causes that overlap between front and back. The main cause of neck pain is a disorder of the cervical spine, which usually manifests as neck pain but can refer pain to the head, shoulders and chest. Such pain usually originates from the facet (apophyseal) joints but can arise from other musculoskeletal structures such as the intervertebral discs and the muscles or ligaments (Fig. 56.1). The other major symptom is limited movement or stiffness.

General causes of neck pain are presented in Table 56.1.

Key facts and checkpoints

- At any time approximately 10% of the adult population are experiencing[1] an episode of neck pain.

Fig. 56.1 *Transverse section illustrating the functional unit and nervous network of the cervical spine*

spinal cord

facet joint

posterior primary ramus

nerve root

sinuvertebral nerve

vertebral artery

sympathetic chain

nucleus pulposus } intervertebral
annulus fibrosus } disc

Table 56.1 *Causes of neck pain (a pathological classification)*

Musculoskeletal

Joint dysfunction
• apophyseal
• intervertebral disc
Muscular/ligamentous strains or sprains
Trauma
• 'whiplash'
• fracture
• other disorders

Inflammation
• osteoarthritis*
• rheumatoid arthritis
• ankylosing spondylitis
• psoriasis
• inflammatory bowel disorders
• Reiter's disease/reactive arthritis
• polymyalgia rheumatica
• thyroiditis

Infective

Spinal
• osteomyelitis
• tuberculosis
• herpes zoster
Extraspinal
• cervical adenitis
• poliomyelitis
• tetanus
Extracervical
• meningitis
• febrile states:
   — meningism
   — malaria

Degenerative
• spondylosis*

Neoplasia
• benign
• malignant

Fibromyalgia syndrome

Psychogenic

Referred visceral
• heart
• oesophagus
• carcinoma lung

Referred cranial
• haemorrhage, e.g. subarachnoid
• tumour
• abscess

---

* Osteoarthritis, or spondylosis, is inflammatory and degenerative.

• The commonest cause of neck pain is dysfunction of the facet joints with or without a history of injury.
• Disorders of the intervertebral discs are common, especially in the lower cervical spine, and may cause unilateral pain, paraesthesia or anaesthesia in the arm.
• In a UK study radiological cervical disc degeneration was present in 40% of males and 28% of females[1] between 55 and 64 years.
• Strains, sprains and fractures of the facet joints, especially after a 'whiplash' injury, are difficult to detect and are often overlooked as a cause of persistent neck pain.
• Cervical spondylosis is a disorder of ageing: radiological signs occur in 50% of people over the age of 50 and in 75% over the age of 65.[2]
• In cervical spondylosis, osteophytic projections may produce nerve root and spinal cord compression, resulting in radiculopathy and myelopathy respectively.
• Radiculopathy can be caused by a soft disc protrusion (usually unilateral), a hard calcified lump and osteophytes (may be bilateral).
• Cervical disorders are aggravated by vibration, e.g. riding in a motor vehicle.
• Always determine the C2, C6 and C7 levels by finding the relevant spinous processes (easily palpable landmarks) prior to palpation.
• Palpation of the neck is the cornerstone of cervical management. Palpate gently—the more one presses the less one feels.
• Most episodes of neck pain, including acute torticollis, are transient, lasting from about 2 to 10 days.
• In one study 70% of people with neck pain who sought medical attention had recovered or were recovering within one month.[1]
• Effective management of neck pain is based on the principle that stiff dysfunctional joints are painful and restoration of normal movement may be associated with resolution of pain.
• The optimal treatment for dysfunctional joints (without organic disease or radiculopathy) is active and passive mobilisation, especially as exercises.

A diagnostic approach

A summary of the safety diagnostic model is presented in Table 56.2.

Probability diagnosis

The main causes of neck pain are vertebral dysfunction, especially of the facet joints, and traumatic strains or sprains affecting the musculoligamentous structures of the neck. The

Table 56.2 *Neck pain: diagnostic strategy model*

Q. *Probability diagnosis*
A. Vertebral dysfunction
Traumatic 'strain' or 'sprain'
Cervical spondylosis

Q. *Serious disorders not to be missed*
A. Cardiovascular
• angina
• subarachnoid haemorrhage
Neoplasia
• primary
• metastasis
• Pancoast's tumour
Severe infections
• osteomyelitis
• meningitis
Vertebral fractures or dislocation

Q. *Pitfalls (often missed)*
A. Disc prolapse
Myelopathy
Cervical lymphadenitis
Fibromyalgia syndrome
Outlet compression syndrome, e.g. cervical rib
Polymyalgia rheumatica
Ankylosing spondylitis
Rheumatoid arthritis
Oesophageal foreign bodies and tumours
Paget's disease

Q. *Seven masquerades checklist*
Depression   √
Diabetes   —
Drugs   —
Anaemia   —
Thyroid disease   √ Thyroiditis
Spinal dysfunction   √√
UTI   —

Q. *Is the patient trying to tell me something?*
A. Highly probable. Stress and adverse occupational factors relevant.

so-called myofascial syndrome is mainly a manifestation of dysfunction of the facet joints. Acute wry neck (torticollis), which is quite common, is yet another likely manifestation of apophyseal joint dysfunction. Spondylosis, known also as degenerative osteoarthrosis and osteoarthritis, is also a common cause, especially in the elderly patient.

Intervertebral disc disruption is also a relatively common phenomenon in the cervical spine, especially at the lower levels C5–6 and C6–7.[3]

Serious disorders not to be missed

Conditions causing neck pain and stiffness may be a sign of meningitis or of cerebral haemorrhage, particularly subarachnoid haemorrhage, or of a cerebral tumour or retropharyngeal abscess.

Angina and myocardial infarction should be considered in anterior neck pain. Other visceral disorders can refer pain to the neck.

Tumours are relatively rare in the cervical spine but metastases do occur and should be kept in mind, especially with persistent neck pain present day and night.

Metastasis to the spine occurs in 5–10% of patients with systemic cancer, making it the second most common neurological complication of cancer. The cervical spine accounts for some 15% of spinal metastases.[2] The commonest primary tumours are the breast, prostate or lung. Other primaries include the kidney, thyroid and melanoma.

Pitfalls

There are many pitfalls in the clinical assessment of causes of neck pain and many of them are inflammatory.

Rheumatoid arthritis is the prime severe inflammatory arthropathy that involves the neck but the neck can be affected by the seronegative spondyloarthropathies, particularly ankylosing spondylitis, psoriasis and the inflammatory bowel disorders.

While polymyalgia rheumatica affects mainly the shoulder girdle, pain in the lower neck, which is part of the symptom complex, is often overlooked. Diffuse neck pain in myofascial soft tissue with tender trigger areas is part of the uncommon but refractory fibromyalgia syndrome.

General pitfalls

• Failing to appreciate how often the benign problem of facet joint dysfunction occurs in the neck, causing pain and limited movement. This involves failure to appreciate the value of physical therapy, especially exercise programs, in alleviating the problem.
• Failing to adhere to the idiom: one disc—one nerve root. Involvement of more than one nerve root in the upper limb may mean a neoplastic disorder such as metastatic disease, lymphoma in the thoracic outlet and similar serious diseases.
• Missing the insidious onset of myelopathy, especially the spasticity component, caused by rheumatoid arthritis, osteophytic overgrowth or, rarely, a soft disc prolapse.

Seven masquerades checklist

Cervical spinal dysfunction is the obvious outstanding cause. Thyroiditis may cause neck pain, as in the extremely rare cases of acute specific infection in the thyroid (e.g. syphilis, pyogenic infections), which causes severe pain; non-specific thyroiditis (de Quervain's thyroiditis) produces painful swelling with dysphagia. The association between depression and neck pain is well documented.

Psychogenic considerations

The neck is one of the commonest areas for psychological fixation following injury. This may involve perpetuation or exaggeration of pain because of factors such as anxiety and depression, conversion reaction and secondary gain.

The psychological sequelae that can follow a whiplash injury and chronic neck problems such as spondylosis serve as a reminder that the state of the patient's cervical spine can profoundly affect his or her life and that we should always be aware of the whole person. A feeling of depression is a very common sequel to such an injury and these patients demand our dutiful care and understanding.

The clinical approach

History

It is important to analyse the pain into its various components, especially the nature of its onset, its site and radiation, and associated features. The diurnal pattern of the pain will provide a lead to the diagnosis (refer to Fig. 33.3: the patterns are similar to low back pain).

Key questions

- Can you point to exactly where in your neck you get the pain?
- Do you wake up with pain in the morning?
- Does the pain come on when you have to look up for a while?
- Do you have trouble reversing your car?
- Can you recall an injury to your head or neck such as hitting your head on an overhead bar?
- Does your neck grate or get stiff?
- Do you get headaches or feel dizzy?
- Is the pain present day and night?
- Do you get pain or pins and needles or numbness in your arms?
- Does the pain come on with activity?
- Does the pain wake you at night?

- Do you feel pain on both sides of your neck and over your shoulders?
- Do your hands or arms feel weak or clumsy?

Physical examination

It is appropriate to follow the traditional rule for examination of any joint or complex of joints: LOOK, FEEL, MOVE, MEASURE, TEST FUNCTION and X-RAY. Careful examination of the cervical spine is essential for the correct diagnosis and for specific treatment at the painful level.

Three objectives of the examination are to:

- reproduce the patient's symptoms
- identify the level of lesion or lesions
- determine the cause (if possible)

A neurological examination is essential if radicular pain is present, or weakness or other upper limb symptoms, including any pain or paraesthesia that extends below the elbow.

Inspection

The patient should be examined sitting on a couch, rather than on a chair. The body should be fully supported with the hands resting on the thighs. The following should be noted:
- willingness to move the head and neck
- level of the shoulders
- any lateral flexion
- contour of the neck from the side

In the patient with torticollis the head is held laterally flexed with, perhaps, slight rotation to one side—usually away from the painful side. Patients suffering from whiplash injury and severe spondylosis tend to hold the neck stiff and the head forward, and tend to turn the trunk rather than rotate the neck.

Palpation

For this vital component of the examination it is essential to know the surface anatomy of the neck so that the affected level can be determined.

Method

The patient lies prone on the examination couch with the forehead resting on the hands (palms up). The neck should be flexed forward and the shoulders relaxed.

1. *Central digital palpation*

   Systematically palpate the first spinous processes of the cervical vertebrae.
   - C2 (axis) is the first spinous process palpable beneath the occiput.
   - C7 is the largest 'fixed' and most prominent process—situated at the base of the neck.
   - C6 is also prominent but usually 'disappears' under the palpating finger with extension of the neck.
   - the spinous processes of C3, C4 and C5 are difficult to palpate because of cervical lordosis but their level can be estimated (Fig. 56.2).

   Standing at the patient's head, place opposed pulps of the thumbs on the spinous processes (starting at C2) and then move down the middle line to C7. Press firmly over each and with arms straight oscillate with moderate firmness three or four times to assess pain, stiffness or muscle spasm.

2. *Lateral digital palpation*

   The facet joints lie in sequence (called the articular pillar) about 2 to 3 centimetres from the midline. Press with opposed thumbs against this pillar in a systematic manner on either side of the midline (top to base) to determine any painful area.

   Palpation should be extended to include the anterior neck, searching for evidence of lymphadenitis, muscle spasm, thyroid disease and other problems.

Movement

Active movements are observed with the patient sitting on the couch. The movements are as follows with normal range indicated.

- flexion—45°
- extension—50°
- lateral flexion (R and L)—45°
- rotation (R and L)—75°

If there is a full range of pain-free movement, apply overpressure slowly at the end range and note any pain.

The range of movements can be plotted on a special grid called a direction of movement diagram (Fig. 56.3). This provides a ready reference for serial assessments.

Neurological examination

A neurological examination for nerve root lesions (C5 to T1) is indicated if the clinical assessment identifies the presence of neurological symptoms and signs such as pain, paraesthesia or anaesthesia in the arm. Nerve root pressure is indicated by:

- pain and paraesthesia along the distribution of the dermatome
- localised sensory loss
- reduced muscular power (weakness or fatigue or both)
- hyporeflexia (reduced amplitude or fatigue or both)

It is necessary to know the sensory distribution for each nerve root and the motor changes. This is summarised in Table 56.3. The dermatomes are illustrated in Figure 56.4.

Fig. 56.2 *Relative sizes of spinous processes of the cervical spine*

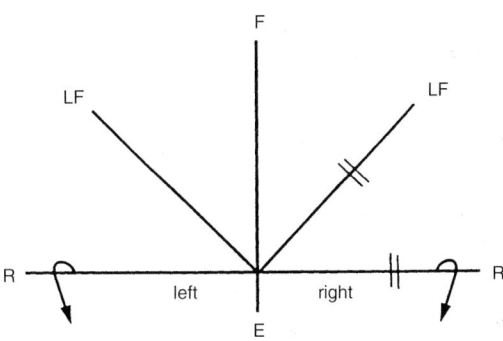

Fig. 56.3 *Direction of movement diagram to record movements of the neck. This record shows restricted and painful movements (indicated by II) in right lateral flexion and right rotation; the other movements are free*

Fig. 56.4 *Dermatomes of the upper limb, head and neck*

Investigations

The investigations are directed to diagnosing the painful condition and determining if suspected or true organic disease is present in the spine. It is inappropriate to perform sophisticated investigations such as CT scans on most patients. Scanning should be reserved where surgery is contemplated and serious disease is suspected but not confirmed by plain X-ray.

Investigations include:

- haemoglobin, film and WCC
- ESR
- rheumatoid arthritis factor
- HLA-B$_{27}$ antigen
- radiology

- plain X-ray
- plain CT scan
- CT scan and myelogram (if cervical disc surgery contemplated)
- radionuclide bone scan
- MRI

These should be selected conservatively.

Neck pain in children

In children and adolescents neck pain, often with stiffness, may be a manifestation of infection or inflammation of cervical lymph nodes, usually secondary to an infected throat—for example, tonsillitis or pharyngitis. However, it is vital to consider the possibility of meningitis. Sometimes a high fever associated with a systemic infection or pneumonia can cause meningism. In the presence of fever the rare possibility of poliomyelitis should be kept in mind. In both children and adults the presence of cerebral pathology such as haemorrhage, abscess or tumour are uncommon possibilities.[5] Acute torticollis is quite common in this age group and the neck may be involved in chronic juvenile arthritis.

Neck pain in the elderly

In adults the outstanding causes are dysfunction of the joints and spondylosis, with the acute febrile causes encountered in children being rare. However, cerebral and meningeal disorders may cause pain and stiffness in the neck.[5]

Rheumatoid arthritis is the prime severe inflammatory arthropathy that involves the neck, but the neck can be affected by the spondyloarthropathies, e.g. ankylosing spondylitis. The painful acute wry neck can affect all ages and is considered to be caused mainly by acute disorders of the apophyseal joints rather than disc prolapse. However, disc lesions do occur and

Table 56.3 *Cervical nerve root syndromes*

Nerve root	Sensory change	Muscle power	Power loss	Reflex
C5	Outer arm	Deltoid	Abduction arm	Biceps jerk
C6	Outer forearm/thumb/ index finger	Biceps	Elbow flexion Extension wrist	Biceps + brachioradialis
C7	Hand/middle and ring fingers	Triceps	Elbow extension	Triceps
C8	Inner forearm/ little finger	Long flexors finger, long extensors thumb	Grip	
T1	Inner arm	Interossei	Finger spread	

can cause referred pain or radicular pain. In the elderly radicular pain can be caused also by impingement of the nerve root in the intervertebral foramen that has become narrowed from the degenerative changes of long-standing spondylosis.

Problems with a higher probability with increasing age include:

- cervical spondylosis with radiculopathy or myelopathy
- atlantoaxial subluxation complicating rheumatoid arthritis
- polymyalgia rheumatica
- metastatic cancer
- Pancoast's tumour of the lung
- angina and myocardial infarction
- pharyngeal and retropharyngeal infection and tumour

Clinical problems of cervical spinal origin

Pain originating from disorders of the cervical spine is usually, although not always, experienced in the neck. The patient may experience headache, or pain around the ear, face, arm, shoulder, upper anterior or posterior chest.[6]

Possible symptoms:

- neck pain
- neck stiffness
- headache
- 'migraine'-like headache
- facial pain
- arm pain (referred or radicular)
- myelopathy (sensory and motor changes in arms and legs)
- ipsilateral sensory changes of scalp
- ear pain (periauricular)
- scapular pain
- anterior chest pain
- torticollis
- dizziness/vertigo
- visual dysfunction

Figure 56.5 indicates typical directions of referred pain from the cervical spine. Pain in the arm (brachialgia) is common and tends to cover the shoulder and upper arm as indicated.

Cervical dysfunction

Dysfunction of the 35 intervertebral joints that comprise the cervical spine complex is responsible for most cases of neck pain. The problem

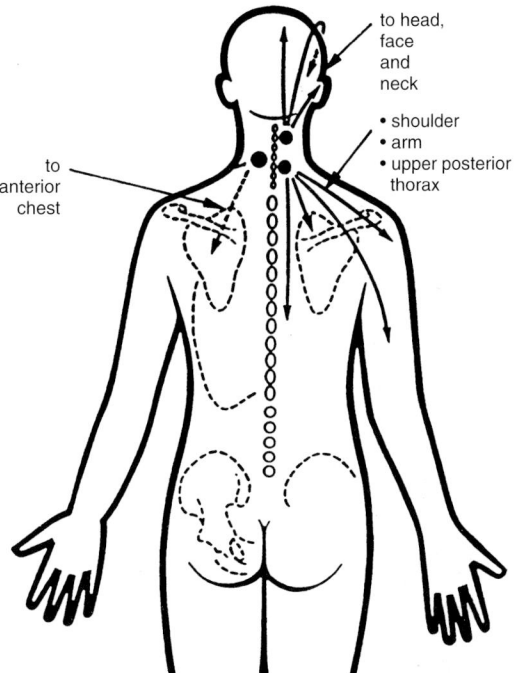

Fig. 56.5 *Possible directions of referred pain from the cervical spine*

can occur at all ages and appears to be caused by disorder (including malalignment) of the many facet joints, which are pain-sensitive. Dysfunction of these joints, which may also be secondary to intervertebral disc disruption, initiates a reflex response of adjacent muscle spasm and myofascial tenderness. Dysfunction can follow obvious trauma such as a blow to the head or a sharp jerk to the neck, but can be caused by repeated trivial trauma or activity such as painting a ceiling or gentle wrestling. People often wake up with severe neck pain and blame it on a 'chill' from a draught on the neck during the night. This is incorrect because it is usually caused by an unusual twist on the flexed neck for a long period during sleep.

Typical clinical features:

- typical age range 12–50 years
- dull ache (may be sharp) in neck
- may radiate to occiput, ear, face and temporal area (upper cervical)
- may radiate to shoulder region, especially suprascapular area (lower cervical)
- rarely refers pain below the level of the shoulder
- pain aggravated by activity, improved with rest
- various degrees of stiffness

- neck tends to lock with specific movements, usually rotation
- localised unilateral tenderness over affected joints
- variable restriction of movement but may be normal
- X-rays usually normal

Management

- Provide appropriate reassurance, information and support.
- Give advice to the patient about rules of living including the following:

Do
— Keep your neck upright in a vertical position for reading, typing and so on.
— Keep a good posture—keep the chin tucked in.
— Sleep on a low firm pillow or a special conforming pillow.
— Sleep with your painful side on the pillow.
— Use heat and massage: massage your neck firmly three times a day using an analgesic ointment.

Don't
— Look up in a strained position for long periods.
— Twist your head often towards the painful side, e.g. when reversing a car.
— Lift or tug with your neck bent forwards.
— Work, read or study with your neck bent for long periods.
— Become too dependent on 'collars'.
— Sleep on too many pillows.

- Monitor the patient's progress without overtreatment.
- Use basic analgesics, e.g. paracetamol.
- Prescribe an exercise program as early as possible.
- Refer to an appropriate therapist for cervical mobilisation. Mobilisation combined with exercises is very effective treatment. Occasionally, manipulation may help with a stubborn 'locked' neck but should be left to an expert.

Chronic pain

Additional treatment modalities to consider include:

- a course of antidepressants
- transcutaneous electrical nerve stimulation (TENS), especially when drugs are not tolerated

- hydrotherapy
- acupuncture
- corticosteroid facet injections (ideally under image intensification)
- facet joint denervation

Cervical spondylosis

Cervical spondylosis following disc degeneration and apophyseal joint degeneration is far more common than lumbar spondylosis and mainly involves the C5–6 and C6–7 segments. The consequence is narrowing of the intervertebral foramen with the nerve roots of C6 and C7 being at risk of compression.

Cervical spondylosis is generally a chronic problem but it may be asymptomatic. In some patients the pain may lessen with age, while stiffness increases.

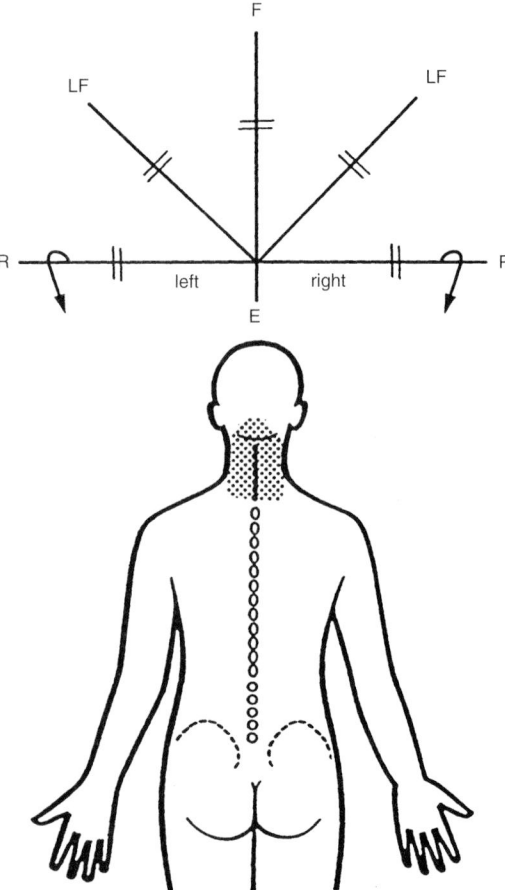

Fig. 56.6 *Cervical spondylosis: typical pain distribution with DOM diagram indicating painful and restricted movements*

The main clinical features are as follows:

- dull, aching suboccipital neck pain (Fig. 56.6)
- stiffness
- worse in morning on arising and lifting head
- improves with gentle activity and warmth, e.g. warm showers
- deteriorates with heavy activity, e.g. working under car, painting ceiling
- usually unilateral pain—may be bilateral
- pain may be referred to head, arms and scapulae
- may wake patient at night with paraesthesia in arms
- C6 nerve root most commonly involved
- acute attacks on chronic background
- aggravated by flexion (reading) and extension
- associated vertigo or unsteadiness
- restricted tender movements, especially rotation/lateral flexion
- joints tender to palpation
- X-ray changes invariable

Treatment

- Provide appropriate reassurance, information and support.
- Refer for physiotherapy, including warm hydrotherapy.
- Use regular mild analgesics, e.g. paracetamol.
- Use NSAIDs: a trial for two weeks and then review.
- Prescribe gentle mobilising exercises as early as possible.
- Give passive mobilising techniques.
- Outline general rules to live by, including advice regarding sleeping and pillows, and day-to-day activities.

Complications

- radiculopathy (unilateral or bilateral)
- myelopathy—pressure on spinal cord.

Acute torticollis

Torticollis (acute wry neck) means a lateral deformity of the neck. This is usually a transient self-limiting acutely painful disorder with associated muscle spasm of variable intensity.

The typical features include:

- age of patient between 12 and 30 years
- patient usually awakes with the problem
- pain usually confined to neck but may radiate
- deformity of lateral flexion and slight flexion/ rotation

- deformity usually away from the painful side
- loss of extension
- mid-cervical spine (C2–C3, C3–C4, C4–C5)
- any segment between C2 and C7 can cause torticollis
- usually no neurological symptoms or signs

The exact cause of this condition is uncertain, but both an acute disc lesion and apophyseal joint lesion are implicated, with the latter the more likely cause. Management by mobilisation and muscle energy therapy is very effective.

Muscle energy therapy

This amazingly effective therapy relies on the basic physiological principle that the contracting and stretching of muscles leads to automatic relaxation of agonist and antagonist muscles.[4] Lateral flexion or rotation or a combination of movements can be used but treatment in rotation is preferred. The direction of contraction can be away from the painful side (preferred) or towards the painful side, whichever is most comfortable for the patient.

Method

1. Explain the method to the patient, with reassurance that it is not painful.
2. Rotate the patient's head passively and gently towards the painful side to the limit of pain (the motion barrier).
3. Place your hand against the head on the side opposite the painful one. The other (free) hand can be used to steady the painful level—usually C3–C4.
4. Request the patient to push the head (in rotation) as firmly as possible against the resistance of your hand. The patient should therefore be producing a strong isometric contraction of the neck in rotation away from the painful side (Fig. 56.7(a)). Your counter-force (towards the painful side) should be firm and moderate (never forceful) and should not 'break' through the patient's resistance.
5. After 5–10 seconds (average 7 seconds) ask the patient to relax; then passively stretch the neck gently towards the patient's painful side (Fig. 56.7(b)).
6. The patient will now be able to turn the head a little further towards the painful side.
7. This sequence is repeated at the new improved motion barrier. Repeat 3 to 5 times until the full range of movement returns.

(a)

motion barrier

resisted
contraction

limit of movement

(b)

reduced motion barrier

Fig. 56.7 *Muscle energy therapy for acute torticollis:* **(a)** *isometric contraction phase for problem on the left side;* **(b)** *relaxation phase towards the affected (left) side*

8. Ask the patient to return the following day for treatment although the neck may be almost normal.

The patient can be taught self-treatment at home using this method.

Whiplash syndrome

Patients with the whiplash syndrome present typically with varying degrees of pain-related loss of mobility of the cervical spine, headache and emotional disturbance in the form of anxiety and depression. The problem can vary from mild temporary disability to a severe and protracted course.

The injury occurs as a consequence of hyperextension of the neck followed by recoil hyperflexion, typically following a rear-end collision between motor vehicles. There is reversal of sequence of these movements in a head-on collision. In addition to hyperextension, there is prolongation or anterior stretching plus longitudinal extension of the neck.[4]

Whiplash causes injury to soft tissue structures including muscle, nerve roots, the cervical sympathetic chain, ligaments, apophyseal joints and their synovial capsules and intervertebral discs. Damage to the apophyseal joints appears to be severe, with possible microfractures (not detectable on plain X-ray) and long-term dysfunction.

Pain and stiffness of the neck are the most common symptoms. The pain is usually experienced in the neck and upper shoulders but may radiate to the suboccipital region, the interscapular region and down the arms. The stiffness felt initially in the anterior neck muscles shifts to the posterior neck.

Headache is a common and disabling symptom that may persist for many months. It is typically occipital but can be referred to the temporal region and the eyes.

Nerve root pain can be caused by a traction injury of the cervical nerve roots or by inflammatory changes or direct pressure subsequent to herniation of a disc.

Paraesthesia of the ulnar border of the hand, nausea and dizziness are all relatively common symptoms.

Delayed symptoms are common. A patient may feel no pain until 24 (sometimes up to 96) hours later; most experience symptoms within six hours. Complications of whiplash are summarised in Table 56.4.

Management principles

The objective of treatment is to obtain a full range of free movement of the neck without pain by attending to both the physical and the psychological components of the problem. Other objectives include an early return to work and discouragement of unnecessary and excessive reliance on cervical collars and legal action.

Treatment

• Establish an appropriate empathy and instil patient confidence with a positive professional approach. Discourage multiple therapists.

Table 56.4 *Complications of whiplash*

Referred pain (headache, arm pain)
Visual problems
Vertigo
Dysphagia
Depression
Compensation neurosis
Disc rupture increasing to nerve root pain
Osteoarthritis becomes symptomatic

- Provide appropriate reassurance and patient education.
- Compare the problem with a sprained ankle, which is a similar injury.
- Inform that an emotional reaction of anger, frustration and temporary depression is common (lasts about 2 weeks).
- X-ray is required.
- Prescribe rest.
- Use a cervical collar (limit to 2 days).
- Use analgesics, e.g. paracetamol (avoid narcotics).
- Use NSAIDs for 14 days.
- Use tranquillisers, mild—up to 2 weeks.
- Refer for physiotherapy.
- Provide neck exercises (as early as possible).
- Use heat and massage; 'spray and stretch'.
- Give passive mobilisation (not manipulation).

Cervical disc disruption

Disruption of a cervical disc can result in several different syndromes.

Fig. 56.8 *Zone of possible referred pain distribution caused by a cervical disc lesion on the right side*

1. Referred pain over a widespread area due to pressure on adjacent dura mater.

   Note: A disc disruption is capable of referring pain over such a diffuse area (Fig. 56.8) that the patient is sometimes diagnosed as functional, e.g. hysterical.

2. Nerve root or radicular pain (radiculopathy). The pain follows the dermatomal distribution of the nerve root in the arm.
3. Spinal cord compression (myelopathy).

Radiculopathy

Apart from protrusion from an intervertebral disc, nerve root pressure causing arm pain can be caused by osteophytes associated with cervical spondylosis. The pain follows neurological patterns down the arm, being easier to localise with lower cervical roots, especially C6, C7 and C8.

Note: 1. The cervical roots exit above their respective vertebral bodies. For example, the C6 root exits between C5 and C6 so that a prolapse of C5–C6 intervertebral disc or spondylosis of the C5–C6 junction affects primarily the C6 root (Fig. 56.9).
2. One disc—one nerve root is the rule.

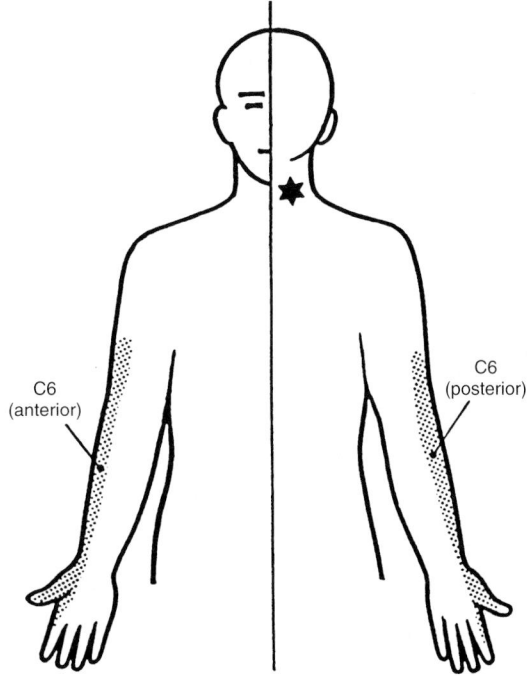

Fig. 56.9 *Typical C6 nerve root (radicular) pain*

3. Spondylosis and tumours tend to cause bilateral pain, i.e. more than one nerve root.

Clinical presentation
- a sharp aching pain in the neck, radiating down one or both arms
- onset of pain may be abrupt, often precipitated by a sudden neck movement on awakening
- stiffness of neck with limitation of movement
- nocturnal pain, waking patient during night
- pain localised to upper trapezius and possible muscle spasm

Investigations
- plain X-ray (A–P, lateral E and F, oblique views to visualise foramina); good for diagnosis, not for surgery
- plain CT scan
- CT scan and myelogram—excellent visualisation of structures but invasive
- MRI—excellent but expensive, sometimes difficult to distinguish soft disc from osteophytes
- electromyography—may help delineate lesions requiring surgery

Treatment
Many patients respond to conservative treatment, especially from a disc prolapse:
- bed rest
- soft cervical collar
- analgesics
- tranquillisers, especially at night
- traction
- careful mobilisation (manipulation is contraindicated)

Myelopathy
Clinical features:
- older patients, typically men > 50
- insidious onset: symptoms over 1–2 years
- numbness and tingling in fingers
- leg stiffness
- numb clumsy hands, especially with a high cervical lesion
- signs of UMN: spastic weakness, increased tone and hyper-reflexia (arms > legs)
- neurological deficit, which predicts the level with reasonable accuracy
- bowel and bladder function usually spared

Note: LMN signs occur at the level of the lesion, and UMN signs and sensory changes occur below this level.

Causes
- cervical spondylosis
- atlantoaxial subluxation
  — rheumatoid arthritis
  — Down syndrome
- primary spinal cord tumours, e.g. meningiomas
- metastasis to cervical spine → epidural spinal cord compression

Investigations
- MRI scan
- CT scan with myelogram (most accurate)

Central cord syndrome[7]
This rather bizarre condition occurs classically in a patient with a degenerative cervical spine following a hyperextension injury that causes osteophytes to compress the cord anteriorly and posteriorly simultaneously.

The maximum damage occurs in the central part of the cord leading to sensory and motor changes in the upper limbs with relative sparing of the lower limbs due to the arrangements of the long tracts in the cord.

Fortunately, the prognosis is good with most patients achieving a good neurological recovery.

Anterior cord syndrome
The anterior cord syndrome occurs with hyperflexion injuries that produce 'tear drop' fractures of the vertebral bodies or extrusion of disc material. The syndrome can also be produced by comminuted vertebral body fractures.

It is characterised by complete motor loss and the loss of pain and temperature discrimination below the level of the injury, but deep touch, position and vibration sensation remain intact.

Because it is probably associated with obstruction of the anterior spinal artery, early surgical intervention to relieve pressure on the front of the cord may enhance recovery. Otherwise the prognosis for recovery is poor.

Down syndrome
One of the more sinister problems with trisomy 21 syndrome is hypoplasia of the odontoid process, leading to C1–2 subluxation and dislocation. If unrecognised in the early stages,

sudden death can occur in these children. If suspected, flexion-extension lateral views of the cervical spine will highlight the developing instability and the need for early specialist opinion.

Rheumatoid arthritis

Involvement of the cervical spine is usually a late manifestation of RA. It is important to be aware of the potentially lethal problem of C1–C2 instability due to erosion of the major odontoid ligaments in the rheumatoid patient. These patients are especially vulnerable to disasters when under general anaesthesia and when involved in motor vehicle accidents. Early cervical fusion can prevent tragedies, especially with inappropriate procedures such as cervical manipulation. It is imperative to X-ray the cervical spine of all patients with severe RA before major surgery to search for C1–C2 instability.

Treatment of spondylotic myelopathy

Conservative (may help up to 50%):[1]

- soft cervical collar
- physiotherapy for muscle weakness
- analgesics and/or NSAIDs

Surgery is indicated when the myelopathy interferes with daily activities. One procedure is the 'Cloward' method, which is anterior decompression with discectomy and fusion.

When to refer

- Persisting radicular pain in an arm despite conservative treatment
- Evidence of involvement of more than one nerve root lesion in the arm
- Evidence of myelopathy such as weakness, numbness or clumsiness of the upper limbs
- Evidence, clinical or radiological, of cervical instability in post-accident victims, Down syndrome or rheumatoid arthritis.

Practice tips

- 'One disc—one nerve root' is a working rule for the cervical spine.
- The patient should sit on the couch with the thighs fully supported for inspection and movements of the neck.
- Beware of patients with rheumatoid arthritis

and Down syndrome who have cervical instability. Physical treatments such as cervical manipulation may easily cause quadriplegia.

- All acutely painful conditions of the cervical spine following trauma should be investigated with a careful neurological examination of the limbs, sphincter tone and reflexes. Plain film radiology is mandatory.
- In conscious patients, flexion and extension lateral cervical spinal plain films are useful for diagnosing instability of spinal segments with or without associated spinal fractures.
- The so-called 'whiplash' syndrome is a diagnosis of exclusion of spinal fractures or severe ligamentous disruption causing instability, and even then, for medicolegal and psychological reasons, would best be termed a 'soft tissue injury of the cervical spine'.
- Most 'soft tissue cervical spine injuries' heal within 3 months with conservative treatment. If severe pain persists, follow-up investigations may be required.
- Dysfunction of the cervical spine is an underestimated cause of headache.
- Always consider dysfunction of the cervical spine as a possible cause of shoulder pain.
- Strains and fractures of the apophyseal joints, especially after a whiplash injury, are difficult to detect, and are often overlooked causes of neck and referred pain.

References

1. Cohen ML. Neck pain. Mod Med Aust, November 1989; 44–53.
2. Payne R. Neck pain in the elderly: A management review. Mod Med Aust, July 1988, 56–67.
3. Bogduk N. Neck pain. Aust Fam Physician, 1984; 13:26–29.
4. Kenna C, Murtagh J. *Back pain and spinal manipulation* (2nd edn). Oxford: Butterworth-Heinemann, 1997, 83–99.
5. Hart FD. *Practical problems in rheumatology*. London: Dunitz, 1985, 10–14.
6. Sloane PD, Slatt LM, Baker RM. *Essentials of family medicine*. Baltimore: Williams and Wilkins, 1988, 236–240.
7. Young D, Murtagh J. Pitfalls in orthopaedics. Aust Fam Physician, 1989; 18:645–646.

57
Shoulder pain

—

It is important to realise that patients' perception of pain in the 'shoulder' may be amazing. For example, pain in the lower border of the scapula may be referred to as shoulder pain.

Text, page 570

The painful shoulder is a relatively common and sometimes complex problem encountered in general practice. The diagnostic approach involves determining whether the disorder causing the pain arises from within the shoulder structures or from other sources such as the cervical spine (Fig. 57.1), the acromioclavicular joint or diseased viscera, especially heart, lungs and subdiaphragmatic structures.[1]

Key facts and checkpoints

- Virtually all shoulder structures are innervated by the fifth cervical vertebra (C5) nerve root. Pain present in the distribution of C5 can arise from:
  - cervical spine
  - upper roots of brachial plexus
  - glenohumeral joint
  - rotator cuff tendons, especially supraspinatus
  - biceps tendon
  - soft tissue, e.g. polymyalgia rheumatica
  - viscera, especially those innervated by the phrenic nerve (C3, C4, C5)
- The visceral diseases causing a painful shoulder include cardiac disorders such as angina and pericarditis; lung diseases, especially Pancoast's tumour; mediastinal disorders; and diaphragmatic irritation, as from intra-abdominal bleeding or a subphrenic abscess.

Fig. 57.1 *Typical pain zone arising from disorders of the shoulder joint and the lower cervical spine (C5 level)*

- A careful history should generally indicate whether the neck or the shoulder is responsible for the patient's pain.
- By the age of 50 about 25% of people have some wear and tear of the rotator cuff, making it more injury-prone.[2]

568

- Disorders of the rotator cuff are common, especially supraspinatus tendinitis. The most effective tests to diagnose these problems are the resisted movement tests.[3]
- Injections of local anaesthetic and long-acting corticosteroid produce excellent results for inflammatory disorders around the shoulder joint, especially for supraspinatus tendinitis.

Functional anatomy of the shoulder

A working knowledge of the anatomical features of the shoulder is essential for the understanding of the various disorders causing pain or dysfunction of the shoulder. Apart from the acromioclavicular (AC) joint there are two most significant functional joints—the glenohumeral (the primary joint) and the subacromial complex (the secondary joint) (Fig. 57.2). The glenohumeral joint is a ball and socket joint enveloped by a loose capsule. It is prone to injury from traumatic forces and develops osteoarthritis more often than appreciated. Two

other relevant functional joints are the scapulothoracic and stenoclavicular joints.

The clinically important subacromial space lies above the glenohumeral joint between the head of the humerus and an arch formed by the bony acromion, the thick coracoacromial ligament and the coracoid process. This relatively tight compartment houses the subacromial bursa and the rotator cuff, particularly the vulnerable supraspinatus tendon.[4] Excessive friction and pinching in this space renders these structures prone to injury.

There is a critical zone of relative ischaemia that appears to affect the rotator cuff about 1 cm medial to the attachment of the supraspinatus tendon,[5] and this area is compromised during adduction and abduction of the arm due to pressure on the rotator cuff tendons from the head of the humerus.

Such factors are largely responsible for the many rotator cuff syndromes, bicipital tendinitis, subacromial bursitis and lesions of supraspinatus tendon.

Fig. 57.2 *The basic anatomical structures of the shoulder joint*

A diagnostic approach

A summary of the safety diagnostic model is presented in Table 57.1.

Probability diagnosis

The commonest causes of pain in the shoulder zone (Fig. 57.1) are cervical disorders and periarthritis, i.e. soft tissue inflammation involving the tendons around the glenohumeral joint. The outstanding common disorders of the shoulder joint are the various disorders of the tendons comprising the rotator cuff and biceps tendon. Of these, supraspinatus tendon disorders, which include tendinitis, calcific degeneration and tearing, are the commonest. It is obvious that the supraspinatus tendon is subjected to considerable friction and wear and tear.

Serious disorders not to be missed

As usual it is important to exclude any malignancy or septic infection, be it septic arthritis or

Table 57.1 *Shoulder pain: diagnostic strategy model*

Q. *Probability diagnosis*
A. Cervical spine dysfunction
Supraspinatus tendinitis ± a tear
Adhesive capsulitis

Q. *Serious disorders not to be missed*
A. Cardiovascular
  • angina
  • myocardial infarction
Neoplasia
  • Pancoast's tumour
  • primary or secondary in humerus
Severe infections
  • septic arthritis (children)
  • osteomyelitis
Rheumatoid arthritis

Q. *Pitfalls (often missed)*
A. Polymyalgia rheumatica
Cervical dysfunction
Osteoarthritis of acromioclavicular joint
Winged scapula—muscular fatigue pain

Q. *Seven masquerades checklist*
A. Depression   √
Diabetes   √
Drugs   √
Anaemia   –
Thyroid dysfunction   rarely
Spinal dysfunction   √
UTI   –

Q. *Is the patient trying to tell me something?*
A. Shoulder is prone to psychological fixation for secondary gains, depression and conversion reaction.

osteomyelitis. Carcinoma of the lung (Pancoast's syndrome) should be kept in mind. For pain in the region of the left shoulder the possibility of myocardial ischaemia (MI) has to be considered. Referred pain to the right shoulder from MI is rare, occurring about once for every 20 episodes of left shoulder referral.

With an acute onset of painful capsulitis the possibility of rheumatoid arthritis (or even gout) is worth considering.

Pitfalls

The shoulder is notorious for diagnostic traps, especially for referred pain from visceral structures, but polymyalgia rheumatica is the real pitfall. A good rule is to consider it foremost in any older person (over 60) presenting with bilateral shoulder girdle pain that is worse in the morning.

Specific pitfalls include:

• misdiagnosing posterior dislocation of the shoulder joint
• misdiagnosing recurrent subluxation of the shoulder joint
• overlooking an avascular humeral head (post fracture)
• misdiagnosing rotator cuff tear or degeneration

Seven masquerades checklist

Of the seven primary masquerades spinal dysfunction and depression are those most likely to be associated with shoulder pain. The degree to which cervical spondylosis is associated with shoulder pain is not always appreciated.

It is important to realise that patients' perception of pain in the 'shoulder' may be amazing. For example, pain in the lower border of the scapula may be referred to as shoulder pain.

Diabetics have a higher incidence of adhesive capsulitis. Drugs are relevant as cortiocosteroids can cause avascular necrosis of the humeral head and anabolic steroids (weightlifters) can cause osteolysis of the AC joint.

Psychogenic considerations

The shoulder is closely connected with psychological factors. Cyriax emphasises this fact with the interesting comment that:

'the outstretched arm is a symbol of pleasure and welcome. The arm held into the side is a symbol of rejection. Hence, those who feel withdrawn from the world or view it with disgust readily develop an inability to abduct the arm'.[6]

The clinical approach

History

In analysing the pain pattern it is appropriate to keep the various causes of shoulder pain in mind (Table 57.2). Many of these conditions, such as

Table 57.2 *Causes of shoulder pain (excluding trauma, fractures and dislocations*

Cervical
- dysfunction
- spondylosis

Cervical radiculopathy

Polymyalgia rheumatica (bilateral)

Acromioclavicular joint
- dysfunction
- osteoarthritis

Shoulder complex
  Extracapsular
- subacromial bursitis
- rotator cuff disorders
  — supraspinatus lesions
  — infraspinatus tendinitis
  — subscapularis tendinitis
- bicipital tendinitis

  Intracapsular (glenohumeral joint)
- adhesive capsulitis
  — idiopathic
  — blunt trauma
  — diabetes
  — others
- rheumatoid inflammation
  — rheumatoid arthritis
  — ankylosing spondylitis
  — psoriatic arthropathy
- osteoarthritis
- avascular necrosis
- septic arthritis

Winged scapula—muscular fatigue pain

Malignant disease
- primary or secondary in humerus
- Pancoast (ref. lung)

Referred pain
Cardiac
- ischaemic heart disease
- pericarditis
Lung
Mediastinum, including oesophagus
Diaphragmatic irritation

Herpes zoster

rheumatoid arthritis, osteoarthritis and gout, are uncommon.

A careful history should generally indicate whether the neck or the shoulder (or both) is responsible for the patient's pain. However, once the shoulder joint is implicated as the source of pain the history is often unrewarding, and the diagnosis is dependent on the physical examination.

Key questions
- Did you have any injury, even very minor, before your pain started?
- Does the pain keep you awake at night?
- Do you have pain or stiffness in your neck?
- Do you have pain or restriction when clipping or handling your bra or touching your shoulder blades? (indicates painful internal rotation and a problem of capsular restriction or a disorder of the acromioclavicular joint)
- Do you have trouble combing or attending to your hair? (indicates problematic external rotation and also a disorder of the capsule, e.g. adhesive capsulitis)
- Do you get the pain on walking or with some stressful activity?
- Is the pain worse when you wake in the morning? (indicates inflammation)
- Do you have aching in both your shoulders or around your hips?
- Do you get pain associated with sporting activity, including weight training, or with housework, dressing or other activities?

Physical examination

The diagnosis is based on systematic examination of the cervical spine followed by examination of the shoulder joint. For details of examination of the cervical spine, refer to Chapter 56.

Examination of the shoulder

For the examination of the shoulder it is important to understand the functional anatomy of all important tendons.

The tendon disorders are diagnosed by pain on resisted movement (Table 57.3). A knowledge of the anatomical attachments of the rotator cuff tendons to the head of the humerus (Fig. 57.3) provides an understanding of the shoulder movements powered by these muscles.

With tendon disorders (rotator cuff tendons or biceps) there is painful restriction of movement

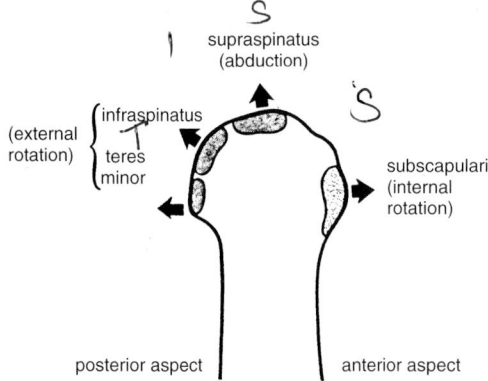

Fig. 57.3 *The attachments of the rotator cuff tendons to the head of the humerus* REPRODUCED FROM C. KENNA AND J. MURTAGH, *BACK PAIN AND SPINAL MANIPULATION*, BUTTERWORTHS, SYDNEY, 1989, WITH PERMISSION

in one direction, but with capsulitis and subacromial bursitis there is usually restriction in most directions.

Inspection

Observe the shape and contour of the shoulder joints and compare both sides. Note the posture and the position of the neck and scapulae. The position of the scapulae provides considerable clinical information. Note any deformity, swelling or muscle wasting.

Palpation

Stand behind the patient and palpate significant structures such as the acromioclavicular (AC) joint, the subacromial space, the supraspinatus tendon and the long head of biceps. The subacromial bursa is one area where it is possible to localise tenderness with inflammation. Feel also over the supraspinatus and infraspinatus muscles for muscle spasm and trigger points. The axilla should be palpated for lymphadenopathy.

Table 57.3 *Tendon disorders: determining resisted movements*

Painful resisted movement at shoulder	Affected tendon
1. Abduction	Supraspinatus
2. Internal rotation	Subscapularis * Teres minor
3. External rotation	Infraspinatus * Biceps
4. Adduction	Pectoralis major * Latissimus dorsi

* lesser role

Movements

The movements of the shoulder joint are complex and involve the scapulothoracic joint as well as the glenohumeral joint, with each joint accounting for about half the total range. Significant signs of a painful capsular pattern can be gained by determining the movements of flexion, abduction, external rotation and internal rotation.

For each movement, note:
- the range of movement
- any pain reproduction
- any trick movement by the patient
- scapulothoracic rotation

Movements should be tested bilaterally and simultaneously wherever possible.

1. *Active movements*

- Flexion (anterior elevation) 180°
- Extension (posterior elevation) 45°

With the palm facing medially the patient moves the arm upwards through 180° to a vertical position above the head and then backwards through this plane.
- Abduction—180°
- Adduction— 80° (from neutral position)

Abduction is possible only if the arm is fully externally rotated. It is a key combined glenohumeral and scapulothoracic movement, which should reach 180°, and these components should be differentiated if the movement is limited. This is done by fixing the scapula with one hand holding the scapula at its inferior angle and noting the degree of movement of each component (initial glenohumeral range 85–100°). Look for the presence of a painful arc, which occurs usually between 60° and 120° of abduction (Fig. 57.4). The commonest cause is

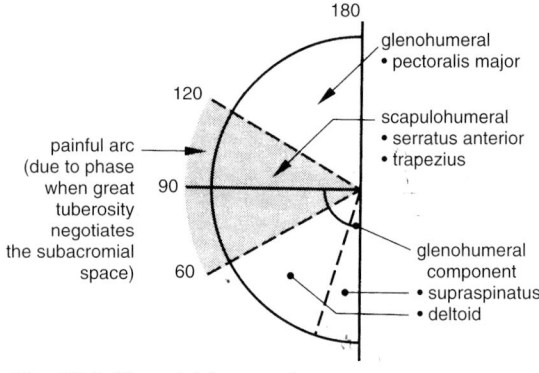

Fig. 57.4 *The painful arc syndrome*

supraspinatus tendinitis. Other causes include infraspinatus tendinitis and subacromial bursitis (milder degree).
- Internal rotation—90°
- External rotation—90°

These movements are tested with the arm by the side and the elbow flexed to 90° with palm facing medially. The hand is carried outwards to test external rotation and inwards towards the abdomen for internal rotation.

2. Resisted movements

Resisted movements (isometric contractions of a muscle) are important ways of testing capsulitis and for pinpointing tenderness of muscle insertions around the shoulder joint, and no examination of the shoulder is complete without them (see Table 57.3).

Abduction (supraspinatus test). With the arm abducted to no more than 15° the patient pushes the elbow away from the side while the examiner's hands resist and prevent the movement, holding for 5 seconds. Compare both sides and note any reproduction of the patient's pain.

A better and more specific test for supraspinatus is testing resisted elevation in the 'emptying the can' position (90° of abduction, 30° horizontal flexion and full internal rotation).

Internal rotation (subscapularis test). The examiner stands behind the patient and grasps the palmar surface of the patient's wrists (with the arm by the side and elbow at 90°). The patient attempts to move the forearm internally (medially) against resistance.

External rotation (infraspinatus test). With the examiner and patient adopting a similar position to that for internal rotation, the examiner grasps the dorsal surface of the forearm near the wrist and asks the patient to press outwards, using the forearm as a lever to produce external rotation. This test is also positive for a C5 nerve root lesion.

3. Special tests

Supraspinatus/infraspinatus rapid differentiation test. A quick test that helps to differentiate between a lesion of either of these tendons causing a painful arc syndrome is the 'thumbs up/thumbs down' abduction test. To test supraspinatus, perform abduction with thumbs pointing upwards, and then with the thumbs pointing downwards to test infraspinatus.

Long head of biceps test. The best test is opposed forward elevation of the arm with the elbow at right angles. A positive test is reproduction of pain in the bicipital groove. Another useful test is resisted supination at the wrist (Yergason's test).

The brachial plexus tension test. This test devised by Elvey[7] tests the nerve roots and sheaths of the brachial plexus without implicating the cervical spine and the glenohumeral joint. The upper cervical roots of the plexus are sometimes injured in accidents; so this test is an effective differentiation test.

Impingement test for supraspinatus lesions. Refer to page 575.

Investigations

Appropriate investigations for shoulder pain include:
- ESR (especially for polymyalgia rheumatica)
- rheumatoid factor
- serum uric acid (acute pain)
- ECG
- radiology
  — X-ray of a specific part of the shoulder, e.g. AC joint, axillary view of glenohumeral joint (best view to show osteoarthritis)
  — X-ray of cervical spine and chest (if relevant)
  — radionuclide bone scan
  — shoot through axillary views (posterior dislocation)
  — high-resolution ultrasound: modern techniques make this the ideal test to assess shoulder pain due to rotator cuff lesions and capsulitis, especially if surgery is contemplated.
  — arthrogram of shoulder (beware of false negatives)
  — CT scan (limited use)
  — MRI: the best imaging method but not routinely required

Shoulder tip pain

Pain at the shoulder tip may be caused by local musculoskeletal trauma or inflammation or can be referred. Referred causes include:
- peptic ulceration
- diaphragmatic irritation
- ruptured viscus, e.g. perforated ulcer
- intraperitoneal bleeding, e.g. ruptured spleen

- pneumothorax
- myocardial infarction

Shoulder pain in children

Shoulder pain in children is not a common presenting problem but the following require consideration:

- septic arthritis/osteomyelitis
- swimmer's shoulder

Swimmer's shoulder

Although it occurs in adults, shoulder pain is the most common complaint in swimmers in the teenage years (over 12 years of age). American studies of college and national competition swimmers showed 40–60% had suffered significant pain.[8]

The problem, which is considered to be associated with abnormal scapular positioning and cervicothoracic dysfunction, occurs in the supraspinatus tendon where an avascular zone is compressed by the greater tuberosity when the arm is adducted and relieved when abducted. Swimmers' shoulders are forced through thousands of revolutions each day; so the susceptible area tends to impinge on the coraco-acromial arch, leading to the impingement syndrome, which can progress with continued stress and age.[9]

Symptoms

- Stage 1: pain only after activity
- Stage 2: pain at beginning only, then after activity
- Stage 3: pain during and after activity, affects performance

Management

- Early recognition is important.
- Discuss training program with coach.
- Consider alteration of technique.
- Application of ICE after each swim.
- Use NSAIDs.
- Avoid corticosteroid injections.
- Refer for physiotherapy for scapular stabilisation and cervicothoracic mobilisation.

Shoulder pain in the elderly

As a rule most of the shoulder problems increase with age. Special features in the elderly are:

- polymyalgia rheumatica (increased incidence with age)
- supraspinatus tears and persistent 'tendinitis'
- other rotator cuff disorders
- stiff shoulder due to adhesive capsulitis
- osteoarthritis of acromioclavicular and gleno-humeral joints
- cervical dysfunction with referred pain
- the avascular humeral head

Since the rotator cuff is prone to degeneration with age there is a high incidence of rotator cuff tears in the elderly that are mostly asymptomatic.

The avascular humeral head

The humeral head may become avascular after major proximal humeral fractures. With experience, it is usually possible to predict the fractures at special risk. Early humeral head replacement with a prosthesis can lead to excellent pain relief and to a return of good function. Once the head has collapsed, there is secondary capsular contracture. Prosthetic replacement of the head is then rarely associated with an adequate return of joint movement. Thus early referral of comminuted proximal humeral fractures for an expert opinion in all age groups is good practice. Early replacement can improve the functional outcome.[11]

Supraspinatus tendinitis

Supraspinatus tendinitis is the commonest inflammatory problem encountered around the shoulder joint and can vary in intensity from mild to extremely severe. The severe cases usually involve calcification (calcific periarthritis) of the tendon and spread to the subacromial bursa.

Typical pain profile

- Site: The shoulder and outer border of arm; maximal over deltoid insertion
- Radiation: to elbow
- Quality: throbbing pain, can be severe
- Frequency: constant, day and night
- Duration: constant
- Onset: straining the shoulder (e.g. dog on leash, working under car, fall onto outstretched arm)
- Offset: nil
- Aggravation: heat, putting on shirt, toilet activity, lying on shoulder

- Relief: analgesics only
- Associated   trigger point over
  features: supraspinatus origin
- Examination   — painful resisted abduction
  (typical   — painful arc
  features):   — painful resisted external
                rotation
               — positive impingement test
               — positive 'emptying the can'
                sign

The impingement test

This is an effective test for supraspinatus lesions as it forces impingement of the greater tuberosity under the acromion.

Method

- The patient places the arms in the position of semiflexion (90° of forward flexion) and internal rotation with the forearms in full pronation.
- You then test resisted flexion by pushing down as the patient pushes up against this movement (Fig. 57.5).
- If pain is reproduced, this is called a positive 'impingement sign' and is a very sensitive test for the upper components of the rotator cuff, especially supraspinatus.

The 'emptying the can' resistance test

This effective test is described on page 573.

Treatment of supraspinatus tendinitis

- rest during the acute phase
- analgesics
- peritendon injection

Injection technique

The ideal injection is a specific injection onto the tendon rather than general infiltration into the subacromial space. As a rule the therapeutic result is quite dramatic after one or two days of initial discomfort (often severe). The tendon can be readily palpated as a tender cord anterolaterally as it emerges from beneath the acromion to attach to the greater tuberosity of the humerus. This identification is assisted by depressing the shoulder via a downward pull on the arm and then externally and internally rotating the humerus. This manoeuvre allows the examiner to locate the tendon readily.

Method

- Identify and mark the tendon.
- Place the patient's arm behind the back, with the back of the hand touching the far waistline. This locates the arm in the desired internal rotation and forces the humeral head anteriorly.
- Insert a 23-gauge 32 mm needle under the acromion along the line of the tendon, and inject around the tendon just under the acromion (Fig. 57.6). If the gritty resistance of the tendon is encountered, slightly withdraw the needle to ensure that it lies in the tendon sheath.
- The recommended injection is 1 mL of a soluble or long-acting corticosteroid with 5 mL of 1% lignocaine.

Fig. 57.5 *The impingement test: resisted flexion in semiflexion, internal rotation and pronation*

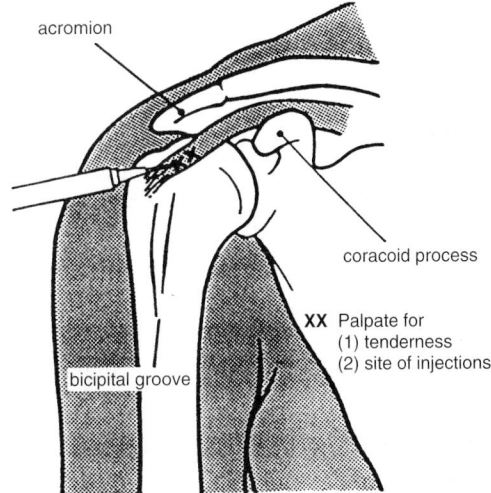

acromion

coracoid process

XX Palpate for
(1) tenderness
(2) site of injections

bicipital groove

Fig. 57.6 *Injection placement for supraspinatus tendinitis*

Persistent supraspinatus tendinitis

There are three factors to consider with this problem:

1. *A very tight subacromial space.* Refer for subacromial decompression by division of the thickened coracoacromial ligament. Even in younger patients this procedure (with or without acromioplasty) may be indicated for those with pain persisting beyond 12 months.
2. *Rotator cuff tear or degeneration.* In middle-aged and elderly patients persisting tendinitis is usually due to rotator cuff tear and degeneration, an underdiagnosed condition. Excellent clinical and functional results can be achieved if surgery is performed when the tear is small.
3. *Calcification of the tendon.* This problem usually settles but occasionally surgical intervention is necessary.

Other rotator cuff lesions

The patient may present with dominant signs of subscapularis or infraspinatus, or a combination of two or three tendinous lesions including supraspinatus. This problem could be confused with milder adhesive capsulitis, hence the value of investigations such as ultrasound.

Management

A subacromial space injection of 1 mL of corticosteroid and 2–3 mL of 1% local anaesthetic, using the posterior approach, generally achieves a good result.

| Method |

With the patient sitting upright the large posterior gap between the medial acromial ridge and the humeral head is identified by palpation from behind. The needle (23 gauge, 32 or 38 mm long) is inserted into this gap just inferior to the acromion. The solution should flow into this space without resistance.

Subacromial bursitis

Subacromial (subdeltoid) bursitis is the more severe association of the frozen shoulder and may require hospital admission for pain control. It is the only inflammatory disorder around the shoulder joint where localised tenderness is a reliable sign.

Typical pain profile

- Site: outer shoulder, outer arm
- Radiation: to outer elbow and upper forearm
- Quality: intense pain
- Frequency: constant
- Duration: constant
- Onset: either spontaneous or following unaccustomed work
- Offset: nil
- Aggravation: heat, brushing hair, most activities
- Relief: very strong analgesics only
- Examination (typical features):   — 'frozen' shoulder
  - — difficult to undress and dress
  - — marked tenderness below acromion over deltoid
  - — all active movements limited and painful

Management

- strong analgesics, e.g. paracetamol and codeine
- large local injection of 5–8 mL of LA into and around the bursa, followed immediately by 1 mL of corticosteroid (long-acting) into the focus of the lesion

Adhesive capsulitis

Adhesive capsulitis is an acute inflammation affecting the glenohumeral joint. Differential diagnoses include monoarticular rheumatoid arthritis, a crystal arthropathy such as gout, and septic arthritis. It is worse in diabetics.

It generally occurs in three stages:

1. 'freezing, frozen and thawing'—an inflammatory painful phase of 2–9 months
2. a fibrotic contracted phase of 4–12 months
3. partial or complete resolution of 5–26 months

Typical pain profile

- Site: around the shoulder and outer border of arm
- Radiation: to elbow
- Quality: deep throbbing pain
- Frequency: constant, day and night
- Duration: constant
- Onset: spontaneous or following minor fall onto shoulder, wakes the patient from sleep
- Offset: nil

- Aggravation: activity, dressing, combing hair, heat
- Relief: analgesics only (partial relief)
- Associated features: stiffness of arm, may be frozen
- Examination (typical features):
  — 'frozen' shoulder (some cases)
  — various active and passive movements painful and restricted, especially extension
  — resisted movements pain-free
  (Patient compensates with scapulo-humeral movements)
- Diagnosis: high-resolution ultrasound

Treatment

This problem, which can persist for at least 12 months, can be treated with an intra-articular injection of corticosteroid. The modern treatment is hydrodilation of the joint with a large quantity of sterile solution (to stretch the capsule) ± corticosteroid. Another important treatment is severing adhesions under arthroscopic control. The rule is: if very stiff use arthroscopy; if more mobile use a distension procedure. Active exercises are important to restore function. Fifty per cent of people with adhesive capsulitis do not regain normal movement if untreated.

Bicipital tendinitis

Bicipital tendinitis is a tenosynovitis of the long head of biceps. Important signs include pain on restricted flexion of the elbow joint and on resisted supination. A painful arc may be present when the intrascapular part is affected. Hence it is often confused with one of the rotator cuff lesions. Sometimes it is possible to elicit local tenderness along the course of the tendon in the bicipital groove. Most active shoulder movements, especially external rotation, bring on the pain.

Bicipital tendinitis is not a common problem. It usually follows chronic repetitive strains in young to middle-aged adults, e.g. home decorating, tennis, swimming freestyle, cricket and baseball pitching. Two complications are complete rupture and subluxation of the tendon out of its groove.

Typical pain profile

- Site: in front of shoulder
- Radiation: outside and middle of upper arm to just below elbow
- Quality: dull pain, sharp with certain movements
- Frequency: daily, after activity
- Duration: hours
- Onset: can follow activity such as painting and wallpapering
- Offset: rest
- Aggravating factors: tennis, swimming, housework
- Relief: rest
- Examination (typical features):
  — tender external rotation
  — painful resisted flexion of elbow
  — painful resisted supination of elbow
  — positive Yergason's test
  — may be painful arc
  — tender along tendon in bicipital groove
- Diagnosis: detecting abnormal tenderness over tendon in bicipital groove when the arm is externally rotated

Injection method

- The patient sits with arm hanging by the side and palm facing forwards.
- Find and mark the site of maximal tenderness. This is usually in the bicipital groove and more proximal than expected.
- Insert a 23-gauge needle at the proximal end of the bicipital groove above the tender area.
- Slide the needle down the groove to reach the tender area (Fig. 57.7).

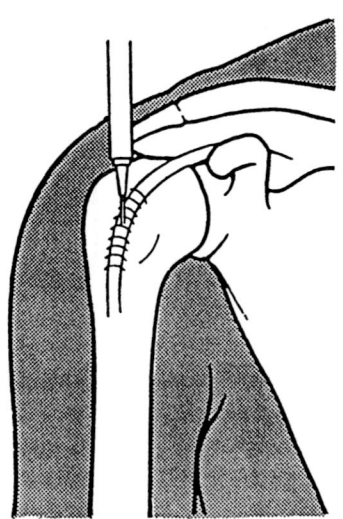

Fig. 57.7 *Injection placement for bicipital tendinitis*

- Inject 1 mL of long-acting corticosteroid and 2 mL of LA around this site.

Polymyalgia rheumatica

It is very important not to misdiagnose polymyalgia rheumatica in the older person (over 50 years) presenting with bilateral pain and stiffness in the shoulder girdle. It may or may not be associated with hip girdle pain. Polymyalgia rheumatica sometimes follows an influenza-like illness. The patients seem to complain bitterly about their pain and seem flat and miserable. In the presence of a normal physical examination they are sometimes misdiagnosed as 'rheumatics' or 'fibrositis'.

Typical pain profile
- Site: shoulders and upper arms (Fig. 57.8)
- Radiation: towards lower neck
- Quality: a deep intense ache
- Frequency: daily
- Duration: constant but easier in afternoon and evening
- Onset: wakes with pain at greatest intensity
- Offset: nil

- Aggravating factors: staying in bed, inactivity
- Relieving factors: activity (slight relief)
- Associated features: severe morning stiffness 'in muscles'; malaise; ± weight loss, depression
- Diagnosis: greatly elevated ESR (can be normal)
- Treatment: corticosteroids give dramatic relief but long-term management can be problematic; regular review and support is essential

Posterior dislocation of the shoulder

This is a rare form of shoulder instability, which is often misdiagnosed. On first inspection there may not be an obvious abnormality of the shoulder contour. Consider this condition if there is a history of electric shock or a tonic-clonic convulsion. The major clinical sign is painful restriction of external rotation, which is usually completely blocked. Routine shoulder X-rays following trauma should always include the 'axillary shoot through' view and then the diagnosis becomes obvious. Early diagnosis and management can prevent a poor outcome and perhaps litigation.[11]

Recurrent subluxation

Recurrent anterior or inferior subluxations, or both, are probably more common than recurrent dislocations, yet frequently are not diagnosed. Patients complaining of attacks of sudden weakness and even a 'dead arm feeling' lasting for a few minutes with overhead activities of the arm should be investigated for this condition.

The disorder is usually apparent on careful stress testing of the shoulder. Air-contrast computerised tomography (CT) arthrography is considered the best investigation. Surgery is usually curative while conservative treatment often fails for younger patients.

Acromioclavicular osteoarthritis

This condition is usually traumatic or degenerative and is relatively common in builders and sports people, especially rowers. It is treated with rest and support. Intra-articular injections of corticosteroids can be used for resistant or severe cases.

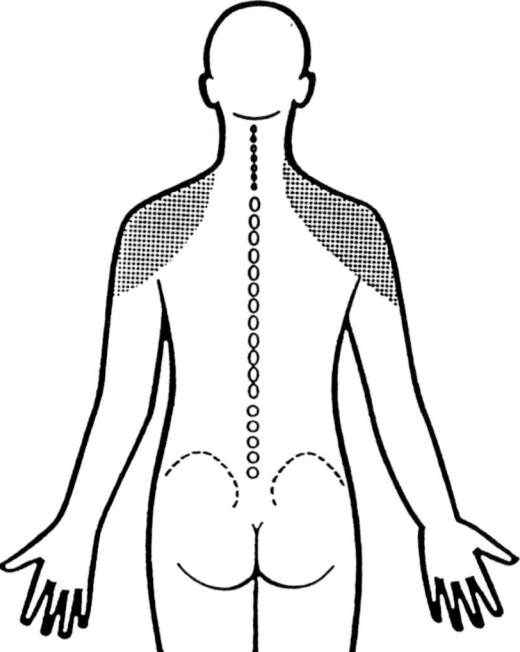

Fig. 57.8 *Polymyalgia rheumatica: typical area of pain around the shoulder girdle*

When to refer

- Persisting night pain with shoulder joint stiffness
- Persisting supraspinatus tendinitis; consider possibility of rotator cuff tear or degeneration, especially in the elderly
- Persisting restriction of movement, e.g. restricted cross-body flexion (indicates capsular constriction)
- Persisting supraspinatus tendinitis or other rotator cuff problem, because decompression of the subacromial space with division of the coracoacromial ligament ± acromioplasty gives excellent results
- Confirmed or suspected posterior dislocation of the shoulder—the most commonly missed major joint dislocation
- Confirmed or suspected recurrent subluxation or avascular humeral head
- Children with shoulder joint instability
- Swimmer's shoulder refractory to changes in technique and training schedule
- Severe osteoarthritis of the glenohumeral joint (which usually follows major trauma) for consideration of prosthetic replacement
- Severe osteoarthritis of acromioclavicular joint

Practice tips

- Consider dysfunction of the cervical spine, especially C4–C5 and C5–C6 levels, as a cause of shoulder pain.
- Tendinitis and bursitis are very refractory to treatment and tend to last for several months. One well-placed injection of local anaesthetic and corticosteroid may give rapid and lasting relief.
- Test for supraspinatus disorders (including swimmer's shoulder) with the impingement tests, including the 'emptying the can' test.
- Modern ultrasound is the investigation of choice for painful disorders of the rotator cuff, especially to investigate tears in tendons.
- An elderly person presenting with bilateral shoulder girdle pain has polymyalgia rheumatica until proved otherwise. Relief from corticosteroids is dramatic. Although bilateral it may start as unilateral discomfort.

- Dysfunction of the cervical spine can coexist with dysfunction of the shoulder joints.
- Correlation between clinical symptoms and the degree of tendon injury or failure is not reliable.[12]

References

1. Corrigan B. Painful shoulder. Patient Management, 1978; 2:23.
2. Sloane PD, Slatt LM, Baker RM. *Essentials of family medicine*. Baltimore: Williams & Wilkins, 1988, 242.
3. Cormack J, Marinker M, Morrell D. *Practice: A handbook of primary health care*. London: Kluwer-Harrap, 1980, 3.62: 1–4.
4. Kenna C, Murtagh J. *Back pain and spinal manipulation* (2nd edn). Oxford: Butterworth-Heinemann, 1997, 109–133.
5. Rathburn JB, Macnab I. The microvascular pattern of the rotator cuff. J Bone and Joint Surg, 1970; 52B:540.
6. Cyriax J. *Textbook of orthopaedic medicine*, Vol. 1 (6th edn). London: Bailliere Tindall, 1976, 202.
7. Elvey R. The investigation of arm pain. In: Grieve GP. *Modern manual therapy of the vertebral column*. London: Churchill Livingstone, 1986, 530–535.
8. Dominguez RH. Shoulder pain in swimmers. Physician and Sportsmedicine, 1980; 8:36.
9. McLean ID. Swimmers' injuries. Aust Fam Physician, 1984; 13:499–500.
10. Reeves B. The natural history of the frozen shoulder syndrome. Scand J Rheumatol, 1975; 4:193–196
11. Young D, Murtagh J. Pitfalls in orthopaedics. Aust Fam Physician, 1989; 18:645–648.
12. Sher JS et al. Abnormal findings on magnetic resonance images of asymptomatic shoulders. J Bone Joint Surg Am, 1995; 77:10–15.

58

Pain in the arm and hand

—

A pain in the hand is worth a look at the neck.
By heck don't forget the neck!

Orthopaedic surgeon to students 1965

Pain in the arm and hand is a common problem
in general practice, tending to affect the middle
aged and elderly in particular.

Overview of causes of a painful arm and hand

Like pain in the shoulder, pain originating from
the cervical spine and shoulder disorders can
extend down the arm. While pain from disorders
of the shoulder joint (because of its C5 innervation) does not usually extend below the elbow,
radiculopathies originating in the cervical spine
can transmit to distal parts of the arm (Fig. 56.4).

Important causes are illustrated in Figure 58.1.
Myocardial ischaemia must be considered,
especially for pain experienced down the inner
left arm.

Soft tissue disorders of the elbow are
extremely common, especially tennis elbow.
Two types of tennis elbow are identifiable: 'backhand' tennis elbow, or lateral epicondylitis, and
'forehand' tennis elbow, or medial epicondylitis,
which is known also as golfer's or pitcher's
elbow.

Other significant elbow disorders include
inflammatory disorders of the elbow joint such
as rheumatoid arthritis, osteoarthritis and olecranon bursitis, which may follow recurrent
trauma, gout, rheumatoid arthritis or infection.

Another important group of disorders are the
various regional pain syndromes around the

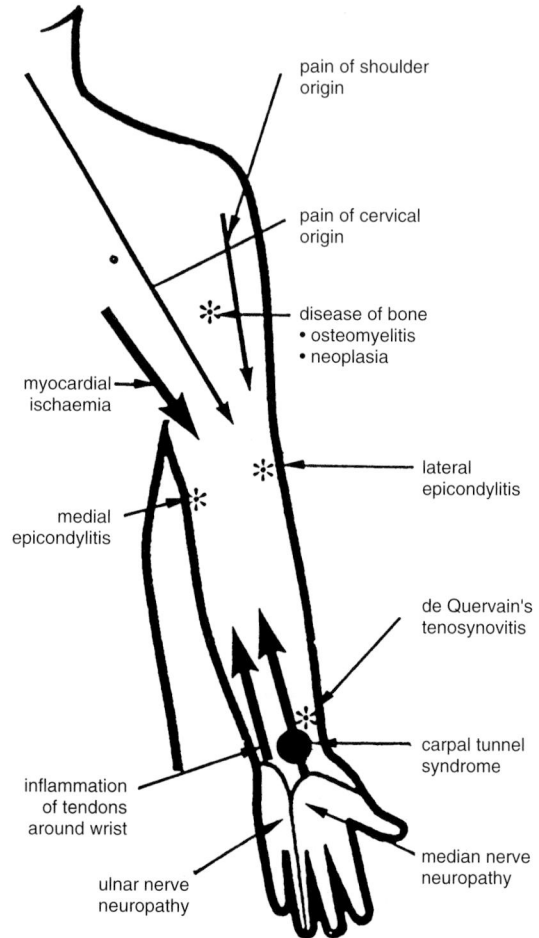

Fig. 58.1 *Important causes of arm pain (excluding trauma and arthritis)*

wrists, including the common de Quervain's tenosynovitis (affecting the tendons of extensor
pollicis brevis and abductor pollicis longus) and
to a lesser extent the extensor tendons to the

fingers. Pain from these overuse syndromes can be referred in a retrograde manner into the forearm.

A fascinating and poorly understood syndrome is that related to dysfunction of the upper four vertebral segments of the thoracic spine, which can cause referred pain in the arm that does not correspond to the dermatomes. This syndrome is often confused with the more common regional pain disorders such as tenosynovitis and tennis elbow.

The various causes of the painful arm can be considered with the diagnostic model (Table 58.1).

Table 58.1 *Pain in the arm and hand: diagnostic strategy model*

Q.	*Probability diagnosis*
A.	Dysfunction of cervical spine (lower)
	Disorders of the shoulder
	Medial or lateral epicondylitis
	Overuse tendinitis of the wrist
	Carpal tunnel syndrome
	Osteoarthritis of thumb and DIP joints
Q.	*Serious disorders not to be missed*
A.	Cardiovascular
	• angina (referred)
	• myocardial infarction
	Neoplasia
	• Pancoast's tumour
	• bone tumours (rare)
	Severe infections
	• septic arthritis (shoulder/elbow)
	• osteomyelitis
	• infections of tendon sheath and fascial spaces of hand
Q.	*Pitfalls (often missed)*
A.	Entrapment neuropathies
	e.g. median nerve, ulnar nerve
	Pulled elbow—children
	Foreign body, e.g. elbow
	Rarities
	• Polymyalgia rheumatica (for arm pain)
	• Reflex sympathetic dystrophy
	• Thoracic outlet syndrome
	• Arm claudication (left arm)
	• Kienböck's disease
Q.	*Seven masquerades checklist*

A.		
Depression	√
Diabetes	√
Drugs	—
Anaemia	—
Thyroid disease	—
Spinal dysfunction	√
UTI	—

Q.	*Is the patient trying to tell me something?*
A.	Highly likely, especially with so-called RSI syndromes.

A diagnostic approach
Probability diagnosis

The commonest causes of arm pain are referred pain and radiculopathies caused by disorders of the cervical spine, the tennis elbows (lateral and, to a lesser extent, medial epicondylitis), carpal tunnel syndrome and regional pain syndromes caused by inflammation of the tendons around the wrist and thumb.

Disorders of the shoulder, particularly supraspinatus tendinitis, should be considered if the pain is present in the C5 dermatome distribution. Pain in the hand is commonly caused by osteoarthritis of the carpometacarpal joint of the thumb and the distal interphalangeal (DIP) joints, and also by the carpal tunnel syndrome.

Serious disorders not to be missed

Like any other presenting problem it is vital not to overlook malignant disease or severe infection. In the case of the arm, possible malignant disease includes tumours in bones, lymphoma involving axillary glands and Pancoast's syndrome.

Neoplastic tumours of the hand are uncommon and usually benign. Benign tumours include giant cell tumour of the tendon sheath, pigmented villonodular synovitis, neurilemmoma and neurofibroma. Malignant tumours are exceptionally rare but can include synovioma and rhabdomyosarcoma.

In addition, myocardial ischaemia, especially infarction in the case of pain of sudden onset, should be considered for left arm pain.

Sepsis can involve joints, the olecranon bursa and the deeper compartments of the hand, the latter leading to serious sequelae if not rapidly diagnosed and treated.

Pitfalls

Such conditions may include entrapment syndromes for peripheral nerves. If in doubt the patient should be referred for electromyography. Variations of peripheral nerve entrapments include the pronator syndrome (compression of the median nerve by the pronator teres or a fibrous band near the origin of the deep flexor muscles) and ulnar nerve entrapment at the elbow in the cubital fossa and, rarely, in Guyon's canal in the wrist.

Lesions of the nerve roots comprising the brachial plexus can also cause arm pain, especially in the C5 and C6 distribution. These can be detected by the brachial plexus tension tests.

Rarer causes of arm pain

These include polymyalgia rheumatica, although the pain typically involves the shoulder girdle, reflex sympathetic dystrophy (Sudek's atrophy) and the thoracic outlet syndromes.

The thoracic outlet syndromes include problems arising from compression or intermittent obstruction of the neurovascular bundle supplying the upper extremity, for example cervical rib syndrome, costoclavicular syndrome, scalenus anterior and medius syndrome, 'effort thrombosis' of axillary and subclavian veins and the subclavian steal syndrome.

The commonest cause of the thoracic outlet syndrome is sagging musculature related to ageing, obesity, and heavy breasts and arms, aptly described by Swift and Nichols as 'the droopy shoulder syndrome'.[1]

Cervical ribs are relatively common and may, or may not, contribute to the thoracic outlet syndrome. Often the cause is a functional change in the thoracic outlet due to the 'droopy shoulder syndrome' with no significant anatomical fault.[2]

Arm claudication is also rare. It can occur with arterial obstruction due to occlusion of the proximal left subclavian artery or the innominate artery. Exercise of the arm may be associated with central nervous system symptoms as well as claudication.

Seven masquerades checklist

Of the seven primary masquerades, spinal dysfunction and depression are those most likely to be associated with arm pain. Nerve root pain arising from entrapment in intervertebral foramina of the cervical spine or from a disc prolapse frequently leads to pain and/or paraesthesia in the arm.

Although diabetic neuropathy primarily manifests in the lower limbs it may be associated with neuropathies in the hands, including erythermalgia (redness and burning related to heat). Hypothyroidism may cause a carpal tunnel syndrome.

Psychogenic considerations

The hand can be regarded as a highly emotive 'organ' that is frequently used to give outward expression to inner feelings. These can range from grossly disturbed psychiatric behaviour, manifested as a hysterical conversion disorder by a non-functioning hand, to occupational neuroses such as repetition strain injury (RSI) and malingering.[3] Experienced occupational physicians and surgeons[3] find the hand and arm a source of functional disability most often as a result of industrial injury. Of great concern are the various so-called RSI disorders, which in some people may be a means of work avoidance or a 'ticket' for compensation or both.

The clinical approach

History

The painful arm represents a real diagnostic challenge; so the history is very relevant.

It is common for arm pain to cause sleep disturbances and three causes are cervical disorders, carpal tunnel syndrome and the thoracic outlet syndrome. The working rule is:

- thoracic outlet syndrome—patients cannot fall asleep
- carpal tunnel syndrome—patients wake in the middle of the night
- cervical spondylosis—wakes the patient with pain and stiffness that persists well into the day.[4]

The history should include an analysis of the pain and a history of trauma, particularly unaccustomed activity. In children evidence should be obtained about the nature of any injury, especially pulling the child up by the arms or a fall on an outstretched hand, which can cause potentially serious fractures around the elbow.

Physical examination

As part of the physical examination of the painful arm it may be necessary to examine a variety of joints including the cervical spine (Chapter 56), shoulder (Chapter 57), elbow, wrist and the various joints of the hand. The arms should be inspected as a whole and it is very important to have both arms free of clothing and compare both sides.

> **Elbow joint**

Inspection (from anterior, lateral and posterior aspects). Hold elbow in an anatomical position to measure the carrying angle of forearm— elbow fully extended, forearm supinated (palm facing forwards) normal 5–15° (greater in females). Note any swellings:

- olecranon bursitis (bursa over olecranon)
- nodules
  - RA (subcutaneous border ulna)
  - gout
  - SLE (rare) and rheumatic fever (very rare)
  - granulomas, e.g. sarcoid

Palpation. Perform with patient supine and elbow held in approximately 70° flexion. Palpate bony landmarks and soft tissue. Note especially any tenderness over lateral epicondyle (tennis elbow) and medial epicondyle (golfer's elbow).

Movement (test active and passive). Hinge joint:

- extension—flexion (0° to 150°)
  - the arc for daily living is 30–130°
  - limitation of extension is an early sign of synovitis
- pronation–supination (rotation)
  - occurs at radiohumeral joint
  - test in two positions:
    - 90° flexion (held to side of body)
    - at full extension
  - supination 85° plus
  - pronation 75° plus

Resisted movements
- Painful resisted flexion at wrist = medial epicondylitis.
- Painful resisted extension at wrist = lateral epicondylitis.

| Wrist joint |

Follow the usual rules: LOOK, FEEL, MOVE, TEST FUNCTION, MEASURE and X-RAY. Note swellings or deformities, including the anatomical snuff box and distal end of radius. Feel for heat, tenderness and swelling, especially over the radial aspect of the wrist.

Movements. With elbow fixed at 90° and held into the waist:

1. Compare dorsiflexion and palmar flexion on both sides (normal range 80–90°).
2. Compare ulnar deviation (normal to 45°) and radial deviation (30°).
3. Compare pronation and supination (normal to 90° for both).

Neurological examination
Test sensation, motor power and reflexes where indicated.

Summary of tests for motor power:

C5—test resisted movement deltoid

C6—test resisted movement biceps
C7—test resisted movement triceps
C8—test resisted EPL and FDL
T1—test resisted interossei

Sensory patterns are presented in Figure 56.4.

Investigations
Pain in the arm and hand can be difficult to diagnose but the rule to follow is: 'If in doubt, X-ray and compare both sides'. This applies particularly to elbow injuries in children. The presence of a foreign body in the hand or arm also requires consideration.

Investigations to consider include:

- blood film and WCC
- ESR
- ECG
- X-rays
  - cervical spine
  - upper thoracic spine
  - elbow/forearm/shoulder
  - wrist and hand
  - ultrasound
  - arthrograms (shoulder, elbow, wrist)
  - CT scanning
  - technetium bone scan
- nerve conduction studies
- electromyography

Note: Modern sophisticated ultrasound examination is becoming a vital diagnostic modality for soft tissue disorders.

Arm pain in children
The main concerns with children are the effects of trauma, especially around the elbow. Considerable awareness of potential problems and skilful management are required with children's elbow fractures. Foreign bodies in the arm also have to be considered.

Pulled elbow
This typically occurs in children under 8 years of age, usually at 2–5 years, when an adult applies sudden traction to the child's extended and pronated arm: the head of the radius can be pulled distally through the annular radioulnar ligament (Fig. 58.2a).[5]

Symptoms and signs
- The crying child refuses to use the arm.
- The arm is limp by the side or supported in the child's lap.

- The elbow is flexed slightly (any flexion will be strenuously resisted).
- The forearm is pronated or held in mid-position (Fig. 58.2b).
- The arm is tender around the elbow (without bruising or deformity).

Note: An X-ray is not necessary.

Treatment method

1. Gain the child's confidence.
2. The child stands facing the doctor with the parent holding the non-affected arm.
3. Place one hand around the child's elbow to give support, pressing the thumb over the head of the radius.

4. With the other hand, firmly and smoothly flex the elbow and suddenly and firmly twist the forearm into full supination (Fig. 58.2c). A faint click (which will be painful) will be heard. After a few minutes the child will settle and resume full pain-free movement. Warn parents that recurrences are possible up to 6 years.

Note: Spontaneous resolution can occur eventually.

Fractures and avulsion injuries around the elbow joint, which are a major problem in children, are discussed in more detail in Chapter 117.[6]

Fig. 58.2 *Pulled elbow:* **(a)** *mechanism of injury;* **(b)** *annular ligament displaced over head of radius;* **(c)** *reduction by supination*

Arm pain in the elderly

Elderly patients are more likely to be affected by problems such as referred pain, radiculopathy or myelopathy from cervical spondylosis, tumours, polymyalgia rheumatica, entrapment neuropathies such as carpal tunnel syndrome and ulnar nerve entrapment. The latter can be related to trauma such as Colles' fractures. In addition the elderly are more prone to suffer from the thoracic outlet syndrome as previously described under 'Pitfalls'. Osteoarthritis of the hand and tenosynovitis, such as trigger thumb or finger, are more common with advancing age.

Tennis elbow

Tennis elbow is caused by overuse or overload of the muscles of the forearm, especially in the middle aged. Two types are identifiable: 'backhand' tennis elbow, or lateral epicondylitis, and 'forehand' tennis elbow, or medial epicondylitis, which is known also as golfer's, or pitcher's elbow. 'Backhand' tennis elbow, which will be termed lateral tennis elbow, is the common classic variety. It is caused by excessive strain on the extensor muscles of the forearm resulting from wrist extension.

Lateral tennis elbow (lateral epicondylitis)

The patient who presents with this common and refractory problem is usually middle aged (between 40 and 60 years of age) and only about 1 in 20 plays tennis. It is common in golfers, carpenters, bricklayers, squash players, violinists and housewives.

The disorder is obviously an overuse sporting or occupational injury, being common in those who are relatively unfit or those commencing an unaccustomed activity. Tennis elbow is an overload injury following mainly minor and often unrecognised trauma (microtrauma), involving the extensor muscles of the forearm. It may be provoked by any exercise that involves repeated and forcible extension movements of the wrist, such as playing tennis, using a screwdriver, wringing wet clothes, carrying buckets or picking up bricks.

Symptoms

Tennis elbow usually has a gradual onset but occasionally it can be sudden. At the moment the tear occurs the patient feels nothing. Several days after this event, an ache in the forearm is noticed when movements involve extension of the wrist. The ache gets worse and a tennis player is unable to play. The typical clinical profile is presented in Table 58.2.

Table 58.2 *Lateral tennis elbow: typical clinical profile*

Age:	40–60 years
Occupation:	Carpenter, bricklayer, housewife, gardener, dentist, violinist
Sport:	Tennis, squash
Symptoms:	• pain at outer elbow, referred down back of forearm • rest pain and night pain (severe cases) • pain in the elbow during hand movements, e.g. turning on taps, turning door handles, picking up objects with grasping action, carrying buckets, pouring tea, shaking hands
Signs:	• no visible swelling • localised tenderness over lateral epicondyle, anteriorly • pain on passive stretching wrist • pain on resisted extension wrist • normal elbow movement
Course:	6 to 24 months
Management:	Basic • rest from offending activity • RICE and oral NSAIDs if acute • exercises—stretching and strengthening Additional (if refractory) • corticosteroid/LA injection (maximum two) • manipulation • surgery

RICE: rest, ice, compression, elevation
LA: local anaesthetic

Signs

On examination the elbow looks normal, and flexion and extension are painless.

There are three important positive physical signs:
1. localised tenderness to palpation over the anterior aspect of the lateral epicondyle
2. pain on passive stretching at the wrist with the elbow held in extension and the forearm prone (Fig. 58.3)
3. pain on resisted extension of the wrist with the elbow held in extension and the forearm prone (Fig. 58.4).

Fig. 58.3 *Lateral tennis elbow test: reproducing pain on passive stretching at the wrist*

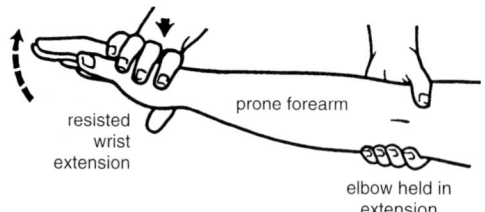

Fig. 58.4 *Lateral tennis elbow test: reproducing pain on resisted extension of the wrist*

Management

Although there are a myriad of treatments the cornerstones of therapy are rest from the offending activity and exercises to strengthen the extensors of the wrist.

Exercises

Stretching and strengthening exercises for the forearm muscles represent the best management for tennis elbow. Three options are presented.

1. *The wringing exercise.* Chronic tennis elbow can be cured by a simple wringing exercise using a small hand towel.[7]

Method
- Roll up the hand towel.
- With the arm extended, grasp the towel with the affected side placed in neutral.
- Then exert maximum wring pressure:
  — first flexing the wrist for 10 seconds
  — then extending the wrist for 10 seconds

  This is an isometric 'hold' contraction.

This exercise should be performed only twice a day, initially for 10 seconds in each direction. After each week increase the time by 5 seconds in each twisting direction until 60 seconds is reached (week 11). This level is maintained indefinitely.

Note: Despite severe initial pain, the patient must persist, using as much force as possible. Review at 6 weeks to check progress and method.

2. *'Weights' exercise.* The muscles are strengthened by the use of hand-held weights or dumbbells. A suitable starting weight is 0.5 kg, building up gradually (increasing by 0.5 kg) to 5 kg, depending on the patient.

Method
- To perform this exercise the patient sits in a chair beside a table.
- The arm is rested on the table so that the wrist extends over the edge.
- The weight is grasped with the palm facing downwards (Fig. 58.5).
- The weight is slowly raised and lowered by flexing and extending the wrist.
- The flexion/extension wrist movement is repeated 10 times, with a rest for 1 minute, and the program is repeated twice.

3. *The pronating exercise.* A suitable stretching exercise is to rhythmically rotate the hand and wrist inwards with the elbow extended and the forearm pronated (Fig. 58.6). Another proven exercise program is that outlined by Nirschl[9] and this can be provided by referral to a physiotherapist familiar with the program.

Injection therapy

The injection of 1 mL of corticosteroid and 1 mL of local anaesthetic should be reserved for more severe cases when pain occurs on most activities, and not used initially for those patients with only intermittent pain. The key to a successful injection is to have the tender lesions pinpointed

Fig. 58.5 *Lateral tennis elbow: the dumbbell exercise with the palm facing down*

Fig. 58.6 *Tennis elbow stretching exercise: the hand and wrist are rhythmically rotated inwards until the painful point is reduced*

precisely. The point of maximal tenderness is usually on or just distal to the lateral epicondyle.

Method
- The patient sits with the elbow resting on a table, flexed to a right angle and fully supinated.
- Using an anterior approach, palpate the tender area and mark it with a pen.
- With the thumb (of the non-dominant hand) over the patient's lateral epicondyle to stretch the skin and the fingers spread out around the elbow to steady it, insert the needle (25 or 23 gauge) vertically downwards to touch the periosteum of the tender point (Fig. 58.7).
- After introducing about 0.5 mL of the mixed solution, partly withdraw the needle and re-insert it to ensure that the tender area is covered both deeply and superficially.

vertical approach for injection

supinated forearm

tender lateral epicondyle

thumb stretches skin around epicondyle

Fig. 58.7 *Lateral tennis elbow: injection technique*

Postinjection:
- Ask patient to 'work it in' during the next few hours with repeated extensions of the elbow joint and pronation of the wrist.
- Warn the patient that the area will be very painful for the next 24 hours and recommend moderately strong analgesics.
- Repeat the injection in 2–4 weeks unless all the symptoms have been abolished.
- A maximum of two injections only is recommended.

Surgery
Severe and refractory cases can be referred for surgery but this is rarely indicated. It appears to have about a 70% success rate. The usual procedure is the stripping of the common extensor origin combined with debridement of any granulation tissue.[3]

Medial tennis elbow (medial epicondylitis)
In 'forehand' tennis elbow, or golfer's elbow, the lesion is the common flexor tendon at the medial epicondyle. The pain is felt on the inner side of the elbow and does not radiate far. The main signs are localised tenderness to palpation and pain or resisted flexion of the wrist.

In tennis players it is caused by stroking the ball with a bent forearm action or using a lot of top spin, rather than stroking the ball with the arm extended.

The treatment is similar to that for lateral epicondylitis except that in a dumbbell exercise program that palm must face upwards.

A similar injection method is used to that for lateral epicondylitis. The elbow is flexed and supinated with full external rotation of the shoulder of the affected arm. The anterior approach is used, and the tender area of the medial epicondyle injected as for lateral epicondylitis.

After-care and prevention
Tennis should be resumed gradually. Players recovering from tennis elbow should start quietly with a warm-up period and obtain advice on style, including smooth stroke play. During a game they should avoid elbow bending and 'wristy' shots. A change to a good quality racket (wooden or graphite frame) with a medium-sized head and suitable grip size may be appropriate.[9] The patient should be advised not to use a tightly strung, heavy racket or heavy tennis

balls. It is worthwhile to advise the use of a non-stretch band or brace situated about 7.5 cm (3 in) below the elbow.

Olecranon bursitis

Olecranon bursitis presents as a swelling locali-sed to the bursa (which has a synovial membrane) over the olecranon process. The condition may be caused by trauma, arthritic conditions (rheumatoid arthritis and gout) or infection.

Traumatic bursitis may be caused by a direct injury to the elbow or by chronic friction and pressure as occurs in miners (beat elbow), truck drivers or carpet layers. Acute olecranon bursitis with redness and warmth can occur in rheuma-toid arthritis, gout, pseudogout, haemorrhage and infection (sepsis).[10] Septic bursitis must be considered where the problem is acute or sub-acute in onset, and hence aspiration of the bursa contents with appropriate laboratory examina-tion is necessary (smear, gram stain, culture and crystal examination). Treatment depends on the cause.

Simple aspiration/injection technique

Chronic recurrent traumatic olecranon bursitis with a synovial effusion may require surgery but most cases can resolve with partial aspiration of the fluid and then injection of corticosteroid through the same needle. Sepsis must be ruled out.

Carpal tunnel syndrome

Patients with carpal tunnel syndrome (CTS) complain of 'pins and needles' affecting the pulps of the thumb, and index, middle and half of the ring finger (Fig. 58.8). They usually notice these symptoms after, rather than during, rapid use of the hands. They may also complain of pain, which may even radiate proximally as far as the shoulder, from the volar aspect of the wrist. Causes or associations of carpal tunnel syn-drome are presented in Table 58.3.

The pathognomonic symptom

Patients complain of awakening from their sleep at night with 'pins and needles' affecting the fingers. They get out of bed, shake their hands, the 'pins and needles' subside and they return to sleep. In severe cases, the patient may awaken

median nerve

transverse carpal ligament

ulnar tunnel

carpal tunnel

Fig. 58.8 *Carpal tunnel syndrome (median nerve compression syndrome)*

two or three times a night and go through the same routine.

Work-related CTS

CTS is seen in many work situations requiring rapid finger and wrist motion under load such as meat workers and process workers. A type of flexor tenosynovitis develops and thus nerve compression in the tight tunnel. It is advisable to arrange confirmatory investigations by nerve conduction studies and electromyography for this work-induced overuse disorder. This testing is also indicated where the diagnosis is uncertain

Table 58.3 *Carpal tunnel syndrome: causes or associations*

Idiopathic
Trauma
Fibrosis
Granulomatous disorders (TB, etc.)
Rheumatoid arthritis
Acromegaly
Amyloidosis
Pregnancy
Premenstrual oedema
Hypothyroidism
Paget's disease
Diabetes mellitus
Tophaceous gout

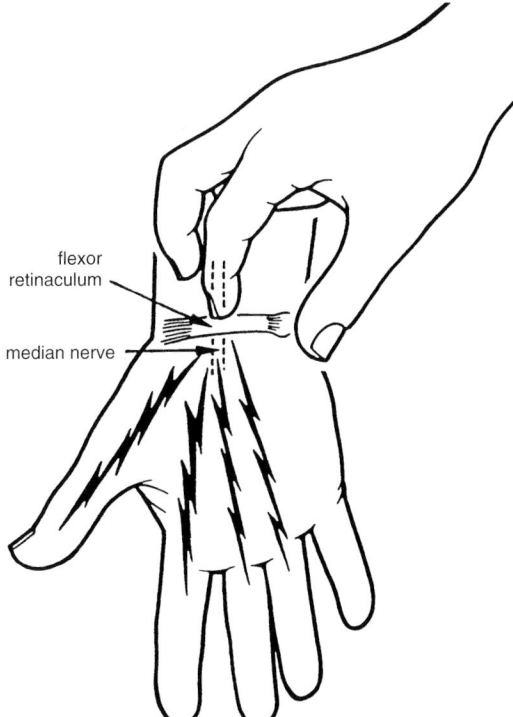

Fig. 58.9 *Carpal tunnel syndrome: Tinel sign*

or if the condition persists and numbness or weakness develops.

Simple clinical tests

In the physical examination a couple of simple tests can assist with confirming the diagnosis. These are Tinel's test and Phalen's test. However, they are 'soft' signs with a relatively low sensitivity and specificity.[11]

The Tinel test

• Hold the wrist in a neutral or flexed position and tap over the median nerve at the flexor surface of the wrist. This should be over the retinaculum just lateral to the palmaris longus tendon (if present) and the tendons of flexor digitorium superficialis (Fig. 58.9).
• A positive Tinel's sign produces a tingling sensation (usually without pain) in the distribution of the median nerve.

The Phalen test

• The patient approximates the dorsum of both hands, one to the other, with wrists maximally flexed and fingers pointing downwards (Fig. 58.10).
• This position is held for 60 seconds.
• A positive test reproduces tingling and numbness along the distribution of the median nerve.

Two point discrimination

The test that has the highest specificity of all basic clinical tests is two point discrimination, but it has low sensitivity for CTS.[11]

Fig. 58.10 *Carpal tunnel syndrome: Phalen's sign*

Treatment

The treatment is determined by the severity. For mild cases simple rest and splinting (particularly at night) is sufficient. Carpal tunnel cortico-steroid infiltration is frequently of diagnostic as well as therapeutic value. Ultrasound therapy has been used with some success. Surgical release is necessary for patients with sensory or motor deficits and those with recalcitrant CTS.

| Injection into the carpal tunnel |

Injections may relieve symptoms permanently or, more commonly, temporarily. The injections may be repeated. Do *not* use local anaesthetic in the injection.

Method
- The patient sits by the side of the doctor with the hand palm upwards, the wrist slightly extended.
- Identify the palmaris longus tendon and ulnar artery.
- Insert the needle (23 g) at a point about 2.5–3 cm proximal to the main transverse crease of the wrist and between the palmaris longus tendon and the artery (Fig. 58.11). Take care to avoid the superficial veins.
- Advance the needle distally, parallel to the tendons and nerve at about 5° to the horizontal. It should pass under the transverse carpal

ligament (flexor retinaculum) and come to lie in the carpal tunnel.
- Inject 1 mL of corticosteroid. This is usually painless and runs freely. Ensure the patient feels no severe pain or paraesthesia during the injection.
- Withdraw the needle and ask the patient to flex and extend the fingers for 2 minutes.

Trigger finger/thumb

In the fingers the common work-induced condition is stenosing flexor tenosynovitis, also known as trigger thumb and finger. It is caused by the same mechanism as de Quervain's stenosing tenosynovitis. In middle age these tendons, which are rapidly and constantly being flexed and extended, can undergo attrition wear and tear, and fibrillate and fragment; this causes swelling, oedema and painful inflammation and the formation of a nodule on the tendon that triggers back and forth across the thick, sharp edge of the 'pulley' (of the fibrosseous tunnel in the finger) (Fig. 58.12).

These patients may present with a finger locked in the palm of the hand; the finger can only be extended passively (manually) with the other hand. It is easily diagnosed by triggering. If the pulp of the finger is placed over the 'pulley' crepitus can be felt and tenderness elicited. The

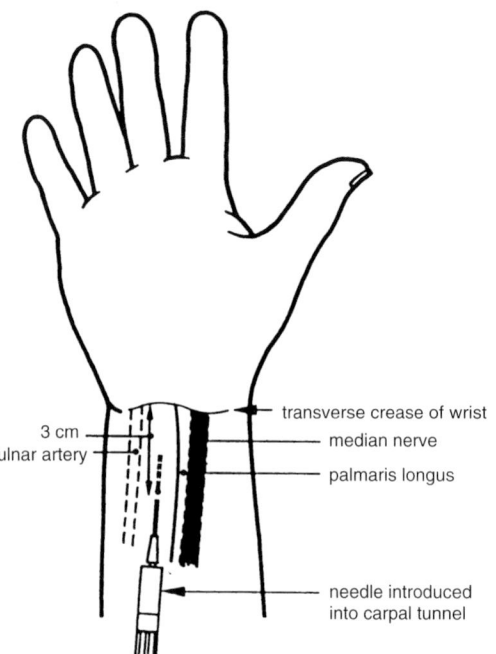

3 cm
ulnar artery
transverse crease of wrist
median nerve
palmaris longus
needle introduced
into carpal tunnel

Fig. 58.11 *Injection technique for carpal tunnel syndrome*

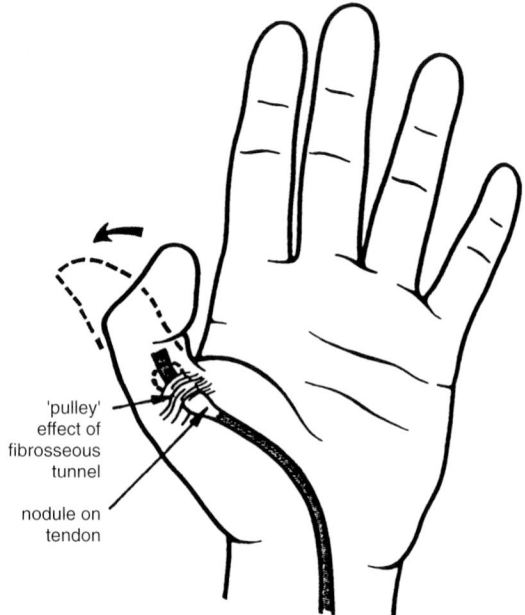

'pulley'
effect of
fibrosseous
tunnel
nodule on
tendon

Fig. 58.12 *Trigger thumb*

thumb and fourth (ring) finger are commonly affected.

Treatment

Although surgery is simple and effective, treatment by injection is often very successful. The injection is made under the tendon sheath and not into the tendon or its nodular swelling.

Method

- The patient sits facing the doctor with the palm of the affected hand facing upwards.
- Draw 1 mL of long-acting corticosteroid solution into a syringe and attach a 25-gauge needle for the injection.
- Insert the needle at an angle distal to the nodule and direct it proximally within the tendon sheath (Fig. 58.13). This requires tension on the skin with free fingers.
- By palpating the tendon sheath, you can (usually) feel when the fluid has entered the tendon sheath.
- Inject 0.5–1 mL of the solution, withdraw the needle and ask the patient to exercise the fingers for 1 minute.

Postinjection

Improvement usually occurs after 48 hours and may be permanent. The injection can be repeated after 3 weeks if the triggering is not completely relieved. If triggering recurs, surgery is indicated. This involves division of the thickened tendon sheath only.

De Quervain's tenosynovitis (washerwoman's sprain)

At the wrist a not uncommon work-induced condition is de Quervain's stenosing tenosynovitis of the first dorsal extensor compartment tendons (extensor pollicus brevis and abductor pollicis longus), which pass along the radial border of the wrist to the base of the thumb. It is usually seen when the patient is required to engage in rapid, repetitive movements of the thumb and the wrist, especially for the first time, and thus is common in assembly line workers, such as staple gun operators.

Clinical features

- typical age 40–50 years
- pain at and proximal to wrist on radial border
- pain during pinch grasping
- pain on thumb and wrist movement
- dull ache or severe pain (acute flare-up)
- can be disabling with inability to use hand, e.g. writing

Triad of diagnostic signs

- tenderness to palpation over and just proximal to radial styloid
- firm tender localised swelling in area of radial styloid (may be mistaken for exostosis)
- positive Finklestein's sign (the pathognomonic test)

Finkelstein's test

- The patient folds the thumb into the palm with the fingers of the involved hand folded over the thumb, thus making a fist.
- Rotate the wrist in an ulnar direction to stretch the involved tendons as you stabilise the forearm with the other hand (Fig. 58.14).
- A positive test is indicated by reproduction of or increased pain.

Treatment

- Rest and avoid the causative stresses and strains on the thumb abductors.
- Use a custom-made splint that involves the thumb and immobilises the wrist.
- Local long-acting corticosteroid injection can

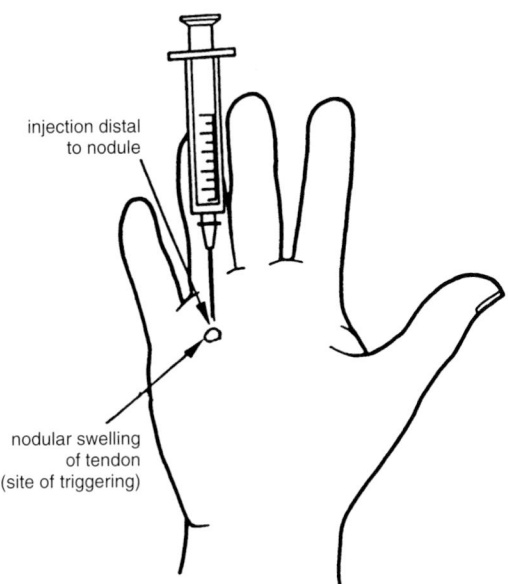

injection distal to nodule

nodular swelling of tendon (site of triggering)

Fig. 58.13 *Injection site for trigger finger*

Fig. 58.14 *Finkelstein's test*

relieve and may even cure the problem but care should be taken to inject the suspension within the tendon sheath rather than into the tendon.
• Surgical release is required for chronic cases.

Method of tendon sheath injection
• Identify and mark the most tender site of the tendon and the line of the tendon. Identify and avoid the radial artery.
• Thoroughly cleanse the skin with an antiseptic such as povidone iodine 10% solution.
• Insert the tip of the needle (23 g) about 1 cm distal to the point of maximal tenderness (Fig. 58.15).
• Advance the needle almost parallel to the skin along the line of the tendon.
• Inject about 0.5 mL of the corticosteroid suspension within the tendon sheath. If the needle is in the sheath very little resistance to the plunger should be felt, and the injection causes the tendon sheath to billow out.

Fig. 58.15 *Tendon sheath injection*

Tendinitis/tenosynovitis

After excluding carpal tunnel syndrome, trigger thumb/finger, de Quervain's tenosynovitis, rheumatoid and related disease, tendinitis is uncommon in the hand.[12] Tendinitis may occur in other extensor compartments of the wrist and hand with unusual repetitive stressful actions such as power drills jamming, and in conveyer quality control where an object is picked up with the forearm prone, supinating to examine it and pronating to replace it.

Treatment is rest from the provoking activity, splintage and tendon sheath injection with long-acting corticosteroid in a manner similar to that described for de Quervain's tenosynovitis.

Neurovascular disorders of the hand

Painful vascular disorders, which are more likely to occur in women in cold weather, include Raynaud's phenomenon, erythermalgia, chilblains and acute blue fingers syndrome. Acrocyanosis is not a painful condition.

Raynaud's phenomenon and disease

The basic feature of Raynaud's phenomenon, which is a vasospastic disorder, is sequential discolouration of the digits from pallor to cyanosis to rubor upon exposure to cold and other factors (a useful mnemonic is WBR, namely white → blue → red). The rubor is a reactive hyperaemia when fingers become red and tender. It is possible to get loss of tissue pulp at the ends of the fingers and subsequent necrotic ulcers.

Causes
• Raynaud's disease (idiopathic)
• occupational trauma (vibrating machinery)
• connective tissue disorders
  — rheumatoid arthritis
  — SLE
  — systemic sclerosis, CREST
  — polyarteritis nodosa
• arterial disease
  — Buerger's disease
• haematological disorders
  — polycythaemia
  — cold agglutinin disease
  — leukaemia
• drugs
  — beta-blockers
  — ergotamine

Investigations

Exclude underlying causes with appropriate tests.

Treatment

- total body protection from cold
- gloves and thick woollen socks
- avoid smoking
- vasodilators, e.g. amlodipine (o) 5 mg/day during cold weather
- topical glyceryl trinitrate 2% ointment, applied to the base of the affected finger/s, 2 to 4 times daily
- consider sympathectomy

Erythermalgia

This condition is characterised by erythema (redness), a burning sensation and swelling of the hands (and feet) after exposure to heat and exercise. It may be primary or secondary to a disease such as diabetes, haematological disorders[10] and connective tissue disease. Treatment of primary erythermalgia includes trials of aspirin, phenoxybenzamine (Dibenyline), methysergide or sympathectomy.

Acute blue fingers in women syndrome

This unusual syndrome involves the sudden onset of pain and cyanosis of the ventral aspect of the digit initially, and then the entire digit. It lasts for two or three days and the attacks recur one or more times per year. No abnormalities are found on physical or laboratory examination.

The cause is probably spontaneous rupture of a vein at the base of the finger.

Chilblains (perniosis)

Refer Chapter 123.

Reflex sympathetic dystrophy

Sudek's atrophy is a form of reflex sympathetic dystrophy in which the patient presents with severe pain, swelling and disability of the hand. It may occur spontaneously or, more usually, it follows trauma that may even be trivial. It can occur after a Colles' fracture, especially with prolonged immobilisation.

Clinical features

- throbbing burning pain, worse at night
- paraesthesia
- initial: red, swollen hand; warm, dry skin
- later: cold, cyanosed and mottled, moist skin; shiny and stiff fingers

- wasting of small muscles
- X-rays—patchy decalcification of bone (diagnostic)

The problem eventually settles but may take years. Patients need considerable support, encouragement, basic pain relief, mobility in preference to rest and perhaps referral to a pain clinic.

Kienböck's disease

Kienböck's disease is avascular necrosis of the carpal lunate bone (Fig. 58.16), which may

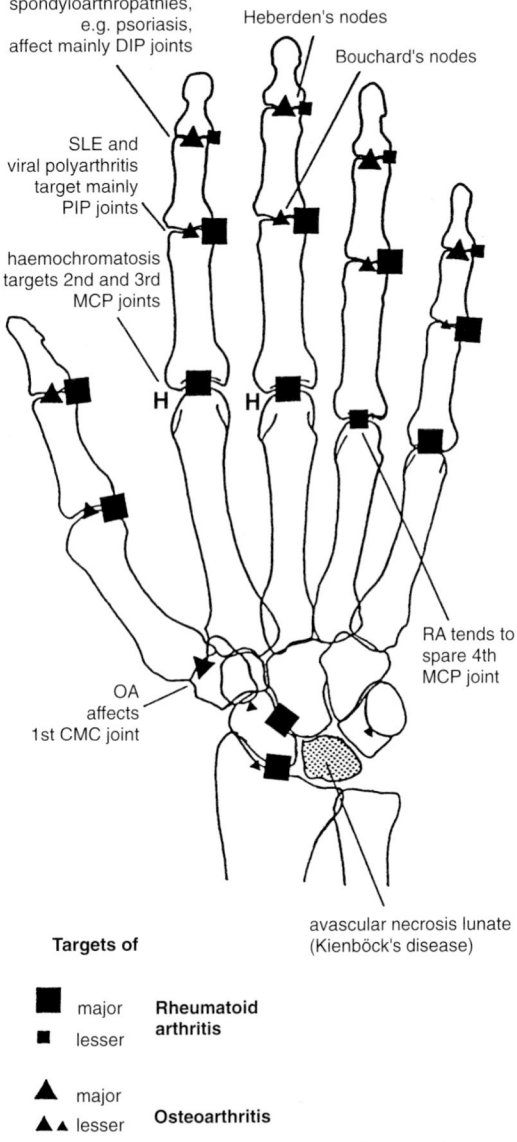

Fig. 58.16 *Typical sites of arthritic conditions and osteochondritis in the hand*

fragment and collapse, eventually leading to osteoarthritis of the wrist.

It presents usually in young adults over the age of 15 as insidious, progressive wrist pain and stiffness that limits grip strength and hand function. Males are affected more often than females and the right hand more than the left indicating the relationship to trauma.

Arthritic conditions of the wrist and hand

Arthritis of the hand is an inappropriate diagnosis and specificity is required to highlight the various joints that are the targets of the specific arthritides, which include osteoarthritis, rheumatoid arthritis, spondyloarthropathies, gout, haemochromatosis, and connective tissue disorders. Typical target areas in the hand are shown in Figure 58.16.

Osteoarthritis

Osteoarthritis commonly involves the interphalangeal joints of the fingers (especially the DIP joints)[13] and the carpometacarpal joint of the thumb. Degenerative changes produce bony swellings around the margins of the joints— Heberden's nodes of the DIP joints and less commonly Bouchard's nodes of the PIP joints. A patchy distribution occurs in metacarpophalangeal, intercarpal and wrist joints, usually related to trauma.

Rheumatoid arthritis

In rheumatoid arthritis the DIP joints are often spared (only about 30% involved) but the metacarpophalangeal and proximal interphalangeal joints and wrist joints are generally affected symmetrically and bilaterally. Rheumatoid arthritis tends to affect the metacarpophalangeal joints of the fourth finger less commonly.

Gout

Gout may involve normal joints of the hand but is encountered more frequently in osteoarthritic joints of the hand (especially DIP joints) in elderly people taking diuretics. This clinical feature is known as nodular gout.

Seronegative arthropathies

A similar appearance to rheumatoid arthritis occurs except that with psoriatic arthritis the terminal joints are often involved with swelling, giving the appearance of 'sausage digits'.

Infections of the hand

Although not encountered as frequently as in the past, serious suppurative infections of the deep fascial spaces of the hand and tendon sheath can still occur, especially with penetrating injuries and web space infection.

Infections of the hand include:

- Infected wounds with superficial cellulitis or lymphangitis (*Streptococcus pyogenes*)
- Subcutaneous tissues
  — nail bed (paronychia)
  — pulp (whitlow, e.g. herpes simplex)
- Erysipeloid—this is a specific infection in one finger of fishers or meat handlers, caused by *Erysipelothrix insidiosa*. There is a purplish erythema that gradually extends over days. It is rapidly cured by penicillin.
- Tendon sheath infection (suppurative tenosynovitis)—this is a dangerous and painful infection that can cause synovial adhesions with severe residual finger stiffness. The affected finger is hot and swollen and looks like a sausage.
- Deep palmar fascial space infection—infection from an infected tendon sheath or web space may spread to one of the two deep palmar spaces: the medial (midpalmar space) or lateral (thenar) space.
- Sporotrichosis (gardener's arm)—a chronic fungal infection from contaminated spikes of wood or rose thorns presenting as hard nontender nodules in skin of hand and extending along lymphatics of arm.

Management of serious infection

- Early appropriate antibiotic treatment for infection and early surgical referral where necessary.
- Antibiotics (adult doses)[14]
  — *Streptococcus pyogenes* (cellulitis, lymphangitis)
- procaine penicillin 1 g IM daily
  or
- phenoxymethyl penicillin 500 mg (o) 6 hourly
  — *Staphylococcus aureus* infection (suspected or proved)
- flucloxacillin/dicloxacillin 500 mg to 1 g (o) 6 hourly
  or
- cephalexin 500 mg (o) 6 hourly
  or
- erythromycin 500 mg (o) 12 hourly

When to refer

- Disabling osteoarthritis of carpometacarpal joint for possible surgical repair
- Myelopathy (motor weakness) and persistent radiculotherapy (nerve root pain and sensory changes) in the arm
- Unresolving nerve entrapment problems such as median and ulnar nerves
- Elbow injuries in children with proven or possible supracondylar fracture or avulsion epicondylar fractures
- Evidence or suspicion of suppurative infection of the tendon sheaths or deep palmar fascial spaces
- Septic arthritis and osteomyelitis
- Reflex sympathetic dystrophy
- Other conditions not responding to conservative measures

Practice tips

- With elbow injuries in children, X-ray both elbows and compare one side with the other; this helps to determine whether there is displacement of fragments or a disturbance in the normal anatomy of the elbow.
- Tendinitis and other entheseal problems of the arm are common and tend to take 1–2 years to resolve spontaneously, yet they resolve rapidly with rest, an exercise program or corticosteroid injections. Surgical relief is effective for refractory cases.
- The so-called thoracic outlet syndrome is probably most often caused by 'the droopy shoulder syndrome' rather than by a cervical rib.
- Consider corticosteroid injections for the carpal tunnel syndrome and stenosing tenosynovitis (de Quervain's and trigger finger or thumb). They are very effective and often curative.
- The site of arthritis in the hand provides a reasonable guide as to the cause.
- Always keep reflex sympathetic dystrophy in mind for persistent burning pain in the hand following injury—trivial or severe.

References

1. Swift TR, Nichols FT. The droopy shoulder syndrome. Neurol, 1984; 34: 212–215.
2. Bertelsen S. Neurovascular compression syndromes of the neck and shoulder. Acta Chir Scand, 1969; 135:137–148.
3. Ireland D. The hand (part two). Aust Fam Physician, 1986; 15:1502–1513.
4. Dan NG. Entrapment syndromes. Med J Aust, 1976; 1:528–531.
5. Corrigan B, Maitland GP. *Practical orthopaedic medicine.* Sydney: Butterworths, 1986, 75–77.
6. Young D, Murtagh J. Pitfalls in orthopaedics. Aust Fam Physician, 1989; 18:645–653.
7. White ADN. Practice tip. A simple cure for chronic tennis elbow. Aust Fam Physician, 1987; 16:953.
8. Oakes B, Fuller P, Kenihan M, Sandor S. *Sports injuries.* Melbourne: Pitman, 1985, 51–55.
9. Brinbaum AJ. Tennis elbow: Don't worry, it can be avoided and it can be cured. Tennis, April 1978, 96–103.
10. Sheon R, Moskowitz R, Goldberg V. *Soft tissue rheumatic pain.* Philadelphia: Lea and Febiger, 1987, 134–140.
11. Buch-Jaeger N, Foucher G. Carpal tunnel syndrome, Journal of Hand Surgery. 1994; 19B:72–74.
12. Ireland D. The hand (part one). Aust Fam Physician, 1986; 15:1162–1171.
13. Corrigan B, Maitland G. *Practical orthopaedic medicine.* Sydney: Butterworths, 1986, 97–100.
14. Mashford ML. *Antibiotic guidelines* (9th edn). Melbourne: Victorian Medical Postgraduate Foundation: 1996–97, 137–138.

59

Hip and buttock pain

—

Which of your hips has the most profound sciatica?

William Shakespeare (1564–1616),
Measure for Measure

Pain in the hip, buttock, groin and upper thigh tend to be interrelated. Patients often present complaining of pain in the hip yet are referring to pain in the buttock or lower back. Most pain in the buttock has a lumbosacral origin. Pain originating from disorders of the lumbosacral spine (commonly) and the knee (uncommonly) can be referred to the hip region, while pain from the hip joint (L3 innervation) may be referred commonly to the thigh and the knee. Disorders of the abdomen and retroperitoneal region may cause hip and groin pain, sometimes mediated by irritation of the psoas muscle.

Key facts and checkpoints

- Hip troubles have a significant age relationship (Fig. 59.1).
- Children can suffer from a variety of serious disorders of the hip, e.g. developmental dysplasia (DDH), Perthes' disorder, tuberculosis, septic arthritis and slipped capital femoral epiphysis (SCFE), all of which demand early recognition and management.
- SCFE typically presents in the obese adolescent (10–15 years) with knee pain and a slight limp.
- Every newborn infant should be tested for DDH, which is the most graphic orthopaedic disability that can be prevented.

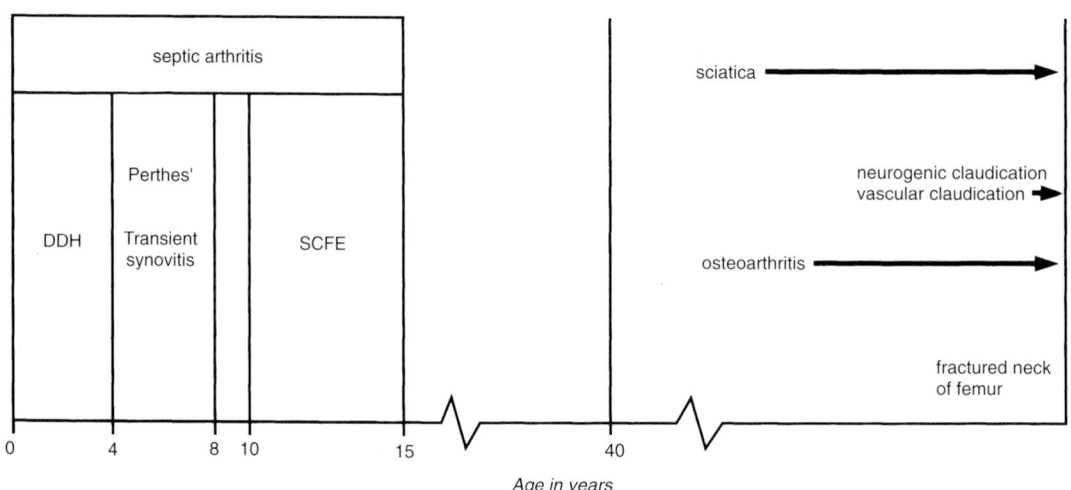

Fig. 59.1 *Typical ages of presentation of hip disorders*

Table 59.1 *Hip and buttock pain: diagnostic strategy model*

Q. Probability diagnosis
A. Traumatic muscular strains
    Referred pain from spine
    Osteoarthritis of hip

Q. Serious disorders not to be missed
A. Cardiovascular
    • buttock claudication
    Neoplasia
    • metastatic carcinoma
    Septic infections
    • septic arthritis
    • osteomyelitis
    • tuberculosis
    • pelvic and abdominal infections
        — pelvic abscess
        — PID
    Childhood disorders
    • DDH
    • Perthes' disease
    • slipped femoral epiphysis
    • synovitis (irritable hip)
    • juvenile chronic arthritis

Q. Pitfalls (often missed)
A. Polymyalgia rheumatica
    Fractures
    • stress fractures femoral neck
    • subcapital fractures
    • sacrum
    Avascular necrosis femoral head
    Sacroiliac joint disorders
    Inguinal or femoral hernia
    Bursitis or tendinitis
    • gluteus medius tendinitis
    • trochanteric bursitis
    • ischial bursitis
    Neurogenic claudication
    Chilblains
    Rarities
    • Haemarthrosis, e.g. haemophilia
    • Paget's disease
    • Nerve entrapments
        — sciatica 'hip pocket nerve'
        — obturator
        — lateral cutaneous nerve thigh

Q. Seven masquerades checklist
A. Depression   √
 . Diabetes   —
    Drugs   —
    Anaemia   —
    Thyroid disease   —
    Spinal dysfunction   √
    UTI   —

Q. Is this patient trying to tell me something else?
A. Non-organic pain may be present. Patient with arthritis fearful of being crippled.

• Limp has an inseparable relationship with painful hip and buttock conditions, especially those of the hip.
• The spine is the most likely cause of pain in the buttock in adults.
• Disorders of the hip joint commonly refer pain to the knee.
• Disorders of the knee joint can (but rarely do) refer pain to the hip joint.
• If a woman, especially one with many children, presents with bilateral buttock or hip pain, consider dysfunction of the sacroiliac joints as the cause.
• If a middle-aged or elderly woman presents with hip pain, always consider the under-diagnosed conditions of trochanteric bursitis or gluteus medius tendinitis.

A diagnostic approach

A summary of the diagnostic model is presented in Table 59.1.

Probability diagnosis

The commonest cause of hip and buttock pain presenting in general practice is referred pain from the lumbosacral spine and the sacroiliac joints.[1] The pain is invariably referred to the outer buttock and posterior hip area (Fig. 59.2). The origin of the pain can be the facet joints of the lumbar spine, intervertebral disc disruption or, less commonly, the sacroiliac joints. Much of this pain is inappropriately referred to as 'lumbago', 'fibrositis' and 'rheumatism'.

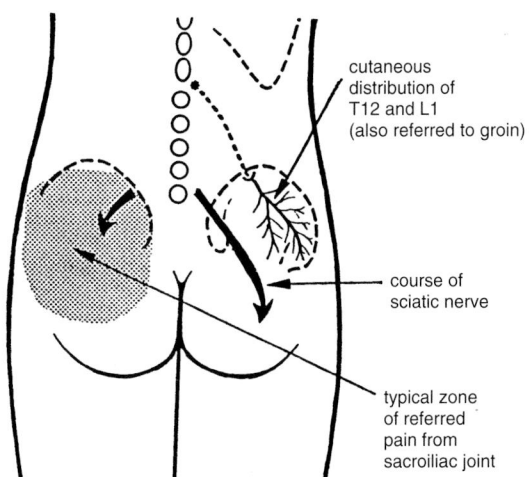

Fig. 59.2 *Referral patterns of pain from the lumbosacral spine and the sacroiliac joints*

Trauma and overuse injuries from sporting activities are also common causes of muscular and ligamentous strains[2] around the buttock and hip.

The hip joint is a common target of osteoarthritis. This usually presents after 50 years but can present earlier if the hip has been affected by another condition.

Serious disorders not to be missed

The major triad of serious disorders—cardiovascular, neoplasia and severe infections—are applicable to this area albeit limited in extent.

Aortoiliac occlusion

Ischaemic muscle pain including buttock claudication secondary to aortoiliac arterial occlusion is sometimes confused with musculoskeletal pain. An audible bruit over the vessels following exercise is one clue to diagnosis.

Neoplasia

Primary tumours including myeloma and lymphosarcoma can arise rarely in the upper femur and pelvis (especially the ilium). However, these areas are relatively common targets for metastases, especially from the prostate and breast.

Infection

Some very important, at times 'occult', infections can develop in and around the hip joint.

Osteomyelitis is prone to develop in the metaphysis of the upper end of the femur and must be considered in the child with intense pain, a severe limp and fever. Tuberculosis may also present in children (usually under 10 years) with a presentation similar to Perthes' disease.

Transient synovitis or 'irritable hip' is the most common cause of hip pain and limp in childhood.

Inflammation of the side wall of the pelvis as in a deep pelvic abscess (e.g. from appendicitis), pelvic inflammatory disease (PID) including pyosalpinx, or an ischiorectal abscess can cause deep hip pain and a limp. This pain may be related to irritation of the obturator nerve.

Retroperitoneal haematoma can cause referred pain and femoral nerve palsy.

Childhood disorders that must not be missed include:

- developmental dysplasia of the hip and acetabular dysplasia
- Perthes' disorder

- slipped capital femoral epiphysis (SCFE)
- stress fractures of the femoral neck

Inflammatory disorders of the hip joint that should be kept in mind include:

- rheumatoid arthritis
- juvenile chronic arthritis (JCA)
- rheumatic fever (a flitting polyarthritis)
- spondyloarthropathy

Pitfalls

There are many pitfalls associated with hip and buttock pain and these include the various childhood problems. Fractures can be a pitfall, especially subcapital fractures.

Sacroiliac joint disorders are often missed, whether it be the inflammation of sacroiliitis or mechanical dysfunction of the joint.

Inflammatory conditions around the hip girdle are common and so are often misdiagnosed. These include the common gluteus medius tendinitis and trochanteric bursitis.

Polymyalgia rheumatica commonly causes shoulder girdle pain in the elderly but pain around the hip girdle can accompany this important problem.

Chilblains around the upper thighs occur in cold climates and are often known as 'jodhpur' chilblains because they tend to occur during horse riding in very cold weather.

Nerve entrapment syndromes require consideration. Meralgia paraesthetica is a nerve entrapment causing pain and paraesthesia over the lateral aspect of the hip (Fig. 59.3).

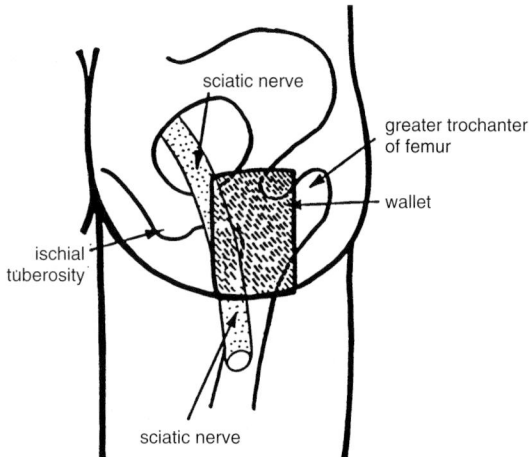

Fig. 59.3 *'Hip pocket nerve' syndrome: location and relations of sciatic nerve in the buttock*

An interesting modern phenomenon is the so-called 'hip pocket nerve' syndrome. If a man presents with 'sciatica', especially confined to the buttock and upper posterior thigh (without local back pain), consider the possibility of pressure on the sciatic nerve from a wallet in the hip pocket. This problem is occasionally encountered in people sitting for long periods in cars (e.g. taxi drivers). It appears to be related to the increased presence of plastic credit cards in wallets (Fig. 59.3).

Paget's disease can involve the upper end of the femur and the pelvis.

General pitfalls

- Failure to test the hips of neonates carefully and follow up developmental dysplasia of the hip.
- Misdiagnosis of arthritis and other disorders of the hip joint because of referred pain.
- Overlooking a SCFE or a stress fracture of the femoral neck in teenage boys, especially athletes. If an X-ray shows that the epiphysis is fusing or has fused, arrange a technetium bone scan. Stress fractures are associated with a significant incidence of avascular necrosis.

Seven masquerades checklist

The one outstanding masquerade is spinal dysfunction, which is the most likely cause of pain in the buttock. Many dermatomes meet at the buttock and theoretically pain in the buttock can result from any lesion situated in a tissue derived from L1, L2, L3, S2, S3, S4.[1] Symptoms from L3 can spread from the outer buttock to the front of the thigh and down the leg, over the medial aspect of the knee to the calf. Such a distribution is common to an L3 nerve root lesion and arthritis of the hip.

Furthermore, dysfunction of the facet joints and sacroiliac joints can refer pain to the buttock. The relatively common L1 lesion due to dysfunction at the T12–L1 spinal level can lead to referred pain over the outer upper quadrant of the buttock (Fig. 59.2) and also to the groin (Fig. 60.1).

Psychogenic considerations

Cyriax[1] claims that the hip shares with the back and the shoulder 'an enhanced liability to fixation' for psychological reasons. This problem is often related to work compensation factors and overpowering stresses at home. A common finding in psychoneurotic patients complaining of buttock and thigh pain is 90° limitation of flexion at the hip joint. The importance of testing passive movements of the hip joint is obvious, for often such limitation of flexion is combined with a full range of rotation. In arthritis of the hip joint internal rotation is invariably affected first.

Such patients often walk into the office with a marked limp and leaning on a thick stick. It requires great skill to evaluate and manage them tactfully and successfully.

On the other hand, patients with genuine osteoarthritis fear being crippled and ending in a wheelchair. They require considerable education and reassurance.

The clinical approach
History

Pain associated with hip joint pathology is usually described as a deep aching pain, aggravated by movement[2] and felt in the groin and anteromedial aspect of the upper thigh, sometimes exclusively around the knee (Fig. 61.1). A limp is a frequent association.

An obstetric history in a woman may be relevant for sacroiliac pain.

Key questions

- Can you tell me how the pain started?
- Could you describe the pain?
- Point to where the pain is exactly.
- Does the pain come on after walking for a while and stops as soon as you rest?
- Is there any stiffness, especially first thing in the morning?
- Do you get any backache?
- Do your movements feel free?
- Do you have a limp?
- Do you have a similar ache around the shoulders?
- Have you had an injury such as a fall?
- Have you lost any weight recently?

Physical examination

Follow the traditional methods of examination of any joint: LOOK, FEEL, MOVE, MEASURE, TEST FUNCTION, LOOK ELSEWHERE and X-RAY. The patient should strip down to the pants to allow maximum exposure.

Inspection

Ask the patient to point exactly to the area of greatest discomfort. Careful observation of the patient, especially walking, provides useful diagnostic information. If walking with a limp, the leg adducted and foot somewhat externally rotated, osteoarthritis of the hip joint is the likely diagnosis.

If called to a patient who has suffered an injury such as a fall or vehicle accident, note the position of the leg. If shortened and externally rotated (Fig. 59.4a), a fractured neck of femur is the provisional diagnosis; if internally rotated, suspect a posterior dislocation of the hip (Fig. 59.4b). With anterior dislocation of the hip, the hip is externally rotated.

Get the patient to lie supine on the couch with ASISs of the pelvis placed squarely and note the shape and position of the limbs.

Palpation

Feel one to two finger-breadths below the midpoint of the inguinal ligament for joint tenderness. Check for trochanteric bursitis, gluteus medius tendinitis and other soft tissue problems over the most lateral bony aspect of the upper thigh.

Movements

* Passive movements with *patient supine* (normal range is indicated):
  — flexion (compare both sides) 140°
  — external rotation (knee and hip extended in adults) 45–50°

— internal rotation (knee and hip extended in adults) 45°
— abduction (stand on same side—steady pelvis) 45°
— adduction (should see the patella of the opposite leg) 25°

In children it is most important to measure rotation and abduction/adduction with the knee and hip flexed to detect early Perthes' or SCFE.
* *Patient prone*:
* extension (one hand held over SIJ) 25°

Note: Osteoarthritis of the hip affects IR, extension and abduction first.

Measurements

* true leg length (ASIS to medial malleolus)
* apparent leg length (umbilicus to medial malleolus)

Note: • Unequal true leg length = hip disease on shorter side.
• Unequal apparent leg length = tilting of pelvis.

Feel the height of the greater trochanters relative to the ASIS to determine if shortening is in the hip or below.

Test function and special tests

Gait:
* Trendelenburg test—tests hip abductors (gluteus medius)
* Thomas test—tests for fixed flexion deformity

Look elsewhere

Examine lumbosacral spine, sacroiliac joints, groin and knee. Consider hernias and possibility of PID.

Investigations

These can be selected from:
* serological tests
  — RA factor
  — FBE
  — ESR
  — C-reactive protein
* radiological
  — plain AP X-ray of pelvis showing both hip joints
  — lateral X-ray ('Frog' lateral best in children)
  — X-ray of lumbosacral spine and sacroiliac joints
  — isotope bone scan; useful if plain X-rays normal for:

(a)   (b)

Fig. 59.4 (a) *General configuration of the legs for a fractured neck of femur;* **(b)** *general configuration for a posterior dislocated hip*

- stress fracture
- early avascular necrosis
- early osteomyelitis
- metastases
— CT scan; hip joint, pelvis, lumbosacral spine
— MRI scan
  - early avascular necrosis
  - labial tears of hip joint
  - soft tissue tumours
- needle aspiration of joint

Role of ultrasound. Ultrasound diagnosis is now sensitive in children (and adults) in detecting fluid in the hip joint, and can diagnose septic arthritis and also localise the site of an osteomyelitic abscess around a swollen joint. It can accurately assess the neonatal hip joint and confirm the position of the femoral head.

Hip pain in children

Hip disorders have an important place in childhood and may present with a limp when the child is walking. These important disorders include:

- developmental dysplasia of the hip (DDH)
- congenital subluxation of hip and acetabular dysplasia
- transient synovitis
- Perthes' disorder (pseudocoxalgia or coxa plana)
- septic arthritis
- slipped capital femoral epiphysis (adolescent coxa vara)
- pathological fractures through bone cyst

The important features of hip pain in children are summarised in Table 59.2.

Developmental dysplasia of the hip

In DDH, previously known as congenital dislocation of the hip, the underdeveloped femoral head dislocates posteriorly and superiorly. DDH is described as dislocatable (1 in 80 hips at birth, which stabilise in a few days) and frankly dislocated (1 in 800 hips).[3]

Clinical features
- females: males = 6:1
- bilateral in one-third
- tight adductors and short leg evident
- diagnosed early by Ortolani and Barlow tests (abnormal thud or clunk on abduction); test usually negative after 2 months
- ultrasound excellent (especially up to 3–4 months) and probably more sensitive than clinical examination
- X-ray usually normal

Note: 1. When diagnosed and treated from birth it is possible to produce a normal joint after a few months in an abduction splint.
2. Every baby should be examined for DDH during the first day of life and before discharge from hospital or after care.[3] The Ortolani and Barlow tests remain important means of detecting the congenitally unstable or dislocated hip, but ultrasound is becoming more important and is recommended for

Table 59.2 *Comparison of important causes of hip pain in children*

	DDH	Transient synovitis	Perthes'	SCFE	Septic arthritis
Age (years)	0–4	4–8	4–8	10–15	Any
Limp	+	+	+	+	Won't walk
Pain	−	+	+	+	+++
Limited movement	Abduction	All, especially abduction and IR	Abduction and IR	All, especially IR	All
Plain X-ray	• Normal or dislocation • No diagnostic value in neonatal period (use ultrasound)	• Normal	• Subchondral fracture • Dense head • Pebble stone epiphysis	• AP may be normal • Frog view shows slip	Normal Use ultrasound

high-risk babies, e.g. breech, family history DDH.

Screening examination

Carry out the examination on a large firm bench with the baby stripped. Relaxation is essential; give the baby a bottle if necessary. Be gentle and have warm hands.

With the legs extended any asymmetry of the legs or skin creases is noted.

- Hold the leg in the hand with knee flexed—thumb over groin (lesser trochanter) and middle finger over greater trochanter—see Fig. 59.5.
- Flex hips to about 90°, abduct to 45° (note any clunk).
- Gently rock the femur backwards and forwards on the pelvis by pressing forward with the middle finger and backwards with the thumb.

Note any jerk or clunk. If the femoral head displaces, there is dislocation. Plain X-ray has little or no place in the diagnosis of DDH in the neonatal period.[4] Early referral for treatment is essential. If not detected early the femoral head stays out of the acetabulum and after the age of 1 year the child may present with delay in walking or a limp. The diagnosis is then detected by X-ray.

Treatment (guidelines)

- DDH must be referred to a specialist[3]
- 0–6 months—Pavlik harness; double nappies may suffice for milder cases
- 8–18 months—reduction (closed or open) and cast (pelvic spica)
- 18 months—open reduction and osteotomy

Fig. 59.5 *Examination of the infant for DDH: demonstrating Ortolani's sign on left side*

Note: Despite early treatment some hip conditions progress to acetabulum dysplasia (underdevelopment of the 'roof' of the hip joint) and to premature osteoarthritis. Thus a follow-up X-ray of the pelvis during teenage years should be considered for anyone with a history of DDH.

Perthes' disorder

Perthes' disorder is one of the group of juvenile osteochondroses in which the femoral head becomes partly or totally avascular, i.e. avascular necrosis.

Clinical features

- males:females = 4:1
- usual age 4–8 years (rarely 2–18 years)
- sometimes bilateral
- presents as a limp and aching
- 'irritable' hip early
- limited movement in abduction and IR

X-ray. Joint space appears increased and femoral head too lateral: typical changes of sclerosis, deformity and collapse of the femoral capital epiphysis may be delayed.

Management

- Refer urgently.
- Aim is to keep femoral head from becoming flat.
- Choice of treatment dependent on consultant.

If untreated, the femoral head usually becomes flat over some months, leading to eventual osteoarthritis. Some untreated Perthes' heal and have a normal X-ray.

Transient synovitis

This common condition is also known as 'irritable hip' or observation hip[5] and is the consequence of a self-limiting synovial inflammation.

Clinical features

- child aged 4–8 years
- sudden onset of hip pain and a limp
- child can usually walk (some may not)
- may be history of trauma
- painful limitation of movements especially abduction and IR
- blood tests and X-rays normal (may be soft tissue swelling); ESR may be mildly elevated
- ultrasound shows fluid in the joint

Differential diagnosis. This includes septic arthritis, JCA, Perthes' disease.

Outcome. It settles to normal within 7 days, without sequelae.

Treatment. This is bed rest and analgesics. Follow-up X-ray is needed in 4 to 6 months to exclude Perthes' disease. Aspiration under GA may be needed to exclude septic arthritis.

Slipped capital femoral epiphysis (SCFE)

A most distressing aspect of the displaced capital epiphysis of the femoral head is the significant number of patients who develop avascular necrosis despite expert treatment. Therefore diagnosis of the condition before major slipping is important. This necessitates early consultation with the teenager experiencing hip or knee discomfort and then accurate interpretation of X-rays.

Clinical features

- adolescent 10–15 years, often obese
- most common in the oversized and undersexed (e.g. the heavy prepubertal boy)
- bilateral in 20%
- limp and irritability of hip on movement
- knee pain
- hip rotating into external rotation on flexion and often lies in external rotation
- most movements restricted, especially IR

Any adolescent with a limp or knee pain should have X-rays (AP and frog view) of both hips (Fig. 59.6). Otherwise, this important condition will be overlooked.

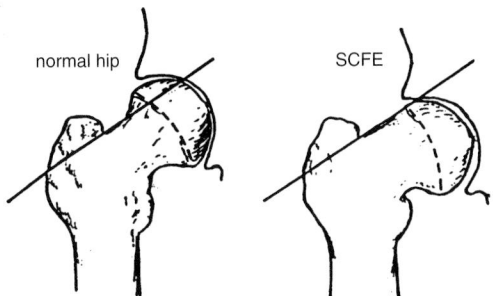

Fig. 59.6 *Appearance of a slipped capital femoral epiphysis. Note that, in the normal state, a line drawn along the superior surface of the femoral neck passes through the femoral head, but passes above it with SCFE*

Management

- Cease weight bearing and refer urgently.
- If acute slip, gentle reduction via traction is better than manipulation in preventing later avascular necrosis.
- Once reduced, pinning is performed.

Septic arthritis

Septic arthritis of the hip should be suspected in all children with acutely painful or irritable hip problems. These patients may not be obviously sick on presentation. A negative needle aspiration does not exclude septic arthritis. If sepsis is suspected it is better to proceed to an arthrotomy if clinically indicated.

The irritable hip syndrome should be diagnosed only after negative investigations, including plain films and ultrasound, full blood examination, ESR and bone scan. Needle aspiration has to be considered but irritable hip is often diagnosed without it, by observing in hospital in traction. If a deterioration or elevated temperature develops, needle aspiration with or without arthrotomy is indicated.

The little athlete

The most common problem in the little athlete is pain or discomfort in the region of the iliac crest or anterior or superior iliac spines, usually associated with traction apophysitis or with acute avulsion fractures.[6] There is localised tenderness with pain on stretching and athletes should rest until they can compete without discomfort.

If there are persistent signs, pain in the knee, hip irritability or restricted range of motion, X-rays should be ordered to exclude serious problems such as SCFE or Perthes' disorder.

Hip and buttock pain in the elderly

The following conditions are highly significant in the elderly:

- osteoarthritis of the hip
- aortoiliac arterial occlusion → vascular claudication
- spinal dysfunction with nerve root or referred pain
- degenerative spondylosis of lumbosacral spine → neurogenic claudication
- polymyalgia rheumatica
- trochanteric bursitis

- fractured neck of femur
- secondary tumours

Subcapital fractures

The impacted subcapital fractured femoral neck can often permit weight bearing by an elderly patient. No obvious deformity of the leg is present. Radiographs are therefore essential for the investigation of all painful hips in the elderly. Patients often give a story of two falls—the first[7] very painful, the second with the hip just 'giving way' as the femoral head fell off.

The displaced subcapital fracture has at least a 40% incidence of avascular necrosis and usually requires prosthetic replacement in patients over 70 years. Bone scans or tomograms are useful if the plain X-rays are equivocal.

Osteoarthritis of the hip

Osteoarthritis of the hip is the most common form of hip disease. It can be caused by primary osteoarthritis, which is related to an intrinsic disorder of articular cartilage, or to secondary osteoarthritis. Predisposing factors to the latter include previous trauma, DDH, acetabular dysplasia, SCFE and past inflammatory arthritis.

Clinical features

- equal sex incidence
- usually after age 50, increases with age
- may be bilateral: starts in one, other follows
- insidious onset
- at first, pain worse with activity, relieved by rest, and then nocturnal pain and pain after resting
- stiffness, especially after rising
- characteristic deformity
- stiffness, deformity and limp may dominate (pain mild)
- pain usually in groin—may be referred to medial aspect of thigh, buttock or knee

Physical examination

- abnormal gait
- usually gluteal and quadriceps wasting
- first hip movements lost are IR and extension
- hip held in flexion and ER (at first)
- eventually all movements affected
- order of movement loss is IR, extension, abduction, adduction, flexion, ER

Treatment

- careful explanation: patients fear OA of hip
- weight loss if overweight
- relative rest
- complete RIB for acute pain
- analgesics and NSAIDs (judicious use)
- aids and supports, e.g. walking stick
- physical therapy, including isometric exercises
- hydrotherapy—very useful

Surgery

This is an excellent option for those with severe pain or disability unresponsive to conservative measures. Total hip replacement is the treatment of choice in older patients but a femoral[8] osteotomy may be considered in younger patients in selected cases. The development of cementless total hip replacement has allowed surgery in more patients in their twenties and thirties.

Sacroiliac pain

Pain arising from sacroiliac joint disorders is normally experienced as a dull ache in the buttock but can be referred to the groin or posterior aspect of the thigh. It may mimic pain from the lumbosacral spine or the hip joint. The pain may be unilateral or bilateral.

There are no accompanying neurological symptoms such as paraesthesia or numbness but it is common for more severe cases to cause a heavy aching feeling in the upper thigh.

Causes of sacroiliac joint disorders

- inflammatory (the spondyloarthropathies)
- infections, e.g. TB, *Staphylococcus aureus* (rare)
- osteitis condensans ilii
- degenerative changes
- mechanical disorders
- post-traumatic, after sacroiliac disruption or fracture

Examination of the sacroiliac joints

The SIJs are difficult to palpate and examine but there are several tests that provoke the SIJs.

Direct pressure. With the patient lying prone a rhythmic springing force is applied directly to the upper and lower sacrum respectively.

Winged compression test. With the patient lying supine and with arms crossed, 'separate' the iliac crests with a downwards and outwards pressure. This compresses the SIJs.

Lateral compression test. With hands placed on the iliac crests, thumbs on the ASISs and heels of hand on the rim of the pelvis, compress the pelvis. This distracts the SIJs.

Patrick or Fabere test. This method can provoke the hip as well as the SIJ. The patient lies supine on the table and the foot of the involved side and extremity is placed on the opposite knee (the hip joint is now flexed, externally rotated and abducted). The knee and opposite ASIS are pressed downwards simultaneously (Fig. 59.7). If low back or buttock pain is reproduced the cause is likely to be a disorder of the SIJ.

Unequal sacral 'rise' test. Squat behind the standing patient and place hands on top of the iliac crests and thumbs on the posterior superior iliac spines. Ask the patient to bend slowly forwards and touch the floor. If one side moves higher relative to the other a problem may exist in the SIJs, e.g. a hypomobile lesion in the painful side if that side's PSIS moves higher.

Fig. 59.7 *The Patrick (Fabere) test for right-sided hip or sacroiliac joint lesions, illustrating directions of pressure from the examiner*

Mechanical disorders of the SIJ

These problems are more common than appreciated and can be caused by hypomobile or hypermobile problems.

Hypomobile SIJ disorders are usually encountered in young people after some traumatic event, especially women following childbirth (notably multiple or difficult childbirth), and in those with structural problems, e.g. shortened leg. Pain tends to follow rotational stresses of the SIJ, e.g. tennis, dancing. Excellent results are obtained by passive mobilisation or manipulation, such as the non-specific rotation technique with the patient lying supine as described in *Practice Tips* by the author.[9]

Hypermobile SIJ disorders are sometimes seen in athletes with instability of the symphysis pubis, in women after childbirth and in those with a history of severe trauma to the pelvis, e.g. MVAs, horse riders with foot caught in the stirrups after a fall. The patient presents typically with severe aching pain in the lower back, buttocks or upper thigh. Such problems are difficult to treat and manual therapy usually exacerbates the symptoms. Treatment consists of relative rest, analgesics and a sacroiliac supportive belt.

Gluteus medius tendinitis and trochanteric bursitis

Pain around the lateral aspect of the hip is a common disorder, and is usually seen as lateral hip pain radiating down the lateral aspect of the thigh in older people engaged in walking exercises, tennis and similar activities. It is analogous in a way to the shoulder girdle, where supraspinatus tendinitis and subacromial bursitis are common wear-and-tear injuries.

The two common causes are tendinitis of the gluteus medius tendon, where it inserts into the lateral surface of the greater trochanter of the femur, and bursitis of one or both of the trochanteric bursae. Distinction between these two conditions is difficult, and it is possible that, as with the shoulder, they are related. The pain of bursitis tends to occur at night; that of tendinitis occurs with such activity as long walks and gardening.

Treatment

Treatment for both conditions is similar.

1. Determine the points of maximal tenderness over the trochanteric region and mark them.

(For tendinitis, this point is immediately above the superior aspect of the greater trochanter—see Fig. 59.8).

2. Inject aliquots of a mixture of 1 mL of long-acting corticosteroid with 5–7 mL of LA into the tender area, which usually occupies an area similar to that of a standard marble.

The injection may be very effective. Follow-up management includes sleeping with a small pillow under the involved buttock and stretching the gluteal muscles with knee–chest exercises. Advise the patients to walk with the feet turned out—'the Charlie Chaplin gait'. One or two repeat injections over 6 or 12 months may be required. Surgical intervention is rarely necessary.

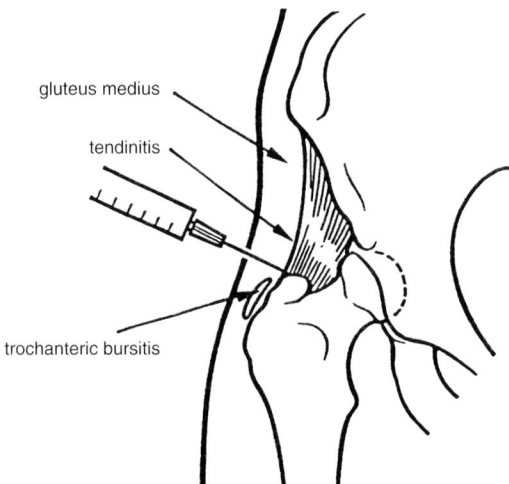

Fig. 59.8 *Injection technique for gluteus medius tendinitis (into area of maximal tenderness)*

gluteus medius

tendinitis

trochanteric bursitis

Snapping or clicking hip

Some patients complain of a clunking, clicking or snapping hip. This represents a painless, but annoying, problem.

Causes

- a taut iliotibial band (tendon or tensor fascia femoris) slipping backwards and forwards over the prominence of the greater trochanter
or

- the iliopsoas tendon snapping across the ilio-pectineal eminence
- the gluteus maximus sliding across the greater trochanter
- joint laxity

Treatment

The two basics of treatment are:
- explanation and reassurance
- exercises to stretch the iliotibial band[10]

Exercises

1. The patient lies on the 'normal' side and flexes the affected hip, with the leg straight and a weight around the ankle (Fig. 59.9), to a degree that produces a stretching sensation along the lateral aspect of the thigh.
2. This iliotibial stretch should be performed for 1–2 minutes, twice daily.

weight around ankle

Fig. 59.9 *Treatment for the clicking hip*

When to refer

- Clinical evidence or suspicion of severe childhood disorders: DDH, Perthes' disorder, septic arthritis, slipped capital femoral epiphysis or osteomyelitis
- Undiagnosed pain, especially night pain
- Any fractures or suspicion of fractures such as impacted subcapital fracture or stress fracture of the femoral neck
- Patients with true claudication in buttock whether it is vascular from aortoiliac occlusion or neurogenic from spinal canal stenosis
- Patients with disabling osteoarthritis of the hip not responding to conservative measures; excellent results are obtained from surgery to the hip
- Any mass or lump

Practice tips

- Training on a plastic DDH model should be essential for all neonatal practitioners in order to master the manoeuvres for examining the neonatal hip.

- True hip pain is usually groin pain or is referred to the medial aspect of the knee.[10]
- The name of the Fabere test is an acronym for *F*lexion, *Ab*duction, *E*xternal *R*otation and *E*xtension of the hip.
- Night pain adds up to inflammation, bursitis or tumour.
- The hip joint can be the target of infections such as *Staphylococcus aureus* or tuberculosis or inflammatory disorders such as rheumatoid and the spondyloarthropathies, but these are rare numerically compared with osteoarthritis.

References

1. Cyriax J. *Textbook of orthopaedic medicine*, vol 1 (6th edn). London: Balliere Tindall; 1976, 568–594.

2. Cormack J, Marinker M, Morell D. Hip problems. *Practice*. London: Kluwer-Harrap Handbooks, 1980, 3.65:1–6.

3. Anonymous. *The Eastern Seal guide to children's orthopaedics*. Toronto: Eastern Seal Society, 1982.

4. Robinson M.J. *Practical paediatrics*. Melbourne: Churchill Livingstone, 1990, 72–74.

5. Corrigan B, Maitland G. *Practical orthopaedic medicine*. Sydney: Butterworths, 1986, 103–124.

6. Larkins PA. The little athlete. Aust Fam Physician, 1991; 20:973–978.

7. Young D, Murtagh J. Pitfalls in orthopaedics. Aust Fam Physician, 1989; 18:654–655.

8. Corrigan B., Maitland G. *Practical orthopaedic medicine*. Sydney: Butterworths, 1986, 324–331.

9. Murtagh J. *Practice tips* (2nd edn). Sydney: McGraw-Hill, 1995, 143.

10. Sheon RP, Moskowitz RW, Goldberg VM. *Soft tissue rheumatic pain* (2nd edn). Philadelphia: Lea and Febiger, 1987, 211–212.

60
Pain in the leg

—

Pain in the leg has many causes, varying from a simple cramp to an arterial occlusion. Overuse of the legs in the athlete can lead to a multiplicity of painful leg syndromes, ranging from simple sprains of soft tissue to compartment syndromes. A major cause of leg pain lies in the source of the nervous network to the lower limb, namely the lumbar and sacral nerve roots of the spine. It is important to recognise radicular pain, especially from L5 and S1 nerve roots, and also the patterns of referred pain such as from apophyseal (facet) joints and sacroiliac joints.

Illustrative case histories

Mrs PJ, aged 38, housewife
This previously well person was walking briskly when she felt intense pain in the area of the lateral aspect of her left calf. It persisted and she visited a casualty department where a diagnosis of a torn lateral head of gastrocnemius was made. The pain then spread to the outer area of the ankle and to the outer foot, which started to feel numb.

On review the diagnosis was changed to a sural nerve lesion. Two days later she was found to have persistent severe pain in the leg and anaesthesia corresponding to S1. She had no back pain. Examination showed there was no ankle jerk, and loss of eversion of the left foot.

Diagnosis and outcome: progressive S1 nerve palsy due to an L5–S1 disc prolapse. The disc was removed 6 days after the onset of pain.

Mr LR, aged 67, farmer
A middle-of-the-night home visit was made to this upset non-English-speaking man because of the sudden onset of severe pain in his right leg. A provisional diagnosis of arterial occlusion was made over the phone but the problem was in fact a simple nocturnal cramp. Smiles of relief and embarrassment all round.

Mrs CM, aged 63, librarian
This obese patient complained of a dull ache in the middle of her thigh for 2 months. Examination was normal. She was reassured but an X-ray ordered if the pain persisted. A house call 2 weeks later found the patient lying on the kitchen floor with a fractured femur.

Diagnosis and outcome: pathological fracture due to a single metastasis from a breast primary (removed 9 years previously).

These case histories illustrate some of the difficulties experienced by patients and doctors with diagnosing leg pain.

Key facts and checkpoints

- Always consider the lumbosacral spine, the sacroiliac joints and hip joints as important causes of leg pain.
- Hip joint disorders may refer pain around the knee only (without hip pain).
- Nerve root lesions may cause pain in the lower leg and foot only (without back pain).

- Nerve entrapment is suggested by a radiating burning pain, prominent at night and worse at rest.
- Older people may present with claudication in the leg from spinal canal stenosis or arterial obstruction or both.
- Think of the hip pocket wallet as a cause of sciatica from the buttocks down.
- Acute arterial occlusion to the lower limb requires relief within 4 hours (absolute limit of 6 hours).
- The commonest site of acute occlusion is the common femoral artery.
- Varicose veins can cause aching pain in the leg.

A diagnostic approach

A summary of the safety diagnostic model is presented in Table 60.1.

Probability diagnosis

Many of the causes, such as foot problems, ankle injuries and muscle tears (e.g. hamstrings and quadriceps), are obvious and common. There is a wide range of disorders related to overuse syndromes in athletes.

A very common cause of acute severe leg pain is cramp in the calf musculature, the significance of which escapes some patients as judged by middle-of-the-night calls.

One of the commonest causes is nerve root pain, invariably single, especially affecting the L5 and S1 nerve roots. Tests of their function and of the lumbosacral spine for evidence of disc disruption or other spinal dysfunction will be necessary. Should multiple nerve roots be involved other causes such as compression from a tumour should be considered. Remember that a spontaneous retroperitoneal haemorrhage in a patient on anticoagulant therapy can cause nerve root pain and present as intense acute leg pain. The nerve root sensory distribution is presented in Figure 60.1

Other important causes of referred thigh pain include ischiogluteal bursitis (weaver's bottom) and gluteus medius tendinitis or trochanteric bursitis.

Serious disorders not to be missed

Neoplasia

Malignant disease, although uncommon, should be considered, especially if the patient has a

Table 60.1 *Pain in the leg: diagnostic strategy model*

Q. Probability diagnosis
A. Cramps
Nerve root 'sciatica'
Muscular injury, e.g. hamstring
Osteoarthritis (hip, knee)
Overuse injury, e.g. Achilles tendinitis

Q. Serious disorders not to be missed
A. Vascular
  - arterial occlusion (embolism)
  - thrombosis popliteal aneurysm
  - deep venous thrombosis
  - iliofemoral thrombophlebitis
  Neoplasia
  - primary, e.g. myeloma
  - metastases, e.g. breast to femur
  Infection
  - osteomyelitis
  - septic arthritis
  - erysipelas
  - lymphangitis
  - gas gangrene

Q. Pitfalls (often missed)
A. Osteoarthritis hip
Osgood-Schlatter's disease
Spinal canal stenosis
Herpes zoster (early)
Nerve entrapment
'Hip pocket nerve'
Iatrogenic: injection into nerve
Sacroiliac disorders
Gluteus medius tendinitis
Sympathetic dystrophy (causalgia)
Peripheral neuropathy

  Rarities
  - Osteoid osteoma
  - Polymyalgia rheumatica (isolated)
  - Paget's disease
  - Popliteal artery entrapment
  - Tabes dorsalis
  - Ruptured Baker's cyst

Q. Seven masquerades checklist
A. Depression   √
Diabetes   √
Drugs   √ (indirect)
Anaemia   √ (indirect)
Thyroid disease   –
Spinal dysfunction   √√
UTI   –

Q. Is this patient trying to tell me something else?
A. Quite possible. Common with work-related injuries.

history of one of the primary tumours such as breast, lung or kidney. Such tumours can metastasise to the femur. Consider also osteogenic sarcoma and multiple myeloma, which is usually seen in the upper half of the femur. The possibility of an osteoid osteoma should be considered with pain in a bone relieved by aspirin.

Fig. 60.1 *Dermatomes of the lower limb, representing approximate cutaneous distribution of the nerve roots*

Infections

Severe infections are not so common, but septic arthritis and osteomyelitis warrant consideration. Superficial infections such as erysipelas and lymphangitis occur occasionally.

Vascular problems

Acute severe ischaemia can be due to thrombosis or embolism of the arteries of the lower limb. Such occlusions cause severe pain in the limb and associated signs of severe ischaemia, especially of the lower leg and foot.

Chronic ischaemia due to arterial occlusion can manifest as intermittent claudication or rest

pain in the foot due to small vessel disease.[1]

Various pain syndromes are presented in Figure 60.2. It is important to differentiate vascular claudication from neurogenic claudication (Table 60.2).

Venous disorders

The role of uncomplicated varicose veins as a cause of leg pain is controversial. Nevertheless, varicose veins can certainly cause a dull aching 'heaviness' and cramping, and can lead to painful ulceration.

Superficial thrombophlebitis is usually obvious, but it is vital not to overlook deep venous thrombosis. These more serious conditions of the veins can cause pain in the thigh or calf.

Pitfalls

There are many traps and pitfalls in the painful leg. Herpes zoster at the pre-eruption phase is an old trap and more so when the patient develops only a few vesicles in obscure parts of the limbs.

In future we can expect to encounter more cases of spinal canal stenosis (secondary to the degenerative changes) in the elderly. The early diagnosis can be difficult, and buttock pain on walking has to be distinguished from vascular claudication due to a high arterial obstruction.

The many disorders of the sacroiliac joint and hip region can be traps, especially the poorly diagnosed yet common gluteus medius tendinitis. Another more recent phenomenon is the 'hip pocket nerve syndrome', where a heavy wallet crammed with credit cards can cause pressure on the sciatic nerve.

One of the biggest traps, however, is when hip disorders, particularly osteoarthritis, present as leg pain, especially on the medial aspect of the knee.

Nerve entrapments (Fig. 60.3) are an interesting cause of leg pain, although not as common as in the upper limb. Some entrapments to consider include:

- lateral cutaneous nerve of thigh, known as meralgia paraesthetica
- common peroneal nerve
- posterior tibial nerve at ankle (the 'tarsal tunnel' syndrome)
- obturator nerve, in obturator canal
- femoral nerve (in inguinal region or pelvis)

Then there are the rare causes. One overlooked problem is sympathetic dystrophy, which may

Fig. 60.2 *Arterial occlusion and related symptoms according to the level of obstruction*

follow even minor trauma to the limb. This 'causalgia' syndrome manifests as burning or aching pain with vasomotor instability in the limbs. The essential feature is the disparity between the intensity of the pain and the severity of the inciting injury.

General pitfalls
- overlooking beta-blockers and anaemia as a precipitating factor for vascular claudication
- overlooking hip disorders as a cause of knee pain
- mistaking occlusive arterial disease for sciatica
- confusing nerve root syndromes with entrapment syndromes

Seven masquerades checklist
The outstanding cause of leg pain in this group is spinal dysfunction. Apart from nerve root pressure due to a disc disruption or foraminal entrapment, pain can be referred from the apophyseal (facet joints). Such pain can be referred as far as the mid-calf (Fig. 60.4).

The other checklist conditions—depression, diabetes, drugs and anaemia—can be associated with pain in the leg. Depression can reinforce any painful complex.

Diabetes can cause discomfort through a peripheral neuropathy that can initially cause localised pain before anaesthesia predominates. Drugs such as beta-blockers, and anaemia, can precipitate or aggravate intermittent claudication in a patient with a compromised circulation.

Psychogenic considerations
Pain in the lower leg can be a frequent complaint (maybe a magnified one) of the patient with non-organic pain, such as the malingerer, the conversion reaction patient (hysteria) and the depressed. Sometimes sympathetic dystrophy (reflex or post-traumatic) is incorrectly diagnosed as functional.

The clinical approach
Careful attention to basic detail in the history and examination can point the way of the clinical diagnosis.

Table 60.2 *Clinical features of neurogenic and vascular claudication*

	Neurogenic claudication	**Vascular claudication**
Cause	• Spinal canal stenosis	• Aortoiliac arterial occlusive disease
Age	• Over 50 • Long history of backache	Over 50
Pain site and radiation	• Proximal location, initially lumbar, buttocks and legs • Radiates distally	• Distal location • Buttocks, thighs and calves (especially) • Radiates proximally
Type of pain	Weakness, burning, numbing or tingling (not cramping)	Cramping, aching, squeezing
Onset	• Walking (uphill and downhill) • Distance walked varies • Prolonged standing	Walking a set distance each time, especially uphill
Relief	• Lying down • Flexing spine, e.g. squat position • May take 20–30 minutes	• Standing still—fast relief • Slow walking decreases severity
Associations	• Bowel and bladder symptoms	• Impotence • Rarely, paraesthesia or weakness
Physical examination • Peripheral pulses	• Present	• Present (usually) • Reduced or absent in some, especially after exercise
• Lumbar extension	• Aggravates	• No change
• Neurological	• Saddle distribution • Ankle jerk may be reduced after exercise	• *Note:* abdominal bruits after exercise
Diagnosis confirmation	• Radiological studies	• Duplex ultrasound • Ankle brachial index • Arteriography

History

In the history it is important to consider several distinctive aspects, outlined by the following questions.

- Is the pain of acute or chronic onset?
- If acute, did it follow trauma or activity?
  - If not, consider a vascular cause: vein or artery; occlusion or rupture.
- Is the pain 'mechanical' (related to movement)?
  - If it is unaltered by movement of the leg or a change in posture, it must arise from a soft tissue lesion, not from bone or joints.
- Is the pain postural?
  - Analyse the postural elements that make it better or worse.
  - If worse on sitting, consider a spinal cause (discogenic) or ischial bursitis.
  - If worse on standing, consider a spinal cause (instability) or a local problem related to weight bearing (varicose veins).

- If worse lying down, consider vascular origin such as small vessel peripheral vascular disease.
- Pain unaffected by posture is activity-related.
- Is the pain related to walking?
  - *No:* Determine the offending activity, e.g. joint movement with arthritis.
  - *Yes:* If immediate onset, consider local cause at site of pain, e.g. stress fracture. If delayed onset, consider vascular claudication or neurogenic claudication.
- Is the site of pain the same as the site of trauma?
  - If not, the pain in the leg is referred. Important considerations include lesions in the spine, abdomen or hip and entrapment neuropathy.
- Is the pain arising from the bone?
  - If so, the patient will point to the specific

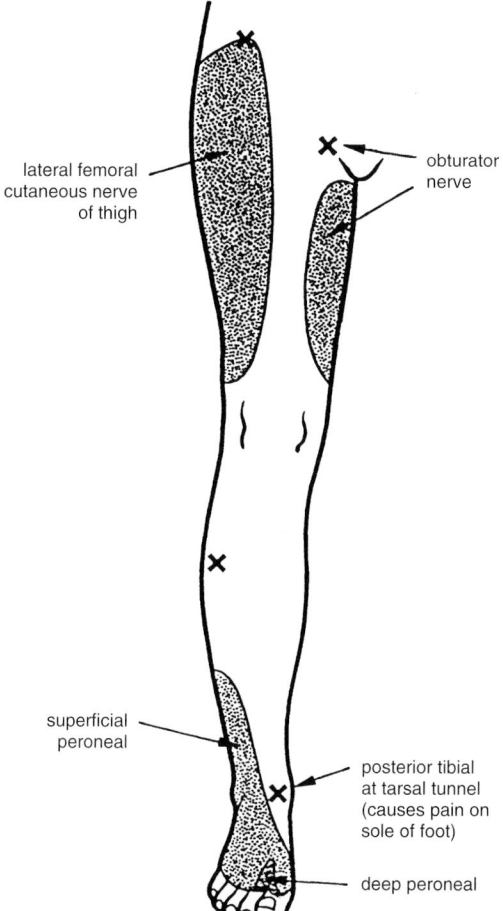

lateral femoral cutaneous nerve of thigh

obturator nerve

superficial peroneal

posterior tibial at tarsal tunnel (causes pain on sole of foot)

deep peroneal

Fig. 60.3 *Distribution of pain in the leg from entrapment of specific nerves; the sites of entrapment are indicated by an* **X**

site and indicate a 'deep' bone pain (consider tumour, fracture or, rarely, infection) compared with the more superficial muscular or fascial pain.
• Is the pain arising from the joint?
— If so, the clinical examination will determine whether it arises from the joint or juxtaposed tissue.

Physical examination

The first step is to watch the patient walk and assess the nature of any limp.

Note the posture of the back and examine the lumbar spine. Have both legs well exposed for the inspection.

Inspect the patient's stance and note any asymmetry and other abnormalities such as swellings, bruising, discolouration, or ulcers and

rashes. Note the size and symmetry of the legs and the venous pattern. Look for evidence of ischaemic changes, especially of the foot.

Palpate for local causes of pain and if no cause is evident examine the spine, blood vessels (arteries and veins) and bone. Areas to palpate specifically are the ischial tuberosity, trochanteric area, hamstrings and tendon insertions. Palpate the superficial lymph nodes. Note the temperature of the feet and legs. Perform a vascular examination including the peripheral pulses and the state of the veins if appropriate.

If evidence of PVD, remember to auscultate the abdomen and adductor hiatus, and the iliac, femoral and popliteal vessels.

A neurological examination may be appropriate, particularly to test nerve root lesions or entrapment neuropathies.

Examination of the joints, especially the hip and sacroiliac joints, is very important.

Fig. 60.4 *Possible referred pain patterns from dysfunction of an apophyseal joint, illustrating pain radiation patterns from stimulation by injection of the right L4–L5 apophyseal joint*
REPRODUCED FROM C. KENNA AND J. MURTAGH, *BACK PAIN AND SPINAL MANIPULATION,* BUTTERWORTHS, SYDNEY, 1989, WITH PERMISSION

Investigations

A checklist of investigations that may be necessary to make the diagnosis is as follows:

- Full blood examination and ESR
- X-rays: — leg, especially knee, hip
  - plain X-ray of lumbosacral spine
  - CT scan of lumbosacral spine
  - MRI scan of lumbosacral spine
  - bone scan
- Electromyography
- Vascular — arteriography
  - duplex ultrasound scan
  - ankle brachial index
  - venous pool radionuclide scan
  - contrast venography
  - air plethysmograph (varicose veins)

Leg pain in children

Aches and pains in the legs are a common complaint in children. The most common cause is soreness and muscular strains due to trauma or unaccustomed exercise.

It is important to consider child abuse, especially if bruising is noted on the backs of the legs.

Growing pains

So-called 'growing pains', or idiopathic leg pain, is thought to be responsible for up to 20% of leg pain in children.[2] Such a diagnosis is vague and often made when a specific cause is excluded. It is usually not due to 'growth' but related to excessive exercise or trauma from sport and recreation, and probably emotional factors.

The pains are typically intermittent and symmetrical and deep in the legs, usually in the anterior thighs or calves. Although they may occur at any time of the day or night, typically they occur at night, usually when the child has settled in bed. The pains usually last for 30 to 60 minutes and tend to respond to attention such as massage with an analgesic balm or simple analgesics.

Serious problems

It is important to exclude fractures (hence the value of X-rays if in doubt), malignancy (such as osteogenic sarcoma, Ewing's tumour or infiltration from leukaemia or lymphoma), osteoid osteoma, osteomyelitis, scurvy and berri-berri

(rare disorders in developed countries) and congenital disorders such as sickle-cell disease, Gaucher's disease and Ehlers-Danlos syndrome.

Leg pain in the elderly

The older the patient the more likely it is that arterial disease with intermittent claudication and neurogenic claudication due to spinal canal stenosis will develop. Other important problems of the elderly include degenerative joint disease such as osteoarthritis of the hips and knees, muscle cramps, herpes zoster, Paget's disease, polymyalgia rheumatica (affecting the upper thighs) and sciatica.

Spinal causes of leg pain

Problems originating from the spine are an important, yet at times complex, cause of pain in the leg.

Important causes are:

- nerve root (radicular) pain from direct pressure
- referred pain from:
  - disc pressure on tissues in front of the spinal cord
  - apophyseal joints
  - sacroiliac joints
- spinal canal stenosis causing claudication

Various pain patterns are presented in Figures 60.1 and 60.4.

Nerve root pain

Nerve root pain from a prolapsed disc is a common cause of leg pain. A knowledge of the dermatomes of the lower limb (Fig. 60.1) provides a pointer to the involved nerve root, which is usually L5 or S1 or both. The L5 root is invariably caused by an L4–L5 disc prolapse and the S1 root by an L5–S1 disc prolapse. The nerve root syndromes are summarised in Table 60.3.

A summary of the physical examination findings for the most commonly involved nerve roots is presented in Figure 60.5.

Sciatica

Sciatica is defined as pain in the distribution of the sciatic nerve or its branches (L4, L5, S1, S2, S3) that is caused by nerve pressure or irritation. Most problems are due to entrapment neuropathy of a nerve root, either in the spinal canal (as outlined above) or the intervertebral foramen.

Table 60.3 *Nerve root syndromes*

Nerve root	Pain distribution	Sensory loss	Motor weakness changes	Reflex
L3	Front of thigh, inner aspect of thigh, knee and leg	Anterior aspect of thigh	Extension of knee	Knee jerk
L4	Anterior thigh to front of knee	Lower outer aspect of thigh and knee, inner great toe	Flexion, adduction of knee, inversion of foot	Knee jerk
L5	Lateral aspect of leg, dorsum of foot and great toe	Dorsum of foot, great toe, 2nd and 3rd toes, anterolateral aspect of lower leg	Dorsiflexion of great toe	Tibialis posterior (clinically impractical)
S1	Buttock to back of thigh and leg, central calf, lateral aspect of ankle and sole of foot	Lateral aspect of ankle, foot (4th and 5th toes)	Plantar flexion of ankle and toes, eversion of foot	Ankle jerk

Fig. 60.5 *Comparison of neurological findings of the neurologic levels L4, L5 and S1* REPRODUCED FROM S. HOPPENFELD, *PHYSICAL EXAMINATION OF THE SPINE AND EXTREMITIES,* APPLETON AND LANGE, NORWALK, CT, USA, WITH PERMISSION

It should be noted that back pain may be absent and peripheral symptoms only will be present.

Treatment of sciatica

Acute sciatica. A protracted course can be anticipated, in the order of 12 weeks. The patient should be reassured that spontaneous recovery can be expected. A trial of conservative treatment would be recommended thus:

- back care education
- relative bed rest (2 days is optimal)—a firm base is ideal
- analgesics (avoid narcotic analgesics)
- NSAIDs (2 weeks is recommended)
- basic exercise program, including swimming
- traction can help, even intermittent manual

Referral to a therapist of your choice, e.g. physiotherapist, might be advisable. Conventional spinal manipulation is usually contraindicated for radicular sciatica. If the patient is not responding or the circumstances demand more active treatment, an epidural anaesthetic injection is appropriate. Surgical intervention may be necessary.

Chronic sciatica. If a trial of NSAIDs, rest and physiotherapy has not brought significant relief, an epidural anaesthetic (lumbar or caudal) using half-strength local anaesthetic only (e.g. 0.25% bupivacaine HCl) is advisable.

Referred pain

Referred pain in the leg can arise from disorders of the sacroiliac joints or from spondylogenic disorders. It is typically dull, heavy and diffuse. The patient uses the hand to describe its distribution compared with the use of fingers to point to radicular pain.

Spondylogenic pain

Non-radicular or spondylogenic pain is that which originates from any of the components of the vertebrae (spondyles) including joints, the intervertebral disc, ligaments and muscle attachments. An important example is distal referred pain from disorders of the apophyseal joints, where the pain can be referred to any part of the limb as far as the calf and ankle but most commonly to the gluteal region and proximal thigh (Fig. 60.4).

Another source of referred pain is that caused by compression of a bulging disc against the posterior longitudinal ligament and dura. The pain is typically dull, deep and poorly localised. The dura has no specific dermatomal localisation, and so the pain is usually experienced in the low back, sacroiliac area and buttocks. Less commonly it can be referred to the coccyx, groin and both legs to the calves. It is not referred to the ankle or the foot.

Sacroiliac dysfunction

This causes typically a dull ache in the buttock but it can be referred to the iliac fossa, groin or posterior aspects of the thighs. It rarely radiates to or below the knee. It may be caused by inflammation (sacroiliitis) or mechanical dysfunction. The latter must be considered in a postpartum woman presenting with severe aching pain present in both buttocks and thighs.

Nerve entrapment syndromes

Entrapment neuropathy can result from direct axonal compression or can be secondary to vascular problems, but the main common factor is a nerve passing through a narrow rigid compartment where movement or stretching of that nerve occurs under pressure.

Clinical features of nerve entrapment:

- pain at rest (often worse at night)
- variable effect with activity
- sharp, burning pain
- radiating and retrograde pain
- clearly demarcated distribution of pain
- paraesthesia may be present
- tenderness over nerve
- may be positive Tinel's sign

Meralgia paraesthetica

This is the commonest lower limb entrapment and is due to the lateral femoral cutaneous nerve of the thigh being trapped under the lateral end of the inguinal ligament, 1 cm medial to the anterior superior iliac spine.[3]

The nerve is a sensory nerve from L2 and L3. It occurs mostly in middle-aged people, due mainly to thickening of the fibrous tunnel beneath the inguinal ligament, and is associated with obesity, pregnancy, ascites or local trauma such as belts, trusses and corsets. Its entrapment causes a burning pain with associated numbness and tingling (Fig. 60.3).

The distribution of pain is confined to a localised area of the lateral thigh and does not cross the midline of the thigh.

Differential diagnosis
- L2 or L3 nerve root pain (L2 causes buttock pain also)
- femoral neuropathy (extends medial to midline)

Treatment options
- injection of corticosteroid medial to the ASIS, under the inguinal ligament
- surgical release (neurolysis) if refractory

Note: Meralgia paraesthetica often resolves spontaneously.

Peroneal nerve entrapment
The common peroneal (lateral popliteal) nerve can be entrapped where it winds around the neck of the fibula or as it divides and passes through the origin of the peroneus longus muscle 2.5 cm below the neck of the fibula. It is usually injured, however, by trauma or pressure at the neck of the fibula.

Symptoms and signs:
- pain in the lateral shin area and dorsum of the foot
- sensory symptoms in the same area
- weakness of eversion and dorsiflexion of the foot (described by patients as 'a weak ankle')

Differential diagnosis
L5 nerve root (similar symptoms)

Treatment
- shoe wedging or other orthotics to maintain eversion
- neurolysis is the most effective treatment

Tarsal tunnel syndrome
This is an entrapment neuropathy of the posterior tibial nerve in the tarsal tunnel beneath the flexor retinaculum on the medial side of the ankle (Fig. 60.6a). The condition is due to dislocation or fracture around the ankle or tenosynovitis of tendons in the tunnel from injury, rheumatoid arthritis, and other inflammations.

Symptoms and signs
- a burning or tingling pain in the toes and sole of the foot, occasionally the heel
- retrograde radiation to calf, perhaps as high as the buttock
- numbness is a late symptom
- discomfort often in bed at night and worse after standing
- removal of shoe may give relief
- sensory nerve loss variable, may be no loss
- Tinel test (finger or reflex hammer tap over nerve below and behind medial malleolus) may be positive
- tourniquet applied above ankle may reproduce symptoms

The diagnosis is confirmed by electrodiagnosis.

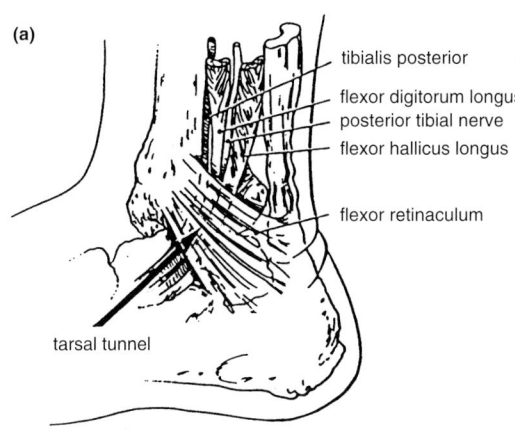

(a)

tibialis posterior
flexor digitorum longus
posterior tibial nerve
flexor hallucis longus
flexor retinaculum
tarsal tunnel

(b)

Fig. 60.6 (a) *Anatomy of the tarsal tunnel syndrome;* **(b)** *showing injection sites*

Treatment
- relief of abnormal foot posture with orthotics
- corticosteroid injection
- decompression surgery if other measures fail

Injection for tarsal tunnel syndrome
Using a 23-gauge 32 mm needle, a mixture of triamcinolone 10 mg/mL or 40 mg methylprednisolone in 1% xylocaine or procaine is injected into the tunnel either from above or below the flexor retinaculum. The sites of injection are shown in Figure 60.6b; care is required not to inject the nerve.

Vascular causes of leg pain
Occlusive arterial disease
Risk factors for peripheral vascular disease (for development and deterioration):

- smoking
- diabetes mellitus
- hypertension
- hypercholesterolaemia
- family history
- atrial fibrillation (embolism)

Aggravating factors:

- beta-blocking drugs
- anaemia

Acute lower limb ischaemia
Sudden occlusion is a dramatic event that requires immediate diagnosis and management to save the limb.
   Causes:

- embolism—peripheral arteries
- thrombosis — major artery
                — popliteal aneurysm
- traumatic contusion, e.g. postarterial puncture

The symptoms and signs of acute embolism and thrombosis are similar, although thrombosis of an area of atherosclerosis is often preceded by symptoms of chronic disease, e.g. claudication. The commonest site of acute occlusion is the common femoral artery (Fig. 60.7).

Signs and symptoms—the 6 P's
- Pain
- Pallor
- Paraesthesia or numbness
- Pulselessness
- Paralysis
- 'Perishing' cold

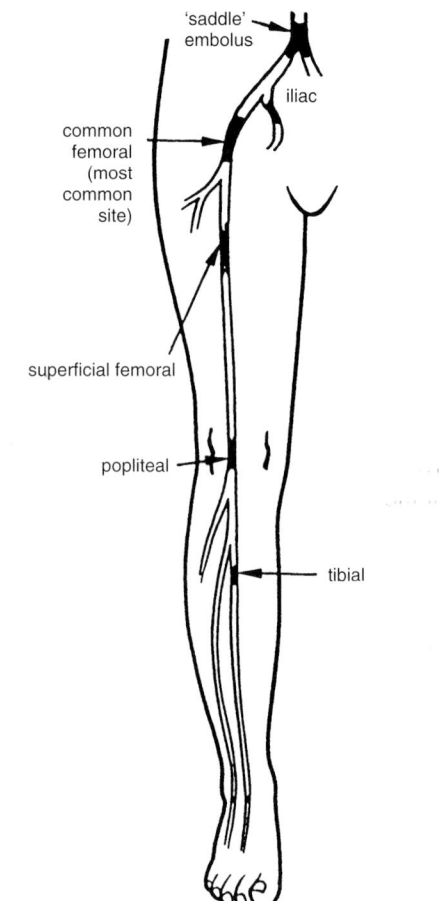

Fig 60.7 *Common sites of acute arterial occlusion*

The pain is usually sudden and severe and any improvement may be misleading. Sensory changes initially affect light touch, not pinprick. Paralysis (paresis or weakness) and muscle compartment pain or tenderness is a most important and ominous sign.
   Other signs include mottling of the legs, collapsed superficial veins, and no capillary return. *Note:* Look for evidence of atrial fibrillation.

Examination of arterial circulation
This applies to chronic ischaemia and also to acute ischaemia.

Skin and trophic changes
Note colour changes, hair distribution and wasting. Note the temperature of the legs and feet with the backs of your fingers.

Palpation of pulses

It is important to assess four pulses carefully (Fig. 60.8). Note that the popliteal and posterior tibial pulses are difficult to feel, especially in obese subjects.

Femoral artery. Palpate deeply just below the inguinal ligament, midway between the anterior superior iliac spine and the symphysis pubis. If absent or diminished, palpate over abdomen for aortic aneurysm.

Popliteal artery. Flex the leg to relax the hamstrings. Place fingertips of both hands to meet in the midline. Press them deeply into the popliteal fossa to compress artery against the upper end of the tibia, i.e. just below the level of the knee crease. Check for a popliteal aneurysm (very prominent popliteal pulsation).

Posterior tibial artery. Palpate, with curved fingers, just behind and below the tip of the medial malleolus of the ankle.

Fig. 60.8 *Sites of palpation of peripheral pulses in the leg*

Dorsalis pedis artery. Feel at the proximal end of the first metatarsal space just lateral to the extensor tendon of the big toe.

Oedema

Look for evidence of oedema: pitting oedema is tested by pressing firmly with your thumb for at least 5 seconds over the dorsum of each foot, behind each medial malleolus and over the shins.

Postural colour changes (Buerger's test)

Raise both legs to about 60° for about 1 minute, when maximal pallor of the feet will develop. Then get the patient to sit up on the couch and hang both legs down.[4] Note, comparing both feet, the time required for return of pinkness to the skin (normally less than 10 seconds) and filling of the veins of the feet and ankles (normally about 15 seconds). Look for any unusual rubor (dusky redness) that takes a minute or more in the dependent foot. A positive Buerger's test is pallor on elevation and rubor on dependency and indicates severe chronic ischaemia.

Auscultation for bruits after exercise

Listen over abdomen and femoral area for bruits.
Note: Neurological examination (motor, sensory, reflexes) is normal unless there is associated diabetic peripheral neuropathy.

Management of acute ischaemia

Golden rules. Occlusion is usually reversible if treated within 4 hours, i.e. limb salvage. It is often irreversible if treated after 6 hours, i.e. limb amputation.

Treatment

- Intravenous heparin (immediately) 5000 U
- Emergency embolectomy (ideally within 4 hours)
  — under general or local anaesthesia
  — through an arteriotomy site in the common femoral artery
  — embolus extracted with Fogarty balloon or catheter
                                    or
- Arterial bypass if acute thrombosis in chronically diseased artery
- In selected cases thrombolysis with streptokinase or urokinase appropriate
- Amputation (early) if irreversible ischaemic changes

- Lifetime anticoagulation with warfarin will be required

Note: An acutely ischaemic limb is rarely life threatening in the short term. Thus, even in the extremely aged, demented or infirm, a simple embolectomy not only is worthwhile but also is usually the most expedient treatment option.

Chronic lower limb ischaemia

Chronic ischaemia caused by gradual arterial occlusion can manifest as intermittent claudication, rest pain in the foot, or overt tissue loss—ulceration, gangrene.

Intermittent claudication is a pain or tightness in the muscle on exercise (Latin *claudicare*, to limp), relieved by rest. Rest pain is a constant severe burning-type pain or discomfort in the forefoot at rest, typically occurring at night when the blood flow slows down.

The main features are compared in Table 60.4.

Intermittent claudication

The level of obstruction determines which muscle belly is affected (Figs 60.2 and 60.7).

Proximal obstruction, e.g. aortoiliac

- pain in the buttock, thigh and calf, especially when walking up hills and stairs
- persistent fatigue over whole lower limb
- impotence is possible (Leriche syndrome)

Obstruction in the thigh

- superficial femoral (the commonest) causes pain in the calf, e.g. 200–500 metres, depending on collateral circulation
- profunda femoris → claudication about 100 metres
- multiple segment involvement → claudication 40–50 metres

Causes:

- atherosclerosis (mainly men over 50, smokers)
- embolisation (with recovery)
- Buerger's disease: affects small arteries, causes rest pain and cyanosis (claudication uncommon)
- popliteal entrapment syndrome (< 40 years of age)

Note: The presence of rest pain implies an immediate threat to limb viability.

Management of occlusive vascular disease

Prevention (for those at risk)

- Smoking is *the* risk factor and must be stopped.
- Other risk factors, especially hyperlipidaemia, must be attended to and weight reduction to ideal weight is important.
- Exercise is excellent, especially walking.

Diagnostic plan

- Check if patient is taking beta-blockers.
- General tests: blood examination, random blood sugar, urine examination, ECG.
- Measure blood flow by duplex ultrasound examination or ankle brachial index.
- Arteriography should be performed *only* if surgery contemplated.

Treatment

- General measures (if applicable): control obesity, diabetes, hypertension, hyperlipidaemia, cardiac failure.
- Achieve ideal weight.
- There must be absolutely no smoking.
- Exercise: daily graduated exercise to the level of pain. About 50% will improve with walking; so advise as much walking as possible.

Table 60.4   *Comparison between intermittent claudication and ischaemic rest pain*

	Intermittent claudication	Ischaemic rest pain
Quality of pain	Tightness/cramping	Constant ache
Timing of pain (typical)	Daytime; walking, other exercise	Night-time; rest
Tissue affected	Muscle	Skin
Site	Calf > thigh > buttock	Forefoot, toes, heels
Aggravation	Walking, exercise	Recumbent, walking
Relief	Rest	Hanging foot out of bed; dependency
Associations	Beta-blockers Anaemia	Night cramps Swelling of feet

- Try to keep legs warm and dry.
- Maintain optimal foot care (podiatry).
- Drug therapy: aspirin 150 mg daily.

Note: • Vasodilators and sympathectomy are of little value.
- About one-third progress, while the rest regress or don't change.[5]

When to refer to a vascular surgeon

- 'Unstable' claudication of recent onset; deteriorating
- Severe claudication—unable to maintain lifestyle
- Rest pain
- 'Tissue loss' in feet, e.g. heel crack, ulcers on or between toes, dry gangrenous patches, infection

Surgery. Reconstructive vascular surgery is indicated for progressive obstruction, intolerable claudication and obstruction above the inguinal ligament.

- endarterectomy—for localised iliac stenosis
- bypass graft (iliac or femoral artery to popliteal or anterior or posterior tibial arteries)

Percutaneous transluminal dilation: This angioplasty is performed with a special intra-arterial balloon catheter for localised limited occlusions. An alternative to the balloon is laser angioplasty.

Venous disorders

Varicose veins

Varicose veins are dilated, tortuous and elongated superficial veins in the lower extremity.

The veins are dilated because of incompetence of the valves in the superficial veins or in the communicating or perforating veins between the deep and superficial systems. The cause is a congenital weakness in the valve and the supporting vein wall but there are several predisposing factors (Table 60.5), the most important being family history, female sex (5:1), pregnancy and multiparity. Previous deep venous thrombosis (DVT) can also damage valves, especially calf perforators, and cause varicose veins.

Dilated superficial veins, which can mimic varicose veins, may be caused by extrinsic compression of the veins by a pelvic or intra-abdominal tumour (e.g. ovarian carcinoma, retroperitoneal fibrosis). Uncommonly, but importantly, superficial veins dilate as they

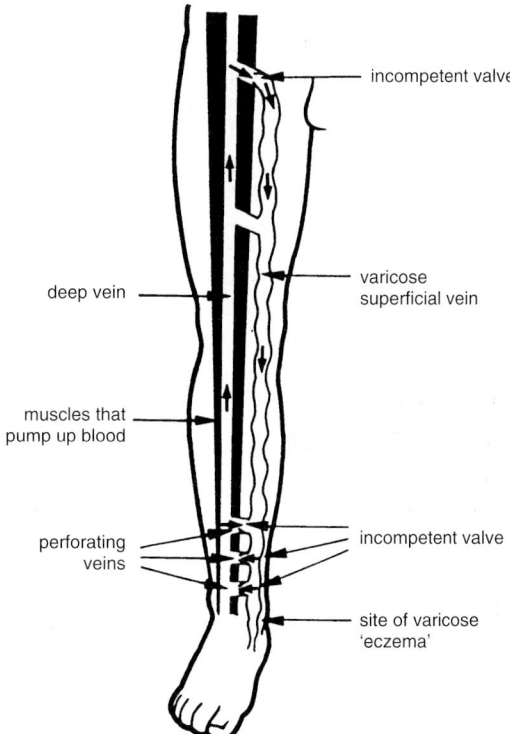

Fig. 60.9 *The common sites of varicose veins*

become collaterals following previous DVT, especially if the ilio-femoral segment is involved.

Symptoms

Varicose veins may be symptomless, the main complaint being their unsightly appearance. Symptoms include swelling, fatigue, heaviness in the limb, an aching discomfort and itching.

Varicose veins and pain

They may be painless even if large and tortuous. Pain is a feature where there are incompetent perforating veins running from the posterior tibial vein to the surface through the soleus muscle.

Table 60.5 *Risk factors for varicose veins*

Female sex
Family history
Pregnancy
Multiparity
Age
Occupation
Diet (low-fibre)

Severe cases lead to the lower leg venous hypertension syndrome[6] characterised by pain that is worse after standing, cramps in the leg at night, irritation and pigmentation of the skin, swelling of the ankles and loss of skin features such as hair.

A careful history will usually determine if the aching is truly due to varicose veins and not to transient or cyclical oedema, which is a common condition in women.[7]

The complications of varicose veins are summarised in Table 60.6.

Table 60.6 *Complications of varicose veins*

Superficial thrombophlebitis

Skin 'eczema' (10%)

Skin ulceration (20%)

Bleeding

Calcification

Marjolin's ulcer (squamous cell carcinoma)

Fig. 60.10a *Trendelenburg test: the leg is elevated to 45° to empty the veins and a tourniquet applied*

Examination

The following tests will help determine the site or sites of the incompetent valves.

Venous groin cough impulse. This helps determine long saphenous vein incompetence.

Place the fingers over the line of the vein immediately below the fossa ovalis (4 cm below and 4 cm lateral to the pubic tubercle).[8] Ask the patient to cough—an impulse or thrill will be felt expanding and travelling down the long saphenous vein. A marked dilated long saphenous vein in the fossa ovalis (saphena varix) will confirm incompetence. It disappears when the patient lies down.

Trendelenburg test. In this test for long saphenous vein competence the patient lies down and the leg is elevated to 45° to empty the veins (Fig. 60.10a). Apply a tourniquet with sufficient pressure to prevent reflux over the upper thigh just below the fossa ovalis. (Alternatively, this opening can be occluded by firm finger pressure, as originally described by Trendelenburg.)

The patient then stands. The long saphenous system will remain collapsed if there are no incompetent veins below the level of the fossa ovalis. When the pressure is released the vein will fill rapidly if the valve at the saphenofemoral junction is incompetent (Fig. 60.10b). This is a positive Trendelenburg test.

Fig. 60.10b *Trendelenburg test: test for competence of long saphenous venous system (medial aspect of knee)*

Note: A doubly positive Trendelenburg test is when the veins fill rapidly before the pressure is released and then with a 'rush' when released. This indicates coexisting incompetent perforators and long saphenous vein.

Short saphenous vein incompetence test. A similar test to the Trendelenburg test is performed with the pressure (tourniquet or finger) being applied over the short saphenous vein just below the popliteal fossa (Fig. 60.11).

Incompetent perforating vein test. Accurate clinical tests to identify incompetence in the three common sites of perforating veins on the medial aspect of the leg, posterior to the medial border of the tibia, are difficult to perform. The general appearance of the leg and palpation of the sites give some indication of incompetence here.

Note: Venous duplex ultrasound studies will accurately localise sites of incompetence and determine the state of the functionally important deep venous system.

Fig. 60.11 *Testing for competence of the short saphenous vein*

Management of varicose veins

Prevention
• Maintain ideal weight.
• Eat a high-fibre diet.
• Rest and wear supportive stockings if at risk (pregnancy, a standing occupation).

Treatment
• Keep off legs as much as possible.
• Sit with legs on a footstool.
• Use supportive stockings or tights (apply in morning before standing out of bed).
• Avoid scratching itching skin over veins.

Compression sclerotherapy
• Use a small volume of sclerosant, e.g. sodium tetradecyl sulfate (Fibro-vein 3%).
• It is ideal for smaller isolated veins particularly below the knee joint.

Surgical ligation and stripping
• This is the best treatment when a clear association exists between symptoms and obvious varicose veins, i.e. long saphenous vein incompetence.
• Remove obvious varicosities and ligate perforators.

Superficial thrombophlebitis
• usually occurs in superficial varicose veins
• presents as a tender, reddened subcutaneous cord in leg
• usually localised oedema
• no generalised swelling of the limb or ankle
• requires symptomatic treatment only (see below) unless there is extension above the level of the knee when there is a risk of pulmonary embolism
• venous duplex scan is diagnostic and also determines:
    1. extent of superficial thrombosis, and
    2. if coexisting, unsuspected DVT is present

Treatment
The objective is to prevent propagation of the thrombus by uniform pressure over the vein.

• Cover whole tender cord with a thin foam pad.
• Apply a firm elastic bandage (preferable to crepe) from foot to thigh (well above cord).
• Leave pad and bandage on for 7–10 days.
• Bed rest with leg elevated is recommended.

- Prescribe an NSAID, e.g. indomethacin, for 10 days.

Note:
- No anticoagulants are required.
- The traditional glycerin and ichthyol dressings are still useful.
- Consider association between thrombophlebitis and deep-seated carcinoma.
- If the problem is above the knee, ligation of the vein at the saphenofemoral junction is indicated.

Deep venous thrombosis (DVT)
There is an up to 20% association with pulmonary emboli, of which 30% may be fatal. DVT may be asymptomatic but usually causes tenderness in the calf. One or more of the following features may be present.

Clinical features
- ache or tightness in calf
- acute diffuse leg swelling
- pitting oedema
- tender 'doughy' consistency to palpation
- increased warmth
- pain on extension of foot (Homan's sign)

Differential diagnosis
- Pseudophlebitis from ruptured popliteal (Baker's) cyst—this must be excluded before anticoagulation.

Investigations
- duplex ultrasound
- contrast venography

Management
Prevention (cases at risk):
- elastic stockings
- physiotherapy
- pneumatic compression
- electrical calf muscle stimulation during surgery
- unfractionated heparin 5000 U (sc) bd or tds (LMW heparin for orthopaedic surgery)

Treatment
- collect blood for APTT, INR and platelet count
- bed rest with leg elevated
- one-way-stretch elastic bandages (both legs to above knees)
- IV heparin 5000 U statim, then continuous monitored infusion (at least 10 days); aim for partial thromboplastin time 1.5 to 2 normal

or

LMW heparin e.g. enoxaparin 1.5 mg/kg subcutaneously daily
- oral anticoagulant (warfarin) for 3 to 6 months
- do not give aspirin
- mobilisation upon resolution of pain, tenderness and swelling

Surgery is necessary in extensive and embolising cases.

Iliofemoral thrombophlebitis (phlegmasia dolens)[10]
This rare but life-threatening condition is when an extensive clot obstructs the iliofemoral veins so completely that subcutaneous oedema and blanching occurs. This initially causes a painful 'milky white leg' previously termed phlegmasia alba dolens. It may deteriorate and become cyanotic—phlegmasia cerulea dolens. Massive iliofemoral occlusion is an emergency as such patients may develop 'shock', gangrene and pulmonary embolus.

Management of other painful conditions
Cellulitis and erysipelas
- Rest in bed.
- Elevate limb (in and out of bed).
- Use aspirin for pain and fever.

Streptococcus pyogenes (the common cause)[10]
- severe
  — benzylpenicillin 1.2 g IV 4 hourly
- less severe
  — procaine penicillin 1 g IM 12 hourly
      or
  — phenoxymethyl penicillin 500 mg (o) 6 hourly
- if penicillin sensitive
  — cephalothin IV or cephalexin 0.5 mg (o) 6 hourly
      or
  — erythromycin 500 mg (o) 12 hourly

Staphylococcus aureus[11]
- severe, may be life-threatening
  — flucloxacillin/dicloxacillin 2 g IV 6 hourly
- less severe
  — flucloxacillin/dicloxacillin 500 mg (o) 6 hourly
      or
  — cephalexin 500 mg (o) 6 hourly
      or
  — erythromycin 500 mg (o) 12 hourly

Nocturnal cramps

Note: Treat cause (if known) e.g. tetanus, drugs, sodium depletion, hypothyroidism.

Physical measures

- Muscle stretching and relaxation exercises: calf stretching for 3 minutes before retiring,[12] then rest in chair with the feet out horizontal to the floor with cushion under tendoachilles for 10 minutes.
- Massage and apply heat to affected muscles.
- Try to keep bedclothes off feet and lower part of legs—a doubled-up pillow at the foot of the bed can be used.

Medication

- Tonic water before retiring may help.
- Drug treatment:
  — quinine sulphate 300 mg nocte
    or
  — biperiden 2–4 mg nocte

Roller injuries to legs

A patient who has been injured by a wheel passing over a limb, especially a leg, can present a difficult problem. A freely spinning wheel is not so dangerous, but serious injuries occur when a non-spinning (braked) wheel passes over a limb and these are compounded by the wheel then reversing over it. This leads to a 'degloving' injury due to shearing stress. The limb may look satisfactory initially, but skin necrosis may follow.

- Admit to hospital for observation.
- Fasciotomy with open drainage may be an option.
- Surgical decompression with removal of necrotic fat is often essential.

When to refer

- The sudden onset of pain, pallor, pulselessness, paralysis, paraesthesia and coldness in the leg
- Worsening intermittent claudication
- Rest pain in foot
- Presence of popliteal aneurysm
- Superficial thrombophlebitis above knee
- Evidence of deep venous thrombosis
- Suspicion of gas gangrene in leg
- Worsening hip pain
- Evidence of disease in bone, e.g. neoplasia, infection, Paget's
- Severe sciatica with neurological deficit, e.g. floppy foot, absent reflexes

Practice tips

- Always X-ray the legs (including hips) of a patient complaining of unusual deep leg pain, especially a child.
- Pain that does not fluctuate in intensity with movement, activity or posture has an inflammatory or neoplastic cause.
- Hip disorders such as osteoarthritis and slipped femoral epiphysis can present as pain in the knee (usually medial aspect).
- Consider retroperitoneal haemorrhage as a cause of acute severe nerve root pain, especially in people on anticoagulant therapy.
- Avoidance of amputation with acute lower limb ischaemia depends on early recognition (surgery within 4 hours—too late if over 6 hours).

References

1. House AK. The painful limb: is it intermittent claudication? Mod Med Aust, November 1990; 16–26.
2. Tunnessen WW. *Signs and symptoms in paediatrics* (2nd edn). Philadelphia: Lippincott, 1988, 483.
3. Hart FD. *Practical problems in rheumatology*. London: Dunitz, 1983, 120.
4. Bates B. *A guide to physical examination and history taking* (5th edn). New York: Lippincott, 1991, 450.
5. Fry J, Berry H. *Surgical problems in clinical practice*. London: Edward Arnold, 1987, 125–134.
6. Ryan P. *A very short textbook of surgery* (2nd edn). Canberra: Dennis and Ryan, 1990, 61.
7. Hunt P, Marshall V. *Clinical problems in general surgery*. Sydney: Butterworths, 1991, 172.
8. Davis A, Bolin T, Ham J. *Symptom analysis and physical diagnosis* (2nd edn). Sydney: Pergamon, 1990, 179.
9. Mashford ML (Chairman). *Cardiovascular drug guidelines* (2nd edn). Melbourne: Victorian Medical Postgraduate Foundation 1995–96, 158–160.
10. Colucciello SA. Evaluation and management of deep venous thrombosis. Primary care reports, 1996; 2(12):105.
11. Mashford ML (Chairman). *Antibiotic guidelines* (9th edn). Melbourne: Victorian Medical Postgraduate Foundation 1996–97, 137–138.
12. Murtagh JE. *Practice tips* (2nd edn). Sydney: McGraw-Hill, 1995, 244.

61

The painful knee

—

The human knee is a joint and not a source of entertainment.

Percy Hammond 1912
Review of a play

The knee, which is a gliding hinge joint, is the largest synovial joint in the body. Its small area of contact of the bone ends at any one time makes it dependent on ligaments for its stability. Although this allows a much increased range of movement it does increase the susceptibility to injury, particularly from sporting activities. Finding the cause of a knee problem is one of the really difficult and challenging features of practice. It is useful to remember that peripheral pain receptors respond to a variety of stimuli. These include inflammation due either to inflammatory disease or chemical irritation such as crystal synovitis, traction pain, e.g. trapped meniscus stretching the capsule, tension on the synovium capsule, e.g. effusion or haemarthrosis, and impact loading of the subchondral bone.

Key facts and checkpoints

- Disorders of the knee account for about one presentation per fifty patients per year.[1]

- The commoner presenting symptoms in order of frequency are pain, stiffness, swelling, clicking and locking.[1]

- The age of presentation of a painful knee has varied significance as many conditions are age-related.

- Excessive strains across the knee, such as a valgus-producing force, are more likely to

cause ligament injuries, while twisting injuries tend to cause meniscal tears.

- A ruptured anterior cruciate ligament (ACL) is a commonly missed injury of the knee.[2] It should be suspected with a history of either a valgus strain or a sudden pivoting of the knee, often associated with a cracking or popping sensation. It is often associated with the rapid onset of haemarthrosis or inability to walk or weight bear.

- A rapid onset of painful knee swelling (minutes to 1–4 hours) after injury indicates blood in the joint—*haemarthrosis*.

- Swelling over 1–2 days after injury indicates synovial fluid—*traumatic synovitis*.

- Any collateral ligament repair should be undertaken early but, if associated with ACL injuries, early surgery may result in knee stiffness. Thus, surgery is often delayed. With isolated ACL ruptures, early reconstruction is appropriate in the high-performance athlete; otherwise, delayed reconstruction is appropriate if there is clinical instability.[3]

- Acute spontaneous inflammation of the knee may be part of a systemic condition such as rheumatoid arthritis, rheumatic fever, gout, pseudogout (chondrocalcinosis), a spondyloarthropathy (psoriasis, ankylosing spondylitis, Reiter's disease, bowel inflammation), Lyme disease and sarcoidosis.

- Consider Osgood-Schlatter disorder in the prepubertal child (especially a boy aged 10–14) presenting with knee pain.

- Disorders of the lumbosacral spine (especially L3 to S1 nerve root problems) and of the hip joint (L3 innervation) refer pain to the region of the knee joint.

The knee and referred pain—key knowledge

Pain from the knee joint

Disorders of the knee joint give rise to pain felt accurately at the knee, often at some particular part of the joint, and invariably in the anterior aspect, very seldom in the posterior part of the knee. An impacted loose body complicating osteoarthritis and a radial tear of the lateral meniscus[1] are the exceptional disorders liable to refer pain proximally and distally in the limb, but the problems obviously originate from the knee.

Pain referred to the knee

Referred pain to the knee or the surrounding region is a time-honoured trap in medicine. The two classic problems are disorders of the hip joint and lumbosacral spine.

- The hip joint is mainly innervated by L3, hence pain is referred from the groin down the front and medial aspects of the thigh to the knee (Fig. 61.1). Sometimes the pain can be experienced on the anteromedial aspect of the knee only. It is not uncommon for children with a slipped upper femoral epiphysis to present with a limp and knee pain.
- Knee pain can be referred from the lumbosacral spine. Patients with disc lesions may notice that sitting, coughing or straining hurts the knee, whereas walking does not.

L3 nerve root pressure from an L2–L3 disc prolapse (uncommon) and L4 nerve root pain will cause anteromedial knee pain; L5 reference from an L4–L5 disc prolapse can cause anterolateral knee pain, while S1 reference from an L5–S1 prolapse can cause pain at the back of the knee (Fig. 61.1).

A diagnostic approach

A summary of the safety diagnostic model is presented in Table 61.1.

Probability diagnosis

A UK study[1] has highlighted the fact that the commonest cause of knee pain is simple ligamentous strains and bruises due to overstress of the knee or other minor trauma. Traumatic synovitis may accompany some of these injuries. Some of these so-called strains may include a variety of recently described syndromes such as the synovial plica syndrome, patellar tendinitis and infrapatellar fat-pad inflammation (Fig. 61.2).

Low-grade trauma of repeated overuse such as frequent kneeling may cause prepatellar bursitis known variously as 'housemaid's knee' or 'carpet layer's knee'. Infrapatellar bursitis is referred to as 'clergyman's knee'.

Osteoarthritis of the knee, especially in the elderly, is a very common problem. It may arise spontaneously or be secondary to previous trauma with associated internal derangement and instability.

The most common overuse problem of the knee is the patellofemoral joint pain syndrome (often previously referred to as chondromalacia patellae).

Serious disorders not to be missed

Neoplasia in the bones around the knee is relatively uncommon but still needs consideration. The commonest neoplasias are secondaries from the breast and lung. Uncommon examples include osteoid osteoma, osteosarcoma and Ewing's disease. Septic arthritis and infected bursitis are prone to occur in the knee joint, especially following contaminated lacerations

Fig. 61.1 *Possible area of referred pain from disorders of the hip joint*

Table 61.1 *The painful knee: diagnostic strategy model*

Q. *Probability diagnosis*
A. Ligament strains and sprains
   ± traumatic synovitis
   Osteoarthritis
   Patellofemoral syndrome
   Prepatellar bursitis

Q. *Serious disorders not to be missed*
A. Acute cruciate ligament tear
   Vascular disorders
   • deep venous thrombosis
   • superficial thrombophlebitis
   Neoplasia
   • primary in bone
   • metastases
   Severe infections
   • septic arthritis
   • tuberculosis
   Rheumatoid arthritis
   Juvenile chronic arthritis
   Rheumatic fever

Q. *Pitfalls (often missed)*
A. Referred pain: back or hip
   Foreign bodies
   Intra-articular loose bodies
   Osteochondritis dissecans
   Osteochondrosis
   Osgood-Schlatter disorder
   Meniscal tears *J*
   Fractures around knee
   Pseudogout (chondrocalcinosis)
   Gout → patellar bursitis

   Rarities
   Sarcoidosis
   Paget's disease
   Spondyloarthropathy
   Ruptured popliteal cyst

Q. *Seven masquerades checklist*
A. Depression   √
   Diabetes   √
   Drugs   (indirect)
   Anaemia   —
   Thyroid disease   —
   Spinal dysfunction   √
   UTI   —

Q. *Is this patient trying to tell me something?*
A. Psychogenic factors relevant, especially with possible injury compensation.

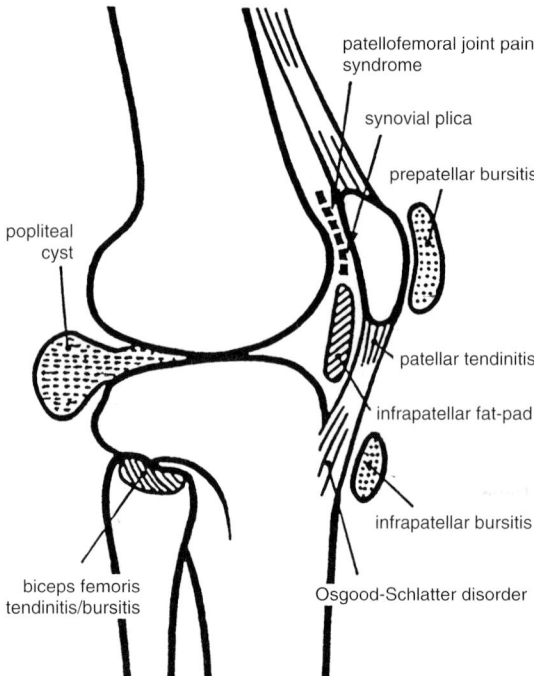

Fig. 61.2 *Lateral view of knee showing typical sites of various causes of knee pain*

crystal arthropathy due to calcium pyrophosphate dihydrate in the elderly), gout and juvenile chronic arthritis have to be considered in the differential diagnosis.

Pitfalls

There are a myriad pitfalls in knee joint disorders, often arising from ignorance, because there are a myriad problems that are difficult to diagnose. Fortunately, many of these problems can be diagnosed by X-ray. A particular trap is a foreign body such as a broken needle acquired by kneeling on carpet.

The presence of a spontaneous effusion demands careful attention because it could represent osteochondritis dissecans (more common in the young) or osteonecrosis of the femoral condyle (a necrotic problem in the elderly) and perhaps a subsequent loose body in the joint.

A ruptured Baker's cyst will cause severe pain behind the knee and can be confused with deep venous thrombosis. It is important to bear in mind complications of varicose veins which can cause pain or discomfort around the knee joint.

and abrasions. Septic arthritis from blood-borne infection can be of the primary type in children, where the infection is either staphylococcal or due to *Haemophilus influenzae*, or gonococcal arthritis in adults. Rheumatic fever should be kept in mind with a fleeting polyarthritis that involves the knees and then affects other joints.

Inflammatory disorders such as spondyloarthropathies, sarcoidosis, chondrocalcinosis (a

General pitfalls
- Overlooking referred pain from the hip or low back as a cause of knee pain.
- Failing to realise that meniscal tears can develop due to degeneration of the menisci with only minimal trauma.
- Failing to X-ray the knee joint and order special views to detect specific problems such as a fractured patella or osteochondritis dissecans.

Seven masquerades checklist
Of these, spinal dysfunction is the prime association. Diabetes may cause pain through a complicating neuropathy and drugs such as diuretics may cause gout in the elderly.

Psychogenic considerations
Patients, young and old, may complain of knee pain, imaginary or exaggerated, to gain attention especially if compensation for an injury is involved. This requires discreet clinical acumen to help patients work through the problem.

The clinical approach
History
The history is the key to diagnosis. If any injury is involved careful description of the nature of the injury is necessary. This includes past history. A special problem relates to the elderly who can sustain knee injuries after a 'drop attack', but attention can easily be diverted away from the knee with preoccupation with the cerebral pattern.

It is relevant to define whether the pain is acute or chronic, dull or sharp, and continuous or recurring. Determine its severity and position and keep in mind age-related causes.

Key questions
Related to an injury
- Can you explain in detail how the injury happened?
- Did you land awkwardly after a leap in the air?
- Did you get a direct blow? From what direction?
- Did your leg twist during the injury?
- Did you feel a 'pop'or hear a 'snap'?
- Did your knee feel wobbly or unsteady?
- Did the knee feel as if the bones separated momentarily?
- How soon after the injury did the pain develop?

- How soon after the injury did you notice swelling?
- Have you had previous injury or surgery to the knee?
- Were you able to walk after the injury or did you have to be carried off the ground or court?
- Does this involve work care compensation?

No history of injury
- Does the pain come on after walking, jogging or other activity?
- How much kneeling do you do? Scrubbing floors, cleaning carpets?
- Could there be needles or pins in the carpet?
- Does your knee lock or catch?
- Does swelling develop in the knee?
- Does it 'grate' when it moves?
- Does the pain come on at rest and is there morning stiffness?

Significance of symptoms
Swelling after injury
The sudden onset of painful swelling (usually within 60 minutes) is typical of haemarthrosis. Bleeding occurs from vascular structures such as torn ligaments, torn synovium or fractured bones, while injuries localised to avascular structures such as menisci do not usually bleed. About 75% of cases are due to anterior cruciate ligament tears.[5] If a minor injury causes acute haemarthrosis suspect a bleeding diathesis. The causes of haemarthrosis are listed in Table 61.2. Swelling of intermediate rate of onset, stiffness and pain in the order of hours, e.g. 6–24 hours, is typical of an effusion of synovial fluid. Causes include meniscal tears and milder ligamentous injuries. Swelling gradually developing over days and confined to the anterior knee is typical of bursitis such as 'housemaid's knee'.

Table 61.2 *Causes of haemarthrosis*

Torn cruciate ligaments, esp. ACL
Capsular tears with collateral ligament tears
Peripheral meniscal tears
Dislocation or subluxation of patella
Osteochondral fractures
Bleeding disorders, e.g. haemophilia

Recurrent or chronic swelling
This indicates intra-articular pathology and includes:
- patellofemoral pain syndrome

* osteochondritis dissecans
* degenerative joint disease
* arthritides

Locking

Locking usually means a sudden inability to extend the knee fully (occurs at 10–45°, average 30°) but ability to flex fully.[6]

| Causes |

True locking:

* torn meniscus (bucket handle)
* loose body, e.g. bony fragment from osteo-chondritis dissecans
* torn anterior cruciate ligament (remnant)
* avulsed anterior tibial spine
* dislocated patella
* synovial osteochondromatosis

Pseudo-locking:

* first or second degree medial ligament tear
* strain of ACL
* gross effusion
* pain and spasm of hamstrings

Catching

'Catching' of the knee implies that the patient feels that something is 'getting in the way of joint movement' but not locking. Causes include any of the conditions that cause locking, but a sub-luxing patella and loose bodies in particular must be considered.

| Causes of loose bodies |

* osteochondritis dissecans (usually lateral side of medial femoral condyle)
* retropatellar fragment, e.g. from dislocation of patella
* dislodged osteophyte
* osteochondral fracture—post injury

Clicking

Clicking may be due to an abnormality such as patellofemoral maltracking or subluxation, a loose intra-articular body or a torn meniscus, but can occur in normal joints when people climb stairs or squat.

Physical examination

The provisional diagnosis may be evident from a combination of the history and simple inspection of the joint but the process of testing palpation, movements (active and passive) and

specific structures of the knee joint helps to pin-point the disorder.

Inspection

Inspect the knee with the patient walking, standing erect and lying supine. Get the patient to squat to help localise the precise point of pain. Get the patient to sit on the couch with legs hanging over the side and note any abnormality of the patella. Note any deformities, swelling or muscle wasting.

The common knee deformities are genu valgum 'knock knees' (Fig. 61.3a), genu recurvatum 'back knee' (Fig. 61.3b) and genu varum 'bowed legs' (Fig. 61.3c). A useful way of remembering the terminology is to recall that the 'l' in valgus stands for 'l' in lateral.[7] In the normal knee the tibia has a slight valgus angulation in reference to the femur, the angulation being more pronounced in women.

Palpation

Palpate the knee generally concentrating on the patella, patella tendon, joint lines, tibial tubercle, bursae and popliteal fossa.

Palpate for presence of any fluid; warmth; swelling; synovial thickening; crepitus; clicking and tenderness. Feel for a popliteal (Baker's) cyst in the popliteal fossa. Draw the fingers upwards over the suprapatellar pouch: synovial thickening, a hallmark of chronic arthritis, is most marked just above the patella—it feels warm, boggy, rubbery and has no fluid thrill.

Flex the knees to 45° and check for a pseudocyst, especially of the lateral meniscus (Fig. 61.4).

Fig. 61.3 *Knee deformities;* **(a)** *genu valgum ('knock knees'): tibia deviates laterally from knee;* **(b)** *genu recurvatum ('back knee');* **(c)** *genu varum ('bowed legs')*

Fig. 61.4 *Pseudocyst of the lateral meniscus: flex the knees to 45° to force lump (if present) to appear*

Fig. 61.6 *The patellar tap test*

Fluid effusion

The bulge sign: compress the suprapatellar pouch and evacuate any fluid out of the medial side of the joint. The test is positive when the lateral side of the joint is then stroked and the fluid is displaced across the joint, creating a visible bulge or filling of the medial depression (Fig. 61.5). The test will be negative if the effusion is gross and tense, in which case the *patellar tap test* (Fig. 61.6) is used by sharply tapping the lower pole of the patella against the femur with the index finger. A positive tap is when the patella can be felt to tap against the femur and then float free.

suprapatellar pouch
compressed

lateral compartment
tapped with fingers

Fig. 61.5 *The bulge sign with a knee effusion: fluid bulges into the medial compartment*

Movements

Extension: normal is 0–5°. The loss of extension is best measured by lifting the heel off the couch with the knee held down. In the normal knee the heel will lift 2.5–4 cm off the couch, that is, into hyperextension.

Flexion (supine or prone): normal to 135°. The normal knee flexes heel to the buttock but in locking due to medial meniscus tears there is a gap of 5 or more centimetres between the heel and buttock.

Rotation: normal 5–10°. Test at 90° with patient sitting over the edge of the couch; rotate the feet with the hand steadying the knee.

Note: Normally, no abduction, adduction or rotation of the tibia on the femur is possible with the leg fully extended.

Ligament stability tests

Collateral ligaments. Adduction (varus) and abduction (valgus) stresses of tibia on femur are applied in full extension and then at 30° flexion with the leg over the side of the couch. With ligament strains there is localised pain when stressed. With a complete (third degree) tear the joint will open out. This end-point feel should be carefully noted: firmness indicates stability, 'mushiness' indicates damage (Figs 61.7a, b).

Cruciate ligaments. Stability of the ACL can be tested with the anterior drawer test. This is done with the patient supine and the knee flexed to 90°. The tibia is pulled forwards off the femur and in the presence of a cruciate ligament injury there will be increased gliding of the tibia on the femur. An aberrant positive sign can occur in the presence of posterior cruciate ligament insufficiency · in which case the knee is actually

Fig. 61.7 *Medial and lateral ligament instability:* **(a)** *medial instability of knee joint;* **(b)** *lateral instability of knee joint*

brought back to its normal site from a dropped-back position. This gives the appearance of a positive anterior drawer sign. In that situation, a Lachman's test will be negative. In the presence of medial ligament injury, the increased external rotation of the tibia against the femur may add to the positive drawer sign.

Specific provocation tests
The simplest menisci function tests are those outlined in Table 61.4.

• *McMurray's test.* The patient lies on the couch and the flexed knee is rotated in varying degrees of abduction as it is straightened into extension. A hand over the affected knee feels for 'clunking' or tenderness.

• *Apley grind/distraction test.* The patient lies prone, the knee is flexed to 90° and then rotated under a compression force. Reproduction of painful symptoms may indicate meniscal tear. Then repeat the rotation under distraction—tests ligament damage.

Patella apprehension test. At 15–20° flexion, attempt to push the patella laterally and note the patient's reaction.

Patellar tendinitis. Palpate patellar tendon (refer Fig. 61.16).

Patellofemoral pain test. Refer Fig. 61.15.

Examine the lumbosacral spine and the hip joint of the affected side.

Measurements
Quadriceps. For suspected quadriceps wasting, measure the circumference of the thighs at equal points above the tibial tuberosity. It is helpful to assess quadriceps function by feeling the tone.

Static Q angle (Fig. 61.8). If the Q angle is > 15° in men and > 19° in women there is a predisposition to patellofemoral pain and instability.[8]

Investigations
Investigation for the diagnosis of knee pain can be selected from:

• Blood tests
  — RA factor tests
  — ESR
  — blood culture (suspected septic arthritis)
• Radiology
  — plain X-ray
  — special views
    • intercondylar (osteochondritis dissecans, loose bodies)
    • tangential (or skyline view for suspected patella pathology)
    • oblique (to define condyles and patella)
  — bone scan: for suspected tumour, stress fracture, osteonecrosis, osteochondritis dissecans
  — MRI: excellent for diagnosing cartilage disorders and ligament damage
  — arthrography (generally superseded by arthroscopy)
  — ultrasound: good for assessment of patellar tendon, Baker's cyst and bursae.
• Special
  — examination under anaesthesia

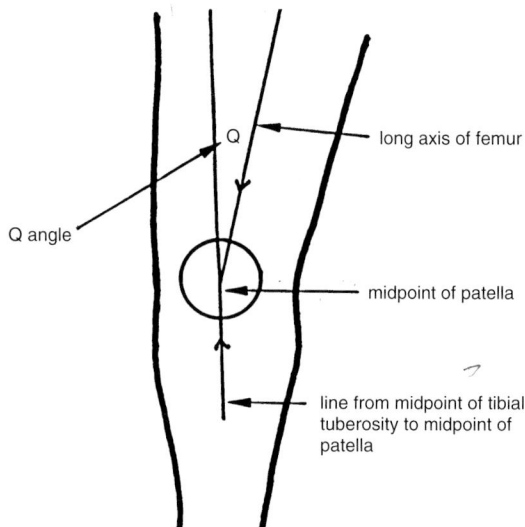

Fig. 61.8 *The Q angle of the knee gives a measure of patellar alignment*

— arthroscopy
— knee aspiration: culture or crystal examination

Knee pain in children

Children may present with unique conditions that are usually related to growth, including epiphyseal problems. Their tendency towards muscle tightness, especially in the growth spurt, predisposes them to overuse injuries such as patellar tendinitis and patellofemoral pain syndrome.

First decade

A painful knee during the first decade of life (0–10 years) in non-athletes is an uncommon presenting symptom, but suppurative infection and juvenile chronic arthritis have to be considered.

Genu valgum or varum is a common presentation but usually not a source of discomfort for the child. However, genu valgum, which is often seen around 4–6 years, may predispose to abnormal biomechanical stresses which contribute to overuse-type injuries if the child is involved in sport.

Second decade

Pain in the knee presents most frequently in this decade and is most often due to the patellofemoral syndrome[9] which is related to the retropatellar and peripatellar regions and usually anterior to the knee. It occurs in the late teenage years of both sexes.

An important problem is subluxation of the patella, typically found in teenage girls. It is caused by maltracking of the patellofemoral mechanism without complete dislocation of the patella (Fig. 61.9). On examination, the patella is usually in a high and lateral position. Surgery may be required if symptoms persist.

Osgood-Schlatter disorder (OSD) is common in prepubertal adolescent boys but can occur in those aged 10–16 years.

Other conditions found typically in this age group include:

- slipped upper femoral epiphysis—usually in middle teenage years after a growth spurt
- anserinus ('goose foot') bursitis
- osteochondritis dissecans

Age-related causes of the painful knee are presented in Table 61.3.[9]

Fig. 61.9 *Lateral subluxation of the patella*

The little athlete

Children competing in sporting activities, especially running and jumping, are prone to overuse injuries such as the patellofemoral pain syndrome, traumatic synovitis of the knee joint and OSD. Haemarthrosis can occur with injuries, sometimes due to a synovial tear without major joint disruption. If knee pain persists, especially

Table 61.3 *Age-related causes of painful knee*

First decade (0–10 years)
Infection
Juvenile chronic arthritis

Second decade (10–20 years)
Patellofemoral syndrome
Subluxation/dislocation of patella
Slipped femoral epiphysis (referred)
'Hamstrung' knee
Osteochondritis dissecans
Osgood-Schlatter disorder
Anserinus tendinitis

Third decade (20–30 years)
Bursitis
Mechanical disorders

Fourth and fifth decades (30–50 years)
Cleavage tear of medial meniscus
Radial tear of lateral meniscus

Sixth decade and older (50 years and over)
Osteoarthritis
Osteonecrosis
Paget's disease (femur, tibia or patella)
Anserinus bursitis
Chondrocalcinosis and gout
Osteoarthritis of hip (referred pain)

in the presence of an effusion, X-rays should be performed to exclude osteochondritis of the femoral condyle.[10]

Osgood-Schlatter disorder

OSD results from repetitive traction stresses at the insertion of the patellar tendon into the tibial tubercle, which is vulnerable to repeated traction in early adolescence.

Clinical features

- commonest ages 10–14
- boys: girls—3:1
- bilateral in about one-third of cases
- common in sports involving running, kicking and jumping
- localised pain in region of tibial tubercle during and after activity
- aggravated by kneeling down and going up and down stairs
- development of lump in area
- localised swelling and tenderness at affected tubercle
- pain reproduced by attempts to straighten flexed knee against resistance

X-ray to confirm diagnosis (widening of the apophysis and possible fragmentation of bone) and exclude tumour or fracture.

Management

This is conservative as it is a self-limiting condition (6–18 months: average 12 months).

- If acute, use ice packs and analgesics.
- Main approach is to abstain from or modify active sports.
- Localised treatments such as electrotherapy are unnecessary.
- Corticosteroid injections should be avoided.[11]
- Plaster cast immobilisation should also be avoided.
- Surgery may be used (rarely) if an irritating ossicle persists[12] after ossification.

Prevention

Promote awareness and early recognition of OSD.

Program of stretching exercises for quadriceps mechanism in children in sport.

Osteochondritis dissecans

This commonly occurs in adolescent boys whereby a segment of articular cartilage of the femoral condyle (85%) undergoes necrosis and may eventually separate to form an intra-articular loose body (Fig. 61.10). It then usually presents as pain, effusion and locking.

Knee pain in the elderly

Rheumatic disorders are very common and responsible for considerable pain or discomfort, disability and loss of independence in the elderly.

Osteoarthritis is also very common and excellent results are now being obtained with total knee replacement in those severely affected.

The elderly are particularly prone to crystal-associated joint diseases including monosodium urate (gout), calcium pyrophosphate dihydrate (CPPD)(pseudogout) and hydroxyapatite (acute calcific periarthritis).

Chondrocalcinosis of knee (pseudogout)

The main target of CPPD is the knee where it causes chondrocalcinosis. Unlike gout, chondrocalcinosis of the knee is typically a disease of the elderly with about 50% of the population having evidence of involvement of the knee by the ninth decade.[13] Most cases remain asymptomatic but patients (usually aged 60 or older) can present with an acutely hot, red, swollen joint resembling septic arthritis.

Investigations include aspiration of the knee to search for CPPD crystals, and X-ray. If positive, consider an associated metabolic disorder such as haemochromatosis, hyperparathyroidism or diabetes mellitus. Acute episodes respond well

Fig. 61.10 *Osteochondritis dissecans: on X-ray, sclerosis of the lateral aspect of the medial condyle*

to NSAIDs or intra-articular corticosteroid injection.

Osteonecrosis

Osteonecrosis is more common after the age of 60; it can occur in either the femoral (more commonly) or tibial condyles. The sudden onset of pain in the knee, with a normal joint X-ray, is diagnostic of osteonecrosis. It can take three months for the necrotic area to show radiologically although a bone scan may be positive at an early stage (Fig. 61.11). Surgery in the form of subchondral drilling may be required for persistent pain in the early stages.

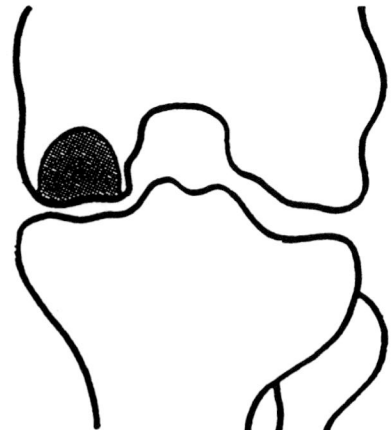

Fig. 61.11 *Osteonecrosis: necrosis in the medial femoral condyle can take three months to show radiologically*

Acute injuries

Meniscal tears

Medial and lateral meniscal tears are usually caused by abduction and adduction forces causing the meniscus to be compressed between the tibial and femoral condyles and then subjected to a twisting force.

The medial meniscus is three times more likely to be torn than the lateral. These injuries are common in contact sports and are often associated with ligamentous injuries. Suspect these injuries when there is a history of injury with a twisting movement with the foot firmly fixed on the ground.

However, pain in the knee can present in the patient aged 30–50 years as the menisci degenerate, with resultant cleavage tears from the posterior horn of the medial meniscus and 'parrot beak' tears of the mid-section of the lateral meniscus. These problems cause pain because these particular deformities create tension on the joint capsule and stretch the nerve ends.

Clinical features

- General symptoms[8]
  — joint line pain (49%)
  — locking (17%)
  — swelling (14%)
- Parrot beak tear of lateral meniscus
  — pain in the lateral joint line
  — pain radiating up and down the thigh
  — pain worse with activity
  — a palpable and visible lump when the knee is examined at 45°

Arthroscopic partial meniscectomy offers relief.
- Cleavage tear of medial meniscus
  — pain in medial joint line
  — pain aggravated by slight twisting of the joint
  — pain provoked by patient lying on the side and pulling the knees together
  — pain worse with activity

Arthroscopic meniscectomy is appropriate treatment.

A diagnostic memoire

Table 61.4 is a useful aid in the diagnosis of these injuries. There is a similarity in the clinical signs between the opposite menisci, but the localisation of pain in the medial or lateral joint lines helps to differentiate between the medial and lateral menisci.

Note: The diagnosis of a meniscal injury is made if three or more of the five examination findings ('signs' in Table 61.4) are present.

Ligament injuries

Tears of varying degrees may occur in the

- anterior cruciate ligament
- posterior cruciate ligament
- medial collateral ligament
- lateral collateral ligament

Table 61.4 *Typical symptoms and signs of meniscal injuries*

	Medial meniscus tear	*Lateral meniscus tear*
Mechanism	• Abduction (valgus) force • External rotation of lower leg on femur	• Adduction (varus) force • Internal rotation of leg on femur
Symptoms		
1. Knee pain during and after activity	Medial side of knee	Lateral side of knee
2. Locking	yes	yes
3. Effusion	+ or −	+ or −
Signs		
1. Localised tenderness over joint line (with bucket handle tear)	Medial joint line	Lateral joint line (may be cyst)
2. Pain on hyperextension of knee	Medial joint line	Lateral joint line
3. Pain on hyperflexion of knee joint	Medial joint line	Lateral joint line
4. Pain on rotation of lower leg (knee at 90°)	On external rotation	On internal rotation
5. Weakened or atrophied quadriceps	May be present	May be present

Anterior cruciate ligament (ACL) rupture

This is a very serious and disabling injury which may result in chronic instability. Chronic instability can result in degenerative joint changes if not dealt with adequately. Early diagnosis is essential but there is a high misdiagnosis rate. Sites of ACL rupture are shown in Figure 61.12.

Mechanisms
• sudden change in direction with leg in momentum
• internal tibial rotation on a flexed knee (commonest)
• valgus force, e.g. a rugby tackle
• may be associated with collateral ligament tears and meniscus injuries

Clinical features
• onset of severe pain after a sporting injury such as landing from a jump, or a forced valgus rotational strain of the knee when another player falls across the abducted leg
• immediate effusion of blood, usually within 30 minutes
• common sports: contact sports, e.g. rugby, football and soccer, basketball, volleyball, skiing
• differential diagnosis is a subluxed or dislocated patella
• subsequent history of pain and 'giving way' of the knee

Examination
• gross effusion
• diffuse joint line tenderness
• joint may be locked due to effusion, anterior

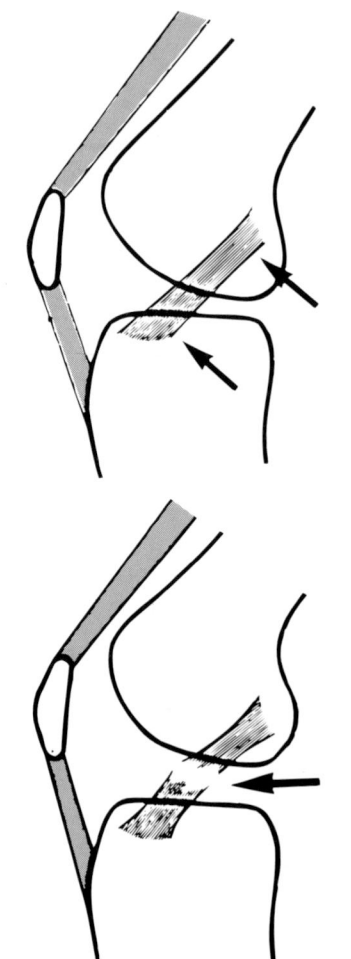

Fig. 61.12 *Sites of rupture of the anterior cruciate ligament*

cruciate tag or associated meniscal (usually medial) tear
• ligament tests
    — anterior drawer: negative or positive
    — pivot shift test: positive (only if instability)
    — Lachman test: lacking an end-point

Note: It may be necessary to examine the knee under anaesthesia, with or without arthroscopy, to assess the extent of injury.

The Lachman test

This test is emphasised because it is a sensitive and reliable test for the integrity of the ACL. It is an anterior drawer test with the knee at 15–20° of flexion. At 90° of flexion, the draw may be negative but the anterior cruciate torn.

Method
1. The examiner should be positioned on the same side of the examination couch as the knee to be tested.
2. The knee is held at 15–20° of flexion by placing a hand under the distal thigh and lifting the knee into 15–20° of flexion.
3. The patient is asked to relax, allowing the knee to 'fall back' into the steadying hand and roll slightly into external rotation.
4. The anterior drawer is performed with the second hand grasping the proximal tibia from the medial side (Fig. 61.13) while the thigh is held steady by the other hand. The examiner's knee can be used to steady the thigh.
5. The feel of the end-point of the draw is carefully noted. Normally there is an obvious jar felt as the anterior cruciate tightens. In an anterior cruciate deficient knee there is

sharp 'draw'

supporting knee under patient's thigh (optional)

Fig. 61.13 *The Lachman test*

excess movement and no firm end point. The amount of draw is compared with the opposite knee. Movement greater than 5 mm is usually considered abnormal.

Note: Functional instability due to anterior cruciate deficiency is best elicited with the pivot shift test. This is more difficult to perform than the Lachman test.

Pivot shift test

This is an important test for anterolateral rotatory instability. It is positive when anterior cruciate injuries are sufficient to produce a functional instability.

• The tibia is held in internal rotation by grasping the ankle firmly, with the knee in full extension.
• A valgus force is applied to the knee with the hand placed on the lateral aspect of the knee just below it (this maximises subluxation in the presence of an ACL tear).
• The knee is then flexed from 0–90°, listening for a 'clunk' of reduction. The test is positive when there is a sudden change of rhythm during flexion which corresponds to relocation of the subluxed knee. This usually occurs between 30° and 45° of flexion.
• From this flexed position the knee is extended, seeking a click into subluxation. This is called a positive jerk test.

Management

The management depends on the finding by the surgeon. Surgical repair is reserved for complete ligament tears. This usually involves reconstruction of the tendon. Early reconstruction is appropriate in younger patients who participate in high levels of sporting activity in which it can be predicted that functional instability will be a problem. In less active people, a conservative approach is appropriate. Cruciate reconstruction can then be undertaken if the knee becomes clinically unstable. The presence of an ACL injury with a significant medial ligament injury will necessitate reconstructive surgery but this is probably best delayed for some weeks as the subsequent incidence of knee stiffness is high.

Posterior cruciate ligament rupture

Mechanisms
• direct blow to the anterior tibia in flexed knee
• severe hyperextension injury

Clinical features
- posterior (popliteal) pain, radiating to calf
- usually no or minimal swelling
- minimal disability apart from limitation of running or jumping
- pain running downhill
- recurvatum
- posterior sag or draw

Management
- usually managed conservatively with immobilisation and protection for six weeks
- graduated weight bearing and exercises

Medial collateral ligament rupture

Mechanisms
- direct valgus force to knee (lateral side knee), e.g. rugby tackle from side
- external tibial rotation, e.g. two soccer players kicking ball simultaneously

Clinical features
These depend on the degree of tear (1st, 2nd or 3rd degree):

- pain on medial knee
- aggravated by twisting
- localised swelling over medial aspect
- pseudo-locking—hamstring strain
- ± effusion
- no end point on valgus stress testing (3rd degree) (Fig. 61.7a)

Note: Check lateral meniscus if MCL tear.
Pellegrini-Stieda disease—calcification in haematoma at upper (femoral) origin of MCL may follow.

Management
If an isolated injury, this common injury responds to conservative treatment with early limited motion bracing to prevent opening of the medial joint line. Six weeks of limited motion brace at 20–70° followed by knee rehabilitation usually returns the athlete to full sporting activity within 12 weeks.

Note: The same principles of diagnosis and management apply to the less common rupture of the lateral collateral ligament which is caused by a direct varus force to the medial side of the knee.

Overuse syndromes

The knee is very prone to overuse disorders. The pain develops gradually without swelling, is aggravated by activity and relieved with rest. It can usually be traced back to a change in the sportsperson's training schedule, footwear or technique, or to related factors. It may also be related to biomechanical abnormalities ranging from hip disorders to feet disorders.

Overuse injuries include:
- patellofemoral pain syndrome ('jogger's knee', 'runner's knee')
- patellar tendinitis ('jumper's knee')
- synovial plica syndrome
- infrapatellar fat-pad inflammation
- anserinus bursitis/tendinitis
- biceps femoris tendinitis
- semimembranous bursitis/tendinitis
- quadriceps tendinitis/rupture
- popliteus tendinitis
- iliotibial band friction syndrome ('runner's knee')
- the hamstrung knee

It is amazing how often palpation identifies localised areas of inflammation (tendinitis or bursitis) around the knee, especially from overuse in athletes and in the obese elderly (Figs 61.14a,b).

Patellofemoral pain syndrome
This syndrome, also known as chondromalacia patellae and referred to as 'jogger's knee', 'runner's knee' or 'cyclist's knee', is the most common overuse injury of the knee. There is usually no specific history of trauma. It may be related to biomechanical abnormalities and abnormal position and tracking of the patella, e.g. patella alta.

Clinical features
- pain behind patella or deep in knee
- pain aggravated during activities that require flexion of knee under loading
  — climbing stairs
  — walking down slopes or stairs
  — squatting
  — prolonged sitting
- the 'movie' sign: using aisle seat to stretch knee
- crepitus around patella may be present

Signs of chondromalacia patellae
Patellofemoral crepitation during knee flexion and extension is often palpable, and pain may

Fig. 61.14 *Typical painful areas around the knee for overuse syndromes:* **(a)** *anterior aspect;* **(b)** *medial aspect*

be reproduced by compression of the patella onto the femur as it is pushed from side to side with the knee straight or flexed (Perkins' test).

Method for special sign (Fig. 61.15)
- Have the patient supine with the knee extended.
- Grasp the superior pole of the patella and displace it inferiorly.
- Maintain this position and apply patellofemoral compression.
- Ask the patient to contract the quadriceps (it is a good idea to get the patient to practise

quadriceps contraction before applying the test).
- A positive sign is reproduction of the pain under the patella and hesitancy in contracting the muscle.

Treatment
- Correct any underlying biomechanical abnormalities by use of orthotics and correct footwear.
- Give reassurance and supportive therapy.
- Employ quadriceps exercises.

Patellar tendinitis ('jumper's knee')
'Jumper's knee', or patellar tendinitis (Fig. 61.2), is a common disorder of athletes involved in repetitive jumping sports, such as high jumping, basketball, netball, volleyball and soccer.

Clinical features
- gradual onset of anterior pain
- pain localised to below knee
- pain eased by rest, returns with activity

The diagnosis is often missed because of the difficulty of localising signs. The condition is best diagnosed by eliciting localised tenderness at the inferior pole of the patella with the patella tilted. There may be localised swelling.

Method
- Lay the patient supine in a relaxed manner with the head on a pillow, arms by the side and quadriceps relaxed (a must).
- The knee should be fully extended.
- Tilt the patella by exerting pressure over its superior pole. This lifts the inferior pole.
- Now palpate the surface under the inferior

Fig. 61.15 *Special sign of the patellofemoral pain syndrome*

pole. This allows palpation of the deeper fibres of the patellar tendon (Fig. 61.16).

- Compare with the normal side.
- Very sharp pain is usually produced in the patient with patellar tendinitis.

Management

Early conservative treatment including rest from the offending stresses is effective. This includes adequate warm-up and warm-down. Training modification includes calf, hamstring and quadriceps muscle stretching. Modified footwear and a patellar tendon strap may be helpful in some cases. The use of NSAIDs and corticosteroid injections is disappointing. Chronic cases invariably require surgery.

Anserinus tendinitis/bursitis

Localised tenderness is found over the medial tibial condyle where the tendons of sartorius, gracilis and semitendinosus insert into the bone. It is a common cause of knee pain in the middle aged or elderly, especially the overweight woman. Pain is aggravated by resisted knee flexion.

Semimembranous tendinitis/bursitis

This inflamed area is sited either at the tendon insertion or in the bursa between the tendon and the medial head of gastrocnemius. It is an uncommon problem.

Biceps femoris tendinitis/bursitis

The tendon and/or the bursa which lies between the tendon insertion and the fibular collateral ligament at the head of the fibula may become inflamed due to overuse. It is usually encountered in sprinters.

patella

Fig. 61.16 *Patellar tendinitis: method of palpation*

Popliteus tendinitis

Tenosynovitis of the popliteus tendon may cause localised pain in the posterior or the posterolateral aspect of the knee. Tenderness to palpation is elicited with the knee flexed to 90°.

Iliotibial tract tendinitis

Inflammation develops over the lateral aspect of the knee where the iliotibial band passes over the lateral femoral condyle. The problem, which is caused by friction of the iliotibial band on the bone, is common in long-distance runners, especially when running up and down hills.

> *Treatment of tendinitis and bursitis (small area)*

Generally (apart from patellar tendinitis), the treatment is an injection of local anaesthetic and long-acting corticosteroids into and deep to the localised area of tenderness. In addition it is important to restrict the offending activity with relative rest and refer for physiotherapy for stretching exercises. Attention to biomechanical factors and footwear is important.

If conservative methods fail for iliotibial tract tendinitis, surgical excision of the affected fibres may cure the problem.

Prepatellar bursitis

Repetitive low-grade direct trauma such as frequent kneeling can cause inflammation with swelling of the bursa which lies between the anterior surface of the patella and the skin. 'Housemaid's knee', or 'carpet layer's knee', can be difficult to treat if rest from the trauma does not allow it to subside. If persistent, drain the fluid with a 23 g needle and then introduce 0.5–1 mL of long-acting corticosteroid. The presence of a bursa 'mouse', which is a pedunculated fibrous tumour arising from the bursa wall, and persistent bursitis usually means that surgical intervention is required.

Acute bursitis may also be caused by acute infection, or one of the inflammatory arthropathies, e.g. gout, Reiter's disease.

Infrapatellar bursitis

'Clergyman's knee' is produced by the same mechanisms as patellar bursitis and can be involved with inflammatory disorders or infection. Treatment is also the same.

The hamstrung knee

Cross describes this condition in young active sportspeople (second decade)[9] as one that causes bilateral knee pain and possibly a limp. It is caused by a failure to warm up properly and stretch the hamstring muscles, which become tender and tight during the growth spurt. A six week program of straight leg raising and hamstring stretching will alleviate the pain completely.

Synovial plica syndrome

This syndrome results from a synovial fold (an embryological remnant) being caught between the patella and the femur during walking or running. It causes an acute 'catching' knee pain of the medial patellofemoral joint (Fig. 61.2) and sometimes a small effusion. It generally settles without treatment.

Infrapatellar fat-pad inflammation

Acute compression of the fat-pad, which extends across the lower patella deep to the patellar tendon and into the knee joint (Fig. 61.2), during a jump or other similar trauma, produces local pain and tenderness similar to the sensation of kneeling on a drawing pin.[14]

The pain usually settles without therapy over a period of days or weeks. There is localised tenderness and it can be confused with patellar tendinitis.

Arthritic conditions

Osteoarthritis

Osteoarthritis is a very common problem of the knee joint. Symptoms usually appear in middle life or later. It is more common in women, the obese, and in those with knee deformities, e.g. genu varum, or previous trauma, especially meniscal tears. The degenerative changes may involve either the lateral or medial tibiofemoral compartment, the patellofemoral joint or any combination of these sites.

Clinical features

- slowly increasing joint pain and stiffness
- aggravated by activities such as prolonged walking, standing or squatting
- descending stairs is usually more painful than ascending stairs (suggestive of patellofemoral OA)
- pain may occur after rest, especially prolonged flexion
- minimal effusion and variable crepitus
- restricted flexion but usually full extension
- often quadriceps wasting and tender over medial joint line
- diagnosis confirmed by X-ray (weight-bearing view)

Management

- relative rest
- weight loss
- analgesics and/or judicious use of NSAIDs
- walking aids and other supports
- physiotherapy, e.g. hydrotherapy, quadriceps exercises, mobilisation and stretching techniques
- intra-articular injections of corticosteroids are generally not recommended but a single injection for severe pain can be very effective
- surgery is indicated for severe pain and stiffness; includes arthroscopic debridement and washout, osteotomy, arthrodesis and total joint replacement (Fig. 61.17).

Rheumatoid arthritis

The knee is frequently affected by RA although it rarely presents as monoarticular knee pain. RA shows the typical features of inflammation—pain and stiffness that is worse after resting. Morning stiffness is a feature.

Note: The spondyloarthropathies have a similar clinical pattern to RA.

Synovectomy is a useful option with persistent boggy thickening of synovial membrane but without destruction of the articular cartilage.[2]

Septic arthritis

Tends to be more common in the knee than other joints. Septic (pyogenic) arthritis should be suspected when the patient complains of intense joint pain, malaise and fever. In the presence of acute pyogenic infection the joint is held rigidly. The differential diagnosis includes gout and pseudogout (chondrocalcinosis).

Principles of management

Most painful knee conditions are not serious and, providing a firm diagnosis is made and internal knee disruption or other serious illness

Fig. 61.17 *Total joint replacement of knee*

discounted, a simple management plan as outlined leads to steady relief. For more serious injuries the primary goal is to minimise the adverse consequences of forced inactivity.

- First aid: RICE.
- Lose weight if overweight.
- Adequate support for ligament sprains, e.g. supportive elastic tubular (tubigrip) bandage or a firm elastic bandage over Velband.
- Simple analgesics, e.g. paracetamol (acetaminophen).
- Judicious use of NSAIDs and corticosteroid injections.
- Physiotherapy to achieve strength and stability.
- Attend to biomechanical abnormalities, inappropriate footwear and athletic techniques.
- Orthotics and braces to suit the individual patient.
- Specialised exercise techniques, e.g. the McConnell technique.[2]
- Quadriceps exercises: these simple exercises are amazingly effective.

Quadriceps exercises (examples)
- Instruct the patient to tighten the muscles in front of the thighs (as though about to lift the leg at the hip and bend the foot back but keeping the leg straight). The patient should hold the hand over the lower quads to ensure

it is felt to tighten. This tightening and relaxing exercise should be performed at least 6 times every 2 hours or so until it becomes a habit. It can be done sitting, standing or lying (Fig. 61.18).
- Sitting on a chair the patient places a weight of 2–5 kg around the ankle (e.g. a plastic bag with sand or coins in a sock) and lifts the leg to the horizontal and then gently lowers it (avoid in patellofemoral problems).

Fig. 61.18 *A quadriceps exercise: with outstretched legs the quadriceps muscle is slowly and deliberately tightened by straightening the knee to position **(a)** from the relaxed position **(b)***

When to refer
- Early referral is required for knees 'at risk' following acute injuries where one or more of the following are present:
  — locked knee
  — haemarthrosis
  — instability
- Clinical evidence of a torn cruciate ligament, third degree tear of the collateral ligaments or torn meniscus.
- Undiagnosed acute or chronic knee pain.
- Recurrent subluxation or dislocation of the patella.
- Suspected septic arthritis.
- Presence of troublesome intra-articular loose body.

Practice tips
- The absence of an effusion does not rule out the presence of severe knee injury.
- Examine the hip and lumbosacral spine if examination of the knee is normal but knee pain is the complaint.
- Always think of an osteoid osteoma in a young boy with severe bone pain in a leg (especially at night) that responds nicely to aspirin or paracetamol or other NSAID.
- Tears of the meniscus can occur, especially in middle age, without a history of significant preceding trauma.
- If a patient presents with a history of an audible 'pop' or 'crack' in the knee with an immediate effusion (in association with trauma) he or she has an anterior cruciate ligament tear until proved otherwise.
- Haemarthrosis following an injury should be regarded as an anterior cruciate tear until proved otherwise.
- The 'movie' sign whereby the patient seeks an aisle seat to stretch the knee is usually due to patellofemoral pain syndrome.
- The 'bed' sign, when pain is experienced when the knees touch while in bed, is suggestive of a medial meniscal cleavage tear.
- A positive squat test (medial pain on full squatting) indicates a tear of the posterior horn of the medial meniscus.
- Joint aspiration should not be performed on the young athlete with an acute knee injury.
- Reserve intra-articular corticosteroid injections for inflammatory conditions such as rheumatoid arthritis or a crystal arthropathy: regular injections for osteoarthritis are to be avoided. Do not give the injections when the inflammation is acute and diffuse or in the early stages of injury.
- Many inflammatory conditions around the knee joint, such as bursitis or tendinitis, respond to a local injection of local anaesthetic and corticosteroid but avoid giving injections into the tendon, especially the patellar tendon.

References
1. Knox JDE. Knee problems. In: *Practice.* London: Kluwer-Harrap Handbooks, 1982; 3.66:01–05.
2. Selecki Y, Helman T. How to treat knee pain. Australian Dr Weekly, 1993.
3. McLean I. Assessment of the acute knee injury. Aust Fam Physician, 1984; 13:575–580.
4. Cyriax J. *Textbook of orthopaedic medicine Volume 1* (6th edn). London: Bailliere Tindall, 1976, 594.
5. Noyes FR. Arthroscopy in acute traumatic haemarthrosis of the knee. J Bone and Joint Surgery, 1980:624–687.
6. Corrigan B, Maitland GD. *Practical orthopaedic medicine.* Sydney: Butterworths, 1986, 126–161.
7. Hoppenfeld S. *Physical examination of the spine and extremities.* Englewood Cliffs: Prentice-Hall, 1976, 172–173.
8. Cross MJ, Crichton KJ. *Clinical examination of the injured knee.* London: Harper & Row, 1987, 21–46.
9. Cross MJ. The painful knee. Aust Fam Physician, 1984; 13:166–168.
10. Larkins P. The little athlete. Aust Fam Physician, 1991; 20:973–978.
11. Rostrom PKM, Calver RF. Subcutaneous atrophy following methyl prednisolone injection in Osgood-Schlatter epiphysitis. J Bone and Joint Surgery, 1979; 61A: 627–628.
12. Mital MA, Matza RA, Cohen J. The so-called unresolved Osgood-Schlatter's lesion. J Bone and Joint Surgery, 1980; 62A:732–739.
13. Wilkins E et al. Osteoarthritis and articular chondrocalcinosis in the elderly. Ann Rheum Dis, 1983; 42(3):280–284.
14. Fricker P. Anterior knee pain. Aust Fam Physician, 1988; 17:1055–1056.

62

Pain in the foot and ankle

—

The victim goes to bed and sleeps in good health. About two o'clock in the morning he is awakened by a severe pain in the great toe; more rarely in the heel, ankle, or instep . . . The part affected cannot bear the weight of the bed clothes nor the jar of a person walking in the room. The night is spent in torture.

Thomas Sydenham (1624–89)

Pain in the foot (podalgia) and ankle problems are a common occurrence in general practice. Various characteristics of the pain can give an indication of its cause, such as the description of gout by Thomas Sydenham. There are many traumatic causes of podalgia and ankle dysfunction, especially fractures and torn ligaments, but this chapter will focus mainly on everyday problems that develop spontaneously or through overuse. The main causes of foot pain are presented in Table 62.1.[1]

Key facts and checkpoints

- Foot deformities such as flat feet (pes planus) are often painless.
- Foot strain is probably the commonest cause of podalgia.[2]
- A common deformity of the toes is hallux valgus, with or without bunion formation.
- Osteoarthritis is a common sequel to hallux valgus.

Table 62.1 *Causes of foot pain (after Johnson)*[1]

General
Arthritis—OA, gout, RA, seronegative spondyloarthropathies.
Diabetes—neuropathy [sensory (Charcot), motor, autonomic, single nerve], sepsis, vasculopathy.
Peripheral neuritis—alcohol, B_{12} deficiency.
Vascular—arteriosclerosis (claudication, gangrene), hemiplegia, Raynaud's, RSD (Sudeck's).
Infections—cellulitis, septic arthritis, TB, actinomyces.
   Other: Paget's disease of bone, osteoid osteoma, hypermobility syndrome (including Marfan's).

Ankle and hindfoot
Tendoachilles (bursitis, tendinitis, tear), posterior tibial tendinitis, rupture or subluxation, plantar fasciitis, sprain, bruised heel, phlebitis, cellulitis.

Midtarsal
Acute or chronic foot strain, synovitis of subtaloid, tarsal coalition, hypomobility of transverse tarsal joints, osteochondritis of navicular (Kohler's), dorsal exostosis, peroneus brevis tendinitis, flexor hallucis longus tendinitis.

Forefoot
Bunion, bunionette, Tailor's bunion, intermetatarsal bursitis, traumatic synovitis of MTP, sesamoiditis, march fracture, Freiberg's infraction.

Toes
Hallux valgus, hallux rigidus, varus little toe, mallet toe, clawed toe, corn, wet corn, ingrown toenail, onychogryphosis, subungual exostosis, deep peroneal nerve entrapment, digital nerve entrapment (Morton's neuralgia).

Sole
Callus, plantar wart, epidermoid cyst, foreign body, tarsal tunnel syndrome, Dupuytren's (Ledderhose's) contracture.

OA: osteoarthritis   **RA:** rheumatoid arthritis   **MTP:** metatarsophalangeal

- Osteoarthritis affecting the ankle is relatively rare.
- All the distal joints of the foot may be involved in arthritic disorders.
- Many foot and ankle problems are caused by unsuitable footwear and lack of foot care.
- Ankle sprains are the most common injury in sport, representing about 25% of injuries.
- Severe sprains of the lateral ligaments of the ankle due to an inversion force may be associated with various fractures.
- Bunions and hammer toes are generally best treated by surgery.

A diagnostic approach

A summary of the safety diagnostic model is presented in Table 62.2.

Probability diagnosis

Common causes include osteoarthritis, especially of the first metatarsophalangeal joint, acute or chronic foot strain, plantar fasciitis, plantar skin conditions such as warts, corns and calluses and various toenail problems.

Serious disorders not to be missed

The very important serious disorders to consider include:

- vascular disease—affecting small vessels
- diabetic neuropathy
- osteoid osteoma
- rheumatoid arthritis
- reflex sympathetic dystrophy

Vascular causes

The main problem is ischaemic pain that occurs only in the foot. The commonest cause is atheroma. Vascular causes include:

- acute arterial obstruction
- chilblains
- atherosclerosis, especially small vessel disease
- functional vasospasm (Raynaud's)—rare

Symptoms:

- claudication (rare in isolation)
- sensory disturbances, especially numbness at rest or on walking
- rest pain—at night, interfering with sleep, precipitated by elevation, relieved by dependency.

For treatment refer to page 620.

Table 62.2   *The painful foot and ankle: diagnostic strategy model*

Q. *Probability diagnosis*
A. Acute or chronic foot strain
Sprained ankle
Osteoarthritis, esp. great toe
Plantar fasciitis
Achilles tendinitis
Wart, corn or callus
Ingrowing toenail/paronychia

Q. *Serious disorders not to be missed*
A. Vascular insufficiency
  • small vessel disease
Neoplasia
  • osteoid osteoma
  • osteosarcoma
Severe infections (rare)
  • septic arthritis
  • actinomycosis
  • osteomyelitis
Rheumatoid arthritis
Peripheral neuropathy
Reflex sympathetic dystrophy
Ruptured Achilles tendon
Ruptured tibialis posterior tendon

Q. *Pitfalls (often missed)*
A. Foreign body (especially children)
Gout
Nerve entrapment
  • Morton's neuroma
  • tarsal tunnel syndrome
  • deep peroneal nerve
Chilblains
Stress fracture, e.g. navicular
Erythema nodosum

Rarities
Spondyloarthropathies
Reflex sympathetic dystrophy
Osteochondritis
  • navicular (Köhler's)
  • metatarsal head (Freiberg)
  • calcaneum (Sever's)
Glomus tumour (under nail)
Paget's disease

Q. *Seven masquerades checklist*
A. Depression   ?
Diabetes   √
Drugs   √
Anaemia   ?
Thyroid disease   –
Spinal dysfunction   √
UTI   –

Q. *Is the patient trying to tell me something?*
A. A non-organic cause warrants consideration with any painful condition.

Reflex sympathetic dystrophy (RSD)

RSD, also known as Sudeck's atrophy, is characterised by severe pain, swelling and disability of the feet. It is a neurovascular disorder resulting in hyperaemia and osteoporosis that may be a sequela of trauma (often trivial) and prolonged immobilisation. RSD usually lasts two years and recovery to normality usually follows.

The clinical features include sudden onset in middle-aged patients, pain worse at night, stiff joints and skin warm and red. X-rays that show patchy decalcification of bone are diagnostic. Treatment includes reassurance, analgesics, mobility in preference to rest, and physiotherapy.

Osteoid osteoma

Osteoid osteomas are rare but important little 'brain teasers' of benign tumours that typically occur in older children and adolescents. Males are affected twice as often as females. Any bone (except those of the skull) can be affected but the tibia and femur are the main sites. Nocturnal pain is a prominent symptom with pain relief by aspirin being a feature.

Diagnosis is dependent on clinical suspicion and then X-ray which shows a small sclerotic lesion with a radiolucent centre. Treatment is by surgical excision.

Pitfalls

There are many traps in the diagnosis and management of problems presenting with a painful foot. Common problems require consideration—these include gouty arthritis, chilblains, a stress fracture and a foreign body in the foot, especially in children. Nerve entrapment, as outlined in Chapter 60, is uncommon but Morton's neuroma is reasonably common.

Less common disorders include RSD which is often misdiagnosed, the spondyloarthropathies (psoriasis, Reiter's disease, ankylosing spondylitis and the inflammatory bowel disorders) and osteochondritis of the calcaneus, navicular bone and metatarsal head. If there is an exquisitely tender small purple-red spot beneath a toenail, a glomus tumour (a benign hamartoma) is the diagnosis. It is worth noting that most of these conditions are diagnosed by X-rays.

General pitfalls

• Failing to order X-rays of the foot.
• Failing to order X-rays of the ankle following injury.
• Failing to appreciate the potential for painful problems caused by diabetes—neuropathy and small vessel disease.
• Neglecting the fact that most of the arthritides can manifest in joints in the foot, especially the forefoot.

• Regarding the sprained ankle in adults and children as an innocuous injury: associated injuries include chondral fractures to the dome of the talus, impaction fractures around the medial recess of the ankle, avulsion fractures of the lateral malleolus and base of fifth metatarsal.
• Misdiagnosing a stress fracture of the navicular which, like the scaphoid fracture, causes delayed union and non-union. Cast immobilisation for 8 weeks initially may prevent the need for surgery.
• Misdiagnosing a complete rupture of the Achilles tendon because the patient can plantar flex the foot.

Seven masquerades checklist

The checklist has four conditions that should be considered, especially diabetes and spinal dysfunction. Diabetes may be responsible for a simple type of atherosclerotic pattern, possibly complicated by infection and ulceration. The neuropathy of diabetes can cause a burning pain with paraesthesia. It has a 'sock'-type pattern as opposed to the dermatome pattern of nerve root pressure arising from the lumbosacral spine. The common S1 pain is experienced on the outer border of the foot, into the fifth toe and on the outer sole and heel of the foot.

Drugs and anaemia could indirectly cause pain through vascular insufficiency. The drugs that could cause vasospasm include beta-blockers and ergotamine. An alcoholic neuropathy also has to be considered.

Psychogenic considerations

Any painful condition can be closely associated with psychogenic disorders, including depression.

The clinical approach
History

This is very important, as always, since various characteristics of the pain can give an indication of its cause. Questions should address the quality of the pain, its distribution, mode of onset, periodicity, relation to weight bearing, and associated features such as swelling or colour change. It is relevant to enquire about pain in other joints such as the hand and spine, including the sacroiliac joints, which might indicate that the foot pain is part of a polyarthritis. A history of diarrhoea, psoriasis, urethritis or iritis may suggest that one of the spondyloarthropathies has to be excluded.

Key questions

The practitioner should address the following questions:

- Does the pain arise from a local condition or is it part of a generalised disease?
- Is there a history of psoriasis, chronic diarrhoea or colitis, urethritis or iritis?
- Is pain also present in other joints, thus indicating the foot pain is part of a polyarthritis, such as rheumatoid arthritis?
- Is the problem related to unsuitable footwear?
- Does the nature of the pain point to the cause?
  - throbbing pain → inflammation
  - burning pain → nerve entrapment, diabetic neuropathy or RSD
  - severe episodic pain → gout
  - pain worse at night → ischaemia (small vessel disease), RSD, cramps or osteoid osteoma
  - pain worse at night, relieved by aspirin → osteoid osteoma
  - pain worse on standing after sitting and getting out of bed → plantar fasciitis

For ankle injuries it is important to ask about the nature of the injury:

- Did the foot twist in (invert) or twist out (evert)?
- Was the foot pointing down or up at the time of injury?
- Point with one finger to where it hurts (the finger-pointing sign)
- What happened immediately after the injury?
- Were you able to walk straight away?
- What happened when you cooled off?

If there has been a fall onto the foot from a height, consider the possibility of a fracture of the calcaneus or talus or disruption of the syndesmosis between the tibia and fibula.

Physical examination

Inspection

Inspect the feet with the patient standing, sitting, walking (in shoes and bare-footed) and lying down (note plantar surfaces). Inspect the footwear (normally, a shoe wears first on the outer posterior margin of the heel).

Note:

- any gait abnormalities including limping and abnormal toe in or toe out

- deformities, e.g. hammer toes, bunions—medial (hallux valgus) and lateral (Tailor's bunion)—and claw toes
- swellings including callosities
- muscle wasting
- skin changes and signs of ischaemia

Palpation

Systematic palpation is very useful as most structures in the foot are accessible to palpation.

Movements (active and passive)

- plantar flexion (normal—50°) and dorsiflexion (20°) of ankle
- inversion and eversion of hindfoot (mainly subtalar joint)—hold heel and abduct and adduct (Fig. 62.1)
- inversion and eversion of forefoot (midtarsal joint)—hold heel in one hand to fix hindfoot, hold forefoot in the other and abduct and adduct (rotation movement) (Fig. 62.2)
- test other joints individually, e.g. metatarsophalangeal, midtarsal

Fig. 62.1 *Testing inversion and eversion of the hindfoot*

Fig. 62.2 *Testing inversion and eversion of the forefoot*

Special tests

- Achilles tendon including calf squeeze (Thompson's or Simmond's test) (Fig. 121.11)
- compress metatarsophalangeal joints from above and below
- compress metatarsals mediolaterally between thumb and forefinger
- check circulation—test dorsalis pedis and posterior tibial pulses
- neurological examination including tests for L4, L5 and S1 nerve root function

Investigations

The choice of investigations depends on the clinical features elicited by the history and examination. Select from the following list:

- For systemic diseases
  - blood glucose
  - RA tests
  - ESR/C reactive protein
  - HLA B27
- Serum uric acid
- Radiology
  - X-ray ± stress and weight-bearing views
  - radionuclide scans
  - CT scans
  - ultrasound
- Nerve condition studies

Note: High-resolution ultrasound is used to diagnose disorders of the Achilles tendon and to locate foreign bodies such as splinters of wood and glass.

Radionuclide scanning may detect avascular necrosis in bones, stress fractures, osteoid osteomas, inflammatory osteoarthritis and similar lesions.[4]

Foot and ankle pain in children

Apart from the common problem of trauma, special problems in children include:

- foreign bodies in the foot
- tumours, e.g. osteoid osteoma, osteosarcoma, Ewing's tumour
- plantar warts
- osteomyelitis/septic arthritis
- ingrowing toenails
- osteochondritis/aseptic necrosis
- osteochondritis dissecans of talus (in adolescents)
- pitted keratolysis and juvenile plantar dermatosis (adolescents)
- stress fractures

Osteochondritis/aseptic necrosis

Three important bones to keep in mind are:
- the calcaneum—Sever's disease
- the navicular—Köhler's disease
- the head of the second metatarsal—Freiberg's disease

Sever's disease is traction osteochondritis while the other disorders are a 'crushing' osteochondritis with avascular necrosis.

Sever's disease of the heel

This is calcaneal apophysitis which presents in a child (usually a boy) aged 8–12 (average of 10 years) with a painful tender heel at the insertion of tendoachilles. It is diagnosed by X-ray. The only treatment is to ensure that the child avoids wearing flat-heeled shoes and wears a slightly raised heel. Strenuous sporting activities should be restricted for 12 weeks.

Köhler's disease of the navicular

This disorder causes a painful limp (usually mild) with some swelling and tenderness around the navicular in a child (usually a boy) aged 3–6 years, although it is seen sometimes in older children. Complete recovery occurs with temporary resting. Sometimes a supportive strapping is helpful.

Freiberg's disease

This problem affects the head of the second metatarsal (rarely the third) which feels tender and swollen on palpation. It is more common in girls aged 12–16 and can present in young adults. Plain X-ray shows the characteristic collapse of the metatarsal head. The treatment is restriction of activity and protective padding.

Sprained ankle in a child

Children rarely sprain ligaments so it is important to assess apparent strains carefully, including an X-ray.

Skin disorders

Two conditions commonly seen in teenagers are pitted keratolysis and juvenile plantar dermatosis.

Pitted keratolysis

This malodorous condition known as 'stinky feet' or 'sneakers feet' is related to sweaty feet. Treatment includes keeping the feet dry and using an ointment such as Whitfield's or an imidazole or sodium fusidate to remove the responsible Corynebacterium organism. Change to all-leather shoes with charcoal liners.

Juvenile plantar dermatosis
'Sweaty sock dermatitis' is a painful condition of weight-bearing areas of the feet. The affected skin is red, shiny, smooth and often cracked. It is rare in adults. The treatment is to change to leather or open shoes and to cotton socks. A simple emollient cream gives excellent relief.

The little athlete
The 'little athlete' can suffer a variety of injuries from accidents and overuse. Diffuse heel pain, which is common, is most often related to Sever's apophysitis of the calcaneum. Occasionally, a juvenile-type plantar fasciitis may occur. Little athletes can develop tendinitis around the ankle, either on the lateral side (peroneals) or medially (tibialis posterior). Occasionally, a stress fracture of the metatarsals or other bones can occur.[3] Special attention must be paid to any developmental structural abnormalities and to footwear.

Foot and ankle problems in the elderly

Foot problems are more prevalent in old age. Some are due to a generalised disease such as diabetes or peripheral vascular disease, while others, such as bunions, hammer toes, calluses and corns, atrophy of the heel fat-pad and Morton's neuroma, increase with ageing. The transverse arch may flatten out and the protective pads under the metatarsals may atrophy, resulting in painful callosities.

Unfortunately, many elderly people regard foot problems as a normal process but these problems actually require considerable care and attention, especially in the presence of peripheral vascular disease, diabetes or rheumatoid arthritis. Deformed toenails (onychogryphosis) is also common albeit not a painful condition.

Flat foot occurring in middle age is usually due to stretching or rupture of the tibialis posterior tendon.[5]

Sprained ankle

There are two main ankle ligaments that are subject to heavy inversion or eversion stresses,

namely the lateral ligaments and the medial ligaments respectively. Most of the ankle 'sprains' or tears involve the lateral ligaments (up to 90%) while the stronger, tauter medial (deltoid) ligament is less prone to injury. It is important not to misdiagnose a complete rupture of the lateral ligaments.

Most sprains occur when the ankle is plantar flexed and inverted, such as when landing awkwardly after jumping or stepping on uneven ground. It is a very common sporting injury and is presented in more detail in Chapter 121.

Clinical features of sprained lateral ligaments
Common features:
- ankle 'gives way'
- difficulty in weight bearing
- discomfort varies from mild to severe
- bruising (may take 12–24 hours) indicates more severe injury
- may have functional instability: ankle gives way on uneven ground

Physical examination (perform as soon as possible):
- note swelling and bruising
- palpate over bony landmarks and three lateral ligaments (Fig. 121.9)
- test general joint laxity and range of motion
- a common finding is a rounded swelling in front of lateral malleolus (the 'signe de la coquille d'oeuf')
- test stability in A–P plane (anterior draw sign)

Is there an underlying fracture?
For a severe injury the possibility of a fracture—usually of the lateral malleolus or base of fifth metatarsal—must be considered. If the patient is able to walk without much discomfort straight after the injury a fracture is unlikely. However, as a rule, ankle injuries should be X-rayed.

Heel pain

Important causes of heel pain in adults (Fig. 62.3)[6] include:
- Achilles tendon disorders
  — tendinitis/peritendinitis (Chap. 121)
  — bursitis • postcalcaneal
      • retrocalcaneal
  — tendon tearing (Chap. 121) • partial
      • complete

- bruised heel
- tender heel pad—usually atrophy
  —also inflammation
- neuropathies, e.g. diabetic, alcoholic
- tenosynovitis (FHL, FDL)
- 'pump bumps'
- plantar fasciitis
- periostitis
- calcaneal apophysitis
- peroneal tendon dislocation
- nerve entrapments
  — tarsal tunnel
  — medial calcaneal nerve
  — nerve to abductor digiti minimi

Ultrasound examination is useful to differentiate the causes of Achilles tendon disorders.

Achilles tendinitis/peritendinitis

The inflammation is a combination of degenerative and inflammatory changes due to overuse and may occur either in the tendon itself or in the surrounding paratendon. The latter is called peritendinitis rather than tenosynovitis because there is no synovial sheath.

Achilles tendon bursitis

Bursitis can occur at two sites:

- posterior and superficial—between skin and tendon
- deep (retrocalcaneal)—between calcaneus and tendon (Fig. 62.3)

The former occurs mainly in young women from shoe friction and is readily palpated. Tenderness from the deep bursitis is elicited by squeezing in front of the tendon with the thumb and index finger: a swelling may be seen bulging on either side of the tendon.

Treatment

- avoid shoe pressure, e.g. wear sandals
- 1–2 cm heel raise inside the shoe
- apply local heat and ultrasound
- NSAIDs
- inject corticosteroid into bursa with a 25 g needle

Fat-pad disorders

The fat-pad, which consists of globules of fat encapsulated in multiple U-shaped scepti, acts as a hydraulic shock absorber on heel strike. It also contains significant nerve endings.[7] It can undergo atrophy, especially in the elderly, and also become inflamed. Problems are treated with an orthotic or an insert. Corticosteroids should be avoided as they can accelerate the atrophy.[6]

Plantar fasciitis

This common condition (also known as 'policeman's heel') is characterised by pain on the plantar aspect of the heel, especially on the medial side; it usually occurs about 5 cm from

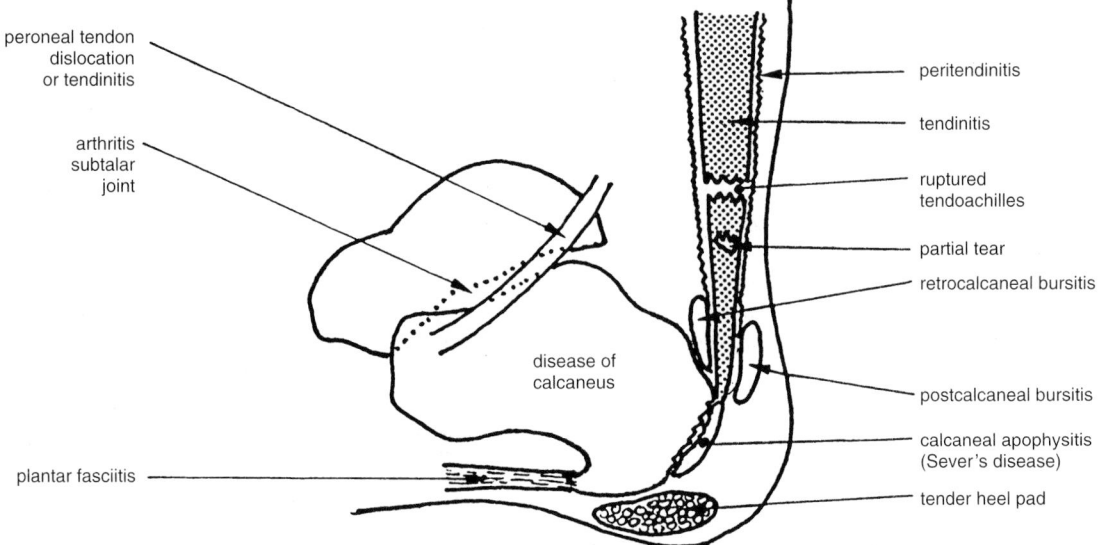

Fig. 62.3 *Important causes of the painful heel*

the posterior end of the heel although it can be experienced over a wide area beneath the heel. The pain radiates into the sole.

History
- Pain:
  - under the heel
  - first steps out of bed
  - relieved after walking about
  - increasing towards the end of the day
  - worse after sitting
- May be bilateral—usually worse on one side
- Typically over 40 years
- Both sexes
- Sometimes history of injury or overuse
- No constant relationship to footwear

Signs[8]
- Tenderness:
  - localised to medial tuberosity
  - may be more posterior
  - may be lateral
  - may be widespread
  - not altered by tensing fascia (but this action may cause pain)
- Heel pad may bulge or appear atrophic
- Crepitus may be felt
- No abnormality of gait, heel strike, or foot alignment
- Patient often obese

Treatment
Plantar fasciitis tends to heal spontaneously in 12–24 months. It has a variable response to treatment with NSAIDs, injections, ultrasound and insoles. Rest from long walks and from running is important.

Protection
Symptomatic relief is obtained by protecting the heel with an orthotic pad to include the heel and arch of the foot, e.g. Rose insole. Otherwise, a pad made from sponge or sorbo rubber that raises the heel about 1 cm is suitable. A hole corresponding to the tender area should be cut out of the pad to avoid direct contact with the sole.

Injection technique
Plantar fasciitis can be treated by injecting local anaesthetic and long-acting corticosteroid into the site of maximal tenderness in the heel. An alternative is to inject the corticosteroid into the anaesthetised heel.

Method

1. Perform a tibial nerve block. (The area of maximal tenderness should be marked prior to nerve block.)
2. When anaesthesia of the heel is present (about 10 minutes after the tibial nerve block), insert a 23 gauge needle with 1 mL of long-acting corticosteroid (e.g. methylprednisolone acetate) perpendicular to the sole of the foot at the premarked site (Fig. 62.4). Insert the needle until a 'give' is felt as the plantar fascia is pierced.
3. Inject half the steroid against the periosteum in the space between the fascia and calcaneus.
4. Reposition the needle to infiltrate into the fascial attachments over a wider area.

Arthritic conditions
Arthritis of the foot or ankle is a rather meaningless diagnosis and specificity is required. Typical sites of arthritic targets are shown in Figure 62.5.

Osteoarthritis
Osteoarthritis may occur in any of the joints of the foot but it commonly involves the first metatarsophalangeal joint (MTP), leading to hallux rigidus. It can affect the subtalar joint, but the ankle joint proper is usually not affected by osteoarthritis.

Hallux rigidus
Osteoarthritis of the first MTP joint can lead to gradual loss of motion of the toe and considerable discomfort. Roomy protective footwear and relative rest is the basis of treatment, coupled with daily self-mobilisation (stretching toe into

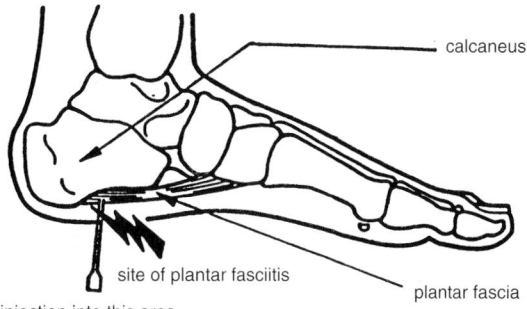

Fig. 62.4 *Injection approach for plantar fasciitis*

spondyloarthropathies ●
rheumatoid arthritis ■

gout

Osteoarthritis
(including hallux
rigidus)

Osteoarthritis
talonavicular joint
subtalar joint

Fig. 62.5 *Typical sites of arthritic causes of podalgia on skeleton of right foot (plantar aspect)*

plantar flexion morning and night). Other measures include manipulation under general anaesthesia or surgery (arthrodesis or arthroplasty) for severe cases.

Rheumatoid arthritis

Rheumatoid arthritis is typically a symmetrical polyarthritis presenting with pain in the metatarsophalangeal joints. It may also affect the ankle, mid-tarsal and tarsometatarsal joints. The interphalangeal joints are seldom affected primarily. It causes pain and stiffness under the balls of the feet, especially first thing in the morning.

Gout

Gout typically affects the first MTP and should be considered with the sudden onset of pain, especially in the presence of redness, swelling and tenderness. It can affect any synovial joint and occasionally may be polyarticular. Gout is often dismissed by the patient as a 'sprain'. A history of alcohol consumption or diuretic treatment is relevant.

Spondyloarthropathies

This group of arthritic disorders (Reiter's disease, ankylosing spondylitis, psoriatic arthritis and arthritides associated with chronic bowel disorders) may involve peripheral joints. Other foot involvement includes plantar fasciitis, Achilles tendinitis and sausage-shaped toes due to tenosynovitis, and arthritis of the proximal interphalangeal joints.

Foot strain

Foot strain is probably the commonest cause of podalgia. A foot may be strained by abnormal stress, or by normal stress for which it is not prepared. In foot strain the supporting ligaments become stretched, irritated and inflamed. It is commonly encountered in athletes who are relatively unfit or have a disorder such as flat feet, or in obese adults.

Symptoms and signs
- aching pain in foot and calf during or after prolonged walking or standing
- initial deep tenderness felt on medial border of plantar fascia (Fig. 62.6)
- worse with new shoes, especially a change to high heels

Acute foot strain

Acute ligamentous strain, such as occurs to the occasional athlete or to the person taking long unaccustomed walks, is usually self-limiting. It recovers rapidly with rest.

Chronic foot strain

Foot strain will become chronic with repeated excessive stress or with repeated normal stress on a mechanical abnormality. A common consequence is an everted foot leading to flattening of the longitudinal arch on weight bearing. It is important to establish whether the symptoms commenced after the patient began wearing a different type of footwear.

Treatment

The treatment is basically the same as that of the adult flat foot. Acute strain is treated with rest and by reducing walking to a minimum. Try the application of cold initially and then heat. The management of chronic strain is based on an exercise program and orthotics, including arch supports, to correct any deformity.

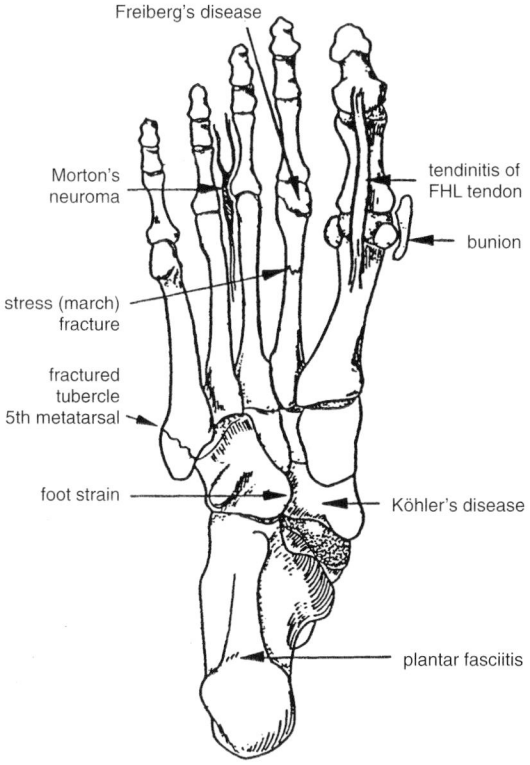

Freiberg's disease

Morton's
neuroma

stress (march)
fracture

fractured
tubercle
5th metatarsal

foot strain

tendinitis of
FHL tendon

bunion

Köhler's disease

plantar fasciitis

FHL: flexor hallucis longus

Fig. 62.6 *Typical sites of important causes of podalgia (other than arthritis)—right foot*

Sesamoiditis[10]

The two sesamoids that lie beneath the head of the first metatarsal may develop painful conditions such as chondromalacia, osteoarthritis and stress fractures. A special 'sesamoid' X-ray assists diagnosis. Painful callus can develop over here in the elderly. Well designed insoles are usually effective as is surgical excision for persistent problems.

Metatarsalgia

Metatarsalgia is not a disease but refers to pain and tenderness over the plantar heads of metatarsals. Causes include foot deformities (especially with depression of the transverse arch), arthritis of the MTP joints, trauma, Morton's neuroma, Freiberg's disease and entrapment neuropathy.

Depression of the transverse arch results in abnormal pressure on the second, third and fourth metatarsal heads with possible callus formation. Repetitive foot strain, pes cavus and high heels may cause a maldistribution of weight to the forefoot.

Treatment involves treating any known cause, advising proper footwear and perhaps a metatarsal bar. Flat-heeled shoes with ample width seldom cause problems in the metatarsal region.

Tibialis posterior tendon rupture

Rupture of the tibialis posterior tendon after inflammation, degeneration or trauma[9] is a relatively common and misdiagnosed disorder, especially in middle-aged females. It causes collapse of the longitudinal arch of the foot, leading to a flat foot.[5]

It is uncommon for patients to feel obvious discomfort at the moment of rupture. They may subsequently present with the sudden appearance of an 'abnormal' flat foot. There is gross eversion of the foot.

A simple test is the 'too many toes' test whereby more toes are seen on the affected side when the feet are viewed from about 3 metres behind the patient (Fig. 62.7).[5] The single heel raise test is also diagnostic. The most useful investigation is an ultrasound examination. Minor cases can be treated conservatively but severe problems respond well to surgical correction.

Fig. 62.7 *Tibialis posterior rupture (right foot): the 'too many toes' posterior view*

Stress fractures

Clinical features:

• The aches or pains may be slow in onset or sudden.

- Common in dancers, especially classical ballet, and in unfit people taking up exercise.
- Examination is often unhelpful: swelling uncommon.[11]
- Routine X-rays often unhelpful.
- A bone scan is the only way to confirm the suspected diagnosis.
- Basis of treatment is absolute rest for six or more weeks with strong supportive footwear.
- A walking plaster is not recommended.

Avulsion fracture of base of fifth metatarsal
Known also as a Jones fracture; it is usually a traumatic fracture but can be a stress fracture and associated with severe ankle sprains.

March fracture of metatarsal
Stress or fatigue fracture of the forefoot usually involves the neck of the second metatarsal (sometimes the third).

Tarsals, especially navicular
Stress fracture of the navicular, which is a disorder of athletes involved with running sports, presents as poorly localised midfoot pain during weight bearing. Examination and plain X-ray are usually normal. It is a recently recognised serious disorder due to the advent of nuclear bone scans and CT scans. A protracted course of treatment can be expected.

Calcaneum
Stress fractures of the os calcis usually have an insidious onset. Osteoporosis is a predisposing factor as is an increased training program.[6]

Morton's neuroma
Morton's neuroma is probably misdiagnosed more often than any other painful condition of the forefoot. It is not a true neuroma and its aetiology is still uncertain. The diagnosis is made on clinical grounds and special investigations are of no help. An ultrasound examination may exclude a cyst or ganglion but rarely shows a neuroma.

Clinical features
- usually presents in adults < 50
- four times more common in women
- bilateral in 15% of cases

- commonest between third and fourth metatarsal heads (Fig. 62.8), then 2–3 (otherwise uncommon)
- severe burning pain between third and fourth toes
- worse on weight bearing on hard surfaces (standing and walking)
- aggravated by wearing tight shoes
- relieved by taking off shoe and squeezing the forefoot
- localised tenderness between metatarsal heads

Treatment
Early problems are treated conservatively by wearing loose shoes with a low heel and using a sponge rubber metatarsal pad. An orthosis with a dome under the affected interspace helps to spread the metatarsals and thus takes pressure off the nerve. Most eventually require surgical excision, preferably with a dorsal approach.

Hallux valgus
Hallux valgus with associated bunion formation and splaying of the forefoot is common. It may be a consequence of poor-fitting footwear.

A bunionette, also caused by pressure, may form over the fifth metatarsal.

Pain, if present, may be due to shoe pressure on an inflamed bunion, a hammer toe, metatarsalgia or secondary arthritis of the first metatarsophalangeal joint.

Hallux valgus with bunions should be treated by correcting footwear prior to any surgical correction.

Fig. 62.8 *Morton's neuroma: typical site and pain distribution*

Callus, corn and wart

The diagnosis of localised, tender lumps on the sole of the foot can be difficult. The differential diagnosis of callus, corn and wart is aided by an understanding of their morphology and the effect of paring these lumps (Table 62.3).

A callus (Fig. 62.9) is simply a localised area of hyperkeratosis related to some form of pressure and friction. It is very common under the metatarsal heads, especially the second.

A corn (Fig. 62.10) is a small, localised, conical thickening. It may resemble a plantar wart but gives a different appearance on paring.

A wart (Fig. 62.11) is more invasive, and paring reveals multiple small, pinpoint bleeding spots.

Fig. 62.9 *Callus*

Fig. 62.10 *Corn*

Fig. 62.11 *Plantar wart*

Treatment

Calluses

No treatment is required if asymptomatic. Remove the cause. Proper footwear is essential—wide enough shoes and cushioned pads over ball of foot. Proper paring gives relief, also filing with callus files. If severe, apply daily applications of 10% salicylic acid in soft paraffin with regular paring.

Corns

Remove cause of friction and use wide shoes to allow the foot to expand to its full width. Soften corn with a few daily applications of 15% salicylic acid in collodion and then pare. For soft corns between the toes (usually last toe-web) keep the toe-webs separated with lamb's wool at all times and dust with a foot powder.

Plantar warts

There are many treatments for this common and at times frustrating problem. A good rule is to avoid scalpel excision, diathermy and electrocautery because of the problem of scarring. One of the problems with the removal of plantar warts is the 'iceberg' configuration—not all the wart may be removed.

Table 62.3 *Comparison of the main causes of a lump on the sole of the foot*

	Typical site	*Nature*	*Effect of paring*
Callus	where skin is normally thick: beneath heads of metatarsals, heels, inframedial side of great toe	hard, thickened skin	normal skin
Corn	where skin is normally thin: on soles, fifth toe, dorsal projections of hammer toes	white, conical mass of keratin, flattened by pressure	exposes white, avascular corn with concave surface
Wart	anywhere, mainly over metatarsal heads, base of toes and heels; has bleeding points	viral infection, with abrupt change from skin at edge	exposes bleeding points

Methods of removal

- Liquid nitrogen
  — pare wart (a 21g blade is recommended)
  — apply liquid nitrogen
  — repeat weekly

Can be painful and the results are often disappointing.

- Topical chemotherapy
  — pare wart (particularly in children)
  — apply Upton's paste to wart each night and cover
  — review if necessary

(Upton's paste comprises trichloracetic acid 1 part, salicylic acid 6 parts, glycerin 2 parts.)

- Topical chemotherapy and liquid nitrogen
  — pare wart
  — apply paste of 70% salicylic acid in raw linseed oil
  — occlude for 1 week
  — pare on review, then apply liquid nitrogen and review
- Curettage under local anaesthetic
  — pare the wart vigorously to reveal its extent
  — thoroughly curette the entire wart with a dermal curette
  — hold the foot dependent over kidney dish until bleeding stops (this always stops spontaneously and avoids a bleed later on the way home)
  — apply 50% trichloracetic acid to the base
- Occlusion with topical chemotherapy: a method of using salicylic acid in a paste under a special occlusive dressing is described.

Equipment
  — 2.5 cm (width) elastic adhesive tape
  — 30% salicylic acid in Lassar's paste of plasticine consistency

Method
  — Cut two lengths of adhesive tape, one about 5 cm and the other shorter.
  — Fold the shorter length in half, sticky side out (Fig. 62.12a).
  — Cut a half-circle at the folded edge to accommodate the wart.
  — Press this tape down so that the hole is over the wart.
  — Roll a small ball of the paste in the palm of the hand and then press it into the wart.

(a)

sticky side

(b)

wart and salicylic acid paste

long strip

short strip

Fig. 62.12 *Treatment of plantar wart:* **(a)** *'window' to fit the wart is cut out of shoulder of elastic adhesive tape;* **(b)** *larger strip covers the wart and shoulder strip*

  — Cover the tape, paste and wart with the longer strip of tape (Fig. 62.12b).
  — This paste should be reapplied twice daily for 2–3 weeks. The reapplication is achieved by peeling back the longer strip to expose the wart, adding a fresh ball of paste to the wart and then re-covering with the upper tape.

The plantar wart invariably crumbles, and vanishes. If the wart is particularly stubborn, 50% salicylic acid can be used.

Ingrown toenail (onychocryptosis)

Ingrown toenail is a very common condition, especially in adolescent boys. Although not so common in adults, it may follow injury or deformity of the nail bed. It is typically located along the lateral edges of the great toenail and represents an imbalance between the soft tissues of the nail fold and the growing nail edge. The basic cause is a redundant skin fold. It is exacerbated by faulty nail trimming, constricting shoes and poor hygiene. A skin breach is followed by infection, then oedema and granulation tissue of the nail fold.[5]

Treatment

Prevention

All patients should be instructed on correct foot and nail care. Foot hygiene includes foot baths, avoiding nylon socks, and frequent changes of cotton or wool socks. Cotton wool pledgets can be placed beneath the nail edge to assist separation.

It is important to fashion the toenails so that the corners project beyond the skin (Fig. 62.13). The end of the nail (not the corners) should be cut squarely so that the nail can grow out from the nail fold. Then each day, after a shower or bath, use the pads of both thumbs to pull the nail folds as indicted.

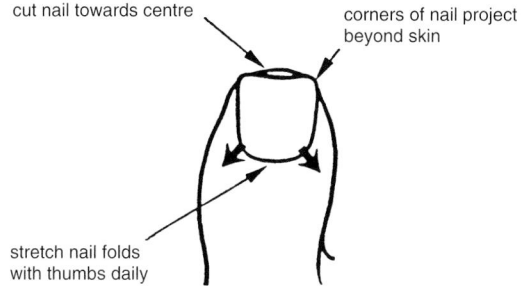

cut nail towards centre
corners of nail project beyond skin
stretch nail folds with thumbs daily

Fig. 62.13 *Method of fashioning toenails*

Surgical methods

1. *Excision of ellipse of skin.* This 'army method' transposes the skin fold away from the nail. The skin heals, the nail grows normally and the toe retains its normal anatomy.

   Under digital block, an elliptical excision is made such that the skin fold is forced off the nail with a blunt instrument and held there by the wound closure (Fig. 62.14). Any granulation tissue and debris should be removed with a curette.

2. *Electrocautery.* This is similar in principle to the preceding method but is simple, quick and very effective with minimal after-pain, especially for severe ingrowing with much granulation tissue. Under digital block the electrocautery needle removes a large wedge of skin and granulation tissue so that the ingrown nail stands free of skin (Fig. 62.15).

3. *Skin wedge excision.* Another similar method under digital block is to dissect away all the skin fold adjacent to the nail, starting from the nail base, extending proximally for about

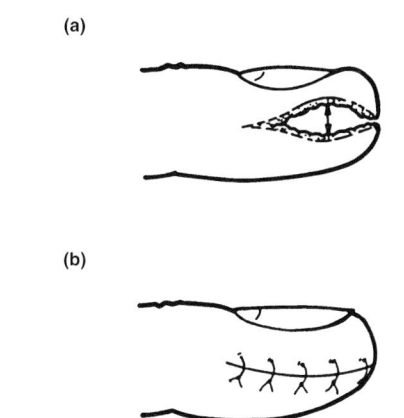

(a)

(b)

Fig. 62.14 *Treatment of ingrown toenail: excision of ellipse of skin*

4 mm and then sweeping around the side of the nail to under its tip, using a 3–4 mm margin all the way. Removal includes granulation and subcutaneous tissue. Bleeding points are cauterised and the raw area dressed. Dressings are necessary for the next 4–6 weeks.

4. *Wedge of nail excision and phenolisation.* This method uses 80% phenol (concentrated solution) to treat the nail bed following excision with scissors of a wedge for about one quarter of the length (rather than a standard wedge resection) of the ingrown nail. A cotton wool stick soaked in phenol is introduced deep into the space of the nail bed (Fig. 62.16). Leave the stick in this site for 3 minutes (by the clock). Then remove and flush this pocket with isotonic saline or alcohol, then dry with a cotton wool stick. Dress with paraffin gauze, then with dry gauze. Re-dress as appropriate. The success rate is almost 100%.

electrocautery needle

ingrowing nail lies free

cauterised wedge of tissue

Fig. 62.15 *Treatment of ingrown toenail: electrocautery of wedge of tissue*

Fig. 62.16 *Phenolisation method*

Warning: Take care not to spill the phenol onto the surrounding skin as it is very corrosive.

Paronychia

Initial treatment:

- antiseptic (e.g. Betadine)-soaked dressing
- elevation of nail fold to drain pus
- application of petroleum gauze dressing
- antibiotics if extensive or cellulitis developing

Sometimes the nail requires avulsion to establish free drainage of a periungual abscess.

Practice tips

- Good-quality X-rays are mandatory in all severely sprained ankle injuries.
- If in doubt about the diagnosis of a painful foot—X-ray.
- Children rarely sprain ligaments. All joint injuries causing pain and swelling in children need to be X-rayed.
- Think of the rare problem of a dislocating peroneal tendon if a sharp click and stab of pain is experienced just behind and below the lateral malleolus.
- Paraesthesia of part or whole of the foot may be caused by peripheral neuropathy, tarsal tunnel syndrome, mononeuritis, e.g. diabetes mellitus, rheumatoid arthritis or a nerve root lesion from the lumbosacral spine.

- Avoid giving injections of corticosteroids into the Achilles tendon.
- Avoid invasive procedures such as surgical excision, diathermy or electrocautery for plantar warts. Be aware of the limitations of liquid nitrogen.
- High-resolution ultrasound can help diagnose Achilles tendon disorders.
- Keep in mind the possibility of pain around the sesamoid bones of the first metatarsal.

References

1. Johnson FL. The painful foot: an overview of podalgia. Aust Fam Physician, 1987; 16:1086.
2. Cailliet R. *Foot and ankle pain*. Philadelphia: FA Davis, 1983, 105–115.
3. Larkins PA. The little athlete. Aust Fam Physician, 1991; 20:973–978.
4. de Jager JP. Problems with the shoulder, knee, ankle and foot. Med J Aust, 1996; 165: 570–571.
5. Quirk R. Flat foot in middle age: diagnosis and treatment. Mod Med Aust, 1995; 38(11): 44–47.
6. Brown CH. A review of subcalcaneal heel pain and plantar fasciitis. Aust Fam Physician, 1996; 25: 875–885.
7. Jahss MH et al. Investigations into the fat-pads of the sole of the foot: anatomy and histology. Foot and Ankle, 1992; 13: 233–242.
8. Harbison S. Plantar fasciitis. Aust Fam Physician, 1987; 16:113.
9. Masterton E et al. The planovalgus rheumatoid foot—is tibialis tendon rupture a factor? Br J Rheumatol, 1995; 34: 645–646.
10. Quirk R. Metatarsalgia. Aust Fam Physician, 1996; 25: 863–869.
11. Quirk R. Stress fractures of the foot. Aust Fam Physician, 1987; 16:1101–1102.

63
Walking difficulty

—

The clinical evaluation of the patient presenting with difficulty walking can be very complex especially for abnormal gaits caused by neurological conditions. Not all gaits fall into a single category; gait disturbances may be multifactorial especially in the elderly.

Non-neurological conditions are the most common cause of walking difficulties. They include various arthritic conditions of the lower limbs, usually presenting as a limp, other mechanical factors such as swelling of the legs, disorders of circulation such as intermittent claudication, and general debility, e.g. malignancy, anaemia and endocrine disorders such as hyperparathyroidism.

It is important for the general practitioner not to overlook hypokalaemia and drugs or the myopathies as a cause of walking difficulty. The drugs that require special consideration include alcohol, corticosteroids, chloroquine, colchicine, clofibrate, bretylium, HMG-CoA reductase inhibitors (the statins), gemfibrozil, clofibrate, penicillamine, diuretics, beta-blockers and general anaesthetic agents.

Abnormal gaits

It is convenient to classify abnormal gaits as painless or painful (antalgic). With antalgic gaits the rhythm is disturbed; with painless abnormal gaits the contour is affected. One type of skeletal mechanical abnormality is described as arthrogenic (due particularly to hip disorders) and a second type as osteogenic (due to a shortened limb).

Neurogenic gaits and myogenic gaits are considered together below, under the heading 'Neurological disorders of gait'.

Psychogenic or 'hysterical' gait may have to be considered if the gait is bizarre or seems greatly exaggerated. On the other hand, loss of confidence, especially in the elderly, is an important cause of gait disturbance. However, many abnormal gaits that are caused by neurological disease may also appear bizarre, and caution is advised. Doubtful cases should be referred for an expert opinion.

Examination of gait and posture[1]

Disorders of gait and posture go hand in hand because of a common physiological process.

The source of the abnormality is indicated.

1. Ask the patient to stand.

   Note any difficulty in reaching a standing position. Difficulty = proximal muscle weakness.

2. Ask the patient to stand with eyes closed (Romberg's test).

   If positive (sways or falls) = loss of proprioception, e.g. peripheral neuropathy.

3. Ask the patient to walk (ensure sufficient testing length).

   - Gait initiation — hesitancy = basal ganglia or frontal cortex
   - Stride length — very short = basal ganglia or frontal cortex
     irregular = cerebellar
   - Narrow or broad base — narrow = UMN, muscle weakness, basal ganglia
     broad = cerebellum, proprioception, vestibular

- Stiff or 'sloppy'   stiff = UMN, basal ganglia sloppy = LMN, muscle weakness
- Heel strike   loss of normal strike = UMN, LMN, myopathy
- High stepping   positive = LMN (distal), proprioception, muscle weakness
- Arm swing   decreased = basal ganglia, UMN (frontal lobes)
- Pelvis control   Trendelenburg gait = proximal muscle weakness

4. Ask the patient to walk using provocation tests.
   - 'Tightrope' walk   tests proprioception
   - Stand on tiptoes and back on the heels   tests distal muscle weakness

Note: Peripheral neuropathy is a common cause of an LMN lesion.

Neurological disorders of gait

Cerebellar gait

The patient has difficulty standing, has a broad-based stance and an unsteady gait, with swaying from side to side. It has been described as the 'dirty diaper' gait. The patient may stagger or bump into walls and may be accused of being drunk. When asked to walk in a straight line the patient tends to veer towards the side of the lesion. Ask the patient to walk 'heel to toe' in a straight line and perform a heel-knee-shin test to demonstrate cerebellar ataxia. Significant causes are multiple sclerosis, alcoholic cerebellar degeneration and space-occupying lesions.

Basal ganglia gait (Parkinson's type)

Identifying this disorder in its early stages can be difficult as the first sign may be a limp with one leg being described as weak or stiff or slow.[2] However, the typical gait is a shuffling of the feet with small steps in a forward flexed posture. This leads to a hurrying (festinant) gait as though there is an impending feeling of falling forward.

Spastic gait

Spastic gait may be regarded as the typical bilateral or paraplegic gait, or as a hemiplegic gait. With the former the gait affects both legs—they are stiff or weak, leading to slow, jerking walking, dragging of the feet and scraping of the toes. This scuffing can be heard as the front of the shoe drags along the ground. Every step can be a struggle and the patient may appear as though walking through glue on the floor.

A scissor-type gait will develop with bilateral hip adduction. Spasticity is caused by an upper motor neurone lesion, including multiple sclerosis and spinal cord compression. The typical UMN posture is of a flexed upper limb and an extended lower limb.

With hemiplegia the patient drags the affected leg stiffly with the hips adducted, the knee extended and the foot plantar flexed, leading to scraping of the toes. Mounting stairs can be very difficult especially if clonus is induced with dorsiflexion of the foot.

Foot drop gait

The patient cannot dorsiflex the foot, leading to a high-stepping gait with extra flexion of the hip and knees to lift the foot off the ground. The foot then slaps down on the ground.

Vestibular gait

If unilateral the patient tends to veer off to the side of the lesion.

Apraxia

With apraxia of gait (due to a prefrontal lobe lesion) there is a failure of control of the legs. The patient may stand up and try to walk but looks with bewilderment at the legs and moves them in an inappropriate manner with a broad-based, small-stepping unsteady gait. Turning is difficult. Apraxia is caused by bilateral cortical involvement such as hydrocephalus, multi-infarct states and tumours of the corpus callosum.[2]

Neurogenic claudication

With intermittent claudication of the cauda equina, due to spinal canal stenosis, the patient develops pain in the leg after walking a certain distance. However, weakness and numbness are usually more prominent than pain.

Drop attacks

In a drop attack the patient suddenly falls to the ground, without other symptoms, and gets up almost immediately. There is no loss of consciousness. Drop attacks can be caused by disorders such as epilepsy, Parkinson's disease and vertebrobasilar insufficiency. However, in most cases, particularly middle-aged and elderly women, there is no obvious cause.

Waddling gait

A waddling gait is usually caused by muscular dysfunction affecting the pelvic girdle muscles and trunk. There is a wide-based gait with a marked 'rocking and rolling' body swing from side to side and related compensatory movements of the pelvis, that is a bilateral Trendelenburg gait.

Proximal muscle weakness

The patient may complain when getting out of a low chair or going up or down stairs. The weakness can be demonstrated by asking the patient to squat down and, after a second, rise from the squatting position.[2] Waddling of gait reflects extreme cases. Causes include myopathies, motor neurone disease and Guillain-Barré syndrome.

Distal muscle weakness

This causes a high-stepping gait as the foot is floppy and tends to flap, with walking similar to foot drop gait. Causes include peripheral neuropathy, myotonic dystrophy and peroneal muscular atrophy.

Limp

Limp is a symptom commonly associated with painful disorders of the lower limb, especially of the hip and knee joints. A limp implies an asymmetrical gait pattern caused by one of four general factors:

1. unequal leg length
2. antalgic (painful) gait, e.g. hip disorder
3. restricted joint movement, e.g. ankylosed knee
4. neuromuscular weakness, e.g. poliomyelitis

Limp has an inseparable relationship with painful hip and buttock conditions, especially those of the hip. Painful hip and pelvic conditions that cause limp are presented on pages 601–603.

Limp in adults

In adults the cause of limp is usually more obvious than in children and is commonly due to degenerative osteoarthritis of the hip or knee, to spinal disorders, especially sciatica caused by a disc prolapse, or to overuse disorders of the knee, ankle or foot.

Limp in children

The child who limps presents an interesting diagnostic dilemma. The limp must be considered to be due to a definite organic cause, although conversion reactions can be a factor.[3] It is appropriate to focus initially on the hip. The diagnostic strategy is presented in Table 63.1.

Table 63.1 *Limp in children: diagnostic strategy (modified)*

Q. *Probability diagnosis*
A. Post trauma/intense exercise causing strain syndromes
Ill-fitting shoes
Hip disorders, esp. transient synovitis
Heel disorders (12–14 years)

Q. *Must not be missed*
A. Toddlers: developmental dysplasia hip
child abuse
septic arthritis
foreign body, e.g. needle in foot
Adolescents: SCFE
avulsion injuries, e.g. ischial tuberosity
osteochondritis dissecans of knee
4–8 years: Perthes' disorder
transient synovitis
All groups: septic infections
• septic arthritis
• osteomyelitis
• tuberculosis
tumour, e.g. osteosarcoma
juvenile chronic arthritis
spinal disorders
• discitis
• fracture

Q. *Pitfalls (often missed)*
A. Foreign body, e.g. in foot
Osteochondritis (aseptic necrosis)
• femoral head—Perthes' disorder
• knee—Osgood-Schlatter's disorder
• calcaneum—Sever's disorder
• navicular—Köhler's disorder
Myalgia = 'growing pains'
Overuse syndrome (esp. adolescent)
• patellar tendinitis (jumper's knee)
Stress fractures, e.g. tibia, femoral neck, navicular

Limp can be considered as acute, subacute or chronic. An acute limp may be due to injury, infection (osteomyelitis, septic arthritis), spinal injuries, a fracture or an irritable hip (transient synovitis). Subacute causes include juvenile rheumatoid arthritis and tumour or leukaemia. Chronic causes include cerebral palsy, developmental dysplasia of the hip, Perthes' disease and chronic SCFE.

Key checkpoints

- Trauma, sepsis and developmental dysplasia (formerly congenital dislocation) of the hip (DDH) are perhaps the most common reasons for an infant to limp and refuse to walk. However, a painless waddling gait suggests DDH or Perthes' disease, which usually begins with a painless limp.
- Multiple fractures and epiphyseal separations in toddlers are highly suggestive of child battering; a skeletal survey should be ordered if this is suspected.
- Perthes' disorder can present from ages 4 to 12 but is usually found from 4–8 years with a peak age of 5–7.
- Infections of and around the hip joints are most common in infancy. Classically, the hip is held immobile in about 30° of flexion with slight abduction and external rotation. The commonest organism is *Staphylococcus aureus*, followed by *Haemophilus influenzae*.
- Tuberculosis may also occur in children (usually under 10 years) with a presentation similar to Perthes' disease.
- Slipped capital femoral epiphysis (SCFE) typically presents in the obese adolescent (10–15 years) with knee pain and a slight limp.
- Growing pains are a controversial issue but do appear to exist as an aching myalgia usually manifest in the leg muscles (anterior thigh, calf, posterior knee). The pain is bilateral, non-articular and usually unrelated to activity.

Diagnostic approach

History
The age of the patient gives a diagnostic pointer. A careful history, especially of trauma, may lead to the diagnosis. A history of injury is usually but not always available. The relationship of the limp to exercise and footwear is significant. The location of any associated pain is relevant: low back pathology can refer to the buttocks and hip pathology can cause knee pain.

Examination
The hip and knee joints should be carefully examined if the source of limp has no specific localisation. Get the child to walk and run on the toes and heels (if appropriate). Note the gait and check whether it is antalgic (painful), hemiplegic (the arm is held out in a balancing action) or Trendelenburg (classic for DDH). Look for evidence of muscular dystrophy.

Investigations
The following have to be considered:
- FBE and ESR
- blood culture
- needle aspiration of joint
- radiological investigations
  — plain X-ray
  — ultrasound
  — bone scan
  — CT scan

Management
Management is based on the cause. Surgical drainage supplemented with antibiotics is essential for septic arthritis. If the child initially has a limp and cannot walk, admit to hospital for:
- skin traction
- FBE and ESR
- ultrasound of hip
- blood culture

| Specific conditions |

Osteomyelitis
Osteomyelitis should be suspected in a child with an acute febrile illness and metaphyseal tenderness and the child admitted to hospital. Blood should be collected for an FBE, ESR and culture. An IV line should be inserted and IV antibiotics commenced.
> 5 years: flucloxacillin
< 5 years: flucloxacillin + cefotaxime or ceftriaxone

Septic arthritis
Septic arthritis should be suspected in a child with pyrexia and an acute arthritis with limited motion. Manage as for osteomyelitis.

Bone tumour

Chronic limp is a common presentation of malignant bone tumours. Radiological investigation is mandatory.

Irritable hip syndrome (transient synovitis)

Typical age is 3–8 years and the child presents with an acute limp with restricted hip motion. Plain X-ray is normal. Orthopaedic assessment is recommended.

Perthes' disorder, SCFE and DDH

Refer to Chapter 59.

Paget's disease

Paget's disease of bone (osteitis deformans) is a chronic disorder of the adult skeleton in which new soft bone replaces localised areas of normal bone. The cause is unknown but a viral aetiology is suspected. There is a great increase in bone turnover with osteoclastic resorption followed by increased osteoblastic activity. The disorder is quite common:

1 in 200 of the population at age 40
1 in 10 of population at age 90

Paget's disease is usually asymptomatic but some patients may present with deep aching pain in the lower back and lower limbs. They may also present with a disturbance of gait due to unequal leg length, osteoarthritis of associated joints such as the knee or hip, or a change in the distribution of mechanical forces in the lower extremities.

Features

- M:F ratio = 2:1.
- 95% asymptomatic (discovered by X-ray or raised serum alkaline phosphatase).
- Symptoms may include joint pain and stiffness (e.g. hips, knees), bone pain (usually spine), deformity, headache and deafness.
- Bone pain is typically deep and aching; it occurs at rest, particularly at night.
- Signs may include deformity, enlarged skull ('hats don't fit any more'), bowing of tibia, waddling gait, hyperdynamic circulation (Fig. 63.1).
- Bones most commonly affected, in decreasing order, are the pelvis, femur, skull, tibia, vertebrae, clavicle and humerus.

Diagnosis

- Raised serum alkaline phosphatase (often very high > 1000 U/L).

Note: calcium and phosphate normal.
- Plain X-ray: dense expanded bone—best seen in skull and pelvis.
Note: can mimic prostatic secondaries so every male Pagetic patient should have a DRE and serum PSA.
- Bone isotopic scans: useful in locating specific areas.

Treatment[4]

The two major goals are relief of pain and prevention of long-term complication, e.g. deafness, deformities.

Localised and asymptomatic disease requires no treatment.

Three groups of drugs are currently available:

- the calcitonins
- the biphosphonates, i.e. etidronate, pamidronate disodium (APD), alendronate
- various antineoplastic agents, e.g. mithramycin

Biphosphonates have become the preferred drugs for first-line therapy and include[4]

- alendronate 40 mg (o) daily for 6 months (oesophagitis can be problematic)
- pamidronate disodium 45–60 mg IV infused over 4–8 hours (usually the preferred option)
- risedronate 30 mg (o) daily for 2 months

Repeated doses may rarely be required in severe cases as judged by symptoms and disease activity, e.g. monitoring with serum ALP.

Leg swelling

Diagnostic features and pitfalls

- Not all swollen legs require investigation and treatment.
- The significance of leg swelling varies according to the age group, to whether it is bilateral or unilateral, and whether the onset is sudden or gradual.
- Deep venous thrombosis (DVT) must be considered in all unilateral cases and ultrasound examination performed if appropriate.
- If a DVT is present, consider occult malignancy, e.g. Ca pancreas.
- Consider pelvic cancer causing lymphatic obstruction in a woman >40 years presenting with painless unilateral leg oedema.
- A drug history is essential as several drugs can cause oedema.
- Pitting oedema is a feature of venous thrombosis or insufficiency, not lymphatic obstruction.

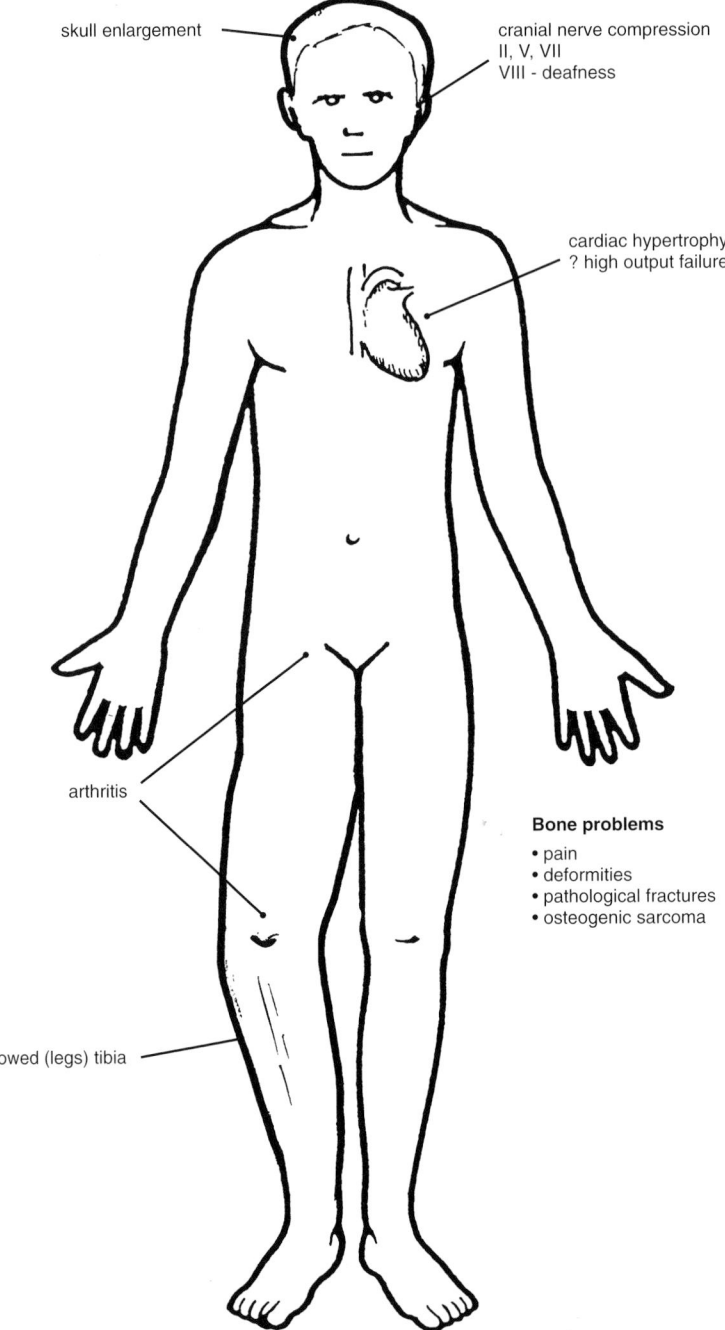

Fig. 63.1 *Paget's disease: possible clinical features*

Investigations

Select from these first-line tests:

- urinalysis (? albumin)
- FBE and ESR
- serum urea/creatinine
- serum albumin/LFTs
- ultrasound (DVT screen)
- other radiographs, e.g. CT scan, venogram

Table 63.2 *Causes of swollen legs*

Physiological
- prolonged standing or walking
- prolonged sitting, e.g. elderly on long journey
- pregnancy
- hot weather
- mechanical factors, e.g. constricting garters/pantyhose

Local disorders
- skin, e.g. allergy
- arthritis with particular oedema
- infection, e.g. cellulitis, filariasis
- trauma
- thrombophlebitis
- vascular obstruction
  - — venous, e.g. DVT, varicose veins
  - — lymphatic → lymphoedema

Generalised disease
- cardiac, e.g. CCF
- renal, e.g. nephrotic syndrome
- hepatic, e.g. cirrhosis

Drugs
- NSAIDS, antihypertensives (e.g. nifedipine), oestrogens, others

Lipoedema

Lymphoedema: primary or secondary

Idiopathic (periodic) oedema

Table 63.3 *Swollen legs: diagnostic perspective*

Probability diagnosis
Chronic venous insufficiency (varicose veins)
Physiological, e.g. dependency

Must not be missed
Deep venous thrombosis
Thrombophlebitis
Obstruction from pelvic cancer

Pitfalls
Drugs (sodium retention)
Idiopathic (cyclical) oedema

Calf swelling of sudden onset

Causes to consider:
- acute arterial occlusion
- ruptured Baker's cyst
- ruptured medial head gastrocnemius
- DVT (usually gradual)
- cellulitis/erysipelas
- compartment syndrome

Pain accompanies most of these conditions but the absence of pain does not exclude DVT or thrombophlebitis.

Lipoedema

Lipoedema is the development of bilateral leg swelling that does not involve the feet (in lymphoedema the swelling develops in the most distal part of the foot).

Features
- exclusive to obese women
- spares the feet
- bilateral and symmetrical distribution of fat

References

1. Horne M. Gait and postural disorders. Monash University Neurology Notes 1996; 1–4.
2. Kincaid-Smith P, Larkins R, Whelan G. *Problems in clinical medicine.* Sydney: MacLennan & Petty, 1990; 190–194.
3. Efron D, Nolan T. *Paediatric handbook* (5th edn). Melbourne: Blackwell Science, 1996: 237–251.
4. Moulds RFW (Chairman). Therapeutic guidelines: endocrinology. Melbourne VMPF 1997–98; 103–106.

64

Palpitations

Palpitations are an unpleasant awareness of the beating of the heart. By definition it does not always imply 'racing' of the heart but any sensation in the chest such as 'pounding', 'flopping', 'skipping', 'jumping', 'thumping' or 'fluttering' of the heart. The problem requires careful attention and reassurance (if appropriate) because heartbeat is regarded as synonymous with life. To the practitioner it may simply represent anxiety or it could be a prelude to a cardiac arrest.

Key facts and checkpoints

- The symptom of palpitations is suggestive of cardiac arrhythmia but may have a non-cardiac cause.
- Palpitations not related to emotion, fever or exercise suggest an arrhythmia.
- Perhaps the commonest arrhythmia causing a patient to visit the family doctor is the symptomatic premature ventricular beat (ventricular ectopic).
- The commonest cause of an apparent pause on the ECG is a blocked premature atrial beat (atrial ectopic).
- A 12 lead electrocardiographic diagnosis is mandatory. If the cause is not documented, an ambulatory electrographic monitor (e.g. Holter) may be used.
- Consider myocardial ischaemia as a cause of the arrhythmia.

- Consider drugs as a cause, including prescribed drugs and non-prescribed such as alcohol, caffeine and cigarettes.
- Common triggers of paroxysmal supraventricular tachycardia (PSVT) include anxiety and cigarette smoking.
- The commonest mechanism of any arrhythmia is re-entry.
- Get patients to tap out the rate and rhythm of their abnormal beat.

A diagnostic approach

A summary of the safety diagnostic model is presented in Table 64.1, which includes significant causes of palpitations.

Probability diagnosis

If the palpitations are not caused by anxiety or fever, the common causes are sinus tachycardia and premature beats (atrial or ventricular). Sinus tachycardia, which by definition is a rate of 100–160/minute, may be precipitated by emotion, stress, fever or exercise.

Paroxysmal supraventricular tachycardia (PSVT) and atrial fibrillation are also quite common arrhythmias. Some cardiologists claim that the commonest arrhythmia causing a patient to visit the family doctor is the symptomatic ventricular ectopic.[1]

Sinus tachycardia can be differentiated clinically from PSVT in that it starts and stops more gradually than PSVT (abrupt) and has a lower rate of 100–150 compared with 160–220.

Serious disorders not to be missed

It is vital not to overlook myocardial infarction or other myocardial ischaemia, such as unstable angina, as a cause of the arrhythmia manifesting

Table 64.1 *Palpitations: diagnostic strategy model*

Q. *Probability diagnosis*
A. Anxiety
   Premature beats (ectopics)
   Sinus tachycardia
   Drugs, e.g. stimulants

Q. *Serious disorders not to be missed*
A. Myocardial infarction/angina
   Arrhythmias
   • ventricular tachycardia
   • bradycardia
   • sick sinus syndrome
   • torsade de pointes
   WPW syndrome
   Electrolyte disturbances
   • hypokalaemia
   • hypomagnesaemia
   • hypoglycaemia (IDDM)

Q. *Pitfalls (often missed)*
A. Fever/infection
   Pregnancy
   Menopause
   Drugs, e.g. caffeine, cocaine
   Mitral valve disease
   Aortic incompetence
   Hypoxia/hypercapnia

   Rarities
   Tick bites (T_1–T_5)
   Phaeochromocytoma

Q. *Seven masquerades checklist*
A. Depression   √
   Diabetes   indirect
   Drugs   √√
   Anaemia   √
   Thyroid disease   √
   Spinal dysfunction   √
   UTI   possible

Q. *Is the patient trying to tell me something?*
A. Quite likely. Consider cardiac neurosis, anxiety.

as palpitations. About 25% of infarcts are either silent or unrecognised.

Sinister life-threatening arrhythmias are:
• ventricular tachycardia
• atypical ventricular tachycardia (torsade de pointes)
• sick sinus syndrome
• complete heart block

It is also important not to miss:
• hypokalaemia
• hypomagnesaemia

Pitfalls

There are many pitfalls in the diagnosis and management of arrhythmias, especially in the elderly where symptoms of infection may be masked.

Palpitations associated with the menopause can be overlooked. Valvular lesions, usually associated with rheumatic heart disease, such as mitral stenosis, and aortic incompetence may cause palpitations. The rare tumour, phaeochromocytoma, presents with palpitations and the interesting characteristic of postural tachycardia (a change of more than 20 beats/minute). The toxin from tick bites in dermatomes T1–T5 can cause palpitations.

General pitfalls
• Misdiagnosing PSVT as an anxiety state
• Overlooking a cardiac arrhythmia as a cause of syncope or dizziness
• Overlooking atrial fibrillation in the presence of a slow heartbeat
• Overlooking mitral valve prolapse in a patient, especially a middle-aged woman, presenting with unusual chest pains and palpitations (auscultate in standing position to accentuate click(s) ± murmurs)

Seven masquerades checklist

Surprisingly, all the masquerades have to be considered, either as direct or indirect causes: depression, especially with anxiety and in the postpartum period; diabetes, perhaps as an arrhythmia associated with a silent myocardial infarction or with hypoglycaemia; drugs as a very common cause (Table 64.2); anaemia, causing

Table 64.2 *Drugs that cause palpitations*

alcohol
aminophylline
amphetamines
anti-arrhythmic drugs
antidepressants
• tricyclics
• MAO inhibitors
caffeine
cocaine
class 1_A and 1_C drugs
digitalis
diuretics
   → K ↓, Mg ↓
glyceryl trinitrate
sympathomimetics
• in decongestants
• salbutamol
• terbutaline
thyroxine

a haemodynamic effect; hyperthyroidism; spinal dysfunction of the upper thoracic vertebrae T1–T5; and urinary tract infection, especially in the elderly.

Paroxysmal supraventricular tachycardia has been described as resulting from injury or dysfunction of the upper thoracic spine (especially T4 and T5) in the absence of organic heart disease.[2] The author has personally encountered several cases of PSVT alleviated by normalising function of the spine.

Psychogenic considerations

Emotional factors can precipitate a tachycardia which in turn can exaggerate the problem in an anxious person. Some people have a cardiac neurosis, often related to identification with a relative or friend. A family history of cardiac disease can engender this particular anxiety. Evidence of anxiety and depression should be sought in patients presenting with palpitations without clinical evidence of cardiovascular disease.

The clinical approach

Careful attention to basic detail in the history and examination can point the way clearly to the clinical diagnosis.

History

Ask the patient to describe the onset and offset of the palpitations, the duration of each episode and any associated features. Then ask the patient to tap out on the desk the rhythm and rate of the heartbeat experienced during the 'attack'. If the patient is unable to do this, tap out the cadence of the various arrhythmias to find a matching beat.

An irregular tapping 'all over the place' suggests atrial fibrillation, while an isolated thump or jump followed by a definite pause on a background or a regular pattern indicates premature beats (ectopics/extrasystoles) usually of ventricular origin. The thump is not the abnormal beat but the huge stroke volume of the beat following the compensatory pause.

Key questions

- Do the palpitations start suddenly? How long do they last?
- What do you think brings them on?
- Are they related to stress or worry or excitement?

- What symptoms do you notice during an attack?
- Do you have pain in the chest or breathlessness during the attack?
- Do you feel dizzy or faint during the attack?
- What medications do you take?
- How much coffee, tea, Coke do you drink?
- Have you been using nasal decongestants?
- Did you eat Chinese food before the attack?
- Do you smoke cigarettes, and how many?
- Do you take any of the social drugs such as cocaine or marijuana?
- Have you ever had rheumatic fever?
- Have you lost weight recently or do you sweat a lot?

Chest pain may indicate myocardial ischaemia or aortic stenosis; breathlessness indicates anxiety with hyperventilation, mitral stenosis or cardiac failure; dizziness or syncope suggests severe arrhythmias such as the sick sinus syndrome and complete heart block, aortic stenosis and associated cerebrovascular disease.

Physical examination

The ideal time to examine the patient is while the palpitations are being experienced. Often this is not possible and the physical examination is normal. Measurement of the heart rate may provide a clue to the problem.

As a working guide, a rate estimated to be about 150 beats per minute suggests PSVT, atrial flutter/fibrillation or ventricular tachycardia (Fig. 64.1). A rate less than 150 beats per minute is more likely to be sinus tachycardia which may be associated with exercise, fever, drugs or thyrotoxicosis.[3]

The nature of the pulse, especially the pulse pressure and rhythm, should be carefully evaluated (Fig. 64.2). Look for evidence of fever and infection and features of an anxiety state or depressive illness. Have the patient hyperventilate for 3 minutes to determine whether the arrhythmia is induced. Evidence of underlying disease such as anaemia, thyroid disease, alcohol abuse or cardiac disease should be sought. Also look for evidence of a mitral valve prolapse (mid-systolic click; late systolic murmur). Possible signs in the patient presenting with palpitations are shown in Figure 64.3.[4]

Diagnostic investigations

The number and complexity of investigations should be selected according to the problem

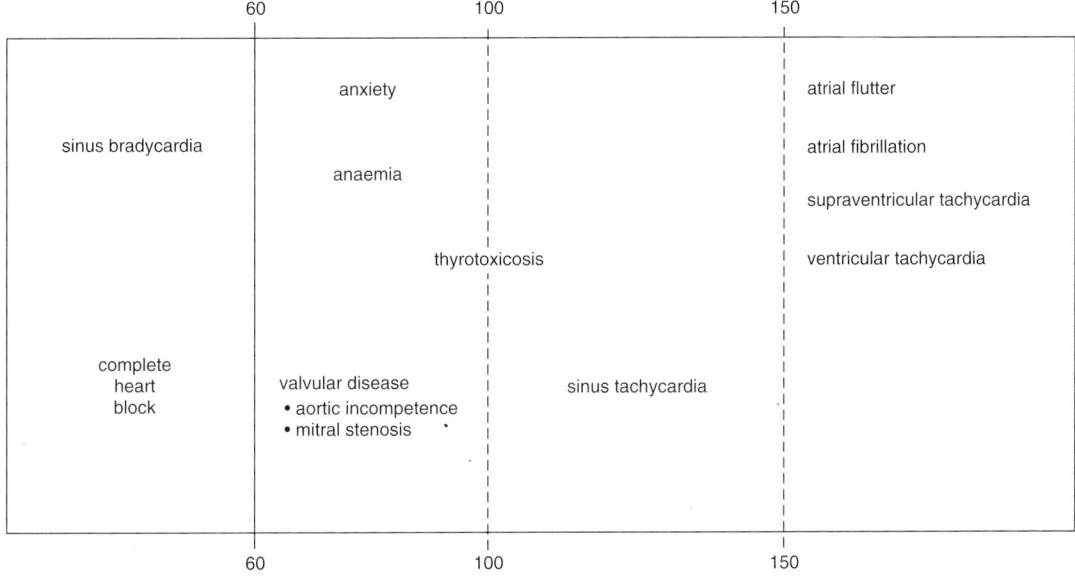

Fig. 64.1 *Heart rate guide to causes of various arrhythmias*

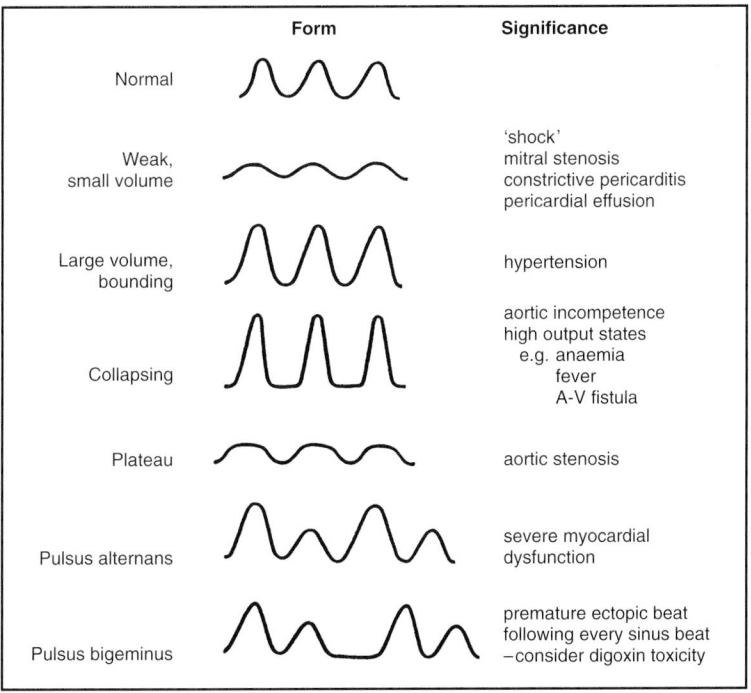

Fig. 64.2 *Various pulse forms*

and test availability. A checklist would include:

• Blood tests (for underlying disease)
  — haemoglobin and film
  — thyroid function tests
  — serum potassium and magnesium
  — serum digoxin ? digitalis toxicity
  — virus antibodies ? myocarditis
• Chest X-ray
• Cardiac (ischaemia and function)
  — ECG (12 lead)

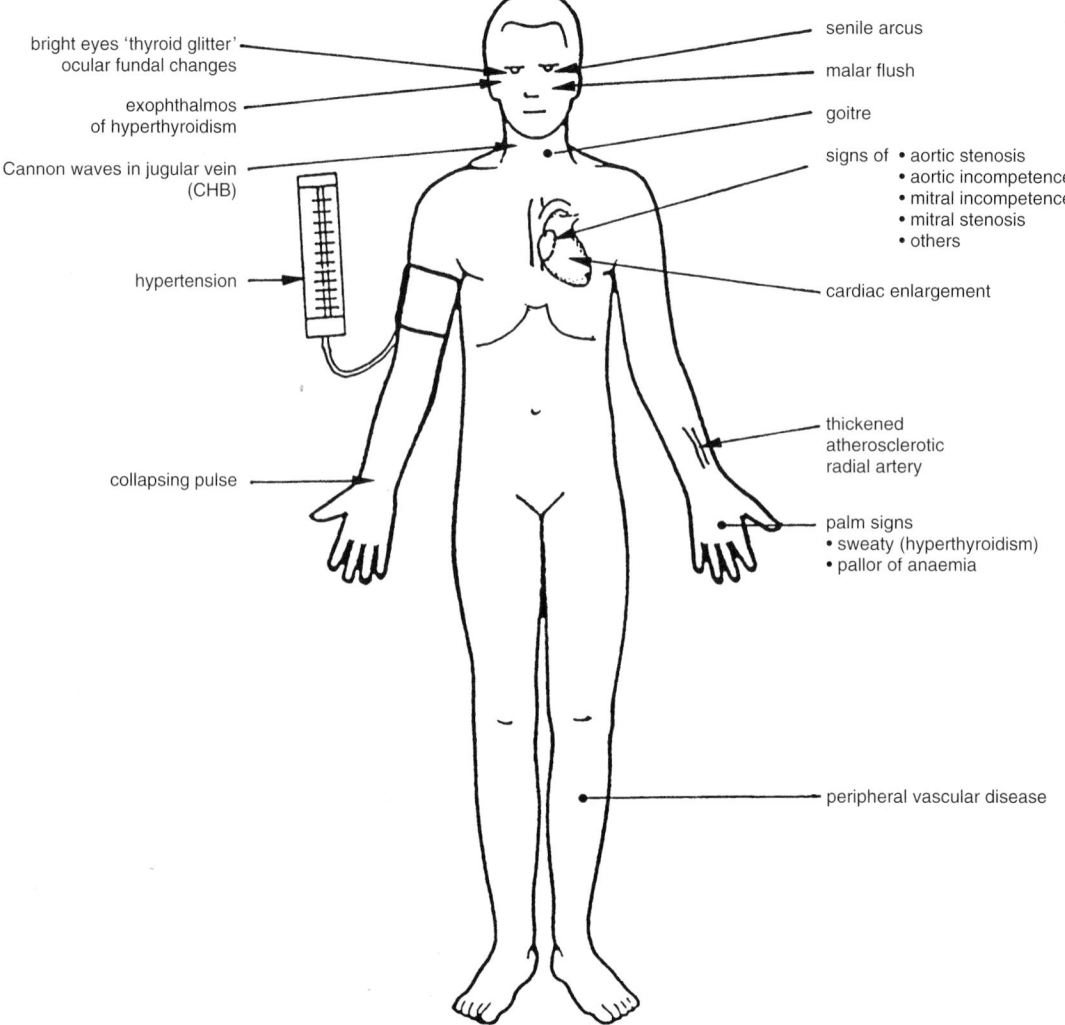

Fig. 64.3 *Signs to consider in a patient with palpitations*

— ambulatory 24 hour ECG monitoring
— echocardiography (to look for valvular heart disease and assess left ventricular function)
— electrophysiology studies

Palpitations in children

Children may complain of palpitations which may be associated with exercise, fever or anxiety. Various arrhythmias can occur with three requiring special consideration—paroxysmal supraventricular tachycardia, heart block and ventricular arrhythmias.[5]

PSVT is characterised by beats at 160–300 per minute, the fastest rates occurring in infants. The cause is often not found but some children have ECG abnormalities compatible with the Wolff-Parkinson-White syndrome. The recommended first-line treatment of PSVT is vagal stimulation via the application of ice packs to the upper face (forehead, eyes and nose) of the affected infant.

Palpitations in the elderly

The older the patient the more likely the onset of palpitations due to cardiac disease such as myocardial infarction/ischaemia, hypertension, arrhythmias and drugs, especially digoxin. Occasional atrial and ventricular arrhythmias, especially premature beats (ectopics), occur in 40%

of old people[6] and treatment is rarely required. Atrial fibrillation occurs in 5–10% of patients over 65 years of age, 30% of whom have no clinical evidence of cardiovascular disease. A rapid ventricular rate with symptoms is the only indication for digoxin in the elderly but beware of the sick sinus syndrome, especially if dizziness or syncope accompanies the fibrillation.

In the elderly, thyrotoxicosis may present as sinus tachycardia or atrial fibrillation with only minimal signs—the so-called 'masked thyrotoxicosis'—so it is easy to overlook it. The only clue may be bright eyes ('thyroid glitter') due to conjunctival oedema.

Arrhythmias
Facts and figures
- Cardiac arrhythmias account for about 25% of management decisions in cardiology (Table 64.3).
- Commonest are premature (ectopic) ventricular beats and atrial fibrillation.
- PSVT is next most common—6 per 1000 of population.
- The commonest mechanism of paroxysmal tachycardias is re-entry (Fig. 64.4).
- Electrophysiological studies are the gold standard investigation for tachycardias but are rarely needed for diagnosing most arrhythmias.

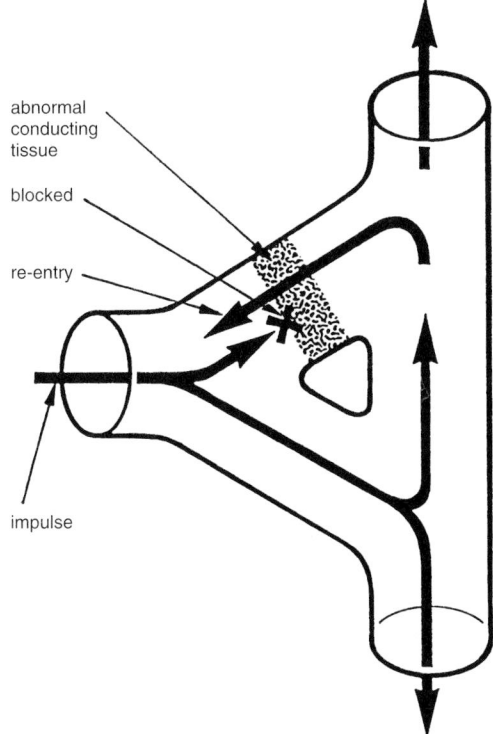

Fig. 64.4 *Diagrammatic mechanism of re-entry tachycardia*

Table 64.3 *Types of arrhythmias*

Non-pathological sinus rhythms
- sinus arrhythmia
- sinus bradycardia
- sinus tachycardia

Pathological bradycardias
- sinus node disease (sick sinus syndrome)
- atrioventricular (AV) block
  - first degree AV block
  - second degree AV block
  - third degree (complete) AV block

Pathological tachyarrhythmias
1. *Atrial*
   - atrial premature (ectopic) beats
   - paroxysmal tachycardia (PSVT)
   - atrial flutter
   - atrial fibrillation

2. *Ventricular*
   - ventricular premature beats
   - ventricular tachycardia
   - ventricular fibrillation
   - torsade de pointes (twisting of points)

- Almost all antiarrhythmic drugs have a pro-arrhythmic potential, i.e. they may worsen existing arrhythmias or provoke new arrhythmias in some patients (refer Table 64.4).
- Avoid digoxin in cases with an accessory pathway.
- If 'quinidine syncope' occurs, consider torsade de pointes as the cause.
- The two main indications for permanent pacemaking are sick sinus syndrome (only if symptomatic) and complete heart block.

Management strategies
- Treat the underlying cause.
- Give appropriate reassurance.
- Provide clear patient education.
- Explain about the problems of fatigue, stress and emotion.
- Advise moderation in consumption of tea, coffee, caffeine-containing soft drinks and alcohol.
- Advise about cessation of smoking and other drugs.

Table 64.4 *Electrophysiological classification of common antiarrhythmic drugs (after Vaughan Williams)*

Class	Drug	Usual dosage	Common side effects
1_A	Disopyramide	100–200 mg qid	Blurred vision, dry mouth, urinary problems in males (avoid in men > 50)
	Procainamide	1g qid IV use	Anorexia, nausea, urticaria
	Quinidine	2–3 SR tabs (0.25 g) bd	Diarrhoea, headache, tinnitus
1_B	Lignocaine	IV use	Nausea, dizziness, tremor
	Mexiletine	200 mg tid	Nausea, vomiting, tremor, dizziness
1_C	Flecainide	100 mg bd	Nausea, dizziness, rash
II	Beta-blockers	various	Fatigue, insomnia, nightmares, hypotension, bronchospasm. Avoid in asthmatics
III	Amiodarone	SVT: 200 mg daily VT: 400 mg daily	Rash, pulmonary fibrosis, thyroid, hepatic and CNS effects
	Bretylium	IV use only	Nausea, vomiting, hypotension
	Sotalol	160 mg bd	As for beta-blockers
IV	Verapamil	80 mg tid	Constipation, dizziness, hypotension
	Diltiazem	30–60 mg qid	Hypotension, headache

Note: Sotalol is a beta-blocker and thus is a class II and III agent. Adenosine and digoxin are not classified.

Premature (ectopic) beats
Atrial premature beats
- These are usually asymptomatic.
- Management is based on reassurance.
- Check lifestyle factors such as excess alcohol, caffeine, stress and smoking; avoid precipitating factors.
- Treatment is rarely required and should be avoided if possible.
- At present there is no ideal antiectopic agent.
- They may be a forerunner of other arrhythmias, e.g. PSVT, atrial fibrillation.

Ventricular premature beats
- These are also usually asymptomatic (90%).
- They occur in 20% of people with 'normal' hearts.
- Symptoms are usually noticed at rest in bed at night.
- Check lifestyle factors as for atrial premature beats.
- Drugs that can cause both types of premature beats include digoxin and sympathomimetics.
- Look for evidence of ischaemic heart disease, mitral valve prolapse (especially women), thyrotoxicosis and left ventricular failure.
- Ventricular premature beats may be a forerunner of other arrhythmias, e.g. ventricular tachycardia.

- If symptomatic but otherwise well with a normal chest X-ray and ECG, reassure the patient.
- Drug therapy: Never commence drug therapy without performing an echocardiograph. This will help to guide the choice of agent. Class 1 agents can make the arrhythmia worse or even life-threatening if there is reduced ventricular function. If this is the case, the patient should be referred to a cardiologist.

Supraventricular tachycardia
- SVT can be paroxysmal or sustained.
- Rate is 150–220/minute.
- There are at least eight different types of SVT with differing risks and responses to treatment.
- PSVT commonly presents with a sudden onset in otherwise healthy young people.
- Passing copious urine after an attack is characteristic of PSVT.
- Look for predisposing factors such as an accessory pathway and thyrotoxicosis.
- Approximately 60% are due to AV node re-entry and 35% due to accessory pathway tachycardia, e.g. Wolff-Parkinson-White syndrome (WPW).[7]
- Look for evidence of accessory pathways after reversion because accessory pathways can lead to sudden death (avoid digoxin in WPW).

normal sinus rhythm

sinus bradycardia and sinus arrhythmia—rate approx. 55 per minute

sinus tachycardia—rate approx. 100 per minute

complete heart block

atrial flutter

atrial fibrillation

Fig. 64.5 *Tracings of important arrhythmias*

(continues)

atrial premature beats

ventricular premature beats

supraventricular tachycardia

ventricular tachycardia

ventricular fibrillation

Fig. 64.5 *Tracings of important arrhythmias (cont.)*

- Consider sick sinus syndrome in a patient with SVT and dizziness.

Management of PSVT

1. Vagal stimulation can be attempted. Carotid sinus massage is the first treatment of choice. Other methods of vagal stimulation include:
   - Valsalva manoeuvre (easiest for patient)
   - self-induced vomiting
   - ocular pressure (avoid)
   - cold (ice) water to face
   - immersion of the face in water
2. If vagal stimulation fails, give adenosine IV (try 3 mg first, then 6 mg in 2 minutes if unsuccessful, then 12 mg every 2 minutes if necessary). Second-line treatment is verapamil IV 1 mg/min up to 10–15 mg (provided patient is not on a beta-blocker).

Precautions
- adenosine causes less hypotension than verapamil but may cause bronchospasm in asthmatics
- use only if narrow QRS and BP > 80
- carefully monitor blood pressure
- **AVOID** verapamil if on beta-blockers
  and
  persistent tachycardia with QRS complexes > 0.14s (suggests ventricular tachycardia)
3. In the rare event of failure of medical treatment, consider DC cardioversion or overdrive pacing.

Prophylaxis
To prevent recurrences use flecainide (only if no structural heart damage) or sotalol. If these agents fail, consider amiodarone. Do an echocardiograph first to exclude structural heart disease. Radiofrequency catheter ablation which is usually curative is indicated for frequent attacks.

Carotid sinus massage
Carotid sinus massage causes vagal stimulation and its effect on SVT is all or nothing. It has no effect on ventricular tachycardia. It slows the sinus rate and breaks the SVT by blocking AV nodal conduction.

Method
- Locate the carotid pulse in front of the sternomastoid muscle just below the angle of the jaw (Fig. 64.6).
- Ensure that no bruit is present.
- Rub the carotid with a circular motion for 5–10 seconds.
- Rub each carotid in turn if the SVT is not 'broken', but never both together.

In general, right carotid pressure tends to slow the sinus rate[8] and left carotid pressure tends to impair AV nodal conduction.

Precautions
In the elderly (risk of embolism or bradycardia).

Atrial fibrillation
Facts and figures
- A common problem (9% incidence in the over 70 age group).
- Remember to look for the underlying cause: myocardial ischaemia (15% of cases), mitral

sternomastoid muscle

site for carotid sinus massage

Fig. 64.6 *Carotid sinus massage*

valve disease, thyrotoxicosis, hypertension, cardiomyopathy including chronic alcohol dependence, alcohol binge.
- All patients should have thyroid function tests and an echocardiograph to help find a cause.
- With sustained atrial fibrillation there is a 5% chance per annum of embolic episodes. There is a fivefold risk of CVA overall.
- The risk of CVA is greater in those with previous CVA, valvular heart disease, prosthetic mitral valve and cardiac failure.
- For reversion anticoagulate with warfarin for 2–4 weeks beforehand and maintain for 4 weeks after.
- Digoxin controls the ventricular rate but does not terminate or prevent attacks.
- Sotalol (preferred) and amiodarone are used for conversion of atrial fibrillation and maintenance of sinus rhythm.

Treatment for atrial fibrillation/flutter
Medical treatment
For rapid urgent control of ventricular rate:
- digoxin   0.5–1.0 mg (o) immediately then 0.25–0.5 mg (o) every 4–6 hours to maximum of 1.5–2.0 mg in first 24 hours
  or

• verapamil   1 mg/min IV up to maximum 15 mg
(provided no evidence of heart failure and well monitored BP)

Routine control:
• digoxin 0.0625–0.25 mg (o) daily according to age, plasma creatinine and digoxin level

Maintenance:
• digoxin (as above)
±
• verapamil 40–160 mg (o) 8 hourly
• beta-blockers

Medical cardioversion

sotalol (preferred) or amiodarone

If the rate cannot be well controlled despite maximal medical therapy, consider AV node ablation and a permanent pacemaker. Atrial fibrillation with a rapid ventricular response over a long period gradually causes LV dysfunction.

Electrical DC cardioversion

For failed medical conversion.

The use of warfarin in atrial fibrillation

Warfarin is effective in preventing stroke in patients with lone or non-rheumatic atrial fibrillation. The decision to use it or an antiplatelet agent, especially in the younger patient, is difficult and should be made in consultation with a cardiologist. As a general rule all patients should start on warfarin unless < 65 years old or have a major contraindication to its use. If using warfarin, start with a low dose, e.g. 2–4 mg, and maintain a relatively low INR of 2–3 with regular checks.

Advances in treatment of arrhythmias

Apart from special rate responsive pacemakers for bradycardia, there are several new modalities of treatment for complex arrhythmias, including means of blocking the re-entry phenomenon.

Surgery

Guided by electrophysiologic monitoring, surgeons can dissect a small section of the atrioventricular ring to ensure that all aberrant connections between the atria and the underlying ventricular muscle are severed.

Catheter electrode ablation

Specific abnormal foci in the conducting pathways can be ablated using direct current electrical surgery or radiofrequency 'burns' via a catheter electrode. Radiofrequency ablation, which will probably supplant surgery as a form of treatment, is indicated for AV junction (His bundle) dysfunction, accessory pathways, nodal re-entry tachycardia and ventricular tachycardia.

Automatic implantable cardiac defibrillator (AICD)

This expensive implant is the most effective therapy yet devised for the prevention of sudden cardiac death in patients with documented sustained VT or VF. Operative mortality should be less than 10% after which survival at 1 year is over 90%. These new defibrillators incorporate an antitachycardia pacemaker. Patients can either be paced out of arrhythmia or, if they develop ventricular fibrillation, they can be defibrillated using higher energy.

When to refer

Patients should be referred to a cardiologist[9] when:
• a sustained supraventricular tachycardia is suspected
• a sustained ventricular tachycardia is suspected
• an ECG shows sustained delta waves of WPW syndrome, even if asymptomatic
• syncope or dizziness suggests a cardiovascular cause
• a paroxysmal arrhythmia may be the cause of unexplained cardiovascular symptoms
• anticoagulation has to be considered

Practice tips

• Atrial fibrillation and dizziness (even syncope) are suggestive of the sick sinus syndrome (bradycardia–tachycardia syndrome), which is made worse by digoxin.
• Consider thyrotoxicosis as a cause of atrial fibrillation or sinus tachyardia even if clinical manifestations are not apparent.
• Check for a history of palpitations in a patient complaining of dizziness or syncope (and vice versa). Consider an arrhythmia, especially in the elderly.
• PSVT is rarely caused by organic heart disease in young patients.

Table 64.5 *Summary of treatment of arrhythmias*

Arrhythmia	First line	Second line	Third line
Sinus tachycardia	Treat cause	Metoprolol or atenolol or Verapamil (rarely indicated)	
Bradycardias			
Sick sinus syndrome	Permanent pacing if symptomatic		
AV block			
first degree	No treatment		
second degree			
• Mobitz I	No treatment	Pacing if problematic	
• Mobitz II	Consider pacing		
third degree			
• acute, e.g. MI	Temporary pacing or Isoprenaline IV		
• chronic	Permanent pacing		
Atrial tachyarrhythmias			
PSVT	Valsalva Carotid sinus massage	Adenosine IV or Verapamil IV	DC cardioversion Class III drug ? Ablation
Atrial fibrillation	Digoxin (to control rate)		
Atrial flutter	and/or Verapamil	Consider beta-blocker (with care, to control rate)	DC cardioversion or sotalol, amiodarone
Atrial premature beats	Treat cause Check lifestyle	Metoprolol or atenolol or Verapamil	
Ventricular tachyarrhthmias			
Ventricular premature beats	Treat cause Check lifestyle	Beta-blocker (especially mitral valve prolapse)	Class I or III drugs (rarely needed)
Ventricular tachycardia			
• non-sustained	Lignocaine IV	Procainamide IV	Class III drug
• sustained	Lignocaine IV if stable — if not: DC shock	Class III drug	DC cardioversion
Ventricular fibrillation	DC cardioversion	IV adrenaline if fine VF then DC cardioversion	Lignocaine IV (maintenance) Class III (if recurrent)

- Arrhythmia of sudden onset suggests PSVT, atrial flutter/fibrillation or ventricular tachycardia.
- A normal ECG in sinus rhythm does not exclude an accessory pathway.
- Consider conduction disorders such as the WPW syndrome in PSVT. Avoid digoxin in WPW syndrome.
- Common triggers of premature beats and PSVT are smoking, anxiety and caffeine (especially 8 or more cups a day).
- Many antiarrhythmic drugs have proarrhythmic potential:
  — never use digoxin in WPW syndrome and SSS (without pacemaker back-up)
  — never use digoxin or verapamil for atrial fibrillation in WPW syndrome
  — beware of quinidine or disopyramide causing torsade de pointes VT
  — beware of using verapamil with a beta-blocker
  — beware of giving quinidine without digoxin for atrial flutter
- There is no ideal antiarrhythmic agent for ventricular premature beats.

Table 64.5 presents a summary of the treatment of arrhythmias.

References

1. Boxall J. Annual update course for general practitioners. Course abstracts. Melbourne: Monash University, 1991, 16.

2. Lewit K. *Manipulative therapy in rehabilitation of the motor system*. London: Butterworths, 1985, 338–339.

3. Davis A, Bolin T, Ham J. *Symptom analysis and physical diagnosis* (2nd edn). Sydney: Pergamon, 1985.

4. Sandler G, Fry J. *Early clinical diagnosis*. Lancaster: MTP Press, 1986, 327–359.

5. Robinson MJ. *Practical paediatrics*. Melbourne: Churchill Livingstone, 1990, 318–319.

6. Merriman A. *Handbook of international geriatric medicine*. Singapore: PG Publishing, 1989, 99–100.

7. Stafford W. Arrhythmias. Medical Observer: 13 September 1991, 33–34.

8. Kumar P, Clarke M. *Clinical medicine* (2nd edn). London: Bailliere Tindall, 1990, 554.

9. Ross DL. Cardiac arrhythmias. In: MIMS Disease Index (2nd edn). Sydney: IMS Publishing, 1996, 93–96.

65

Sore throat

I believe there are hundreds of young adults who
have erroneously suffered tonsillectomy because of the
tonsillitis of undiagnosed glandular fever.

Sceptical GP (anonymous)

A sore or painful throat is one of the commonest symptoms encountered in general practice. The most usual cause is viral pharyngitis.

Definitions

pharyngitis = inflammation of pharynx ± tonsils
  tonsillitis = inflammation of tonsils only

Key facts and checkpoints

- In the National Morbidity Survey (UK)[1] nine episodes per annum of acute pharyngitis or acute tonsillitis were diagnosed for every 100 patients.
- Sore throats account for about 5% of consultations in general practice per annum.[2]
- In one United Kingdom general practice it was the third most common new presenting symptom—5.4% of presenting problems.
- Although throat infections are common from infancy, children under 4 years of age rarely complain of a sore throat.
- Complaints of a sore throat are prevalent in children between 4 and 8 and in teenagers.
- Sore throats continue to be common up to the age of 45 and then decline significantly.
- The common causes are viral pharyngitis and tonsillitis due to *Streptococcus pyogenes*.
- The sore throat may be the presentation of serious and hidden systemic diseases, such as blood dyscrasias, HIV infection and diabetes (due to moniliasis).

- A very important cause is tonsillitis caused by Epstein-Barr mononucleosis. Treating this cause with penicillin can produce adverse effects.

Presentation

Sore throat may be present as part of a complex of the common upper respiratory infections, such as the common cold and influenza. However, sore throat often presents as a single symptom. The pain is usually continuous and aggravated by swallowing. In those under 4 years old the presentation of acute pharyngitis or tonsillitis may be confusing as the presenting complaints may be vomiting, abdominal pain and fever rather than sore thoat and swallowing difficulty.

It is appropriate to consider sore throat as acute or chronic. Most presentations come as acute problems, the causes of which are listed in Table 65.1.

A diagnostic approach

A summary of the safety diagnostic model is presented in Table 65.2.

Probability diagnosis

At least 50% of sore throats, mainly pharyngitis, will be caused by a virus. The commonest cause of tonsillitis is considered to be Group A beta-haemolytic *Streptococcus pyogenes*[3] (GABHS) which is more likely in children between the ages of 4 and 15 years. A viral infection is supported by the presence of coryza prodromata, hoarseness and nasal stuffiness.

Serious disorders not to be missed

It is vital to be aware of *Haemophilus influenzae* infection in children, especially between 2 and 4

Table 65.1 *Causes of acute sore throat*

BACTERIA
B haemolytic streptococci
Diphtheria (rare)
Gonococcal pharyngitis
Haemophilus influenzae
Quinsy
Staphylococcus aureus (rare)
Syphilis (rare)
Vincent's angina

VIRAL
Severe–moderate soreness

Epstein-Barr mononucleosis
Herpangina
Herpes simplex pharyngitis

Mild–moderate soreness

Adenovirus
Coronavirus
Enterovirus
Influenza virus
Picornavirus
Rhinovirus
Human immunodeficiency virus
Varicella (chicken pox)

OTHER INFECTIONS
Candida albicans, especially in infants
Mycoplasma pneumoniae
Chlamydia pneumoniae

BLOOD DYSCRASIAS
Agranulocytosis
Leukaemia

IRRITANTS
Tobacco smoke
Antiseptic lozenges (oral use)

Table 65.2 *Sore throat: diagnostic strategy model*

Q. *Probability diagnosis*
A. Viral pharyngitis
    Chronic sinusitis with postnasal drip

Q. *Serious disorders not to be missed*
A. Cardiovascular
    • angina
    • myocardial infarction
    Neoplasia
    • carcinoma of oropharynx, tongue
    Blood dyscrasias, e.g. agranulocytosis
                                         acute leukaemia
    Severe infections
    • acute epiglottitis (children and adults)
    • peritonsillar abscess (quinsy)
    • pharyngeal abscess
    • diphtheria (very rare)
    • HIV/AIDS

Q. *Pitfalls (often missed)*
A. Foreign body
    Epstein-Barr mononucleosis
    Monilia
    • common in infants
    • steroid inhalers
    STDs
    • gonococcal pharyngitis
    • herpes simplex (type II)
    • syphilis
    Irritants, e.g. cigarette smoke,chemicals
    Reflux oesophagitis
    Mouth breathing
    Thyroiditis

    Rarities
    Systemic sclerosis
    Sarcoidosis
    Malignant granuloma
    Tuberculosis

Q. *Seven masquerades checklist*
A. Depression   √
    Diabetes   √ (monilia)
    Drugs   √
    Anaemia   √ possible
    Thyroid disease   √ thyroiditis
    Spinal dysfunction √ cervical
    UTI   –

Q. *Is the patient trying to tell me something?*
A. Unlikely, but the association with depression is significant.

years, when the deadly problem of epiglottitis can develop suddenly. These patients present with a short febrile illness, respiratory difficulty (cough is not a feature) and are unable to swallow.

Apart from acute epiglottitis it is important not to overlook carcinoma of the oropharynx or tongue, or the blood dyscrasias including acute leukaemia. The severe infections not to be missed include streptococcal pharyngitis with its complications, including quinsy, diphtheria and HIV infection (including AIDS).

Pitfalls

There are many pitfalls, the classic being to diagnose the exudative tonsillitis of Epstein-Barr mononucleosis as streptococcal tonsillitis and prescribe one of the penicillins, which may precipitate a severe rash. Primary HIV infection can present with a sore throat along with other symptoms. Adenovirus pharyngitis can also mimic streptococcal pharyngitis, especially in young adults.

Traumatic episodes are important but are often not considered, especially in children. They include:

• a foreign body—may cause a sudden onset of throat pain then drooling and dysphagia
• vocal abuse—excessive singing or shouting can cause a sore throat and hoarseness
• burns—hot food and drink, acids or alkalis

Various irritants, especially cigarette smoke in the household and smoke inhalation from fires, can cause pharyngeal irritation with sore throat, especially in children.

The mouth and pharynx may become dry and sore from mouth breathing which is often associated with nasal obstruction, e.g. adenoid hypertrophy, allergic rhinitis.

Seven masquerades checklist

Depression may be associated with a sore throat. Diabetes and aplastic anaemia and drugs are indirectly associated through candidiasis, neutropenia and agranulocytosis respectively. NSAIDs can cause a sore throat. The possibility of thyroiditis presenting as a sore throat should be kept in mind.

Making a diagnosis

The issues of making a reliable diagnosis and prescribing antibiotics are rather contentious and at times difficult, a situation not usually appreciated by some academics. The main issue is to determine whether the sore throat has a treatable cause by interpretation of the clinical and epidemiological data.

The appearance of the pharynx and tonsils is not always discriminating. A generalised red throat may be caused by a streptococcal or a viral infection, as may tonsils that are swollen with follicular exudates. On probability, most sore throats are caused by a virus and generally do not show marked inflammatory changes or purulent looking exudates (Fig. 65.1). Such throats should be treated symptomatically.

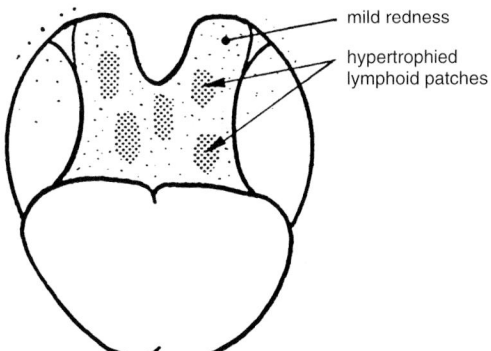

Fig. 65.1 *Viral pharyngitis: the signs may be minimal but mild redness of pharynx and prominent lymphoid patches on the oropharynx are typical*

mild redness

hypertrophied lymphoid patches

The clinical approach
History

It is necessary to determine whether the patient has a sore throat, a deep pain in the throat or neck pain. Instruct the patient to point to exactly where the pain is experienced. Enquire about relevant associated symptoms such as metallic taste in mouth, fever, upper respiratory infection, other pain such as ear pain, nasal stuffiness or discharge and cough.

Note whether the patient is an asthmatic and uses a corticosteroid inhaler, or is a smoker, or exposed to environmental irritants. Check the immunisation history, enquiring especially about diphtheria.

The history should give a clue to the remote possibility that the painful throat is a manifestation of angina.

Examination

An inspection should note the general appearance of the patient, looking for 'toxicity', the anaemic pallor of leukaemia, the nasal stuffiness of infectious mononucleosis, the characteristic halitosis of a streptococcal throat.

Palpate the neck for soreness and lymphadenopathy, inspect the ears and check the sinus areas.

Then inspect the oral cavity and pharynx. Look for ulcers, abnormal masses and exudates. Note whether the uvula and soft palate, tonsils, fauces or pharynx are swollen, red or covered in exudate. The typical appearances of various conditions causing a sore throat are shown in Figures 65.1 to 65.7, and important causes to exclude in Figure 65.8.

Guidelines
- Small patches of exudate on the palate or other structure indicate *Candida albicans* (oral thrush) (Fig. 65.2).
- A large whitish-yellow membrane virtually covering both tonsils indicates Epstein-Barr mononucleosis (Fig. 65.3).
- A generalised red, swollen appearance with exudate indicates Group A beta-haemolytic streptococcus (GABHS) infection (Figs 65.4 and 65.5).

Investigations

Investigations can be selected from:
- throat swab
- haemoglobin, blood film and white cell count

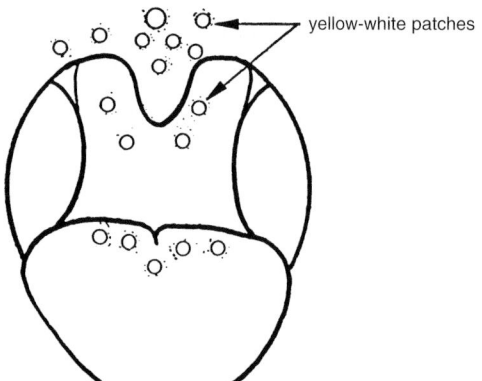

Fig. 65.2 *Oral thrush due to* Candida albicans: *small patches of whitish-yellow exudate on the palate, dorsum of tongue, pharynx and mucosa are typical*

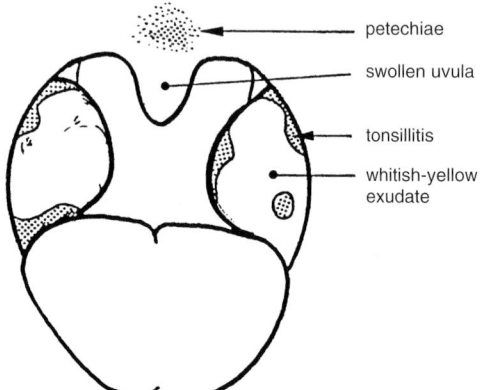

Fig. 65.3 *Epstein-Barr mononucleosis: swollen red tonsils with a whitish-yellow membranous exudate are usually seen; petechiae on the soft palate may be present*

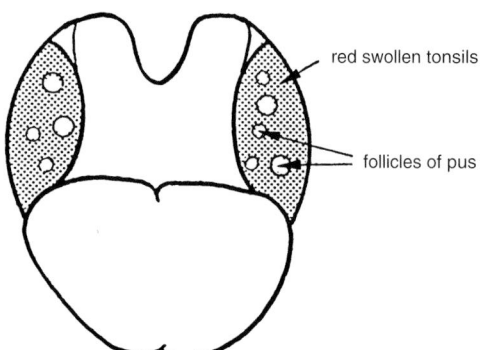

Fig. 65.4 *Follicular tonsillitis due to* Streptococcus pyogenes: *the tonsils are swollen and red with pockets of pus*

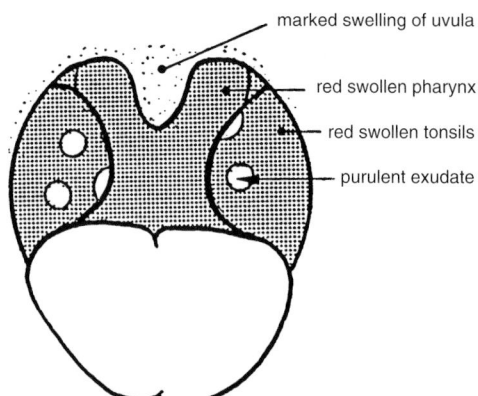

Fig. 65.5 *Streptococcal tonsillopharyngitis: severe inflammation involves both tonsils and pharynx with marked redness, swelling and exudate. Consider herpes simplex and mononucleosis as alternative diagnoses*

- mononucleosis test
- random blood sugar (? diabetes)

To swab or not to swab

Throat swabs are about 90% effective in isolating GABHS from the infected throat. Authorities are divided about management. Some recommend that throat cultures be performed for all sore throats and antibiotics given only when GABHS is found. Others regard throat cultures as being unnecessary and recommend therapy based on clinical judgments. Still others recommend throat cultures for selected patients only.[4]

Generally, throat cultures are not necessary except to verify the presence of *Streptococcus pyogenes*, especially in closed institutions such as boarding schools, or if diphtheria is suspected in the non-immunised. A positive culture and a fourfold rise in the ASOT titre is necessary for a precise diagnosis.

Epstein-Barr mononucleosis (EBM) screening

It is important initially if tonsillar exudate is present to consider the possibility of EBM. If suspected, a blood film and a Paul Bunnell heterophile antibody titre should be ordered. However, neither may be positive for EBM during the first few days of illness.[4]

Sore throat in children

A sore throat in a child usually means a viral or, less commonly, bacterial infection of the tonsillopharynx. Other causes to consider are:

- gingivostomatitis, especially primary herpes simplex
- epiglottitis
- laryngotracheobronchitis (croup)
- laryngitis
- oral moniliasis (more a bad taste than pain)
- aphthous ulcers
- foreign bodies
- postnasal drip, e.g. allergic rhinitis
- irritation
  — low environmental humidity
  — smoke (e.g. household smoke)

Sore throat in the elderly

Sore throat in the elderly may be caused by a viral infection but otherwise needs to be treated with considerable respect. It is important to exclude pharyngeal carcinoma which can present with the classic triad—pain on swallowing, referred ear pain and hoarseness.

Oropharangeal lesions may occur with herpes zoster but vesicles are usually present on the face.

A metallic taste in the mouth with or without a complaint of a sore throat indicates *Candida albicans* and hence diabetes must be excluded.

Streptococcal tonsillopharyngitis

This infection may involve the pharynx only and vary from mild to severe, or it may involve both tonsils and pharynx. It is uncommon under age 2 or over age 40.[5]

Typical clinical features:

- abrupt onset sore throat
- severe pain
- extreme difficulty in swallowing
- pain on talking
- foul-smelling breath
- constitutional symptoms
  — fever $\geq$ 38°C
  — toxicity

Examination

Pharynx very inflamed and oedematous. Tonsils swollen with pockets of yellow exudate on surfaces (Figs 65.4 and 65.5). Very tender enlarged tonsillar lymph nodes.

Treatment

It should be treated with penicillin or an alternative antibiotic (Table 65.3).[6] Antibiotic treatment has a variable effect on the resolution of symptoms. It does not protect against glomerulonephritis but does protect against rheumatic

Table 65.3   *Treatment for streptococcal throat (proven or suspected)*[6]

Children
  phenoxymethyl penicillin 50 mg/kg/day (o) in
  2 divided doses for 10 days (to maximum 1 g/day)
                    or
              (if sensitive to penicillin)
  roxithromycin 150 mg (o) bd for 10 days (if > 40 kg)

Adults
  phenoxymethyl penicillin 500 mg (o) 12 hourly for 10 days
  (can initiate treatment with one injection of procaine penicillin)
                    or
  roxithromycin 300 mg (o) daily for 10 days

In severe cases:
  procaine penicillin 1–1.5 mg IM daily for 3–5 days
                   plus
  phenoxymethyl penicillin (as above) for 10 days

Note: Although symptoms and most evidence will disappear within 1–2 days of treatment, a full course of 10 days should be given to provide an optimal chance of eradicating *Streptococcus pyogenes* from the nasopharynx and thus minimising the risk of recurrence or complications such as rheumatic fever.[6]

fever.[5] Amoxycillin should be avoided in tonsillitis because of confusion caused should mononucleosis be present.

Supportive measures include:
- adequate soothing fluids, including icy poles
- analgesia: adults—2 soluble aspirin
        children—paracetamol elixir (not alcohol base)
- rest with adequate fluid intake
- soothing gargles, e.g. soluble aspirin used for analgesia
- advice against overuse of OTC throat lozenges and topical sprays which can sensitise the throat; limited use (3 days) of decongestants for nasal decongestion is helpful

Quinsy

Quinsy is a peritonsillar abscess characterised by marked swelling of the peritonsillar area with medial displacement of tonsillar tissue (Fig. 65.6). It is usually caused by GABHS or anaerobes, occasionally Haemophilus sp. and *Staphylococcus aureus*. A typical picture of tonsillitis is followed by increasing difficulty in swallowing and trismus.

Treatment
Antibiotics, e.g. procaine penicillin IM or clindamycin plus drainage under local anaesthetic if it is pointing. Oral penicillin treatment is likely to fail. Subsequent tonsillectomy may, but not always, be necessary.

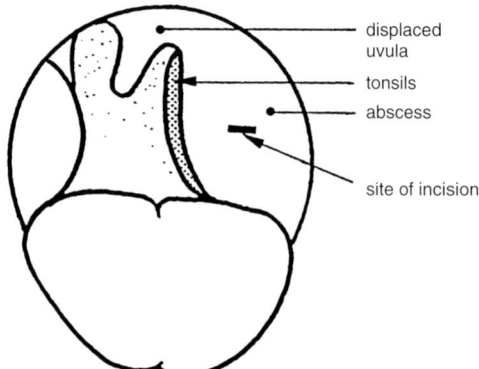

Fig. 65.6 *Peritonsillar abscess (quinsy): a tense red bulging mass is noted and the uvula is displaced from the midline; a site of incision for drainage is indicated*

Acute epiglottitis

In children this is a life-threatening infection (p. 788). It may be overlooked in adults where, unlike children, the airway is usually not obstructed and the patient presents with a severe sore throat, dysphagia, drooling of saliva and a tender neck. Examination of the throat may appear quite normal. However, it is a severe infection requiring hospitalisation and parenteral antibiotics, e.g. cefotaxime.

Viral causes of sore throat
Epstein-Barr mononucleosis
The angiose form of EBM is a real trap and must be considered in 15–25 year old patients (peak incidence) with a painful throat that takes about 7 days to reach its peak.

Clinical features
- sore throat
- prodromal fever, malaise, lethargy
- anorexia, myalgia
- nasal quality to voice
- skin rash

Examination
- petechiae on palate (not pathognomonic)
- enlarged tonsils with or without white exudates (looks, but isn't, purulent)
- periorbital oedema
- lymphadenopathy, especially posterior cervical
- splenomegaly (50%)
- jaundice ± hepatomegaly (5–10%)

The rash
- primary rash (5%)
- secondary rash
    — with ampicillin, amoxycillin (90–100%)
    — with penicillin (50%)

Diagnosis
- blood film—atypical lymphocytes
- white cell count—absolute lymphocytosis
- heterophil antibodies
        or
    Monospot test
        or
    EBV IgM test (more specific)

Herpangina
An uncommon infection caused by Coxsackie virus. Presents as small vesicles on soft palate,

uvula and anterior fauces. These ulcerate to form small ulcers. The problem is benign and rapidly self-limiting.

Herpes simplex pharyngitis
In adults primary infection is similar to severe streptococcal pharyngitis but ulcers extend beyond the tonsils.

Other viral pharyngitis
Typically, the signs are fewer than with other causes. The typical case has mild redness without exudate and prominent (sometimes pale) lymphoid patches on the posterior pharynx (Fig. 65.1). Tonsillar lymph nodes are usually not enlarged or tender. This picture is the commonest encountered in general practice.

Diphtheria

The potentially fatal form of this disease almost always occurs in non-immunised people. The clinical presentation may be modified by previous immunisation or by antibiotic treatment.

Typical clinical features
- insidious onset
- mild to moderate fever
- mild sore throat and dysphagia
- patient looks pale and ill
- enlarged tonsils
- pharynx inflamed and oedematous
- membrane (any colour but usually grey-green) can spread beyond tonsils to fauces, soft palate, lateral pharyngeal wall and downwards to involve larynx (Fig. 65.7)

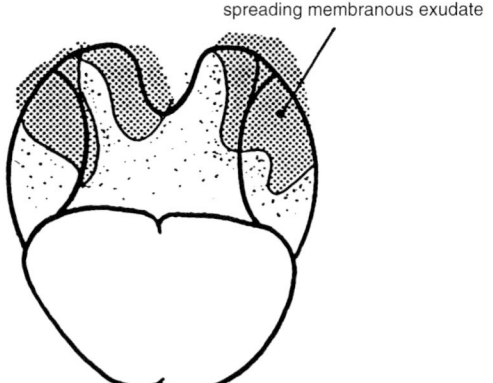
spreading membranous exudate

Fig. 65.7 *Diphtheria: tonsils and pharynx are red and swollen; a thick grey-green exudate forms on the tonsils as a spreading membrane*

- enlarged cervical lymph nodes
- soft tissue swelling of neck → 'bull neck' appearance

Management
- throat swabs
- antitoxin
- penicillin or erythromycin 500 mg qid for 10 days
- isolate patient

Candida pharyngitis

Oral candidiasis typically presents as milky-white growths on the palate, buccal and gingival mucosae, pharynx and dorsum of the tongue (Fig. 65.2). If scraped away, a bleeding ulcerated surface remains. A bad (metallic) taste is a feature but the patient may complain of a sore throat and tongue and dysphagia.

Causes or predisposing factors to consider:
- HIV infection
- diabetes mellitus
- broad spectrum antibiotics
- corticosteroids, including inhalers
- dentures
- debility

Management
- Determine underlying cause.
- Nystatin suspension, rinse and swallow qid
                    or
  amphotericin 10 mg lozenge dissolved slowly in oral cavity, 6 hourly, for 7–14 days.

When to refer
- Acute epiglottitis in children (a medical emergency).
- Inaccessible foreign body.
- Abscess: peritonsillar or retropharangeal.
- Recurrent attacks of tonsillitis and adenoid hypertrophy for an opinion about tonsillectomy and/or adenoidectomy.
- Suspicion or evidence of HIV infection or diphtheria.
- Patients not responding to treatment.
- Patients with more generalised disorders that are not yet diagnosed.

Practice tips
- Consider severe tonsillitis with a covering membrane as Epstein-Barr mononucleosis.

- If an adult presents with an intensely painful throat with a heavy exudate and seems toxic, consider primary herpes simplex as well as streptococcal throat.
- Reserve swabs of the throat for verification of a strep throat where it is important to do so, for suspected diphtheria and for suspicion of other serious infections such as tuberculosis.
- Be aware of possible complications such as febrile convulsions in children and abscess formation.
- Do not misdiagnose unusual causes of a sore throat, such as carcinoma (Fig. 65.8).
- The triad: hoarseness, pain on swallowing and referred ear pain = pharyngeal carcinoma.
- The two major considerations in managing the acute sore throat are:
  — Can diphtheria be excluded?
  — Should the patient be treated with an antibiotic?[7]

Antibiotic treatment is aimed primarily at streptococcal pharynitis and this is often based on clinical judgment.

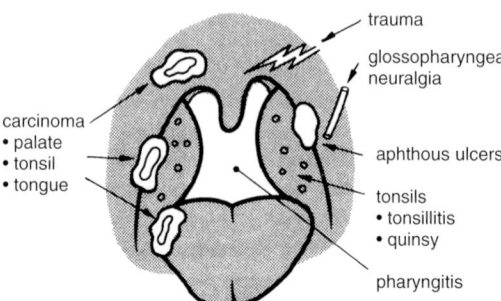

Fig. 65.8 *General causes of a sore throat: note the importance of excluding carcinoma*

References

1. Office of Population Censuses and Surveys. *Morbidity statistics from general practice studies on medical and population subjects. No 26.* London: HSMO, 1974, 33–40.

2. Cormack J, Marinker M, Morrell D. *Practice: a handbook of primary medical care.* London: Kluwer-Harrap, 1980; 3(25):1–7.

3. Fry J. *Common diseases, their nature, incidence and care.* Lancaster: MTP Press, 1987, 74–77.

4. Yung AP, Stanley PA. The patient with the acute sore throat. Current Therapeutics, 1985; 26:54–55.

5. Shires D, Hennen B, Rice D. *Family medicine* (2nd edn). New York: McGraw-Hill, 1987, 97–103.

6. Mashford ML. *Antibiotic guidelines* (9th edn). Victorian Medical Postgraduate Foundation Inc, 1996, 100–103.

7. Kincaid-Smith P, Larkins R, Whelan G. *Problems in clinical medicine.* Sydney: MacLennan & Petty, 1990, 340–347.

66

Tiredness

Chronic fatigue syndrome is not tiredness: there is a difference between feeling tired and 'fatiguey'. Fatigue involves a heaviness in the limbs, a sense of inability to think or move, pain in muscles and joints, nausea etc. Please understand the difference.

CFS patient to author
January 1995

Tiredness or chronic fatigue is not a diagnosis but rather a symptom of illness: it may occur as either a presenting or a supporting symptom. Tiredness is interchangeable with terms such as weariness, loss of energy, listlessness and exhaustion. It is a common and difficult presenting symptom. The symptom of tiredness is likely to be 'hidden' behind the request for a tonic or a physical check-up.[1]

Tiredness can be a symptom of a great variety of serious and uncommon diseases including malignant disease. The challenge for the family doctor is to diagnose such disorders quickly without extravagant investigation.

Key facts and checkpoints

- The commonest cause of tiredness is psychological distress including anxiety states, depression and somatisation disorder.
- The study by Hickie et al.[2] showed that 25% of a sample of attendees visiting general practices had chronic fatigue. Of these, 70% had psychological distress. The others were more likely to have a current depressive disorder.
- In Jerrett's study[3] no organic cause was found in 62.3% of his patients presenting with lethargy; the constant factors were sleep disturbance and the presence of stress in their lives. Many of them turned out to be suffering from

psychological problems or psychiatric illnesses, including depression, anxiety state or bereavement.
- An important cause of daytime tiredness is a sleep disorder such as obstructive sleep apnoea which results in periodic hypoventilation during sleep. It occurs in 2% of the general population in all age groups and in about 10% of middle-aged men.[3] A history of snoring is a pointer to the problem.
- Underlying disorders that need to be considered as possible causes of chronic fatigue are endocrine and metabolic disorders, malignancy, chronic infection, autoimmune disorders, primary psychiatric disorders, neuromuscular disorders, anaemia, drugs and cardiovascular disorders.
- Prolonged or chronic tiredness is characterised clinically by disabling tiredness, typically lasting more than 2 weeks, associated with non-restorative sleep, headaches and a range of other musculoskeletal and neuropsychiatric symptoms.[2]
- Sociodemographic correlates are concurrent psychological distress, female sex, lower socio-economic status and fewer total years of education.[2]
- Chronic fatigue syndrome (CFS) is defined as debilitating fatigue, persisting or relapsing over six months, associated with a significant reduction in activity levels of at least 50%, and for which no other cause can be found.

Causes of tiredness

Analysing the symptom and reaching a diagnosis demands considerable skill since tiredness may indicate the first subtle manifestation of a serious physical disease or, more commonly, may represent a patient's inability to deal with the problems of everyday life. Chronic tiredness or fatigue is a feature of the 'high pressure' nature of many people's lifestyles.

Careful consideration must be given to the differentiation of physiological tiredness, which results from excessive physical activity, from psychological tiredness. Furthermore, before diagnosing tiredness as psychological, pathological as well as physical causes must be excluded.

A summary of causes of chronic tiredness is presented in Table 66.1.

Table 66.1 *Causes of chronic tiredness/ fatigue*

Psychogenic/non-organic

Psychiatric disorders
• anxiety states
• depression
• other primary disorders
• bereavement
• somatisation disorder

Lifestyle factors
• workaholic tendencies and 'burnout'
• lack of exercise/sedentary lifestyle
• mental stress and emotional demands
• exposure to irritants, e.g. carbon monoxide, 'lead' fumes
• inappropriate diet
• obesity
• sleep deprivation

Organic

Congestive cardiac failure
Anaemia
Malignancy
HIV/AIDS
Subacute to chronic infection, e.g. hepatitis, malaria, Lyme disease
Endocrine
• thyroid (hyper- and hypo-)
• adrenal (Cushing's disease, Addison's disease)
• hyperparathyroidism
• diabetes mellitus
Nutritional deficiency
Renal failure
Liver disorders—chronic liver failure, chronic active hepatitis
Respiratory conditions, e.g. chronic bronchitis
Neuromuscular, e.g. MS, myasthenia gravis, Parkinson's disease
Metabolic, e.g. hypokalaemia, hypomagnesaemia
Drug toxicity, addiction or side effects (see Table 66.3)
Autoimmune disorders
Sleep-related disorders
Postinfectious fatigue syndrome, e.g. influenza, mononucleosis

Unknown

Fibromyalgia
Chronic fatigue syndrome

A diagnostic approach

A summary of the safety diagnostic model is presented in Table 66.2.

Probability diagnosis

The most probable diagnoses to consider are:

• tension, stress and anxiety
• depression
• viral or postviral infection
• sleep-related disorders

Table 66.2 *Tiredness/chronic fatigue: diagnostic strategy model*

Q. *Probability diagnosis*
A. Stress and anxiety
   Depression
   Viral/postviral infection
   Sleep-related disorders, e.g. sleep apnoea

Q. *Serious disorders not to be missed*
A. Malignant disease
   Cardiac arrhythmia, e.g. sick sinus syndrome
   Cardiomyopathy
   Anaemia
   HIV infection

Q. *Pitfalls (often missed)*
A. 'Masked' depression
   Chronic infection, e.g. Lyme disease
   Incipient CCF
   Fibromyalgia
   Lack of fitness
   Drugs: alcohol; prescribed; withdrawal
   Menopause syndrome
   Pregnancy
   Neurological disorders
   • Post head injury
   • CVA
   • Parkinson's disease
   Renal failure
   Metabolic, e.g. hypokalaemia, hypomagnesaemia
   Chemical exposure e.g. occupational

   Rarities
   Hyperparathyroidism
   Addison's disease
   Cushing's disease
   Narcolepsy
   Multiple sclerosis
   Autoimmune disorders

Q. *Seven masquerades checklist*
A. Depression   √
   Diabetes   √
   Drugs   √
   Anaemia   √
   Thyroid disease   √
   Spinal dysfunction √
   UTI   √

Q. *Is the patient trying to tell me something?*
A. Highly likely.

Research studies have reported that over 50% (and in some cases as many as 80%) of reported cases of fatigue have been of psychological causation.[2,4] Overwork is a common cause of fatigue and is often obvious to everyone but the patient. The modern approach to sleep-related disorders has revealed several important factors causing excessive tiredness.

Serious disorders not to be missed
Many serious disorders such as anaemia, malignant disease and subacute or chronic infections such as hepatitis, bacterial endocarditis and tuberculosis can be 'hidden' or masked in the initial stages or not readily apparent. Neuromuscular diseases such as myasthenia gravis and multiple sclerosis, connective tissue disorders and HIV infection also have to be excluded.

Pitfalls
The symptom of tiredness is fraught with pitfalls. Common ones include depression and other psychoneurotic disorders, and incipient congestive cardiac failure. Drug intake is a very common pitfall whether it be by self-administration (including alcohol) or iatrogenic.

Tiredness is a feature of pregnancy in many women, so this association is worth keeping in mind, especially in the early stages when a change in menstrual history is not given or a young single woman will attempt to conceal the fact. It is also a presenting symptom of the menopause syndrome which should not be misdiagnosed.

Seven masquerades checklist
All these important problems are capable of being responsible for tiredness, especially depression, diabetes, drugs, anaemia and urinary infection. Thyroid disease could certainly be responsible. Spinal pain can indirectly cause tiredness. Drugs that commonly cause tiredness are listed in Table 66.3. Antihypertensives require special consideration. Drug withdrawal, especially for illicit drugs such as amphetamines, marijuana, cocaine and heroin, has to be considered.

Psychogenic considerations
Tiredness is a symptom that may represent a 'ticket of entry': a plea for help in a stressed, anxious or depressed patient. Any of the primary psychiatric disorders can present as tiredness.

Table 66.3 *Drugs that can cause tiredness*

Alcohol
Analgesics
Antibiotics
Anticonvulsants
Antiemetics
Antidepressants
Antihistamines
Antihypertensives
Anxiolytics
Corticosteroids
Ergot alkaloids
Digoxin
Hormones, e.g. oral contraceptives
Hypnotics
Nicotine
NSAIDs
Vitamins A and D (early toxic symptoms)
Note: Most drugs have a considerable capacity to cause tiredness.

The clinical approach
In routine history taking, it is mandatory that questions be asked about the following if the information is not volunteered by the patient.

- Sleep pattern (it is not uncommon for patients to say they sleep well and yet on questioning it is found they have initial insomnia, or middle insomnia, or both, with or without early morning waking). It is most relevant to talk to any sleeping partners to obtain a history of sleep disturbance.
- Weight fluctuations.
- Energy—performance—ability to cope.
- Sexual activity.
- Suicidal ideas.
- Self-medication—OTC preparations, e.g. bromides, stimulants, analgesics, alcohol, cigarettes, other drugs. This is particularly important in the drug addiction-prone group: doctors, chemists, nurses, workers in the liquor industry, truck drivers.
- Fears (including phobic symptoms, hypochondriasis).
- Precipitating factors (present in over 50% of patients with depressive illness):
  — postpartum
  — postoperative
  — associated with chronic physical illness

— bereavement
— pain—chronic pain conditions
— retirement
— medication
— post trauma, e.g. motor vehicle accident
— postviral infections, especially hepatitis, mononucleosis, influenza.
• Work history—determine whether the patient is a workaholic.
• Dietary history—determine pattern, including fad diets or skipped meals.
• Menstrual history and symptoms related to the menopause syndrome.
• Self-question: 'Is this patient depressed?'

Physical examination

A routine physical examination is important, followed by a more detailed specific examination relevant to the individual patient. In particular, it is important to ascertain the presence of hepatosplenomegaly and lymphadenopathy. In general the physical examination is unrewarding. In the chronic fatigue syndrome the relevant abnormal findings are muscle tenderness, mild pharyngitis and tender slightly enlarged cervical lymph nodes. When an alternative underlying medical illness is responsible for the tiredness there will usually be evidence for this on physical examination, e.g. positive Babinski reflex in multiple sclerosis, postural hypotension in Addison's disease, right ventricular lift with an ASD. A mental state assessment should be considered.

Investigations

Investigations should be selected judiciously from the following (tests that most patients should have when the examination is completely normal are marked*):
• Haemoglobin, blood count and film*
• ESR*
• ECG and Holter monitor
• Thyroid function tests*
• Liver function tests*
• Urea/renal function tests*
• Serum electrolytes (including calcium and magnesium)*
• Blood sugar*
• Plasma cortisol
• Serum iron and ferritin
• Micro and culture of urine*
• Tests for autoimmune disorders
— antinuclear antibodies
— rheumatoid factor

• HIV screening
• Chest X-ray and spirometry
• Chronic infection screening (consider): hepatitis A, B, C, D, E, cytomegalovirus, EBM, Ross River virus, Lyme disease, brucellosis, Q fever, tuberculosis, malaria, infective endocarditis, toxoplasmosis
• Primary neuromuscular disorders
— muscle enzyme assay
— electromyography
• Tissue markers for malignancy
• Referral to a sleep disorder laboratory for sleep apnoea studies

The diagnosis of CFS can only be made when the minimum investigations (listed *) have been shown to be normal or to demonstrate minor abnormalities in liver function or blood film (atypical lymphocytes).

Tiredness in children

Tiredness in children is caused by a range of predictable conditions such as physiological factors (excessive exercise, lack of sleep, poor diet), infections, allergies including asthma, drugs, depression and various illnesses in general.

Overweight children are likely to fatigue more rapidly than children of normal weight.[5] Any bacterial, viral or other infection may be associated with tiredness, with Epstein-Barr mononucleosis being very significant in adolescents. Chronic Epstein-Barr virus infection causing recurrent episodes of fever, pharyngitis, malaise and adenopathy can occur, especially in teenagers, who present with chronic exhaustion which is frequently mistaken for malignancy.[5]

Tiredness is a presenting feature of depression in adolescents, a serious problem that often goes unrecognised. Tonsillar–adenoidal hypertrophy may be large enough to compromise air exchange, particularly during sleep. Snoring may be a feature plus tiredness and lethargy in the waking state.

Tiredness in the elderly

Elderly people tend to tire more quickly and recover more slowly and incompletely than younger ones. Sleep in older people is generally shorter in duration and of lesser depth, and they feel less refreshed and sometimes irritable on awakening.

Fatigue may be present as a result of emotional frustration. Whenever the prospect of gratification is small, a person tends to tire quickly and to remain so until something stimulating appears. Since the prospects for gratifying experience wane with the years, easy 'fatigueability' or tiredness is common in this age group.

Bereavement

Although a bereavement reaction is common and a normal human response that occurs at all ages, it is more frequently encountered in the elderly, with the loss of a spouse or a child (young or middle-aged!). Fatigue that occurs during the initial mourning period is striking and might represent a protective mechanism against intense emotional stress. With time, usually around 6 to 12 months, a compensated stage is reached, fatigue gradually abates, and the patient resumes normal activities as the conflicts of grief are gradually resolved. Freud pointed out the complexities of mourning as the bereaved person slowly adjusts to the loss of the loved one. In others, various symptoms persist as an 'abnormal grief reaction' including persistence of fatigue. Some factors that may lead to this include:

- unexpected death
- high dependence upon the dead person
- guilt feelings, especially in a love/hate relationship

Studies in general practice have shown that widows see their family doctors for psychiatric symptoms at three times the usual rate in the first 6 months after bereavement. The consultation rate for non-psychiatric symptoms also increases, by almost 50%.

Role of the family doctor

Following bereavement it is important to watch for evidence of depression, drug dependency, especially on alcohol, and suicidal tendencies. In cases of expected death, management should, if possible, start before the bereavement. Supportive care and ongoing counselling are very important.

Sleep-related disorders

Disorders of sleep are a common and significant contribution to community illness and death. For example, it is now known that untreated moderate to severe obstructive sleep apnoea has an 11–13% five-year mortality and a 37% eight-year mortality, mainly from cardiovascular and motor vehicle accident related deaths.[7,8]

A classification of sleep disorders is presented in Table 66.4.[6]

Many conditions may disturb breathing during the night (Fig. 66.1). Nocturnal dyspnoea may result from cardiac causes (mitral stenosis, ischaemic cardiomyopathy, cardiac arrhythmias, fluid overload or retention) which usually present with orthopnoea, pulmonary crepitations and peripheral oedema. Asthma is another common cause of nocturnal dyspnoea, cough (with or without wheeze) occurring classically between 2 a.m. and 5 a.m. Gastro-oesophageal reflux with or without aspiration may disturb respiration at night, but it usually presents with daytime or postural reflux. All these conditions can usually be differentiated from sleep apnoea clinically or with further investigation.

The sleep apnoea syndromes are a common group of disorders that result in periodic hypoventilation during sleep. They occur in about 2% of the general population in all age groups, and in about 10% of middle-aged men.

Sleep apnoea

The term 'sleep apnoea' is used to describe cyclical brief interruptions of ventilation, each cycle lasting 15–90 seconds and resulting in hypoxaemia, hypercapnia and respiratory acidosis, terminating in an arousal from sleep (often not recognised by the patient). The interruption is then followed by the resumption of normal ventilation, a return to sleep, and further interruption of ventilation.

Sleep apnoea is broadly classified into obstructive and central types.

Table 66.4 *Classification of sleep disorders*[6]

Disorders of initiating or maintaining sleep
e.g. nocturnal myoclonus
     sleep apnoea syndromes
Disorders of excessive somnolence
e.g. sleep apnoea syndromes
     narcolepsy
     hypothyroidism
Disorders of sleep/wake cycle
e.g. jet lag
     shift work
Dysfunctions associated with sleep
e.g. night terrors
     sleepwalking

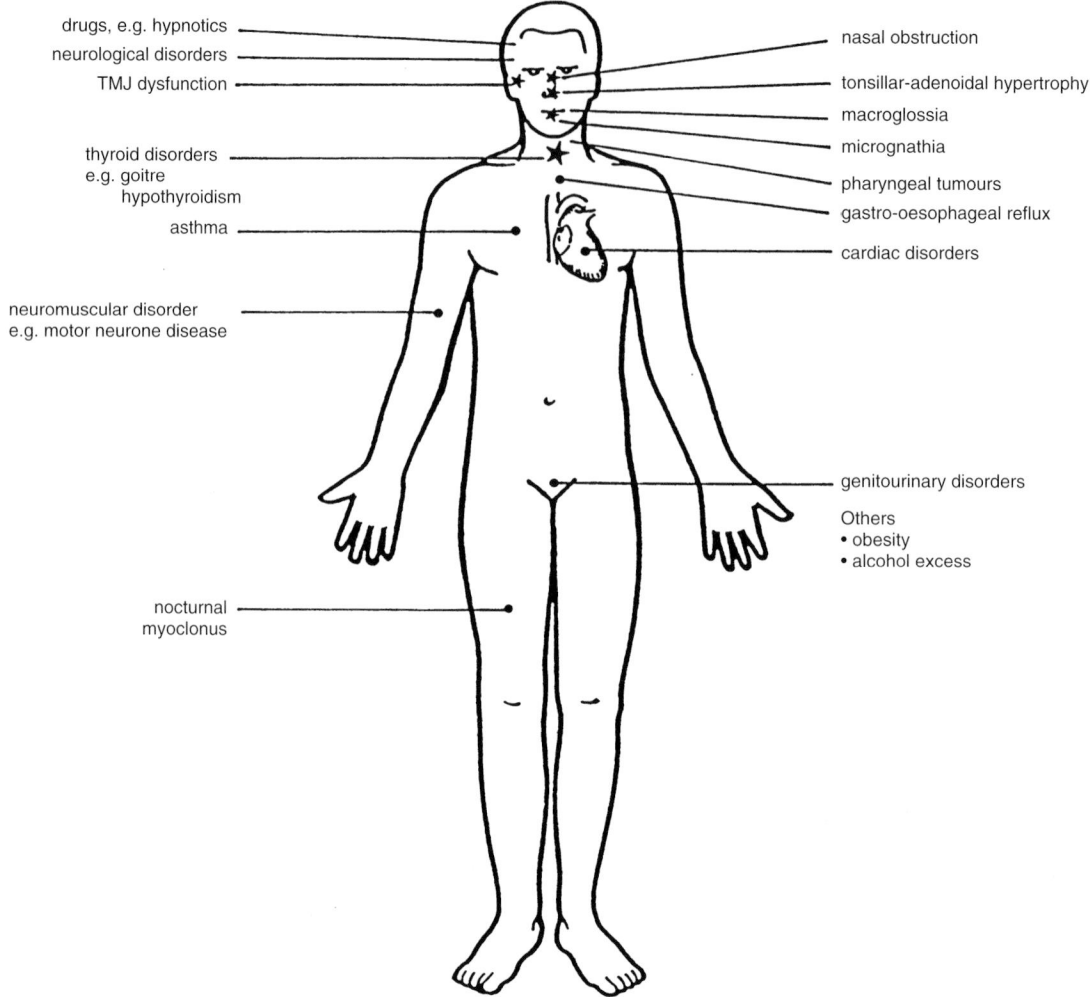

Fig. 66.1 *Significant causes of sleep disturbance*

Obstructive sleep apnoea (OSA) is the commonest type and involves an intermittent narrowing or occlusion of the pharyngeal area of the upper airway. The effects include snoring and hypopnoea, sometimes apnoea.

Predisposing causes include:

- diminished airway size, e.g. macroglossia, obesity, tonsillar-adenoidal hypertrophy
- upper airway muscle hypotonia, e.g. alcohol, hypnotics, neurological disorders
- nasal obstruction

Central sleep apnoea is less common and is due mainly to neurological conditions such as brain stem disorders leading to reduced ventilatory drive, and neuromuscular disorders such as motor neurone disease.

Clinical effects of sleep apnoea syndromes[7]

Important clinical presentations include:

- excessive daytime sleepiness and tirdness
- nocturnal problems, e.g. loud snoring, thrashing, 'seizures', choking, pain reactions
- morning headache
- subtle neuropsychiatric disturbance—learning difficulties, loss of concentration, personality change, depression
- sexual dysfunction

Causes of excessive daytime sleepiness are presented in Table 66.5. In OSA, sleepiness results from repeated arousals during sleep and the effects of hypoxaemia and hypercapnia on the brain. Physical examination may reveal few or no signs.

Table 66.5 *Causes of excessive somnolence*

Sleep apnoea syndromes
Narcolepsy
Endocrine, e.g. hypothyroidism
Drug induced
Purposeful sleep deprivation
Nocturnal myoclonus
Bereavement
Idiopathic

Referral to a comprehensive sleep disorder centre is appropriate if this disorder is suspected.

Narcolepsy

Narcolepsy is a condition where periods of irresistible sleep occur in inappropriate circumstances and consists of a tetrad of symptoms:

- Sudden brief sleep attacks (15–20 minutes).
- Cataplexy—a hidden loss of muscle tone in the lower limbs that may cause the person to slump to the floor, unable to move. These attacks are usually triggered by sudden surprise or emotional upset.
- Sleep paralysis—a frightening feeling of inability to move while drowsy (between sleep and waking).
- Hypnagogic (terrifying) hallucinations on falling asleep or waking up.

Narcolepsy usually begins in early adult life and tends to improve at about 30 years of age. Treatment includes methylphenidate (Ritalin) or amphetamines or small doses of tricylic antidepressants (for cataplexy).

Burnout

Definition
Burnout is a clinical syndrome with:

- emotional exhaustion
- depersonalisation of others
- lack of personal accomplishment

It is similar to stress-related depression but mood lowering is temporary and work-specific.

Patients sometimes claim that they feel 'burnout'. Burnout can mean many things and include a whole constellation of psychogenic symptoms such as exhaustion, boredom and cynicism, paranoia, detachment, heightened irritability and impatience, depression and psychosomatic complaints such as headache and tiredness. Ellard[8] defines burnout as the syndrome that arises when a person who has a strong neurotic need to succeed in a particular task becomes confronted with the impossibility of success in that task. This seems a realistic explanation, but the important factor is to clarify the nature of the problem with care and determine whether the patient has a psychoneurotic disorder, such as hypomania, anxiety state or depression, or a personality disorder or simply unrealistic goals.

Chronic fatigue syndrome

This complex syndrome, which causes profound and persistent tiredness, is also referred to as myalgic encephalomyelitis, chronic neuromuscular viral syndrome,[9] postviral syndrome, chronic Epstein-Barr viral syndrome, viral fatigue state, epidemic neuromyasthenia, neurasthenia, Icelandic disease, Royal Free disease and Tapanui disease. Chronic fatigue syndrome (CFS) is not to be confused with the tiredness and depression that follow a viral infection such as infectious mononucleosis, hepatitis or influenza. These postviral tiredness states are certainly common but resolve within 6 months or so.

Typical features of CFS:[10]

- extreme exhaustion (with minimal physical effort)
- headache or a vague 'fuzzy' feeling in the head
- aching in the muscles and legs
- poor concentration and memory
- hypersomnia or other sleep disturbance
- waking feeling tired
- emotional lability
- depressive-type illness
- arthralgia
- sore throat
- subjective feeling of fever (with a normal temperature)
- tender swollen lymph glands
- usually occurs between 20 and 40 years of age

Epidemiologically it has been related to Coxsackie B virus infections.[10] The responsible organism is referred to as a slow virus infection by some authorities.[9]

In approximately two-thirds of patients the illness follows a clearly defined viral illness.

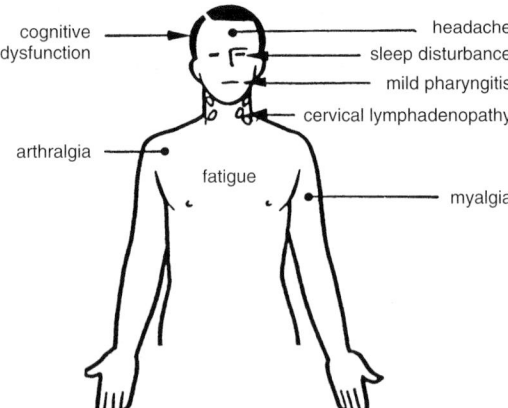

Fig. 66.2 *Chronic fatigue syndrome: characteristic symptoms*

Table 66.6 *Criteria for the diagnosis of chronic fatigue syndrome*

Major criteria (must meet both)
1. New onset of persistent or relapsing debilitating fatigue (of a muscular type) that impairs daily activity to below 50% of the premorbid level for at least 6 months
2. Complete exclusion of other physical or psychiatric disorders that may produce similar symptoms

Minor criteria (must have 6+2 physical criteria or 8 of 11 symptoms)

Symptom criteria
1. mild fever (37.5–38.6°C)
2. sore throat
3. painful cervical or axillary lymph nodes
4. unexplained generalised muscle weakness
5. myalgia
6. prolonged fatigue after exercise
7. generalised headaches
8. neuropsychiatric complaints, e.g. poor concentration
9. migratory arthralgias (no joint swelling)
10. sleep disturbance
11. rapid onset of the symptom complex

Physical criteria
1. low-grade fever
2. non-exudative pharyngitis
3. palpable or tender cervical or axillary nodes

However, no single virus has been consistently associated with the development of the syndrome which is known to develop following a wide range of viral and non-viral infective illness. Immune system dysfunction with chronic overproduction of cytokines (e.g. interferon) is a possible pathogenetic mechanism.

Every family doctor probably has patients with this disorder and the syndrome has been observed in isolated endemics from time to time. Hickie et al.[2] found that only 0.3% of those with prolonged fatigue had been diagnosed with chronic fatigue syndrome by their family doctor.

There is no doubt that the syndrome is real in these patients. One of the major problems confronting clinicians is that there is no diagnostic test for this illness, so it remains a clinical diagnosis backed up by normal baseline investigations.

Diagnostic criteria for CFS have been published[11] (Table 66.6), which emphasise the positive clinical features of the syndrome and the chronicity of symptoms (greater than 6 months), in addition to the need for careful exclusion of alternative diagnoses by history, physical examination and laboratory investigation.

Physical examination and investigation

Apart from mild pharyngeal infection, cervical lymphadenopathy or localised muscle tenderness, the physical examination is normal.

Investigations should be directed towards excluding possible diagnoses for that patient, such as chronic infection, autoimmune disorders, endocrine and metabolic disorders, primary neuromuscular disorders, malignancy and primary psychiatric disorders. The last mentioned is the most difficult of the differential diagnoses and psychiatric referral will often need to be considered.

Management

Patients who have CFS are really suffering and unhappy people, similar to those with fibromyalgia. They require considerable understanding and support. Symptoms last approximately 2½ years.

Management strategies include:[12]

• CFS recognition—explain that the illness is real but the cause unknown and tests are likely to be normal.
• Explanation and reassurance that the illness is usually self-limiting with no permanent complications; and that a slow steady improvement can be anticipated with most CSF patients returning to normal health.
• Provide continued psychological support.
• Review for diagnostic reappraisal (examine at least every 4 months).
• Avoid telling patients they are depressed.
• Regular rest is the key to recovery.
• Treat symptomatically—pain relief, consider NSAIDs.

- Refer to counselling and support groups.
- Provide a realistic, regular, graduated exercise program.
- Reduce relevant stress factors (map a realistic living program).
- Psychiatric referral if appropriate.
- Ask the patient to keep a diary of exercise/stress and symptom severity, in particular.
- Avoid long-distance travel, which is poorly tolerated.

Cognitive therapy appears to help some patients, as do relaxation therapy, meditation, stress management and psychotherapy, where indicated.

The emphasis should be placed on caring, rather than curing, until a scientific solution is found.

Medication options

Consider:

- low-dose tricylic or SSRI antidepressants (trial if depression significant)
- NSAIDs, with or without low-dose tricyclics when necessary, especially for aches and pains
- domperidone for nausea

Some individual patients benefit from evening primrose oil and injections of immunoglobulin or Vitamin B_{12}, but such therapies lack hard evidence-based criteria to justify general acceptance.

Fibromyalgia

The fibromyalgia syndrome (see Chap. 34) bears a clinical resemblance to CFS. Musculoskeletal pain is more prominent although tiredness (fatigue) and sleep disturbance are features. According to Schwenk,[13] fibromyalgia affects 5% of the American population with a peak age of 35 (range 20–60) and the F:M sex ratio 10:1. The management is similar to CFS but the prognosis less optimistic.

Practice tips

- Always consider underlying psychological distress, especially depressive disorder.
- Do not overlook a sleep disorder.
- Believe the patient's symptoms.
- Be careful of labelling a patient as having CFS.
- Key investigations are:

— FBE and ESR
— S urea and creatinine
— S electrolytes, including calcium
— liver function tests
— blood sugar
— thyroid function tests
— micro and culture of urine.

References

1. Marinker M, Watter CAH. The patient complaining of tiredness. In: Cormack J, Marinker M, Morrell D eds, *Practice*. London: Kluwer Medical, 1982, Section 3.1.
2. Hickie IB et al. Sociodemographic and psychiatric correlates of fatigue in selected primary care settings. Med J Aust, 1996; 164:585–588.
3. Jerrett WA. Lethargy in general practice. Practitioner, 1981; 225:731–737.
4. French MA. The clinical significance of tiredness. Can Med Assoc J, 1960; 82: 665–671.
5. Tennessen WW. *Signs and symptoms in paediatrics*. Philadelphia: Lippincott, 1988, 37–40.
6. Pierce R, Naughton M. Sleep-related breathing disorders: recent advances. Aust Fam Physician, 1992; 21:397–405.
7. Partinen M, Guilleminault C. Daytime sleepiness and vascular morbidity: a seven year follow-up in obstructive sleep apnoea patients. Chest, 1990, 97:27–32.
8. Ellard J. A note on burnout. Mod Med Aust, 1987 (January), 32–35.
9. Simpson G. Persistent neuromuscular viral syndrome. Aust Fam Physician, 1987; 16:978–981.
10. Blaiklock DA. The chronically tired patient. Patient Management, 1986; 10 (July): 89–96.
11. Holmes G et al. Chronic fatigue syndrome: a working class definition. Ann Intern Med, 1988; 108: 387–389.
12. Wakefield D, Lloyd A, Hickie I. The chronic fatigue syndrome. Mod Med Aust, July 1990, 16–22.
13. Schwenk TL. Fibromyalgia and chronic fatigue syndrome: solving diagnostic and therapeutic dilemmas. Modern Medicine (USA), 1992; 60:50–60.

67

The unconscious patient

—

In whatever disease sleep is laborious, it is a deadly
symptom; but if sleep does good, it is not deadly.

Hippocrates

The state of arousal is determined by the function of the central reticular formation which extends from the brain stem to the thalamus. Coma occurs when this centre is damaged by a metabolic abnormality or by an invasive lesion which compresses this centre. Coma is also caused by damage to the cerebral cortex.[1]

The word 'coma' is derived from the Greek *koma*, which is deep sleep. The deeply unconscious patient is not in deep sleep. Coma is best defined as 'lack of self-awareness'.[3]

The various levels of consciousness are summarised in Table 67.1; the levels vary from consciousness, which means awareness of oneself and the surroundings in a state of wakefulness,[2] to coma which is a state of unrousable unresponsiveness. Rather than using these broad terms in clinical practice it is preferable to describe the actual state of the patient in a sentence.

Key facts and checkpoints

- Always consider hypoglycaemia or opioid overdose in any unconscious patient, especially of unknown background.
- If a patient is unconscious and cyanosed consider upper airway obstruction until proved otherwise.
- The commonest causes of unconsciousness encountered in general practice are syncope, expecially postural hypotension, concussion

Table 67.1 *The five conscious levels*

	State	Clinical features	Simplified classification
	1 Consciousness	Aware and wakeful	Awake
	2 Clouded consciousness	Reduced awareness and wakefulness 'Alcohol effect' Confusion Drowsiness	Confused
↑ **Degree of consciousness** ↓	3 Stupor	Unconscious Deep sleep-like state Arousal with vigorous stimuli	Responds to shake and shout
	4 Semicomatose	Unconscious (deeper) Responds only to painful stimuli (sternal rubbing with knuckles) without arousing	Responds to pain
	5 Coma	Deeply unconscious Unrousable and unresponsive	Unresponsive coma

and cerebrovascular accidents. The main causes are presented in Table 67.2.

- Do not allow the person who accompanies the unconscious patient to leave until all relevant details have been obtained.
- Record the degree of coma as a base-line to determine improvement or deterioration.

Table 67.2 *Main causes of loss of consciousness*

Episodic causes—blackouts
- Epilepsy
- Syncope
- Drop attacks
- Cardiac arrhythmias, e.g. Stokes-Adams attacks
- Vertebrobasilar insufficiency
- Psychogenic disorders, including hyperventilation
- Breath holding (children)

Coma
(COMA provides a useful mnemonic for four major groups[1] of causes of unconsciousness)

C = CO_2 narcosis: respiratory failure

O = Overdose of drugs
- alcohol
- opioids
- tranquillisers and antidepressants
- carbon monoxide
- analgesics
- others

M = Metabolic
- diabetes
  — hypoglycaemia
  — ketoacidosis
- hypothyroidism
- hepatic failure
- renal failure (uraemia)
- others

A = Apoplexy
Supratentorial
- intracerebral haemorrhage
- haematoma: subdural or extradural
- head injury
- cerebral tumour
- cerebral abscess

Infratentorial (posterior fossa)
- pressure from above
- cerebellar tumour
- brainstem infarct/haemorrhage
- Wernicke's encephalopathy

Meningismus (neck stiffness)
- subarachnoid haemorrhage
- meningitis

Other
- encephalitis
- overwhelming infection

Trauma

Urgent attention

The initial contact with the unconscious patient is invariably sudden and dramatic and demands immediate action which should take only seconds to minutes. The primary objective is to keep the patient alive until the cause is determined and possible remedial action taken.[2]

Examination	Action
Is the patient breathing? Note chest wall movement	If not, clear airway and ventilate
Check pulse and pupils	Perform cardiopulmonary resuscitation if necessary Consider naloxone
Is there evidence of trauma?	Consider extradural haematoma
Is the patient hypoglycaemic? Evidence of diabetes (discs, etc)	Consider glucometer estimation of blood sugar
Are vital functions present yet immediate correctable causes eliminated?	Place in coma position

History

A history can be obtained from relatives, friends, witnesses, ambulance officers or others. The setting in which the patient is found is important. Evidence of discs or cards identifying an illness such as diabetes or epilepsy should be searched for. Is there a known history of hypertension, heart disease, respiratory disease or psychiatric illness?

Questions to be considered[4]
- Is the patient diabetic?
  Does the patient have insulin injections?
  Has the patient had an infection?
  Has the patient been eating properly?
- Is drug overdose possible?
  Has the patient been depressed? Has the patient experienced recent stress or personal 'mishaps'?
  Has the patient been on any medications?
- Is opioid usage possible in this patient?
  Are the presenting circumstances unusual?
- Is epilepsy possible?
  Was twitching in the limbs observed?
  Did the patient pass urine or faeces?
- Is head injury possible?
  Has the patient been in a recent accident?
  Has the patient complained of headache?

- Has a stroke or subarachnoid haemorrhage occurred?
  Has the patient a history of hypertension?
  Did the patient complain of a severe headache?
  Has the patient complained of weakness of the limbs?

Examination

General features requiring assessment:

- Breathing pattern:
  Cheyne-Stokes respiration (periodic respiration) = cerebral dysfunction
  Ataxic respiration: shallow irregular respiration = brain stem lesion
  Kussmaul respiration: deep rapid hyperventilation = metabolic acidosis
- Breath: characteristic odours may be a feature of alcohol, diabetes, uraemia and hepatic coma.
- Level of consciousness: degree of coma (Table 67.1); the Glasgow coma scale (Table 67.3) is frequently used as a guide to the conscious state.
- Skin features: look for evidence of injection sites (drug addicts, diabetics) and snake bite marks, colour (cyanosis, purpura, jaundice, rashes, hyperpigmentation) and texture.
- Circulation.

Table 67.3 *Glasgow coma scale*

	Score
Eye opening (E)	
• Spontaneous opening	4
• To verbal command	3
• To pain	2
• No response	1
Motor response (M)	
• Obeys verbal command	6
Response to painful stimuli	
• Localises pain	5
• Withdraws from pain stimuli	4
• Abnormal flexion	3
• Extensor response	2
• No response	1
Verbal response (V)	
• Orientated and converses	5
• Disoriented and converses	4
• Inappropriate words	3
• Incomprehensible sounds	2
• No response	1
Coma score = E + M + V	
Minimum 3	
Maximum 15	

- Temperature: consider infection such as meningitis and hyperpyrexia if raised and hypothermia, e.g. hypothyroidism, if low.
- Hydration: dehydration may signify conditions such as a high fever with infections, uraemia, hyperglycaemic coma.

Examination of the head and neck[2,4]
The following should be considered:

- facial asymmetry
- the skull and neck: palpation for evidence of trauma and neck rigidity
- eyes, pupils and ocular fundi
- tongue
- nostrils and ears
- auscultation of the skull

Examination of the limbs
Consider:

- injection marks (drug addicts, diabetics)
- tone of the limbs by lifting and dropping, e.g. flaccid limbs with early hemiplegia
- reaction of limbs to painful stimuli
- reflexes: tendon reflexes and plantar response

General examination of the body
This should include assessment of the pulses and blood pressure.

Urine examination
Catheterisation of the bladder may be necessary to obtain urine. Check the urine for protein, sugar and ketones.

Diagnosing the hysterical 'unconscious' patient
One of the most puzzling problems in emergency medicine is how to diagnose the unconscious patient caused by a conversion reaction (hysteria). These patients really experience their symptoms (as opposed to the pretending patient) and resist most normal stimuli, including painful stimuli.

Method
- Hold the patient's eye or eyes open with your fingers and note the reaction to light.
- Now hold a mirror over the eye and watch closely for pupillary reaction. The pupil should constrict with accommodation from the patient looking at his or her own image.

Investigations

Appropriate investigations depend on the clinical assessment. The following is a checklist.

- Blood tests
  - All patients: blood sugar
                       urea and electrolytes
  - Selected patients: full blood examination
                       blood gases
                       liver function tests
                       blood alcohol
                       serum cortisol
                       thyroid function tests
                       serum digoxin
- Urine tests
  - A urine specimen is obtained by catheterisation.
  - Test for glucose and albumin.
  - Keep the specimen for drug screening.
- Stomach contents: aspiration of stomach contents for analysis.
- Radiology: CT scan or MRI are the investigations of choice (if available). If unavailable, X-ray of the skull may be helpful.
- Cerebrospinal fluid: lumbar puncture, necessary with neck stiffness, has risks in the comatose patient. A preliminary CT scan is necessary to search for coning of the cerebellum. If clear, the lumbar puncture should be safe and will help to diagnose subarachnoid haemorrhage and meningitis.
- Electroencephalograph
- ECG

Blackouts—episodic loss of consciousness

Episodic or transient loss of consciousness is a common problem. The important causes of blackout are presented in Table 67.2. The history is important to determine whether the patient is describing a true blackout or episodes of dizziness, weakness or some other sensation.

The clinical features of various types of blackouts are summarised in Table 67.4.

Epilepsy

Epilepsy is the commonest cause of blackouts. There are various types, the most dramatic being the tonic-clonic seizure in which patients have sudden loss of consciousness without warning.

Table 67.4   *Clinical features of blackouts*

Cause	*Precipitants*	*Subjective onset*	*Observation*	*Recovery*
Vasovagal syncope	posture stress haemorrhage micturition	warning of feeling 'faint', 'distant' 'clammy, sweaty'	very pale sweating	gradual feels 'terrible' fatigue nausea
Respiratory syncope	cough weight-lifting trumpet playing	warning (feels faint)	pale	rapid

Carotid sinus syncope	carotid pressure
	   e.g. tight collar +
	      turning neck
	postendarterectomy
		warning
		(feels faint)
			pale	rapid

Cardiac syncope	various	may be palpitations	pale	rapid may be flushing
Migrainous syncope	foods stress sleep deprivation	scotomas	pale	nausea and vomiting throbbing headache
Autonomic syncope	postural change	warning (feels faint)	pale	rapid

Epilepsy	stress
	sleep deprivation
	alcohol withdrawal
	infection
	menstruation
	drug non-compliance
		aura with complex partial seizures (CPS)	automatism
			   e.g. fidgeting,
			      lip smacking
			with CPS
				slow
				confused

The typical features (in order) of a tonic-clonic convulsion are:

- aura (sensory or psychological feelings)
- initial rigid tonic phase (up to 60 seconds)
- convulsion (clonic phase) (seconds to minutes)
- mild coma or drowsiness (15 minutes to several hours) i.e. post-ictal confusion

Associated features:

- cyanosis, then heavy 'snoring' breathing
- eyes rolling 'back into head'
- ± tongue biting
- ± incontinence of urine or faeces

It should be noted that sphincter incontinence is not firmly diagnostic of epilepsy. In less severe episodes the patient may fall without observable twitching of the limbs.[5]

In atonic epilepsy, which occurs in those with tonic-clonic epilepsy, the patient falls to the ground and is unconscious for only a brief period.

Syncope

In syncope there is a transient loss of consciousness but with warning symptoms and rapid return of alertness following a brief period of unconsciousness (seconds to 3 minutes).

Relevant features of vasovagal or common faint:

- occurs with standing or, less commonly, sitting
- warning feelings of dizziness, faintness or true vertigo
- nausea, hot and cold skin sensations
- fading hearing or blurred vision
- sliding to ground (rather than heavy full-length fall)
- rapid return of consciousness
- pallor and sweating and bradycardia
- often trigger factors, e.g. emotional upset, pain

The patient invariably remembers the onset of fainting. Most syncope is of the benign vasomotor type and tends to occur in young people, especially when standing still, e.g. choir boys.

Other forms of syncope

Micturition syncope
This uncommon event may occur after micturition in older men, especially during the night when they leave a warm bed and stand to void. The cause appears to be peripheral vasodilation

associated with reduction of venous return from straining.

Cough syncope
Severe coughing can result in obstruction of venous return with subsequent blackout. This is also the mechanism of blackouts with breath-holding attacks.

Carotid sinus syncope
This problem is caused by pressure on a hypersensitive carotid sinus, e.g. in some elderly patients who lose consciousness when their neck is touched.

Effort syncope
Syncope on exertion is due to obstructive cardiac disorders such as aortic stenosis and hypertrophic obstructive cardiomyopathy.

Choking

Sudden collapse can follow choking. Examples include the so-called 'cafe coronary' or 'barbecue coronary' when the patient, while eating meat, suddenly becomes cyanosed, is speechless and grasps the throat. This is caused by inhaling a large bolus of meat which obstructs the larynx. To avoid death, immediate relief of obstruction is necessary. An emergency treatment is the Heimlich manoeuvre whereby the patient is grasped from behind around the abdomen and a forceful squeeze applied to try to eject the food. If this fails, the foreign body may have to be manually removed from the throat.

Drop attacks

Drop attacks are episodes of 'blackouts' in which the patient suddenly falls to the ground and then immediately gets up again. They involve sudden attacks of weakness in the legs. Although there is some doubt about whether loss of consciousness has occurred, most patients cannot remember the process of falling. Drop attacks occur typically in middle-aged women and are considered to be brain stem disturbances producing sudden changes in tone in the lower limbs. Other causes of drop attacks include vertebrobasilar insufficiency, Parkinson's disease and epilepsy.[5]

Cardiac arrhythmias

Stokes-Adams attacks and cardiac syncope are manifestations of recurrent episodes of loss of consciousness, especially in the elderly, caused by cardiac arrhythmias. These arrhythmias include complete heart block, sick sinus syndrome and ventricular tachycardia. The blackout is sudden with the patient falling straight to the ground without warning and without convulsive movements. The patient goes pale at first and then flushed.

Twenty-four-hour ambulatory cardiac monitoring may be necessary to confirm the diagnosis.

Patients with aortic stenosis are prone to have exercise-induced blackouts.

Vertebrobasilar insufficiency

Loss of consciousness can occur rarely with vertebrobasilar insufficiency (VBI). Typical preceding symptoms of VBI include dyspnoea, vertigo, vomiting, hemisensory loss, ataxia and transient global amnesia.

Hypoglycaemia

Hypoglycaemia can be difficult to recognise but must be considered as it can vary from a feeling of malaise and lightheadedness to loss of consciousness, sometimes with a convulsion. There are usually preliminary symptoms of hunger, sweating, shaking or altered behaviour. Hypoglycaemic attacks are usually related to diabetes and can occur with oral hypoglycaemics as well as insulin.

Psychogenic factors

Psychogenic factors leading to blackouts represent a diagnostic dilemma, especially if occurring in patients with tonic-clonic epilepsy. If the attacks are witnessed by the practitioner then the possibility of functional origin can be determined.

Hysterical blackouts or fits are not uncommon and have to be differentiated from hyperventilation. It is unusual for hyperventilation to cause unconsciousness but it is possible to get clouding of consciousness, especially if the patient is administered oxygen.

Other features that suggest psychogenic factors rather than organic are:

• labile affect

• rapidly changing levels of consciousness
• well articulated speech
• bizarre thought control

Initial management of the unconscious patient

The first principle of management of a person found unconscious is to keep the patient alive by maintaining the airway and the circulation. The basic management essentials are summarised in Table 67.5.

Before embarking on a secondary survey always consider giving the 'coma cocktail' (also called TONG[3]) which refers to the combination of:

Thiamine	100 mg IM or IV
Oxygenation	
Naloxone	0.1–0.2 mg IV
Glucose	i.e. 50 mL, 50% dextrose

The rapid administration of these agents should be considered for any patient[3, 6] with an altered level of consciousness because they may lessen or reverse metabolic insult to the brain.

In the presence of hypoventilation, constricted pupils[6] or circumstantial evidence of opioid use, naloxone (the specific opiate antagonist) should be given intravenously. If there is no response the patient should be intubated before further naloxone is given.

Use of flumazenil

Flumazenil is a specific benzodiazepine antagonist and may have an important use in the assessment of the unconscious patient. It can have a dramatic effect on benzodiazepine overdosage. After an initial dose of 0.2 mg IV, 0.3–0.5 mg boluses should be given every 1–2 minutes with caution until a response is observed.[6]

Table 67.5 *Basic management essentials*

Keep patient alive
(maintain airway and circulation)

Get history from witnesses

Examine patient

Give 'coma cocktail' (TONG)

Take blood (for investigations)

CT scan (if diagnosis doubtful)

Opioid (heroin) overdose

A known overdose patient should be treated initially with both IV and IM naloxone.

- naloxone 0.4 mg IV (repeat in 3 mins if necessary)
- naloxone 0.4 mg IM (to maintain cover)

Practice tips[3]

- The hypotensive patient is bleeding until proved otherwise.
- The presence of a head injury should not prevent rigorous resuscitation of the hypotensive patient.
- Always suspect cervical injury in the presence of patients who are victims of time-critical trauma.
- Tachypnoea is a sign of inadequate oxygenation and not a sign of central nerve damage.
- Always suspect opioid overdosage in the 'unknown' patient brought in with an altered conscious state.
- Consider administration of TONG—the 'coma cocktail'.

References

1. Talley N, O'Connor S. *Clinical examination* (3rd edn). Sydney: MacLennan & Petty, 1996, 414.
2. Kumer PJ, Clark ML. *Clinical medicine* (2nd edn). London: Bailliere Tindall, 1990, 1.
3. Wassertheil J. Management of neurological emergencies. Monash University. Update for GP's Course notes 1996, 1–10.
4. Davis A, Bolin T, Ham J. *Symptom analysis and physical diagnosis* (2nd edn). Sydney: Pergamon Press, 1990, 276–279.
5. Kincaid-Smith P, Larkins R, Whelan G. *Problems in clinical medicine*. Sydney: MacLennan & Petty, 1990, 156–175.
6. McGirr J, McDonagh T. Management of acute poisoning. Current Therapeutics, 1995; 36(5): 51–59.

68

Urinary disorders

As men draw near the common goal,
Can anything be sadder
Than he who, master of his soul,
Is servant to his bladder?

Anonymous 1938
Speculum

Disturbances of micturition are a common problem in general practice with an annual incidence of about 20 per 1000 patients at risk.[1] Such disturbances include dysuria, frequency of micturition, difficulty or inability to initiate micturition, stress incontinence and haematuria. These symptoms are three times as common in women as in men.[1] The combination of dysuria and frequency is the most common of the symptoms with an incidence of about 14 per 1000 patients and a female to male ratio of 5 to 1.[1]

In children and the elderly the patient may complain of urinary incontinence unassociated with stress. However, with the exception of enuresis (Chap. 73), disturbances of micturition are uncommon in children.

Dysuria and frequency

Dysuria, or difficult and/or painful micturition, which is characterised mainly by urethral and suprapubic discomfort, indicates mucosal inflammation of the lower genitourinary tract, i.e. the urethra, bladder or prostate. The passage of urine across inflamed mucosa causes pain. Frequency can vary from being negligible to extreme. Sometimes haematuria and systemic symptoms can accompany dysuria and frequency.

A summary of the diagnostic strategy model for dysuria is presented in Table 68.1.

Table 68.1 *Dysuria: diagnostic strategy model*

Q. *Probability diagnosis*
A. Urinary infection, esp. cystitis (female)
   Urethritis
   Urethral syndrome (female)
   Vaginitis

Q. *Serious disorders not to be missed*
A. Neoplasia
   • bladder
   • prostate
   • urethra
   Severe infections
   • gonorrhoea
   • NSU
   • genital herpes
   Reiter's disease
   Calculi, e.g. bladder

Q. *Pitfalls (often missed)*
A. Menopause syndrome
   Prostatitis
   Foreign bodies in LUT
   Acidic urine
   Acute fever
   Interstitial cystitis
   Urethral caruncle/diverticuli
   Vaginal prolapse
   Obstruction
   • benign prostatic hyperplasia
   • urethral stricture
   • phimosis
   • meatal stenosis

Q. *Seven masquerades checklist*
A. Depression   √
   Diabetes   √
   Drugs   √
   Anaemia   –
   Thyroid disease   –
   Spinal dysfunction   –
   UTI   √

Q. *Is the patient trying to tell me something?*
A. Consider psychosexual problems; anxiety and hypochondriasis.

Key facts and checkpoints[1,2]

- Strangury = difficult and painful micturition with associated spasm.
- Inflammation usually results in frequent passage of small amounts of urine and a sense of urgency.
- Urethritis usually causes pain at the onset of micturition.
- Cystitis usually causes pain at the end of micturition.
- Suprapubic discomfort is a feature of bladder infection (cystitis).
- Vesicocolonic fistulas (e.g. prostatic cancer) cause severe dysuria, pneumaturia and foul-smelling urine.
- Dysuria and frequency are most common in women aged 15 to 44 years.
- They are four times more common in sexually active women.
- Vaginitis is an important cause and must be considered.
- Dysuria and discomfort is a common feature of postmenopausal syndrome, due to atrophic urethritis. The urethra and lower bladder are oestrogen-dependent.
- Urinary infection and other disorders can be quite asymptomatic.

Is it really a urinary tract infection?

Although urinary tract infections account for the majority of cases of dysuria in women it must be remembered that vaginitis and postmenopausal atrophic vaginitis can cause dysuria (Fig. 68.1).

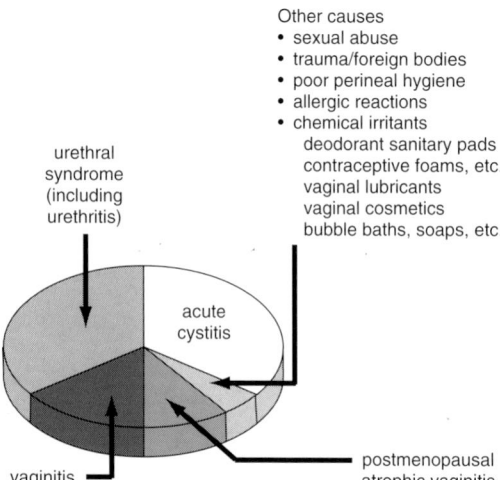

Fig. 68.1 *Relative causes of dysuria in women*

Vaginitis is the most common cause of dysuria in the adolescent age group and is a relatively common cause of dysuria in family practice, estimated at around 15%. Postmenopausal oestrogen deficiency is estimated at 5–10%.[3] In the latter it is worthwhile prescribing oestrogen, either topically or systemically. Acute bacterial cystitis accounts for about 40% of causes of dysuria.

The dysuria associated with vaginitis may be described as burning 'on the outside' with the discomfort usually felt at the beginning or end of micturition. If vaginitis is suspected, a pelvic examination should be carried out to inspect the genitalia and obtain swabs.[3]

The clinical approach

History

It is important to determine whether dysuria is really genitourinary in origin and not attributable to functional disorders such as psychosexual problems. Disturbances of micturition are uncommon in the young male and if present suggest venereal infection.

Key questions

- Could you describe the discomfort?
- What colour is your urine?
- Does it have a particular odour?
- Have you noticed a discharge?
- If so, could it be sexually acquired?
- Do you find intercourse painful or uncomfortable (women)?
- Have you any fever, sweats or chills?

Examination

The general inspection and examination should include measurement of the basic parameters of pulse, temperature and blood pressure. The possibility of underlying renal disease, especially in the presence of an obstructive component, should be kept in mind.

Abdominal palpation is important with a focus on the loins and suprapubic areas. The possibility of sexually transmitted diseases should also be considered and vaginal examination of the female and rectal and genital examination in the male may be appropriate. In the menopausal female a dry atrophic urethral opening, a ureteral caruncle or urethral prolapse may give the clue to this important and neglected cause of dysuria.

Investigations

Basic investigations include:

- dipstick testing of urine
- microscopy and culture (midstream specimen of urine or suprapubic puncture), and possibly urethral swabs for sexually transmitted diseases

Further investigations depend on initial findings and referral for detailed investigation will be necessary if the primary cause cannot be found.

Haematuria

Haematuria is the presence of blood in the urine and can vary from frank bleeding (macroscopic) to the microscopic detection of red cells. Haematuria can occur in a wide variety of disorders but a careful history and examination can often lead to the source of the bleeding and help with the selection of investigations.

Key facts and checkpoints

- Macroscopic haematuria is the presence of blood visible to the naked eye. It is always abnormal except in menstruating women.
- Small amounts of blood (1 mL/1000 mL urine) can produce macroscopic haematuria.
- Microscopic haematuria is the presence of blood in the urine that can only be detected by microscopic or chemical methods.
- Microscopic haematuria includes the presence of red blood cells (RBC) > 8000 per mL of urine (phase contrast microscopy) or > 2000 per mL of urine (light microscopy) representing the occasional RBC on microscopic examination.
- Joggers and athletes engaged in very vigorous exercise can develop transient microscopic haematuria.
- Common sources of macroscopic haematuria are the bladder, urethra, prostate and kidney.[4]
- Macroscopic haematuria occurs in 70% of people with bladder cancer and 40% with kidney cancer.[4]
- Common urological cancers that cause haematuria are the bladder (70%), kidney (17%), renal pelvis or ureter (7%) and prostate (5%).
- It is important to exclude renal damage, so patients should have blood pressure, urinary protein and plasma creatinine measured as a base-line.
- All patients presenting with macroscopic haematuria or recurrent microscopic haematuria require judicious investigation which may involve both radiological investigation of the upper urinary system and visualisation of the lower urinary system to detect or exclude pathology.
- The key radiological investigation is the intravenous urogram (pyelogram), unless there is a history of iodine allergy, severe asthma or other contraindications, when ultrasound is the next choice.

The clinical approach

History

In many patients the underlying disorder may be suspected from a detailed enquiry about associated urinary symptoms. The presence of blood can be verified rapidly by microscopy so that red discolouration due to haemolysis or red food dye can be discounted.

The time relationship of bleeding is useful because, as a general rule, haematuria occurring in the first part of the stream suggests a urethral or prostatic lesion, while terminal haematuria suggests bleeding from the bladder. Uniform haematuria has no localising features.

The possibility of sexually acquired urethritis should be kept in mind. It is most unusual for haematuria to cause anaemia unless it is massive. Massive haematuria is a feature of radiation cystitis.

Painful haematuria is suggestive of infection, calculi or renal infarction, while painless haematuria is commonly associated with infection, trauma, tumours or polycystic kidneys. Loin pain can occur as a manifestation of nephritis and may be a feature of bleeding in carcinoma of the kidney or polycystic kidney.

A drug history is relevant, especially with anticoagulants and cyclophosphamide. A diet history should also be considered.

It is worth noting that large prostatic veins, secondary to prostatic enlargement located at the bladder neck, may rupture when a man strains to urinate.

A summary of the diagnostic strategy model for haematuria is presented in Table 68.2.

Key questions

- Have you had an injury such as a blow to the loin, pelvis or genital area?
- Have you noticed whether the redness is at the start or end of your stream or throughout the stream?
- Have you noticed any bleeding elsewhere such as bruising of the skin or nose bleed?

Table 68.2   *Haematuria: diagnostic strategy*
model

Q. Probability diagnosis
A. Infection[7]
   • cystitis/urethrotrigonitis (female)
   • urethritis (male)
   • prostatitis (male)
   Calculi—renal, ureteric, bladder

Q. Serious disorders not to be missed
A. Cardiovascular
   • renal infarction
   • renal vein thrombosis
   • prostatic varices
   Neoplasia
   • renal tumour
   • urothelial: bladder, renal pelvis, ureter
   • carcinoma prostate
   Severe infections
   • infective endocarditis
   • renal tuberculosis
   • glomerulonephritis
   • Blackwater fever
   Renal papillary necrosis
   Other renal disease

Q. Pitfalls (often missed)
A. Urethral prolapse/caruncle
   Pseudohaematuria, e.g. beetroot, porphyria
   Benign prostatic hyperplasia
   Trauma: blunt or penetrating
   Foreign bodies
   Bleeding disorders
   Exercise
   Radiation cystitis

   Rarities
   • hydronephrosis
   • Henoch-Schönlein purpura
   • bilharzia
   • polycystic kidneys
   • renal cysts
   • endometriosis (bladder)
   • systemic vasculitides

Q. Seven masquerades checklist
A. Depression   –
   Diabetes   –
   Drugs   √ cytotoxics
                             anticoagulants
   Anaemia   –
   Thyroid disease   –
   Spinal dysfunction   –
   UTI   √

Q. Is this patient trying to tell me something?
A. Consider artifactual haematuria.

• Have you experienced any pain in the loin or abdomen?
• Have you noticed any burning or frequency of your urine?
• Have you had any problems with the flow of your urine?

• Have you been having large amounts of beet-root, red lollies or berries in your diet?
• Could your problem have been sexually acquired?
• Have you been overseas recently?
• What is your general health like?
• Have you been aware of any other symptoms?
• Do you engage in strenuous sports such as jogging?
• Have you had any kidney problems in the past?

Physical examination (Fig. 68.2)

The general examination should include looking for signs of a bleeding tendency and anaemia, and recording the parameters of temperature, blood pressure and the pulse. The heart should be assessed to exclude atrial fibrillation or infective endocarditis with emboli to the kidney, and the chest should be examined for a possible pleural effusion associated with perinephric or renal infections.

The abdomen should be examined for evidence of a palpable enlarged kidney or spleen. The different clinical findings for an enlarged left kidney and spleen are shown in Table 68.3. Renal enlargement may be due to renal tumour, hydronephrosis, or polycystic disease. Splenomegaly suggests the possibility of a bleeding disorder.

The suprapubic region should be examined for evidence of bladder tenderness or enlargement. In men the prostate should be examined rectally to detect benign or malignant enlargement or tenderness from prostatitis.

In women a vaginal examination should be performed to search for possible pelvic masses. The urethral meatus should be inspected to exclude a urethral caruncle or urethral prolapse.

Investigations

It is important to identify the cause, especially if a possible sequel is impaired kidney function.

• Urinalysis by dipstick testing, e.g. 'Hemastix' and its derivatives (affected by Vitamin C intake).
• Urine microscopy
   — formed RBCs in true haematuria
   — red cell casts indicate glomerular bleeding
   — deformed (dysmorphic) red cells indicate glomerular bleeding.
• Urinary culture: early culture is important

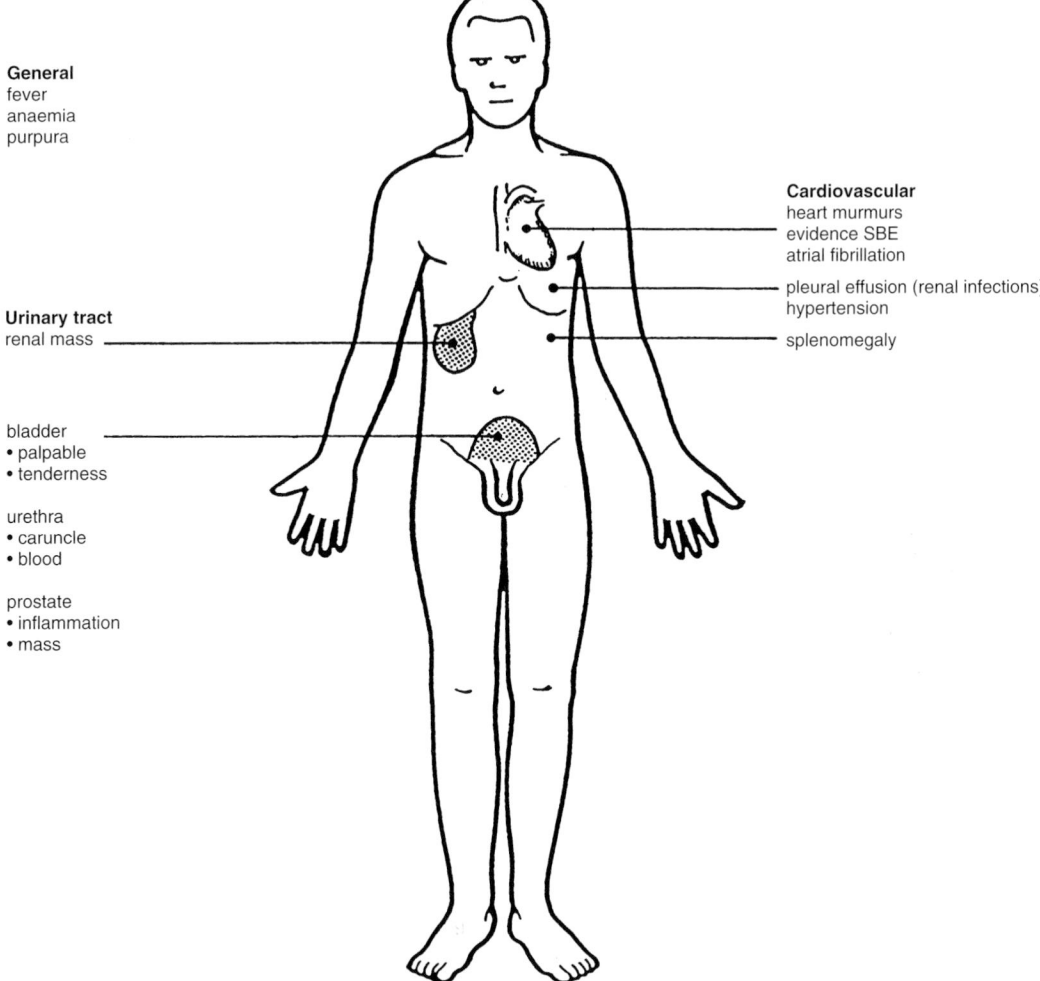

General
fever
anaemia
purpura

Cardiovascular
heart murmurs
evidence SBE
atrial fibrillation

pleural effusion (renal infections)
hypertension

splenomegaly

Urinary tract
renal mass

bladder
• palpable
• tenderness

urethra
• caruncle
• blood

prostate
• inflammation
• mass

Fig. 68.2 *Features to consider in the physical examination of the patient with haematuria*

because of the common association with infection and consideration of early treatment with antibiotics. If tuberculosis is suspected, three early morning urines should be cultured for tubercle bacilli.

• Urinary cytology: this test, performed on a urine sample, may be useful to detect malignancies of the bladder and lower tract but is usually negative with carcinoma of the kidney.
• Blood tests: appropriate screening tests include

Table 68.3 *Differences between spleen and left kidney on abdominal examination*

	Spleen	*Left kidney*
Palpable upper border	Impalpable	Palpable
Movement with inspiration	Inferomedial	Inferior
Notch	Yes	No
Ballotable	No	Yes
Percussion	Dull	Resonant (usually)
Friction rub	Possible	Not possible

a full blood count, ESR and basic renal function tests (urea and creatinine). If glomerulonephritis is suspected, antistreptolysin O titres and serum complement levels should be measured.
- Radiological techniques: available tests include
  - intravenous urography (intravenous pyelogram)—the key investigation
  - ultrasound (less sensitive at detecting lower UT abnormalities)
  - CT scanning
  - renal angiography
  - retrograde pyelography
- Direct imaging techniques: these include urethroscopy, cystoscopy and ureteroscopy. In all patients, regardless of the IVU findings, cystoscopy is advisable.
Renal biopsy: indicated if glomerular disease is suspected, especially in the presence of dysmorphic red cells on microscopic examination.

Pseudohaematuria

Pseudohaematuria is red urine caused by pigments other than red blood cells that simply stain the culture red.
  Causes include:

- anthrocyanins in food, e.g. beetroot, berries
- red-coloured confectionery
- porphyrins
- free haemoglobin, e.g. haemoglobinuria
- myoglobin (red-black colour)
- drugs, e.g. pyridium, phenolphthalein (alkaline urine)

Exercise haematuria

Exercise or sports haematuria is the passage of a significant number of red cells in the urine during or immediately after heavy exercise. It has been recorded in a wide variety of athletes, including swimmers and rowers. Dipstick testing is usually positive in these athletes. Despite the theory that it is largely caused by the posterior wall of the bladder impacting repetitively on the base of the bladder during running, there are other possible factors and glomerular disease must be excluded in the athlete with regular haematuria, especially if dysmorphic red cells are found on microscopy.

Artifactual haematuria

Macroscopic haematuria is a common presenting ploy of people with Munchausen's syndrome and pethidine addicts simulating renal colic. If suspected, it is wise to get these people to pass urine in the presence of an appropriate witness before examining the urine.

Proteinuria

Proteinuria is an important and common sign of renal disease. The protein can originate from the glomeruli, the tubules or the lower urinary tract. Healthy people, however, do excrete some protein in the urine which can vary from day to day and hour to hour; hence the value of collecting it over 24 hours. While proteinuria can be benign, it always requires further investigation. Important causes of proteinuria are presented in Table 68.4.

Key facts and checkpoints[6]
- The amount of protein in the urine is normally less than 100 mg/24 hours.

Table 68.4 *Important causes of proteinuria*

Transient
- Contamination from vaginal secretions ⎫ require
- Urinary tract infection   ⎬ exclusion
- Pre-eclampsia   ⎭ and follow-up

Renal disease
- Glomerulonephritis
- Nephrotic syndrome
- Congenital tubular disease
  e.g. polycystic kidney
      renal dysplasia
- Acute tubular damage
- Renal papilliary necrosis
  e.g. analgesic nephropathy
      diabetic papillary necrosis
- Overflow proteinuria
  e.g. multiple myeloma
- Systemic diseases affecting the glomeruli
  e.g. diabetes mellitus
      hypertension
      systemic lupus erythematosus
      malignancy
      drugs, e.g. penicillamine, gold salts
      amyloid
      vasculitides

No renal disease
- Orthostatic proteinuria
- Exercise
- Fever
- Postoperative
- Heart failure

- Greater than 150 mg protein/24 hours is abnormal in adults.
- Greater than 300 mg/24 hours is abnormal for children and adults.
- Proteinuria > 1g /24 hours indicates a serious underlying disorder.
- If accompanied by dysmorphic haematuria or red cell casts, this tends to confirm glomerular origin.
- Routine dipstick testing will only detect levels greater than 0.3 g/L and thus has limitations.
- In diabetics, microalbuminuria is predictive of nephropathy and an indication for early blood pressure treatment.

If proteinuria is confirmed on repeated dipstick testing it should be measured more accurately by measuring daily protein excretion with a 24 hour urine. High values require referral for investigation. The minimum investigations are micro-urine and assessment of renal function (creatinine clearance). Nephrotic range proteinuria (> 3g/24 hours) is due to one or other form of glomerulonephritis in over 90% of patients.[6] Possible contamination from vaginal secretions or from a low urinary tract infection needs to be excluded.

Orthostatic proteinuria

Orthostatic proteinuria is the presence of significant proteinuria after the patient has been standing but is absent from specimens obtained following recumbency for several hours, such as an early morning specimen.

It occurs in 5–10% of people,[7] especially during their adolescent years. In the majority it is of no significance and eventually disappears without the development of significant renal disease. However, in a small number the proteinuria can foreshadow serious renal disease.

Diabetic microalbuminuria

The presence of protein in the urine is a sensitive marker of diabetic nephropathy, so regular screening for microalbuminuria in diabetics is regarded as an important predictor of nephropathy and other possible complications of diabetes. Dipstick testing for microalbuminuria is now available but more accurate measurement can be performed with radioimmunoassay techniques. The use of ACE inhibitors at the microalbuminuria stage may slow the development of overt nephropathy.

Consequences of proteinuria

While proteinuria is usually simply a marker of renal disease, heavy proteinuria in excess of 3g/24 hours may have severe clinical consequences including oedema, intravascular volume depletion, venous thromboembolism, hyperlipidaemia and malnutrition.

Minimal change glomerulonephritis is the commonest cause of the nephrotic syndrome in childhood and accounts for about 30% of adult nephrotic syndrome.[6] It is steroid responsive.

Urinary incontinence

Definitions

- *Urinary incontinence* is the involuntary loss of urine during the day or night.
- *Nocturnal enuresis*, or bed-wetting, is involuntary urine loss during sleep.
- *Urge incontinence* is an urgent desire to void followed by involuntary loss of urine.
- *Stress incontinence* is the involuntary loss of urine on coughing, sneezing, straining or lifting, or any factor that suddenly increases intra-abdominal pressure.
- *Voiding dysfunction* includes urinary difficulties, detrusor instability and overflow incontinence.
- *Functional incontinence* is loss of urine secondary to factors extrinsic to the urinary tract.

A summary of the types of incontinence and their causes is presented in Table 68.5.

The basic requirements for continence are:
- adequate central and peripheral nervous function
- an intact urinary tract
- a compliant stable bladder
- a competent urethral sphincter
- efficient bladder emptying

Female urinary incontinence

Urinary leakage affects at least 9% of women aged 15–64 and this is a conservative estimate. Successful treatment depends on an accurate assessment of the lower urinary tract storage and emptying functions. The most common contributing factor is weakness of the pelvic floor muscles.

Assessment

The basic assessment of the incontinent patient requires a careful history and examination, exclusion of infection and the keeping of a

Table 68.5 *Types of incontinence and their implied causes*

Type of incontinence	Likely cause
Simple stress incontinence (with cough/sneeze)	Sphincter incompetence
Urge incontinence Giggle incontinence Stress and urge incontinence Enuresis Complex stress incontinence (with exercise)	Unstable bladder, with or without sphincter weakness
Quiet dribble incontinence	Sphincter incompetence and unstable bladder or overflow
Continuous leakage	Fistula, ectopic ureter, patulous urethra
Reflex incontinence	Neuropathic bladder

micturition or bladder chart. Drugs that adversely affect urinary function are presented in Table 68.6. Investigations may be required to dispel doubt about the diagnosis or to exclude intravesical or renal disorders: these include cystometry, uroflowmetry, cystourethroscopy, micturating cystourethrogram, IVU and also residual volume (> 100 ml is abnormal).

Management approach
1. Exclude urinary tract infection and drug causes.
2. Is it stress incontinence?
   - key symptoms: involuntary loss with coughing, jumping, etc.
   - demonstrable, e.g. patient coughs when standing with full bladder

Table 68.6 *Drugs that can cause or aggravate incontinence*

Antihypertensive/vasodilator drugs → stress incontinence
- phenoxybenzamine (Dibenyline)
- prazosin
- labetalol

Bladder relaxants → overflow incontinence
- anticholinergic agents
- tricyclic antidepressants

Bladder stimulants → urge incontinence
- cholinergic agents
- caffeine

Sedatives → urge incontinence
- antidepressants
- antihistamines
- psychotropics
- hypnotics
- tranquillisers

Others → urge incontinence
- alcohol
- loop diuretics, e.g. frusemide
- lithium

Treatment
- weak pelvic floor—exercises
- obesity—weight reduction
- menopause—HRT/vaginal oestrogen
- chronic cough—physiotherapy

If urodynamic studies of lower UT function show genuine stress incontinence (GSI) due to urethral sphincter weakness, consider surgery, e.g. suprapubic urethral suspension (better than vaginal repair)

3. Is it urge incontinence?
   - urge symptoms prominent
   - no residual urine
   Rx neurological signs → neurologist
      abnormal voiding pattern → bladder retraining, e.g. void more urine less frequently
4. Is it voiding dysfunction?
   - symptoms of voiding difficulty, e.g. frequency, urgency, nocturia, incomplete emptying
   - large residual urine
   Rx neurological signs → neurologist
      gynaecological cause, e.g. pelvic mass → gynaecologist
      if bladder atony → anticholinergic drugs may require catheterisation

Pelvic floor exercises
- The mainstay of treatment of most problems, esp. GSI.
- 75% improved and 25% cured.
- Best in motivated young women with bladder GSI.
- At least 3 months trial with supervision (physiotherapist or continence nurse adviser).

References

1. Cormack J, Marinker M, Morrell D. *Practice. A handbook of primary medical care*. London: Kluwer-Harrap Handbooks, 1980; 3.51:1–10.

2. Kincaid-Smith P, Larkins R, Whelan G. *Problems in clinical medicine*. Sydney: MacLennan & Petty, 1990, 105–108.

3. Sloane PD, Slatt PD, Baker RM. *Essentials of family medicine*. Baltimore: Williams & Wilkins, 1988, 169–174.

4. Walsh D. *Symptom control*. Boston: Blackwell Scientific Publications, 1989, 229–233.

5. George C. How to treat haematuria and proteinuria. Australian Dr Weekly, 15 March 1991, I–VIII.

6. Thomson N. Managing the patient with proteinuria. Current Therapeutics, 1996; 9:7–28.

7. Brown R. *Urology*. RACGP: CHECK Programme, unit 226, 1990, 11–12.

69

Visual failure

—

The commonest cause of visual dysfunction is a simple refractive error. However, there are many causes of visual failure including the emergency of sudden blindness, a problem that requires a sound management strategy. Apart from migraine, virtually all cases of sudden loss of vision require urgent treatment.

The 'white' eye or uninflamed eye presents a different clinical problem from the red or inflamed eye.[1] The 'white' eye is painless and usually presents with visual symptoms and it is in the 'white' eye that the majority of blinding conditions occur.

Criteria for blindness and driving

This varies from country to country. The World Health Organisation (WHO) defines blindness as 'best visual acuity less than 3/60, while in Australia eligibility for the blind pension is 'bilateral corrected visual acuity less than 6/60 or significant visual field loss'; e.g. a patient can have 6/6 vision but severely restricted fields caused by chronic open-angle glaucoma. The minimum standard for driving is 6/12.

Key facts and checkpoints

- The commonest cause of blindness in the world is trachoma.
- In western countries the commonest causes are senile cataract, glaucoma, age-related macular degeneration, trauma and the retinopathy of diabetes mellitus.[2]
- The commonest causes of sudden visual loss are transient occlusion of the retinal artery (amaurosis fugax) and migraine.[3]
- 'Flashing lights' are caused by traction on the retina and may have a serious connotation: the commonest cause is vitreoretinal traction which is a classic cause of retinal detachment.
- The presence of floaters or 'blobs' in the visual fields indicates pigment in the vitreous: causes include vitreous haemorrhage and vitreous detachment.
- Posterior vitreous detachment is the commonest cause of the acute onset of floaters, especially with advancing age.
- Retinal detachment has a tendency to occur in short-sighted (myopic) people.
- Suspect a macular abnormality where objects look smaller or straight lines are bent or distorted.

The clinical approach
History
The history should carefully define the onset, progress, duration, offset and the extent of visual loss. An accurate history is important because a longstanding visual defect may only just have been noticed by the patient, especially if it is unilateral. Two questions need to be answered.

1. Is the loss unilateral or bilateral?
2. Is the onset acute, or gradual and progressive?

The distinction between central and peripheral visual loss is useful. Central visual loss presents as impairment of visual acuity and implies defective retinal image formation (through refractive error or opacity in the ocular media) or macular or optic nerve dysfunction. Peripheral field loss is more subtle, especially when the onset is gradual, and implies extramacular retinal disease or a defect in the visual pathway.

It is important to differentiate the central field loss of macular degeneration from the hemianopia of a CVA.

A drug history is very important (Table 69.1). Treatment for tuberculosis with ethambutol or treatment with quinine/chloroquine has to be considered as these drugs are oculotoxic. The family history is relevant for diabetes, migraine, Leber's hereditary optic atrophy, amaurotic familial idiocy and retinitis pigmentosa.

Questions directed to specific symptoms
- presence of floaters → indicates haemorrhage, posterior vitreous detachment, choroiditis
- flashing lights → traction on retina ? retinal detachment, posterior vitreous detachment
- coloured haloes around lights → glaucoma, cataract
- zigzag lines → migraine
- vision worse at night or in dim light → retinitis pigmentosa, hysteria, syphilitic retinitis
- headache → temporal arteritis, migraine, benign intracranial hypertension

- central scotomata → macular disease, optic neuritis
- pain on moving eye → retrobulbar neuritis
- distortion, micropsia (smaller), macropsia (larger) → macular degeneration
- visual field loss:
  - central loss—macular disorder
  - total loss—arterial occlusion

It is worth noting that if a patient repeatedly knocks into people and objects on a particular side (including traffic accidents), a bitemporal or homonymous hemianopia should be suspected.

Diseases/disorders to exclude or consider
- diabetes mellitus
- giant cell (temporal) arteritis
- hypopituitarism (pituitary adenoma)
- cerebrovascular ischaemia/carotid artery stenosis (emboli)
- multiple sclerosis
- cardiac disease, e.g. arrhythmias, and SBE (emboli)
- anaemia (if severe can cause retinal haemorrhage and exudate)
- Marfan's syndrome (subluxated lenses)

Table 69.1 *Visual disorders associated with drugs*

Disorder	Drug
Corneal opacities	Amiodarone Hydroxychloroquine Chlorpromazine Vitamin D Indomethacin Chlorpropamide
Precipitating of acute narrow angle glaucoma	Mydriatic drops Tricyclics Antihistamines
Refractive changes	Thiazides
Lens opacities	Corticosteroids Phenothiazines
Retinopathy	Hydroxychloroquine Chloroquine Thioridazine (other phenothiazines less commonly) Tamoxifen
Papilloedema (secondary to benign intracranial hypertension)	Oral contraceptives Corticosteroids Tetracyclines Nalidixic acid Vitamin A
Optic neuropathy	Ethanol Tobacco Ethambutol Disulfiram

Reprinted from *Central Nervous System: clinical algorithms*, published by the *BMJ*, with permission

Examination

The same principles of examination should apply as for the red eye. Testing should include:

- visual acuity (Snellen chart)—with pinhole testing
- pupil reactions, to test afferent (sensory) responses to light
- confrontation fields (using a red pin)
- colour vision
- Amsler grid (or graph paper)
- fundus examination with dilated pupil (ophthalmoscope), noting
  - the red reflex
  - appearance of the retina, macula and optic nerve
- tonometry

General examination

General examination should focus on the general features of the patient, the nervous system, endocrine system and cardiovascular system.

Perimetry

Various defects in the visual fields are depicted in Figure 69.1.

Investigations

Depending on the clinical examination the following tests can be selected to confirm the diagnosis:

- Blood tests
  - full blood ?anaemia, lead poisoning, leukaemia
  - ESR ? temporal arteritis
  - blood sugar ? diabetes mellitus
- Temporal artery biopsy ? temporal arteritis
- CT scan ? CVA, optic nerve lesions, space-occupying lesions
- Formal perimetry and Bjerrum screen
- Fluorescein angiography ? retinal vascular obstruction, diabetic retinopathy
- Visual evoked responses ? demyelinating disorders
- Carotid Doppler ultrasound

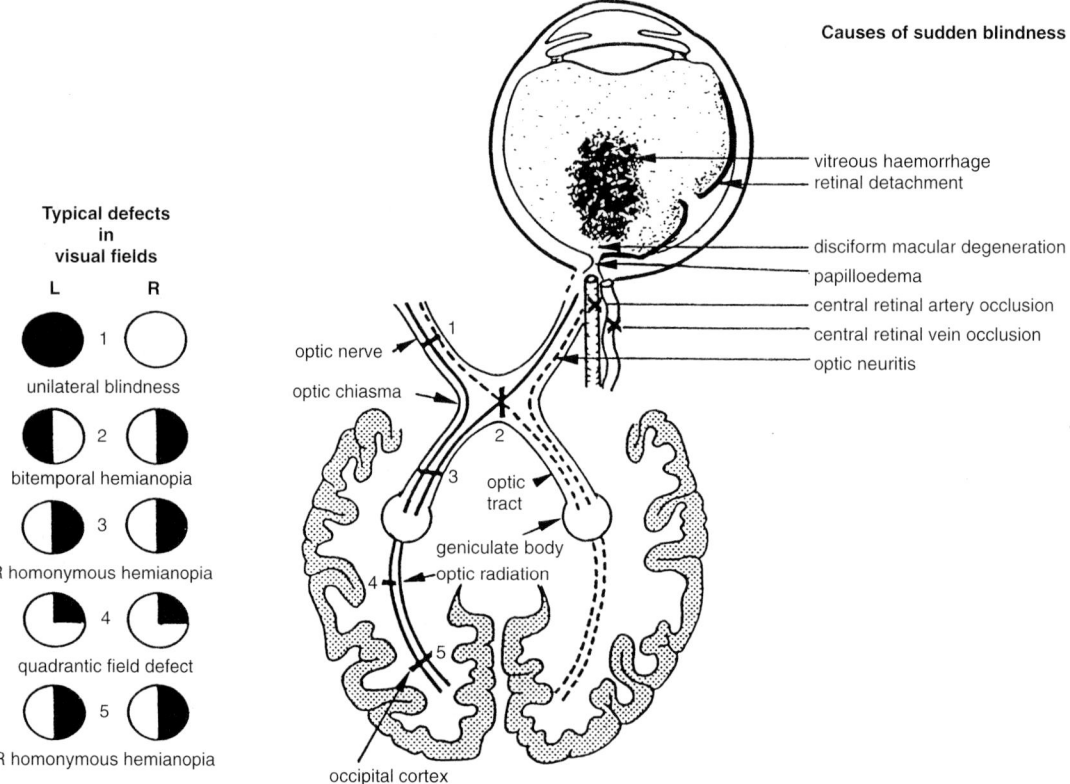

Fig. 69.1 *Diagrammatic representation of important causes of sudden painless loss of vision (right side) and typical defects in the visual fields (left side)*

Visual failure in children

There are long lists of causes for visual failure or blindness in children. An approximate order of frequency of causes of blindness in children is cortical blindness, optic atrophy, choroidoretinal degeneration, cataracts and retinopathy of prematurity. Almost half the causes of blindness are genetically determined, in contrast to the nutritional and infective causes which predominate in Third World countries.[4] About 3% of children will fail to develop proper vision in at least one eye.

Amblyopia

Amblyopia is defined as a reduction in visual acuity due to abnormal visual experience in early childhood. It is the main reason for poor unilateral eyesight until middle age and is usually caused by interference with visual development during the early months and years of life.

The common causes are:
- strabismus
- large refractive defect, especially hypermetropia
- congenital cataract

Principles of management[5]
- Most cases are treatable.
- Early diagnosis and intervention is fundamental to achieving useful vision.
- No child is too young to have the visual system assessed.
- The good eye should be patched in order to utilise the affected eye.
- Remove a remedial cause such as strabismus.
- Correct any refractive error, usually by prescription of glasses.

Some important guidelines in children

Strabismus
- Always refer children with strabismus (squint) when first seen to exclude ocular pathology such as retinoblastoma, congenital cataract and glaucoma, which would require emergency surgery.
- Children with strabismus (even if the ocular examination is normal) need specialist management because the deviating eye will become amblyopic (a lazy eye with reduced vision). The younger the child, the easier it is to treat amblyopia; it may be irreversible if first detected later than school age.

Cataracts

Children with suspected cataracts must be referred immediately; the problem is very serious as the development of vision may be permanently impaired (amblyopia).[2] Cataracts are diagnosed by looking at the red reflex and this should be a routine part of the examination of a young child. Common conditions causing cataracts are genetic disorders and rubella but most causes are unknown. Rarer conditions such as galactosaemia need to be considered.

Refractive errors

Refractive errors, with the error greater in one eye, can cause amblyopia. Detection of refractive errors is an important objective of screening.

Retinoblastoma

Retinoblastoma, although rare, is the commonest intraocular tumour in childhood. It must be excluded in any child presenting with a white pupil. Such children also have the so-called 'cat's eye reflex'. In 30% of patients the condition is bilateral with an autosomal dominant gene being responsible.

Visual failure in the elderly

Most patients with visual complaints are elderly and their failing vision affects their perception of the environment and their ability to communicate effectively. Typical problems are cataracts, vascular disease, macular degeneration, chronic simple glaucoma and retinal detachment. Retinal detachment and diabetic retinopathy can occur at any age, although they are more likely with increasing age. Macular degeneration in its various forms is the commonest cause of visual deterioration in the elderly. For the elderly with cataracts the decision to operate depends on the patients' vision and their ability to cope. Most patients with a vision of $^6/_{18}$ or worse in both eyes usually benefit from cataract extraction, but some can cope with this level of vision and rely on a good, well-placed (above and behind) reading light.[6]

Sudden loss of vision in the elderly is suggestive of temporal arteritis or vascular embolism, so this problem should be checked.

Refractive errors

Indistinct or blurred vision is most commonly caused by errors of refraction.

In the normal eye (emmetropia) light rays from infinity are brought to a focus on the retina by the cornea (contributing about two-thirds of the eye's refractive power) and the lens (one-third). Thus the cornea is very important in refraction and abnormalities such as keratoconus may cause severe refractive problems.[6]

The process of accommodation is required for focusing closer objects. This process, which relies on the action of ciliary muscles and lens elasticity, is usually affected by ageing, so that from the age of 45 close work becomes gradually more difficult (presbyopia).[6]

The important clinical feature is that the use of a simple 'pinhole' in a card will usually improve blurred vision or reduced acuity where there is a refractive error only.[1]

Myopia (short-sightedness)

This is usually progressive in the teens. Highly myopic eyes may develop retinal detachment or macular degeneration.

Management
- glasses with a concave lens
- contact lenses
- consider radial keratotomy or excimer laser surgery

Hypermetropia (long-sightedness)

This condition is more susceptible to closed-angle glaucoma. In early childhood it may be associated with convergent strabismus (squint). The spectacle correction alone may straighten the eyes. It is mostly overcome by the accommodative power of the eye, though it may cause reading difficulty. Typically, the long-sighted person needs reading glasses at about 30 years.

Presbyopia

There is a need for near correction with loss of accommodative power of the eye in the 40's.

Astigmatism

This creates the need for a corrective lens that is more curved in one meridian than another because the cornea does not have even curvature. If uncorrected, this may cause headaches of ocular origin. Conical cornea is one cause of astigmatism.

Pinhole test

The pinhole reduces the size of the blur circle on the retina in the uncorrected eye. A pinhole acts as a universal correcting lens. If visual acuity is not normalised by looking through a card with a 1 mm pinhole, then the defective vision is not solely due to a refractive error. The pinhole test may actually help to improve visual acuity with some cataracts. Further investigation is mandatory.

Cataracts

The term 'cataract' describes any lens opacity. The symptoms depend on the degree and the site of opacity. Cataract causes gradual visual loss with normal direct pupillary light reflex.

The prevalence of cataracts increases with age: 65% at age 50 to 59, and all people aged over 80 have opacities.[3] Significant causes of cataracts are presented in Table 69.2 and causes of progressive visual loss in Table 69.3.

Table 69.2   *Causes of cataracts*

Advancing age
Diabetes mellitus
Steroids (topical or oral)
Radiation
Trauma
Uveitis
Dystrophia myotonia

Table 69.3   *Progressive bilateral visual loss*

Globe	Chronic glaucoma Senile cataracts
Retina	Macular degeneration Retinal disease • diabetic retinopathy • retinitis pigmentosa • choroidoretinitis
Optic nerve	Optic neuropathies Optic nerve compression, e.g. aneurysm, glioma Toxic damage to optic nerves
Optic chiasma	Chiasmal compression: pituitary adenoma, craniopharyngioma, etc.
Occipital cortex	Tumours Degenerative conditions

Note: Unilateral causes, e.g. cataract, refractive errors, uveitis, glaucoma, progressive optic atrophy and tumours can affect the second eye.

Typical symptoms:
• reading difficulty
• difficulty in recognising faces
• problems with driving
• difficulty with television viewing
• reduced ability to see in bright light
• may see haloes around lights

Examination
• reduced visual acuity (sometimes improved with pinhole)
• diminished red reflex on ophthalmoscopy
• a change in the appearance of the lens

The red reflex and ophthalmoscopy
The 'red reflex' is a reflection of the fundus when the eye is viewed from a distance of about 60 cm (2 feet) with the ophthalmoscope using a zero lens. This reflex is easier to see if the pupil is dilated. Commencing with the plus 15 or 20 lens, reduce the power gradually and, at plus 12, lens opacities will be seen against the red reflex which may be totally obscured by a very dense cataract. The setting up of the ophthalmoscope to examine intraocular structures is illustrated in Figure 69.2.

Management
Advise extraction when the patient cannot cope. Contraindications for extraction include intra-ocular inflammation and severe diabetic retin-opathy. There is no effective medical treatment for established cataracts. The removal of the cataractous lens requires optical correction to restore vision and this is usually performed with an intraocular lens implant. Full visual recovery may take 2–3 months. Complications are uncom-mon yet many patients may require YAG laser

capsulotomy to clear any opacities that may develop behind the lens implant.

Postoperative advice to the patient
• Avoid bending for a few weeks.
• Avoid strenuous exercise.
• The following drops may be prescribed:
 — steroids (to reduce inflammation)
 — antibiotics (to avoid infection)
 — dilators (to prevent adhesions)

Glaucoma
Chronic simple glaucoma is the commonest cause of irreversible blindness in middle age.[1] At a very late stage it presents as difficulty in seeing because of loss of the outer fields of vision due to optic atrophy (Fig. 69.3). Acute glaucoma, on the other hand, has a relatively rapid onset over a few days.

Clinical features of chronic glaucoma
• familial tendency
• no early signs or symptoms
• central vision usually normal
• progressive restriction of visual field

Tonometry
• upper limit of normal is 22 mmHg

Ophthalmoscopy
• optic disc cupping > 30% of total disc area

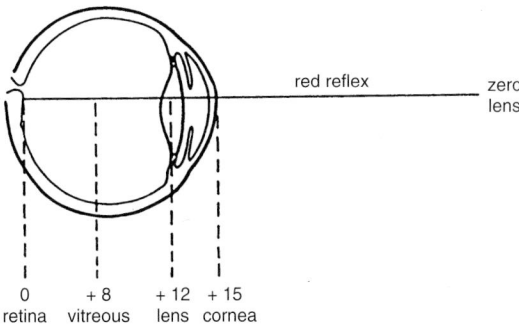

Fig. 69.2 *Settings of the ophthalmoscope used to examine intraocular structures*

Fig. 69.3 *Typical visual field loss for chronic simple glaucoma; a similar pattern occurs with retinitis pigmentosa and hysteria*

Screening
- adults 40 years and over: 2–5 yearly (at least 2 yearly over 60)
- start about 30 years, then 2 yearly if family history

Management
- treatment can prevent visual field loss
- medication (for life) usually selected from
  — timolol or betaxolol drops bd
    (*Note*: These beta-blockers can cause systemic complications, e.g. asthma)
  — pilocarpine drops qid
  — dipivefrine drops bd
  — acetazolamide (oral diuretics)
- surgery or laser therapy for failed medication

Retinitis pigmentosa

Primary degeneration of the retina is a hereditary condition characterised by a degeneration of rods and cones associated with displacement of melanin-containing cells from the pigment epithelium into the more superficial parts of the retina.

Typical features
- begins as night blindness in childhood
- visual fields become concentrically narrowed (periphery to centre)
- blind by adolescence (sometimes up to middle age)

Ophthalmoscopic examination
- irregular patches of dark pigment, especially at periphery

Trauma

Trauma to the eye may cause only a little discomfort so it is important to keep this in mind.

Intraocular foreign body
A small metal chip may penetrate the eye with minimal pain and the patient may not present with an ocular problem until the history of injury is long forgotten.

If infection does not supervene, presentation may be delayed for months or years until vision deteriorates due to metal degradation. The iris becomes rust-brown. It is important to X-ray the eye if it has been struck by a hammered fragment or if in any doubt at all about the mechanism of the injury.[1]

Chronic uveitis

Pain and redness may be minimal with this chronic inflammation. If untreated, visual loss often develops from secondary glaucoma and cataract. The pupil is bound to the lens by synechiae and is distorted.

HIV infection

AIDS may have serious ocular complications, including Kaposi's sarcoma of the conjunctivae, retinal haemorrhage and vasculitis.[3] Another problem is ocular cytomegalovirus infection which presents as areas of opacification with haemorrhage and exudates.

Sudden loss of vision

It is important to remember that the problem is alarming and distressing to the patient; considerable empathy is needed and care must be taken not to diagnose seemingly inappropriate behaviour as of psychogenic origin.

A comparison of bilateral and unilateral causes of sudden loss of vision is presented in Table 69.4, and the diagnostic strategy model in Table 69.5. A simplified classification is:

unilateral:	retinal detachment
	retinal artery occlusion
	retinal vein thrombosis
	temporal arteritis
	optic neuritis
	migraine
bilateral	bilateral optic nerve lesion
	hysteria

A flow chart for the diagnosis of painless loss of vision is presented in Figure 69.4.

Amaurosis fugax
Amaurosis fugax is transient loss of vision (partial or complete) in one eye due to transient occlusion of a retinal artery. It is painless and lasts less than 60 minutes. It is usually caused by an embolus from an atheromatous carotid artery in the neck. The most common emboli are cholesterol emboli which usually arise from an ulcerated plaque.[8] Other causes include emboli from the heart, temporal arteritis and benign intracranial hypertension. Other symptoms or signs of cerebral ischaemia such as transient hemiparesis may accompany the symptom. The source of the problem should be investigated.

Table 69.4 *Causes of sudden loss of vision*[8]

| | BILATERAL | UNILATERAL | |
		Transient	*Permanent*
Vascular causes	Occipital cortex ischaemia Pituitary apoplexy Homonymous hemianopia— vascular	Amaurosis fugax Transient ocular ischaemia Retinal emboli Malignant hypertension	Central retinal artery occlusion Central retinal vein occlusion Vitreous haemorrhage Ischaemic optic neuropathy
Other causes	Bilateral optic neuritis Toxic damage to optic nerve • methanol • ethanol • tobacco • lead Leber's optic atrophy Quinine poisoning of retina Cerebral oedema Occipital lobe trauma Craniopharyngioma Hysteria	Acute angle closure glaucoma Uhthoff's phenomenon Papilloedema Posterior vitreous detachment	Optic neuritis Retinal detachment Optic nerve compression Carcinomatous optic neuropathy Intraocular tumour

Table 69.5 *Acute or subacute painless loss of vision: diagnostic strategy model*

Q. *Probability diagnosis*
A. Amaurosis fugax
   Migraine
   Retinal detachment

Q. *Serious disorders not to be missed*
A. Cardiovascular
   • central retinal artery occlusion
   • central retinal vein occlusion
   • hypertension (complications)
   Neoplasia
   • intracranial tumour
   • intraocular tumour
     — primary melanoma
     — retinoblastoma
     — metastases
   AIDS
   Temporal arteritis
   Acute glaucoma
   Benign intracranial hypertension

Q. *Pitfalls (often missed)*
A. Acute glaucoma
   Papilloedema
   Optic neuritis
   Intraocular foreign body

Q. *Seven masquerades checklist*
A. Depression   –
   Diabetes   √ diabetic retinopathy
   Drugs   √
   Anaemia   –
   Thyroid disease   √ hyperthyroidism
   Spinal dysfunction –
   UTI   –

Q. *Is this patient trying to tell me something?*
A. Consider 'hysterical' blindness, although it is uncommon.

The risk of stroke after an episode of amaurosis fugax appears to be about 2% per year.[8]

Transient ocular ischaemia

Unilateral loss of vision provoked by activities such as walking, bending or looking upwards is suggestive of ocular ischaemia.[8] It occurs in the presence of severe extracranial vascular disease and may be triggered by postural hypotension and stealing blood from the retinal circulation.

Retinal detachment

Retinal detachment may be caused by trauma, thin retina (myopic people), previous surgery (e.g. cataract operation), choroidal tumours, vitreous degeneration or diabetic retinopathy.

Clinical features

• sudden onset of floaters or flashes or black spots
• blurred vision in one eye becoming worse
• 'a curtain came down over the eye', grey cloud or black spot
• partial or total loss of visual field (total if macula detached)

Ophthalmoscopy may show detached retinal fold as large grey shadow in vitreous cavity.

Management

• immediate referral for sealing of retinal tears
• small holes treated with laser or freezing probe
• true detachments usually require surgery

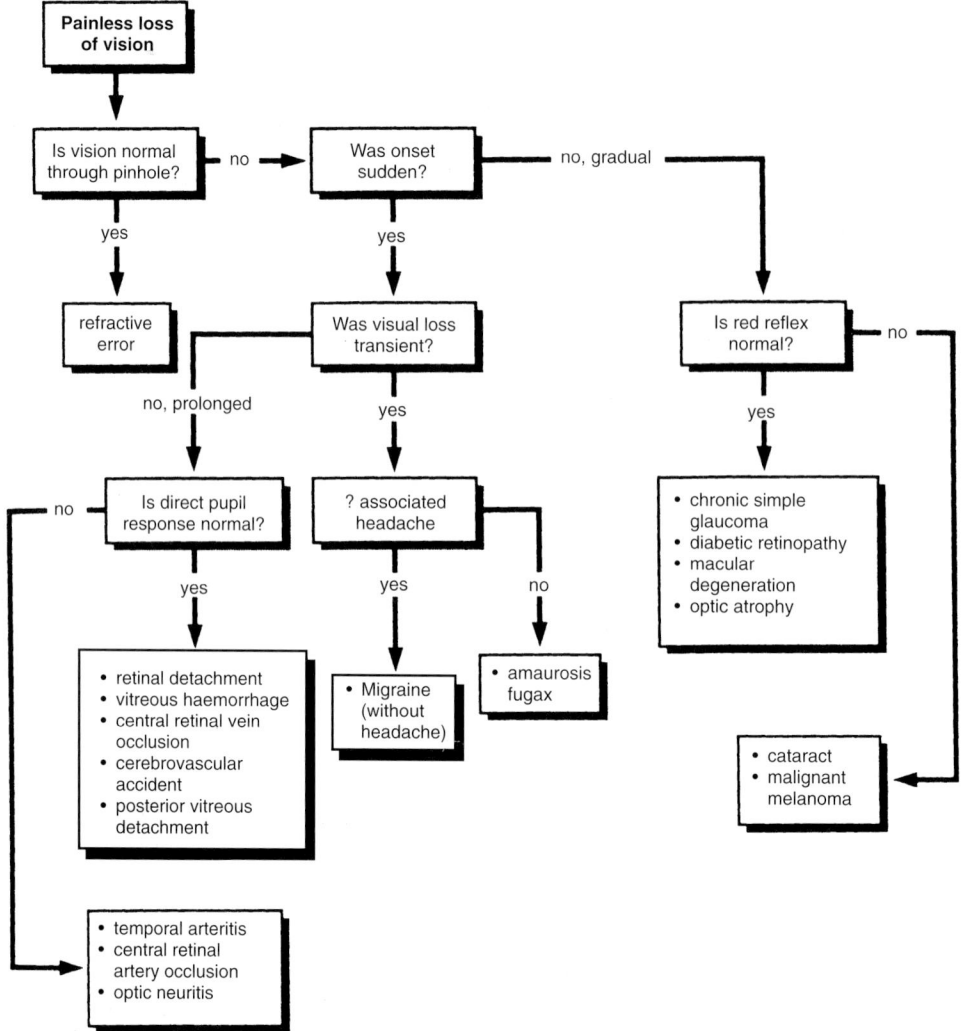

Fig. 69.4 *Diagnosis of painless loss of vision*   REPRODUCED WITH PERMISSION DR J. REICH AND DR J. COLVIN

Vitreous haemorrhage

Haemorrhage may occur from spontaneous rupture of vessels, avulsion of vessels during retinal traction or bleeding from abnormal new vessels.[6] Associations include ocular trauma, diabetic retinopathy, tumour and retinal detachment.

Clinical features

- sudden onset of floaters or 'blobs' in vision
- may be sudden loss of vision
- visual acuity depends on the extent of the haemorrhage; if small, visual acuity may be normal

Ophthalmoscopy may show reduced light reflex:

there may be clots of blood that move with the vitreous (a black swirling cloud).

Management

- urgent referral to exclude retinal detachment
- exclude underlying causes such as diabetes
- ultrasound helps diagnosis
- may resolve spontaneously
- bed rest encourages resolution
- surgical vitrectomy for persistent haemorrhage

Central retinal artery occlusion

The cause is usually arterial obstruction by atherosclerosis, thrombi or emboli. There may be a history of TIAs. Exclude temporal arteritis (perform immediate ESR).

Clinical features
- sudden loss of vision like a 'curtain descending'
- vision not improved with 1mm pinhole
- usually no light perception

Ophthalmoscopy
- initially normal
- may see retinal emboli
- classical 'red cherry spot' at macula

Management
If seen early, use this procedure within 30 minutes:
- massage globe digitally through closed eyelids (use rhythmic direct digital pressure)
- rebreathe carbon dioxide (paper bag) or inhale special CO_2 mixture (carbogen)
- intravenous acetazolamide (Diamox) 500 mg
- refer urgently (less than 6 hours)

Prognosis is poor. Significant recovery is unlikely unless treated immediately (within 30 minutes).

Central retinal vein thrombosis
Thrombosis is associated with several possible factors such as hypertension, diabetes, anaemia, glaucoma and hyperlipidaemia.

Clinical features
- sudden loss of central vision (if macula involved)
- vision not improved with 1 mm pinhole

Ophthalmoscopy shows swollen disc and multiple retinal haemorrhages.

Management
No immediate treatment is effective. The cause needs to be found first and treated accordingly. Some cases respond to fibrinolysin treatment. Laser photocoagulation may be necessary in later stages to prevent thrombotic glaucoma.

Macular degeneration
There are two types: exudative (acute) and pigmentary (slow onset).
- caused by neovascular membranes which develop under the retina of the macular area and leak fluid or bleed
- more common with increasing age (usually over 60) and those with myopia (relatively common)
- may be familial

Clinical features
- sudden fading of central vision
- distortion of vision
- straight lines may seem wavy and objects distorted
- use a grid pattern (Amsler chart): shows distorted lines
- central vision eventually completely lost
- peripheral fields normal

Ophthalmoscopy
- white exudates, haemorrhage in retina
- macula may look normal or raised

Management
Urgent referral for fluorescein angiography and laser photocoagulation where indicated. There is some evidence that the chronic pigmentation type responds to free-radical treatment with antioxidants such as vitamins A, C or E, zinc and selenium.

Temporal arteritis
With temporal arteritis (giant cell arteritis) there is a risk of sudden and often bilateral occlusion of the short ciliary arteries supplying the optic nerves, with or without central retinal artery involvement.[7]

Clinical features
- usually older person: over 65 years
- sudden loss of central vision in one eye (central scotoma)
- can rapidly become bilateral
- associated temporal headache (not invariable)
- temporal arteries tender, thickened and non-pulsatile (but often normal)
- visual acuity severely impaired
- afferent pupil defect on affected side
- usually elevated ESR > 40

Ophthalmoscopy shows optic disc swollen at first, then atrophic. The disc may appear quite normal.

Management
- other eye must be tested
- immediate corticosteroids (100 mg prednisolone daily for at least one week)
- biopsy temporal artery (if there is a localised tender area)

Migraine

Migraine may present with symptoms of visual loss. Associated headache and nausea may not be present.

Clinical features

- zigzag lines or lights
- multicoloured flashing lights
- unilateral or bilateral field deficit
- resolution within a few hours

Posterior vitreous detachment

The vitreous body collapses and detaches from the retina. It may lead to retinal detachment.

Clinical features

- sudden onset of floaters
- visual acuity usually normal
- flashing lights indicate traction on the retina

Management

- Refer to an ophthalmologist urgently.
- An associated retinal hole or detachment needs exclusion.

Optic (retrobulbar) neuritis

Causes include multiple sclerosis, neurosyphilis and toxins. A significant number of cases eventually develop multiple sclerosis.

Clinical features

- usually a woman 20–40 years
- loss of vision in one eye over a few days
- retro-ocular discomfort with eye movements
- variable visual acuity
- usually a central field loss (central scotoma)
- afferent pupil defect on affected side

Ophthalmoscopy

- optic disc swollen if 'inflammation' anterior in nerve
- optic atrophy appears later
- disc pallor is an invariable sequel

Management

- Test visual field of other eye.
- Consider magnetic resonance imaging.
- Most patients recover spontaneously but are left with diminished acuity.
- Intravenous steroids hasten recovery and have a protective effect against the development of further demyelinating episodes.

Pitfalls

- Mistaking the coloured haloes of glaucoma for migraine.
- Failing to appreciate the presence of retinal detachment in the presence of minimal visual impairment.
- Omitting to consider temporal arteritis as a cause of sudden visual failure in the elderly.
- Using eyedrops to dilate the pupil (for fundal examination) in the presence of glaucoma.

When to refer

- Most problems outlined need urgent referral to an ophthalmologist.
- Acute visual disturbance of unknown cause requires urgent referral.
- Any blurred vision—sudden or gradual, painful or painless—especially if 1 mm pinhole fails to alter visual acuity.
- Refer all suspicious optic discs.

Practice tips

- Tonometry is advised routinely for all people over 40; those over 60 should have tests every two years.
- Any family history of glaucoma requires tonometry at earliest age.
- Sudden loss of vision in the elderly suggests temporal arteritis (check the ESR and temporal arteries). It requires immediate institution of high-dose steroids to prevent blindness in the other eye. A time-scale guide showing the rate of visual loss is presented in Table 69.6.
- Temporal arteritis is an important cause of retinal artery occlusion.
- Suspect field defect due to chiasmal compression if people are misjudging when driving.
- Pupillary reactions are normal in cortical blindness.
- Central retinal artery occlusion may be overcome by early rapid lowering of intraocular pressure.
- Retinal detachment and vitreous haemorrhage may require early surgical repair.
- Keep in mind antioxidant therapy (vitamins and minerals) for chronic macular degeneration.
- Consider multiple sclerosis foremost if there is a past history of transient visual failure, especially with eye pain.
- If the patient has been using a hammer, always X-ray if a fragment of metal has hit the eye but nothing can be seen.

Table 69.6 *Time-scale guide for rate of visual loss*[3,8]

Sudden: less than 1 hour
- amaurosis fugax
- central retinal artery occlusion
- hemianopias from ischaemia (emboli)
- migraine
- vitreous haemorrhage
- acute angle glaucoma
- papilloedema

Within 24 hours
- central retinal vein occlusion
- hysteria

Less than 7 days
- retinal detachment
- optic neuritis
- acute macular problems

Up to several weeks (variable)
- choroiditis
- malignant hypertension

Gradual
- compression of visual pathways
- chronic glaucoma
- cataracts
- diabetic maculopathy
- retinitis pigmentosa
- macular degeneration
- refractive errors

References

1. Colvin J, Reich J. CHECK Programme, Unit 219–220. Melbourne: RACGP, 1990, 1–32.
2. Beck ER, Francis JL, Souhami RL. *Tutorials in differential diagnosis* (2nd edn). Edinburgh: Churchill Livingstone, 1988, 141–144.
3. Enoch B. Painless loss of vision in adults. Update, 5 June 1987, 22–30.
4. Robinson MJ. *Practical paediatrics* (2nd edn). Melbourne: Churchill Livingstone, 1990, 120–122.
5. Cole GA. Amblyopia and strabismus. In: MIMS Disease Index (2nd edn). Sydney: IMS Publishing, 1996, 20–24.
6. Elkington AR, Khaw PT. *ABC of eyes*. London: British Medical Association, 1990, 20–38.
7. Warne R, Prinsley D. *A manual of geriatric care*. Sydney: Williams and Wilkins, 1988, 191–195.
8. King J. Loss of vision. Mod Med Aust, May 1990, 52–61.

70
Weight gain

Persons who are naturally very fat are apt to die earlier than those who are slender.

Hippocrates

Obesity is the most common nutrition-related disorder in the western world; as Tunnessen puts it, 'Obesity is the most common form of malnutrition in the United States'.[1] Most overweight adults and children who are obese have exogenous obesity, which tends to imply that 'they ate too much', but the problem is more complex than relative food input. Physical activity, environmental and genetic influences must also be taken into account. There is still a persisting tendency of affected families to blame 'glandular' problems as a cause of obesity. It is now considered that there is a strong genetic basis to obesity and that attributing it to overeating and lack of exercise is an oversimplistic viewpoint.

Key facts and figures

- The cause of exogenous obesity is multifactorial, the end result being increased body fatness (greater than 30% of total body weight in females and greater than 25% in males).[2]
- Abdominal obesity gives a higher cardiovascular risk at any weight.
- The onset of obesity can occur at any age.
- Secondary or pathologic causes are rare.
- Less than 1% of obese patients have an identifiable secondary cause of obesity.[3]
- Two conditions causing unexplained weight gain that can be diagnosed by the physical examination are Cushing's syndrome and hypothyroidism.
- After pregnancy, obesity may result from a failure to return to prepartum energy requirements.

A diagnostic approach

A summary of the safety diagnostic model is presented in Table 70.1.

Table 70.1 *Weight gain: diagnostic strategy model*

Q. *Probability diagnosis*
A. Exogenous obesity

Q. *Serious disorders not to be missed*
A. Cardiovascular
  • cardiac failure
  Hypothalamic disorders
  • craniopharyngiomas
  • optic gliomas
  Liver failure
  Nephrotic syndrome

Q. *Pitfalls (often missed)*
A. Pregnancy (early)
  Endocrine disorders
  • hypothyroidism
  • Cushing's syndrome
  • insulinoma
  • acromegaly
  • hypogonadism
  • hyperprolactinaemia
  • polycystic ovarian disease
  Idiopathic oedema syndrome
  Klinefelter's syndrome
  Congenital disorders
  • Prader-Willi syndrome
  • Laurence-Moon-Biedl syndrome

Q. *Seven masquerades checklist*
A. Depression   √
  Diabetes   –
  Drugs   –
  Anaemia   –
  Thyroid disease   √ hypothyroid
  Spinal dysfunction –
  UTI   –

Q. *Is the patient trying to tell me something?*
A. Yes: the reasons for obesity should be explored.

Probability diagnosis

The outstanding cause of weight gain in exogenous obesity is excessive calorie intake coupled with lack of exercise. Overweight people often deny overeating but the true situation can be determined by recording actual food intake and energy expenditure, and by interviewing reliable witnesses.

Serious causes not to be missed

It is important not to misdiagnose hypothalamic disorders which may result in hyperphagia and obesity. Injury to the hypothalamus may occur following trauma and encephalitis and with a variety of tumours including craniopharyngiomas, optic gliomas and pituitary neoplasms. Some of these tumours may cause headaches and visual disturbances.

It is important not to overlook major organ failure and renal disorders as a cause of increased body weight, especially cardiac failure, liver failure and the nephrotic syndrome. The associated increase in body water needs to be distinguished from increased body fat.

Pitfalls

Endocrine disorders

The endocrine disorders that cause obesity include Cushing's syndrome, hypothyroidism, insulin-secreting tumours and hypogonadism. They should not represent difficult diagnostic problems.

An insulin-secreting tumour (insulinoma) is a very rare adenoma of the B cells of the islets of Langerhans. The main features are symptoms of hypoglycaemia and obesity.

Congenital disorders

The rare congenital disorders that cause obesity such as Prader-Willi and Laurence-Moon-Biedl syndromes should be easy to recognise in children (see pp. 726–727).

Chromosomal abnormalities

An important abnormality to bear in mind is Klinefelter's syndrome (XXY karyotype) which affects one out of every 400–500 males. The boys show excessive growth of long bones and are tall and slim. Without testosterone treatment they become obese as adults.

Some girls with Turner's syndrome (XO karyotype) may be short and overweight.

Some gender pointers

Consider polycystic ovarian disease in women and obstructive sleep apnoea in obese men.

Seven masquerades checklist

The important masquerades include hypothyroidism and drug ingestion. Hypothyroidism is usually not associated with marked obesity. Drugs that can be an important contributing factor include tricyclic antidepressants, corticosteroids, pizotifen, thioridazine, and the contraceptive pill. Obesity (overeating) may be a feature of depression, especially in the early stages. Prescribed tricyclic antidepressants may compound the problem.

Psychogenic considerations

An underlying emotional crisis may be the reason for the overweight patient to seek medical advice. It is important to explore diplomatically any hidden agenda and help the patient to resolve any conflict.

The clinical approach

A careful history is very valuable in ascertaining food and beverage intake and perhaps giving patients insight into their calorie intake, since some deny overeating or will underestimate their food intake.[4]

Relevant questions

- Do you feel that you have an excessive appetite?
- Tell me in detail what you ate yesterday.
- Give me an outline of a typical daily meal.
- Tell me about snacks, soft drink and alcohol that you have.
- What exercise do you get?
- Do you have any special problems, such as getting bored, tense and upset or depressed?
- What drugs are you taking?

Physical examination

In the physical examination it is very important to measure body weight and height and calculate the BMI, and assess the degree and distribution of body fat and the overall nutritional status. Record the blood pressure and test the urine for sugar. Keep in mind that a standard blood pressure cuff on a large arm may give falsely elevated values. Remember the rare possibilities of Cushing's disease, acromegaly and hypothyroidism. Search for evidence of athero-sclerosis and diabetes and for signs of alcohol abuse.

An extensive working up of the CNS is not indicated in obesity without the presence of sus-picious symptoms such as visual difficulties.

Investigations

It is essential to perform two measurements:
- weight and height (to calculate BMI)
- waist–hip ratio

Important investigations
- cholesterol/triglycerides
- glucose (fasting)
- liver function tests
- electrolytes and urea

Investigations to consider
- thyroid function tests
- cortisol (if hypertensive)
- testosterone (suspected sleep apnoea)
- ECG and chest X-ray (older than 40)

Anthropometric measurements

Useful measuring instruments include:
- body mass index (BMI): 'healthy' range is between 20 and 25
- waist–hip circumference ratio (W/H ratio): healthy range < 0.9
- single skinfold thickness (> 25 mm suggests increased body fat)
- upper arm circumference
- 4 skinfold thickness (sum of suprailiac, sub-scapular, triceps and biceps skinfolds)—for calculation of percentage body fat

Abdominal fatness is defined as a W/H ratio of > 0.85 in women and > 0.95 in men.

Body mass index

The easiest and possibly most accurate assess-ment of obesity is the BMI (refer Appendix VI):

$$BMI = \frac{weight\ (kg)}{height\ (M^2)}$$

Garrow[5] has produced a simple classification of the BMI associated with the relative degree of risk increase and suggested therapy (Table 70.2).

Weight gain in children

Various studies have found that approximately 10% of prepubertal and 15% of adolescent age groups are obese.[1]

Parents often blame obesity in children on their 'glands', but endocrine or metabolic causes are rare and can be readily differentiated from exogenous obesity by a simple physical exami-nation and an assessment of linear growth. Chil-dren with exogenous obesity tend to have an accelerated linear growth whereas children with secondary causes are usually short.

Congenital or inherited disorders associated with obesity

Prader-Willi syndrome

The characteristic features are bizarre eating habits (e.g. binge eating), obesity, hypotonia, hypogonadism, mental retardation, small hands and feet and a characteristic facial appearance (narrow bifrontal diameter, 'almond-shaped' eyes and a 'tented' upper lip). Progressive

Table 70.2 *Classification of obesity (after Garrow 1988)[5]*

BMI	Grading	Suggested therapy
< 18	very underweight	diet and counselling
18–20	underweight	diet (and counselling)
20–25	0. healthy weight	
25–30	I. overweight	more exercise diet : less alcohol
30–40	II. obesity	combined program: • behaviour modification • diet • exercise consider medical therapy if > 35
> 40	III. morbid obesity	combined program plus medical therapy consider gastric surgery

obesity results from excessive intake in addition to decreased caloric requirements.

Laurence-Moon-Biedl syndrome
The characteristic features are obesity, mental retardation, polydactyly and syndactyly, retinitis pigmentation and hypogonadism.

Beckwith-Wiedemann syndrome
Characteristics include excessive growth, macrosomia, macroglossia, umbilical hernia and neonatal hypoglycaemia. Children appear obese as they are above the 95th percentile by 18 months of age. Intelligence is usually in the normal range.

Endocrine disorders
Endocrine disorders in children that can rarely cause obesity include hypothyroidism (often blamed as the cause but seldom is), Cushing's syndrome, insulinomas, hypothalamic lesions, Fröhlich's syndrome (adiposogenital dystrophy) and Stein-Leventhal syndrome in girls.

Managing obesity in children
Childhood obesity usually reflects an underlying problem in the family system. It can be a very difficult emotional problem in adolescents, who develop a poor body image. An important strategy is to meet with family members, determine whether they perceive the child's obesity as a problem and whether they are prepared to solve the problem. The family dynamics will have to be assessed and strategies outlined. This may involve referral for expert counselling. It is worth pointing out that children eat between one-third and two-thirds of their meals at school so schools should be approached to promote special programs for children who need weight reduction.

Cushing's syndrome

Cushing's syndrome is the term used to describe the chemical features of increased free circulating glucocorticoid. The most common cause is iatrogenic with the prescribing of synthetic corticosteroids. The spontaneous primary forms such as Cushing's disease (pituitary dependent hyperadrenalism) are rare. As the disease progresses the body contour tends to assume the often quoted configuration of a lemon with matchsticks (Fig. 70.1).

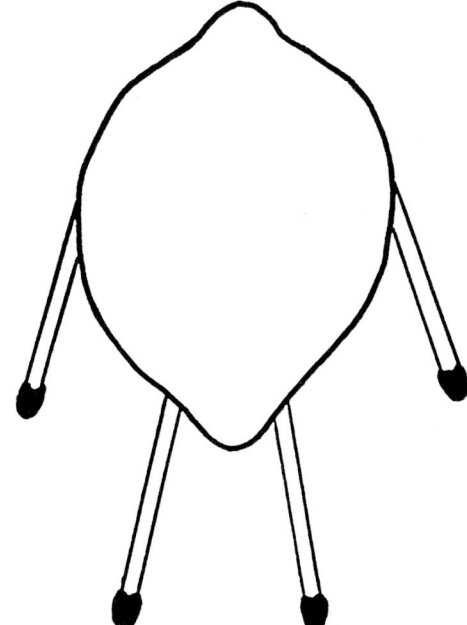

Fig. 70.1 *The traditional 'lemon with matchsticks' configuration of Cushing's syndrome*

Typical clinical features
- change in appearance
- central weight gain (truncal obesity)
- hair growth and acne in females
- muscle weakness
- amenorrhoea/oligomenorrhoea (females)
- thin skin/spontaneous bruising
- polymyalgia/polydypsia (diabetes mellitus)
- insomnia
- depression

Signs
- moon face
- 'buffalo bump'
- purple striae
- large trunk and thin limbs

The patient should be referred for diagnostic evaluation including plasma cortisol and overnight dexamethasone suppression tests.

Untreated Cushing's syndrome has a very poor prognosis, with premature death from myocardial infarction, cardiac failure and infection; hence early diagnosis and referral is essential.

Obesity

Obesity and overweight are the most common pathological conditions in our society and are caused by an accumulation of adipose tissue

Table 70.3 *Factors predisposing to primary obesity*

Genetic	— familial tendency
Sex	— women more susceptible
Activity	— lack of physical activity
Psychogenic	— emotional deprivation; depression
Social class	— poorer classes
Alcohol	— problem drinking
Smoking	— cessation of smoking
Prescribed drugs	— tricyclic derivatives

(Table 70.3). It is not the extra weight *per se* that causes problems but excess fat. The calculation of the BMI gives a better estimate of adiposity and it is convenient and preferable to use this index when assessing the overweight and obese. However, recent data suggest that the distribution of body fat is as important a risk factor as its total amount. Abdominal fat (upper body segment obesity, or 'apple' obesity, is considered a greater health hazard than fat in the thighs and buttocks (lower body segment obesity, or 'pear' obesity) (Fig. 70.2).

Obese patients with high waist–hip ratios (> 1.0 in men and > 0.9 in women) have a significantly greater risk of diabetes mellitus, stroke, coronary artery disease and early death than equally obese people with lower waist–hip ratios.[3]

In regard to the BMI reference scale it is worth noting that the risks follow a J-shaped curve (Fig. 70.3) and are only slightly increased in the overweight range but increase with obesity so that a BMI of > 40 carries a threefold increase in mortality.

The consequences of obesity include:

upper body segment obesity (android/visceral obesity) *v* lower body segment obesity (gynoid obesity)

Fig. 70.2 *Comparison of two types of obesity according to distribution of body fat*

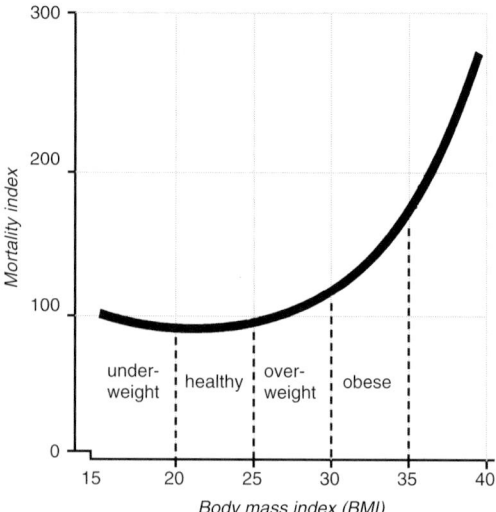

Fig. 70.3 *Body mass index (BMI) reference scale*

- cardiovascular
  - — increased mortality
  - — hypertension
  - — varicose veins
- metabolic
  - — dyslipidaemia
  - — non-insulin dependent diabetes
  - — hyperinsulinaemia
  - — infertility
- mechanical
  - — osteoarthritis
  - — obstructive sleep apnoea
  - — spinal dysfunction

Management

Treatment is based on four major interventions, the choice of which depends on the degree of obesity, the associated health problems and the health risk posed.[2]

1. reduction in energy intake
2. change in diet composition
3. increased physical activity
4. behavioural therapy

Pharmacological agents are not used for first-line therapy although they may have a place in management, especially at grade III level of obesity. Surgery is an option for the treatment of morbid obesity.

There is no single effective method for the treatment of obesity, which is a difficult and frustrating problem. A continuing close therapist/patient contact has a better chance of success than any single treatment regimen.

Most successful programs involve a multidisciplinary approach to weight loss, embracing the four major interventions. Emphasis must be on maintenance of weight loss. Behaviour modification is important and the most valuable strategy is to emphasise planning and record keeping with a continuous weekly diary of menus, exercise and actual behaviour.

Social support is essential for a successful weight loss program. A better result is likely if close family members, especially the chief cook, are involved in the program, preferably striving for the same goals.[3]

A doctor–patient strategy

A close therapeutic supportive relationship with a patient can be effective using the following methods.[6]

1. *Promote realistic goals.* Lose weight at the same rate that it was gained, i.e. slowly. For example, 5–10 kg a year. A graph can be used for this purpose with an 'exaggerated' scale on the vertical axis so that small variations appear highly significant and encouraging (Fig. 70.4).

   Promote the equation:

   ENERGY IN = ENERGY OUT + ENERGY STORED

   The only way to reduce the stored energy (fat) is either to reduce energy in (eat less) or increase energy out (exercise).

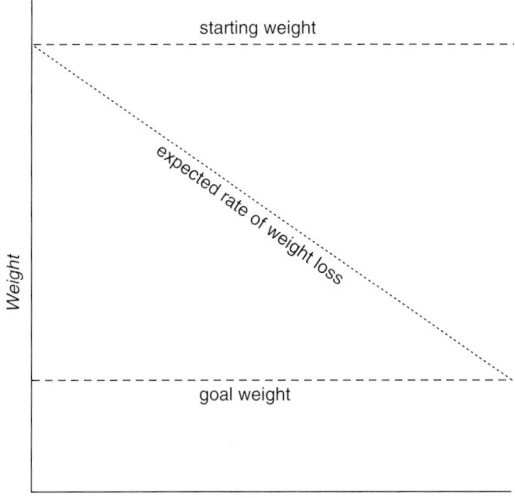

Fig. 70.4 *Weight loss chart to encourage patient*
AFTER KACZMARCZYK[6]

2. *Dietary advice.* It is important to be realistic and allow patients to eat their normal foods but advise them about quantity and frequency. Give advice on simple substitutions, e.g. fortified skim milk in place of whole milk, high-fibre wholemeal bread instead of white bread, and fruit and vegetables instead of biscuits and cakes as in-between snacks.[6] A strategy that seems to work effectively is to advise patients, especially those who are overweight (grade I obesity), to eat one-third less than they usually do and discipline themselves not to 'pick' and to avoid second helpings.

3. *Counselling* is simple and common sense. It involves being supportive, interested and encouraging. A list of tips on coping is provided (see following 'a practical plan' for grade II and III obesity) and the patient advised to keep a food, exercise and behaviour diary.

4. *Review.* 'Review is the most vital part of the weight loss programme as it stimulates and revitalises motivation and enables assessment of progress'.[6] It should be frequent initially, e.g. fortnightly, then monthly until the goal weight has been achieved and then 3-monthly. It is important never to be judgmental or critical if progress is unsatisfactory.

A practical plan

The following patient education sheet to be handed to patients represents useful advice to offer the obese patient.[7]

Physical activity
- A brisk walk for 20–30 minutes each day is the most practical exercise.
- Other activities such as tennis, swimming, golf and cycling are a bonus.

Dietary advice
Breakfast:
- oatmeal (soaked overnight in water); after cooking, add fresh or dried fruit; serve with fat-reduced milk or yoghurt

   or

- muesli (homemade or from a health food store)—medium serve with fat-reduced milk, perhaps add extra fruit (fresh or dried)
- slice of wholemeal toast with a thin scraping of margarine, spread with Vegemite, Marmite or sugar-free marmalade

- fresh orange juice or herbal tea or black tea/coffee

Morning and afternoon tea:
- piece of fruit or vegetable (e.g. carrot or celery)
- freshly squeezed juice or chilled water with fresh lemon

Midday meal:
- salad sandwich with wholemeal or multigrain bread and thin scraping of margarine (for variety use egg, salmon, chicken or cheese fillings)
- drink as for breakfast

Evening meal:
Summer (cold)—lean meat cuts (grilled, hot or cold), poultry (skin removed) or fish; fresh garden salad; slices of fresh fruit
Winter (hot)—lean meat cuts (grilled), poultry (skin removed) or fish; plenty of green, red and yellow vegetables and small potato; fruit for sweets

Weight-losing tips
- Have sensible goals; do not 'crash' diet, but have a 6–12 month plan to achieve your ideal weight.
- Go for natural foods; avoid junk foods.
- Avoid alcohol, sugary soft drinks and high-calorie fruit juices.
- Strict dieting without exercise fails.
- If you are mildly overweight, eat one-third less than you usually do.
- Do not eat biscuits, cakes, buns, etc. between meals (preferably at no time).
- Use high-fibre foods to munch on.
- A small treat once a week may add variety.
- Avoid seconds and do not eat leftovers.
- Eat slowly—spin out your meal.

Pharmacological agents
A variety of these are available or imminent but have limitations and need to be used with caution, if at all.

The agents are:[8]
Local acting on GIT
- bulking agents, e.g. methylcellulose
- tetrahydrolipstatin

Centrally acting agents
- amphetamine derivatives (reduce hunger)
- serotonin analogues (enhance satiety)
  — fenfluramine

  — dexfenfluramine (the d-isomer of above)
  — fluoxetine
- thermogenic agents (in development)
  — β3-receptor agonists

Surgery
In those with morbid obesity (about 2% of the population) unresponsive to behaviour modification therapy and a course of dexfenfluramine for 3 months or so, gastric banding has a place. One example is Lap-Band which is inserted laparoscopically and can be adjusted and eventually removed with no significant residual adverse defect left in the stomach.[9] Gastric stapling and gastric bypass are other techniques to consider.

Oedema
Oedema (dropsy) is an excessive accumulation of fluid in tissue spaces. It may be generalised or localised—periorbital, peripheral or an arm (lymphoedema).

Generalised oedema
The site of generalised oedema is largely determined by gravity. It is due to an abnormal excess of sodium in the body which leads to accumulation of water. The causes can be generally divided into two groups—oedema associated with a decreased plasma volume and oedema associated with an increased plasma volume (see Table 70.4).

Diagnosis
Clinical examination including urinalysis is usually sufficient to establish the cause of the oedema. In other cases, investigation of renal or liver function may be required.

Treatment of generalised oedema
- Treat the cause where known
- Salt (sodium) restriction

Table 70.4 *Causes of generalised oedema*

Decreased plasma volume
- Hypoalbuminaemia, e.g. nephrotic syndrome, chronic liver disease, malnutrition

Increased plasma volume
- Congestive cardiac failure
- Chronic renal failure
- Drugs, e.g. corticosteroids, NSAIDs, certain antihypertensives, oestrogens, lithium, others

Idiopathic oedema

- Diuretics—a loop diuretic, e.g. frusemide
  —a potassium-sparing diuretic,
  e.g. spironolactone

Idiopathic oedema

Idiopathic oedema, also known as cyclical or periodic oedema, is a common problem and the diagnosis is made on a characteristic history:

- exclusive to women
- may be cyclical or persistent
- usually unrelated to menstrual cycle
- excessive diurnal weight gain (worse on prolonged standing)
- abdominal bloating
- may affect hands and face as well as feet
- often made worse by diuretics
- may be associated with headache, depression, tension

Treatment of this condition is difficult. Most diuretics can aggravate the problem. Supportive stockings and a nutritious diet (with restricted sodium intake) is recommended as first-line treatment. A trial of spironolactone is often recommended.

Swelling (puffiness) of the face and eyelids

The causes are similar to those for generalised oedema. Important specific causes to consider are:

- renal disease, e.g. nephrotic syndrome, acute nephritis
- hypothyroidism
- Cushing's disease and corticosteroid treatment
- mediastinal obstruction
- angio-oedema
- skin sensitivity, e.g. drugs, cosmetics, hair dryers

Swelling of the legs

Refer to page 663.

When to refer

- Patients with grade II or III obesity (BMI > 30) who are resistant to simple weight control measures.[2]
- Patients with associated medical problems such as angina or severe osteoarthritis who require rapid weight reduction.
- Possibility of endocrine cause of obesity.

- Suspicion of congenital or inherited disorder in children.

Practice tips

- Avoid a critical or judgmental attitude to the overweight patient.[10]
- Seek diplomatic independent information from a spouse or parent about food and beverage intake.
- Obtain a chronological history of the patient's weight from infancy onwards and attempt to correlate any significant changes to stressful life events.
- Central or visceral obesity carries a large risk factor for medical complications. People are advised to keep the waist circumference to less than 100 cm.

References

1. Tunnessen WW jnr. *Signs and symptoms in paediatrics* (2nd edn). Philadelphia: JB Lippincott, 1988, 33–41.
2. Marks S, Walqvist M. Obesity. In: MIMS Disease Index (2nd edn). Sydney: IMS Publishing, 1996, 354–356.
3. Schroeder SA et al. *Current medical diagnosis and treatment.* East Norwalk: Appleton and Lange, 1990, 874–875.
4. Sloane PD, Slatt PD, Baker RM. *Essentials of family medicine.* Baltimore: Williams and Wilkins, 1988, 200–208.
5. Garrow J. *Treat obesity seriously.* Edinburgh: Churchill Livingstone, 1988.
6. Kaczmarczyk W. The obese patient. In: How I manage my difficult problems. Aust Fam Physician, 1991; 20:417–421.
7. Murtagh JE. Obesity: how to lose weight wisely. In: *Patient Education* (2nd edn). Sydney: McGraw-Hill, 1996, 62.
8. Caterson ID. Obesity: effective management in general practice. Mod Med Aust, 1996: 39(6): 70–80.
9. O'Brien P. Advances in gastrointestinal surgery. Update Course handbook. Monash University, 1996: 29.
10. Kincaid-Smith P, Larkins R, Whelan G. *Problems in clinical medicine.* Sydney: MacLennan & Petty, 1990: 105–108.

71
Weight loss

—

*Among young women dieters in modern society about
1 in 20 will become preoccupied with their
appearance and progress to the eating disorders of
anorexia nervosa and bulimia.*

In family practice complaints of loss of weight
are more frequent than complaints about being
too thin. Of great significance is the problem of
recent loss of weight. A very analytical history is
required to determine the patient's perception of
weight loss. The equivalent problem in children
is failure to gain weight or thrive.

Weight loss is an important symptom because
it usually implies a serious underlying disorder,
either organic or functional. It may or may not
be associated with anorexia and thus diminished
food intake.

Key facts and checkpoints

- Any loss of more than 5% of normal body
  weight is significant.
- The most common cause in adults of recent
  weight loss is stress and anxiety.[1]
- Serious organic diseases to consider are:
  — malignant disease
  — diabetes mellitus
  — chronic infections, e.g. tuberculosis
  — thyrotoxicosis
- The most important variable to consider in
  evaluating weight loss is appetite. Eating and
  weight go hand in glove.
- Two conditions commonly associated with
  weight loss are anaemia and fever; they must
  be excluded.
- Early detection of eating disorders improves
  outcome.

A diagnostic approach

A summary of the safety diagnostic model is presented in Table 71.1.

Probability diagnosis

Excluding planned dietary restriction, psychological factors are the most common cause, particularly recent stress and anxiety.[1] Elderly people
with adverse psychological factors, neglect and
possibly drug effects can present with wasting.

Serious disorders not to be missed

Many of the problems causing weight loss are
very serious, especially malignant disease.

Malignant disease

Weight loss may be a manifestation of any malignancy. With carcinoma of the stomach, pancreas
and caecum, malignant lymphomas and
myeloma, weight loss may be the only symptom.
Occult malignancy must be regarded as the most
common cause of weight loss in the absence of
major symptoms and signs. The mechanisms
may be multiple, with anorexia and increased
metabolism being important factors.

Chronic infections

These are now less common but tuberculosis
must be considered, especially in people from
less developed countries. Some cases of infective endocarditis may progress only very slowly
with general debility, weight loss and fever as
major features.[2]

Other infections to consider are brucellosis,
and protozoal and systemic fungal infection.
Infection with HIV virus must be considered,
especially in high-risk groups.

Table 71.1 *Weight loss: diagnostic strategy model (other than deliberate dieting or malnutrition)*

Q. Probability diagnosis
A. Stress and anxiety
   Non-coping elderly

Q. Serious disorders not to be missed
A. Congestive cardiac failure
   Malignant disease
   • stomach
   • pancreas
   • lung
   • myeloma
   • caecum
   • lymphoma
   Chronic infection
   • HIV infections (AIDS, ARC)
   • tuberculosis
   • hidden abscess
   • infective endocarditis
   • brucellosis
   • others

Q. Pitfalls (often missed)
A. Drug dependence, esp. alcohol
   Malabsorption states
          ? intestinal parasites
   Other GIT problems
   Chronic renal failure
   Connective tissue disorders, e.g. SLE

   Rarities
   Addison's disease
   Hypopituitarism

Q. Seven masquerades checklist
A. Depression   √
   Diabetes   √
   Drugs   √
   Anaemia   √
   Thyroid disease   √
   Spinal dysfunction −
   UTI   −

Q. Is the patient trying to tell me something?
A. A possibility. Consider stress, anxiety and depression. Anorexia nervosa and bulimia are special considerations.

Pitfalls

Drug dependency, including alcohol and narcotic drugs, must be considered especially when the problem may result in inappropriate nutrition. Apart from malignant disease there is a whole variety of gastrointestinal disorders that require consideration—these include malabsorption states, gastric ulceration, and intestinal infestations that should be considered especially in people returning from a significant stay in tropical and underdeveloped countries.

Addison's disease can be very difficult to diagnose. Symptoms include excessive fatigue, anorexia, nausea and postural dizziness. Hyperpigmentation is a late sign.

Seven masquerades checklist

Depression and the endocrine disorders, diabetes mellitus and hyperthyroidism, are important causes.

Diabetes

The diabetic who presents with weight loss will be young and insulin-dependent. The initial presentation may be ketoacidosis. The triad of symptoms is *thirst—polyuria—weight loss*.

Hyperthyroidism

This is usually associated with weight loss although in some, such as an elderly male, it may not be obvious. An important clue will be weight loss in the presence of an excellent appetite and this helps to distinguish it from a psychoneurotic disturbance.

Depression

Weight loss is a common feature of depression and is usually proportional to the severity of the disease. In the early stages of depression weight gain may be present but when the classical loss of the four basic drives (appetite, energy, sleep and sex) becomes manifest, weight loss is a feature.

Drugs

Any prescribed drugs causing anorexia can cause weight loss. Important drugs include digoxin, narcotics, cytotoxics, NSAIDs, some antihypertensives and theophylline.

Psychogenic considerations

Weight loss is a feature of anxiety as well as depression. Some patients with psychotic disturbances, including schizophrenia and mania, may present with weight loss.

Anorexia nervosa is quite common and is almost entirely confined to females between the ages of 12 and 20. The main differential diagnosis is hypopituitarism, although anorexia nervosa can cause endocrine disturbances through the hypothalamic pituitary axis.

The clinical approach

History

It is important to document the weight loss carefully and evaluate the patient's recordings. The same set of scales should be used. It is also important to determine the food intake. However, in the absence of an independent witness such as a spouse or parent, this can be difficult. Food intake may be diminished with psychogenic disorders and carcinoma but increased or steady with endocrine disorders such as diabetes and hyperthyroidism and with steatorrhoea.

General questions

- Exactly how much weight have you lost and over how long?
- Have you changed your diet in any way?
- Has your appetite changed? Do you feel like eating?
- Have your clothes become looser?
- What is your general health like?
- How do you feel in yourself?
- Do you feel uptight (tense), worried or anxious?
- Do you get very irritable or tremulous?
- Do you feel depressed?
- Do you ever force yourself to vomit?
- Are you thirsty?
- Do you pass a lot of urine?
- Do you have excessive sweating?
- Do you experience a lot of night sweats?
- What are your motions like?
- Are they difficult to flush down the toilet?
- Do you have a cough or bring up sputum?
- Do you get short of breath?
- Do you have any abdominal pain?
- Are your periods normal (for females)?
- What drugs are you taking?
- How many cigarettes do you smoke?

Physical examination

A careful general examination is essential with special attention to:

- vital parameters
- the thyroid and signs of hyperthyroidism
- the abdomen (check liver, any masses and tenderness)
- rectal examination (test stool for occult blood)
- reflexes

Investigations

Basic investigations include:

- haemoglobin, red cell indices and film
- white cell count
- ESR
- thyroid function test
- random blood sugar
- chest X-ray
- urine analysis

Others to consider:

- upper GIT (endoscopy or barium meal)
- ultrasound of abdomen (or CT if suspected abnormality not found)
- colonoscopy
- LFTs

Weight loss in children

Weight loss in children can be considered as:

1. Failure to thrive (FTT): the child up to 2 years below 3rd percentile.
2. Weight loss in a child after normal development.

Failure to thrive

The long list of possible causes includes malfunction of any of the organ systems of the body as well as nutritional, environmental, social and psychological factors.

FTT is best determined by sequentially plotting the weight, length and head circumference on growth charts (see growth charts in appendix). The infant with FTT has a decreased growth rate or is losing weight, and may be below the 3rd percentile. The percentile charts mean little without considering the context of the baby's growth, e.g. premature babies, children of small parents.

On an average, babies put on 150–200 g a week.[3] A classification of FTT is presented in Table 71.2, divided into organic and non-organic causes. The distinction is not always easy. Psychosocial problems may coexist with organic problems. Feeding problems are common to both.

Non-organic failure to thrive

Non-organic FTT can be caused by emotional deprivation or by poor nutrition from inadequate intake. Emotional deprivation might be anticipated by a knowledge of the mother, her family background, marital relationships, attitude to the

Table 71.2 *Failure to thrive: general causes (after Robinson)*

Non-organic causes
1. Inadequate parenting
2. Poor nutrition

Organic causes
1. Failure of intake
   - underfeeding, e.g. nipple disorders
   - congenital abnormalities, e.g. cleft palate
   - dyspnoea, e.g. congenital heart disease
   - neurological lesions, e.g. cerebral birth injuries
   - behavioural factors
2. Abnormal losses
   - vomiting, e.g. pyloric stenosis, galactosaemia
   - stools, e.g. steatorrhoea
   - urine, e.g. renal disease
3. Failure of utilisation
   - chronic infection, e.g. cystic fibrosis
   - metabolic disorders, e.g. phenylketonuria
   - endocrine disorders, e.g. hypothyroidism
   - constitutional, e.g. Down syndrome

pregnancy, delivery and early bonding experience. In her book *The Abused Child*, Martin lists factors influencing such bonding.[4]

Factors in the parent
- expectation of the child
- desire for the child
- capacity to give
- ego-strength to adapt to stress
- ability to accept imperfection
- realistic fantasies of the child

Factors in the child
- absence of defects
- the ability to match the parent's expectations
- good health
- loving behaviour, including smiling, cuddling and thriving

Disturbance of any of these factors may lead to relationship difficulties. The management of FTT due to psychological factors may be complex.[5] At the simplest level the recognition by the mother that she is having difficulty in relating to her baby is essential, and the reassurance that not all babies are as lovable and easy to manage as portrayed may help. A home visit to evaluate the home environment will provide invaluable information. These mothers require considerable caring support and encouragement.

Organic failure to thrive
Any chronic disease will cause FTT. Serious organic diseases include renal failure, cystic

hypothyroidism, cystic fibrosis, other causes of malabsorption such as coeliac disease, and various inborn errors of metabolism such as galactosaemia (Table 71.2).

Poor developmental progress may indicate mental retardation. Babies born to mothers who are HIV carriers present with FTT in the first 5 months, with or without other signs of disease, such as infections.[3] Another possible cause of growth failure in a baby who has a good intake may be sleep apnoea and this requires investigation.

Examination of the baby
Examine for developmental problems including cerebral palsy, cleft palate, respiratory disorders and abdominal abnormalities.

Investigations
Simple screening tests should be performed if either the history or physical examination suggests organic disease. Tests include routine blood counts, urinalysis and urine culture, Guthrie test for PKU, IVP, thyroid function tests and chromosomal and hormone analysis.

Main causes of FTT (account for up to 90%):[6]

- normal variants, and
- nutritional deprivation

Most important considerations
- manner of feeding
- home visit
- environmental factors
- parental problems
- admission to hospital

Rare possibilities
- HIV infection
- sleep apnoea
- hypopituitarism (growth hormone↓)
- chromosomal abnormalities

Loss of weight in the older child
Acute or chronic infections are the most common causes of weight loss in children beyond infancy.[6] In acute infections the weight loss is transient, and once the infection clears the child generally regains the lost weight. In chronic infections signs may be more difficult to detect; for example, urinary tract infection, pulmonary infection, osteomyelitis, chronic hepatitis. In common with the younger child who fails to thrive, the older may be suffering from

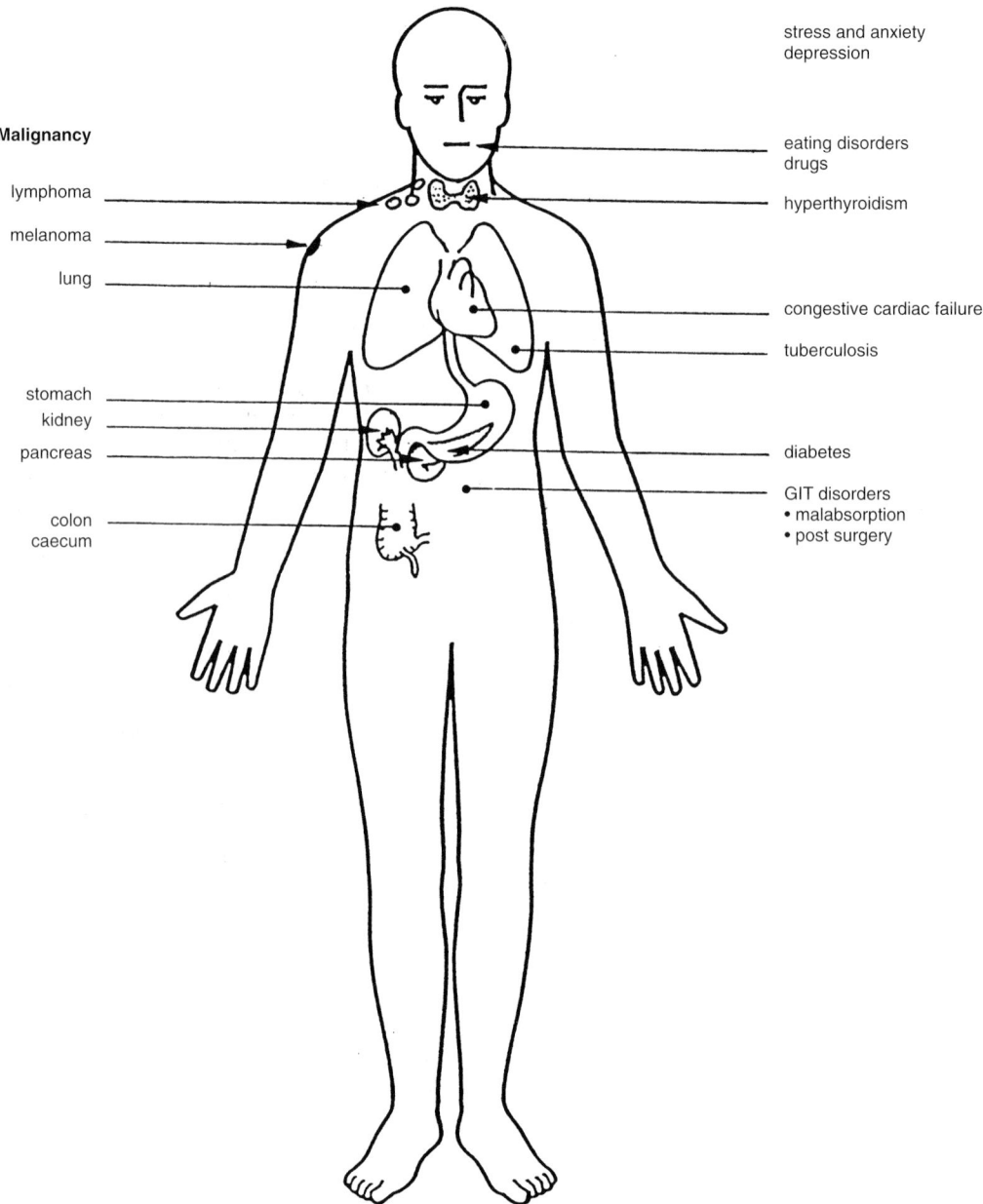

Fig. 71.1 *Weight loss: causes to consider*

malabsorption syndrome, chronic infection of the urinary tract or a rare chromosomal or metabolic disorder.[7] Tuberculosis, diabetes and malignant disease may present as weight loss and it is necessary to exclude organic disease before considering the more common emotional disorders.

Eating disorders in the adolescent

Concerns about body image and dieting are very common among young women in modern society. Among these dieters 5–10% become abnormally preoccupied with dieting and slimness and progress to the eating disorders of anorexia nervosa and bulimia.

The DSM III criteria for diagnosing these disorders, which have serious physical and psychological consequences, are presented in Table 71.3. The differential diagnosis of anorexia nervosa includes most of the problems listed in Table 71.1.

Anorexia nervosa

Anorexia nervosa is a syndrome characterised by the obsessive pursuit of thinness through dieting with extreme weight loss and disturbance of body image.[8] The mortality rate may be as high as 18%.

Typical features
- adolescent and young adult females
- up to 1% incidence among schoolgirls aged 16[9]
- bimodal age of onset: 13 to 14 and 17 to 18 years[8]
- unknown cause
- severe emaciation
- amenorrhoea
- loss of body fat
- dry and scaly skin
- increased lanugo body hair
- BMI < 17.5

Bulimia

Bulimia is episodic secretive binge eating followed by self-induced vomiting, fasting or the use of laxatives or diuretics. This binge–purge

Table 71.3   *DSM III criteria for diagnosing anorexia nervosa and bulimia*

Anorexia nervosa
1. Refusal to maintain normal body weight
2. Loss of more than 25% of original body weight
3. Disturbance of body image
4. Intense fear of becoming fat
5. No known medical illness leading to weight loss

Bulimia
1. Recurrent episodes of binge eating
2. At least three of the following:
   a. consumption of high-calorie, easily ingested food during binge
   b. termination of binge by abdominal pain, sleep or vomiting
   c. inconspicuous eating during a binge
   d. repeated attempts to lose weight
   e. frequent fluctuations of more than 4.5 kg
3. Awareness of abnormal eating pattern and fear of not being able to stop voluntarily
4. Depressed mood after binge
5. Not due to anorexia or any physical disorder

syndrome is also referred to as bulimarexia. It is more difficult to detect than anorexia nervosa but has a higher incidence.

Typical clinical features
- young females
- begins at later age, usually 17–25 years
- associated psychoneurotic disorders
- fluctuations in body weight
- periods irregular—amenorrhoea rare
- physical complications of frequent vomiting, e.g. dental decay, effects of hypokalaemia
- recurrent laxative, stimulant or enema abuse

Management of eating disorders

Early detection and intervention are essential to reduce the risk of chronicity. Treatment can be conducted on an outpatient basis but if there are marked trends, such as severe weight loss, a family crisis, severe depression and a suicide risk, the patient requires hospital admission. There are often problematic family interrelationships which require exploration.

Important goals are:

- establish a good and caring relationship with the patient
- resolve underlying psychological difficulties
- restore weight to a level between ideal and the patient's concept of optimal weight
- provide a balanced diet of at least 3000 calories per day (anorexia nervosa)

Structured behavioural therapy, intensive psychotherapy and family therapy may be tried but supportive care by physicians and allied health staff appears to be the most important feature of therapy.[10] Antidepressants, especially of the SSRI group, may be helpful for selective patients. It is important to provide ongoing support for both patient and family.

Weight loss in the elderly

General weight loss is a relatively common physiological feature of many elderly people. However, abnormal weight loss is commonly encountered in the socially disadvantaged elderly, especially those who live alone and lack drive and interest in adequate food preparation. Other factors include relative poverty and poor dentition, including ill-fitting and painful false teeth. An important cause that should always be considered is malignant disease.

Congestive cardiac failure, especially secondary to ischaemic heart disease, is a common cause of weight loss. This is due to visceral congestion.

Gastrointestinal causes of weight loss

The following conditions may lead to weight loss:

- poor oral hygiene
- chronic vomiting or diarrhoea, e.g. pyloric stenosis
- gastric ulcer
- carcinoma of the stomach, oesophagus, large bowel
- problem alcohol drinking
- partial or total gastrectomy
- other GIT surgery
- inflammatory bowel disease, e.g. Crohn's disease, ulcerative colitis
- steatorrhoea
- lymphoma of the gut
- parasitic infestation
- cirrhosis of the liver

The mechanisms of weight loss include anorexia, malabsorption, obstruction with vomiting and inflammation.

When to refer

- Any unexplained weight loss, especially if an endocrine cause or malignancy is suspected.
- Weight loss related to a serious psychological illness.
- A serious eating disorder.
- Failure to thrive in a child where a normal variant or simple mismanagement is excluded.

Practice tips

- Ask patients what they really believe is the cause of their weight loss.
- An anxiety state and hyperthyroidism can be difficult to differentiate. Consider the latter and perform thyroid function tests.
- Laboratory tests are rarely needed to establish the diagnosis of an eating disorder. Hormonal levels return to normal following weight gain.
- A high index of suspicion by the family doctor is required to diagnose eating disorders. Think of it in a mid-teen female; weight loss through dieting; wide fluctuation in weight; amenorrhoea and hyperactivity.

References

1. Cormack J, Marinker M, Morrell D. *Practice: A handbook of primary health care.* London: Kluwer-Harrap Handbooks, 1980; 3.42:1–2.
2. Beck ER, Francis JL, Souhami RL. *Tutorials in differential diagnosis* (2nd edn). Edinburgh: Churchill Livingstone, 1988, 117–120.
3. Caswell A, Hutchins P. How to treat failure to thrive. Aust Dr Weekly, 13 April 1990, I–VIII.
4. Martin HP. *The abused child.* Cambridge, Mass: Ballinger, 1976.
5. Cormack J, Marinker M, Morrell D. *Practice: A handbook of primary health care.* London: Kluwer-Harrap Handbooks, 1980; 3.70A:1–8.
6. Tunnessen WW. *Symptoms and signs in paediatrics* (2nd edn). Philadelphia: Lippincott, 1988, 25–28.
7. Robinson MJ. *Practical paediatrics.* Melbourne: Churchill Livingstone, 1990, 140–144.
8. Young D. Eating disorders in the adolescent. Aust Fam Physician, 1988; 17:334–336.
9. Crisp AH, Palmer RL, Kalucy RS. How common is anorexia nervosa? A prevalence study. Br J Psychiatry, 1976; 128, 549–554.
10. Tierney LM et al. *Current medical diagnosis and treatment.* Stamford: Appleton and Lange, 1996, 1096.

PART 4

CHILD AND ADOLESCENT HEALTH

72

An approach to the child

—

In every child who is born, under no matter the circumstances, and of no matter what parents, the potentiality of the human race is born again; and in him, too, once more, and of each of us, our terrific responsibility towards human life; towards the utmost idea of goodness, of the horror of error, and of God.

James Agee

The diagnostic approach to the child is based on the ability to achieve good lines of communication with both the child and the parent. In the diagnostic approach, the relative importance of the various components is clinical history 80%, physical examination 15%, special investigations 5%.[1]

The establishment of rapport can be achieved by showing a genuine interest in the child with strategies such as:

- asking them what they like to be called
- passing a compliment about the child such as a clothing item or a toy or book they are carrying
- taking time to converse with them
- asking them if they would like to be a doctor when they grow up
- asking about their teacher or friends

This process will help set the scene for easier history taking and a sound physical examination.

Children's general behaviour patterns and personality can be classified into broad identifiable categories according to age group. Although there is considerable variation and generalisations can be inappropriate, the following stereotypes are helpful guidelines for parents.

- terrible 2's   mischievous, explorative, dangerous activity, conflicts
- trusting 3's   friendly, amenable to reason, loving
- frustrating 4's   cheeky, inquisitive, hard to reason, no social graces
- fascinating 5's   more co-ordinated and independent
- sociable 6's   enjoys tasks for temporary interests, loves to be wooed
- problematic 7's   tendency to wrongdoing, stubborn, searching for independence
- steady 8's
- noisy and adventurous 9's

History

Obtaining information in the following sequence is recommended:

- presenting problem (focus on this first)
  — allow the parents to elaborate without interruption
  — be a listener and believe the story
- state of health prior to the present complaint
- past history
  — general features
  — pregnancy and neonatal features
  — feeding and diet
  — immunisation
  — toilet training
- family history
  — inherited disorders
  — other
- systems review
  — general features, e.g. fever, energy
  — feeding and elimination
  — hearing
  — vision
- developmental history
  — check list of milestones (Table 72.1)
- social history

Table 72.1 *Developmental milestones (m=months) (after Jarman and Oberklaid[2])*

Gross motor	Expressive language
Chin up (1 m)	Coos (3 m)
Lifts head (4 m)	Babbles (6 m)
Rolls—prone to supine (4 m)	Da-Da—inappropriate (8 m)
Rolls—supine to prone (5 m)	Da/Ma—appropriate (10 m)
Sits unsupported (8 m)	First word (11 m)
Pulls to stand (9 m)	Two to six words (15 m)
Cruises (10 m)	Two-word phrases (21 m)
Walks alone (13 m)	Speech all understandable (27 m)
Walks up stairs (20 m)	Names one colour (30 m)
Kicks ball forward (24 m)	Uses plurals (36 m)
Walks up stairs—alternate feet (30 m)	Names four colours (42 m)
Rides tricycle (36 m)	Gives first and last names (44 m)
Two-wheeler bike (36 m)	Names two opposites (50 m)
Hops on one foot (60 m)	Strings sentences together (60 m)
Fine motor	**Receptive language**
Unfisting (3 m)	Gesture games (9 m)
Reach and grasp (5 m)	Understands 'no' (9 m)
Transfer (6 m)	Follows one-step command (12 m)
Thumb-finger grasp (9 m)	Points to animal pictures (19 m)
Tower of 2 cubes (16 m)	Points to 6 body parts (20 m)
Handedness (24 m)	Follows two-step command (24 m)
Scribbles (24 m)	
Tower of 4 cubes (26 m)	
Tower of 8 cubes (40 m)	
Social/self help	**Cognitive**
Social smile (6 weeks)	Shows anticipatory excitement (3 m)
Recognises mother (3 m)	Plays with rattle (4 m)
Stranger anxiety (9 m)	Plays peek-a-boo (8 m)
Finger feeds (10 m)	Finds hidden object (9 m)
Uses spoon (15 m)	Pulls string to obtain toy (14 m)
Uses fork (21 m)	Activates mechanical toy (20 m)
Assists with dressing (12 m)	Pretend play (24 m)
Pulls off socks (15 m)	Seeks out other for play (36 m)
Unbuttons (30 m)	
Buttons (48 m)	
Ties shoelaces (60 m)	
Dresses without supervision (60 m)	

- psychological history
  — behavioural problems
  — reaction to other people and situations

Parent–child interaction

It is advisable to observe carefully the parent–child interaction at all times, including in the waiting room. The parent's manner in talking to and handling the child will provide useful clues about possible problems related to the parent's ability to nurture the child adequately.

Physical examination

It is convenient to consider the physical examination for two main groups:[1]

- the infant and child up to the age of 3 years

- the child from 3 years onwards

An important aspect of assessment is to note the development of the child by comparing its growth with standard developmental charts (Appendices I to IV). Developmental milestones are summarised in Table 72.1[2] and the incidence of developmental problems under 5 years in Table 72.2.[3] The examination includes attention to any unusual appearance, which is the beginning of the process of diagnosis of the dysmorphic child.

Achieving co-operation of infants

A good aphorism is 'Never examine the child until you have made the mother laugh'.

Table 72.2 *Incidence of developmental problems under 5 years (after Hutchins)*[3]

More common, less severe	Less common, more severe
10–20% behaviour problems	3.0% intellectual handicap (IQ < 70)
10% specific learning deficits	1% intellectual handicap (IQ < 50)
10% conductive hearing loss	0.3% cerebral palsy
10% eye problems, e.g. squint	0.2% neural tube defects
5% isolated speech problems	0.17% severe deafness
3% attention deficit disorder	0.06% blind
1% specific language disorder, e.g. comprehension	0.1% autistic spectrum features
	0.05% classical autism

Children, especially if sick and irritable, can be very difficult to examine and may be most unco-operative, particularly if distressed by past experience. However, they can be readily distracted, a characteristic that the family doctor can use effectively to achieve some degree of co-operation for examination, especially for the ears, throat and chest.

Children respond very positively to playing games such as a flashing light, tickling or peek-a-boo, and to any type of noise, particularly animal noises, and good humour from a friendly patient practitioner. Some doctors have strategies such as small animal images on stethoscopes to distract attention.

Distracting children[4]

In the consulting room, a small duck with a rattle inside it can be used for palpating the abdomen of young children. This seems more acceptable to them, as it becomes a game and you obtain the same information as if you had palpated with your hand. When examining the ears of young children sitting on their mother's lap, difficulty is encountered when the child follows the auroscope light and moves its head. A small rabbit or other animal on the desk which, at the press of a button under the desk, will play a drum, distracts the child to the right and enables you to get a good look into the left ear.

Similarly, a clockwork revolving musical toy over the examination couch will distract the child for examination of the ear. It is also a distraction for the general examination of children on the couch, and can become a most useful instrument.

Spatula sketches for children[5]

Many young patients have quickly forgotten any inspection of their throats while observing the preparation of a 'present' in the form of a drawing on the wooden spatula used for the examination.

After the examination they are informed of their special present, and you can then proceed to draw on the unused end of the spatula. The drawings take about 15 seconds. Figure 72.1 illustrates three sketches from one repertoire: a penguin (with optional bow tie), a caterpillar, and a racing car.

Fig. 72.1 *Spatula sketches for children*

Recognition of serious illness in infancy

It is vital to diagnose serious life-threatening disease in children, especially in early infancy. Certain symptoms and signs which provide a reliable indicator to such a problem are:[6]

• drowsiness

- decreased activity (lies quietly)
- child moves eyes (rather than head) to follow you
- pallor
- whimpers and lies quietly (as opposed to crying lustily)
- reduced feeding (<50% normal intake—over 24 hour period)
- less than four wet nappies in 24 hours
- chest wall reaction

Serious illnesses to consider include:

- haemophilus influenza type B (HiB) infection
  — acute epiglottitis
  — meningitis
  — pneumonia
  — septicaemia
  — septic arthritis/osteomyelitis
- meningococcal infection
  — septicaemia
  — meningitis
- other forms of meningitis
- acute myocarditis
- asthma/bronchitis
- intussusception

The child as a barometer of the family

A disturbed child is a very common indicator of family disharmony. There is a saying that 'love is to a child what sunlight is to a flower'.

Children need from their parents:[7]

- affection (acceptance for what they are, not for what they might have been)
- security (freedom from fighting parents, child abuse and sibling problems)
- consistent discipline
- stable figures to act as role models (parents are their heroes)
- freedom to develop a personality without emotional entanglements
- play (a need to be active and creative)
- honesty

Parents with their own problems and conflicts will have difficulty meeting the needs of their children. Family tensions, financial problems, marital disharmony, separation and divorce have a major effect on children. Parent frustration may eventuate in child abuse. Depressive illness in a parent can have a profound effect on the child.

The child's reaction to the family disharmony may manifest in three ways (with significant overlap):[7]

- behavioural problems
- psychosomatic symptoms
- school difficulties

The importance of the family doctor

The family doctor is in an important position to detect disharmony in the family through presenting problems that give subtle clues; for example, several uncharacteristic visits from parent and child, inappropriate non-verbal behaviour such as a trembling hand or voice, or somatic symptoms incompatible with physical findings.

It is important to consider the environment of the disturbed child. Search for a possible source of disturbances at home such as parental quarrelling, economic hardship, drug abuse including alcohol, physical or sexual abuse and maternal depression. If detected and addressed, the family dysfunction may be resolved satisfactorily.

Personal health record

Many family practices issue a personal health record to the child's parents as a means of improving health care delivery, including the enhancement of preventive care. The personal health record (PHR), also referred to as the 'parent-held health record' or 'health passport', is distributed in several states and research has shown it to be well received by both health practitioners and parents.[8]

The PHR is a small, loose-leaf booklet with a sturdy plastic cover which can be easily carried around by the parent. The contents can vary from one producer to another but generally it contains:

- records of birth details and newborn examination
- percentile charts for weight gain
- visual check
- hearing check
- developmental check
- immunisation schedules and recordings (Table 72.3)
- progress notes
- advice on accident prevention (Table 72.4)
- other health educational material

The PHR provides a very practical method of promoting communication between various

Table 72.3 *Typical page in the personal health record*

IMMUNISATION RECORD—to be completed by doctor/nurse giving immunisation

Age	Immunisations	Date given	Batch no.	Date next dose	Signature/stamp/notes
Birth					
2 months					
4 months					
6 months					
12 months					
18 months					
Preschool (4–5 years)					
Prior to leaving school (15–19 years)					

Table 72.4 *Accidents don't have to happen*

Six to eighteen months

- Have cupboards made child-resistant for the storage of medicinals and household chemicals. Pesticides and petroleum products should be locked away in the shed. Don't store in ordinary food and drink containers.
- Fires and radiators should be adequately guarded.
- Cords on electrical food and drink heaters need to be shortened or hooked up out of a toddler's reach. Do not use tablecloths. Put hot food and drinks into the centre of the table. Take care with buckets of hot water.
- Fit dummy plugs in unused power points.
- From 9 kg (20 lb) body weight, baby's car rides should be in an ASA approved child seat.
- Supervise your toddler at all times in or near water. The swimming pool needs to be adequately fenced.
- Keep matches in the child-resistant cupboard in the kitchen. Put scissors, needles and pins well out of reach.
- Have the play yard safely fenced from the street.
- Parents: Walk right round the car before reversing down the drive, or place your child in the car first.
- Do not allow your small child to be unsupervised in the bathroom.
- Never give the child nuts to eat because it cannot chew them properly. Peanuts present a particular hazard because of their shape and hardness. They can cause the child to choke.

health professionals involved in the child's care and also between the family and their doctor. It promotes the concept of 'self-care' by encouraging a sense of responsibility by parents for the child's health and is also a medium for enhancing preventive care, especially with immunisation, hearing tests and development.[8]

References

1. Robinson MJ. *Practical paediatrics* (2nd edn). Melbourne: Churchill Livingstone, 1990, 61–70.

2. Jarman FC, Oberklaid F. The detection of developmental problems in children. Aust Fam Physician, 1992; 21:1079–1088.

3. Hutchins P. The young child with developmental problems. Australian Dr Weekly: How to treat series, 20 July 1990, i–viii.

4. Trollor J. Distracting children. Aust Fam Physician, 1987; 16:1372.

5. Malcher G. Spatula sketches for children. Aust Fam Physician, 1990; 19:1441.

6. Hewson P. Recognition of serious illness in early infancy. Aust Paed Review, 1992, No.2(6): 1.

7. Connell HM. The child as a barometer of the family. Aust Fam Physician, 1980; 9:759–763.

8. Jeffs D, Harris M. The personal health record—making it work better for general practitioners. Aust Fam Physician, 1993; 22:1417–1427.

73
Specific problems of children

—

Children are not simply micro-adults, but have their own specific problems.

Bela Schick (1877–1967)

The family doctor usually treats children for common minor complaints such as skin disorders and respiratory infections, and for preventive measures such as immunisation. However, in many instances, parents consult their doctor for advice on normal or abnormal behavioural disorders so doctors need to be well versed in normal behaviour in order to provide appropriate advice and reassurance. Many of these everyday problems are discussed in this chapter. Childhood management of problems such as constipation, anaemia, diarrhoea and cough are included in the relevant chapter on problem solving.

Crying and fussing in infants

Crying and fussing is a common problem in the first 3 months but is now considered to be a normal physiological aspect of a maturing central nervous system.[1]

Crying is excessive if it lasts for long periods when the baby should be sleeping or playing. It usually occurs 6–9 p.m. In most instances an organic cause such as infection, milk allergy or reflux cannot be demonstrated.

Parents should be made aware of a checklist of common causes:

- hunger (underfeeding is the main feeding problem causing crying)
- wet or soiled nappy
- loneliness: crying usually ceases when the baby is picked up

- infant colic: a possibility at 2–16 weeks
- individual temperament
- teething (more likely to cause discomfort after 12 months)

Management
- Perform careful physical examination including assessment of child's temperament.
- Give parental reassurance and education.
- Reassure parents that extra attention will not affect the baby but overstimulation should be avoided.
- Provide soothing alternatives, e.g. use of dummy (pacifier); extra cuddling and carrying; gentle massage.

Diet and medications do not have a significant place in management.

Infantile colic
Refer to page 254.

Typical features
- baby 2–16 weeks old, esp. 10 weeks
- prolonged crying—at least 3 hours
- crying during late afternoon and early evening
- child flexing legs and clenching fists because of the 'stomach ache'

Management
- Reassurance and explanation to the parents
- Pacifying methods

Medication
Avoid medications if possible, but consider:
   simethicone preparations, e.g. Infacol wind drops

                                    or

   dicyclomine syrup

747

Teething

Baby teeth (milk or deciduous teeth)

- Babies usually cut their teeth from age 6 months until 2–3 years.
- The first teeth to appear (which seldom cause discomfort) are the lower incisors (during first year).
- The first and second molars (ages 1–3) tend to cause problems.
- Usually the first set (20 teeth) is complete soon after the second birthday (Fig. 73.1)

Symptoms

- The gum is slightly swollen and red.
- This may cause little or no discomfort but may be quite painful.
- The child is more clinging, fretful and dribbling than usual.
- Chews on something such as fingers.
- Irritability and crying (on and off for no more than a few days).
- Difficulty with sleeping.

Note: Teething does not cause fever.

Treatment

Reassure the parents that the problem will soon settle.

Soothing methods

- Gentle massaging of the gum with the parent's forefinger wrapped in a soft cloth or gauze pad is comforting. A gel such as Oro-Sed can be massaged into the gums every 3 hours if extremely troublesome.

or

- Allow the baby to chew on a clean, cold, lightly moistened facewasher (a piece of apple can be placed inside the facewasher).

or

- Give the baby a teething ring (kept cold in the refrigerator) or a teething biscuit.

Medication

Medicine is usually not necessary for teething. Paracetamol mixture should be used for any discomfort. For more severe problems, especially affecting sleep, an antihistamine can be given at night or a combined mixture of antihistamine and analgesic.

Pitted dark teeth

Some children who are breast-fed for long periods (e.g. 3 years) may develop unsightly pitting of the front surface of their teeth. This will not go away but parents should be reassured that the adult teeth will be normal when they appear.

Thumb sucking

Thumb sucking involves placing the thumb or finger on the roof of the mouth behind the teeth (hard palate) and sucking with the mouth closed. It is basically a habit and should be regarded as normal. It is one of the first pleasurable acts that the infant can manage. It occurs in children up to the age of 12 years but is most common under the age of 4 years. It usually settles by age 6 or 7. If it persists beyond this age it can cause problems with the permanent teeth which begin to appear at about age 7. One effect

Fig. 73.1 *The lower set of primary teeth with average times of eruption*

is that the pressure on the front teeth may cause protrusion of these teeth, i.e. buck teeth.

Prevention
Provide alternative comfort measures such as a dummy (pacifier) if the habit is developing. If it persists, avoid making an issue and drawing attention to it.

Treatment (advice to parents)
- No special diet or medication is necessary.
- For a child over 6 years, carefully observe trigger factors and find ways of avoiding them. Provide extra attention and organise pleasant distractions.
- Help the child explore other solutions.
- Give praise and rewards for efforts to stop.

Referral for specialised treatment may be necessary for a persistent problem.

Snuffling infant
Snuffling in infants is usually caused by rhinitis due to an intercurrent viral infection. The presence of yellow or green mucus should not usually be cause for concern.

Treatment
Reassure the parents.
- Paracetamol mixture or drops for significant discomfort.
- Get the parents to perform nasal toilet with a salt solution (one teaspoon of salt dissolved in some boiled water); using a cotton bud, gently clear out nasal secretions every 2 waking hours.
- Once the nose is clean, saline nose drops or spray (e.g. Narium nasal mist) can be instilled.
- Stronger decongestant preparations are not advised unless the obstruction is causing a significant feeding problem when they can be used for up to 4–5 days.

Enuresis
Enuresis can be defined as daytime wetting (diurnal enuresis) after age 4 years or night-time wetting (nocturnal enuresis) after 6 years.[2] These are primary enureses and appear to be due to delayed maturation of achieving bladder continence. Secondary enuresis is wetting after normal continence of at least 3 months.

Nocturnal enuresis
Nocturnal enuresis refers to the involuntary passage of urine during sleep in the absence of any identified physical abnormality in children (or adults) at a time when control of urine could reasonably be expected (usually the age of 5).

What is normal?
Bed-wetting at night is common in children up to the age of 5. About 50% of 3 year olds wet the bed, as do 20% of 4 year olds and 15% of 5 year olds. It is considered a problem if regular bed-wetting occurs in children 6 years and older, although many boys do not become dry until about 8 years. About 2% of 14 year olds are affected.[3] Of children with diurnal enuresis, 60% also have nocturnal enuresis while only 10% with nocturnal enuresis also have diurnal enuresis.

Aetiology
There is usually no obvious cause and most of the children affected are normal in every respect but seem to have a delay in development of bladder control. Others may have a small bladder capacity or a sensitive bladder. It tends to be more common in boys and has a genetic predisposition. The cause of secondary enuresis can be psychological; it commonly occurs during a period of stress or anxiety, such as separation from a parent or the arrival of a new baby.

Underlying disorders to be excluded:
- urinary tract infection
- diabetes mellitus
- diabetes insipidus
- neurogenic bladder
- urinary tract abnormality

After the age of 6, investigations including an intravenous urogram or ultrasound are necessary to exclude urinary tract abnormalities.

Advice for parents on managing the child
If no cause is found, reassure the child that there is nothing wrong and that it is a common problem that will eventually go away (spontaneous resolution rate is 15% per year). There are some important ways of helping the child to adjust to the problem.
- Do not scold or punish the child.
- Praise the child often, when appropriate.
- Do not stop the child drinking after the evening meal.
- Do not wake the child at night to visit the toilet.
- Use a night-light to help the child who wakes.

Some parents use a nappy to keep the bed dry, but special absorbent pads beneath the bottom sheet are more appropriate. Make sure the child has a shower or bath before going to kindergarten or school.

Treatment

Many methods have been tried, but the bed-wetting alarm system is generally regarded to be the most effective. If the child has emotional problems, counselling or hypnotherapy may be desirable. Tricyclic antidepressants can be used and may be effective in some children, but they do not always achieve a long-term cure and have limitations. Enuresis clinics currently favour two trials of the alarm system and, if persistent, desmopressin acetate nasal spray.

The bed alarm. There are various types of alarms: some use pads in the pyjama pants and under the bottom sheet, but recently developed alarms use a small bakelite chip, which is attached to the child's briefs by a safety pin. A lead connects to the buzzer outside the bed, which makes a loud noise when urine is passed. The child wakes, switches off the buzzer and visits the toilet. This method works especially well in older children.

Tricyclic antidepressants. The most widely used drug is imipramine in doses of 1–2.5 mg/kg as a single night-time dose.[2]

Desmopressin acetate. This is the treatment of choice after failed trial of bed alarm. The dose is one spray to the lower part of each nostril per night. Avoid water loading before bed.

The persistent problem. For the 1–2% of patients whose bed-wetting persists beyond adolescence, a formal urodynamic assessment is advisable. Many of these patients also have daytime symptoms.

Diurnal enuresis

Suggested management program[2]

- Urinary containment exercises: visit toilet upon urge but sit and hold urine stream for 1 minute. Then stop and start urine flow on three occasions before emptying bladder.
- Structural toilet program: the child sits on the toilet and urinates at scheduled intervals during the day irrespective of urge. Start at 1 hour intervals increasing to 2–3 hours as control is obtained.
- Medication: useful short-term drugs include the anticholinergics—oxybutynin, imipramine.

Secondary enuresis

Secondary enuresis can develop at any age and should always be fully investigated. It is often caused by urinary infection, especially in the elderly, and may be associated with some neurological disorders and chronic retention of urine associated with prostatic enlargement. Treatment is directed at the cause, which may be a psychologically traumatic event.

Encopresis

Encopresis is the involuntary passage of formed or semi-formed stools into underwear, occurring repeatedly for at least one month in children over 4 years.

Features

- incidence 1–2 per 100 children
- more prevalent in boys 3:1
- inadequate toileting
- poor diet
- faecal retention (in most)
- rectal dilatation and insensitive urge to stool
- unawareness of passage of stools
- enuresis common

The key feature is significant chronic faecal retention leading to rectal dilatation and insensitivity to normal defecation reflex.

Assessment

- history
- examination
- abdominal X-ray (serves as base-line)

Management

A structured toileting program is the basis of management and the initial task is to empty the bowel of faeces.

The majority are cured with the following:

- ongoing interest and support (critical)
- education and counselling
- a good normal diet, adequate fluids and exercises
- structured toileting program, e.g. regular sitting on toilet for at least 10 minutes, 3 times per day after each meal
- laxative medication
  - e.g. 3 day cycle: repeated 3–4 times after initial cleanout[4]
    Day 1. Microlax enema
    Day 2. Durolax rectal suppository

Day 3. Oral bowel stimulant, e.g. Senokot (1–2 doses)

Then lubricant or softener, e.g. paraffin oil preparation

- encourage keeping a star chart diary of sitting on toilet and successful results
- regular follow-up with encouragement (maintain program for at least 6 months)
- consider encopresis clinic if problematic

Once the colon and rectum are emptied and of normal size, the frequency of accidents and soiling usually decreases gradually.

Common skin problems[5,6]

Many of the common problems (e.g. acne, psoriasis, atopic dermatitis) are covered in more detail in Chapter 101. The following are disorders of the neonatal period and early infancy.

Toxic erythema of newborn

This is a self-limiting benign condition with onset usually 24–48 hours after birth (up to 14 days). Erythematous macules mainly on face and trunk. Resolves spontaneously in a few days.

Transient neonatal pustular dermatosis

This is a blistering eruption with pustules presenting at birth or in the first few hours of life. Occurs mainly on the trunk and buttocks. No treatment is required.

Naevus flammeus

Dilated capillaries form on the face and eyelids (about 50% of babies) and nape of neck (almost 100%). Fades over 6–12 months.

Sebaceous hyperplasia

Hyperplastic sebaceous glands appear as tiny yellow-white papules on the nose, especially at the tip. Disappear in several weeks.

Milia

Blocked sebaceous glands, especially on the face, are present in 50% of neonates. The firm white papules are about 1–2 mm in diameter and differ from the yellowish papules of sebaceous hyperplasia. Also disappear after several weeks.

Miliaria

This is related to overheating and appears as two types:

- 'crystallina'—beads of sweat trapped under the epidermis, mainly on the forehead
- 'rubia' or 'heat rash'—mainly on forehead, scalp, face and trunk

It is a benign condition that disappears after a few weeks.

If problematic:

- keep skin dry and cool, e.g. fan, air conditioner
- dress in loose-fitting cotton clothing
- reduce activity
- avoid frequent bathing and overuse of soap
- Rx: salicyclic acid 2%, menthol 1%, chlorhexidine 0.5% in alcohol
- prevention: Ego Prickly Heat Powder

Sucking blisters

These are common on upper lip. Reassure that these will settle.

Umbilical granuloma

Gently apply a caustic pencil daily for about 5 days.

Breast hyperplasia

A breast 'bud' is common in most term babies and may enlarge with breast-feeding. Milk may discharge from some ('witches milk') but reassurance is all that is required.

Childhood skin problems (treatment regimens)

Atopic dermatitis (eczema)

Mild atopic dermatitis

- soap substitutes, such as aqueous cream
- emollients—choose from
  — aqueous cream
  — sorbolene with 10% glycerol
  — bath oils, e.g. Alpha-Keri
- 1% hydrocortisone (if not responding to above)

Moderate atopic dermatitis

- as for mild
- topical corticosteroids (twice daily)
  — vital for active areas
  — moderate strength, e.g. fluorinated, to trunk and limbs
  — weaker strength, e.g. 1% hydrocortisone, to face and flexures
- oral antihistamines at night for itch

Severe dermatitis
- as for mild and moderate eczema
- potent topical corticosteroids to worse areas (consider occlusive dressings)
- consider hospitalisation
- systemic corticosteroids (rarely used)

Chronic dermatitis (on limbs)
- zinc and tar combinations
- corticosteroids (short course)

Pityriasis alba
- These are white patches on the face of children and adolescents.
- Can occur on the neck and upper limbs, occasionally on trunk.
- Full repigmentation occurs eventually.

Treatment
- reassurance
- simple emollients
- restrict use of soap and washing
- may prescribe hydrocortisone ointment (rarely necessary)

Seborrhoeic dermatitis
Medication: children
Scalp
- 1% sulphur and 1% salicylic acid in sorbolene cream.
- Apply overnight to scalp, shampoo off next day with a mild shampoo.
- Use 3 times a week.

Face, flexures and trunk
- 2% sulphur and salicylic acid in aqueous or sorbolene cream
- hydrocortisone 1% (for irritation on face and flexures)
- betamethasone 0.02 – 0.05% (if severe irritation on trunk)

Napkin area
- Mix equal parts 1% hydrocortisone with nystatin or ketoconazole 2% cream

Napkin rash
Irritant dermatitis (commonest cause)
- Keep the area dry.
- Change wet or soiled napkins often—disposable ones are good.
- Wash gently and pat dry (do not rub).

- Avoid excessive bathing and soap.
- Avoid powders and plastic pants.
- Use emollients to keep skin lubricated, e.g. zinc oxide and castor oil cream.

If:

Atopic dermatitis	1% hydrocortisone
Seborrhoeic dermatitis	1% hydrocortisone and ketoconazole ointment
Candida albicans	topical nystatin at each nappy change
Widespread nappy rash	1% hydrocortisone and nystatin ointment or clotrimazole cream (qid after changes)

Impetigo
- Remove crusts with gentle washing (antibacterial soap and water).
- If mild and limited: antiseptic cleaning with chlorhexidine or povidone-iodine; then mupirocin (Bactroban) tds for 10 days (avoid around mouth).
- If extensive: oral cephalexin or flucloxacillin or erythromycin for 10 days.

Head lice
Pyrethrins/piperonyl butoxide (Lyban) foam or shampoo
- massage well into wet hair
- leave at least 10 minutes but preferably overnight
- wash off thoroughly
- comb with a fine-toothed comb
- repeat after 7 days
- treat all household contacts

Scabies
Permethrin 5% cream (preferable)
- apply to whole body from jawline down
- leave overnight, then wash off
- single application

or

benzyl benzoate 25% emulsion (dilute with water if under 10 years)
Use either for all ages except children under 2 months.

Tinea capitis
Griseofulvin   10 mg/kg/day (max. 250 mg)
4–6 week course or until non-fluorescent
Take hair plucking and scale for culture.

Papular urticaria (hives)
- Prevent bites by using insecticide sprays and repellents, and treating pets.
- Lukewarm baths with Pinetarsol or similar soothing bath oil.
- Topical Liquor Picis Carb 2% in calamine lotion or 0.5% hydrocortisone—apply every 4 hours for itching.
- Antihistamine, e.g. cyproheptadine, promethazine.

Henoch-Schönlein purpura
- Characteristic rash over buttocks and back of legs.
- Prognosis is generally excellent.
- Consider analgesia (paracetamol), bed rest and crutches if symptoms a problem.
- No specific therapy; follow-up required.

Molluscum contagiosum
There are many methods but aim to provoke an immune response by applying benzyl peroxide 2.5% gel/ointment and then hypoallergenic sticking paper (Micropore) cover on a daily basis.

Warts
Spontaneous resolution may occur so avoid invasive treatment including painful procedures. Do not freeze warts in children under 10 years old.[6]

If problematic and causing embarrassment, use a simple method, e.g.

Common warts	pare every 2–3 days; apply a keratolytic agent with salicylic and lactic acid, e.g. Dermatech Wart Treatment, daily
Plane warts	treat as for common warts but beware of facial lesions
Plantar warts	pare, then apply one of the preparations on pages 655–656

Neonatal leg and foot abnormalities
Developmental dysplasia of hip (congenital dislocation of hip)
- Detected by clinical examination (Ortolani and Barlow tests) and ultrasound examination (see pages 601–602).
- Most cases are treated successfully by abduction bracing with a Pavlik harness.
- Open reduction may be required.

Bow legs (genu varum)
- Most are physiological (which are symmetrical) and improve with age.
- Toddlers are usually bow-legged until 3 years of age.
- Monitor intercondyler separation (ICS): distance between medial femoral condyles.
- Refer when ICS > 6 cm, not improving or asymmetric (Fig. 73.2).

Knock knees (genu valgum)
- Most are physiological and children are usually knock-kneed from 3–8 years.
- Monitor intermalleolar separation (IMS): distance between medial malleoli.
- Refer if IMS > 8 cm (Fig. 73.2).

In-toeing
Causes of in-toeing (Fig. 73.3) are metatarsus varus, internal tibial torsion and medial femoral torsion. These features are compared in Table 73.1.[7]

Out-toeing
Infants
- have restricted internal rotation of hip due to an external rotation contracture
- exhibit a 'Charlie Chaplin' posture between 3 and 12 months
- child weight bears and walks normally
- no treatment required as spontaneous resolution occurs

Surgery may be necessary in older children.

Fig. 73.2 *Postural variance of lower limbs* REPRINTED FROM D. EFRON, *PAEDIATRIC HANDBOOK*, BLACKWELL SCIENCE, MELBOURNE, 1996, WITH PERMISSION

Fig. 73.3 *Causes of in-toeing*   REPRINTED FROM D. EFRON, *PAEDIATRIC HANDBOOK*, BLACKWELL SCIENCE, MELBOURNE, 1996, WITH PERMISSION

Club foot (congenital talipes equinovarus)

Most abnormal-looking feet in infants are not a true club foot deformity; the majority have postural problems such as talipes calcaneovalgus, metatarsus varus and postural talipes equinovarus. Such conditions are usually quite mobile and mild, and all resolve spontaneously without treatment. True club foot deformity is usually stiff and severe, and requires orthopaedic correction.[7]

Flat feet (pes plano valgus)

The majority are physiological. All newborns have flat feet but 80% develop a medial arch by their sixth birthday.[7] No treatment is required unless painful and stiff.

Developmental disability and delay

The family doctor is in an ideal position to recognise and initiate evaluation of the child with a developmental disability, whether it is a physical disability or delay, an intellectual disability or a learning disability.

Many developmental problems will be obvious but others, such as Fragile X syndrome, are subtle. Several disabilities may evade a diagnosis. Success depends on the ability of the family doctor, early referral and the level of sophistication of genetic services.

Transient developmental delay may be associated with factors such as prematurity, family stress, physical illness and learning opportunities while persistent delay can be caused by intellectual disability, cerebral palsy, autism, and hearing and visual impairment.

There are many rare dysmorphic syndromes which are becoming more recognised and referral to genetic disorder units will help in appropriate evaluation.

Evaluation

An appropriate history includes a careful look at developmental milestones and family history.

Table 73.1 *In-toeing in childhood*[7]

	Metatarsus varus	Internal tibial torsion	Medial femoral torsion
Synonyms	Metatarsus adductus		Inset hips
Age at presentation	Birth	Toddler	Child
Site of problem	Foot	Tibia	Femur
Examination	Sole of foot bean-shaped	Thigh–foot angle is inwards	Arc of hip rotation favours internal rotation
Management	Observe or cast	Observe and measure	Observe, rarely surgery
When to refer if not resolved	3 months after presentation	6 months after presentation	8 years after presentation

Reprinted from D. Efron *Paediatric Handbook*[2] with permission from Blackwell Science

The physical examination includes testing of hearing and vision.

Investigations to consider:

- screen for congenital infection, e.g. rubella, toxoplasmosis, cytomegalovirus
- chromosome (karyotyping) studies
- urinary metabolic screen, e.g. PKU
- creatinine phosphokinase in males
- thyroid function studies
- DNA specific tests, e.g. Fragile X, Prader-Willi, Williams syndrome
- CT scan or MRI

Intellectual disability

This is regarded as a component of developmental disability and refers to significant substandard intellectual functioning (2 SD's < mean IQ) with deficits in adaptive behaviour and manifested during the development period. Presentation includes learning difficulties, language delay and behavioural problems.

The two most common causes are trisomy 21 and Fragile X.

Cerebral palsy

Definition

A persistent motor disorder of movement and posture resulting from prenatal developmental abnormalities or perinatal or postnatal CNS damage (to the immature brain).

Facts

- Cerebral palsy is not a diagnosis but a diverse group of disorders.
- In most cases the cause is unknown.
- Fewer than 1 in 10 cases result from hypoxia.
- Prevalence is about 2 per 1000 live births.

Classification of syndrome

- the type of motor disorder, e.g. spasticity (70% of cases), athetosis, mixed
- the distribution, e.g. hemiplegia, paraplegia, diplegia
- the severity of the motor disorder

Associated disorders

- seizures (30% of cases)
- visual problems, e.g. strabismus
- hearing defects
- intellectual disability
- perceptual problems

Management

- accurate diagnosis
- genetic counselling

- assessment of child's capabilities
- referral to several agencies for assessment e.g. hearing, vision, dietitian, speech pathologist, various other allied health professionals
- monitor problematic areas, e.g. constipation
- orthopaedic assessment with special attention to legs, e.g. hips, knees, hamstrings

Down syndrome

Down syndrome (Trisomy 21) is based on typical facial features (flat facies, slanting eyes, epicanthic folds, small ears), hypotonia and single palmar crease.

Facts

- 95% have extra chromosome of maternal origin (Trisomy 21)
- remainder due to either unbalanced translocations or mosaicism
- prenatal diagnostic tests include the triple test in first trimester and karyotyping

Associated disorders

- seizures (usually later onset)
- impaired hearing
- leukaemia
- hypothyroidism
- congenital anomalies, e.g. heart, duodenal atresia, Hirschsprung's, TOF
- Alzheimer-like dementia (4–5th decade)
- prevalence 1:650 live births

Management

- Assess child's capabilities.
- Refer to agencies for assessment, e.g. hearing, vision, developmental disability unit.
- Advise on sexuality, especially for females, i.e. menstrual management, contraception, as fertility must be presumed.

Fragile X syndrome (FXS)

FXS presents as a classical physical phenotype with large prominent ears, long narrow face, macro-orchidism and intellectual disability. It is the most common inherited cause known of developmental disability and should always be considered. The cause is the result of an increase in size of a trinuclotide repeat in the FMR-I gene on the X chromosome (the number of sequences determines carrier or full mutant status).

Facts[8]

- M:F ratio 2:1
- prevalence 1:1000–4000

- variable spectrum of characteristic features, making detection difficult in some cases
- up to 1/300 females may be carriers
- family history of intellectual disability
- affects all ethnic groups

Diagnosis
- cytogenetic test (karyotyping)
- DNA test (specific for full mutation as well as carriers)

Associated disorders
- intellectual disability (IQ < 70)
- autism or autistic-like behaviour
- attention deficit in 10% (with or without hyperactivity)
- seizures (20%)
- connective tissue abnormalities
- learning disability and speech delay
- co-ordination difficulty

Management
- careful genetic appraisal and counselling
- assessment of child's capabilities
- multidisciplinary assessment including developmental disability unit
- referral for integration of speech and language therapy, special education, behaviour management
- pharmacological treatment of any epilepsy, or attention or mood behaviour disorders
- medications may determine whether the child remains in the community or not[8]

Prader-Willi syndrome
This uncommon disorder (1 in 10 000 to 15 000) has classical features, especially a bizarre appetite and eating habits, of which the GP should be aware. The most common cause is deletion of the short arm of chromosome 15.

The features are:
- hypotonic infants with failure to thrive, then
- voracious appetite causing morbid obesity
- mental retardation
- narrow forehead and turned-down mouth
- small hands and feet
- hypogonadism

Management
- early diagnosis and referral
- multidisciplinary approach
- expert dietetic control

Williams syndrome
Williams syndrome[9] (idiopathic hypercalcaemia or elfin face syndrome) is of unknown cause.

The children have a distinctive elfin facial appearance, mild pre- and post-natal growth retardation, mild microcephaly and mild to moderate developmental delay. In the first 2 years of life feeding problems, vomiting, irritability, hyperacusis, constipation and failure to thrive may lead to presentation, but the children are rarely diagnosed at this stage.

Specific learning disabilities
A specific learning disability is an unexpected and unexplained condition, occurring in a child of average or above intelligence, with a significant delay in one or more areas of learning. These areas include reading, spelling, writing, arithmetic, language (comprehension and expression), attention and organisation, co-ordination and social and emotional development. An SLD can vary from very mild to quite severe. It may, in turn, cause a general learning disability. The primary cause is unknown.

Diagnosis
If undetected by parents, any undisclosed SLD will soon be detected in the classroom. Sometimes the disability is not detected until later (8 years or more) when more demanding schoolwork is required. Speech delays, reading difficulties and calculation problems are among the first signs. It is important to check hearing and vision. These children may also present with a behaviour disorder as they are often subject to ridicule by other children and tend to develop a poor self-image and low self-esteem.

Dyslexia

The word 'dyslexia' is derived from the Greek term meaning 'difficulty with words'. The condition was originally called 'word blindness', referring to a specific learning difficulty with reading. Dyslexic children have a normal IQ and no physical problems, but their reading skills are below average. Other SLDs may also be present, particularly in spelling, writing and clear speaking.

The two main features are reading and spelling difficulties because dyslexic children confuse certain letters whose shape is similar, perhaps a mirror image of each other, e.g. confusing *b* with *d* and *p* with *q*. This means that affected children cannot properly use and interpret the knowledge they have acquired.

Characteristics include:

- a reluctance to read aloud

- a monotonous voice when reading
- following the text with the finger when reading
- difficulty repeating long words

These features, of course, are seen in all or most learners but, if they persist in a bright child, dyslexia should be considered. The most important factor in management is to recognise the problem and the earlier the better.

Management of specific learning disabilities

It is important to build the child's self-esteem by explaining the problem carefully, removing any sense of self-blame and encouraging efforts towards progress. Parents can play an important role in building up their child's self-esteem and in helping learning. Parents are the most important teachers.

Children with SLDs are usually referred to an experienced professional or to a clinic (e.g. a dyslexia clinic) for assessment. Management may involve a clinical psychologist, an audiologist, an optometrist or a speech pathologist. A specific method of correcting the problem and promoting learning will be devised. It is also worthwhile seeking the help of a support organisation.

Lead poisoning[10]

It is important to keep in mind that young children are susceptible to lead poisoning. They are more likely than adults to be exposed to lead because of their exploratory behaviour and they absorb more of any ingested dose. The most common source seen in general practice is home renovation involving paint removal in houses built before the 1960s or 1970s.

Children with mild to moderate lead exposure (< 2.17 mmol/L) are usually asymptomatic. When symptoms appear, they are usually non-specific and may include lethargy, intermittent abdominal pain, irritability, headache, abnormal behaviour and encephalopathy. Toxicity may be a cause of unexplained iron deficiency anaemia.

An important feature is that lead poisoning may present insidiously in children with developmental delay, learning difficulties, hyperactivity or other behaviour problems. However, it is a relatively uncommon cause. It is interesting that the Centers for Disease Control in the United States have recommended that all children between 6 months and 6 years of age should be screened with a blood lead measurement.[11]

The following children are at risk of elevated blood lead levels:
- those aged 9–48 months living in, or visiting, older dilapidated houses with peeling paint or such houses undergoing renovation
- those with pica
- those living near lead-contaminated areas such as lead smelters, battery-breaking yards or heavy traffic areas.

High blood lead levels should be considered in the presence of unexplained iron deficiency anaemia.

The treatment of toxicity involves administration of sodium calcium edatate (calcium disodium versenate) or dimercaprol in hospital. The new oral preparation, succimer, is likely to become the drug of choice for less severe degrees of poisoning.

References

1. Oberklaid F. Crying and fussing in infancy. Aust Paed Review, 1995, 5(4):1–2.
2. Jarman F. Common developmental and behavioural problems. In: Efron D, *Paediatric handbook* (5th edn). Melbourne: Blackwell Science, 1996, 183–297.
3. Walsh D. *Symptom control*. Boston: Blackwell Science, 1989, 229–233.
4. Jarman F. Encopresis. Aust Paed Review, 1993, 3(2):1–2.
5. Rogers M. Benign skin conditions of the neonatal period and early infancy. Aust Paed Review, 1994, 4(1):1–3.
6. Varigos G, Phillips R. Dermatologic conditions. In: Efron D, *Paediatric handbook* (5th edn). Melbourne: Blackwell Science, 1996, 113.
7. Kerr G, Barnett P. Orthopaedic conditions. In Efron D, *Paediatric handbook* (5th edn). Melbourne: Blackwell Science, 1996, 237–246.
8. Cohen J. Fragile X syndrome. Course notes. Monash University Update Course for General Practitioners. 1996: 31.
9. Bankier A. Williams syndrome. Syndrome Quiz. Aust Fam Physician, 1990; 19:1758.
10. Campbell B. Lead poisoning. Aust Fam Physician, 1993; 22:1139–1145.
11. Centers for Disease Control. Preventing lead poisoning in young children. Atlanta: Department of Health and Human Services, October 1991.

74

Common childhood infectious diseases (including skin eruptions)

—

The physical signs of measles are nearly the same as those of smallpox, but nausea and inflammation is more severe. The rash of measles usually appears at once, but the rash of smallpox spot after spot. . .

Avicenna (980–1037)

Children are subject to a variety of infectious diseases, mainly causing acute skin eruptions. Fortunately, many of these diseases, such as scarlet fever, measles and rubella, are being seen less frequently by the family doctor.

Reye syndrome and aspirin

The concern about the ingestion of aspirin for febrile illness in children is the suspected causal relationship between it and Reye syndrome, particularly in children with varicella and influenza infections. However, there is some controversy about the connection. Orlowski and colleagues at the Children's Hospital in Sydney found no association between aspirin use and Reye syndrome from 1973–1985.[1] It is possible that the connection is coincidental or at least confounded with other factors.

Despite these doubts, aspirin should not be recommended for the treatment of fever in young children in view of our knowledge of the beneficial effects of fever on the immune response and the availability of a safe alternative antipyretic such as paracetamol.

Reye syndrome

Clinical features:

- A rare complication of influenza, chickenpox and other viral diseases, e.g. Coxsackie virus
- Rapid development of:
  — encephalopathy ⎫ seizures
  — hepatic failure ⎬ and
  — hypoglycaemia ⎭ coma
- 30% fatality rate and significant morbidity
- Treatment is supportive and directed at cerebral oedema

Varicella (chickenpox)

Varicella, a common and highly infectious disease, affects people mainly during childhood, especially between 2 and 8 years, but no age is exempt. The characteristic crops of small vesicles have a central distribution (face, scalp and trunk). It is caused by the varicella zoster virus, one of the human herpes viruses, which remains latent after infection. Clinical reactivation later in life results in herpes zoster.

Epidemiology

Varicella has a worldwide distribution, causing endemic (occasionally epidemic) disease, with little clear evidence of seasonal incidence in temperate climates. About 75% of people in urban communities have had the infection by 15 years of age and at least 90% by young adulthood.

It is one of the most easily transmitted viruses, probably by airborne spread, usually via a person with chickenpox (occasionally with herpes zoster). Varicella is contagious only while the patient has symptoms and vesicles remain; drying of the vesicles indicates that infectivity has stopped. The scabs are not infectious.

The incubation period is 10–21 days (usually 15–16). Laboratory diagnosis is by serology[2] or immunofluorescence of vesicular fluid.

Clinical features

The clinical features of varicella are shown in Table 74.1 and the complications in Table 74.2. Children are not normally very sick but tend to be lethargic and have a mild fever. Adults have an influenza-like illness. The typical distribution is shown in Figure 74.1.

Treatment

Treatment is symptomatic and usually no specific therapy is required. Many people worry about scarring but the lesions invariably heal, leaving normal skin, unless they become infected.

Advice to parents

- The patient should rest until feeling well.
- Give paracetamol for the fever (avoid aspirin).
- Daub calamine or a similar soothing lotion to relieve itching, although the itch is usually not severe.
- Avoid scratching; clean and cut the fingernails

Table 74.1 *Clinical features in varicella*

Onset
- Children: no prodrome
- Adults: prodrome (myalgia, fever, headaches) for 2–3 days

Rash
- Centripetal distribution, including oral mucosa
- Scalp lesions can become infected
- 'Cropping' phenomenon: vesicles, papules, crusting lesions present together
- Pruritic

Degrees of severity
- Number of vesicles can vary from fewer than ten to thousands
- Mild cases can be missed
- More severe in adults, especially the immunocompromised
- Viral pneumonia rare in children, uncommon in adults
- Death rare except in the immunocompromised and neonates with congenital varicella

Table 74.2 *Complications of varicella*

Common
- Bacterial infection of cutaneous lesions (usually staphylococcal or streptococcal); can take form of cellulitis or bullous impetigo
- Can leave pitted scars

Uncommon
- Viral pneumonia
- Thrombocytopenia
- Acute cerebellitis (ataxia, normal mental state)

Rare
- Meningoencephalitis
- Purpura fulminans

of children short. Provide cotton mittens if necessary.
- Keep the diet simple. Drink ample fluids, including orange juice and lemonade.
- Daily bathing is advisable, with the addition of mild antiseptic or sodium bicarbonate if pruritic (half a cup to the bath water). Pat dry with a clean, soft towel; do not rub.

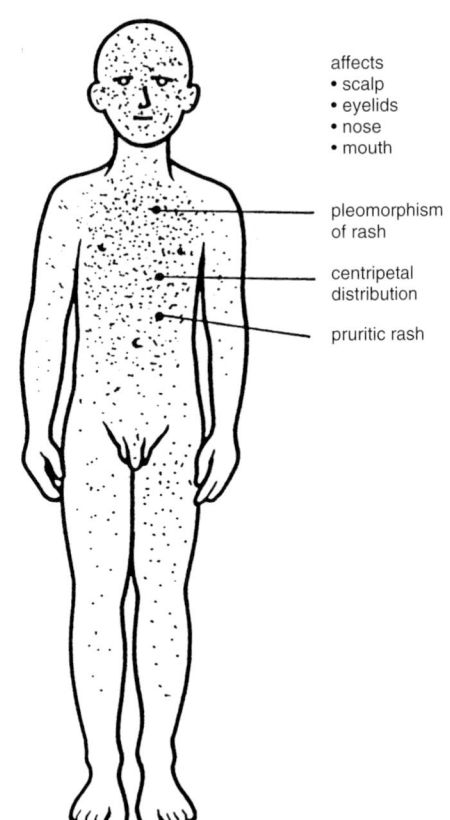

affects
- scalp
- eyelids
- nose
- mouth

pleomorphism of rash

centripetal distribution

pruritic rash

Fig. 74.1 *Chickenpox: typical distribution*

Medication

Antihistamines can be prescribed for itching. Aciclovir or similar agents can be life-saving in the immunocompromised host. Antibiotics (e.g. flucloxacillin/dicloxacillin) are reserved for bacterial skin infection.

Use of antiviral agents for varicella

The antiviral agents, aciclovir and others, have an important place in the management of severe chickenpox. Although generally used in adolescents and adults with a severe eruption or the likelihood of a severe eruption, there is no set age for the use of an antiviral agent. It should be commenced during the first 3 days of the eruption (preferably day 1) and can be introduced in a contact (often the second case in a family) experiencing a severe prodromal syndrome.

In general, it is not used in the very young, or in those with a mild/short prodrome, and in those who are not ill, do not have many spots and are not compromised.

Exclusion from school

Exclusion is recommended until full recovery, usually for 7 days. A few remaining scabs are not an indication to continue exclusion. Except for immunocompromised children, contacts should not be excluded from school.

Exclusion and incubation times are given in Table 74.3.

Prevention

Prevention in contacts who are immunocompromised, or premature infants in contact with varicella, is possible with zoster immune globulin. An attenuated live virus vaccine is now available and suitable for healthy children from the age of 9 months.

Measles

Measles (rubeola) is a highly contagious disease caused by an RNA paramyxovirus. It presents as an acute febrile exanthematous illness with characteristic lesions on the buccal mucosa called Koplik's spots (tiny white spots like grains of salt).

The disease is endemic throughout the world and complications are usually respiratory in nature. If an acute exanthematous illness is not accompanied by a dry cough and red eyes, it is unlikely to be measles. Laboratory diagnosis is by serology, nasopharyngeal aspirate immunofluorescence and culture.[2]

Epidemiology

Measles is transmitted by patient-to-patient contact through oropharyngeal and nasopharyngeal droplets expelled during coughing and sneezing.

The incubation period is 10–14 days and the patient is infectious for about 5 days, but especially just before the appearance of the rash.

Table 74.3 *Basic childhood infectious diseases: incubation periods, minimum exclusion periods from school, preschool and child care centres (times in days)*

	Incubation period (days)	Patient exclusion (least time from onset rash or symptoms) (days)	Contact exclusion (days)
Measles	10–14	5	14 in non-immunised
Mononucleosis	?30–50	Nil	Nil
Mumps	14–21	9	Nil
Pertussis	7–14	5 (after starting antibiotics)	14 in non-immunised
Parvovirus (erythema infectiosum)	4–14	Nil	Nil
Rubella	14–21	5	Nil
Varicella and zoster	10–21	7	Only those immune deficient
Hepatitis			
A	15–45	7 or recovery	Nil
B	40–180	Nil	Nil
C	14–180	Nil	Nil
Infective diarrhoea	varies	until cessation diarrhoea	Nil

Based on NHMRC recommendations

Morbidity and mortality are high in countries with substandard living conditions and poor nutrition.

Immunity appears to be lifelong after infection. Measles, like smallpox, could be eradicated with public health measures.

Clinical features

The clinical presentation can be considered in three stages.

1. *Prodromal stage.* This usually lasts 3–4 days. It is marked by fever, malaise, anorexia, diarrhoea, and 'the three Cs': cough, coryza and conjunctivitis. Sometimes a non-specific rash appears a day before the Koplik's spots (opposite the molars).
2. *Exanthema (rash) stage.* Identified by a typically blotchy, bright red maculopapular eruption; this stage lasts 4–5 days. The rash begins behind the ears and on the first day spreads to the face, the next day to the trunk and later to the limbs. It may become confluent and blanches under pressure. The patient's fever usually subsides within 5 days of the onset of the rash (Fig. 74.2).
3. *Convalescent stage.* The rash fades, leaving a temporary brownish 'staining'. The patient's cough may persist for days, but usually good health and appetite return quickly.

Complications

Respiratory

The patient could develop secondary bacterial otitis media or sinusitis. If pneumonia develops it is more likely to be bacterial superinfection than viral. Laryngotracheobronchitis (croup) is a common complication of measles.

Central nervous system

Encephalitis has an incidence of one in 1500 and although the mortality rate is low there is significant CNS morbidity. Febrile convulsions are another common complication.

Late complications

Two rare complications are bronchiectasis and subacute sclerosing panencephalitis.

Treatment

There is no specific treatment although some symptoms can be relieved, e.g. a linctus for the cough, paracetamol for fever. The patient should rest quietly, avoid bright lights and stay in bed until the fever subsides.

The management of complications is determined by their nature and severity. Children should be kept away from school until they have recovered or for at least 5 days from the onset of the rash.

Prevention

Vaccination programs have been most successful. Live attenuated measles virus vaccinations combined with mumps and rubella (MMR) are recommended at the age of 12 months and then 10–16 years. Consider normal immunoglobulin for infants less than 12 months and the immunocompromised when MMR is contraindicated, given as soon as possible after exposure.

Rubella

Rubella (German measles) is a viral exanthema caused by a togavirus. Because of immunisation programs it is seen less frequently now in family practice. It is a minor illness in children and adults, but devastating when transmitted *in utero*. Congenital rubella is still the most important cause of blindness and deafness in the neonate. It is completely preventable.

Epidemiology

Rubella has been reported from virtually every country and is endemic in heavily populated communities. Epidemics occur every 6–9 years in non-immunised populations, the disease being spread by droplets from the nose and

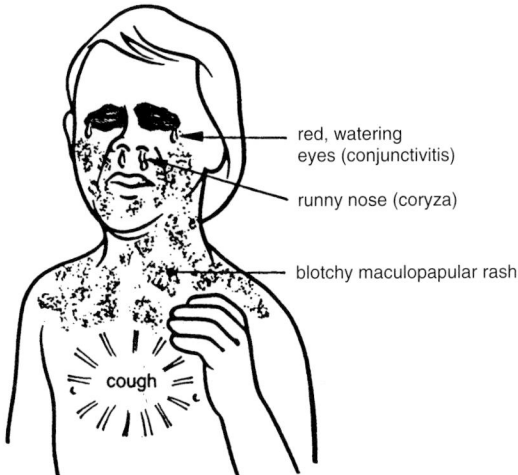

red, watering eyes (conjunctivitis)

runny nose (coryza)

blotchy maculopapular rash

cough

Fig. 74.2 *Measles: typical symptoms. Note the 3C's: cough, coryza, conjunctivitis* throat. It is not as communicable as varicella and measles. Intrauterine infection occurs via the placenta.

Approximately one-third of infections are asymptomatic (subclinical). Infection usually confers lifelong immunity. Infection is proved either by virus culture or by specific serology. Incubation period: 14–21 days.

Clinical features

The clinical features of rubella are presented in Table 74.4 and Figure 74.3 and the complications in Table 74.5.

Congenital rubella

Infection of the mother in the first trimester can lead to abortion or stillbirth, or to foetal malformation, including congenital heart disease, deafness and blindness (cataract or glaucoma). It can also produce lesions (such as microcephaly), mental retardation, retarded growth, thrombocytopenic purpura (with a 30% mortality rate), jaundice/hepatosplenomegaly and bone abnormalities.

Rubella in pregnancy

Ideally all women of child-bearing age should know their rubella immune status by having serology performed. A history of immunisation is

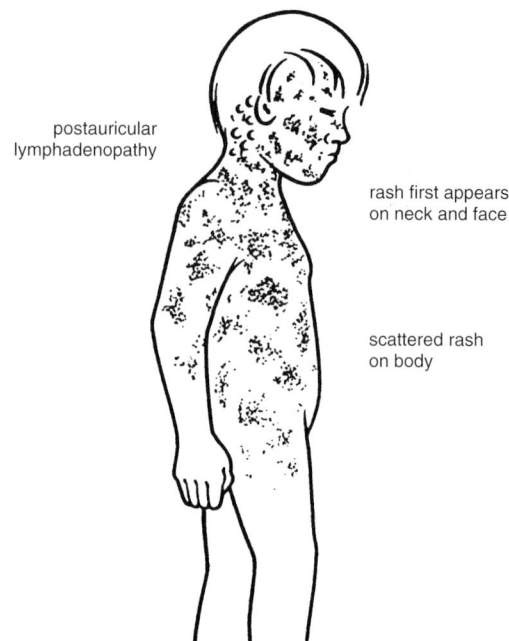

Fig. 74.3 *Rubella: typical symptoms*

[labels in figure:] postauricular lymphadenopathy; rash first appears on neck and face; scattered rash on body

not good enough evidence of immunity. However, in Victoria, Australia, almost 95% of women aged 15–40 are immune.[3]

If the immune status is not known, then serology testing should be ordered at the first antenatal visit. Rubella vaccine, while not shown to be embryopathic, should not be given during pregnancy. If maternal rubella antibodies are in adequate titre, there is no risk to the foetus from rubella infection.

Treatment

Treatment is symptomatic, especially as rubella is a mild disease. Patients should rest quietly until they feel well and take paracetamol for fever and aching joints. Prevention is by vaccine, recommended at 12 months and 10–16 years.

Table 74.4 *Clinical features of rubella*

- There is no prodrome.
- A generalised, maculopapular rash, sometimes pruritic, may be the only evidence of infection.
- Other symptoms are usually mild and short-lived.
- There is often a reddened pharynx but sore throats are unusual. An exudate may be seen as well as palatal exanthem.
- Fever is usually absent or low-grade.
- Other features: headache, myalgia, conjunctivitis and polyarthritis (small joints).
- Lymphadenopathy may be noted; usually postauricular, suboccipital and postcervical.
- The patient is infectious for up to 10 days from onset of rash (this aspect is often not appreciated as the patient is asymptomatic by that time).

The rash
- A discrete pale pink maculopapular rash (not confluent as in measles).
- Starts on the face and neck—spreads to the trunk and extremities.
- Variable severity: may be absent in subclinical infection.
- Exaggerated on skin exposed to sun.
- Brief duration—usually fades on the third day.
- No staining or desquamation.

Table 74.5 *Complications of rubella*

- Encephalitis (one in 5000)
- Polyarthritis, espcially in adult women (this complication abates spontaneously)
- Thrombocytopenia with bleeding (one in 3000)
- Congenital rubella

School exclusion

The child is usually excluded until fully recovered or for at least 5 days from the onset of the rash.

Viral exanthema (fourth disease)

This mild childhood infection may be caused by a number of viruses, especially the enteroviruses, and produces a rubella-like rash which may be misdiagnosed as rubella. The rash, which is usually non-pruritic and mainly confined to the trunk, does not desquamate and often fades within 48 hours. The child may appear quite well or can have mild constitutional symptoms including diarrhoea.

Erythema infectiosum (fifth disease)

Erythema infectiosum, also known as 'slapped face' syndrome or fifth disease, is a childhood exanthem caused by parvovirus B19. It occurs typically in young school-aged children. Incubation period is 4–14 days. The bright macular rash erupts on the face first then, after a day or so, a maculopapular rash appears on the limbs.[4] The rash lasts for only a few days but may recur for several weeks.

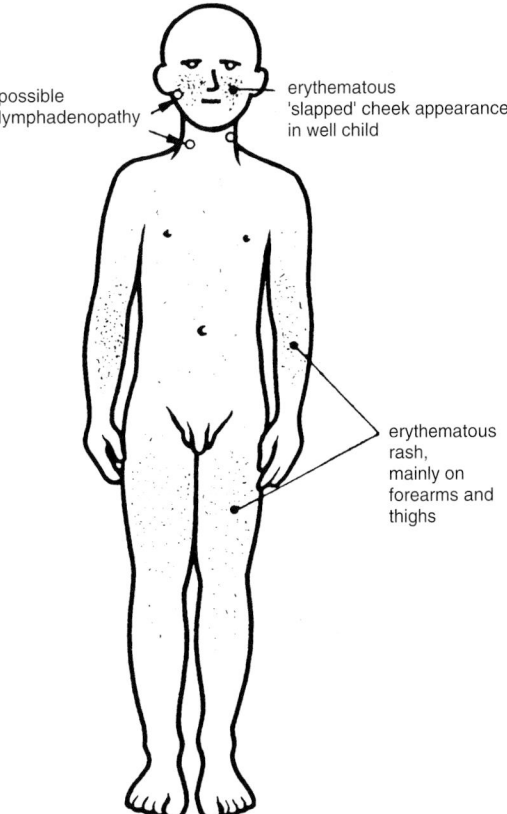

Fig. 74.4 *Erythema infectiosum: typical distribution of rash*

Clinical features

- mild fever (30%) and malaise
- possible lymphadenopathy (esp. cervical)

The rash (Fig. 74.4):

- bright red flushed cheeks with circumoral pallor for 2–3 days
- maculopapular rash on limbs (especially) and trunk (sparse)
- reticular appearance on fading
- may be pruritic

Typically, the cheeks become reddened again for the next few weeks on exposure to sunlight or wind or after a hot bath.[2] Erythema infectiosum is a mild illness but, if the parvovirus infection occurs during pregnancy, foetal complications including death *in utero* can occur.[3] Adults can be infected and the side effects, especially arthritis, can be quite severe. Diagnosis is by serology. Treatment is symptomatic.

Roseola infantum (exanthema subitum or sixth disease)

Roseola infantum is a viral infection (human herpes virus6) of infancy, affecting children at the age of 6–18 months; it is rare after this time. Constitutional symptoms are generally mild.

Clinical features

- high fever (up to 40°)
- runny nose
- temperature falls after 3 days (or so)
              then
- red macular or maculopapular rash appears

The rash:

- largely confined to trunk
- usually spares face and limbs
- appears as fever subsides
- disappears within 2 days
- no desquamation
- mild cervical lymphadenopathy

The infection runs a benign course, although a febrile convulsion can occur. Diagnosis is by serology and treatment is symptomatic.

Scarlet fever

Scarlet fever results when a Group A *Streptococcus pyogenes* organism produces erythrogenic toxin. The prodromal symptoms prior to the acute exanthem comprise about 2 days of malaise, sore throat, fever (may be rigors) and vomiting.

Features of the rash

- appears on second day of illness
- first appears on neck
- rapidly generalised
- punctuate and red
- blanches on pressure
- prominent on neck, in axillae, groin, skinfolds (Fig. 74.5)
- absent or sparse on face, palms and soles
- circumoral pallor
- feels like fine sandpaper

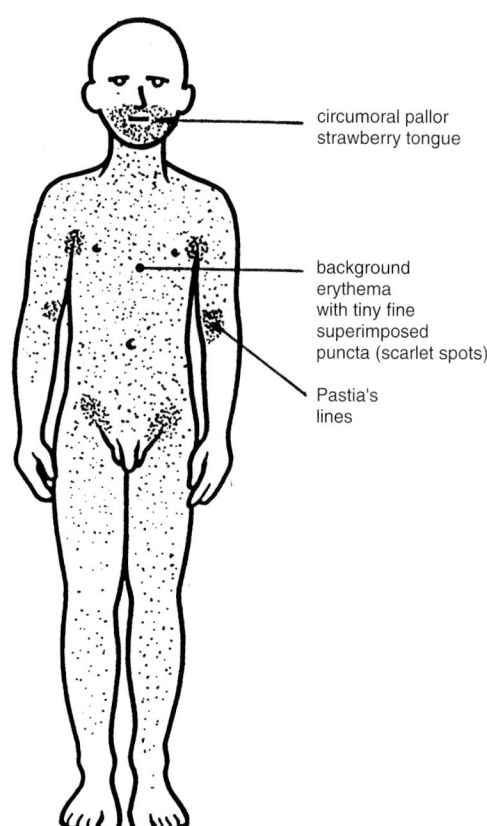

circumoral pallor
strawberry tongue

background
erythema
with tiny fine
superimposed
puncta (scarlet spots)

Pastia's
lines

Fig. 74.5 *Scarlet fever: typical presentation of rash*

- lasts about 5 days
- fine desquamation

Treatment

Phenoxymethylpenicillin (dose according to age) with rapid resolution of symptoms.

Kawasaki's disease (mucocutaneous lymph node syndrome)

This is an uncommon acute multisystemic disorder in children, characterised by an acute onset of fever of 5 days or more and accompanied by the following features:

- bilateral conjunctivitis
- maculopapular polymorphous rash
- ± cervical lymphadenopathy > 1.5 cm
- dryness, redness and cracking of the lips
- erythema of the oral cavity
- erythema of palms and soles with induration and oedema
- desquamation of fingertips (a characteristic)
- tender mass in right hypochondrium

Kawasaki's disease can be elusive as there are variations with incomplete manifestations. There is no specific test but the ESR is usually elevated.

The disease is generally benign and self-limiting but it is important to make an early diagnosis because early treatment may prevent complications. The major complication is vasculitis, which causes coronary aneurysms in 17–31% of cases, with an overall case fatality rate of 0.5–2.8%[5] due to the aneurysm that usually develops between the second week and the second month of the illness. Early treatment with immunoglobulin and aspirin has been shown to be effective in reducing the prevalence of coronary artery abnormalities. Echocardiography is indicated to detect these aneurysms and determine prognosis. Avoid corticosteroids in these patients.

Mumps (epidemic parotitis)

Mumps is an acute infectious disease caused by a paramyxovirus, with an affinity for the salivary glands and meninges. Although it most often affects children (90% present before adolescence), no one is exempt.[3]

Mumps has a worldwide prevalence. Most adults have antibodies to it, whether or not they have had the clinical infection. Because the antibody crosses the placenta in pregnancy, the infant will be immune for the first 6–9 months of life. One episode of the illness is sufficient to confer permanent immunity.

The patient is most infective during the prodrome, less so by the time the parotid glands are enlarged. Spread of infection is by aerosol droplets from the saliva and nasopharynx and can be rapid in school classrooms and throughout a household.

Mumps in a woman in early pregnancy occasionally causes abortion or foetal abnormalities.

General course and symptoms

The incubation period is 2–3 weeks.

The patient might be free of symptoms but a high fever, headache and malaise, for 5–7 days (occasionally 2–3 weeks), is usual. Involvement of the salivary glands is common. Dry mouth and discomfort on eating or opening the mouth occur.

Major manifestations

Unilateral or bilateral inflammation of the parotid gland is usual: one parotid gland swells first and in 70% of cases the opposite side swells after 1–2 days. The submandibular and sublingual glands are less commonly involved. About 6% of patients will have presternal oedema resembling cellulitis of the neck.

Complications

The complications are summarised in Table 74.6.

Orchitis, usually unilateral, occurs in 25% of postpubertal males, developing 3–4 days after parotitis. Subsequent sterility is rare, even if both testes are affected.

Aseptic meningitis is common but benign. Many patients suffer transient abdominal pain and vomiting: severe pancreatitis is a rare complication.

Table 74.6 *Complications of mumps*

Common
- Orchitis
- Aseptic meningitis (benign)
- Abdominal pain (transient)

Rare
- Oöphoritis
- Encephalitis
- Arthritis (one or several joints)
- Deafness (usually transient)
- Pancreatitis

Clinical diagnosis

Enlargement of the cervical lymph glands can be mistaken for parotitis but the correct diagnosis is indicated by the anatomy of this area. Lymph nodes are posteroinferior to the ear lobe; the parotid gland is anterior and, when enlarged, obscures the angle of the mandible.

Bacterial (suppurative) parotitis is associated with toxaemia and results in a high leucocyte count. The skin over the parotid gland is tense and shiny and Stensen's duct might discharge pus.

Rare disorders such as Sjögren's syndrome can be misdiagnosed as mumps.

Virological diagnosis

The diagnosis of mumps is usually clinical; virological confirmation is rarely required but the virus can be isolated from the nasopharynx or saliva during the acute illness (and from cerebrospinal fluid in mumps meningitis).

A serological test for antibodies is available.

Management

Treatment is symptomatic. Paracetamol may be prescribed for fever, meningitis and orchitis. Ample fluid intake and a bland diet is advisable. Bed rest should be taken only according to the symptoms: it does not seem to have an influence on the development of complications.[3]

Children should not return to school until the symptoms subside but contacts need not be excluded.

The patient with orchitis should use supportive underwear. Steroids may be prescribed to relieve severe pain but will have no other effect; nor will they reduce the risk of testicular atrophy.

Prevention

Isolation is generally ineffective. The best protection is immunisation of all children.

Epstein-Barr mononucleosis

Although glandular fever is more common in adolescents and young adults, it can occur in young children but is often asymptomatic or atypical. The differential diagnosis includes cytomegalovirus infection and acute lymphatic leukaemia. Diagnosis is confirmed by the Paul-Bunnell test or the Monospot test.

Pertussis

Pertussis (whooping cough) is a respiratory infection caused by *Bordetella pertussis* and occurs worldwide. The incidence of this infectious disease has diminished because of immunisation programs and improvements in standards of living, but the infection is still seen frequently, often modified by partial immunity.

Pertussis is predominantly an illness of infants under two years of age (up to 50% of all cases). Approximately 70% of unimmunised children will eventually develop pertussis, the majority by their fifth birthday.[3] However, no age is exempt. The source of infection is older children or young adults who have relatively mild disease.

The illness is characterised by three stages: catarrhal, paroxysmal and convalescent, with the person being most infectious during the catarrhal stage.

Suspect pertussis in an illness lasting 2 weeks or more with one of:

paroxysms of coughing
or
inspiratory 'whoop' without other apparent causes
or
post-tussive vomiting

Clinical features

- Incubation period 7–14 days
- Catarrhal stage (7–14 days)
  — anorexia
  — rhinorrhoea
  — conjunctivitis/lacrimation
  — dry cough
- Paroxysmal stage (about 4 weeks)
  — paroxysms of severe coughing with inspiratory 'whoop'
  — vomiting (at end of coughing bout)
  — coughing mainly at night
  — lymphocytosis (almost absolute)
- Convalescent stage
  — coughing (less severe)

Note: Physical findings are minimal or absent.

Diagnosis

The diagnosis is basically a clinical one—virtually no other acute infectious illness in children causes a cough that lasts 4–8 weeks.[3] Confirmed by culture of nasopharyngeal aspirate (within 1 week from onset of cough) or Ig A serology (late in disease), although this can be misleading.

High-grade lymphocytosis (12–25 × 10^9/L) on an FBE is strongly suggestive of pertussis. New methods include immunofluorescence, PCR and ELISA techniques.[6]

Differential diagnosis

Viral pneumonia, acute bronchitis, influenza. Chlamydia respiratory infection can cause a 'pseudopertussis' type of illness in infants.

Complications

These include asphyxia, hypoxia, convulsions and cerebral haemorrhage. Also pulmonary complications, e.g. atelectasis, pneumonia, pneumothorax.

Treatment

Erythromycin estolate for 10 days may help reduce the period of communicability (but not the symptoms) if given early (cough less than 3 weeks). There is no evidence that antibiotics produce an improvement in the patient.[7] Cough mixtures are ineffective.[3] Good ventilation is important: avoid dust and smoke, and also emotional excitement and overfeeding during the paroxysmal phase.

Almost all infants under 6 months and some who are older require admission to hospital.[2] School exclusion until at least 5 days of antibiotics.

Prevention

Active immunisation with pertussis vaccine.

Prophylaxis

A 10 day course of erythromycin (cotrimoxazole if contraindicated) is recommended for household and other close contacts, regardless of immunisation status, commenced within 3 weeks of onset of cough in the patient.[6]

Herpes simplex

Herpes simplex virus infection is common and widespread. Primary HSV infection is basically a disease of childhood, presenting as severe acute gingivostomatitis. However, the infection may be subclinical in children; based on antibody studies, approximately 90% of the population acquire herpes simplex infection before the age of 4 or 5 years.[5]

The primary infection

Typical clinical features:

- children 1–3 years
- fever and refusal to feed
- ulcers on gums, tongue and palate
- prone to dehydration
- may be lesions on face and conjunctivae
- resolution over 7–10 days

These children are generally very miserable and ill, and some may require hospitalisation for intravenous therapy to correct fluid and electrolyte loss. Treatment is usually symptomatic, e.g. oral lignocaine gel. Careful nursing and prevention of secondary infection is important. The latter includes gentle mouth toilets. Children with severe infections, those who are immunosuppressed and those with eczema herpeticum can have aciclovir IV or orally.

Serious complications:

- encephalitis can develop in otherwise healthy children
- eczema herpeticum—children with eczema can get widespread herpetic lesions
- disseminated HSV infection in neonates

Herpes zoster

Herpes zoster (shingles) is caused by reactivation of varicella zoster virus (acquired from the primary infection of chickenpox) in the dorsal root ganglion. It occurs at all ages and can occur in children, including infants, who have been exposed to varicella *in utero*.[3]

Recurrences are uncommon except in immunocompromised patients. The diagnosis is a clinical one but can pose difficulties, especially as it is not so common in childhood and may present with only a few vesicles.

Impetigo

Impetigo (school sores) is a contagious superficial bacterial skin infection caused by *Streptococcus pyogenes* or *Staphylococcus aureus* or a combination of these two virulent organisms.

There are two common forms:

1. vesiculopustular with honey-coloured crusts (either *Strep* or *Staph*)
2. bullous type, usually *Staph aureus*

Ecthyma is a deeper form of impetigo, usually on the legs and other covered areas.

If mild with small lesions and a limited area:

- Topical antiseptic cleansing with gentle removal of crusts, using antibacterial soap, chlorhexidine or povidone-iodine. Then mupirocin (Bactroban), a small amount tds for 10 days. Topical antibiotics other than mupirocin (Bactroban) are not recommended.[7]

If extensive and causing systemic symptoms:[7]

- Cephalexin 6.25 mg/kg up to adult dose (250 mg) (o) 6 hourly for 10 days (first choice)

  or
- Flucloxacillin/dicloxacillin 6.25 mg/kg up to adult dose (250 mg) (o) 6 hourly for 10 days

  or
- Erythromycin 10 mg/kg up to adult dose (500 mg) (o) 12 hourly for 10 days

Boils (furunculosis) and carbuncles—same treatment as impetigo.

The child should be excluded from childcare settings until sores have healed fully.

Head lice

Head lice is an infestation caused by the louse *Pediculus humanus capitis*. The female louse lays eggs (or 'nits') which are glued to the hairs; they hatch within 6 days, mature into adults in about 10 days and live for about a month. Head lice spread from person to person by direct contact, such as sitting and working very close to one another. They can also spread by the sharing of combs, brushes and headwear, especially within the family. Children are the ones usually affected, but people of all ages and from all walks of life can be infested. It is more common in overcrowded living conditions. Resistance to the usual agents is becoming a problem.

Clinical features

- asymptomatic or itching of scalp
- white spots of nits can be mistaken for dandruff
- unlike dandruff, the nits cannot be brushed off
- diagnosis by finding lice (or 'nits')

Treatment (topical)

- pyrethrins/piperonyl foam or shampoo, e.g. Lyban foam

  or
- permethrin 1% or maldison 0.5%

Method

Massage well into wet hair, leave for at least 10 minutes but preferably overnight, then wash off thoroughly. Repeat treatment at one week.

Treat household child contacts at the same time.

Note: The hair does not have to be cut short. All members of the family must be treated whether or not lice, or nits, can be found. There is no need to treat clothing, pillows or other items. School exclusion should not be necessary after proper treatment. For eyelash involvement, apply petrolatum bd for 8 days and then pluck off remaining nits.

References

1. Jarman R. A word about aspirin in children. Aust Ped Review, 1991; 1(6):2.

2. Efron D. *Paediatric handbook* (5th edn). Melbourne: Blackwell Science, 1996, 69.

3. Robinson MJ. *Practical paediatrics* (2nd edn). Melbourne: Churchill Livingstone, 1990, 217–227.

4. Mansfield F. Erythema infectiosum. Slapped face disease. Aust Fam Physician, 1988; 17:737–738.

5. Wilson JD et al. *Harrison's principles of internal medicine* (12th edn). New York: McGraw-Hill, 1991, 1462–1463.

6. Golledge C. A case of persistent cough. Aust Fam Physician, 1997; 26:1219.

7. Mashford ML. *Antibiotic guidelines* (9th edn). Melbourne: Victorian Medical Postgraduate Foundation, 1996–97, 106–136.

8. Tierney LM et al. *Current medical diagnosis and treatment.* Stamford: Appleton & Lange, 1996, 113–114.

75

Behaviour disorders in children

—

The habit of constantly gratifying every wayward wish and temper under the plea of illness, and the constant indulgence which it meets with in this form from a mother's overkindness, exert a most injurious influence on the child's character, and it grows up a juvenile hypochondriac.

Charles West (1816–98)
Founder of the Great Ormond Street Hospital
for Sick Children

Table 75.1 *The five phases of childhood development*

1. Infancy	sense of trust
2. Early childhood	sense of autonomy (independence)
3. Preschool	sense of initiative
4. School age	sense of industry
5. Adolescence	sense of identity

The prevalence of significant psychiatric disorders in children in western society is at least 12% in the age range 1–14 years, with an increase of 3–4% after puberty.[1] Most of these disorders are behavioural but there is a significant incidence of emotional disorders such as anxiety and depression which tend to be misdiagnosed, as there is a perception that children do not suffer from these psychiatric disorders in the same way as adults.

The author has observed that most of the personality characteristics and behavioural problems of infancy tend to remain throughout childhood and adolescence and form the personality and behavioural disposition of the adult, although many associated problems do not tend to persist into adult life.

Parry, who describes the five phases of childhood development (Table 75.1), emphasises the importance of the first phase of infancy (where the infant is learning to trust the environment) as crucial to overall normal development.

The second phase, in which the child is developing independent skills in the second and third years of life, is also an important phase and

needs to be based on a secure and smooth first phase. It is in this toddler stage that many of the behavioural disorders will be discussed.

Temper tantrums

The tantrum is a feature of the 'terrible twos' toddler whose protestation to frustration is a dramatic reaction of kicking, shouting, screaming, throwing, or banging of the head. They usually start at 15–18 months and often persist until 3–4 years.[2] Tantrums are more likely to occur if the child is tired or bored. This behaviour may be perpetuated if the tantrums are inadvertently rewarded by the parents to seek peace and avoid conflict.

A careful history is required to gain insight into the family stresses; it also allows parents to ventilate their feelings.

Management

Reassure parents that the tantrums are relatively commonplace and not harmful. Explain the reasons for the tantrums and include the concept that 'temper tantrums need an audience'.

Advice[3]

- Ignore what is ignorable: parents should pretend to ignore the behaviour and leave the child alone without comment, including moving to a different area (but not locking the child in its room).
- Stay calm and say nothing.
- Avoid what is avoidable: try to avoid the cause or causes of the tantrums, e.g. visiting the supermarket.
- Distract what is distractable: redirect the child's interest to some other object or activity.
- Praise appropriate behaviour.

When ignored, the problem will probably get worse for a few days before it starts to improve. Medication has no place in the management of temper tantrums.

Breath-holding attacks

The age group for the attack is 6 months to 6 years (peak 2–3 years). There are two distinct types—one occurring with a tantrum and the other a simple faint in response to pain or fright. The precipitating event can be of a minor emotional or physical nature. In the tantrum situation children will emit a loud cry, then hold their breath. They become pale, then cyanosed (this distinguishes it from a seizure disorder). If prolonged it may result in unconsciousness or a fit. The episode lasts 10–60 seconds.

Management

Place the child in the coma position. Reassure parents that the attacks are self-limiting and are not associated with epilepsy or mental retardation. Advise parents to maintain discipline and to resist spoiling the child. Try to avoid incidents known to frustrate the child or to precipitate a tantrum.

Head banging

This behaviour is common, occurring in 5–15% of normal infants and toddlers.[2] It also occurs in developmental disability and severe emotional deprivation.

Features

- occurs in children under 4, especially 3 years old
- usually prior to going to sleep
- head banging occurs 60–80 times/minute
- lasts several minutes to 60 minutes or more per episode
- associated repetitive movements, e.g. body rocking, thumb sucking
- child usually not distressed and rarely self-injurious

Management

- Reassure parents that it's a normal self-limiting behaviour and usually settles by 3–5 years.
- Avoid reinforcing behaviour by excessive attention or punishment.
- Advise distraction or actively ignoring the behaviour.

Oppositional behaviour[2]

Resistant and oppositional behaviour is common and perhaps normal from time to time provided it is not associated with antisocial behaviour. It is a feature of 2–4 year olds as well as school-age children and adolescents. It is important to interview the child and family to determine whether it is normal or abnormal. Generally, supportive counselling and behaviour modification works effectively. This includes looking for and praising or rewarding good behaviour. It is important to praise (or chastise) behaviour rather than the child. 'Time out' is the preferred disciplinary measure for children over 18 months (maximum 1 minute per year of age) while withdrawing privileges is appropriate for children over 6 years.

Conduct disorders

Conduct disorders affect 3–5% of children and represent the largest group of childhood psychiatric disorders.

Clinical features[2]

- antisocial behaviour that is repetitive and persistent
- lack of guilt or remorse for offensive behaviour
- generally poor interpersonal relationships
- manipulative
- tendency to aggressive, destructive, 'criminal' behaviour

- learning problems (about 50%)
- hyperactivity (one-third)

Family and environmental factors[2]
- disrupted childhood care
- socially disadvantaged
- lack of a warm, caring family
- family violence: emotional, physical or sexual abuse
- antisocial peer group exposure

Management
- early intervention and family assistance to help provide a warm, caring family environment
- family therapy to reduce interfamily conflict
- appropriate educational programs to facilitate self-esteem and achievement
- provision of opportunities for interesting, socially positive activities, e.g. sports, recreation, jobs, other skills
- behaviour modification programs
- with physically aggressive behaviour, refer for psychotherapy if repeated, severe, causes injury or is associated with other antisocial behaviour

Stealing[2]

Isolated theft, which is common, is not necessarily an indication of serious psychopathology but may reflect normal risk-taking behaviour, a reaction to stress, low self-esteem, searching for peer group acceptance or a 'cry for help and attention'.[2]

Management
- Insist on retribution—return of goods or payment and personal apologies to the 'victim'.
- 'Punish' with withdrawal of appropriate privileges.
- Refer for psychotherapy if persistent.

Sleep disorders

Sleep problems in children are very common in late infancy, toddlerhood and early preschool age groups. The majority do not sleep throughout the night until 6 months of age. Over 50% of toddlers and preschool children resist going to bed.[4] At least 30% of infants and toddlers wake at least once during the night every night. Toddlers begin to have dreams coinciding with language development in the second year of life.[3]

The child who wakes during the night needs reassurance, protection and the parent's presence, but it must be given discreetly. Although psychosocial stresses can trigger sleep problems, serious psychological problems in children with sleep disorders is uncommon.[2]

Management
Advice to parents:
- Resist taking the child into bed during the night unless they are happy to encourage this.
- Avoid giving attention to the child in the middle of the night—it encourages attention seeking.
- Avoid extra feeding or other pacifiers during the night.
- Return the child to bed promptly and spend only a brief time to give reassurance.
- A rigid series of rituals performed before bedtime helps the child to develop a routine. Settling to sleep may be assisted by soft music, a soft toy and a gentle night-light.
- Take the child into the bedroom while still awake.

Medication has a minimal place in the management of sleep disturbances, although the judicious use of a sedative/hypnotic for a short term may break the sleepless cycle. Such drugs include chloral hydrate 25–50 mg/kg per dose and trimeprazine (Vallergan) 1–2 mg/kg per dose (not for infants under 6 months).[2]

Para-insomnias (night terrors, sleep talking and walking)[2]

These are not true sleep disorders or night-time arousals. They occur in deep sleep. With night terrors, which usually develop within 2 hours of sleep and last 1–2 minutes, the child is usually inconsolable and has no memory for the event. These events cluster in two age ranges, 2–4 and 6–9 years, and are self-limiting over a period of months. Usually, no active treatment is needed but for persistent severe problems a 6 week trial of phenytoin or imipramine is worthwhile.

Poor eating

Some parents may complain that their toddler 'eats nothing'. Apart from taking a careful history about what constitutes 'nothing', it is useful to describe the typical diet for the age group and then match the child's weight on the normal growth chart. The important aspect of management is to point out what is necessary from a nutritional viewpoint as opposed to what is considered normal for the particular culture.

Attention deficit hyperactivity disorder (ADHD)

This disorder, which is characterised by developmentally inappropriate degrees of inattentiveness, overactivity and impulsiveness, has an estimated prevalence of about 2–5%. It is far more common in boys than girls (6:1) and is usually present from infancy.[1] About 60% will carry some degree of the disorder into adulthood. A neurological basis for ADHD has been demonstrated. Accurate diagnosis of ADHD is very important.

Diagnostic criteria

A. Either 1 or 2 (refer to diagnostic criteria for ADHD in DSM IV)
    1. Inattention
    2. Hyperactivity and impulsiveness
B. Onset no later than 7 years of age
C. Symptoms must be present in two or more situations, e.g. at school and at home
D. Disturbance causes clinically significant distress or impairment in social, academic or occupational functioning
E. Not part of a pervasive developmental disability, psychotic disorder, mood disorder, anxiety disorder, associative disorder or a personality disorder

Other clinical features

• irritability and moodiness
• poor co-ordination
• disorganisation

Diagnosis

• no foolproof diagnostic tests available
• psychometric tests available
• questionnaires for parents and teachers

Assessment should include child and family interviews, neurological examination, assessment of vision and hearing levels, serum lead levels (in high-risk groups) and the testing of formal cognitive achievement. 25% of children with ADHD have coexistent learning disabilities.[2]

Management

• Protect child's self-esteem.
• Counsel and support family.
• Involve teachers.
• Refer to appropriate consultant, e.g. child psychiatrist.
• Refer to parent support group.

Diet. Exclusion diet probably ineffective but encourage good diet (consider dietitian's help).
Pharmacological: based on stimulants (2 doses: after breakfast and noon)[2,5]

• methylphenidate (Ritalin) 0.3–0.8 mg/kg/dose(o)

or

    dexamphetamine 0.15–0.4 mg/kg/dose(o)

• antidepressants, second line
• clonidine, especially for sleep disturbance and aggression

Sibling rivalry

Sibling rivalry is a real concern as a toddler acts out apparent jealousy towards a new baby. The baby needs help from the inappropriate prodding, pinching and smothering attempts. The jealous toddler needs attention from the mother and a fair share of the comforts, cuddling and love that the toddler has been used to having.

It is important that the toddler is encouraged to feel that it is his or her baby too and to have opportunities to experience warmth and smiles from the baby, so that a sense of belonging is engendered.

Stuttering and stammering

This interruption of the orderly flow of speech may be accompanied by blinking and various other tics. It tends to be common in the school years but approximately 80% of sufferers become fluent by adulthood.[6]

Features of stuttering

• more common in boys
• usually begins under 6 years of age
• no evidence of neurotic or neurological disorder
• causes anxiety and social withdrawal

Management

Although most stutterers improve spontaneously, speech therapy from a caring empathic therapist may be very helpful.

Tics (habit spasm)

Tics are 'sudden, rapid and involuntary movements of circumscribed muscle groups which serve no apparent purpose'.[6] Most are minor, transient facial tics, nose twitching, or vocal tics such as grunts, throat clearing and staccato semicoughs. Most of these tics resolve spontaneously (usually in less than a year) and reassurance can be given.

Tourette's disorder

Also known as Gilles de la Tourette's syndrome or multiple tic disorder, Tourette's disorder usually first appears in children between the ages of 4 and 15 years (before 18 years) and has a prevalence of 1: 10 000. Diagnosis is based on recurrent tics over a period > 1 year in which there is never a tic free period for more than 3 months.

Clinical features

- more common in boys
- bizarre motor tics
- echolia (repetition of words)
- coprolalia (compulsive utterances of obscene words)
- familial: dominant gene with variable expression

Treatment (if necessary) is haloperidol or pimozide.[5]

Autism

Autism, described first by Kanner in 1943, is a pervasive development disorder commencing early in childhood; it affects at least four children in 10 000, boys four times as commonly as girls. Autism is not due to faulty parenting or birth trauma, but is a biological disorder of the CNS which may have multiple organic aetiologies.

Many autistic children appear physically healthy and well developed although there is an association with a range of other disorders such as Tourette's disorder, tuberous sclerosis, epilepsy (up to 30% onset, usually in adolescence) and rubella encephalopathy. Most have intellectual disability but about 20% function in the normal range.

Autistic children show many disturbed behaviours. The main features are presented in Table 75.2.

The earliest signs of autism in infancy include:[7]

Table 75.2   *A guide to the diagnosis of childhood autism (after Tonge)*[7]

1. Onset during infancy and early childhood.
2. An impairment of social interactions shown by at least two of the following:
   - lack of awarness of the feelings of others
   - absent or abnormal comfort seeking in response to distress
   - lack of imitation
   - absent or abnormal social play
   - impaired ability to socialise, which may include gaze avoidance
3. Impairment in communication as shown by at least one of the following:
   - lack of babbling, gesture, mime or spoken language
   - absent or abnormal non-verbal communication
   - abnormalities in the form or content of speech
   - poor ability to initiate or sustain conversation
   - abnormal speech production
4. A restricted range of activities, interests and imaginative development, shown in at least one of the following:
   - stereotyped body movements
   - persistent and unusual preoccupations and rituals with objects or activities
   - severe distress over changes in routine or environment
   - an absence of imaginative and symbolic play
5. Behavioural problems:
   - tantrums
   - hyperactivity
   - destructiveness
   - risk-taking activity

- excessive crying
- no response to cuddling if crying
- failure to mould the body in anticipation of being picked up
- stiffening the body or resisting when being held
- resistance to a change in routine
- appearing to be deaf
- failing to respond or overacting to sensory stimuli
- persistent failure to imitate, such as waving goodbye
- a need for minimal sleep

The diagnosis of autism remains difficult before the age of 2 years.

Assessment

If a child has delayed and deviant development and autism is suspected, a comprehensive multidisciplinary assessment is necessary. Referral to professionals with experience of autism is essential.

Treatment[8]

Many treatments have been tried and behavioural treatment methods have proved to be the most helpful. Medications are unhelpful for autism *per se* although medications such as tranquillisers, antidepressants and anticonvulsants are helpful for associated disorders.

The best results are achieved by early diagnosis, followed by a firm and consistent home management and early intervention program. Remedial education and speech therapy have an important place in management.

Case histories and 'draw a dream'

A useful strategy for communicating with disturbed children and getting to the source of a behaviour problem is to ask them to 'draw a dream'.[9] Professor Tonge believes that the dream is the royal road to the child's mental processes and the family doctor is ideally placed to use this technique. The following case studies concerning insomnia and nightmares illustrate the importance of these symptoms as reflecting a deep emotional problem in the child.

Case study 1[10]

Steven, aged 6, was a bright, happy little boy until he developed an extraordinary and puzzling episode of insomnia which was solved eventually by his teacher.

He presented to our group practice with his bemused mother who claimed that, suddenly, he would not and could not sleep. His parents would be startled at night by the eerie vision of Steven standing silent and motionless beside their bed. When not in his bed at night he would be found hiding under it or in his wardrobe.

Fig. 75.1 *Steven's drawing*

His behaviour was normal otherwise, but his teacher reported that his schoolwork had deteriorated and that he was constantly falling asleep at his desk. On direct questioning Steven was shy and evasive, claiming nothing was worrying him. We considered it was a temporary phase of abnormal behaviour and advised conservative measures such as hot beverages, baths and exercises before retiring, but this strategy failed. He was referred to a consultant who also failed to find the cause of the insomnia and advised long midnight jogs.

Eventually Steven's teacher had the bright idea of asking all the children to draw the thing that scared or worried them the most, stipulating that it would be a 'make believe' picture.

Looking at the drawing depicting two robbers stealing his moneybox as he slept (Fig. 75.1), she tactfully confronted Steven, who admitted that his playmate had told him robbers would come one night, steal his moneybox and 'bash' him.

The final chapter of this story saw a happy Steven perched on a bank counter watching his money being counted, deposited in a huge safe and exchanged for a bank book. Steven has slept normally ever since.

Case study 2[10]

George, the second child of four children, seemed a normal healthy 3 year old when his mother presented him for assessment.

For about 3 months George had been having nightmares, episodes that fractured the entire household. His mother, Mary, was absolutely frustrated by his nocturnal behaviour and said she was 'at her wit's end'. As she excitedly rattled off details of the family dilemma, I noted that she was intense and rather domineering but obviously a very conscientious and dutiful wife and mother.

She explained that George would wake her at night calling out to her because of a monster in his room or outside his window. She had no idea about any causes for this problem and explained that 'our household is very normal—no problems really'. She said George's behaviour was otherwise normal and he was a healthy boy.

Identifying the monster

I then asked George about his problem but could elicit only very scant information. Recalling the immense value of the 'draw a dream' strategy I asked him to draw the monster. George quickly drew the monster as shown in Figure 75.2. I asked him about the monster and finally confronted him with the question: 'Do you know who or what the monster is?'

'Mum,' replied George, very matter-of-factly.

A shocked Mary looked unbelievingly at George and, for once, seemed stuck for words. Realising the delicacy of the situation, I asked George to tell me what it was about his mother that worried him. He offered the very revealing information: 'I don't think that she loves me. She's always yelling at me.'

Obviously the monster was George's insecurity because George declared how much he did love his mother and was 'scared' of losing her love. With appropriate counselling the outcome was good.

A lesson learned often is that it is important to 'look close to home' for any significant behaviour disorder or other psychological problem. It is important to explore the relationship that is most meaningful to the affected person, e.g. mother–daughter, father–son, student–teacher.

The 'draw a dream' strategy revealed vital information in this case.

Fig. 75.2 *George's drawing*

When to refer[1]

- When child abuse is known or suspected.
- When an underlying medical problem is present.
- For assessment of associated psychological, family and related factors.
- For failed management, including simple behavioural and family support interventions.

References

1. Tonge B.J. Behavioural, emotional and psychosomatic disorders in children and adolescents. In: MIMS Disease Index (2nd edn). Sydney: IMS Publishing, 1996, 52–55.

2. Efron D. *Paediatric handbook* (5th edn). Melbourne: Blackwell Science, 1996, 282–297.

3. Parry TS. Behavioural problems in toddlers. Aust Fam Physician, 1986; 15:1038–1040.

4. Jarman R. Sleep problems. Aust Paed Review, 1992; 2(2):1–2.

5. Moulds RFW. *Psychotropic drug guidelines*. Victorian Medical Postgraduate Foundation, 1996–97, 150–164.

6. Robinson MJ. *Practical paediatrics* (2nd edn). Melbourne: Churchill Livingstone, 1990, 543–549.

7. Tonge BJ. Autism. Aust Fam Physician, 1989; 18:247–250.

8. Curtis J. Autism. Patient Education, 1993; 22:1239.

9. Tonge BJ. 'I'm upset, you're upset and so are my Mum and Dad'. Aust Fam Physician, 1983, 12:497–499.

10. Murtagh J. *Cautionary tales*. Sydney: McGraw-Hill, 1992, 165–174.

76

Child abuse

—

It is customary, but I think it is a mistake, to speak of happy childhood. Children, however, are often overanxious and acutely sensitive. Man ought to be man and master of his fate; but children are at the mercy of those around them.

Sir John Lubbock, Baron Avebury 1834–1913

The description of the 'battered child syndrome' in 1962 provoked an awareness of a problem facing children which continues to increase in prominence. The possibility of both physical and sexual abuse has to be kept in mind by the family doctor. It may surface in families known to us as respectable and where a good trustful relationship exists between parents and doctor. Another aspect of child abuse is neglect.

The various types of abuse are classified as:

• physical
• neglect
• emotional
• sexual
• potential

Physical abuse occurs most often in the first 2 years of life, neglect in the first 5 years and sexual abuse from 5 years of age[1] (Fig. 76.1). In a Community Services of Victoria study[2] the distribution of child abuse was physical 15%, emotional 48%, sexual 9% and neglect 28%.

In another study,[2] the findings were:

• Girls are more likely to be abused than boys.
• Girls are more often assaulted by someone they know.
• Most of the adults who sexually abuse are men (> 90%).
• About 75% of offenders are known to the child.
• Abuse is the misuse of a power situation, e.g. a close relative, coupled with the child's immaturity.

Fig. 76.1 *Typical relative age patterns for child abuse* AFTER BENTOVIN.[1]

Definitions

Child abuse can be defined by the nature of the abusive act or by the result of the abuse. A parent, guardian or other carer can harm a child by a deliberate act or by failure to provide adequate care.

Physical abuse (non-accidental injury)

Physical abuse is defined as 'a child with a characteristic pattern of injuries, the explanation of which is not consistent with the pattern, or where there is definite information through acknowledgment or reasonable suspicion that the injury was inflicted or knowingly not prevented by any person having custody, charge or care of the child'.[1]

Neglect

Neglect is defined as 'the privation of food, drink, medical care, stimulation or affection'.

Emotional abuse

Emotional abuse is the 'systematic destruction of the child's sense of self-esteem and competence, where competence is defined as the ability to act in social contexts'.

Sexual abuse

Sexual abuse in children is defined[3] as 'the involvement of dependent, developmentally immature children and adolescents in sexual activities that they do not fully comprehend, to which they are unable to give informed consent, and which violate the social taboos'.

Incest

Incest is legally defined as 'intercourse between biological family members'.

Abuse: who and why?[2]

The real cause seems to be a combination of several interrelated factors: personal, familial, social/cultural and societal stress. Abused children exist at all levels of society, although the majority of abused children who come to the attention of authorities are from families where there is high mobility, lack of education, loneliness, poverty, unemployment, inadequate housing and social isolation. Sexual abuse, occurring alone, does not follow these patterns and can occur under any socioeconomic circumstances.

Both men and women physically abuse their children. While women are the parents most responsible in cases of neglect and emotional abuse (probably because of a dominant role in child care, social and economic disadvantage and being the only one responsible for the care of children in a single parent arrangement), men are more likely to abuse their children sexually.

The child can be abused at any age (even adolescents can be victims of abuse and neglect). It is important to keep this in mind—*it does happen*.

Underdiagnosing and under-reporting[2]

Although the medical profession remains the foremost focus of child abuse reporting (they are the most likely to encounter injured children and are the most qualified to diagnose abuse), they still contribute only a small percentage of the total reporting to central registries. This could be because there is underdiagnosis of the problem but it could also be because of under-reporting.

Reasons given as to why GPs don't report more cases of child abuse include:

- Concern about drain on time and finances
- Lack of positive feedback about other cases
- Lack of undergraduate education on the topic
- Risk of alienation and stigmatisation to the family
- The feeling by some GPs that they can work on the problem with the family without outside intervention
- Lack of trust or confidence in local officials and agencies
- Uncertainty about *what* to do
- Personal and legal risks, i.e. fear of court, libel suits, irate parents
- Reluctance until absolutely certain of diagnosis

It will always be difficult to take the first step but it is important and it can help, no matter how small that first step is.

Interviewing parents or guardians

A skilled, sensitive, diplomatic interview is fundamental to management. Guidelines include:

- a relaxed non-judgmental approach
- sensitivity to all people involved
- appropriate questions—open-ended, not leading
- use verbatim quotes from the child where possible and wait silently for a reaction.

Physical abuse

Physical abuse should be suspected, especially in a child aged under three, if certain physical or behavioural indicators in either the child or the parents are present. Bruising, especially fingertip bruising, is the most common sign of the physically abused child.

Physical indicators:[2]

- unexplained injury

- different explanations offered
- injury unlikely to have occurred in manner stated
- unreasonable delays between injury and presentation
- finger-shaped bruises
- multiple bruises/welts of different ages, especially on face or buttocks
- fractures (especially if child < 2 years old)
- burns, scalds, dislocations, poisoning, cuts, bites
- cigarette butt type burns
- shaking injuries, e.g. retinal damage, torn frenulum
- subdural haematoma
- internal injuries
- episodes of unconsciousness

> Remember Munchausen syndrome by proxy.

Behavioural indicators[2]
- wariness of adult contacts
- inappropriate clothing, e.g. long sleeves on a hot day
- apprehension when other children cry or shout
- behavioural extremes
- fear of parents
- afraid to go home
- child reports injury by parents or gives inappropriate explanation of injury
- excessive compliance
- extreme wariness
- attaches too readily to strangers

Investigations
The following should be considered:[9]
- FBE, including platelets, if bruising
- coagulation studies (PT, APTT) if bruising
- imaging for fractures: specific X-rays; bone scan (especially < 3 years old); skull X-ray; skeletal survey (skull, thorax, abdomen, pelvis)
- photographs: taken on presentation

Management
The family doctor should diplomatically confront the parent or parents and always act in the best interests of the child. Offer to help the family. An approach would be to say, 'I am very concerned about your child's injuries as they don't add up—these injuries are not usually caused by what I'm told has been the cause. I

will therefore seek assistance—it is my legal obligation. My duty is to help you and, especially, your child.'

Acquiring essential help
- psychosocial assessment of child and family: involves social worker and multidisciplinary assessment
- admission to hospital: for moderate and severe injuries
- case conference (where appropriate)
- mandatory reporting: notify child protection authorities

The stages of management are:[1]
- recognition or disclosure of abuse
- the family separation phase
- working towards rehabilitation
- finding a new family for the child, when rehabilitation fails

Emotional abuse
Physical indicators:
- There are few physical indicators, but emotional abuse can cause delay in physical, emotional and mental development.

Behavioural indicators:
- extremely low self-esteem
- compliant, passive, withdrawn, tearful and/or apathetic behaviour
- aggressive or demanding behaviour
- anxiety
- serious difficulties with peers and/or adult relations
- delayed or distorted speech
- regressive behaviour, e.g. soiling

Neglect
Physical indicators:
- consistent hunger
- failure to thrive, or malnutrition
- poor hygiene
- inappropriate clothing
- consistent lack of supervision
- unattended physical problems or medical needs
- abandonment
- dangerous health or dietary practices

Behavioural indicators:
- stealing food
- extending stays at school

- consistent fatigue, listlessness or falling asleep in class
- alcohol or drug abuse
- child states there is no caregiver
- aggressive or inappropriate behaviour
- isolation from peer group

Sexual abuse

Incest and sexual abuse of children within the family occur more frequently than is acknowledged. One difficulty in recognising sexually abused children is to determine what is appropriate physical contact between adult and child, and what is abusive sexual behaviour.

Sexual abuse presents in three main ways:[4]

- allegations by the child or an adult
- injuries to the genitalia or anus
- suspicious presentations, especially:
  — genital infection
  — recurrent urinary infection
  — unexplained behavioural changes/ psychological disorders

Clinical indicators that may suggest child sexual abuse are presented in Table 76.1.[5,6]

Sexual abuse can take many forms, including:

- genital fondling
- digital penetration
- penetration with various objects
- simulated sexual intercourse (anal in boys)
- full sexual penetration
- pornography
- prostitution

Clinical approach

Ideally, the child should be assessed by experienced medical officers at the regional sexual assault service, so the temptation for the inexperienced GP to have a quick look should be resisted. For the practitioner having to assess the problem, a complete medical and social history, including a behavioural history, should be obtained prior to examination.

 The child's history must be obtained carefully, honestly, patiently and objectively, without leading the child. Use language appropriate to the child and employ aids such as drawings and a model (such as a 'gingerbread man') to help the child illustrate what has happened. The

Table 76.1 *Clinical indicators that may suggest child sexual abuse*

- complaint of abuse (rarely invented)
- vaginal discharge
- other STD
- urinary tract infection
- unexplained genital trauma
- unexplained perianal trauma
- overt sexual play
- pregnancy in an adolescent
- deterioration in school work
- family disruption
- indiscriminate attachment
- abnormal sexual behaviour
- poor self-esteem
- psychological disorders
  — behaviour disturbances
  — regression in behaviour
  — sleep disturbances
  — abnormal fears/reactions to specific places or persons
  — psychosomatic symptoms
  — anxiety
  — lack of trust
  — overcompliance
  — aggressive behaviour
- depression
  — self-destructive behaviour
  — substance abuse
  — suicidal tendencies

Examination (abnormal findings uncommon)
- genital trauma
- perforated hymen/lax vagina
- perianal trauma
- vaginal discharge
- look for semen and STDs

---

history is more important than the physical findings as there are no abnormal physical findings in 40% of confessed cases.[7]

Physical examination[8]

It is recommended that the physical examination of any child suspected of being sexually abused is performed by a paediatrician or forensic physician experienced in the area of sexual abuse.

It is important to spend time explaining the examination process to the child and the accompanying parent. In prepubescent girls and boys, the examination is limited to visual inspection of the external areas using a good light source. Magnification may be used with a colposcope or magnifying glass, and photographs may be taken for documentation or medicolegal purposes.

Speculum examination is limited to post-pubertal girls or used if there is concern about internal injuries (the latter may necessitate general anaesthesia). Rectal examination is usually limited to visualisation.

Three recommended positions are:

1. Supine with legs apart (frog-leg position with soles of feet apposed)
2. Prone knee-chest position (the best position)
3. Lateral decubitus

Always record the findings and note the examination position.

It is useful to remember that examination of urine in female children may show sperm so, if the child is uncharacteristically passing urine at night, get her mother to collect a specimen.

The crisis situation

It is important to realise that the child will be in *crisis*.[5] Children are trapped into the secrecy of sexual abuse, often by a trusted adult, by powerful threats of the consequences of disclosure. They are given the great responsibility of keeping the secret and holding the family together or disclosing the secret and disrupting the family. A crisis occurs when these threats become reality.

Management

It is important to act responsibly in the best interests of the child. When we encounter real or suspected child abuse, immediate action is necessary. The child needs an advocate to act on its behalf and our intervention actions may have to override our relationship with the family.

Some golden rules are:

- Never attempt to solve the problem alone.
- Do not attempt confrontation and counselling in isolation (unless under exceptional circumstances).
- Seek advice from experts (only a phone call away).
- Avoid telling the alleged perpetrator what the child has said.
- Refer to a child sexual assault centre where an experienced team can take the serious responsibility for the problem.

Supporting the child

- Acknowledge the child's fear and perhaps guilt.
- Assure the child it is not his or her fault.
- Tell the child you will help.
- Obtain the child's trust.
- Tell the child it has happened to other children and you have helped them.

Confronting the parents

If certain about the diagnosis the doctor should inform the child's mother and encourage her to notify the protective authority. If abuse is suspected, concerns should be raised that the child may have been sexually abused and that you wonder who the perpetrator could be. Ask who has access to the child, e.g. babysitter, member of a creche or kindergarten, teacher, other males, relatives.

Prevention of child abuse

Prevention of abuse, particularly self-perpetuating abuse, can be helped by creating awareness through media attention, programs in schools and the community in general, and increased knowledge and surveillance by all professionals involved with children. Clear guidelines on reporting and the accessibility of child abuse clinics are important for the strategies to be effective. Teaching children how to protect themselves offers the greatest potential for prevention.[4]

Counselling the secondary victims

Non-offending parents, who are the secondary victims of the abused child, will require help and guidance from their family doctor on how to manage the crisis at home. Parents should be advised to reassure the child of support and safety and to maintain usual routines. The child should be allowed to set the pace, without zealous overattention and pressure from the parents. Siblings should be informed that something has happened but that the child is safe. Ensure that the child will inform if the perpetrator attempts further abuse. Parents need substantial support including alleviation of any guilt.

An unhappy consequence of the crisis is the problem of broken relationships, which may involve the separation of the child from the family. At least one hitherto unsuspecting parent will be devastated if a parent is responsible for the abuse. The sexually abused child needs to be living with a protective parent with the abusive parent living separately.

Support for doctors

The attending doctor also requires support, and sharing the problem with colleagues, mentors and family is recommended. Some helpful guidelines are:

- Carefully record all examination findings (take copious notes).
- Always keep to the facts and be objective.
- Do not become emotionally involved.
- Work with (not for) the authorities.
- Avoid making inappropriate judgments to the authorities; e.g. do not state 'incest was committed', but rather say 'there is evidence (or no evidence) to support penetration of . . .'
- If called to court, be well prepared; rehearse presentation; be authoritative and keep calm without allowing yourself to be upset by personal affronts.

The main difficulty in diagnosing child abuse is denial that it could be possible.

Practice tips and guidelines

- A child's statement alleging abuse should be accepted as true until proved otherwise.
- Children rarely lie about sexual abuse.
- False allegations, however, are a sign of family disharmony and an indication that the child may need help.
- Do not insist that the child 'has got it wrong', even if you find the actions by the alleged perpetrator unbelievable.
- Do not procrastinate—move swiftly to solve the problem.
- The genitalia are normal in the majority of sexually abused children.
- Be supportive to the child by listening, believing, being kind and caring.

Basic rules[9]

- Suspect child abuse.
- Recognise child abuse.
- Consult the child protection authorities.

Mandatory reporting

In most states of Australia and in many areas throughout the world it is mandatory to notify the relevant statutory authorities about suspected child abuse. All family doctors should become familiar with the appropriate local legislation.

When to refer

Unless there are exceptional circumstances, referral to an appropriate child abuse centre where an expert team is available is recommended. If doubtful, relatively urgent referral to a paediatrician is an alternative.

References

1. Bentovin A. Child abuse. Medicine International, 1987; 1851–1857.
2. Lewis D. Child abuse. In: Monash University: Department of Community Medicine. Final year student handbook, 1993, 164–168.
3. Schechter MD, Roberge L. Sexual exploitation. In: Helfer RE, Kempe CH eds, *Child abuse and neglect. The family and the community*. Cambridge, Mass: Ballinger, 1976, 127–142.
4. Valman HD. *ABC of one to seven*. London: British Medical Association, 1988, 112–114.
5. McMichael A. Counselling the victims of child sexual assault. Aust Fam Physician, 1990; 19:481–489.
6. Steven I, Castell-McGregor S, Francis J, Winefield H. Child sexual abuse. Aust Fam Physician, 1988; 17:427–433.
7. Irons TG. *Child sexual abuse*. California: Audio Digest, 1993; 41:2.
8. Murnane M. Child sexual abuse. Aust Fam Physician, 1990; 19:603–606.
9. Efron D. *Paediatric handbook*. Melbourne: Blackwell Science, 1996, 333–338.

77

Emergencies in children

We can say with some assurance that, although children may be the victims of fate, they will not be the victims of our neglect.

John F. Kennedy (1917–63)

Important serious emergencies in children include:

- trauma, especially head injuries and intra-abdominal injuries
- swallowed foreign bodies
- respiratory problems
  - bronchial asthma
  - epiglottitis
  - croup
  - inhaled foreign body
  - acute bronchiolitis
- severe gastroenteritis
- septicaemia, e.g. meningococcal septicaemia
- myocarditis
- immersion
- poisoning
- bites and stings
- seizures
  - absence seizures
  - tonic-clonic epilepsy
  - febrile convulsions
- sudden infant death syndrome (SIDS) and ALTE
- child abuse
  - emotional
  - physical
  - sexual
- psychogenic disturbances
  - anxiety/hyperventilation
  - suicide/parasuicide

Survey by age group

The author's study analysed emergencies into three groups,[1] preschool (0–5 years), primary school (6–12), adolescence (13–17).

The commonest emergency calls in the 0–5 years group were poisoning, accidents and violence, dyspnoea, fever/rigors, convulsions, abdominal pain, earache, vomiting.

In the 6–12 age group—accidents and violence, dyspnoea, abdominal pain, vomiting, acute allergy, bites and stings, earache.

In the 13–17 age group—accidents and violence, abdominal pain, psychogenic disorders, acute allergy, bites and stings, epistaxis.

The signs and symptoms of a serious illness

The busy general practitioner will see many sick children in a day's work, especially in the winter months with the epidemic of upper respiratory tract infections. It is vital to be able to recognise the very sick child who requires special attention, including admission to hospital. It is unlikely that the commonplace robust, lustily crying, hot, red-faced child is seriously ill but the pale, quiet, whimpering child spells danger. These rules are particularly helpful in the assessment of babies under six months of age.[2,3] The presence of a fever in itself is not necessarily an indication of serious illness but rather that the baby has an infection.[2]

The features of a very sick infant include:
- inactive, lying quietly, uninterested
- increased respiratory rate
- increased work of breathing
- noisy breathing
  - chest wall or sternal retraction
  - wheezes, grunting, stridor
- tachycardia
- sunken eyes
- cold, pale skin
- drowsiness

Serious illnesses to consider include:
- Haemophilus influenza type B (Hib) infection
  — acute epiglottitis
  — meningitis
  (now uncommon since Hib immunisation)
- acute bacterial meningitis
- septicaemia
  — meningococcaemia
  — toxic shock syndrome
  — other bacterial sepsis
- acute viral encephalitis
- acute myocarditis
- asthma/bronchitis/bronchiolitis
- pneumonia
- intussusception/bowel obstruction/appendicitis
- severe gastroenteritis

Predictive combinations
- pallor + drowsiness + fever = meningitis
- drowsiness + chest wall recession = pneumonia or severe bronchiolitis
- pallor + inactivity = intussusception

Two main groups of signs are good indicators of serious illness.[2]

Group 1: common features with reasonable risk
'A,B,C, fluids in and out'
A = poor arousal, alertness and activity
B = breathing difficulty
C = poor circulation (persistent pallor, cold legs to knees)
'Fluids in' = feeding less than half normal in 24 hours
'Fluids out' = less than 4 wet nappies in 24 hours
Note: The more signs present, the greater the risk.

Group 2: uncommon features with high risk requiring urgent referral
Resp: apnoea, central cyanosis, respiratory grunt
GIT: persistent bile-stained vomiting, mass > 2 cm other than hydrocele or umbilical hernia, significant faecal blood
CNS: convulsions
Skin: petechial rash

Indications for investigations are presented in Table 77.1.

Collapse in children
Collapse in children is a very dramatic emergency and often represents a life-threatening event. It is important to remember that the child's brain requires two vital factors:
oxygen and glucose
There is only a 2 minute reserve once cerebral blood flow stops. Bacterial meningitis should be considered as a cause.

Table 77.1 *Indications for investigations in the sick child*[2]

urine micro, culture and sensitivity	all with fever
full blood examination	all < 4 weeks risk factors present doctor uncertain
blood micro, culture and sensitivity	all < 3 months risk factors present doctor uncertain
faecal micro, culture and sensitivity	all with diarrhoea
chest X-ray	all with significant respiratory tract S&S
C reactive protein	those on antibiotics doctor uncertain
CSF examination **(lumbar puncture contraindicated in the unresponsive febrile patient)**	Suspected meningitis (infant drowsy, pale and febrile) Convulsion in febrile child and • source of fever unknown • preceding drowsiness and pallor • infant < 6 months child > 5 years • prolonged convulsion (> 10 minutes) • postictal phase longer than usual (> 30 minutes)

Note: Fever measured rectally with thermometer bulb 3 cm past anal verge

Important causes of collapse are presented in Table 77.2. Keep in mind child abuse as a cause of collapse.

Initial basic management[4]

1. Lay child on side.
2. Suck out mouth and nasopharynx.
3. Intubate or ventilate (if necessary).
4. Give oxygen 8–10 L/min by mask.
5. Pass a nasogastric tube:
   - 0–3 years 12FG
   - 4–10 years 14FG.
6. Attend to circulation:
   - ? give blood, Haemaccel or N saline.
7. Take blood for appropriate investigations.
8. Consider 'blind' administration of IV glucose.

Cardiopulmonary resuscitation[4]

Sudden primary cardiac arrest is rare in children. Asystole or severe bradycardia is the usual rhythm at the time of arrest.

The following basic life support plan should be followed.

Table 77.2 *Collapse in children: causes to consider*

Anaphylaxis	penicillin injection stings
Asphyxia	near drowning strangulation
Airways obstruction	asthma epiglottitis croup inhaled foreign body
CNS disorders	convulsions meningitis encephalitis head injury
Severe infection	gastroenteritis → dehydration septicaemia myocarditis
Hypovolaemia	dehydration, e.g. heat blood loss, e.g. ruptured spleen
Cardiac failure	arrhythmias cardiomyopathy
Metabolic	acidosis, e.g. diabetic coma hypoglycaemia hyponatraemia
Poisoning	drug ingestion envenomation
SIDS	near miss
Functional	breath-holding attacks conversion reaction vasovagal

Note: Consider child abuse.

- Check breathing and pulse.
- Inspect oropharynx and clear any debris.
- Tilt head backwards, lift chin and thrust jaw forward (the sniffing position).
- Ventilate lungs at about 20/min with bag-valve-mask or mouth to mask or mouth to mouth. An Air-viva using 8–10 L/min of oxygen is ideal if available.
- Intubate via mouth and secure, if necessary (must preoxygenate).
- If intubation not possible, use a needle crico-thyroidotomy as an emergency.
- Start external cardiac compression if pulseless or < 60/min (see Table 114.2). Use two fingers for infants < 1 year and one hand for children 1–8 years.

Guidelines

Differences in children's airways for intubation:
- epiglottis longer and stiffer, more horizontal
- larynx more anterior → difficult to intubate 'blind'
- cricoid ring is narrowest position → cuffed tube not required
- shorter trachea → increased risk intubating R main bronchus
- narrow airway → increased airway resistance.

Endotracheal size (internal diameter in mm): see Table 77.3.

Rule: $ETT \text{ (mm)} = \dfrac{\text{age in years}}{4} + 4$

or

the size of the child's little finger or nares

$ETT \text{ length (cm) oral} = \dfrac{\text{age in years}}{2} + 12$

nasal — add 3 cm

For basic schedule for CPR refer to Table 114.2.

Cardiac arrest due to asystole

Adrenaline (0.01 mg/kg of 1:1000 = 0.1 mL/kg of 1:10 000 solution) is the drug of choice. Subsequent doses of adrenaline given every 3–5 minutes can be up to 10–20 times the strength of the initial dose, i.e. 0.1–0.2 mg/kg. They can also be sprayed into the endotracheal tube.

Note: Once an endotracheal tube is in place, drugs used in paediatric CPR can be given by this route (exceptions are calcium preparations and sodium bicarbonate). Adrenaline, ligno-caine, naloxone and atropine are readily absorbed. The doses should be at least twice IV

Table 77.3   *Childhood intubation: tube size and insertion distance*[4]

Age	Internal diameter (mm)	Length to lip (cm)
newborn	3.0	8.5
1–6 months	3.5	10
6–12 months	4.0	11
2 years	4.5	12
4	5.0	14
6	5.5	15
8	6.0	16
10	6.5	17
12	7.0	18
14	7.5	19
adult	8.0	20

dosage and diluted in N saline. Rather than squirting in directly, put a feeding tube on the end of the syringe and flush in at least 2 mL volumes. Drugs can also be administered by the intraosseous route.[3]

Poisoning

Poisoning in children is a special problem in toddlers (accidental) and in adolescents (deliberate). Children of 1–2 years old are most prone to accidental poisoning. The most common cause of death in comatose patients is respiratory failure.

The common dangerous poisons in the past were kerosene and aspirin. Excluding household chemicals, camphor/moth balls, pesticides, insecticides and opiates, the dangerous drugs are:

- antidepressants, especially tricyclics
- antihypertensives
- anxiolytics, e.g. benzodiazepines
- chloral hydrate
- digoxin
- iron tablets
- Lomotil (diphenoxylate)
- paracetamol/acetaminophen
- potassium tablets
- quinine/quinidine
- salicylates, e.g. aspirin

In a UK study[5] the main cause of deaths from poisoning were (in order) tricyclics, salicylates, opiates including Lomotil, barbiturates, digoxin, orphenadrine, quinine, potassium and iron.

Principles of treatment[6,7]

The use of activated charcoal has become the key to treatment and is the 'universal antidote'.

- Identify the poison

- Support vital functions—ABCD
  Airway — relieve obstruction
  Breathing — ventilate with oxygen
  Circulation — treat hypotension/arrhythmias
  Dextrose — avoid severe hypoglycaemia
- Dilute the poison — give a cupful of milk or water to drink
- Remove the poison (for witnessed ingestion)
  — induce emesis (rarely employed):
  1. rub back of child's throat with spoon or spatula
  2. give syrup of ipecac (see Table 77.4) (still has limited use in the home in country areas); avoid common salt

Table 77.4   *Guidelines for syrup of ipecacuanha*

Dosage:
  < 1 year: do not give
  1 year: 15 mL
  2 years: 20 mL
  3 years: 25 mL
  4 years: 25 mL
  > 4 years: 30 mL
Follow with 100–200 mL water
Optimal time: within 30 minutes
Mean time to emesis—20 minutes
    (range 15–60 minutes)
If ineffective—repeat with ½ dose after 20 minutes

Contraindications:
  > 1 hour since ingestion
  rapidly acting convulsants
  acid
  alkali
  strychnine
  petroleum products
  • kerosene
  • petrol
  patient cannot sit up and hold a vomit bowl
  impaired consciousness
  • actual
  • anticipated

Note: The modern swing is away from emesis which is useful only for very recent ingestion (< 30 minutes) or for iron/slow K poisoning where concretions form in the stomach.

— gastric lavage: within 1 hour (refer Table 77.5 for guidelines) but also limited place
— gastric aspiration
• Delay absorption
  — activated charcoal (the preferred method)
    • 1 g/kg orally or via gastric tube (best) (refer Tables 77.6 and 77.7)
    • Multiple dose charcoal, 5–10 g every 4 hours or 0.25g/kg per hour for 12 hours, is effective
  — evaporated milk
    aspirin and petroleum products
• Administer antidote early (see Table 77.8)
• Treat any complications
  — respiratory failure
    • hypoventilation
    • apnoea
  — pulmonary aspiration of gastric contents
  — arrhythmias
  — hypotension
  — seizures
  — delayed effects,
    e.g. paracetamol (hepatotoxicity) tricyclics (arrhythmia)

Table 77.5 *Guidelines for gastric lavage*

Do within 60 minutes of ingestion
Ideally indicated for serious poisoning when a child is already intubated

Contraindications:
• stuporose or comatose
• absent gag reflex
  (unless endotracheal tube in situ)
• acid
• alkali

Method:
• child on left side
• head of bed tilted down
• insert orogastric tube (lubricated)

< 2 years	12–14 size FG
2–4	14–18 size FG
5–12	18–22 size FG
> 12	22–30

• check in stomach by aspiration
• instil 50–100 mL lukewarm tap water or saline via large syringe or funnel
• brief pause, then drain into bucket
• repeat often until washings clear
• use about 2–3 litres
• restrict the total volume to 40 mL/kg
• be careful of water intoxication

Table 77.6 *Drugs not absorbed by active charcoal*

Acids	Alcohols, e.g. ethanol
Alkalis	Iron
Boric acid	Iodines
Bromides	Lithium
Cyanide	Other heavy metals

Whole bowel irrigation
This is performed with a solution of polyethylene glycol and electrolytes (Golytely) via a nasogastric tube. It is usually limited to iron and lead, and slow-release drug preparations that don't bind to charcoal.

Investigations
• drug levels, e.g. paracetamol, aspirin, iron
• blood gas analysis
• X-ray
  — chest
  — abdomen, e.g. radiopaque iron tablets
  — skull
• ECG

Psychosocial care
The reasons for the poisoning need to be carefully evaluated and proper support and advice given.

Table 77.7 *Drugs successfully treated by repeated doses of activated charcoal*

Carbamazepine
Chlorpropamide
Cyclosporin
Dextropropoxyphene
Digoxin
Methotrexate
Phenobarbital
Phenytoin
Salicylate
Theophylline
Tricyclic antidepressant

Swallowed foreign objects
A golden rule
The natural passage of most objects entering the stomach can be expected.

Table 77.8 *Important antidotes for poisons*

Poison	Antidote
Benzodiazepines	flumazenil
Carbon monoxide	oxygen 100% hyperbaric oxygen
Cyanide	dicobalt edetate sodium nitrite sodium thiosulphate
Digoxin	digoxin-specific antibodies
Heavy metals, e.g. Pb, As, Hg, Fe	dimercaprol
Iron	desferrioxamine
Isoniazid	pyridoxine
Methanol, ethylene glycol	ethanol (ethyl alcohol)
Narcotics/opiates	naloxone (Narcan)
Organophosphates	atropine pralidoxamine (2-PAM)
Paracetamol (acetaminophen)	acetylcysteine (IV) (effective within 12 hours) consider up to 36 hours
Phenothiazines	benztropine

This includes:
- coins
- buttons
- sharp objects
- open safety pins
- glass (e.g. ends of thermometers)

Special cases are:
- very large coins: watch carefully
- hair clips (usually cannot pass duodenum if under 7 years)

Management
- Manage conservatively.
- X-ray all children (mouth to anus) on presentation.
- Investigate unusual gagging, coughing and retching with X-rays of the head, neck, thorax and abdomen (check nasopharynx and respiratory tract).
- Watch for passage of the foreign body in stool (usually 3 days).
- If not passed, order X-ray in one week.
- If a blunt foreign body has been stationary for 1 month without symptoms, remove at laparotomy.

Febrile convulsions

Diagnosis based on presence of fever, short duration and no clinical evidence of CNS pathology.
  Features:
- The commonest cause is an upper respiratory infection, e.g. the common cold or similar viral syndrome.
- About 5 per 100 incidence in children.
- Rare under 6 months and over 5 years.
- Commonest age range 9–20 months.
- Recurrent in up to 50% of children.
- Consider meningitis and lumbar puncture after first convulsion if less than 2 years or cause of fever not obvious.
- Epilepsy develops in about 2–3% of such children.

Management of the convulsion (if prolonged)
- Undress the child to singlet and underpants to keep cool.
- Maintain the airway and prevent injury.
- Place patient chest down with head turned to one side.
- Oxygen 8 L/min by mask.
- Give diazepam by one of two routes:
  IV 0.2 mg/kg, undiluted or diluted (10 mg in 20 ml N saline)
                or
  rectally 0.5 mg/kg (dilute with saline or in pre-prepared syringe) up to 10 mg or with suppository or rectal gel.

Note: Although the IV route is preferred, the rectal route is ideal in a home or office situation; e.g. consider a 2 year old child (weight 12 kg) with a persistent febrile convulsion. The dose of diazepam injectable is 0.5 mg/kg so 6 mg (1.2 mL) of diazepam is diluted with isotonic saline (up to 10 mL of solution) and the nozzle of the syringe pressed gently but firmly into the anus and injected slowly. *Observe carefully for respiratory depression.*

- Rectal paracetamol 15 mg/kg statim.

Meningitis or encephalitis

Diagnosing meningitis and encephalitis requires a high level of clinical awareness and watchfulness for the infective problem that appears more serious than normal. *Bacterial meningitis* is basically a childhood infection. Neonates and children aged 6–12 months are at the greatest risk. Most cases begin as septicaemia, usually via the nasopharynx.

Clinical presentations (typical)
Infancy:
- fever, pallor, vomiting, ± altered conscious state
- lethargic

- increasing irritability, with drowsiness
- refusing to feed, indifferent to mother
- neck stiffness
- Kernig's sign unreliable
- may be bulging fontanelle

Children over 3 years:
- meningeal irritation more obvious, e.g. headache, fever, vomiting, neck stiffness
- later: delirium, altered conscious state

Note: Antibiotics may mask symptoms.
Suspect meningitis if fever > 3 days in reasonably well child on antibiotics.[2]

Fulminating:
- dramatic sudden onset shock, purpura ± coma
- usually due to meningococcal septicaemia, also *Haemophilus influenzae* type B, *Streptococcus pneumoniae*

Treatment

If bacterial meningitis suspected, consider IV ceftriaxone or cefotaxime ± IV benzylpenicillin and admit to hospital for lumbar puncture and ongoing management. Consider dexamethasone.

Meningococcaemia[8,9]

Note: Treatment is urgent once suspected, e.g. petechial or purpuric rash on trunk and limbs.

- take blood culture if time and facilities permit (often impractical)
      then
- ceftriaxone 100 mg/kg IV (max 4 g) statim[9]
      or
   benzylpenicillin 60 mg/kg IV (max 2 g)
- admit to hospital

Treat contacts who:
- live in the household and < 24 months
- have kissed patient in the previous 10 days
- have attended the same daycare centre

For prophylaxis: rifampicin

   dose: adult — 600 mg
         child < 1 month — 5 mg/kg
         child > 1 month — 10 mg/kg
   give bd for 2 days

Acute epiglottitis

Acute epiglottitis due to *Haemophilus influenzae* is a life-threatening emergency in a child. A toxic febrile illness, with sudden onset of expiratory

stridor, should alert one to this potentially fatal condition. A high index of suspicion of epiglottitis is always warranted in such presentations.

Differential diagnosis

The main alternative diagnosis is viral laryngo-tracheobronchitis (croup). There are, however, significant clinical differences.

Epiglottitis is characterised by fever, a soft voice, lack of a harsh cough, a preference to sit quietly (rather than lie down) and especially by a soft stridor with a sonorous expiratory component (Fig. 77.1).

Croup is distinguished by a harsh inspiratory stridor, a hoarse voice and brassy cough.

Other differential diagnoses include tonsillitis, infectious mononucleosis and bacterial tracheitis. The clinical features of croup and epiglottitis are compared in Table 77.9.

Diagnostic tip

The child with epiglottitis usually sits still and the eyes follow you around the room because limited head movement protects the compromised airway.

Physical examination

DO NOT EXAMINE THE THROAT.
A swollen cherry-red epiglottis recognised on examination of the nasopharynx confirms the

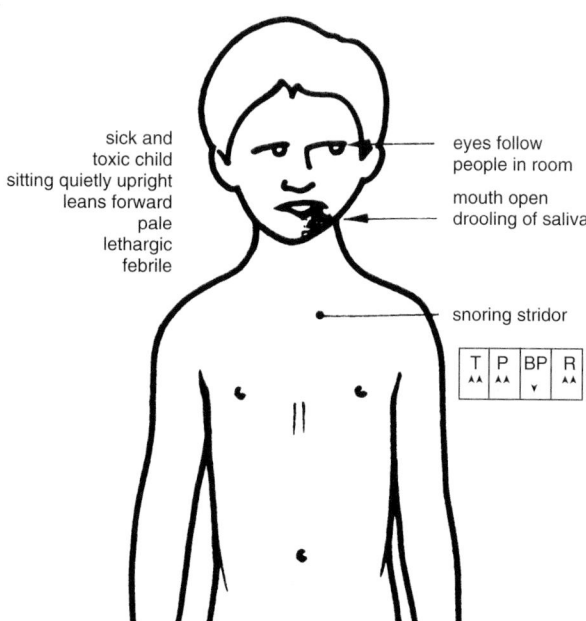

sick and toxic child
sitting quietly upright
leans forward
pale
lethargic
febrile

eyes follow people in room

mouth open drooling of saliva

snoring stridor

T	P	BP	R
▲▲	▲▲	▼	▲▲

Fig. 77.1 *Typical features of acute epiglottitis*

Table 77.9   *Comparison of clinical features of croup and acute epiglottitis*

	Croup	Epiglottitis
Epidemiology		
Periodicity	winter months, late autumn	any time of the year
Age	6 months to 6 years occasionally older	6 months to 6 years
Incidence	common	infrequent
Clinical		
Onset	prodrome of URTI or coryza 2 days	rapid 2–6 hours
Fever	variable, rarely above 39°C	usually above 39°C
Toxicity	often not anorexic drinking fluids looks like URTI	very lethargic looks ill, pale, drooling
Stridor	loud inspiratory, increased if upset harsh brassy cough	soft stridor, often barely audible expiratory 'flutter'
Pathology		
Causative organism	viral—mostly Parainfluenza 1	bacterial, mostly *H.influenzae* some B haemolytic streptococcus
Site	larynx, trachea, bronchi	epiglottis
Laboratory		toxic FBC, increased WCC +ve blood culture +ve epiglottis culture

Treatment
(refer to detailed notes)
	mild cases:
	• at home with moist air
	moderate:
	• admit to hospital
	• cool humified air
	• oral steroids
	• observe
	severe:
	• nurse in intensive care
	• dexamethasone IV 0.2 mg/kg
	• oral steroids
	• nebulised adrenaline 1:1000
	  solution (max. 5 mL)
		• airway support with nasotracheal
		  intubation, e.g. 48 hours
		• blood culture
		
		Antibiotic:
		3rd generation cephalosporin, e.g.
		cefotaxime or ceftriaxone
		
		Prevention
		• Hib vaccine

diagnosis. However, the initial diagnosis should be made on the clinical history and appearance of the child.

Direct examination using a spatula and torch should not be performed in the office but only where there are appropriate facilities for suction, endotracheal intubation and tracheostomy, as this procedure can precipitate laryngeal obstruction.

Almost all children with epiglottitis require nasotracheal intubation.

Management
Transporting the patient to hospital. After ringing the hospital to warn about the emergency the practitioner should escort the child to hospital in an ambulance (with the child sitting propped up on mother's knee) prepared to perform cricothyroidotomy using a large bore cannula in the unlikely event of sudden obstruction.

The primary objective, during transportation, is to keep the child calm. This is enhanced by having mother nurse the child during transfer.

If the child's condition deteriorates, administer 100% oxygen by mask. Most obstructed patients can be bagged and masked which is sufficient to maintain oxygenation. If obstruction occurs, use the cannula to provide an airway.

Method of emergency cricothyroidotomy (last resort)
• Lay the child across your knees with neck fully extended.

• Insert a number 14 needle or angiocath through the cricothyroid membrane.

Always try to intubate once before resorting to cricothyroidotomy.

Hospital treatment

Intubation: in theatre suck away profuse secretions and perform nasotracheal intubation

Antibiotics: chloramphenicol 40 mg/kg IV statim then 75 mg/kg/day IV (max. 3 g in 3 divided doses) 5 days (only if severe penicillin hypersensitivity)[8]
        or (preferable)
cefotaxime 150 mg/kg/day IV (max. 6 g/day in 3 divided doses)
        or
ceftriaxone 100 mg/kg to max. 1 g/day IV as single daily dose

Note: Continue therapy for 5 days. Early transfer to oral therapy, e.g. amoxycillin/clavulanate, is desirable.

Treatment of croup

Mild croup

Mild croup (barking cough, no stridor, hoarse voice):

• manage at home with moist air
• consider oral steroids

Moderate croup

Moderate croup (inspiratory stridor when upset):

• admit to hospital, e.g. emergency department
• cool humidified air
• oral steroids
    dexamethasone 0.15–0.3 mg/kg
        or
    prednisolone (tablets or oral solution) 1 mg/kg (2–3 doses)
     and/or (for children 2 or more years)
    budesonide 100 μg × 20 puffs or 2 mg nebulised
• observe for at least 4 hours

Severe croup

Severe croup (inspiratory stridor at rest, use of accessory muscles, patient restless and agitated):

• nurse in intensive care
• dexamethasone 0.2 mg/kg IV
       or 0.6 mg/kg IM
followed by oral steroids

• nebulised adrenaline 1:1000 solution 0.5 mL/kg/dose (to maximum 5 mL) (beware of possible rebound effect after 2–3 hours)

Note: Can use 5 ampoules of 1:1000 solution in a nebuliser run with oxygen 8 L/min

• have facilities for artificial airway
• may need endotracheal intubation for 48 hours

There is no place for cough medicines or antibiotics.

Bronchiolitis

• an acute viral illness due to RSV
• the commonest acute LRI in infants
• usual age 2 weeks to 9 months (up to 12 months)
• prodromal symptoms for 48 hours, e.g. coryza, irritating cough, then 3–5 days of more severe symptoms
• wheezy breathing—often distressed
• tachypnoea
• hyperinflated chest

Auscultation

• widespread fine crackles (not with asthma)
• frequent expiratory wheezes

X-ray. Hyperinflation of lungs with depression of diaphragm

Management

Admission to hospital is usual, especially with increasing respiratory distress reflected by difficulty in feeding (particularly less than half normal over 24 hours).

• minimal handling/good nursing care
• observation: colour, pulse, respiration, oxygen saturation (pulse oximetry)
• oxygen: to maintain PaO_2 above 90%
• fluids IV or by nasogastric tube if unable to feed orally
• antibiotics not indicated unless secondary bacterial infection

Very severe asthma

Very severe asthma in children should be referred to an intensive care unit.

• continuous nebulised 0.5% salbutamol via mask[4]
• oxygen flow 6 L/min through the nebuliser
• IV infusion of
    salbutamol 5 μg/kg/min
    hydrocortisone 4 mg/kg IV statim then 6 hourly

Common mistakes

- using assisted mechanical ventilation inappropriately (main indications are physical exhaustion and cardiopulmonary arrest—it can be dangerous in asthma)
- not giving high flow oxygen
- giving excessive fluid
- giving submaximal bronchodilator therapy

Breath-holding attacks

This is a dramatic emergency. There are two types: one is related to a tantrum (description follows) and the other is a simple faint.

Clinical features

- age group—usually 6 months to 6 years (peak 2–3 years)
- precipitating event (minor emotional or physical)
- children emit a long loud cry, then hold their breath
- they become pale and then blue
- if severe, may result in unconsciousness or even a brief tonic-clonic fit
- lasts 10–60 seconds

Management

- Reassure the parents that attacks are self-limiting, not harmful and not associated with epilepsy or mental retardation.
- Advise parents to maintain discipline and to resist spoiling the child.
- Try to avoid incidents known to frustrate the child or to precipitate a tantrum.

Note: Important childhood emergency drugs with dosages are presented in Table 77.10.

Aspirated foreign body

Parents or guardians may not give a history of inhalation. One in eight episodes is not witnessed.[4]

Table 77.10 *Important childhood emergency drugs (after Pitt)*

Drug	Route	Dose	Notes
Adrenaline 1:10 000	IV	0.1–0.2 mL/kg/dose	Anaphylaxis, asystole (repeat every 5 minutes until response)
Adrenaline 1:1000	Nebuliser	0.5 mL/kg/dose (maximum 5 mL)	LTB (patient must be admitted)
Aminophylline	IV slowly	5 mg/kg loading	Moderate to severe asthma
Atropine	IV	0.02 mg/kg	Bradycardia producing shock
Dextrose 50%	IV	1 mL/kg	Hypoglycaemia
Diazepam	IV PR	0.2 mg/kg 0.5 mg/kg	Seizures
Glucagon	IV or IM	0.1 mg/kg (maximum 1 mg)	Hypoglycaemia
Hydrocortisone	IV	4–8 mg/kg	Anaphylaxis, asthma
Morphine	IV or IM	0.1–0.2 mg/kg	Sedation, pain relief
Paraldehyde	PR	0.3 mL/kg (dilute 1:2 in peanut oil)	Seizures
Paracetamol	O	15–20 mg/kg loading	Fever
Salbutamol	Nebuliser	0.3 mL/kg	Asthma
Salbutamol	IV	5 µg/kg	
Sodium bicarbonate 8.4%	IV	2 mL/kg	Titrate against blood gases
Soluble insulin	IV infusion	0.1 u/kg/hr	Only if glucose > 14 mmol/L

IV: intravenous injection
PR: per rectum
IM: intramuscular injection
O: orally
LTB: laryngotracheal bronchitis (croup)

Note: Volume resuscitation: IV fluid bolus 20 mg/kg statim of crystalloid, e.g. N saline.

Symptoms

- choking or coughing episodes while eating nuts or similar food or while sucking a small object, e.g. plastic toy
- persistent coughing and wheezing ('all that wheezes is not asthma')
- sudden onset of first wheezing episode in a toddler with no past history of allergy, especially after a choking bout

Signs

- reduced or absent breath sounds over whole or part of a lung
- wheeze

Investigations

Chest X-ray (full inspiration and full expiration) to exclude an area of collapse or obstructive hyperinflation.

Note: Normal X-rays do not absolutely exclude a foreign body.

Management

First aid

- most cough out the FB, so encourage coughing
- a finger sweep helps, as do back blows and the Himlich manoeuvre (take care with viscera)

If complete obstruction—attempt removal of the FB with forceps. If unsuccessful, perform a tracheostomy or cricothyroidotomy.

Note: Once an FB has passed through the larynx it is very rare for there to be an immediate threat to life, so referral is usually quite safe.

Do not instrument the airways if the child is coping.

Bronchoscopy

Bronchoscopy is necessary in almost every child where there is a strong suggestion of an inhaled FB. It is difficult and requires an expert with appropriate facilities.

Anaphylaxis

The management of airway obstruction and hypotension can be summarised as:

- oxygen 6–8 L/min by mask
- adrenaline 0.1 mL/kg of 1:10 000 solution IV slowly

or

    adrenaline 0.01 mL/kg of 1:1000 IM

- nebulised salbutamol for bronchospasm
- colloid or crystalloid solution IV

If necessary: corticosteroid 8–10 mg/kg IV and antihistamine.

If persistent upper airways obstruction—try nebulised 1% adrenaline (max. 4 mL); intubation may be necessary. Admit to hospital and observe for at least 12 hours.

Status epilepticus

Ensure adequate oxygenation: attend to airway (e.g. Guedel tube): give oxygen.

Antiepileptic options include:[4]

- diazepam 0.2 mg/kg IV or 0.5 mg/kg per rectum
- clonazepam 0.25 mg ($<$ 1 year), 0.5 mg (1–5 years), 1 mg ($>$ 5 years)
- phenobarbitone 20 mg/kg slowly, repeated every 15–30 min if required
- phenytoin 15 mg/kg slowly over 20–30 minutes
- thiopentone: titrate the dose (usually 2–5 mg/kg)

If refractory (up to 60 min) use full anaesthetic.

Consider hyponatraemia as the cause of convulsions with meningitis.

Drowning

The differences between salt water and fresh water drowning are usually not clinically significant. If global hypoxic cerebral ischaemia and pulmonary aspiration, treat as follows:[4]

- adequate oxygenation and ventilation
- decompress stomach with nasogastric tube
- support circulation with IV infusion of colloid solution and dopamine 5–20 µg/kg per min
- mannitol 0.25–0.5 g/kg IV if cerebral oedema
- correct electrolyte disturbances, e.g. hypokalaemia
- give prophylactic penicillin

Intraosseous infusion[3]

In an emergency situation where intravenous access in a collapsed person (especially children) is difficult, parenteral fluid can be infused into the bone marrow (an intravascular space). Intraosseous infusion is preferred to a cutdown in children under 5 years. It is useful to practise the technique on a chicken bone.

Site of infusion

- adults and children over 5: distal end of tibia
- children under 5: proximal end of tibia

- the distal femur: 2–3 cm above condyles in midline is an alternative

Avoid growth plates, midshaft and the sternum.

Method for proximal tibia

Note: Strict asepsis is essential (skin preparation and sterile gloves).

- Inject local anaesthetic (if necessary).
- Choose 16 g intraosseous needle (Dieckmann modification) or a 16–18 g lumbar puncture needle (less expensive).
- Hold it at right angles to the anteromedial surface of the proximal tibia about 2 cm below the tibial tuberosity (Fig. 77.2). Point the needle slightly downwards, away from the joint space.

tibial tubercle

Insert midway between level of tibial tubercle and medial border of tibia, and 2 cm distal to the tibial tubercle

Fig. 77.2 *Intraosseous infusion*

- Carefully twist the needle to penetrate the bone cortex; it enters bone marrow with a sensation of giving way.
- Remove the trocar, aspirate a small amount of marrow to ensure its position.
- Hold the needle in place with a small POP splint.
- Fluid, including blood, can be infused with a normal IV infusion—rapidly or slowly.
- The infusion rate can be markedly increased by using a pressure bag at 300 mmHg pressure.

Serious gastroenterological conditions

GIT conditions that cause vomiting require careful evaluation because of potentially fatal outcomes.

Gastroenteritis

This condition should not be treated lightly. Assessment of general signs such as arousal, presence of pallor, degree of weight loss, fluids in and fluids out is important (pp. 401–404). If concerned or in doubt, arrange hospitalisation. The social situation needs to be taken into account.

Intussusception

It is important to recognise this condition as about 50% of infants with intussusception are not diagnosed on initial presentation.[2] Characteristic features include sudden-onset pallor which persists, episodic crying and vomiting. Rectal bleeding and an abdominal mass (see p. 255) are present in only 40% of cases.

Pyloric stenosis

Pyloric stenosis, which appears from 2 weeks to 3 months of age, should be suspected with projectile vomiting, acute weight loss and alkalosis. It must not be confused with projectile vomiting from overfeeding. If in doubt, expert ultrasound-ography of the pylorus will assist diagnosis.

Sudden infant death syndrome

Facts

- SIDS is the major cause of death between 1 and 12 months of age.
- The incidence is around 1 per 500 live births.
- The causes are unknown but risk factors have been identified.
- No investigations have identified susceptible infants.
- Although SIDS can recur in a family, the risk is small.

Risk factors

- Prone sleeping position
- Artificial feeding
- Passive smoking
- Hyperthermia
- Extreme prematurity < 32 weeks
- Parental narcotic/cocaine abuse
- Intercurrent viral infections

Preventive advice

- Place baby to sleep on its back (preferable) or side (unless special reason for placing it on its stomach, e.g. gastro-oesophageal reflux).
- Ensure the head is uncovered.
- Breast-feed.

- Ensure the baby is not exposed to cigarette smoking.
- Ensure the baby does not get overheated (sweating around the head and neck indicates the baby is too hot).

Reactions of bereaved parents
- may be hostility to GP, especially if recent examination
- may 'hear' the baby cry
- distressing dreams
- guilt/self-blame, especially mother
- psychiatric morbidity

Management of SIDS
- Allow parents to see or hold baby.
- Give explanations, including reasons for coroner's involvement.
- Provide bereavement counselling.
- Early contact with counsellors and continuing support.
- Revisit the home.
- Provide hypnotics (limited).
- Offer advice on lactation suppression.
- Remember: siblings can also experience grief reactions.

Apparent life-threatening episode (ALTE)
ALTE, or 'near-miss SIDS', is defined as a 'frightening' encounter of apnoea, colour change or choking. At least 10% will have another episode. Management includes admission to hospital for investigation and monitoring.

Guidelines for home apnoea monitoring
- ALTE
- subsequent siblings of SIDS victims
- twins of SIDS victims
- extremely premature infants

Obstructive sleep apnoea syndrome
A childhood disorder of breathing during sleep characterised by noisy, disturbed breathing and periods of apnoea. Leads to daytime sleepiness, disturbed behaviour and cognitive dysfunction. Requires referral.

References

1. Murtagh J. The anatomy of a rural practice. Aust Fam Physician, 1981; 10:564–567.
2. Hewson P, Oberklaid F. Recognition of serious illness in infants. Mod Med Aust, 1994; 37(7):89–96.
3. Tibballs J. Endotracheal and intraosseous drug administration for paediatric CPR. Aust Fam Physician, 1992; 21:1477–1480.
4. Efron D et al. *Paediatric handbook* (5th edn). Melbourne: Blackwell Science, 1996, 1–81.
5. Fraser NC. Accidental poisoning deaths in British children 1958–77. BMJ, 1980; 280: 1595.
6. Stevenson N. Drug overdose. Aust Fam Physician, 1989; 18:1235–1238.
7. Yuen A. Accidental poisoning in children. Patient Management, Nov. 1991; 39–45.
8. Mashford ML. *Antibiotic guidelines* (9th edn). Victorian Medical Postgraduate Foundation, 1996, 105–133.
9. Patel MS et al. New guidelines for management and prevention of meningococcal disease in Australia. Med J Aust, 1997; 166:598–601.

78
Adolescent health

—

The feeling of apartness from others comes to most with puberty, but it is not always developed to such a degree as to make the difference between the individual and his fellows noticeable to the individual.

W. Somerset Maugham (1874–1965)
Of Human Bondage

Adolescence is the transitional period of development between relatively dependent childhood and relatively independent adulthood.[1] The time of onset and duration varies from one person to another but it is generally considered to occur between the ages of 11 and 19 years. It is a difficult period of considerable physical and mental change in which the young person is trying to cope with an inner conflict of striving for independence while still relying on adult support. There are inevitable clashes with parents, especially during the turbulent years of 13 to 16.

Adolescent patients require special understanding and caring from their doctor. They are often hesitant in approaching adult caregivers but they have a great capacity to appreciate a caring empathic approach. In this setting the family doctor has an excellent opportunity to anticipate their problems, educate them and improve their health.[2]

In recent times reference is made to the young person in the context of health policies and young people are defined as those between the ages of 10 and 24 years.[1]

Adolescent development periods[3]

Early adolescence (puberty: 11–14 years) is dominated by adjustment to the physical and psychosexual changes and by the beginnings of psychological independence from parents. Girls generally advance through this stage more rapidly than boys.

Middle adolescence (the search for independence: 14–17 years) is a time where boys have caught up physically and psychologically with girls, so that peer group sexual attractions and relationships are common preoccupations at this stage. It is a phase of peer group alliances, clothes, music, jargon and food and drink.[3] The average age for first sexual intercourse of both sexes is 16 years. It is a stage where intellectual knowledge' and cognitive processes become quite sophisticated. Experimentation and risk-taking behaviour is a feature.

Late adolescence (maturity: 17–19 years) is the stage of reaching maturity and leads to more self-confidence with relationships and successful rapport with parents. Thought is more abstract and reality-based.

Major areas of health problems[1]

- Psychological health problems including depression, suicide and attempted suicide
- Injuries including sporting injuries, motor vehicle accidents and interpersonal violence
- Risk-taking behaviour including drug abuse
- Sexual adjustment including unsafe sexual practices and teenage pregnancy
- Eating disorders including obesity, fast food, bulimia nervosa and anorexia nervosa (refer to Chaps 70 and 71)
- Chronic illness and disability including survivors of inherited disorders
- Asthma, which is the leading reason for Victorian Public Hospital admissions for both sexes in the 10–14 year age group[1]
- Overexposure to sunlight

Myths about the adolescent patient

The following are myths that some practitioners feel apply to the adolescent:

• different from adults in needs
• 'superficial' thinkers
• represent a 'quick' consultation
• shun personal questions
• resent invasion of space

It is important to treat them as normal human beings.

Hallmarks of the adolescent

The main hallmarks of the adolescent[2] are:

• self-consciousness
• self-awareness
• self-centredness
• lack of confidence

These basic features lead to anxieties about the body, and so many adolescents focus on their skin, body shape, weight and hair. Concerns about acne, curly hair, round shoulders and obesity are very common.

There are usually special concerns about boy–girl relationships and maybe guilt or frustration about sexual matters. Many adolescents therefore feel a lack of self-worth or have a poor body image. They are very private people, and this must be respected. While there are concerns about their identity, parental conflict, school, their peers and the world around them, there is also an innate separation anxiety.

Needs of the adolescent

Adolescents have basic needs that will allow them the optimal environmental conditions for their development:

• 'room' to move
• privacy and confidentiality
• security (e.g. stable home)
• acceptance by peers
• someone to 'lean on' (e.g. youth leader)
• special 'heroes'
• establishment of an adult sexual role
• respect
• at least one close trustworthy friend

Rebelliousness

It is quite normal for normal parents and normal teenagers to clash and get into arguments. Adolescents are usually suspicious of and rebellious against convention and authority (parents, teachers, politicians, police and so on). This attitude tends to fade after leaving school (at around 18 years of age).

Common signs are:

• criticising and questioning parents
• putting down family members or even friends
• unusual, maybe outrageous, fashions and hairstyles
• experimenting with drugs such as nicotine and alcohol
• bravado and posturing
• unusual, often stormy, love affairs

Signs of out-of-control behaviour are:[4]

• refusal to attend school
• vandalism and theft
• drug abuse
• sexual promiscuity
• eating disorders: anorexia, bulimia, severe obesity
• depression

Note: Beware of suicide if there are signs of depression.

The clinical approach

Managing behavioural disorders or out-of-control behaviour demands tact and sensitivity on the part of the family doctor. It is important to interview the adolescent separately. The usual comprehensive medical history including psychosocial features is vital, particularly the family interrelationships (Table 78.1). Specifically it is appropriate to enquire about the adolescent's family relationships (parents and siblings), relationships with peers, drug taking, medical problems in the family, and parental abuse (sexual, physical, emotional or neglect).

Consider the mnemonic HEADS in the history:[2]

   H — home
   E — education, employment, economic situation
   A — activities, affect, ambition, anxieties
   D — drugs, depression
   S — sex, stress, suicide, self-esteem

During this process it is necessary to be aware of the fundamental development tasks of adolescence, namely:[4,5]

Table 78.1 *Basic clinical information (after D. Young)*[4]

History
- General history
- Drug history
- Psychological
  - Personality
    - introverted
    - withdrawn
    - anxious
  - Stress
    - school
    - peers
    - home
  - Depression
- Parent–adolescent relationship
  - Overprotectiveness/distant
  - Separation anxiety
  - Physical or sexual abuse
- Family interrelationships
  - Marital conflict
  - Medical problems
  - Alcohol abuse

Physical examination

Investigations Keep to bare minimum.

- establishing identity and self-image
- emancipation from the family and self-reliance
- establishing an appropriate adult sexual role
- developing a personal moral code
- making career and vocational choices
- ego identity and self-esteem

It is necessary to conduct a physical examination and order very basic investigations if only to exclude organic disease and provide the proper basis for effective counselling. The physical examination should be conducted with sensitivity.

Counselling

Counselling the adolescent involves several important principles and strategies, including:

- seeing the patient alone
- seeing parents and patient together from time to time
- confidentiality and trust
- sensitivity
- engendering the feeling that you are their doctor
- encouraging free talking and then listening carefully
- time and patience
- non-judgmental behaviour
- reassurance
- explanation
- acting as their advocate and friend

- showing genuine respect for their concerns and viewpoint

Intervention strategies on behalf of the adolescent are outlined in Table 78.2.

Areas of counselling and anticipatory guidance that are most relevant are:

- emotional problems/depression
- significant loss, e.g. breakdown of 'first love'
- sexuality
- contraception
- guilt about masturbation or other concerns

Advice to parents

Wise parenting can be difficult, because one cannot afford to be either overprotective or too distant. A successful relationship depends on good communication, which means continuing to show concern and care but being flexible and giving the adolescent 'space' and time.

Important management tips are:

- Treat adolescents with respect.
- Be non-judgmental.
- Stick to reasonable ground rules of behaviour (e.g. regarding alcohol, driving, language).
- Do not cling to them or show too much concern.
- Listen rather than argue.
- Listen to what they are *not* saying.
- Be flexible and consistent.
- Be available to help when requested.
- Give advice about diet and skin care.
- Talk about sex and give good advice, but only when the right opportunity arises.

Healthy distraction

Most authorities say that the best thing to keep adolescents healthy and adjusted is to be active and interested. Regular participation in sporting

Table 78.2 *Intervention strategies on behalf of the adolescent (after D. Young)*[4]

School
- academic assessment (student services)
- pupil welfare co-ordinator

Family
- simple counselling, e.g. letting go
- family therapy

Adolescent
- direct communication about stress
- be the adolescent's advocate, not the parents'
- psychiatric or psychologist referral

---

activities and other hobbies such as bushwalking, skiing and so on with parents or groups is an excellent way to help them cope with this important stage of their lives.

Depression, parasuicide and suicide

When dealing with adolescents it is important always to be on the lookout for depression and the possibility of suicide, which is the second most common cause of death in this group. Males successfully complete suicide four times more often than females, while females attempt suicide 8–20 times more often than males.

The features of depression are presented in Chapter 16 but it is worth looking for the following indicators of depression:

- sleep disturbances
- eating disorders
- apathy towards friends, school and family
- sense of worthlessness
- deterioration of school performance
- crying and emotional lability
- psychosomatic symptoms
- preoccupation with death and dying
- suicide attempts (parasuicide)

It is important not to be afraid to enquire about thoughts of suicide as it gives teenagers a chance to unburden themselves; it is not provoking them to contemplate suicide. Parasuicide is a term coined to differentiate suicide attempts from suicide itself. Identification of risk factors as presented in Table 78.3[6] certainly requires positive intervention in the depressed teenager. Such teenagers are especially vulnerable to a precipitating event, which can be unemployment, significant loss such as death, divorce, separation, relationship break-up, anniversary of a loss or some special celebration, additional stress or conflict and poor health.

Depression and suicidal thoughts can respond very well to basic counselling but psychiatric referral is advisable. Controlled clinical trials have not demonstrated the value of tricyclic antidepressants but some agents may be considered in adolescent depression with psychotic features.[7]

The basic tasks facing the GP in managing suicidal behaviour in adolescents are summarised in Table 78.4.

Table 78.4 *The 4 R tasks of managing suicidal behaviour in adolescents*

Task	Strategies
Recognising the signs	• be aware and alert • ask good questions
Raising the issue	• establish rapport and listen • be direct in questioning • ask directly about suicidal thoughts • do not swear secrecy
Risk assessment (see Table 16.2, sad person's index)	• suicidal ideations • suicidal plan • previous attempts • precipitating events • change in daily routine • mood changes • substance abuse • supports • access to weapons/drugs
Responding	• genuine concern and support • proposed management plan • access supports • antidepressants generally of little value • share the care • appropriate referral • assertive follow-up

Table 78.3 *Risk factors in suicide attempts (after P Birleson)[6]*

- Previous threats or attempts at suicide*
- Limited problem-solving and coping strategies
- Unsupportive families with or without marital conflict
- History of separations, psychiatric disorder, alcohol or drug abuse in family
- Family history or culture of suicide attempts
- Family disorganisation and actual neglect or abuse
- Male*
- Major relationship disturbances with social isolation and/or aggression
- Indicators of psychiatric disorders, especially:
    major depression*
    school refusal
    self-injurious behaviour
    psychosis
    alcohol/drug abuse
    personality disorder
- Availability of guns, psychotropic drugs, ropes, etc.*

* These items are the most lethal risk factors.

Practice tips in handling adolescents

- Adolescents need support and understanding.
- They need just one good personal relationship, that one good friend they can relate to and rely on.
- They also need a good relationship with their family doctor.

- Two good questions to ask the problematic adolescent including the obsessive compulsive:
  — Do you ever have silly thoughts?
  — Do you do silly things?
- Don't be judgmental.
- Confidentiality is of great importance to adolescents.

References

1. Bowes G, Patton G. Adolescent health. In: Efron D. *Paediatric handbook* (5th edn). Melbourne: Blackwell Science, 1996, 309–317.

2. Bennett DL. Understanding the adolescent patient. Aust Fam Physician, 1988; 17:345–346.

3. Clarke S. How to treat the adolescent. Aust Dr Weekly, 1991, 7 June; i–viii.

4. Young D. The troubled adolescent. Aust Fam Physician, 1991; 20:395–397.

5. Abery C. The difficult adolescent. Aust Fam Physician, 1991; 20:383–385.

6. Birleson P. Depression and suicide in adolescence. Aust Fam Physician, 1988; 17:331–333.

7. Moulds RW et al. *Psychotropic guidelines* (3rd edn), Victorian Postgraduate Medical Foundation, 1996–97,156.

PART 5

WOMEN'S HEALTH

———

79

Cervical cancer and Pap smears

—

If all women have regular Pap smears, one every two years, we can prevent 90% of all cervical cancers.

Dr Gabriele Medley
Time, 24 April 1995

Carcinoma of the cervix

Carcinoma of the cervix is the most common malignancy in women worldwide; it is the sixth most common in Australia[1] and seventh in the United States of America.[2] The incidence of invasive cervical cancer rises steadily from age 20 to 50 and then remains relatively steady.

The most common form of cervical cancer is squamous cell carcinoma (SCC) 80–85%, with adenocarcinoma representing 12–15%.[2]

A striking epidemiological feature about cervical cancer is that it is a disorder related to sexual activity. It is almost non-existent in virgins but has an increased incidence in women with multiple partners and those who began sexual activity at an early age. Thus epidemiological studies indicate that cervical cancer is a sexually transmitted disease (Table 79.1).

Facts and figures
- Invasive cervical cancer is almost unknown in women under the age of 20, and very rare before age 25.
- There are two small peaks of incidence, in the late 30s and late 60s.[1]
- The lifetime probability of an Australian woman developing cancer is 1 in 90.[3]
- On average, cervical cancer takes at least a decade to develop from a focus of cervical intraepithelial neoplasia.[4]
- SCC of the cervix occurs almost exclusively in women who have had coitus.

- The earlier the age of first intercourse the greater the chance of developing cervical cancer.
- Invasive cervical cancer is a disease for which definite curable premalignant lesions can be identified using a Papanicolaou's (Pap) smear as a screening test.
- The incidence of cervical cancer has been decreased significantly through the screening procedures of the Pap smear, colposcopy and colposcopically directed cervical biopsy.
- Poor Pap smear technique is a common cause of a false negative result.
- The GP needs to achieve the best possible cervical cell sample and forward it to the best possible cytology laboratory.
- New methods of laboratory examination of the smear include Papnet, which involves computer scanning of the smear, and ThinPrep whereby a liquid-based sample is prepared.

Basic pathology
The focus of attention is the transformation zone (Fig. 79.1) where columnar cells lining the endocervical canal undergo metaplasia to squamous cells—in the region of the squamocolumnar junction. It is important clinically to realise that this transformation zone can extend with progressive metaplasia of columnar epithelium and so the squamocolumnar junction may recede into the endocervical canal. This is a feature in postmenopausal women (Fig. 79.2). As squamous cell carcinoma almost always arises in the transformation zone it is vital that cells are taken from it when performing a Pap smear.

Cervical intraepithelial neoplasia (CIN)
Cellular changes can occur in the transformation zone for a variety of reasons, including invasion

Table 79.1 *Cervical cancer and risk factors*

Age	increased	after 55
Sexuality	increased	• with multiple and or promiscuous sex partners • early age for first intercourse • early age first pregnancy
Viruses	increased	after herpes II or wart virus infection (probable)
Occupation	increased	in prostitutes (decreased in nuns)
Parity	increased	multiparity
Socioeconomic status	increased	with low socioeconomic status

Fig. 79.1 *The transformation zone: it is vital that Pap smears take cells from this zone*

with human papilloma virus (HPV). One such important change is cervical dysplasia, now known as cervical intraepithelial neoplasia (CIN). CIN has the potential to become invasive cervical cancer.

Staging of CIN:

CIN 1   mild dysplasia (outer third of epithelium involved)

CIN 2   moderate dysplasia (two-thirds of epithelium involved)

CIN 3   severe dysplasia/carcinoma *in situ* (full thickness)

Natural history of CIN

CIN may return to normal, persist or eventually progress to invasive cervical cancer. The reported progression times to cervical cancer range from one to 30 years. On average it takes at least 10 years, so it is considered that 2-yearly Pap smears are a reasonable safety margin.

However, women with histologically confirmed CIN require a colposcopic assessment.

Figure 79.3 illustrates the disease spectrum of cervical neoplasia.

Clinical presentation

Many patients with cervical cancer are asymptomatic and when early symptoms do arise they are often dismissed as of little consequence.

Symptoms, if present, may be:
• vaginal bleeding, esp. postcoital bleeding
• vaginal discharge
• symptoms of advanced disease, e.g. vaginal urine or flatus, weakness

Screening recommendations

Routine Pap smears:

• Perform every two years for women with no clinical evidence of cervical pathology (some authorities recommend annual smears).
• Perform from beginning of sexual activity up to 70 years.
• Begin Pap smears at 18–20 years or 1–2 years after first sexual intercourse (whichever is later).
• Cease at 70 years in those who have had two normal Pap smears within the last five years.
• Perform a Pap smear on women over 70 years if they request it or if they have never had a smear.
• Ideally, practices should have a reminder or a recall system.

Women who have never engaged in coitus do not need Pap smears. Six-monthly or 12-monthly screening on young asymptomatic women provides only minimal benefit compared with two-year intervals.

Hysterectomy

Smears are needed if the cervix was not completely removed. Vaginal vault smears are

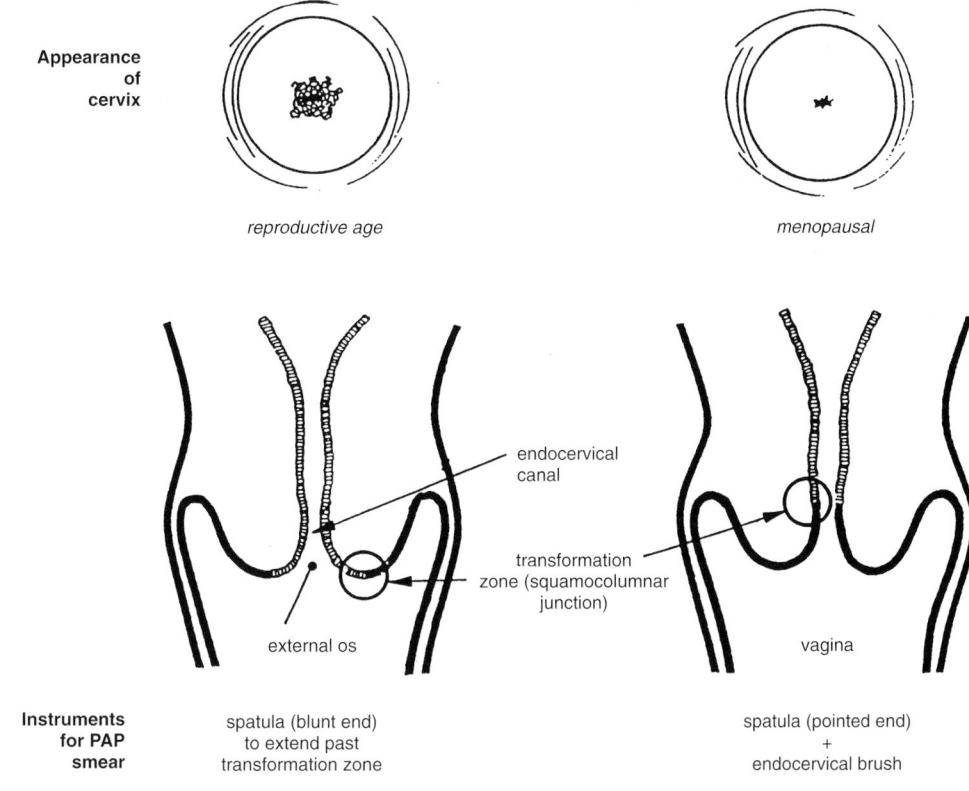

Fig. 79.2 *Changing position of the transformation zone with age, and a selection of sampling instruments according to its position (the Cervex sampler can be used as an alternative to the spatula)*

needed if there is a history of gynaecological dysplasia or malignancy.

Taking a Pap smear[1]
The importance of a good specimen

The optimal Pap smear contains:

- sufficient mature and metaplastic squamous cells to indicate adequate sampling from the whole of the transformation zone
- sufficient endocervical cells to indicate that the upper limit of the transformation zone was sampled; and to provide a sample for screening of adenocarcinoma and its precursors.

Optimal timing of specimens

- The best time is any time after the cessation of the period.
- Avoid smear-taking during menstruation.
- Avoid in the presence of obvious vaginal infection.
- Avoid within 24 hours of use of vaginal creams or pessaries or douching.

Communicating with the pathologist

Good communication with the pathologist is essential. It is important to provide basic details about the reason for the Pap smear and the clinical history on the pathology form sent to the laboratory. Use the opportunity also for breast examination and checking of SBE technique.

The method

1. *Education and explanation*

   Take time to explain the reason for taking the Pap smear, especially if it is the first. Emphasise that it is mainly a preventive measure to detect and treat early cell changes that could develop into cancer. Anatomical models, sample instructions or charts are useful in describing the procedure. Explain that it does not hurt and doesn't take long, that it may be

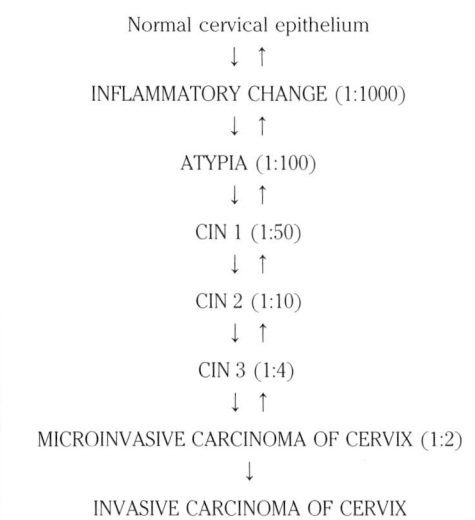

Normal cervical epithelium
↓ ↑
INFLAMMATORY CHANGE (1:1000)
↓ ↑
ATYPIA (1:100)
↓ ↑
CIN 1 (1:50)
↓ ↑
CIN 2 (1:10)
↓ ↑
CIN 3 (1:4)
↓ ↑
MICROINVASIVE CARCINOMA OF CERVIX (1:2)
↓
INVASIVE CARCINOMA OF CERVIX

Fig. 79.3 *Disease spectrum of cervical neoplasia (risk of developing invasive carcinoma of cervix in parenthesis)* ADAPTED FROM CERVICAL NEOPLASIA[5] WITH PERMISSION FROM MIMS AUSTRALIA, A DIVISION OF MEDIMEDIA AUSTRALIA PTY LIMITED

uncomfortable but slow deep breathing will help relaxation and make it easier. It is preferable to talk to the patient during the examination with appropriate explanation. It is advisable for a male doctor to have a chaperone present.

2. *Equipment*
   Prepare the following equipment:
   • adequate light source
   • speculum (preferably bivalve) warmed under lukewarm water
   • glass slide labelled in pencil with the woman's name and date of birth
   • spray fixative
   • plastic gloves for both hands
   • smear-taking instruments; choose from:
     — Ayer's spatula, wooden or plastic
     — Cervex sampler
     — endocervical brush

3. *Positioning*
   The supine position is uually best (Fig. 79.4). The left lateral position can be used if smears are difficult to obtain, e.g. older women with lax anterior vaginal walls, older women with poor hip mobility and the very embarrassed patient. The Sims exaggerated left lateral position (Fig. 79.5) provides better exposure of the vulva but requires more manipulation of the patient.

Fig. 79.4 *The supine or dorsal position is the best position for the speculum examination and subsequent bimanual palpation*

Fig. 79.5 *The Sims exaggerated left lateral position*

4. *Inserting the speculum*[7]

Avoid using lubricating jelly on the speculum blades. Warming the speculum with water should provide adequate lubrication. Gently spread the labia with a gloved hand and introduce the speculum with the blades vertical or at 45° from the vertical. Gently advance the blades with slow firm pressure towards the rectum as far as possible. Rotate the blades during the process until they are horizontal and exerting gentle pressure against the posterior wall of the vagina.

5. *Visualising the cervix*

Good lighting and exposure of the cervix is essential. Note any significant features or abnormalities of the cervix. Reassure the woman if the cervix looks normal with a comment such as 'Your tissues look very healthy'.

A cervical ectropion is normal in most premenopausal women and was formerly incorrectly called an erosion.

6. *Taking the smear*

Choose the sampling instrument that best suits the shape of the cervix and os. Place Ayre's spatula firmly on the os and rotate it through 360°, ensuring that the whole transformation zone is sampled (Fig. 79.6a).

If the squamous columnar junction is not visible (lying within the endocervical canal), use both spatula (first) and the cytobrush (Fig. 79.6b). The cytobrush (tends to cause bleeding) should be advanced until only the lower bristles are still visible, then rotated twice through 360°. The cytobrush should be avoided in pregnant women.

After removing the speculum, perform a bimanual pelvic examination.

7. *Preparing the slide*

Transfer the cervical cell sample on to a glass slide with an even spreading motion (Fig. 79.6c,d). Fix immediately with spray or alcohol (Fig. 79.6e).

8. *Follow-up*

Discuss mutually suitable arrangements to ensure that the woman obtains the result of the smear whether it is positive or negative. Inform her when her next smear is likely to be due (special cards are available) and arrange to send a reminder note.

The explanation of the results, especially if there is CIN present (a variety of abnormal smear), should be crystal clear to the patient.

(a)

(b)

(c)

(d)

(e)

Fig. 79.6 *Method of smear taking and preparing the slide*

Abnormal cervical cytology

Confirmation of the Pap smear result is by colposcopy and/or by a biopsy and appropriate referral should be arranged without delay.

Inaccurate results can be caused by:[7]

- using dirty glass slides
- using lubricants or doing pelvic examinations before taking the smear
- insufficient material
- endocervical cells not being taken in the smear, i.e. taken from the wrong site
- a thick film with an inadequate spread of material
- air-drying before fixing
- smear not being fixed for long enough or the solution of alcohol being too weak
- the slide not being dry before being placed in the cardboard container (this encourages fungal overgrowth).

Abnormal Pap smears

Follow the guidelines in Table 79.2 for the abnormal smear result.

Post-treatment assessment

For a high-grade epithelial abnormality (CIN 2–3), repeat the smear at 6-monthly intervals for 1 year,

then yearly. For a low-grade epithelial abnormality, repeat the smear yearly, reverting to 2-yearly after two successive normal smears.

Prevention of cervical cancer

'In other words, chastity and fidelity are recommended for those who can, and condoms for those who cannot'.[8] This statement is a succinct recommendation for prevention and includes:

- People should have intercourse with only one partner.
- The male should use a condom on each occasion if either sexual partner is unsure of the other's previous behaviour.
- Those at risk should be counselled accordingly.

Other preventive measures include:

- Women should have Pap smears at least two-yearly.
- Use of beta-carotene has a protective effect against cervical cancer, so 'both sexes would be well advised to ensure regular intake of green leaf and orange vegetables in their diet'.[8]

Table 79.2 *Guidelines for abnormal Pap smears*[6]

Pap smear report	Investigation and management
No endocervical cells	Repeat in 2 years
Negative smear—inflammatory cells	Repeat smear in 2 years
Unsatisfactory smear	Repeat smear in 6–12 weeks (allows regeneration of cells)
Low-grade epithelial abnormalities	
Non-specific atypia and minor squamous cell changes	Repeat smear at 12 monthly intervals until reverts to normal
Minor changes in endocervical glandular cells	Repeat smear in 6 months with cytobrush and spatula; if abnormal, refer to gynaecologist
Human papilloma virus (HPV) with associated cell changes	Repeat smear at 6 monthly intervals; if cell changes persist after 12 months, refer for colposcopy
Possible CIN1	As above
CIN1/mild dysplasia	Refer for colposcopy and, if indicated, biopsy
High-grade epithelial abnormalities	
CIN2/moderate dysplasia	Refer for colposcopy and directed biopsy
CIN3/severe dysplasia	Refer for colposcopy and directed biopsy with definitive treatment if confirmed
Invasive squamous cell carcinoma or adenocarcinoma	Refer to appropriate specialist gynaecologist or unit
Inconclusive—raising possibility of high-grade disease	Refer for colposcopy and possible biopsy

Advice and reassurance should be given in a diplomatic way that does not produce guilt feelings. This includes reassurance that not all cervical cancer is sexually transmitted, that women with only one partner may develop cervical cancer and that sexual contact with a male partner who has had the wart virus does not always result in cancer of the cervix.[8]

References

1. Screening for the prevention of cervical cancer. Australia: Department of Health, Housing and Community Services, 1991, 1–26.

2. Rakel RE. *Essentials of family practice.* Philadelphia: Saunders, 1993, 130–131.

3. Giles G, Armstrong GK, Smith LR (eds). *Cancer in Australia.* National Cancer Statistics Clearing House. Scientific Publications No. 1, Australasian Association of Cancer Registries and Australian Institute of Health, Melbourne, 1987.

4. Day NE. Screening for cancer of the cervix. J Epi Comm Health, 1989; 43:103–106.

5. Kennedy L, O'Connor DT. Cervical neoplasia. In: MIMS Disease Index (2nd edn). Sydney: IMS Publishing, 1996, 102–105.

6. Weisberg E. Making the Pap smear better. Mod Med Aust, 1994; 37:52–61.

7. Craig S. The smear test. Aust Fam Physician, 1985; 14:1092–1094.

8. Tattersall M. *Preventing cancer.* Sydney: Australian Professorial Publications, 1988, 182–197.

80
Family planning

—

*The Membranous Envelope (condom) is prepared
from the bladder of a fish caught in the Rhine. Its
extreme thinness does not in the least interfere with
the pleasure of the act . . . [its use] is of the greatest
utility because, while it is a sure preventive of
conception, it also prevents either party from
contracting disease*

Edward Bliss Foote 1864
Medical Common Sense

Effective family planning requires a good understanding of the function of the menstrual cycle,
whether it is for the purpose of conception or
contraception.

The main consultation is the presentation of a
young woman for contraceptive advice. It is a
very critical visit and provides an excellent
opportunity to develop a good rapport with the
patient and provide education and counselling
about important health concerns, such as health
promotion, menses regulation, sexual activity,
planned parenthood, fertility and infertility, pregnancy prevention, STD prevention, immunisation and cervical smears.[1]

In counselling and treating patients, especially
teenagers, confidentiality is of paramount importance. The issues and contraceptive methods
can be confusing so careful education using
charts and other aids is recommended to
enhance the therapeutic relationship and facilitate better compliance.[1]

It is worth discussing the patient's attitude to
pregnancy, including the fear of pregnancy and
the possible reaction to contraceptive failure.

Fertility control

The choice of contraceptive methodology will
be determined not only by individual needs,
personal preference and resources but also by
its safety and incidence of side effects.

It is worth emphasising that the estimated risk
of death associated with child-bearing (1 in
10 000 in developed countries) is higher than the
risk of death associated with all methods of contraception, with two exceptions: women over 35
years of age who smoke and take the combined
oestrogen-progestogen oral contraceptive, and
those over 40 years of age taking this type of
preparation.[2] In developed countries of the
western world the most widely used methods, in
order of preference, are combined oral contraceptives (COC), condoms, diaphragms, intrauterine devices, spermicidal agents and rhythm.[2]

A comparison of the efficacy of the various
contraceptive methods is presented in Table
80.1.

More than half the pregnancies in the United
States are unintended and occur because of non-
use of contraception, failure of a specific
method or discontinuation of contraception.[1,3]

For women at risk of acquiring STDs the
choice of contraception has to consider methods
that protect against both pregnancy and STDs.

Steroidal contraception

Methods of steroidal contraception include:[4]

- combined oral contraceptive pill (COC)
- progestogen-only pill (POP)
- injectables
- postcoital contraception
- implants (Norplant—LNG)
- levonorgestrel-releasing Nova-T
- progestogen-releasing vaginal rings
- oestrogen-progestogen-releasing vaginal rings

Table 80.1 *Effectiveness of contraceptive methods*[3,8]

Method	Effectiveness (pregnancies per 100 years of use) Lowest expected (reliable consistent user)
Natural rhythm methods	20–30
• Billings ovulation (cervical mucus) method	3
Withdrawal (coitus interruptus)	20–25
Spermicides	
• vaginal sponge	10
• diaphragm (with spermicide)	15
• condoms	10–15
Intrauterine devices	3–5
Oral contraceptives	
• combined	1–3
• progestogen only	3
Depomedroxyprogesterone acetate	0.1
Female sterilisation	0.02
Male sterilisation	0.15

Combined oral contraception

Combined oral contraceptives (COCs) usually contain a low-dose oestrogen and a moderate dose of progestogen. The main mode of action of COC is inhibition of hypothalamic and pituitary function leading to anovulation.[2]

Which oestrogen to use[4]

Mestranol and ethinyloestradiol (EO) are about equipotent. Mestranol undergoes metabolic conversion to EO in the liver before it exerts its contraceptive effect. EO is therefore the oestrogen of choice.

Which progestogen to use[4]

All progestogens are nor-testosterone derivatives and exhibit a variety of non-progestogenic actions.

The norethisterone (NET) group includes norethisterone acetate, ethynodiol acetate and lynestrenol. The last three progestogens are converted to NET before exerting any contraceptive activity.

Levonorgestrel (LNG) is ten times more potent than NET. It has less effect on the coagulation system than NET and is therefore the preferred progestogen.

Gestogens are the 'third generation' progestogens and include desogestrel, gestodene, norgestimate and cyproterone acetate. These agents, which are less androgenic than NET and LNG, have been implicated with an increased risk of thromboembolism but the data are of doubtful validity.

Starting the pill: which COC to use[4]

The aim is to provide good cycle control and effective contraception with the least side effects using a pill of the lowest dose. The past menstrual history and contraceptive use of the patient should be documented and taken into account in selecting the appropriate COC. Various COC preparations available in Australia are listed in Table 80.2.[5,6]

A suitable first choice is a pill containing 20–35 µg of oestrogen: either the triphasic or, preferably, the monophasic pill.

- monophasic pills, e.g.   Nordette, Brevinor, Microgynon 30, Levlen ED
- triphasic pills, e.g.   Triphasil, Triquilar

Education and counselling is very important for the woman starting the pill. Suitable patient education should be given. The pill can be used safely up to 50 years of age.

Table 80.2 *Combined oral contraceptive pill formulations*

Oestrogen	Dose (μg)	Progestogen	Dose (μg)	Trade name
Monophasic				
Ethinyloestradiol	20	Levonorgestrel	100	Microgynon 20, Loette
Ethinyloestradiol	30	Levonorgestrel	150	Nordette, Levlen ED
				Microgynon 30, Monofeme 28
Ethinyloestradiol	30	Gestodene	75	Femoden ED, Minulet 28
Ethinyloestradiol	30	Desogestrel	150	Marvelon
Ethinyloestradiol	35	Cyproterone acetate	2000	Diane-35 ED
Ethinyloestradiol	35	Norethisterone	500	Brevinor, Norimin
Ethinyloestradiol	35	Norethisterone	1000	Brevinor-1, Norimin-1
Ethinyloestradiol	50	Levonorgestrel	125	Nordette 50, Microgynon 50
Ethinyloestradiol	50	Levonorgestrel	250	Nordiol
Mestranol	50	Norethisterone	1000	Norinyl-1
Ethinyloestradiol	50	Ethynodiol diacetate	500	Ovulen 0.5/50
Ethinyloestradiol	50	Ethynodiol diacetate	1000	Ovulen 1/50
Biphasic				
Ethinyloestradiol	50	Levonoregestrel	50, 125	Biphasil, Sequilar
Triphasic				
Ethinyloestradiol	30, 40	Levonorgestrel	50, 75, 125	Triphasil, Triquilar
				Trifeme 28, Logynon ED
Ethinyloestradiol	35	Norethisterone	500, 1000	Synphasic, Improvil 28 day
Ethinyloestradiol	30, 40	Gestodene	50, 70, 100	Tri-Minulet 28
				Trioden ED

Specific patient groups[6]

Adolescents. The COC can be prescribed once menstruation has commenced, with appropriate counselling about safe sex and responsibilities. The monophasic low-dose combined preparation should be selected.

Epilespy. Use a COC with a high dose of oestrogen, e.g. 50 μg.

Women with hirsutism. Use a less androgenic preparation, e.g. Diane-35.

Women over 35 years. Use a low-dose monophasic COC provided the woman is a non-smoker. If continued until about 50 years, the hot flushes of the perimenopause are controlled. It is usual to cease the pill at around 50–51, wait several weeks and then measure the serum FSH and oestradiol. If the oestradiol levels are low and FSH high, the woman can be regarded as menopausal and can start HRT if desired.

Menstrual disorders: menorrhagia/dysmenorrhoea. Start with a standard low-dose monophasic COC but a higher-dose oestrogen (50 μg) pill may be necessary.

Acne. For women with acne (not on COC), commence with a less androgenic progestogen, e.g. Diane-35 ED, Marvelon.

The high-dose monophasic (50 μg EO) should be reserved for the following situations:

- breakthrough bleeding on low-dose COCs
- control of menorrhagia
- concomitant use of enzyme-inducing drugs
- low-dose pill failure

Contraindications to COC usage are shown in Table 80.3.

Efficacy of COCs

Under ideal circumstances the pregnancy rate in women taking COCs is 1–3 per 100 women years of use, but in practice varies from 2–6 per 100 women years.[2]

Non-contraceptive advantages of COCs

A number of significant beneficial effects arising from the use of COCs have now been documented.

- reduction in most menstrual cycle disorders
- reduction in the incidence of functional ovarian cysts
- 50% reduction in the incidence of PID
- reduced incidence of ovarian and endometrial carcinoma
- benign breast disease reduced
- fewer sebaceous disorders
- reduced incidence of thyroid disorders

Table 80.3 *Contraindications for use of the COC*[5]

Absolute	Relative
• pregnancy (known or suspected)	• heavy smoking
• first 2 weeks postpartum	• > 35 years and smoking
• history of thomboembolic disease	• > 40 years
• undiagnosed abnormal vaginal bleeding	• breast-feeding
• cerebrovascular disease	• 4 weeks before surgery ⎫
• focal migraine	• 2 weeks after surgery ⎭
• coronary artery disease	• gall bladder or liver disease
• oestrogen-dependent tumours	• hypertension
• recent impaired liver function	• diabetes mellitus
	• long-term immobilisation
	• valvular heart disease
	• hyperlipidaemia
	• chloasma

Serious side effects of COCs

The most serious side effects to be considered are the effects of COCs on the circulatory system and the incidence of cancer.

Cardiovascular effects[4]

The following circulatory disorders have been linked with pill usage:

- Venous   deep vein thrombosis
          pulmonary embolism
          rarely: mesenteric, hepatic and renal thrombosis
- Arterial   myocardial infarction
          thrombotic stroke
          haemorrhagic stroke
          rarely: retinal and mesenteric
          . thrombosis

The risk of circulatory disease has not been related to duration of use and there is no increased risk in perpetual users.

The oestrogen content of the pill is considered to be the aetiological factor and the problem is increased in women taking high-oestrogen-content COCs, but now that the oestrogen content of each pill has been reduced to as low as 30 µg EO, these risks of morbidity and mortality have been reduced.

The progestogen effect on lipid metabolism is not considered significant in the aetiology of circulatory disease. Circulatory diseases have now been recognised as occurring predominantly in certain high-risk groups—the 'at risk female', particularly the smoker over 35 years of age.

Other risk groups include those with hyperlipidaemia, diabetes, hypertension, and a family history of cardiovascular disease or immobilisation.

Provided low-dose COCs are prescribed in low-risk females it would appear safe to use the COC pill up to 50 years of age.

COCs and cancer

There appears to be no overall increase in the incidence of cancer in women using COCs.

Possible effect (not absolutely proven)

- cervix (take regular smears at yearly intervals)
- breast

Protective effect

- endometrial
- epithelial ovarian

No effect

- melanoma
- chorioncarcinoma
- prolactinomas

Common side effects

The relatively minor side effects listed in Table 80.4 may discourage women from persisting with oral contraception in the absence of appropriate explanation and reassurance. Management of these side effects is listed in the same table. It is useful in practice to have this list available as a ready reference for manipulating the COC if necessary.

Important advice for the patient

- Periods tend to become shorter, regular and lighter.
- No break from the pill is necessary.
- Drugs that interact with the pill include vitamin C, antibiotics, griseofulvin, rifampicin and anticonvulsants (except sodium valproate). Warfarin and oral hypoglycaemics requirements may change for those starting the pill.

Table 80.4 *Management of common side effects of COC*[6,7]

Symptom change	Change	Examples of pill change
Acne	Increase oestrogen, reduce or change progestogen	Triphasil/Triquilar to Diane ED/Marvelon
Amenorrhoea	Increase oestrogen or decrease progestogen	Nordette/Microgynon 30 to Nordette 50/Microgynon 50
Breakthrough bleeding		
• early to mid cycle	increase oestrogen	Triphasil/Triquilar to Biphasil/Sequilar
• late cycle	Increase progestogen or change type	Triphasil to Nordette Nordette to Norinyl-1
Breast problems		
• fullness/tenderness	Decrease oestrogen	Biphasil/Sequilar to Triphasil/Triquilar
• mastalgia	Decrease progestogen	Nordette/Microgynon 30 to Triphasil/Triquilar
Chloasma	Stop oestrogen Try progestogen-only pill Avoid direct sun (use blockout)	
Depression	Decrease or change progestogen	Nordette/Microgynon 30 to Triphasil/Triquilar or Brevinor
Dysmenorrhoea/menorrhagia	Increase progestogen	Triphasil/Triquilar to Nordette/Microgynon
Headache		
• focal migraine	Discontinue pill	
• in pill-free week	Add 10–30 μg ethinyloestradiol daily during pill-free week	
Nausea/vomiting	Decrease or change oestrogen or stop oestrogen	Use Nordette, etc. or progestogen-only pill
Weight gain		
• constant	Decrease or change progestogen	Triphasil/Triquilar to Brevinor or Marvelon
• cyclic	Decrease oestrogen	Biphasil/Sequilar to Triphasil/Triquilar or progestrogen-only pill

- Diarrhoea and vomiting may reduce the effectiveness of the pill.
- Yearly return visits are recommended to update the history and examination and repeat the Pap smear.

The seven-day rule for the missed or late pill (more than 12 hours late):

- Take the forgotten pill as soon as possible, even if it means taking two pills in one day. Take the next pill at the usual time and finish the course.
- If you forget to take it for more than 12 hours after the usual time there is an increased risk of pregnancy so use another contraceptive method (such as condoms) for 7 days.
- If these 7 days run beyond the last hormone pill in your packet then miss out on the inactive pills (or 7-day gap) and proceed directly to the first hormone pill in your next packet.

You may miss a period. (At least seven hormone tablets should be taken.)

Progestogen-only contraceptive pill

The progestogen-only contraceptive pill (POP) is perhaps an underutilised method of contraception, although it is not as efficacious as the COC.

The two common formulations are:

levonorgestrel 30 μg/day

and

norethisterone 350 μg/day

Providing the mini-pill is taken regularly at the same time each day, the pregnancy rate is 3 per 100 women years.[2] The failure rate decreases with age. There are no serious side effects but compliance is a problem because of cycle irregularity, especially with irregular bleeding. The mini-pill often reduces the cycle length to less than 25 days or alters the regularity of the bleeding phase.

Indications for the POP include age 45 years or more, smokers aged 45 years or more, contraindications to or intolerance of oestrogens, diabetes mellitus, migraine, chloasma, lactation and well controlled hypertension.

Contraindications include pregnancy, undiagnosed genital tract bleeding, past history of or increased risk of ectopic pregnancy and concomitant use of enzyme-inducing drugs (absolute).

Injectable contraceptives

Medroxyprogesterone acetate ('Depo-Provera') is the only injectable contraceptive available in Australia.

Dose: 150 mg by deep IM injection in first five days of the menstrual cycle. The same dose is given every 12 weeks to maintain contraception.

Failure rate: 1 per 1000 women years.[2]

Side effects include a disrupted menstrual cycle (amenorrhoea rate 70% or irregular or prolonged uterine bleeding), excessive weight gain, breast tenderness, depression and a delay in return of fertility (average 6 months).[4] There is no effect on cardiovascular disease or the incidence of cancer.

There are no absolute contraindications.

The main indication for this form of contraception is the desire for a highly effective method when other methods are contraindicated or disliked. Advantages are avoiding the side effects of oestrogen and overcoming compliance problems, e.g. in the mentally handicapped.

Postcoital contraception

Oestrogens in large doses are effective in preventive contraception after mid-cycle exposure to sexual intercourse by making the endometrium unreceptive to the zygote.[2]

Available methods (NB: must be used within 72 hours)

- Use high-oestrogen-containing COC, e.g. 50 μg EO + 250 μg LNG (Nordiol)—two pills initially then repeated 12 hours later.

Nausea is a common side effect and it is common to prescribe an antiemetic. Failure rate 2.6%.[2]

- Danazol 200 mg tablets, e.g. two initially and repeated 12 hours later.

Reduced incidence of nausea—failure rate 4.6%.

Pill failure

Causes of oral contraceptive failure include errors in administration, decreased absorption, missed pills, drug interactions and high doses of vitamin C. It is possible that the use of triphasics may be a factor.

Management options include using a higher-dose pill, improved education and compliance and an alternative method.

Intrauterine contraceptive devices

Intrauterine contraceptive devices (IUCDs) are usually small devices made of an inert material to which may be added a bioactive substance such as copper, e.g. Multiload-Cu375, or a progestogen.[2] IUCDs probably interfere with the implantation of the zygote.

Efficacy: IUCDs give 96–99% protection against pregnancy.[2]

Contraindications for IUCD use.[4]

- Absolute — known or suspected pregnancy
  — active PID
  — undiagnosed abnormal genital tract bleeding
  — previous ectopic pregnancy
- Relative — menorrhagia
  — dysmenorrhoea
  — uterine cavity distortion
  — very large or very small uterus (> 9.0 or < 5.5 cm)
  — anaemia
  — defective immune system
  — impaired clotting mechanism
  — valvular heart disease
  — acutely anteverted or retroverted uterus
  — increased risk of PID (multiple sex partners)

Problems associated with IUCD usage[2]

Pregnancy/ectopic pregnancy

If pregnancy occurs there is a 40–50% increased risk of abortion and intrauterine sepsis during the second trimester. There is an increased risk of ectopic pregnancy (up to 10 times compared with COC usage) so, if pregnancy occurs, ultrasound examination should be performed to determine the location.

Early removal of the IUCD is essential.

Pelvic inflammatory disease

There is evidence of an increased risk of PID in the first 30 days post-insertion. Prophylactic doxycycline reduces this risk.[4] As this risk is related to sexual activity and the number of partners, those at risk of STDs should avoid using IUCDs.

Extrusion, perforation of uterus and translocation

Spontaneous extrusion is greatest during the first month after insertion and the woman is not always aware of this. Perforation of the uterus occurs once in every 1000 insertions and review at 6 weeks post-insertion is essential. If translocation is proved by X-ray and pelvic ultrasound, removal is mandatory.

Bleeding

Intermenstrual bleeding may follow insertion of an IUCD for 2–3 months and then disappear. If menstrual loss is excessive, the device should be removed.

Pain

Lower abdominal cramp-like pains of uterine origin and backache may occur soon after insertion and persist intermittently for several weeks. Rarely is the pain severe enough to warrant removal of the IUCD.

Checking the IUCD

Women should be taught how to examine themselves vaginally to check if the device remains *in situ* by palpating the strings or threads which protrude from the cervical canal. They should have a medical check 2–3 months after the device has been fitted and again after 12 months.

Barrier methods

Barrier methods include condoms, vaginal diaphragms, cervical caps and vaginal vault caps. If used correctly, some, particularly condoms, are very effective contraceptives with pregnancy rates of 5 or less per 100 women years.[2]

Condoms are also very effective in preventing the spread of STDs including HIV infection.

Diaphragms have to be individually fitted. After being liberally coated on both sides with a spermicidal cream they are inserted at any convenient time before intercourse and removed after six hours have elapsed since the last act of intercourse.

Spermicides

These are useful adjuncts to barrier methods of contraception. When used alone they have a pregnancy rate of less than 10 per 100 women years. They are available as creams, jellies, foams or pessaries containing nonoxynol 9 or octoxinol.

Natural methods

These methods require high motivation and regular menstrual cycles.

Basal body temperature method

Coitus should only occur after there has been a rise in basal body temperature of 0.2°C for 3 days (72 hours) above the basal body temperature measurement during the preceding 6 days, until the onset of the next menstrual period.

Billings ovulation method[8]

This method is based on careful observation of the nature of the mucus so that ovulation can be recognised. Fertile mucus is wet, clear, stringy, increased in amount and feels lubricative. The peak mucus day is the last day with this oestrogenised mucus before the abrupt change to thick tacky mucus associated with the secretion of progesterone. The infertile phase begins on the fourth day after the peak mucus day. Abstinence from intercourse is practised from the first awareness of increased, clearer wet mucus until four days after maximum mucus secretion. If taught correctly and followed as directed, the method is most effective, with a failure rate of only 1–2 (average 3) per 100 women years.[8] There is a failure rate of at least 15 if the rules are not followed properly.

Coitus interruptus

Male withdrawal before ejaculation is still a widely used method of contraception and despite theoretical objections will probably continue to have a definite place in contraceptive practice.

Sterilisation

Vasectomy

With vasectomy it is important to confirm the absence of spermatozoa in the ejaculate 2–3 months after the operation, before ceasing other contraceptive methods. It takes about 12–15 ejaculations to clear all the sperm from the tubes proximal to the surgical division. Vasectomy reversal is successful in up to 80% of patients.[2] There is a 1 in 500–1000 chance of recanalisation.

Tubal ligation

Female sterilisation is usually performed by mini-laparotomy or laparoscopy at which time clips (Filshie or Hulka) or rings (Falope) are applied to each Fallopian tube. These are potentially reversible methods of contraception with a 50–70% success rate of reversal.[2] There is a subsequent pregnancy rate of 3–4 per 1000 women sterilised.

References

1. Sloane PD, Slatt ML, Baker RM. *Essentials of family medicine*. Baltimore: Williams & Wilkins, 1988, 175–189.
2. Walters W. Fertility control. In: MIMS. Sydney: IMS Publishing, 1991–92, 185–190.
3. Stovall TG. *Clinical manual of gynaecology*. New York: McGraw-Hill, 1992, 263–266.
4. Waldron K. *Effective family planning*. Proceedings handbook: Monash University Medical School. Update Course for General Practitioners, 1992, 9–15.
5. Benn M. Prescribing oral contraceptives and the medical record. Aust Fam Physician, 1991; 20:1469–1470.
6. Weisberg E. Choosing an oral contraceptive. Mod Med Aust, 1997; 40(1):18–26.
7. Miller C. The combined oral contraceptive: a practical guide. Aust Fam Physician, 1990; 19:897–905.
8. Billings E, Westmore A. *The Billings method*. Melbourne: Anne O'Donovan, 1992, 11–49.

81
Breast pain (mastalgia)

—

Many women suffer breast pain so severe that it affects their lifestyles, marriages and sexual relationships, and even prevents them from hugging their children.

Breast pain, or mastalgia, is a common problem accounting for at least 50% of breast problems presenting in general practice.[1] Many women suffer breast pain so severe that it affects their lifestyles, marriages and sexual relationships, and even prevents them from hugging their children. If no obvious physical cause is found, the problem is all too often dismissed, without appropriate empathy and reassurance, as a normal physiological effect.

A careful, sympathetic clinical approach, however, followed by reassurance after examination, will be sufficient treatment for most patients.

Symptoms

Mastalgia usually presents as a heaviness or discomfort in the breast or as a pricking or stabbing sensation. The pain may radiate down the inner arm when the patient is carrying heavy objects or when the arm is in constant use, as in scrubbing floors.

Key facts and checkpoints

- The typical age span for mastalgia is 30–50 years.
- The peak incidence is 35–45 years.
- There are four common clinical presentations:
  1. diffuse, bilateral cyclical mastalgia
  2. diffuse, bilateral non-cyclical mastalgia
  3. unilateral diffuse non-cyclical mastalgia
  4. localised breast pain.

- The specific type of mastalgia should be identified.
- The commonest type is cyclical mastalgia.
- Premenstrual mastalgia (part of type 1) is common.
- An underlying malignancy should be excluded.
- Less than 10% of breast cancers present with localised pain.
- Only about 1 in 200 women with mastalgia are found to have breast cancer.
- The problems, especially types 2 and 3, are difficult to alleviate.

A diagnostic approach

A summary of the safety diagnostic model is presented in Table 81.1.

Probability diagnosis

In the non-pregnant patient, generalised pain which may be cyclical or non-cyclical is commonest. Typical patterns are illustrated in Figure 81.1.

Cyclical mastalgia is the commonest diffuse breast pain (see p. 820). It occurs in the latter

Fig. 81.1 *Pain patterns for cyclical and non-cyclical mastalgia*

Table 81.1 *Mastalgia: diagnostic strategy model*

Q. *Probability diagnosis*
A. Pregnancy
   Cyclical mastalgia
   • benign mammary dysplasia

Q. *Serious disorders not to be missed*
A. Neoplasia
   Infection
   • mastitis
   • abscess
   Myocardial ischaemia

Q. *Pitfalls (often missed)*
A. Pregnancy
   Costochondritis
   Pectoralis muscle spasm
   Referred pain, esp. thoracic spine
   Mechanical
   • bra problems
   • weight change
   • trauma

   Rarities
   Hyperprolactinaemia
   Nerve entrapment
   Mammary duct ectasia
   Sclerosing adenosis
   Ankylosing spondylitis

Q. *Seven masquerades checklist*
A. Depression   √
   Diabetes   –
   Drugs   √
   Anaemia   –
   Thyroid disease   –
   Spinal dysfunction   √
   Urinary infection   –

Q. *Is the patient trying to tell me something?*
A. Yes. Fear of malignancy. Consider psychogenic causes.

---

half of the menstrual cycle, especially in the pre-menstrual days, and subsides with the onset of menstruation. It obviously has a hormonal basis, which may be an abnormality in prolactin secretion. The main underlying disorder is benign mammary dysplasia, also referred to as fibro-adenosis, chronic mastitis, cystic hyperplasia or fibrocystic breast disease.

Non-cyclical mastalgia is also quite common and the cause is poorly understood. It may be associated with duct ectasia and periductal mastitis (see page 821).

Serious disorders not to be missed

The three important serious disorders not to be missed with any painful chest condition—neoplasia, infection and myocardial ischaemia—are applicable for breast pain.

Neoplasia

We must avoid the trap of considering that breast pain is not compatible with malignancy. Mastalgia can be a presenting symptom (although uncommon) of breast cancer. 'Mastitis carcinomatosa', which is a rare florid form of breast cancer found in young women, often during lactation, is red and hot but not invariably painful or tender.[2] Pain may also be a symptom in juvenile fibroadenoma, a soft rapidly growing tumour in adolescents, and in the fibroadenoma of adult women.

Infection

Mastitis is common among nursing mothers. It should be regarded as a serious and urgent problem because a breast abscess can develop quickly. Apart from bacterial infection, infection with *Candida albicans* may occur following the use of antibiotics. Candida infection usually causes severe breast pain, producing a feeling like 'hot cords', especially during and after feeding.

Myocardial ischaemia

A constricting pain under the left breast should be regarded as myocardial ischaemia until proved otherwise.

Pitfalls

These include various causes of apparent mastalgia, such as several musculoskeletal chest wall conditions and referred pain from organs such as the heart, oesophagus, lungs and gall bladder and, in particular, from the upper thoracic spine.

Musculoskeletal conditions include costochondritis, pectoralis muscle strains or spasm, and entrapment of the lateral cutaneous branch of the third intercostal nerve. Ankylosing spondylitis can affect the chest wall under the breasts. Mastalgia may be the first symptom of pregnancy. Pregnancy should be excluded before commencing drug treatment.

Seven masquerades checklist

Of these, depression, drugs and spinal dysfunction are probable causes. Drugs that can cause breast discomfort include oral contraceptives, hormone replacement therapy and methylxanthine derivatives such as theophylline. Drugs that cause tender gynaecomastia (more applicable to men) include digoxin, cimetidine, spironolactone and marijuana.

Dysfunction of the upper thoracic spine and even the lower cervical spine can refer pain under a breast. If suspected, these areas of the spine should be examined.

Psychogenic considerations
The symptoms may be exaggerated as a result of an underlying psychogenic disorder, but with a symptom such as breast pain most women fear malignancy and need reassurance.

The clinical approach
History
It is important to relate the pain to the menstrual cycle and determine whether the patient is pregnant or not.

Key questions
- Could you be pregnant?
- Is your period on time or overdue?
- Is the pain in both breasts or only one?
- Do you have pain before your periods or all the time during your menstrual cycle?
- Do you have pain in your back or where your ribs join your chest bone?

Physical examination
The breasts should be systematically palpated to check for soreness or lumps. The underlying chest wall and thoracic spine should also be examined.

Investigations
The following specialised tests could be considered.

Mammography should be considered in older women. It is unreliable in young women. With few exceptions it should not be used under 40 years.

Ultrasound can be complementary to mammography for it is useful to assess a localised mass or tender area. It is inappropriate to evaluate a diffuse area. It is not so useful for the postmenopausal breast which is fatty and looks similar to cancer on ultrasound.

Excision biopsy can be useful for an area of localised pain, especially in the presence of a possible mass.

Mastalgia in children
Breast pain is uncommon in children, including puberty, but it may be a presenting problem in the late teens. Pubertal boys may complain of breast lumps under the nipple (adolescent gynaecomastia) but these are rarely tender and do not require specific treatment.

Mastalgia in the elderly
Breast pain is rare after the menopause but is increasing with increased use of hormone replacement therapy (HRT), where it tends to present as the diffuse bilateral type. If the problem is related to the introduction of HRT, the oestrogen dose should be reduced or an alternative preparation used.

Cyclical mastalgia
The features of cyclical mastalgia are:

- the typical age is 35
- discomfort and sometimes pain are present
- usually bilateral but one breast can dominate
- mainly premenstrual ✓
- breasts diffusely nodular or lumpy
- variable relationship to the pill

It is rare after the menopause.

Management
After excluding a diagnosis of carcinoma and aspirating palpable cysts, various treatments are possible and can be given according to severity.[3]

Mild
- reassurance
- regular review and breast self-examination
- proper brassiere support
- proper low-fat diet, excluding caffeine
- aim at ideal weight
- adjust oral contraception or hormone replacement therapy (if applicable)

Moderate
As for mild, plus options (use one or a combination):

- mefenamic acid 500 mg, three times daily
- vitamin B_1 (thiamine) 100 mg daily, and
- vitamin B_6 (pyridoxine) 100 mg daily
- evening primrose oil 4–6 g daily

If no response

As for mild, plus options (one of the following):

- norethisterone 5 mg daily (for second half of cycle)
- bromocriptine 2.5 mg twice daily
- danazol 200 mg daily

Some of these treatments, particularly vitamin therapy, have not been scientifically tested but some empirical evidence is convincing. The value of diuretics is not proven, and testosterone or tamoxifen treatment is generally not favoured.

Evening primrose oil contains an essential fatty acid claimed to be lacking in the diet, and replacement allows for the production of prostaglandin E, which counters the effect of oestrogen and prolactin on the breast.

Bromocriptine and danazol have significant side effects but clinical trials have proved their efficacy for this condition.[4,5]

A summary of a treatment strategy for cyclical mastalgia is presented in Table 81.2.

Non-cyclical mastalgia

The features of non-cyclical mastalgia are:

- the typical age is the early forties
- bilateral and diffuse
- pain present throughout the cycle
- no obvious physical or pathological basis

Typical pain patterns are presented in Figure 81.1.

Management

Non-cyclical mastalgia is very difficult to treat, being less responsive than cyclical mastalgia. It is worth a therapeutic trial.

Table 81.2 *Management plan for cyclical mastalgia*

Progressive stepwise therapy	
Step 1	Reassurance Proper brassiere support Diet—exclude caffeine Exercises, e.g. aerobics for upper trunk
Step 2	Add Vitamin B$_1$ 100 mg daily Vitamin B$_6$ 100 mg daily
Step 3	Substitute Evening primrose oil 4 g daily
Step 4	Add Danazol 200 mg daily

First-line treatment

- exclude caffeine from diet
- weight reduction if needed
- vitamin B$_1$ 100 mg daily
- vitamin B$_6$ 100 mg daily
- evening primrose oil 4–6 g daily

Second-line treatment

- norethisterone 5 mg daily

Local lesions

Surgical excision may be required for local lesions. If there is no discrete lesion but a tender trigger point (including costochondritis), the injection of local anaesthetic and corticosteroid may relieve the problem.

Costochondritis (Tietze's syndrome)

This is a common cause of referral to a breast pain clinic. The cause is often obscure, but the costochondral junction may become strained in patients with a persistent cough. The pain can appear to be in the breast with intermittent radiation round the chest wall and is initiated or aggravated by deep breathing and coughing.

Features:

- the pain is acute, intermittent or chronic
- the breast is normal to palpation
- palpable swelling about 4 cm from sternal edge due to enlargement of costochondral cartilage
- X-rays are normal
- self-limiting, but may take several months to subside

Treatment. Infiltration with local anaesthetic and corticosteroid.

Mastitis

Mastitis is basically cellulitis of the interlobular connective tissue of the breast. Mostly restricted to lactating women, it is associated with a cracked nipple or poor milk drainage. The infecting organism is usually *Staphlococcus aureus* or more rarely *Escherichia coli* or *Candida albicans*. It is a serious problem and requires early treatment. Breast-feeding from the affected side can continue as the infection is confined to interstitial breast tissue and doesn't usually affect the milk supply.

Clinical features:
- a lump and then soreness (at first)
- a red tender area

possibly
- fever, tiredness, muscle aches and pains

Note: Candida infection usually causes severe breast pain—a feeling like a hot knife or hot shooting pains, especially during and after feeding. It may occur after a course of antibiotics.

Management

Prevention (in lactation):
- maintain free breast drainage
- attend to breast engorgement and cracked nipples

Treatment
- Antibiotics: resolution without progression to an abscess will usually be prevented by antibiotics[6]

  dicloxacillin 500 mg (o) qid for 10 days

  or

  cephalaxin 500 mg (o) qid for 10 days

  If severe cellulitis: flucloxacillin 2 g (IV) 6 hourly
- therapeutic ultrasound ($2W/cm^2$ for 6 minutes) daily for 2–3 days
- aspirin or paracetamol for pain

Instructions to patients
- Keep the affected breast well drained.
- Continue breast-feeding: do frequently and start with the sore side.
- Heat the sore breast before feeding, e.g. with hot shower or hot face washer.
- Cool the breast after feeding: use a cold face washer from the freezer.
- Massage any breast lumps gently towards the nipple while feeding.
- Empty the breast well: hand express if necessary.
- Get sufficient rest.
- Keep to a nutritious diet and drink ample fluids.

Breast abscess

If tenderness and redness persist beyond 48 hours and an area of tense induration develops, then a breast abscess has formed. It requires surgical drainage under general anaesthesia or aspiration with a large bore needle under LA every

second day until resolution, antibiotics, rest and complete emptying of the breast. Temporary weaning of breast-feeding from the affected side is necessary because of the surgical disruption.

Surgical drainage
Method:
1. Make an incision over the point of maximal tenderness, preferably in a dependent area of the breast. A curvilinear transverse incision which does not continue into breast tissue, following Langer's lines, is optimal (Fig. 81.2a).
2. Use artery forceps to separate breast tissue to reach the pus.
3. Take a swab for culture.
4. Introduce a gloved finger to break down the septa that separate the cavity into loculations (Fig. 81.2b).
5. Insert a corrugated drainage tube into the cavity. Fix it to the skin edge with a single suture (Fig. 81.2c).

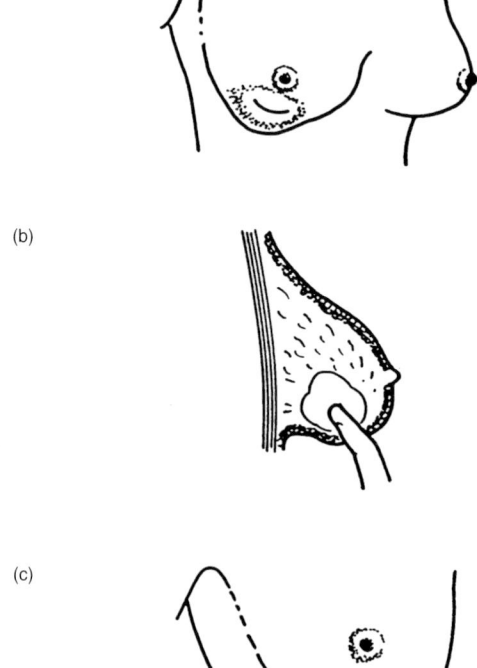

(a)

(b)

(c)

Fig. 81.2 *Surgical drainage of breast abscess:* **(a)** *transverse incision;* **(b)** *exploring abscess cavity;* **(c)** *drainage tube in situ*

Remove the tube two days after the operation. Change the dressings daily until the wound has healed. Continue antibiotics until resolution of the inflammation.

When to refer

- Undiagnosed localised breast pain or lump.

Practice tips

- The basis of management for benign mastalgia is firm reassurance.
- Although breast cancer rarely causes mastalgia, it should be excluded.
- Think of *Candida albicans* if mastitis is very severe with hot shooting pains, especially after antibiotic treatment.
- Look for underlying disorders of the chest wall if examination of the breasts is normal.
- Consider caffeine intake as a cause of benign diffuse mastalgia.
- Mastitis should be treated vigorously—it is a serious condition.
- Fibroadenomas and breast cysts are capable of causing localised pain and tenderness.

References

1. McAvoy PA. Breast problems. In: Cormack J, Marinker M, Morrell D (eds). *Practice*. London: Kluwer Medical, 1982, Section 3.54.
2. Ryan P. *A very short textbook of surgery* (2nd edn). Canberra: Dennis and Ryan, 1990, 10.
3. Barraclough B. The fibrocystic breast—clinical assessment, diagnosis and treatment. Mod Med Aust, 1990; 33(4):16–25.
4. Mansel RE et al. Controlled trial of the antigonadotrophin danazol in painful nodular benign breast disease. Lancet, 1982; 1:928.
5. Hinton CP et al. A double blind controlled trial of danazol and bromocriptine in the management of severe cyclical breast pain. Br J Clin Prac, 1986; 40:326.
6. Mashford L (Chairman). *Antibiotic guidelines* (9th edn). Victorian Medical Postgraduate Foundation, 1996, 140.

Lumps in the breast

—

Neither the cause of breast cancer, one of the most feared and emotion-engendering diseases, nor the means of preventing it are absolutely known.

Lecturer on breast cancer (Anon)

Breast lumps are common and their discovery by a woman provokes considerable anxiety and emotion (which is often masked during presentation) because to many a 'breast lump' means cancer. Many of the lumps are actually areas of thickening of normal breast tissue. Many other lumps are due to mammary dysplasia with either fibrosis or cyst formation or a combination of the two producing a dominant (discrete) lump.[1] However, a good working rule is to consider any lump in the breast as carcinoma until proved otherwise. See Table 82.1 for causes of breast lumps in a specific outpatient study.

Key facts and checkpoints

- The commonest lumps are those associated with benign mammary dysplasia (45%).[2] See Table 82.1.
- There are three types of benign dominant breast lumps: cysts, fibroadenomas and pseudolumps (90% of breast lumps). The other 10% of lumps are carcinomas.
- Benign mammary dysplasia is also a common cause of cysts, especially in the premenopause phase.
- Over 75% of isolated breast lumps prove to be benign but clinical identification of a malignant tumour can only definitely be made following aspiration biopsy or histological examination of the tumour.[3]
- An association between alcohol and breast cancer has been found.

Table 82.1 *Causes of breast lumps[2]*
(a surgical outpatient study)

Common	%
• Benign mammary hyperplasia	45
• Carcinoma	25
• Cysts	15
• Fibroadenoma	10
• Breast abscess/periareolar inflammation	3

Less common
- Mammary duct ectasia
- Duct papilloma
- Lactation cysts (galactocele)
- Paget's disease of the nipple
- Fat necrosis/fibrosis
- Sarcoma
- Lipoma

- Breast cancer is the most common cancer in females, affecting 1 in 12 to 15 women.[3]
- About 25% of all new cancers in women are breast neoplasms.
- A 'dominant' breast lump in an older woman should be regarded as malignant.

The clinical approach

This is based on following a careful history and examination.

History

The history should include a family history of breast disease and the patient's past history, including trauma, previous breast pain, and details about pregnancies (complications of lactation such as mastitis, nipple problems and milk retention).

Key questions[1]
- Have you had any previous problems with your breasts?

- Have you noticed any breast pain or discomfort?
- Do you have any problems such as increased swelling or tenderness before your periods?
- Have you noticed lumpiness in your breasts before?
- Has the lumpy area been red or hot?
- Have you noticed any discharge from your nipple or nipples?
- Has there been any change in your nipples?
- Did your mother or sisters or any close relatives have any breast problems?

Breast symptoms
- lump
- tenderness or pain
- nipple discharge
- nipple retraction
- periareolar inflammation

Nipple discharge[4]
This may be intermittent from one or both nipples. It can be induced by quadrant compression.

- bloodstained   — intraduct papilloma (commonest)
  intraduct carcinoma
  mammary dysplasia
- green-grey   — mammary dysplasia
  mammary duct ectasia
- yellow   — mammary dysplasia
  intraduct carcinoma (serous)
  breast abscess (pus)
- milky white (galactorrhoea)   — lactation cysts
  lactation
  hyperprolactinaemia
  drugs, e.g. chlorpromazine

Periareolar inflammation
This presents as pain around the areola with reddening of the skin, tenderness and swelling. Causes may be inverted nipple or mammary duct ectasia.

Paget's disease of the nipple
This rare but interesting condition usually occurs in middle-aged and elderly women. It starts as an eczematous-looking dry scabbing red rash of the nipple and then proceeds to ulceration of the nipple and areola. It is always due to an underlying malignancy.

Examination of the breasts
Objectives
- Identify a dominant lump (one that differs from the remainder of the breast tissue).
- Identify a lump that may be malignant.
- Screen the breasts for early development of carcinoma.

Time of examination: ideally, 4 days after the end of the period.

Method[1]
1. Inspection: sitting—patient seated upright on side of couch in good light, arms by sides, facing the doctor, undressed to waist.
   (a) Note • Asymmetry of breasts or a visible lump
   - Localised discolouration of the skin
   - Nipples
     — for retraction or ulceration
     — for variations in the level, e.g. elevation on one side
     — for discharge, e.g. blood-stained, clear, yellow
   - Skin attachment or tethering → dimpling of skin (accentuate this sign by asking patient to raise her arms above her head)
   - Appearance of small nodules of growth
   - Visible veins (if unilateral they suggest a cancer)[5]
   - Peau d'orange due to dermal oedema
   (b) Raise arms above the head (renders variations in nipple level and skin tethering more obvious). Hands are pressed on the hips to contract pectoralis major to note if there is a deep attachment of the lump.
2. Examination of lymph glands in sitting position: patient with hands on hips. Examine axillary and supraclavicular glands from behind and front.

   Note: The draining lymphatic nodes are in the axillae, supraclavicular fossae and internal mammary chain.
3. Palpation
   (a) Patient still seated: palpate breast with flat of hand and then palpate the bulk of the breast between both hands.

(b) In supine position:
- patient lies supine on couch with arms above head
- turn body (slight rotation) towards midline so breasts 'sit' as flat as possible on chest wall

Method
- Use the pulps of the fingers rather than the tips with the hand laid flat on the breast.
- Move the hand in slow circular movements.
- Examine up and down the breast in vertical strips beginning from the axillary tail (Fig. 82.1).
- Systematically cover the six areas of the breast (Fig. 82.2)
  — the four quadrants
  — the axillary tail
  — the region deep to the nipple and areola

4. If a suspicious lump is present, inspect liver, lungs and spine.
5. Inspect the bra. Note possible pressure on breast tissue from underwiring of the bra, usually on the upper outer quadrant.

If a solitary lump is present, assess it for:
- position (breast quadrant and proximity to nipple)
- size and shape
- consistency (firm, hard, cystic, soft)
- tenderness
- mobility and fixation
- attachment to skin or underlying muscle

Note:
- 40–50% of carcinomas occur in the upper outer quadrant.[4]
- A hard mass is suspicious of malignancy but cancer can be soft because of fat entrapment.
- The inframammary ridge, which is usually found in the heavier breast, is often nodular and firm to hard.
- Lumpiness (if present) is usually most marked in the upper outer quadrant.
- A useful diagram to record the findings is shown in Figure 82.3.
- Lumps that are usually benign and require no immediate action are: tiny (< 4 mm) nodules in subcutaneous tissue (usully in the areolar margin); elongated ridges, usually bilateral and

Fig. 82.1 *Systematic examination of the breast*

Right breast

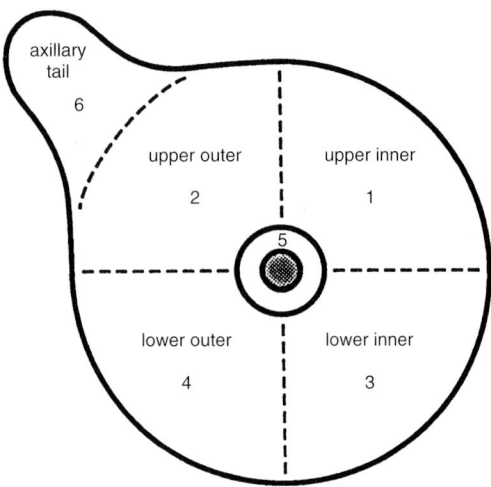

Fig. 82.2 *The six areas of the breast*

in the lower aspects of the breasts; and rounded soft nodules (usually < 6 mm) around the areolar margin.[6]

Investigations
X-ray mammography
Mammography can be used as a screening procedure and as a diagnostic procedure. It is currently the only effective screening tool for breast cancer.[7] Positive signs of malignancy include an

Fig. 82.3 *Diagrammatic scheme for recording the features of breast lumps and any lymphadenopathy (axilla and supraclavicular triangles)*

irregular infiltrating mass with focal spotty microcalcification.

Screening:

- established benefit for women over 50
- possible benefit for women in their 40's
- follow-up in those with breast cancer, as 6% develop in the opposite breast
- localisation of the lesion for fine needle aspiration

Breast ultrasound

This is mainly used to elucidate an area of breast density and is the best method of defining benign breast disease, especially with cystic changes. It is generally most useful in women less than 35 years old (as compared with X-ray mammography).

Useful for:

- pregnant and lactating breast
- differentiating between fluid-filled cysts and solid mass
- palpable masses at periphery of breast tissue (not screened by mammography)
- for more accurate localisation of lump during fine needle aspiration

Note: CT and MRI have limited use. An age-related schemata for likely diagnosis and appropriate investigations is presented in Table 82.2.

Needle aspiration and biopsy techniques

- cyst aspiration
- fine needle aspiration biopsy: this is a very useful diagnostic test in solid lumps, and has an accuracy of 90–95% (better than mammography).[4]

Table 82.2 *Age-related schemata for likely diagnoses and appropriate investigations (after Hirst)*[6]

1. Very young women—12 to 25
   - inflamed cysts or ducts, usually close to areola
   - fibroadenomata, often giant
   - hormonal thickening, not uncommon
   - malignancy rare
   Investigations — mammography contraindicated
            — ultrasound helpful

2. Young women—26 to 35
   - classical fibroadenomata
   - mammary dysplasia with or without discharge
   - cysts uncommon
   - malignancy uncommon
   Investigations — mammography: breasts often
            very dense
            — ultrasound often diagnostic

3. Women—36 to 50 (premenopausal)
   - cysts
   - mammary dysplasia, discharges, duct papillomas
   - malignancy common
   - fibroadenomata occur but cannot assume
   - inflammatory processes not uncommon
   Investigations — mammography useful
            — ultrasound useful

4. Women—over 50 (postmenopausal)
   - any new discrete mass—malignant until proven otherwise
   - any new thickening—regard with suspicion
   - inflammatory lesions—probably duct ectasia (follow to resolution)
   - cysts unlikely
   Investigations — mammography usually diagnostic
            — ultrasound may be useful

5. Women—over 50, on hormones
   - any new mass—regard with suspicion
   - cysts may occur—usually asymptomatic
   - hormonal change not uncommon
   Investigations — mammography usually diagnostic
            but breast may become more
            dense
            — ultrasound may be useful

Reprinted with permission

- large needle (core needle) biopsy
- incision biopsy

Tumour markers

Oestrogen receptors are uncommon in normal breasts but are found in two-thirds of breast cancers, although the incidence varies with age. They are good prognostic indicators. Progesterone receptors can also be estimated.

Fine needle aspiration of breast lump

This simple technique is very useful, especially if the lump is a cyst, and will have no adverse effects if the lump is not malignant. If it is, the needle biopsy will help with the preoperative cytological diagnosis.

Method of aspiration and needle biopsy:

1. Use an aqueous skin preparation without local anaesthesia.
2. Use a 23 gauge needle and 5 mL sterile syringe.
3. Identify the mass accurately and fix it by placing three fingers of the non-dominant hand firmly on the three sides of the mass (Fig. 82.4).
4. Introduce the needle directly into the area of the swelling. Once in subcutaneous tissue, apply gentle suction as the needle is being advanced (Fig. 82.5). If a cyst is involved it can be felt to 'give' suddenly.
5. If fluid is obtained (usually yellowish-green), aspirate as much as possible.
6. If no fluid is obtained, try to get a core of cells from several areas of the lump in the bore of the needle.

7. Make several passes through the lump at different angles, without exit from the skin and maintain suction.
8. Release suction before exit from the skin to keep cells in the needle (not in the syringe).
9. After withdrawal, remove syringe from needle, fill with 2 mL of air, reattach needle and produce a fine spray on one or two prepared slides.
10. Fix to one slide (in Cytofix) and allow one to air dry, and forward to a reputable pathology laboratory to be examined by a skilled cytologist.

Follow-up: the plan for aspiration is outlined in Figure 82.6.

Indications for biopsy or excision of lump:
• The cyst fluid is bloodstained.
• The lump does not disappear completely with aspiration.
• The swelling recurs within one month.

Summary: investigation of a breast lump

If the patient presenting with a breast lump is younger than 35, perform an ultrasound;[8] if older than 35 perform a mammogram and an ultrasound. If the lump is cystic—aspirate; if solid—perform a fine needle biopsy and then manage according to outcomes. If it is suspicious, an excisional biopsy is the preferred option.

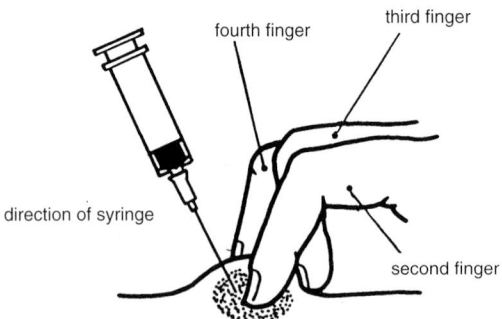

Fig. 82.4 *Aspiration of breast lump: fixation of cyst*

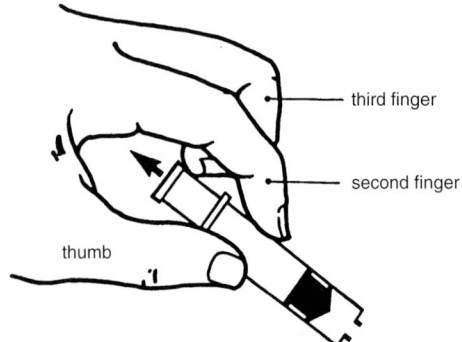

Fig. 82.5 *Aspiration of breast lump: position of the hand—second (index) finger and thumb steady the syringe while the third (middle) finger slides out the plunger to create suction*

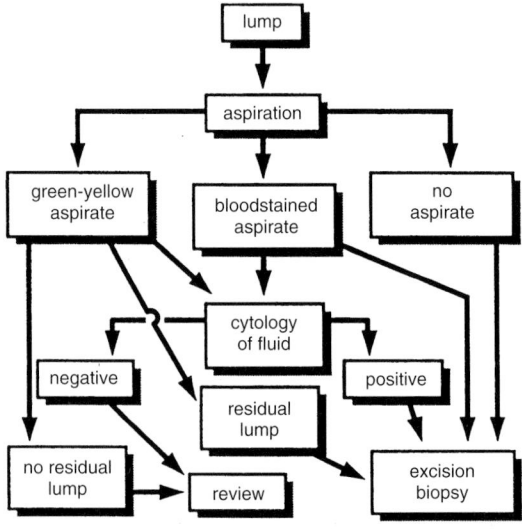

Fig. 82.6 *Scheme for management of a breast lump by fine needle aspiration*

Carcinoma of the breast

Breast carcinoma is uncommon under the age of 30 but it then steadily increases to a maximum at the age of about 60 years.[4] About one-third are premenopausal and two-thirds postmenopausal. About 1 in 12–15 women develop breast cancer. Ninety per cent of breast cancers are invasive duct carcinomas, the remainder being lobular carcinoma, papillary carcinomas, medullary carcinomas and colloid or mucoid carcinomas.[3]

Risk factors include increasing age (> 40 years), Caucasian race, pre-existing benign breast lumps, personal history of breast cancer, family history in a first-degree relative (raises risk about threefold), nulliparity, late menopause (after 53), obesity, childless until after 30 years of age, early menarche,[7] ionising radiation.

Clinical features

- The majority of patients with breast cancer present with a lump.
- The lump is usually painless (16% associated with pain).
- Usually the lump is hard and irregular.
- Other symptoms include breast pain, nipple discharge and nipple retraction.
- Rarely cancer can present with Paget's disease.
- Rarely it can present with bony secondaries, e.g. back pain, dyspnoea, weight loss, headache.

Note: There are basically two presentations of the disease:
  - the vast majority present with a local breast lump[3]
  - some present with metastatic disease

Of those who present with local disease, approximately 50% will develop metastatic disease.

Management

Immediate referral to an expert surgeon on suspicion or proof of breast cancer is essential. The treatment has to be individualised according to the nature of the lump, age of the patient and staging. Accurate staging requires knowledge of whether the draining lymph nodes are involved with the tumour, as this is the single most powerful predictor of subsequent metastases and death. Staging for systemic disease also requires full blood examination and liver function tests (including an alkaline phosphatase). A bone scan may be used as a valuable base-line. Size and histological grading of tumour plus nodal status and receptor status are the most important prognostic factors.

Adjuvant therapy for breast cancer

The consultant will choose the most appropriate surgical and adjuvant treatments for the individual patient.

The National Breast Cancer Consensus report emphasised that 'continuing care should be coordinated through the patient's GP as the impact of treatment may last longer than therapy and support must continue'. The report made the following recommendations:[9]

- Tumour excision followed by whole breast irradiation was the most preferred local therapy for most women with stage I or II cancer.
- Total mastectomy and breast-conservation surgery had an equivalent effect on survival.
- Routine radiotherapy is recommended after breast-conserving surgery, but not after mastectomy.
- Total mastectomy is preferred for a large tumour, multifocal disease, previous irradiation and extensive tumour on mammography.

Guidelines for adjuvant treatments are presented in Table 82.3.

Benign mammary dysplasia

Synonyms: fibroadenosis, chronic mastitis, fibrocystic disease, cystic hyperplasia.

Features

- most common in women between 30 and 50
- hormone-related (between menarche and menopause)
- pain and tenderness and swelling
- premenstrual discomfort or pain and increased swelling
- usually settles after the period
- unilateral or bilateral
- nodularity ± a discrete mass
- ache may extend down inner aspect of upper arm
- nipple discharge may occur (various colours, mainly green-grey)
- most cysts are premenopausal (final 5 years before menopause)

Examination. Look for lumpiness in one or both breasts, usually upper outer quadrant.

Table 82.3 *Adjuvant treatment favoured by trial meta-analyses*[9]

Premenopausal	node-positive	Combination chemotherapy using 6 cycles of CMF (cyclophosphamide, methotrexate and fluorouracil)
	node-negative	As above—in patients with poor prognostic features only*
Postmenopausal	node-positive	*Receptor-positive:* tamoxifen for >2 years (often 5). In younger women (aged <65) or those with poor prognostic features*, additional benefit has been shown by the administration of combination chemotherapy prior to tamoxifen. *Receptor-negative:* combination chemotherapy is recommended.
	node-negative	*Receptor-positive:* tamoxifen for 5 years; *Receptor-negative:* no demonstrated benefit from tamoxifen. Adjuvant chemotherapy should be considered in younger postmenopausal patients.

* Poor prognostic features are defined as tumours >20 mm; or tumours 11–20 mm with additional poor prognostic features such as oestrogen and progesterone receptor negativity, or high histological grade. For patients with good prognostic features (e.g. those with tumours <10 mm diameter) there has been no demonstrated benefit of adjuvant therapy.

Management

- Consider mammography if diffuse lumpiness is present in patient > 40.
- Perform needle biopsy if a discrete lump is present and aspirate palpable cysts.
- Reassure patient that there is no cancer.
- Give medication to alleviate mastalgia (see treatment for cyclical mastalgia in Chap. 81).
- Use analgesics as necessary.
- Surgically remove undiagnosed mass lesions.

Breast cyst

- common in women aged 40–50 years (perimenopausal)
- rare under 30 years
- associated with mammary dysplasia
- tends to regress after the menopause
- pain and tenderness variable
- has a 1 in 1000 incidence of cancer
- usually lined by duct epithelium

Examination. Look for a discrete mass, firm, relatively mobile, that is rarely fluctuant.

Diagnosis
- mammography
- ultrasound (X-ray of choice)
- cytology of aspirate

Lactation cysts

- These present postpartum with similar signs to perimenopausal cysts.
- They vary from 1–5 cm in diameter.
- Treat by aspiration: fluid may be clear or milky.

Fibroadenoma
Clinical features
- a discrete asymptomatic lump
- usually in twenties (range: second to sixth decade, commonly 15–35 years)
- firm, smooth and mobile (the 'breast mouse')
- usually rounded
- usually in upper outer quadrant
- they double in size about every 12 months[8]

Management
Ultrasound and fine needle aspiration with cytology is recommended. The lump may be left in those in the late teens but as a rule it should be removed to be certain of the diagnosis.

Fat necrosis

Fat necrosis is usually the end result of a large bruise or trauma which may be subtle such as protracted breast-feeding. The mass that results is often accompanied by skin or nipple retraction and thus closely resembles carcinoma.

The problem of mammary prostheses[6]

Clinical examination is still necessary and fortunately the residual mammary tissue is usually spread over the prosthesis in a thin easily palpable layer. The areas of clinical difficulty lie at the margin of the prosthesis, especially in the upper outer quadrant where most of the breast tissue is displaced. It should be noted that mammography may be of limited value in the presence of prostheses, especially if a fibrous capsule exists around the prosthesis. Ultrasound examination may be helpful.

Mammary duct ectasia

Synonyms: plasma cell mastitis, periductal mastitis.

In this benign condition a whole breast quadrant may be indurated and tender. The lump is usually located near the margin of the areola and is a firm or hard, tender, poorly defined swelling. There may be a toothpaste-like nipple discharge. It is a troublesome condition with a tendency to repeated episodes of periareolar inflammation with recurrent abscesses and fistula formation. Many cases settle but often surgical intervention is necessary to make the diagnosis.

Breast lumps in children

There are several benign conditions that can cause a breast lump in children, although the commonest presentation is a diffuse breast enlargement.

Neonatal enlargement[10]

Newborn babies of either sex can present with breast hyperplasia and secretion of breast milk. This is due to transplacental passage of lactogenic hormones. The swelling usually lasts 7–10 days if left alone. Any attempts to manipulate the breasts to facilitate emptying will prolong the problem.

Premature hyperplasia[10]

The usual presentation is the development of one breast in girls commonly 7–9 years of age but sometimes younger. The feature is a firm discoid lump 1–2 cm in diameter, situated deep to the nipple. The same change may follow in the other breast within 3–12 months. Reassurance and explanation is the management and biopsy must be avoided at all costs.

Subareolar hyperplasia in boys

A discoid subareolar lesion similar to the premature hyperplasia of girls can occur in boys in one or both breasts at about 12–14 years. No specific treatment is necessary, simply explanation and reassurance.

Gynaecomastia

This is not to be confused with pseudogynaecomastia due to fat in obese preadolescents. However, gynaecomastia in thin boys does occur and requires referral for assessment if it cannot be attributed to drugs such as oestrogen. If no cause is found, simple mastectomy may be performed.

Breast lumps in men

Virtually no breast tissue is palpable in normal men and malignancy is rare.

Gynaecomastia

This is a 'true' enlargement of the male breasts, not to be confused with false enlargement of obese men. Gynaecomastia occurs in up to 50% of adolescent boys.[5]

If present in adult men, look for evidence of hypogonadal states such as Klinefelter's syndrome and secondary testicular failure, e.g. orchitis, orchidectomy, traumatic atrophy. Other causes include drugs, e.g. oestrogen, digoxin, calcium antagonists, marijuana, spironolactone, amiodarone, tricyclic antidepressents, cimetidine; liver failure; testicular feminisation syndrome; and oestrogen-secreting tumours such as adrenal carcinoma and Leydig cell tumour.

Counselling of patients

'Treat the whole woman, not merely her breasts.'[6] Extreme anxiety is generated by the discovery of a breast lump and it is important that women are encouraged to visit their doctor early, especially as they can learn that there is a 90% chance of their lump being benign. It is possible that denial may be a factor or there is a hidden agenda to the consultation. The decision to perform a lumpectomy or a mastectomy should take the patient's feelings into consideration—many do fear that a breast remnant may be a focus for cancer. Longstanding doctor–patient relationships are the ideal basis for coping with the difficulties.

Screening

Screening mammography should be encouraged for women between 50 and 70, and performed at least every 2 years. Technically it is a better diagnostic tool in older women because of the less dense and glandular breast tissue. It has a specificity of around 90%. A management program for women at high risk of breast cancer is presented in Table 82.4.

Breast self-examination is a controversial issue and has no proven benefit in reducing morbidity and mortality. The false positive rate is high, especially in those under 40 years. However, regular BSE is recommended for all women 35 years and over.

When to refer

- Patients with a solitary breast mass.
- Following cyst aspiration:
  — blood in aspirate
  — palpable residual lump
  — recurrence of the cyst
- Patients given antineoplastic drugs, whether for adjuvant therapy or for advanced disease, require skilled supervision.

Lumps that require investigation and referral are presented in Table 82.5.

Table 82.4 *Management program for women at high risk of breast cancer (after Barraclough)*[7]

- Monthly breast self-examination
- At least an annual consultation with general practitioner—if aged 40 or older
- Aspiration of cysts
- Mammography, ultrasound and/or fine needle biopsy to diagnose any localised mass
- Ultrasound alone for further assessment of young, dense breasts
- Regular screening mammography after 50 years of age—every 2 years
- Removal of any undiagnosed mass lesions

Table 82.5 *Lumps that require investigation and referral (after Hirst)*[6]

- A stony hard lump or area, regardless of size, history or position
- A new palpable 'anything' in a postmenopausal woman
- A persisting painless asymmetrical thickening
- An enlarging mass—cyclic or not
- A 'slow-to-resolve' or recurrent inflammation
- A bloodstained or serous nipple discharge
- Skin dimpling, of even a minor degree, or retraction of the nipple
- A new thickening or mass in the vicinity of a scar

Practice tips

- Any doubtful breast lump should be removed.
- Fibroadenomas commonly occur in women in their late teens and twenties, benign breast cysts between 35 years and the menopause, and carcinoma is the most common cause of a lump in women over 50 years.[4]
- Never assume a palpable mass is a fibroadenoma in any woman over 30 years of age.[6]
- Gentle palpation is required. Squeezing breast tissue between finger and thumb tends to produce 'pseudolumps'.
- Any eczematous rash appearing on the nipple or areola indicates underlying breast cancer.
- Mammary duct ectasia and fat necrosis can be clinically indistinguishable from carcinoma of the breast.
- 9 out of 10 women who get breast cancer do not have a strong family history.
- The oral contraceptive pill and HRT have been generally shown *not* to alter the risk of breast cancer.
- Never assume that a lump is due to trauma unless you have seen the bruising and can observe the lump decrease in size.[6]
- Never assume a lesion is a cyst—prove it with ultrasound or successful aspiration.[6]
- Never ignore skin dimpling even if no underlying mass is palpable.[6]
- Never ignore a woman's insistence that an area of her breast is different or has changed.[6]
- Mammography can detect breast cancers which are too small to feel.
- Mammography is not a diagnostic tool.
- Recommended mammography screening for women 50–69 years and those aged 40–49 who request it.

References

1. Davis A, Bolin T, Ham J. *Symptom analysis and physical diagnosis* (2nd edn). Sydney: Pergamon Press, 1990, 118.
2. Fry J, Berry HE. *Surgical problems in clinical practice*. London: Edward Arnold, 1987, 57–67.
3. Green M. Breast cancer. In: MIMS Disease Index (2nd edn). Sydney: IMS Publishing, 1996, 83–85.

4. Hunt P, Marshall V. *Clinical problems in general surgery*. Sydney: Butterworths, 1991, 63–71.

5. Talley N, O'Connor S. *Clinical examination* (3rd edn). Sydney: MacLennan & Petty, 1996, 113–135.

6. Hirst C. Managing the breast lump. Solving the dilemma—reassurance versus investigation. Aust Fam Physician, 1989; 18:121–126.

7. Barraclough B. The fibrocystic breast— clinical assessment, diagnosis and treatment. Mod Med Aust, April 1990; 16–25.

8. Crea P. Benign breast diseases: a management guide for GPs. Mod Med Aust, 1995; 38(8):74–88.

9. Coates A. Breast Cancer Consensus report, Med J Aust, Vol. 161, November 1994; 510–513.

10. Hutson JM, Beasley SW, Woodward AA. *Jones clinical paediatric surgery*. Melbourne: Blackwell Scientific Publications, 1992, 266–267.

83

Abnormal uterine bleeding

—

It is advisable that menstruation begin before the individual ceases to be a virgin.

Soramus of Ephesus (2nd century)
Text on diseases of women

Abnormal uterine bleeding is a common problem encountered in general practice. Heavy menstrual bleeding is the commonest cause of iron deficiency anaemia in the western world. A classification of abnormal uterine bleeding is presented in Table 83.1.

Key facts and checkpoints

- Up to 20% of women in the reproductive age group complain of increased menstrual loss.[1]
- At least 4% of consultations in general practice deal with abnormal uterine bleeding.
- Up to 50% of patients who present with perceived menorrhagia (or excessive blood loss) have a normal blood loss when investigated.[2] Their perception is unreliable.

Table 83.1 *Classification of abnormal uterine bleeding*

Abnormal rhythm
- Irregularity of cycle
- Intermenstrual bleeding (metrorrhagia)
- Postcoital bleeding
- Postmenopausal bleeding

Abnormal amount
- Increased amount = menorrhagia
- Decreased amount = hypomenorrhoea

Combination (rhythm and amount)
- Irregular and heavy periods = metromenorrhagia
- Irregular and light periods = oligomenorrhoea

- The possibility of pregnancy and its complications, such as ectopic pregnancy, abortion (threatened, complete or incomplete), hydatidiform mole or choriocarcinoma should be kept in mind.
- The mean blood loss in a menstrual cycle is 30–40 mL.
- A menstrual record is a useful way to calculate blood loss.
- Blood loss is normally less than 80 mL.
- Menorrhagia is a menstrual loss of more than 80 mL per menstruation.
- Menorrhagia disposes women to iron deficiency anaemia.
- Various drugs can alter menstrual bleeding, e.g. anticoagulants, cannabis, steroids.

Defining what is normal and what is abnormal

This feature is based on a meticulous history, an understanding of the physiology and physiopathology of the menstrual cycle and a clear understanding of what is normal. Most girls reach menarche by the age of 13 (range 10–16).[1] Dysfunctional bleeding is common in the first 2–3 years after menarche due to many anovulatory cycles resulting in irregular periods, heavy menses and probably dysmenorrhoea.

Once ovulation and regular menstruation are established the cycle usually follows a predictable pattern and any deviation can be considered as abnormal uterine bleeding (see Table 83.2). It is abnormal if the cycle is less than 21 days, the duration of loss is more than 8 days, or the volume of loss is such that menstrual pads of adequate absorbency cannot cope with the flow or clots.[3]

Table 83.2 *Normal menstruation in the reproductive age group (after Fung)[1]*

	Mean	**Range**
Length of cycle	26–28 days	21–35 days
Menstrual flow	3–4 days	2–7 days
Normal blood loss	30–40 mL	20–80 mL

Relationship of bleeding to age

Dysfunctional uterine bleeding is more common at the extremes of the reproductive era (Fig. 83.1).[3] The incidence of malignant disease as a cause of bleeding increases with age, being greatest after the age of 45, while endometrial cancer is predicted to be less than 1 in 100 000 in women under the age of 35.[1]

Menorrhagia

Menorrhagia, which is excessive blood loss (> 80 mL per period),[4] is essentially caused by hormonal dysfunction (e.g. anovulation), local pathology (e.g. fibroids), or medical disorder (e.g. blood dyscrasia). Heavy bleeding, possibly with clots, is the major symptom of menorrhagia. Dysmenorrhoea may accompany the bleeding and, if it does, endometriosis or pelvic inflammatory disease (PID) should be suspected. With care a 60–80% accuracy can be achieved in clinical assessment.[4] A summary of the diagnostic strategy model is presented in Table 83.3.

Table 83.3 *Menorrhagia: diagnostic strategy model*

Q. *Probability diagnosis*
A. Dysfunctional uterine bleeding—ovulatory
  Fibroids
  Complications of hormone therapy

Q. *Serious disorders not to be missed*
A. Disorders of pregnancy
  • ectopic pregnancy
  • abortion or miscarriage
  Neoplasia
  • cervical cancer
  • endometrial cancer
  • leukaemia
  • benign tumours
    — polyps, etc.
  Severe infections
  • pelvic inflammatory disease

Q. *Pitfalls (often missed)*
A. Genital tract trauma
  IUCD
  Adenomyosis/endometriosis
  Pelvic congestion syndrome
  SLE

  Rare
  • endocrine disorders (e.g. thyroid disease)
  • bleeding disorder
  • liver disease

Q. *Seven masquerades checklist*
A. Depression   association
  Diabetes   √
  Drugs   √
  Anaemia   association
  Thyroid disease   √ hypothyroidism
  Spinal dysfunction   –
  UTI   –

Q. *Is the patient trying to tell me something?*
A. Consider exaggerated perception. Note association with anxiety and depression.

  By far the most common single 'cause' of menorrhagia is ovulatory dysfunctional uterine bleeding. The most common organic causes are fibromyomatas (fibroids), endometriosis, adenomyosis ('endometriosis' of the myometrium), endometrial polyps and pelvic inflammatory disease.[3]

Clinical approach for menorrhagia

History

Bearing in mind that abnormal uterine bleeding is a subjective complaint, a detailed history is the key initial step in management. The patient's perception of abnormal bleeding may be quite misleading and education about normality is all that is necessary in her management. A meticulous history should include details of the number of

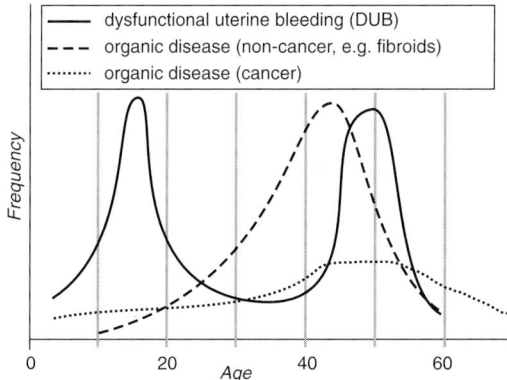

Fig. 83.1 *The relationship between age and various causes of abnormal uterine bleeding*
AFTER MACKAY ET AL[3]
DUB is more common in the extremes of the reproductive era, while the incidence of cancer as a cause of bleeding is greatest in the perimenopausal and postmenopausal phases

Legend within figure:
— dysfunctional uterine bleeding (DUB)
- - - organic disease (non-cancer, e.g. fibroids)
········· organic disease (cancer)

(y-axis: *Frequency*; x-axis: *Age* 0, 20, 40, 60)

tampons or pads used and their degree of saturation. A menstrual calendar (over 3+ months) can be a very useful guide. A history of smoking and other psychosocial factors should be checked. For unknown reasons, cigarette smokers are five times more likely to have abnormal menstrual function.[3]

Questions need to be directed to rule out:[1]

- pregnancy or pregnancy complications, e.g. ectopic pregnancy
- trauma of the genital tract
- medical disorders, e.g. bleeding disorder
- endocrine disorders
- cancer of the genital tract
- complications of the pill

Physical examination [1]

A general physical examination should aim at ruling out anaemia, evidence of a bleeding disorder and any other stigmata of relevant medical or endocrine disease.

Specific examinations include:

- speculum examination: ? ulcers (cervical cancer) or polyps
- Pap smear
- bimanual pelvic examination: ? uterine or adnexal tenderness, size and regularity of uterus.

It is prudent to avoid vaginal examination in selected patients, such as a young virgin girl, as the procedure is unhelpful and unnecessarily traumatic.

Investigations

Investigations, especially vaginal ultrasound scans, should be selected very carefully and only when really indicated. Abnormal pelvic examination findings, persistent symptoms, older patients and other suspicions of disease indicate further investigation to confirm symptoms of menorrhagia and exclude pelvic or systemic pathology.

Consider foremost:

- full blood count (to exclude anaemia and thrombocytopenia)
- iron studies: serum ferritin
- hysteroscopy and endometrial sampling (use directed endometrial biopsy with an instrument such as a Pipelle or Gynoscann, or curettage under general anaesthetic).

Special investigations (only if indicated):

- pregnancy testing
- laparoscopy where endometriosis, PID or other pelvic pathology is suspected

- serum biochemical screen
- coagulation screen
- thyroid function tests
- tests for SLE: antinuclear antibodies

Dysfunctional uterine bleeding

Dysfunctional uterine bleeding (DUB), which is a diagnosis of exclusion, is defined as 'excessive bleeding, whether heavy, prolonged or frequent, of uterine origin, which is not associated with recognisable pelvic disease, complications of pregnancy or systemic disease'.[4]

Features

- It is a working clinical diagnosis based on the initial detailed history, normal physical examination and normal initial investigation.
- Very common: 10–20% incidence of women at some stage.
- Peak incidence of ovulatory DUB in late thirties and forties (35–45 years).
- Anovulatory DUB has two peaks: 12–16 years and 45–55 years.
- The majority complain of menorrhagia.
- Up to 40% with the initial diagnosis of DUB will have other pathology (e.g. fibroids, endometrial polyps) if detailed pelvic endoscopic investigations are undertaken.

Symptoms

- heavy bleeding: saturated pads, frequent changing, 'accidents', 'flooding', 'clots'
- prolonged bleeding
  — menstruation > 8 days
    or
  — heavy bleeding > 4 days
- frequent bleeding—periods occur more than once every 21 days
- pelvic pain and tenderness are not usual[1] prominent features

Management principles [4]

- Establish diagnosis by confirming symptoms and exclude other pathology.
- If no evidence of iron deficiency or anaemia, and significant pathology has been excluded, prospective assessment of the menstrual pattern is indicated using a menstrual calendar.
- Conservative management is usually employed if the uterus is of normal size and there is no evidence of anaemia.

- Drug therapy is indicated if symptoms are persistently troublesome and surgery is contraindicated or not desired by the patient.
- Provide reassurance about the absence of pathology, especially cancer, and give counselling to maximise compliance with treatment.
- Consider surgical management if fertility is no longer important and symptoms cannot be controlled by at least 3–4 months of hormone therapy.
- General rule: < 35 years—medical treatment
  > 35 years—hysteroscopy and direct endometrial sample (diagnostic—sometimes therapeutic)

Drug therapy[4]

Treatment regimens are presented in Tables 83.4 and 83.5. First-line treatment is with fibrinolytic inhibitors or antiprostaglandin agents, given as soon as possible and throughout the menses. These agents are simple to use, generally very safe and can be used over long periods of time.

Table 83.4 *Regimens used in management of menorrhagia*

NSAIDs (prostaglandin inhibitors)
Mefenamic acid 500 mg tds (4 days before menses due to end of menses)
or
Naproxen 500 mg statim then 250 mg tds
or
Ibuprofen 800 mg statim then 400 mg 6–8 hourly

Combined oestrogen-progesterone OC
This is an important first-line therapy.
e.g. 50µg oestrogen + 1 mg norethisterone, e.g. Norinyl

Progestogens (especially for anovulatory patients)
Norethisterone 5–15 mg/day for 14 days (days 15–28)
or
Medroxyprogesterone acetate 20–30 mg/day
Try progestogens from days 5–25 (ovulatory patients) or if no response to days 15–28 therapy.

Danazol
Approved for short-term treatment (6 months or less) of severe menorrhagia—dosage 100–200 mg daily. Stops menstruation.

Antifibrinolytic agents
Tranexamic acid 1 g (o) qid, days 1–4

GnRH agonists
Administer by nasal spray (Synarel) or monthly implant (Zoladex) to induce medical 'menopause' 3–6 months.

Progestogen-releasing IUDs
e.g. Mirena

Table 83.5 *Typical treatment options for acute and chronic heavy bleeding[7]*

Acute heavy bleeding
- curettage/hysteroscopy
- IV oestrogen (Premarin 25 mg)
  or
oral high-dose progestogens
  e.g. norethisterone 5–10 mg 2 hourly until bleeding stops then 5 mg bd or tds for 14 days[3]

Chronic bleeding
- for anovulatory women
  — cyclical oral progestogens for 14 days
  — tranexamic acid
- for ovulatory women
  — cyclical prostaglandin inhibitor e.g. mefenamic acid
    or
  oral contraceptive
  — antifibrinolytic agent, e.g. tranexamic acid 1 g (o) qid, days 1–4
  — progesterone-releasing IUDs, e.g. Mirena

About 60–80% of patients with ovulatory menorrhagia will respond if compliance is good.[4] Such agents include tranexamic acid, mefenamic acid, naproxen, ibuprofen and indomethacin. The agent of first choice is usually mefenamic acid, which reduces blood loss by 20–25% as well as helping dysmenorrhoea. Ideally, it should be started at least 4 days before the menses.

Hormonal agents include progestogens, combined oestrogen-progestogen oral contraceptives and danazol. Oestrogens can be used but generally are not recommended except in the occasional patient with very heavy bleeding, when intravenous conjugated oestrogens 25 mg can be used (repeated in 2 hours if no response) and always followed by a 14 day course of oral progestogen. The COC constitutes important first-line therapy in both ovulatory and anovulatory patients, but at least 20% of patients do not respond. It is preferable to use a pill with a higher oestrogen dose, which works better (50 µg rather than 30 µg or 35 µg of oestrogen), and one that contains norethisterone[1] (e.g. Norinyl-1).

Progestogens can be given via several routes. Oral use is usually of no benefit in ovulatory DUB. In the adolescent with anovulatory DUB, cyclical oral progestogens may be required for 6 months until spontaneous regular ovulation eventuates.[5] Intramuscular medroxyprogesterone acetate (Depo-Provera) will induce amenorrhoea in 50% of users in 1 year.

The most effective agent for both ovulatory and anovulatory DUB is tranexamic acid which inhibits endometrial plasminogen activation. The dose is 1 g orally qid for the first 4 days of the menstrual cycle.[6,7]

Intrauterine progesterone implant systems (Mirena) releasing 20 μg of levonorgestrel/day have shown pleasing effectiveness.[8]

Surgical options

Surgical treatment for menorrhagia is more appropriate if the uterus is enlarged, especially if greater than the size of a 12 week gestation (grapefruit size) or if the patient is anaemic.[1] It is indicated if menorrhagia interferes with lifestyle despite medical (drug) treatment. The surgical options are:

- endometrial ablation or electrodiathermy excision—to produce amenorrhoea
- hysterectomy (up to 25% of Australians will have this before age 50); it requires a very carefully planned approach

Cycle irregularity

For practical purposes patients with irregular menstrual cycles can be divided into those under 35 and those over 35 years.

Patients under 35:

- the cause is usually hormonal, rarely organic, but keep malignancy in mind
- management options[1]
  1. explanation and reassurance (if slight irregularity)
  2. COC pill for better cycle control—any pill can be used
  3. progestogen-only pill (especially anovulatory cycles) norethisterone (Primolut N) 5–15 mg/day from day 5–25 of cycle

Patients over 35 should be referred for investigation for organic pathology, usually by endometrial sampling and/or hysteroscopy. If normal, the above regimens can be instituted.

Intermenstrual bleeding and postcoital bleeding

These bleeding problems are due to factors such as cervical ectropion (often termed cervical 'erosion'), cervical polyps, the presence of an IUCD and the oral contraceptive pill. Cervical cancer and intrauterine cancer must be ruled out, hence the importance of a Pap smear in all age groups and endometrial sampling, especially in the over 35 age group. A Pap smear should be taken, using the speculum carefully so as not to provoke bleeding, if one has not been taken within the previous 3 months, and sent to a laboratory that uses appropriate quality control procedures. Remember that it is only a screening test. Refer women with these bleeding problems with an abnormal smear or even without any unusual features. Those with a friable ectropion that is causing persistent symptoms should also be referred.[10] Thus intermenstrual bleeding should always be investigated.

Cervical ectropion, which is commonly found in women on the pill and post partum, can be left untreated unless intolerable discharge or moderate postcoital bleeding is present. An IUCD should be removed if causing significant symptoms and the causative pill should be changed to one with a higher oestrogen dose (e.g. from 30 μg oestrogen to 50 μg oestrogen).

Amenorrhoea and oligomenorrhoea

Amenorrhoea is classified as primary or secondary.

Primary amenorrhoea is the failure of the menses to start by 16 years of age.[3] Secondary amenorrhoea is the absence of menses for over 6 months in a woman who has had established menstruation.

The main approach in the patient with primary amenorrhoea is to differentiate it from delayed puberty. It is important to keep in mind the possibility of an imperforate hymen. A good rule is to note the presence of secondary sex characteristics.[3] If absent it implies that the ovaries are non-functional. Causes of primary amenorrhoea include genital malformations, ovarian disease, pituitary tumours, hypothalamic disease and Turner's syndrome.

In secondary amenorrhoea, consider a physiological cause such as pregnancy, or the menopause, failure of some part of the hypothalamic–pituitary–ovarian–uterine axis, or a metabolic disturbance. Important causes to consider are emotional, psychiatric and constitutional causes such as anorexia nervosa, hyperprolactinaemia, strenuous exercise, weight loss below 75% of ideal, and drugs/hormone therapy, e.g. oral contraceptives.

Oligomenorrhoea is the term for infrequent and usually irregular periods, where the cycles are between 6 weeks and 6 months.

Postmenopausal bleeding

Postmenopausal bleeding is vaginal bleeding of any amount occurring six months or more after the menopause.[3] It suggests cervical or uterine body cancer (up to 25%).[3] Other causes include polyps, atrophic vaginitis, endometrial hyperplasia and urethral caruncle. Care has to be taken with women on HRT who have irregular bleeding—they require investigation.

Early referral is usually indicated with a view to a diagnostic procedure. If bleeding recurs despite curettage, hysterectomy should be performed since early cancer of the uterus may be missed.

When to refer

- To exclude intrauterine pathology.
- The patient does not respond to initial therapy.
- There is evidence of underlying disease, e.g. endometriosis, SLE.
- Surgery is indicated (minor or major).

Practice tips

- Non-menstrual bleeding suggests cancer until proved otherwise: it may be postcoital (cervical cancer); intermenstrual (common with progestogen-only pill); postmenopausal (endometrial cancer).
- Think of a foreign body, especially an IUCD: if it is an IUCD, remove it.
- Hysteroscopy is more effective than the traditional curettage. Studies have shown that usually less than 50% of the uterine cavity is sampled by curettage.[11]

References

1. Fung P. Abnormal uterine bleeding. Mod Med Aust, May 1992; 58–66.
2. Fraser IS, Pearce C, Shearman RP et al. Efficacy of mefenamic acid in patients with a complaint of menorrhagia. Obstet Gynaecol, 1981; 58:543–551.
3. Mackay EV, Beischer NA, Pepperell RJ, Wood C. Illustrated textbook of gynaecology (2nd edn). Sydney: WB Saunders, 1992, 77–107.
4. Fraser IS. Dysfunctional uterine bleeding. In: MIMS Disease Index. Sydney: IMS Publishing, 1991–92; 165–167.
5. Hickey M. Management options in menorrhagia. Current Therapeutics, 1996; 17–21.
6. Bonnar J, Sheppard BL. Treatment of menorrhagia during menstruation: randomised controlled trial of ethamsylate, mefenamic acid and tranexamic acid. BMJ, 1996; 313:579–582.
7. Gleeson NC, Buggy F et al. The effect of tranexamic acid on measured menstrual blood loss and endometrial fibrinolytic enzymes in dysfunctional uterine bleeding. Acta Obstet Gynaecol Scand, 1994; 73:274–277.
8. Anderson JK, Rybo G. The levonorgestrel-releasing intrauterine contraceptive device in the treatment of menorrhagia. Br J Obstet Gynaecol, 1990; 97:690–694.
9. Hewson A. Menstrual disorders. In: MIMS Disease Index (2nd edn). Sydney: IMS Publishing, 1996, 307–310.
10. RACOG and RACGP. Joint Guidelines for Referral for Investigation of Intermenstrual and Postcoital Bleeding, 1996.
11. Warton B. Gynaecology. Melbourne: CHECK programme, RACGP Unit 240, 1992, 2–20.

84

Lower abdominal and pelvic pain in women

---

*Man endures pain as an undeserved punishment,
woman accepts it as a natural heritage.*

Anonymous

Pain in the lower abdomen and pelvis is one of the most frequent symptoms experienced by women. The diagnostic approach requires a wide variety of consultative skills, especially when the pain is chronic. The examination of acute abdominal pain has been simplified by the advent of sensitive serum pregnancy tests, ultrasound investigation and the increasing use of laparoscopy. However, an accurate history and examination for all types of pain will generally pinpoint the diagnosis. The ever-present problem of pelvic inflammatory disease (PID), the leading cause of infertility in women, demands an early diagnosis and appropriate management.

Key facts and checkpoints

- A distinction has to be made between acute, chronic and recurrent pain.
- Ectopic pregnancy remains a potentially lethal condition and its diagnosis still requires a high index of suspicion.
- Sudden sharp pain in the pelvis which becomes more generalised indicates rupture of an ectopic pregnancy or an ovarian cyst.
- Recurrent sharp self-limiting pain indicates a ruptured Graafian follicle (mittelschmerz).
- Recurrent pain related to menstruation is typical of dysmenorrhoea or endometriosis.
- A UK study[1] of chronic lower abdominal pain

in women showed the causes were adhesions (36%), no diagnosis (19%), endometriosis (14%), constipation (13%), ovarian cysts (11%) and PID (7%). An Australian study found that endometriosis accounted for 30% and adhesions 20%.[2]
- The principal afferent pathways of the pelvic viscera arise from T10,11,12, L1 and S2,3,4. Thus disorders of the bladder, rectum, lower uterus, cervix and upper vagina can refer pain to the low back, buttocks and posterior thigh.[3]

A diagnostic approach

A summary of the safety diagnostic model is presented in Table 84.1.

Probability diagnosis

The commonest causes are primary dysmenorrhoea, the pain of a ruptured Graafian follicle (mittelschmerz), endometriosis and adhesions. In many instances of pain no diagnosis is made as no pathological cause can be found.

Serious disorders not to be missed

The potentially lethal problem of a ruptured ectopic pregnancy must not be missed, hence the axiom 'be ectopic minded'. Pelvic inflammatory disease (PID) can be overlooked, especially if chronic, and requires early diagnosis and aggressive treatment. Neoplasia must be considered, especially malignancy of pelvic structures including the 'silent' carcinoma of the ovary.

Table 84.1 *Lower abdominal and pelvic pain in women: diagnostic strategy model*

Q.	*Probability diagnosis*
A.	Primary dysmenorrhoea
	Mittelschmerz
	Pelvic/abdominal adhesions
	Endometriosis
Q.	*Serious disorders not to be missed*
A.	Ectopic pregnancy
	Neoplasia
	• ovary
	• uterus
	• other pelvic structures
	Severe infections
	• PID
	Acute appendicitis
Q.	*Pitfalls (often missed)*
A.	Endometriosis/adenomyosis
	Torsion of ovary or pedunculated fibroid
	Constipation
	Pelvic congestion syndrome
	Referred pain (to pelvis)
	• appendicitis
	• cholecystitis
	• diverticulitis
	• urinary tract infection
Q.	*Seven masquerades checklist*
A.	Depression $\checkmark$
	Diabetes $-$
	Drugs $\checkmark$
	Anaemia $-$
	Thyroid disease $-$
	Spinal dysfunction $\checkmark$
	UTI $\checkmark$
Q.	*Is the patient trying to tell me something?*
A.	Can be very relevant. Consider various problems and sexual dysfunction.

Pitfalls

There are several disorders that are very difficult to diagnose and these include haemorrhage into the ovary or a cyst, torsion of the ovary or pedunculated fibroid. Endometriosis may be missed so it is important to be familiar with its symptoms. Chronic constipation may be a trap. Another relatively common problem is the so-called 'pelvic congestion syndrome' which tends to occur in somewhat neurotic patients and also tends to be a diagnosis of exclusion.

Seven masquerades checklist

Two important conditions to consider are urinary tract infection and spinal dysfunction. Just as disorders of the pelvic organs, such as endometriosis and PID, can refer pain to the low

back and buttocks so can disorders of the lumbosacral spine cause referred pain to the lower abdomen and groin.

Psychogenic considerations

These can be extremely relevant. Problems in the patient's social, marital or sexual relationships should be evaluated, especially in the assessment of chronic pain. Many patients with undiagnosed chronic pain exhibit psychoneurotic traits and this renders management very complex. Some appear to have the 'pelvic congestion syndrome' and need to be handled with sensitivity and tact, especially if the help of a psychiatrist or psychologist is sought.

The clinical approach
History

The pain should be linked with the menstrual history, coitus and the possibility of an early pregnancy. For recurrent and chronic pain it is advisable to instruct the patient to keep a diary over two menstrual cycles. The severity of the pain can be assessed as follows:[2]

• does not interfere with daily activity
• results in days off work
• results in confinement to bed

In this way the pain can be classified objectively as mild, moderate or severe.

Risk factors in the past history should be assessed, e.g.

• IUCD (salpingitis, ectopic pregnancy)
• infertility (endometriosis, salpingitis)
• tubal surgery (ectopic)

The typical pain patterns in relation to menstruation are shown in Figure 84.1.

Physical examination

One objective is to correlate any palpable tenderness with the patient's statement of the severity of the pain. Use the traditional abdominal and pelvic examination to identify the site of tenderness and rebound tenderness, and any abdominal or pelvic masses. The pelvis should be examined by speculum (preferably bivalve type) and bimanual palpation.

Proper assessment can be difficult if the patient cannot relax or overreacts, if there is abdominal scarring or obesity, or if extreme tenderness is present. It is therefore important, especially in the younger and apprehensive patient, to conduct a gentle caring vaginal examination

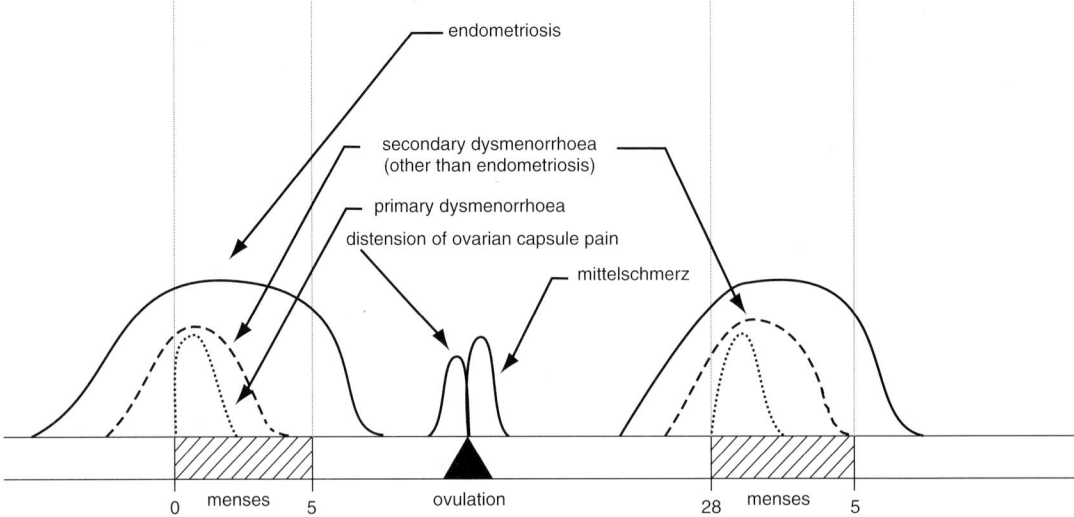

Fig. 84.1 *Typical pain patterns for the menstrual cycle related gynaecological pain*

with appropriate explanation and reassurance. Explanation of the procedure during vaginal examination, preferably using eye contact with the patient, can help her relax and be more confident in the procedure.

Investigations

Investigations may be selected from:

- haemoglobin level
- white blood cell count (limited value)
- haematocrit
- ESR
- microbiology (limited value)
  - — urine from micro and culture
  - — endocervical, urethral, cervical and vaginal swabs
- serum β-HCG assay
- urinary HCG tests (can be negative in the presence of an ectopic pregnancy)

Diagnostic imaging

- vaginal ultrasound—to define a gestation sac
- pelvic ultrasound—to differentiate a cystic from a solid pelvic mass

  Indicated for
  - — pelvic pain
  - — a palpable pelvic mass
  - — a palpable lower abdominal mass
  - — ascites

Laparoscopy is indicated if history and examination are suggestive of ectopic pregnancy and ultrasound fails to confirm an intrauteric pregnancy.

Acute pain

The causes of acute pain are summarised in Table 84.2. The patient is usually young (20–30 years old), sexually active and distressed by the pain, and should be considered foremost to have a bleeding ectopic pregnancy. Important differential diagnoses include acute PID, rupture or torsion of an ovarian cyst and acute appendicitis. Cases of acute ruptured ectopics are obviously easier to diagnose in the presence of circulatory collapse.

Table 84.2 *Causes of acute lower abdominal and pelvic pain in women (after Soo Keat Khoo)*[3]

Genital
- Acute salpingitis
- Pelvic peritonitis
- Bleeding
- Rupture or torsion of ovarian cyst
- Threatened or incomplete abortion
- Rupture or aborting tubal ectopic pregnancy
- Rupture or bleeding endometrioma

Non-genital
- Acute appendicitis
- Bowel obstruction
- Urinary tract infection (cystitis)
- Ureteric colic (calculus)

Functional
- Primary dysmenorrhoea
- Retrograde menstruation

Chronic pain

The common causes of chronic pain are listed in Table 84.3. Chronic pain is more difficult to diagnose and it is often difficult to differentiate between problems such as endometriosis, PID, an ovarian neoplasm and the irritable bowel syndrome. A comparison of the clinical features of endometriosis and PID is presented in Table 84.4. Furthermore it is difficult to distinguish clinically between endometriosis of the uterus (adenomyosis) and pelvic congestion syndrome. Both conditions are associated with dysmenorrhoea and a tender normal-sized uterus.

In pelvic congestion syndrome the patient is usually one who is para 3 or 4, aged 35–40 years, with a multitude of emotional problems.[3] They often undergo hysterectomy, sometimes without relief of symptoms.

Table 84.3 *Causes of chronic lower abdominal and pelvic pain in women*[3]

Genital
- Endometriosis/adenomyosis
- Pelvic inflammatory disease (chronic; adhesions)
- Ovarian neoplasm
- Fibromyomata (rarely)

Non-genital
- Diverticulitis
- Bowel adhesions

Functional
- Pelvic congestion syndrome
- Secondary dysmenorrhoea—IUCD*, polyp
- Irritable bowel, chronic bowel spasm

* intrauterine contraceptive device

Ectopic pregnancy

Ectopic pregnancy occurs approximately once in every 100 clinically recognised pregnancies. If ruptured it can be a rapid, fatal condition so we have to be 'ectopic minded'. It is the commonest cause of intraperitoneal haemorrhage. There is usually a history of a missed period but a normal menstrual history may be obtained in some instances.

Typical clinical features of a ruptured ectopic pregnancy
- average patient in mid-twenties
- first pregnancy in one-third of patients
- patient at risk
  — previous ectopic pregnancy

  — previous PID
  — previous abdominal or pelvic surgery, especially sterilisation reversal
  — IUCD use
  — in-vitro fertilisation/GIFT

> *Classical triad*
> amenorrhoea (65–80%)
> lower abdominal pain (95+%)
> abnormal vaginal bleeding (65–85%)

- pre-rupture symptoms (many cases)
  — abnormal pregnancy
  — cramping pains in one or other iliac fossa
  — vaginal bleeding
- rupture
  — excruciating pain (Fig. 84.2)
  — circulatory collapse

Note: In 10–15% there is no abnormal bleeding.
- pain may radiate to rectum (lavatory sign), vagina or leg
- signs of pregnancy, e.g. enlarged breasts and uterus, usually not present

Examination
- deep tenderness in iliac fossa
- vaginal examination
  — tenderness on bimanual pelvic examination (pain on moving cervix)
  — soft cervix
- bleeding (prune juice appearance)
- temperature and pulse usually normal early

Diagnosis
It is possible to diagnose ectopic pregnancy at a very early stage of pregnancy.
- urine pregnancy test (positive in < 50%)
- serum β-HCG assay (invariably positive if a significant amount of viable trophoblastic tissue present)
- vaginal ultrasound can diagnose at 5–6 weeks (empty uterus, tubal sac)
- laparoscopy (the definitive diagnostic procedure)

Management
Treatment may be conservative (based on ultrasound and β-HCG assays); medical, by injecting methotrexate into the ectopic sac; laparoscopic removal; or laparotomy for severe cases. Rupture with blood loss demands urgent surgery.

Table 84.4 *Comparison of clinical features of PID and pelvic endometriosis*

Feature	Chronic PID	Endometriosis
History	acute pelvic infection, e.g. ruptured appendix IUCD usage	dysmenorrhoea infertility dyspareunia pelvic pain
Pelvic pain	+ to ++ (mild to moderate) premenstrual lower abdominal location	++ to +++ (moderate to severe) premenstrual and menstrual acute pain if rupture of endometrioma
Backache	+ mild	++ moderate low sacral pain with menstruation
Secondary dysmenorrhoea	moderate to severe from onset of acute PID decreases with menstruation	moderate to severe gradual onset increases in severity throughout menstruation
Menstruation	irregular and heavy	heavy
Dyspareunia	moderate	often severe
Infertility	+++	++
Urinary symptoms	—	frequency, dysuria and haematuria if bladder wall involved
Bowel symptoms	—	painful defecation if rectal wall involved
Vaginal symptoms	may be chronic purulent discharge or leucorrhoea	—

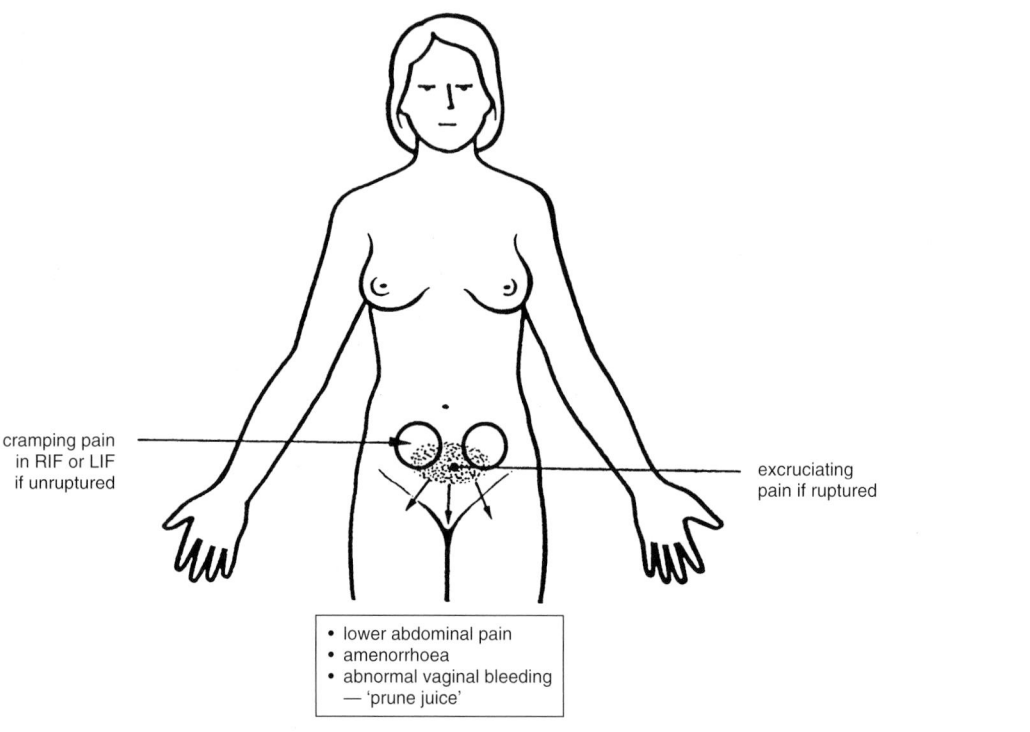

Fig. 84.2 *Clinical features of ectopic pregnancy*

Ruptured ovarian (Graafian) follicle (mittelschmerz)

When the Graafian follicle ruptures a small amount of blood mixed with follicular fluid is usually released into the pouch of Douglas. This may cause peritonism (mittelschmerz) which is different from the unilateral pain experienced just before ovulation due to distension of the ovarian capsule.

Typical clinical features
- onset of pain in mid-cycle
- deep pain in one or other iliac fossa (RIF > LIF)
- often described as a 'horse kick pain'
- pain tends to move centrally (Fig. 84.3)
- heavy feeling in pelvis
- relieved by sitting or supporting lower abdomen
- pain lasts from a few minutes to hours (average 5 hours)
- patient otherwise well

Note: Sometimes it can mimic acute appendicitis.

Management
- explanation and reassurance
- simple analgesics: aspirin or paracetamol (acetaminophen)
- 'hot water bottle' comfort if pain severe

Ovarian tumours

Benign ovarian tumours, particularly ovarian cysts, may be asymptomatic but will cause pain if complicated. They are common in women under 50 years of age. Ovarian cysts are best defined by vaginal ultrasound which can identify whether haemorrhage has occurred inside or outside the cyst.

Symptoms
- pain (usually torsion or haemorrhage)
- pressure symptoms
- menstrual irregularity

Ruptured ovarian cyst
The cysts tend to rupture just prior to ovulation or following coitus.

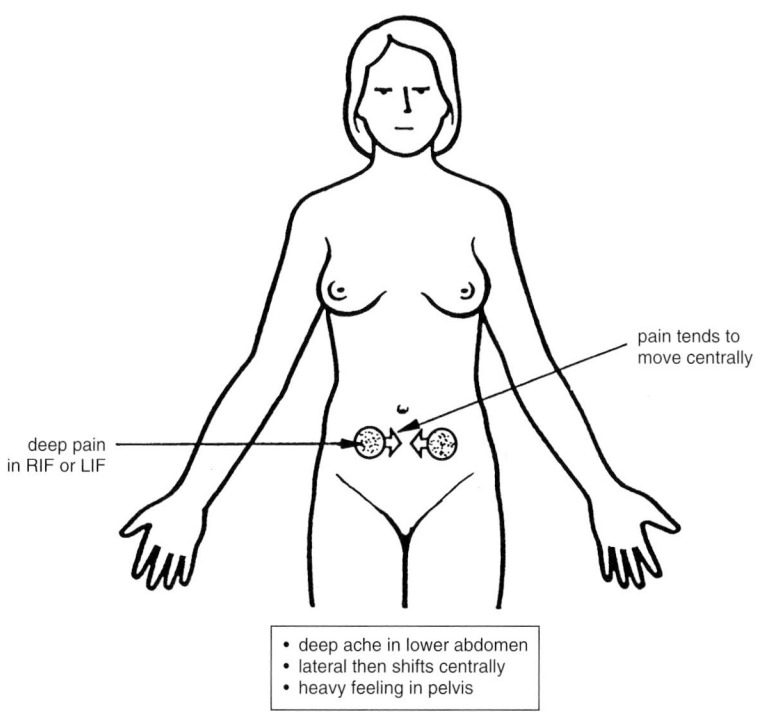

pain tends to move centrally

deep pain in RIF or LIF

- deep ache in lower abdomen
- lateral then shifts centrally
- heavy feeling in pelvis

Fig. 84.3 *Typical clinical features of a ruptured Graafian follicle (mittelschmerz)*

Clinical features
- patient usually 15–25 years
- sudden onset of pain in one or other iliac fossa
- may be nausea and vomiting
- no systemic signs
- pain usually settles within a few hours

Signs
- tenderness and guarding in iliac fossa
- PR: tenderness in rectovaginal pouch

Management
- appropriate explanation and reassurance
- conservative
  — simple cyst < 4 cm
  — internal haemorrhage
  — minimal pain
- needle vaginal drainage by ultrasonography for a simple larger cyst
- laparoscopic surgery
  — complex cysts
  — large cysts
  — external bleeding

Acute torsion of ovarian cyst
Torsions are mainly from dermoid cysts and, when right-sided, may be difficult to distinguish from acute pelvic appendicitis.

Clinical features
- severe cramping lower abdominal pain (Fig. 84.4)
- diffuse pain
- pain may radiate to the flank, back or thigh
- repeated vomiting
- exquisite pelvic tenderness
- patient looks ill

Signs
- smooth, rounded, mobile mass palpable in abdomen
- may be tenderness and guarding over the mass, especially if leakage

Diagnosis
- ultrasound

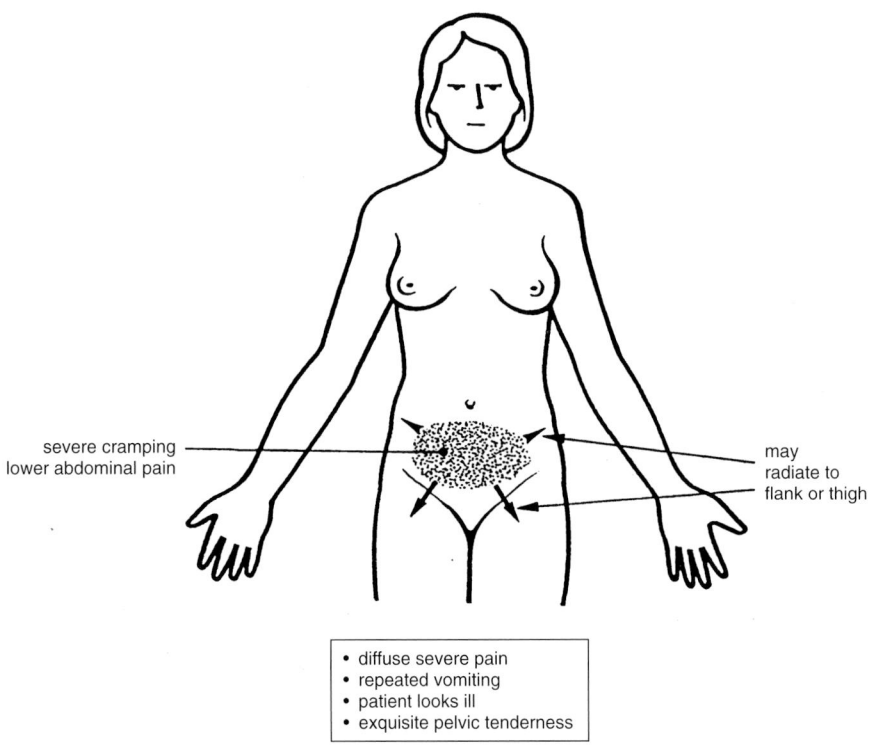

severe cramping lower abdominal pain

may radiate to flank or thigh

- diffuse severe pain
- repeated vomiting
- patient looks ill
- exquisite pelvic tenderness

Fig. 84.4 *Typical clinical features of acute torsion of an ovarian cyst*

Treatment
• laparotomy and surgical correction

Malignant ovarian tumours
Ovarian cancer has an incidence of 10 cases per 100 000 women per year and accounts for 5% of all cancers in women and 20% of all genital cancers. It is responsible for more genital cancer deaths because the tumour is often well advanced at the time of clinical presentation.[4] Earlier discovery may sometimes be made on routine examination or because of investigation of non-specific pelvic symptoms.

Ovarian cancer tends to remain asymptomatic for a long period. No age group is spared but it becomes progressively more common after 45 years.

Clinical features
• ache or discomfort in lower abdomen or pelvis
• gastrointestinal dysfunction, e.g. epigastric discomfort
• sensation of pelvic heaviness
• ± menstrual dysfunction
• dyspareunia and/or dysmenorrhoea (10–20%)
• a combined vaginal–rectal bimanual examination assists diagnosis

Note: Any ovary that is easily palpable is usually abnormal (normal ovary rarely > 4 cm).

Diagnosis
• ultrasound might be useful
• tumour markers such as CA 125, HCG (choriocarcinoma) and alpha fetoprotein are becoming more important in diagnosis and management

Dysmenorrhoea
Dysmenorrhoea (painful periods) may commence with the onset of the menses (menarche) when it is called primary dysmenorrhoea, or later in life when the term secondary dysmenorrhoea is applied.

Primary (functional) dysmenorrhoea
This is menstrual pain associated with ovular cycles without any pathologic findings. The pain usually commences within 1–2 years after the menarche and become more severe with time up to about 20 years. It affects about 50% of menstruating women and up to 95% of adolescents.

Clinical features
• low midline abdominal pain
• pain radiates to back or thighs (Fig. 84.5)
• varies from a dull dragging to a severe cramping pain
• maximum pain at beginning of the period

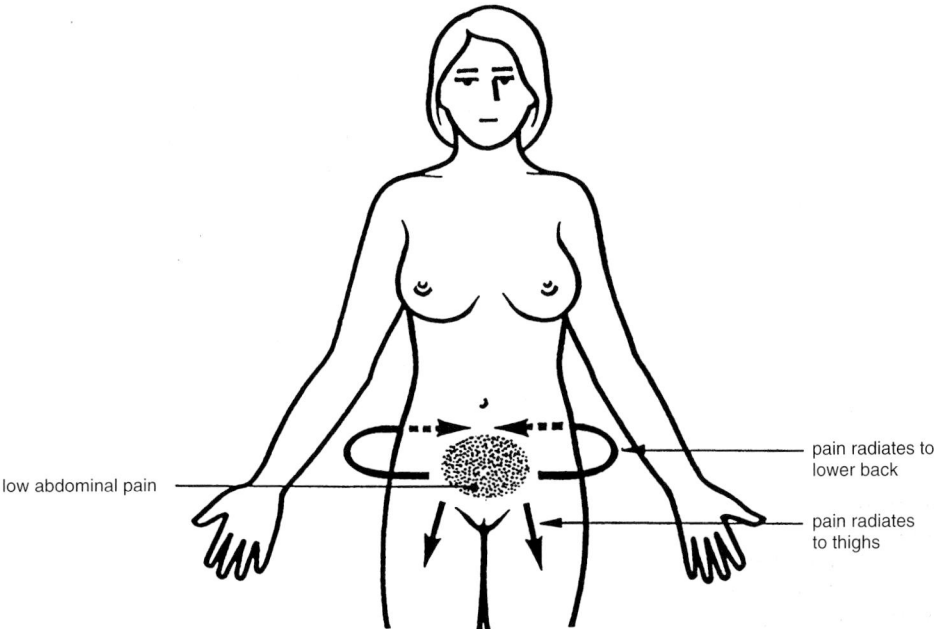

low abdominal pain

pain radiates to lower back

pain radiates to thighs

Fig. 84.5 *Typical pain of dysmenorrhoea*

- may commence up to 12 hours before the menses appear
- usually lasts 24 hours but may persist for 2–3 days
- may be associated with nausea and vomiting, headache, syncope or flushing
- no abnormal findings on examination

Management
- full explanation and appropriate reassurance
- promote a healthy lifestyle
  — regular exercise
  — avoid smoking and excessive alcohol
- recommend relaxation techniques such as yoga
- avoid exposure to extreme cold
- place a hot water bottle over the painful area and curl the knees onto the chest

Medication
Options include (trying in order):
- simple analgesics, e.g. aspirin or paracetamol (acetaminophen)
- prostaglandin inhibitors, e.g. mefenamic acid, 500 mg tds at first suggestion of pain (if simple analgesics ineffective)
- combined oral contraceptive (low-oestrogen triphasic pills preferable)
- progestogen-medicated IUCD

Secondary dysmenorrhoea
Secondary dysmenorrhoea is menstrual pain for which an organic cause can be found. It usually begins after the menarche after years of pain-free menses; the patient is usually over 30 years of age. The pain begins as a dull pelvic ache 3–4 days before the menses and becomes more severe during menstruation.

Commonest causes
- endometriosis ⎫
- PID   ⎬ the major causes
- IUCD   ⎭
- submucous myoma
- intrauterine polyp
- pelvic adhesions

Investigations
Investigations include laparoscopy, ultrasound and (less commonly) assessment of the uterine cavity by dilation and curettage, hysteroscopy or hysterosalpingography.
  Management involves treating the cause.

Pelvic adhesions
Pelvic adhesions may be the cause of pelvic pain, infertility, dysmenorrhoea and intestinal pain. They can be diagnosed and removed laparoscopically when the adhesions are well visualised and there are no intestinal loops firmly stuck together.

Endometriosis
Endometriosis is the condition where ectopically located endometrial tissue (usually in dependent parts of the pelvis and in the ovaries) responds to female sex hormone stimulation by proliferation, haemorrhage, adhesions and ultimately dense scar tissue changes.
  Patients experience varying degrees of symptoms and loss of gynaecological function according to the site and severity of the endometriosis deposits. Pregnancy is beneficial but recurrence can follow.

Clinical features
- 10% incidence[5]
- puberty to menopause, peak 25–35 years
- secondary dysmenorrhoea
- infertility
- dyspareunia
- non-specific pelvic pain
- menorrhagia
- acute pain with rupture of endometrioma
- premenstrual spotting

Possible signs
- fixed uterine retroversion
- tenderness and nodularity in the pouch of Douglas/retrovaginal septum
- uterine enlargement and tenderness

Differential diagnosis
- pelvic inflammatory disease (PID)—see Table 84.4
- ovarian cysts or tumours
- uterine myomas

Diagnosis
- can be made only by direct visual inspection at laparoscopy or laparotomy
- ultrasound scanning helpful

Treatment
- careful explanation
- basic analgesics
- treatment can be surgical or medical

Medical: To induce amenorrhoea (only two-thirds respond to drugs)
- danazol (Danocrine)—current treatment of choice
- combined oestrogen-progestogen oral contraceptive: once daily continuously for about 6 months
- progestogens, e.g. medroxyprogesterone acetate (Depo-Provera)
- GnRH analogues e.g. goserelin, nafarelin

Surgical. Surgical measures depend on the patient's age, symptoms and family planning. Laser surgery and microsurgery can be performed via either laparoscopy or laparotomy.

Pelvic inflammatory disease

There are great medical problems in the serious consequences of PID, namely tubal obstruction, infertility and ectopic pregnancy. PID may be either acute, which causes sudden severe symptoms, or chronic, which can gradually produce milder symptoms or follow an acute episode. Acute PID is a major public health problem and is the most important complication of sexually transmitted disease among young women. The majority are young (less than 25 years) sexually active women who are also nulliparous.

Some patients may experience no symptoms but others may have symptoms that vary from mild to very severe. The clinical diagnosis can be difficult as signs and symptoms can be non-specific and correlate poorly with the extent of the inflammation.

Clinical features

Acute PID
- fever $\geq$ 38°C
- moderate to severe lower abdominal pain

Chronic PID
- ache in the lower back
- mild lower abdominal pain

Both acute and chronic
- dyspareunia
- menstrual problems (e.g. painful, heavy or irregular periods)
- intermenstrual bleeding
- abnormal, perhaps offensive, purulent vaginal discharge
- painful or frequent urination

The diagnostic criteria for acute PID are presented in Table 84.5.[6]

Examination
- In acute PID there may be lower abdominal tenderness $\pm$ rigidity.
- Pelvic examination: in acute PID there is unusual vaginal warmth, cervical motion tenderness and adnexal tenderness. Inspection usually reveals a red inflamed cervix and a purulent discharge.

Causative agents
These can be subdivided into three broad groups:

1. *Exogenous organisms*: those which are community acquired and initiated by sexual activity. They include the classic STDs, *Chlamydia trachomatis* and *Neisseria gonorrhoeae*. This usually leads to salpingitis.
2. *Endogenous infections*: these are normal commensals of the lower genital tract, especially *Escherichia coli* and *Bacteroides fragilis*. They become pathogenic under conditions that interrupt the normal cervical barrier such as recent genital tract manipulation or trauma, e.g. abortion, presence of an IUCD, recent pregnancy or a dilatation and curettage. The commonest portals of entry are cervical lacerations and the placental site. These organisms cause an ascending infection and can spread direct or via lymphatics to the broad ligament, causing pelvic cellulitis (Fig. 84.6).
3. *Actinomycosis*: due to prolonged IUCD use. Look for *Actinomyces Israeli* on culture.

Table 84.5 *Diagnostic criteria for acute PID*[3]

All three of the following should be present:
1. Lower abdominal tenderness (with or without rebound)
2. Cervical motion tenderness
3. Adnexal tenderness (may be unilateral)

plus

One of the following should be present:
1. Temperature $\geq$ 38°C
2. White blood cell count $\geq$ 10 500/mm^2
3. Purulent fluid obtained via culdocentesis
4. Inflammatory mass present on bimanual pelvic examination and/or sonography
5. ESR $\geq$ 15 mm/hr or C-reactive protein > 1.0 mg/dL
6. Evidence for presence of *N.gonorrhoeae* and/or *C.trachomatis* in the endocervix. Gram stain reveals Gram-negative intracellular diplococci. Monoclonal antibody stain for *C.trachomatis*.
7. Presence of > 5 white blood cells per oil immersion field on Gram stain of endocervical discharge.

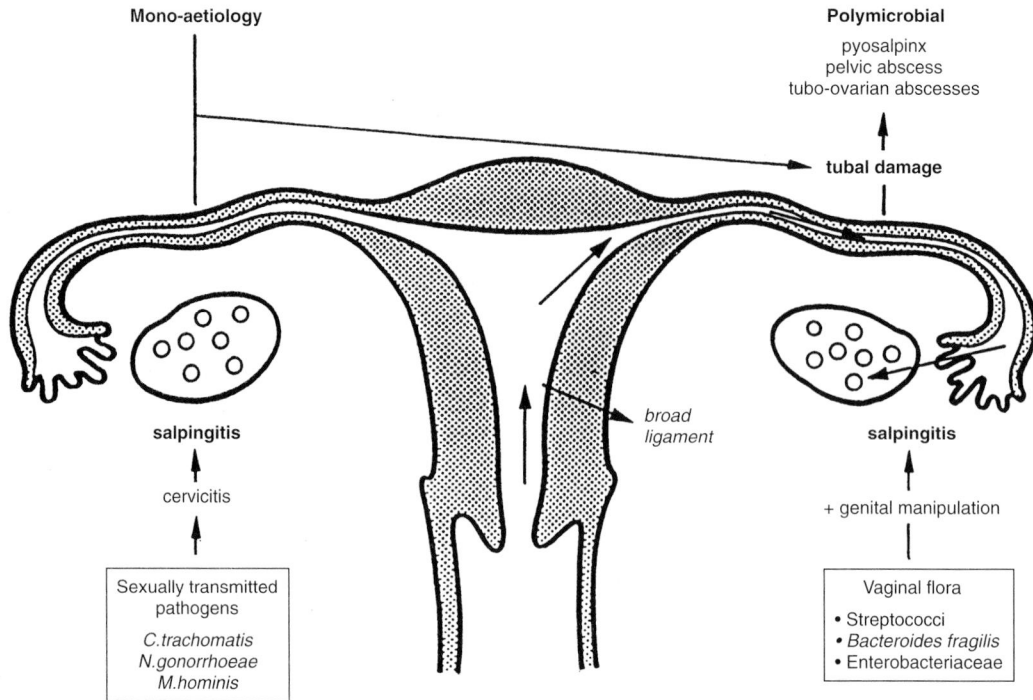

Fig. 84.6 *The pathogenesis of PID*

Investigations

A definitive diagnosis is difficult since routine specimen collection has limitations in assessing the organisms. Definitive diagnosis is by laparoscopy but this is not practical in all cases of suspected PID.

- cervical swab for Gram stain and culture (*N. gonorrhoeae*)
- cervical swab and special techniques for *C. trachomatis*

Treatment of PID

Note: Any IUCD or retained products of contraception should be removed at or before the start of treatment.

Sex partners of women with PID should be treated with agents effective against *Chlamydia trachomatis* and *Neisseria gonorrhoeae*.

| Sexually acquired infection[7] |

Mild infection (treated as an outpatient)
   doxycycline 100 mg (o) 12 hourly for 14 days
                plus either
   metronidazole 400 mg (o) 12 hourly with food for 14 days

                or
   tinidazole 500 mg (o) daily with food for 14 days

Where penicillinase-producing *Neisseria gonorrhoeae* (which is often tetracycline-resistant) is suspected or proven, add:
   ciprofloxacin 500 mg (o) as single dose
For penicillin-susceptible gonorrhoea add:
   amoxycillin 3g (o) + probenecid 1 g (o) as a single dose

Severe infection (treated in hospital)
   cefotaxime 1 g IV 8 hourly or ceftriaxone 1 g IV once daily
                plus
   doxycycline 100 mg (o) 12 hourly
                plus
   metronidazole 500 mg IV 12 hourly

until there is substantial clinical improvement, when the oral regimen above can be used for the remainder of the 14 days. If the patient is pregnant or breast-feeding, doxycyline should be replaced by
   erythromycin 500 mg IV or (o) 6 hourly

| Infection non-sexually acquired |
| (related to genital manipulation) |

Mild infection

amoxycillin 500 mg (o) 8 hourly for 10 days
plus either
metronidazole 400 mg (o) 12 hourly with food
for 10 days
or
tinidazole 500 mg (o) daily with food for 10
days
or (as a single agent)
amoxycillin/potassium clavulanate (500/125
mg) (o) 8 hourly for 10 days

Severe infection (including septicaemia)

(amoxy)ampicillin 1 g IV 6 hourly
together with
gentamicin 1.5 mg/kg IV 8 hourly
together with
metronidazole 500 mg IV 12 hourly
or (as single agents)
cefotaxime 1 g IV 8 hourly or ceftriaxone 1 g
IV once daily

until there is substantial clinical improvement, when the oral regimen above can be used for the remainder of the 14 days.

If infection with *Streptococcus pyogenes* or *Clostridium perfringens* is suspected or proven, then benzylpenicillin 2.4 g IV 4 hourly is the drug of choice.

| Actinomycosis |

Amoxycillin 500 mg tds + metronidazole 400 mg bd for 14 days. Ensure IUCD is removed.

When to refer

- All cases of 'unexplained infertility'.
- All teenagers with dysmenorrhoea sufficient to interfere with normal school, work or recreational activities, and not responding to prostaglandin inhibitors.
- Patients with dysmenorrhoea reaching a crescendo mid menses.
- Patients with dysmenorrhoea and unexplained bowel or bladder symptoms.
- Patients with positional dyspareunia.
- Patients with cyclic pain or bleeding in unusual sites.

Note: Pelvic disease that can be treated by advanced laparoscopy surgery includes ectopic pregnancy, ovarian cysts, endometriosis and endometriomas, fibromyomata, pelvic adhesions and hydrosalpinx.

Practice tips

- Think of endometriosis and ovarian cysts in any woman with lower abdominal pain.
- In any woman whose normal activities are disturbed by dysmenorrhoea unrelieved by NSAIDs, endometriosis should be suspected.
- If an ectopic pregnancy is suspected and there are no facilities for resuscitation, digital vaginal examination should be deferred for it may provoke rupture.[2]
- Acute abdominal and pelvic pain in the presence of a negative β-HCG is most often due to an ovarian cyst.
- A positive β-HCG plus an empty uterus and an adnexal mass are the classic diagnostic features of ectopic pregnancy.

An approach to the management of acute abdominal and pelvic pain in premenopausal women is given on the next page.

References

1. Foy A, Brown R. Chronic lower abdominal pain in gynaecological practice. Update, 27 March 1987, 19–25.
2. Forbes KL. Lower abdominal and pelvic pain in the female: a gynaecological approach. Mod Med Aust, September 1991; 24–31.
3. Soo Keat Khoo. Lower abdominal pain in women. Patient management supplement, August 1990; 13–23.
4. Mackay EV et al. *Illustrated textbook of gynaecology* (2nd edn). Sydney: WB Saunders, Bailliere Tindall, 1992, 514–524.
5. O'Connor DT. Endometriosis. In: MIMS Disease Index (2nd edn). Sydney: IMS Publishing, 1996, 170–172.
6. Hager WD, Eschenbach DA et al. Criteria for diagnosis and grading of salpingitis. Obstet Gynecol, 1983; 61:113–114.
7. Mashford ML et al. *Antibiotic guidelines* (9th edn). Melbourne: Victorian Medical Postgraduate Foundation, 1996–97, 76–77.

Fig. 84.7 *An approach to management of acute abdominal and pelvic pain in premenopausal women*
AFTER FORBES.

85

Premenstrual syndrome

—

Premenstrual syndrome (PMS) is defined as a group of physical, psychological and behavioural changes which begin 2–14 days before menstruation and are relieved immediately the menstrual flow begins.[1]

These symptoms occur in the luteal phase of the menstrual cycle yet the pathogenesis of PMS is still uncertain. Among the proposed causes are pyridoxine deficiency, excess prostaglandin production and increased aldosterone production in the luteal phase.[2] However, PMS is most probably a disorder of ovarian function with a relative excess of oestrogen the main determinant.[3]

Key features

- PMS increases in incidence after 30 years, with a peak incidence in the 30–40 year age group.
- PMS also occurs in the 45–50 year age group when it may alternate with menopausal symptoms, causing clinical confusion.[4]
- The symptoms of PMS decrease in severity just before and during menstruation.
- The symptoms cannot be explained by the presence of various psychological or psychiatric disorders.

Incidence

Up to 90% of women may experience premenstrual symptoms, which can vary from minor to severe. Interestingly, up to 15% of women can

feel better premenstrually.[5] Statistics from countries such as Sweden, the United States and the UK indicate that up to 40% of women are significantly affected.[6] About 5–10% of women experience such severe symptoms that PMS disrupts their quality of life.

Aetiology

Various aetiological factors have been identified as contributing to PMS.[2]
Predisposing factors:

- mental illness
- alcoholism
- sexual abuse
- family history
- stress

Precipitating factors:

- hysterectomy
- tubal ligation
- cessation of the oral contraceptive

Sustaining factors:

- diet containing caffeine, alcohol, sugar
- smoking
- stress
- sedentary lifestyle

Symptoms

Various symptoms from among the 150 reported are summarised in Figure 85.1.

The most common symptoms are depression 71%, irritability 56%, tiredness 35%, headache 33%, bloatedness 31%, breast tenderness 21%, tension 19% and aggression/violence 13%.[7] Other important symptoms include weight gain, lowered performance, decreased libido and feeling out of control.

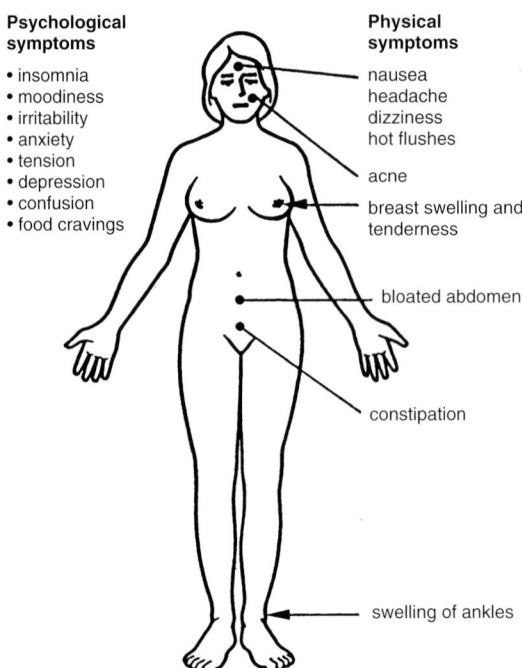

Psychological symptoms

- insomnia
- moodiness
- irritability
- anxiety
- tension
- depression
- confusion
- food cravings

Physical symptoms

nausea
headache
dizziness
hot flushes

acne

breast swelling and tenderness

bloated abdomen

constipation

swelling of ankles

Fig. 85.1 *Symptoms of premenstrual tension*

Classification of PMS

It is convenient to classify PMS in terms of severity of symptoms.[4]

1. *Mild*: symptoms signal onset of menstruation. No medical advice sought or needed.
2. *Moderate*: symptoms annoying but insufficient to interfere with function at home or work. Medical advice sought in about one-third.
3. *Severe*: symptoms are such that functions at work or home are disrupted. Medical advice is usually sought.

Differential diagnosis[4]

- menopause syndrome
- mastalgia
- other causes of fluid retention—renal or adrenal
- thyroid disorder (hyper or hypo activity)
- polycystic ovary syndrome (PMS may be a feature of oestrogen excess)
- psychiatric disorders: depression, mania

Diagnosis

- Thorough history—including diet, exercise habits, psychosocial background, emotional influences and family history.
- Menstrual calendar—for 3 months, showing timing of the three main symptoms.[4]

- Physical examination to exclude gynaecological, endocrine or other systemic disease; and also include:
  — breast examination
  — vaginal examination and Papanicolaou smear
- Investigations (if considered appropriate, perform one or more serological tests):
  — thyroid function tests
  — serum progesterone and oestradiol in mid-luteal phase of three representative cycles
  — electrolytes and creatinine
  — prolactin—if galactorrhoea or oligomenorrhoea present

Management

The basic aim of management is to reassure and treat the woman in such a way that she makes changes in her lifestyle to cope with the hormonal dysfunction rather than rely on medication. The management strategies include the following.

Explanation, reassurance and insight[8]

It is very helpful for the patient to understand the nature of her symptoms and to receive appropriate support and rapport. Advise her to be open about her problem and inform her family and close friends about her symptoms.

Keeping a diary[4]

Advise the patient to keep a daily diary of all her symptoms and when they occur over a 2–3 month period. This information should help her to plan around her symptoms: for example, avoid too many social events and demanding business appointments at the time when PMS symptoms are worst.

Dietary advice[4]

Advise the patient to eat regularly and sensibly; eat small rather than large meals and aim for ideal weight (if necessary).

Increase amount of complex carbohydrates (whole grains, vegetables and fruit), leafy green vegetables and legumes.

Decrease or avoid: refined sugar, salt, alcohol, caffeine (tea, coffee, chocolate), tobacco, red meat and excessive fluid intake during PM phase. Decrease total protein to 1 g/kg/day; decrease fats.

Exercise

Recommend a program of regular exercise such as swimming, aerobics, jogging or tennis. Such exercise has been proven to decrease depression, anxiety and fluid retention premenstrually.[9]

Relaxation

Advise patients to plan activities that they find relaxing and enjoyable at the appropriate time. Consider stress reduction therapy including appropriate counselling.

Appropriate dress

Advise sensible dressing to cope with breast tenderness and a bloated abdomen, such as a firm-fitting brassiere and loose-fitting clothes around the abdomen.

Medication

Pharmaceutical agents that have been used with success in some patients and little or no relief in others include diuretics (e.g. spironolactone), vitamins and minerals (e.g. pyridoxine and evening primrose oil), antiprostaglandin preparations (e.g. mefenamic acid, indomethacin), bromocriptine, danazol (suppresses ovulation), GnRH agonists and hormone preparations such as the oral contraceptive, progestogens and oestradiol implants. A combination of agents may have to be used.

- Oral contraceptives are the ideal first choice if contraception is needed. Select a moderate dose combined OC containing 50 μg ethinyl oestradiol.

Mild to moderate symptoms

- pyridoxine (Vitamin B$_6$) 100 mg daily; if ineffective after 3 cycles, try
- evening primrose oil capsules (gamma lineoleic acid) 1000 mg bd with food (day 12 to first day of next cycle)

A progestogen may be tried after or with evening primrose oil[4]

e.g. dydrogesterone 5 mg bd days 12–25; after 2 months increase to 10 mg bd

Severe symptoms

- fluoxetine 20 mg daily for 10–14 days before menstruation, or 10–20 mg daily continuously[11]

or

non-SSRI: clomipramine 25 mg (o) nocte for 2 cycles, increasing if necessary

Individualised therapy[10]

- PMS + fluid retention—use spironolactone 100 mg daily 3 days before expected onset of symptoms to day 1 of menstruation
- PMS + severe mastalgia—consider bromocriptine 1.25–5 mg (o) nocte on days 10–26 of cycle
- PMS + dysmenorrhoea—mefenamic acid 500 mg tds from onset of symptoms to onset of menses

No matter what medication is taken, up to 70% of women will report an improvement in the early months of treatment, suggesting that a strong placebo factor is involved in management.[12]

When to refer[4]

- Refer to a gynaecologist if underlying disease is suspected or proven, e.g. polycystic ovary disease, endometriosis.
- Consider referral if prescribing of danazol is contemplated.
- Refer to an endocrinologist if an endocrine disorder such as adrenal, pituitary or thyroid is suspected or proven.
- Consider referral if depression or psychosis worsens or is not cyclical.

Practice tips

- Keeping a daily diary of symptoms is very helpful for both patient and clinician.
- Aim for lifestyle changes and common-sense non-pharmacological management.
- Triphasic oral contraceptives do not appear to be as effective as a monophasic OC.[12]
- Allow at least three cycles of treatment to provide a reasonable time for a particular medication.
- Drugs such as danazol or bromocriptine are second-line drugs with significant side effects and should be used with caution.
- High doses of pyridoxine, such as 500 mg a day, are associated with peripheral neuropathy so the dosage should be kept at around 100 mg/day.
- Be careful of overdiagnosing PMS and overlooking disorders such as depression, which may be exacerbated in the premenstrual phase.

References

1. Shreeve CM. *The premenstrual syndrome.* Thorson Publishers Ltd, 1983, 23–24.
2. Smith MA, Yong Kin EQ. Managing the premenstrual syndrome. Clinical Pharm, 1986; 5:788–797.
3. Brush MG. Pharmacological rationale for the management of PMS. Journal of Psychosomatic Obstetrics and Gynaecology, 1983; 2–1:35–39.
4. Smith M. Premenstrual syndrome. In: MIMS Disease Index. Sydney: IMS Publishing, 1991–92, 439–441.
5. Farrell E. How to treat menstrual disorders. Australian Dr Weekly, 25 May 1990; IV–VI.
6. Labrum AH. Hypothalamic, pineal and pituitary factors in the premenstrual syndrome. Journal of Reproductive Medicine, 1983; 28(7):438–445.
7. Dalton K. *The premenstrual syndrome and progesterone therapy.* London: Heinemann, 1984, 3.
8. Murtagh J. Premenstrual syndrome. In: *Patient education* (2nd edn). Sydney: McGraw-Hill, 1996, 52.
9. Tierney LM et al. *Current medical diagnosis and treatment.* Stamford: Appleton and Lange, 1996, 640–641.
10. Roughan P. Premenstrual syndrome. Current Therapeutics, 1995; 36(11):53–59.
11. Stone AB, Perlstein TB, Brown WA. Fluoxetine in the treatment of premenstrual syndrome. Psychopharmacol Bull, 1990; 26:331–335.
12. Abraham S. The premenstrual syndrome. Mod Med Aust, Sept. 1992; 80–86.

86

The menopause and osteoporosis

—

Every woman should use what Mother Nature gave her before Father Time takes it away.

Laurence J. Peter 1977

Definitions

The menopause is the cessation of the menses for longer than 12 months. In most western women it occurs between the ages of 45 and 55, with an average age of 50–51 years.

The World Health Organisation has defined the menopause as signifying the permanent cessation of menstruation, resulting from the loss of ovarian follicular activity.[1] However, the term is used in a broader sense to include the perimenopausal phase when ovarian function waxes and wanes and the periods become irregular. This may last 2–5 years and sometimes longer and involves the premenopausal and menopausal phases.

The postmenopause is the period following the menopause but cannot be defined until after 12 months of spontaneous amenorrhoea, except in women who have had an oöphorectomy.

Surgical menopause is known as bilateral oöphorectomy.

Summary

The climacteric can be subdivided into four phases:

Phase 1 Premenopausal: up to 5 years before the last menstrual period.

Phase 2 Perimenopausal: the presence of early menopausal symptoms with vaginal bleeding (usually irregular)

Phase 3 Menopausal: the last menstrual period

Phase 4 Postmenopausal: approximately 5 years after the menopause

Osteoporosis

Osteoporosis, which literally means porous bone, is reduced bone mass per unit volume. Osteoporosis is usually addressed in the context of the menopause because it is found mainly in postmenopausal middle-aged and elderly women and can be largely prevented by correcting oestrogen deficiency.

Physiology of the menopause

Inspection of Figure 86.1 provides an overview of how menopausal symptoms are related to ovarian follicular activity and hormonal activity.

The number of ovarian primary follicles declines rapidly as the menopause approaches, with few if any being identifiable following the cessation of menstruation. In the postmenopause phase FSH rises to levels 10–15 times that of the follicular phase of the cycle while LH levels rise about threefold. The ovary secretes minimal oestrogen but continues to secrete significant amounts of androgens.

An uncomfortable effect of oestrogen withdrawal, often not appreciated by medical practitioners, involves urogenital problems where the epithelium of the vagina, vulva, urethra and the base of the bladder becomes thin and dry, leading possibly to dysuria and frequency, itching, dyspareunia and atrophic bleeding. Hormone replacement therapy (HRT) can ameliorate these urogenital dysfunctions.

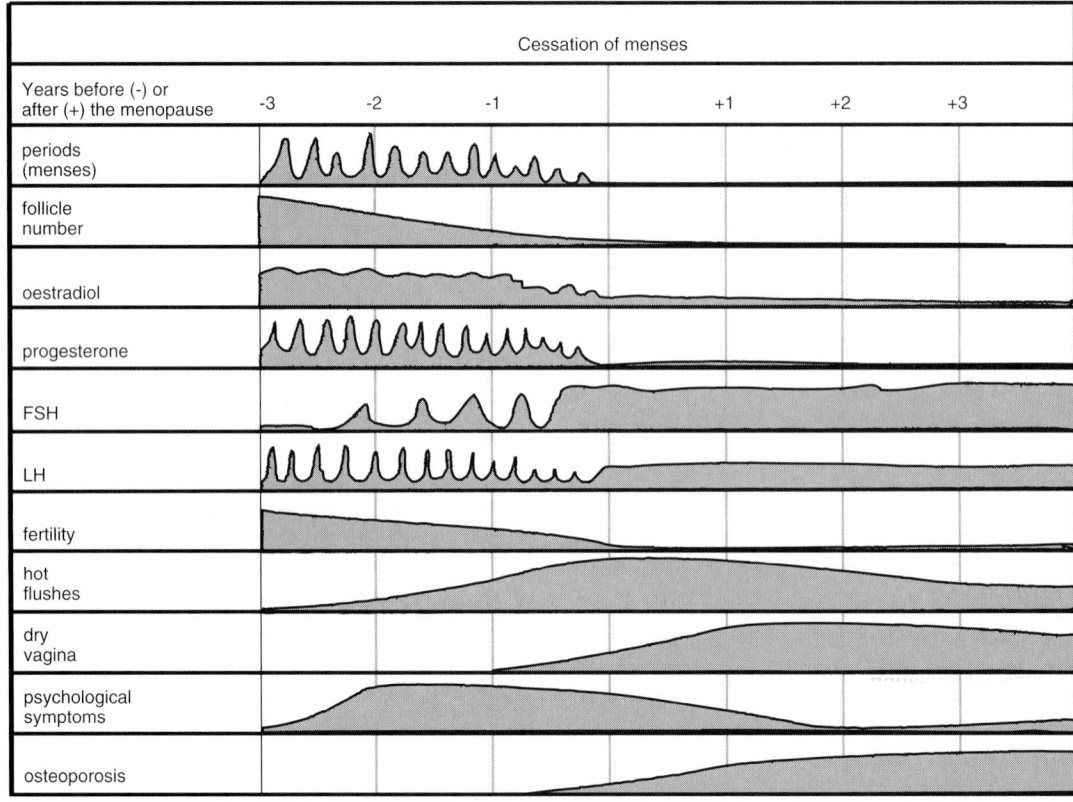

Fig. 86.1 *Schematic representation of some clinical, biological and endocrinological features of the perimenopausal and postmenopausal phases* AFTER BURGER

Clinical features

Because small amounts of oestrogen are still being produced in the adrenal glands, symptoms other than cessation of periods may be mild or absent.

Symptoms

Vasomotor:[2]

- hot flushes (80%)
- night sweats (70%)
- palpitations (30%)
- lightheadedness/dizziness
- migraine

Psychogenic:

- irritability
- depression
- anxiety/tension
- tearfulness
- loss of concentration
- poor short-term memory
- unloved feelings
- sleep disturbances
- mood changes
- loss of self-confidence

Urogenital (60%):

- atrophic vaginitis
- vaginal dryness (45%)
- dyspareunia
- decline in libido
- bladder dysfunction, e.g. dysuria
- stress incontinence/prolapse

Musculoskeletal:

- non-specific muscular aches
- non-specific joint aches and pains

Skin and other tissue changes:

- dry skin
- formication (17%)
- new facial hair
- breast glandular tissue atrophy

Other:
- unusual tiredness
- headache

Clinical approach

A thorough evaluation of the patient is important, including a good history.

History

Enquire about any symptoms related to oestrogen deficiency and about other related symptoms, with an emphasis on the menstrual history and hot flushes. Enquire about mental state symptoms such as anger, irritability, depression, moodiness, loss of self-esteem and other such problems. Ask about sexual history, contraception, micturition and social history, including relationships.

Information on family history of osteoporosis, cancer and cardiovascular disease should be sought.

Physical examination

The general examination should include measurement of blood pressure, weight and height, breast palpation, abdominal palpation, vaginal examination and Pap smear. Note the texture of the vaginal epithelium.

Investigations[2]

Apart from a Papanicolaou smear, the following tests should be considered:
- urinalysis
- full blood count, lipids including HDL
- liver function tests
- mammography (all women, preferably after 3 months on HRT)
- diagnostic hysteroscopy and endometrial biopsy only if undiagnosed vaginal bleeding
- bone density study (if risk factors)

If diagnosis is in doubt, e.g. perimenopause; younger patient < 45 years; hysterectomy:
- serum FSH
- serum oestradiol } Diagnostic

Differential diagnosis of menopause syndrome
- depression
- anaemia
- thyroid dysfunction
- hyperparathyroidism
- gynaecological disorders
  — dysfunctional uterine bleeding

Management

Education and lifestyle

Patients should receive adequate understanding, support and explanation with the emphasis being that the menopause is a natural fact of life. Emphasise the importance of leading a healthy lifestyle.
- correct diet
- avoid obesity
- adequate relaxation
- adequate exercise
- reduced smoking
- reduced caffeine intake
- reduced alcohol intake

Sexual activity

Advise that it is normal and appropriate to continue sexual relations, using a vaginal lubricant for a dry vagina. Contraception is advisable for 12 months after the last period. The OCP can be used up to 50–51 years if there are no risk factors.

Hormone replacement therapy

There is now convincing evidence that hormone replacement therapy at the menopause not only reduces climacteric symptoms and enhances the quality of life but also prevents osteoporosis and fractures, reduces ischaemic heart disease and strokes[3] and the risk of non-genital cancer.

Indications for HRT
- distressing symptoms
- significant cardiovascular risk factors
- significant osteoporosis

HRT has to be tailored to the individual patient and depends on several factors including the presence of a uterus, individual preferences and tolerance.[4]

The hormones to consider are:
- oestrogen
- progestogen, and
- testosterone

If perimenopausal, the OCP or sequential HRT (non-contraceptive) can be used. If menopausal—use HRT.

Oestrogen

Oestrogen comes in various preparations: oral, patches, implants, injections and topical vaginal preparations (Table 86.1). Injectables are not very

Table 86.1 *Oestrogens used in the menopause*[4]

Generic name	Proprietary name/s	Daily dose range	Usual daily protective dose
Oral			
Conjugated equine oestrogen	Premarin	0.3–2.5 mg	0.625 mg
Ethinyl oestradiol	Estigyn	0.01–0.03 mg	0.02 mg
Oestradiol valerate	Progynova	1.0–4.0 mg	2.0 mg
Oestriol	Ovestin	1.0–4.0 mg	2.0 mg
Piperazine oestrone sulphate	Ogen	0.625–5 mg	1.25 mg
Implants			
Oestradiol	Oestradiol implants	20–100 mg	50 mg
Skin patch			
Oestradiol	Various	2–8 mg every 3½ to 7 days	4 mg
Topical gel			
Oestradiol 0.1%	Sandrena	—	—
Vaginal preparations			
Creams			
Conjugated equine oestrogen 0.0625%	Premarin	2–4 g	4 g
Ethinyl oestradiol 0.01%	Dienoestrol	2.5–10 g	5 g
Oestriol 1 mg/g	Ovestin	0.5 g	0.5 g
Tablets			
Oestradiol	Vagifem	25 μg	1 tablet (25 μg)
Pessaries			
Oestrone	Kolpon	100 μg–1 mg	1 mg

Note: Vaginal therapy is usually given continuously for two weeks, then twice weekly.

effective so the common modes of administration are oral, implants or skin patches. Transdermal patches are the most favoured mode worldwide.

Vaginal creams or tablets are usually restricted to women who have mild menopausal symptoms and a dry vagina or urethra, or who cannot tolerate parenteral medication. Most women find the use of vaginal pessaries and creams messy and the older preparations are heavily absorbed, but the new oestradiol tablet, Vagifem, is a very effective topical therapy. The oral oestrogens in common use are Premarin, Ogen and Progynova. Implants of 50–100 mg (usually 50 mg) of oestradiol are given 3–12 monthly; patches (usually 50 μg) are applied weekly or every three and a half days. Continuous daily oestrogen use is recommended; there is no reason to stop therapy for one week.

Progestogen

Progestogen is given to women with a uterus and may be given continuously or cyclically. If it is not given, many women will develop hyperplasia of the uterus and there is a 5–10 times increased risk of endocervical cancer with unopposed oestrogen therapy.[2] If given cyclically (postmenopausal) it is given for the first to the twelfth day of the calendar month, generally as Provera or Primolut N (Table 86.2). A withdrawal bleed will occur which many elderly women find unacceptable. Thus, continuous therapy may be more appropriate. Avoid continuous use in perimenopausal women because of heavy irregular bleeding.

Progestogen alone can be given for menopausal symptoms in a woman with an oestrogen-dependent tumour.

Table 86.2 *Progestogens used in the menopause*[4]

Generic name	Daily dose range	Usual daily protective dose
Dydrogesterone	10–20 mg	10 mg
Levonorgestrel	0.03–0.9 mg	0.03 mg
Medroxyprogesterone acetate	2.5–20 mg	10 mg
Norethisterone	1.25–5 mg	2.5 mg

Progestogens should be given in the smallest possible dose, to prevent endometrial hyperplasia.

Testosterone

Testosterone is usually reserved for women whose libido does not improve with HRT but this indication is controversial. It is given as an implant of 50 mg and will last 3–12 months. An oestrogen implant of 50 mg should be given concurrently.

Contraindications to HRT

Important contraindications to HRT are listed in Table 86.3. The main absolute contraindications are active oestrogen-dependent neoplasms such as endometrial and breast carcinoma, acute thrombophlebitis and undiagnosed abnormal vaginal bleeding. HRT is protective for bowel cancer but not ovarian cancer.

Table 86.3   *Contraindications to HRT*

(Absolute or relative)
Oestrogen-dependent tumour
• endometrial cancer
• breast cancer
Recurrent thromboembolism
Uncontrolled hypertension
Undiagnosed vaginal bleeding
Active liver disease
Active SLE
Otosclerosis
Acute intermittent porphyria

HRT regimens

Some commonly used regimens are presented in Table 86.4 and Figure 86.2. Regimens A and B are in common use. The transdermal system appears to be the most favoured although some women find it unsuitable. A useful regimen, especially for irregular bleeding in the perimenopausal phase, is the combined sequential pill which can be continued for several years if necessary. Sufficient oestrogen should be given to control symptoms and prevent osteoporosis.

There is a proliferation of combination packs with permutations of various oestrogens and progestogens (pills and patches), usually sequential, some combined. These preparations are most suitable for perimenopausal women. The continuous combined preparation is best suited to women at least 1 year postmenopausal. The

Table 86.4   *A summarised regimen for HRT*[4]

Oestrogen
Oral medication
• conjugated oestrogen (Premarin) 0.625 mg
        or
• piperazine oestrone (Ogen) 1.25 mg
        or
• oestradiol valerate (Progynova) 2 mg
  Dosage
• half tablet for 7 days initially, then one tablet daily continuous
Transdermal patches
• oestradiol 4 mg patch

Progestogen
• medroxyprogesterone (Provera) 10 mg
        or
• norethisterone (Primolut N) 2.5 mg,
  one tablet for first 12 days of month
To induce amenorrhoea
  Give progestogen continuously daily, instead of cyclically
• medroxyprogesterone 2.5 mg
        or
• norethisterone 1.25 mg
  Continuous combined preparation, e.g Kliogest

Uterus present
Oestrogen and progestogen

No uterus (hysterectomy)
Oestrogen only

Perimenopausal regimen
Combined oestrogen and progesterone sequential therapy, e.g. Trisequens, Menoprem

Combination patch
e.g. Estracombi
• oestrogen plus progestogen (first half of cycle)
• oestrogen only (second half of cycle)

Fig. 86.2 *Possible HRT regimens for women with a uterus*   AFTER FARRELL[6]

newer progesterone, cyproterone acetate, is regarded as useful in the presence of hirsutism.

Informed consent

HRT should be prescribed only after the woman has been informed of the regimens available, their relative benefits and risks and side effects.[3] It must be emphasised that HRT, especially the combined sequential formulation, is not a contraceptive.

Side effects of therapy[5]

In the first 2–3 months the woman may experience oestrogenic side effects, but these usually resolve or stabilise. Starting with a lower dose may minimise these side effects.

Premenstrual syndrome (in 15%)

Action: decrease progestogen dose
or
change to alternative progestogen

Nausea and breast disorders

Cause: initial sensitivity to oestrogen
Action: reduce oestrogen to starting dose
or
intravaginal oestrogen

Bleeding problems

Heavy bleeding
Action: decrease oestrogen
Breakthrough bleeding
Action: increase progestogen
Irregular bleeding
Action: investigate + endometrial sampling
Intolerance of bleeding
Action: use continuous regimen
No bleeding
Action: reassure that this is not a problem

Leg cramps

Action: decrease oestrogen

Follow-up after commencing HRT[6]

• 3 months (ideal time for mammography)
• then 6 monthly

Allow 6 months to stabilise therapy.

Duration of treatment

The duration of teatment depends on several factors including the severity of symptoms, the response to therapy and the long-term aims, such as the desire for cardioprotection and osteoporosis prevention (at least 10 years) (Fig. 86.3). However, long-term therapy should be an informed decision made by the patient in consultation with the doctor. A useful working rule is to aim for treatment for 5 years and then review.

Some guidelines are:[7]
• 5–10 years for oestrogen deficiency symptoms
• 15–20 years for low bone density
• lifelong for cardiovascular risk factors, strong family history of dementia and significant urogenital symptoms

Non-hormonal therapy regimens

Several non-hormonal regimens have been employed to manage menopausal symptoms. These include medical therapies such as clonidine, tranquillisers and antidepressants and also natural therapies such as evening primrose oil, soy products and other phytoestrogens (plants containing oestrogen-like compounds). Although there is considerable anecdotal evidence about the efficacy of phytoestrogens, evidence from long-term double-blind trials is lacking. However, one study by Murkies et al.[8] showed the positive effect of these foods on hot flushes.

There are three broad classes of phytoestrogens—isoflavones, lignans and coumestans. Isoflavones, which are found almost exclusively in legumes, include soy products, lentils and beans. Lignans are found in varying degrees in a wide variety of plants but particularly in cereals, fruit and vegetables. Coumestans occur mainly in alfalfa and soy bean sprouts.

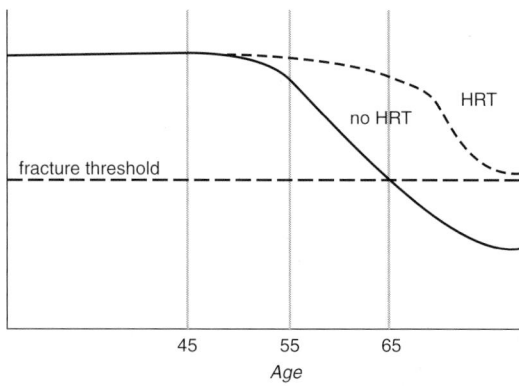

Fig. 86.3 *Graphic illustration of the effects of HRT on the fracture threshold of ageing women*

Dr Murkies advises 'a wholegrain diet with porridge or cereal for breakfast, perhaps a tablespoon of linseed on top, wholemeal bread for lunch with sprouts and fruit, especially apple, and an assortment of vegetables and legumes as part of the evening meal'.

Osteoporosis

Osteoporosis refers to the increased bone fragility that accompanies ageing and many illnesses. Following the menopause, women begin to lose calcium from their bone at a much faster rate than men, presumably as a direct response to low levels of oestrogen. Within 5–10 years of the menopause, women can be seen to suffer from osteoporosis and by the age of 65 the rate of fractures in women has increased to 3–5 times that of men (Fig. 86.4).

Facts and figures

- Osteoporosis is commonest in postmenopausal women.
- Up to 15% of women will develop fractures in their lifetime and 30% of all women reaching 90 years of age will suffer a hip fracture.[9]
- Osteoporosis leads to reduced bone strength and susceptibility to fracture, even with minor trauma.
- Osteoporosis only causes pain when complicated by fracture.
- First presentation is usually a fracture (Colles', femoral neck and vertebra) or height shrinkage.
- Vertebral collapse is the hallmark of osteoporosis.
- The disorder is of bone mass, not calcium metabolism.

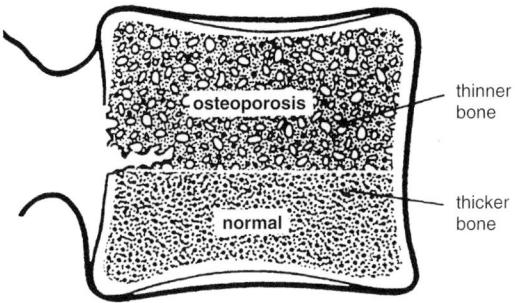

Fig. 86.4 *Osteoporosis is reduced bone mass per unit volume*

- For osteoporosis in a vertebra including a pathological fracture, multiple myeloma may need exclusion.
- The first step in prevention is regular exercise and an adequate dietary intake of calcium (1000 mg per day).

Classification of osteoporosis

Primary

Type 1: postmenopausal (vertebral or distal forearm fractures within first 20 years of menopause)

Type 2: senile osteoporosis (fracture of proximal femur usually 15–30 years after menopause)

Osteopenia is 1–2.5 SD below the young adult standard mean.

Osteoporosis is > 2.5 SD below this mean.

Secondary

To various endocrine disorders, malabsorption and malignancies. Various causes and risk factors are presented in Table 86.5.

Table 86.5 *Osteoporosis: risk factors and/or causes*

Female

Thin build

Race: Asian, caucasian

Family history

Premenopausal oestrogen deficiency
  e.g. amenorrhoea

Early menopause < 45 (natural or surgical)

Cigarette smoking

High caffeine intake > 4 cups per day

High alcohol intake > 2 standard drinks
  per day

Low calcium intake

Physical inactivity

Chronic corticosteroid use

can be modified

Eating disorders, e.g. anorexia nervosa

Endocrine disorders
- Cushing's disease
- diabetes mellitus
- hyperparathyroidism
- thyrotoxicosis
- hypogonadism
- acromegaly

Chronic renal failure

Investigations

- Plain radiography is of limited value. Osteoporosis is not detectable until 40–50% of bone is lost.
- Plasma calcium, phosphate and alkaline phosphatase are all usually normal.
- Consider tests for multiple myeloma in an osteoporotic area.
- Densitometry can predict an increased risk of osteoporosis and fracture, the best current modality being dual energy X-ray absorptimetry (DEXA scan) in a facility with high-standard quality control.[10] The spine and femoral neck are targeted: the femoral neck is the most useful index.

Treatment for osteoporosis

The goal of treatment is to prevent osteoporosis or reduce further loss. No treatment has been shown to replace lost bone effectively. Anabolic agents such as nandrolone deconate may reduce further loss but the side effects are problematic.

Medication of value in decreasing further loss [10]

The following medication may be valuable in preventing further bone loss, possibly reversing the osteoporosis process and preventing further fractures.

- HRT
        or
- Calcitriol (a vitamin D metabolite)
  — use for failed trial HRT
  — very useful for corticosteroid induced osteoporosis
  (avoid calcium supplements during therapy)
        or
- Biphosphonates
  — alendronate 10 mg (o) daily
    (take care with potential side effect of oesophagitis)
  — etidronate
  — risedonate
- Raloxifine (a selective oestrogen receptor modulator) 60 mg (o) daily

The choice depends on the clinical status, such as the age of the patient and the extent of disease, the patient's tolerance of drugs and further clinical trials of these drugs. The one preferable solution is to give prophylaxis for individuals identified as high risk and the only widely accepted proven therapy is oestrogen therapy.

Recommendations for prevention [10]

- HRT within 2 years of the onset of the menopause
- Adequate dietary intake of calcium
    800 mg per day—premenopause
    1000–1500 mg per day—postmenopausal

Calcium-rich foods include low-fat calcium-enriched milk (500 mL contains 1000 mg), other low-fat dairy products (e.g. yoghurt or cheese), fish (including tinned fish such as salmon with the bone), citrus fruits, sesame and sunflower seeds, almonds, brazil nuts and hazel nuts.

Calcium supplements will be necessary in postmenopausal women (except if taking calcitriol). Calcium citrate is better absorbed than carbonate.

- Exercise: moderate exercise against gravity, e.g. walking (brisk walking for 30 minutes four times a week), jogging or tennis, may make a small contribution to retarding bone loss.
- Lifestyle factors: stop smoking and limit alcohol and caffeine intake.

When to refer

- A problem arises in establishing the correct regimens for HRT.
- Complications not corrected by routine measures develop with HRT.
- Osteoporosis appears to be secondary to an underlying illness.
- Advice is required about the management of a patient with pathological osteoporotic fractures or loss of height.

Practice tips on the menopause

- Careful pretreatment assessment is important.
- Encourage conservative self-help management with an emphasis on lifestyle if symptoms are mild.
- Explain benefits and risks and get informed consent.
- Individualise HRT therapy.
- Regular follow-up is essential.
- Allow about 6 months to stabilise with HRT.
- The prime treatment for an oestrogen deficiency disorder is oestrogen.
- Use oestrogen-only therapy for women without a uterus.
- If a uterus is present give combined oestrogen-progestogen therapy (cyclical or continuous).
- Avoid giving progestogen in the presence of continuing ovarian activity.

- Severe side effects of progestogen may necessitate oestrogen-only therapy, with regular yearly endometrial biopsy.
- Always start with a low dose of oestrogen.
- Women who have experienced side effects such as migraine with the combined oral contraceptive may have the same problem with HRT.
- HRT is not a contraceptive and so contraception is advisable in perimenopausal women for 12 months after the last period.
- Problematic loss of libido can be treated with testosterone in the short term, e.g. as a single parenteral dose or as a short course of oral tablets.
- Oestrogen deficiency results in a loss of elasticity and dryness of the vagina which can be partially helped with HRT.
- HRT does not always restore the sex drive but does help make sexual intercourse easier and more pleasant.
- The most practical solution in managing osteoporosis is prevention through HRT and adequate calcium intake. Calcium supplementation by itself is inadequate but appears to have a synergistic effect with HRT.
- HRT needs to be maintained for at least 10 years to achieve full benefit.
- Advantages of long-term HRT:
  — improvement in the quality of life
  — prevention of bone fractures, especially of wrist, hip and spine
  — reduction in coronary artery disease and cerebrovascular disease mortality
- Women taking HRT from the onset of menopause have been shown to live 4 years longer than those who have never received it.[11]

References

1. World Health Organisation Technical Report Series 670. WHO Scientific Group (1981), Research on the Menopause.
2. Wren B. Menopause. In: MIMS Disease Index (2nd edn). Sydney: IMS Publishing, 1996, 303–306.
3. Silberberg S, Burger H. Management of the menopause from an Australian perspective. Mod Med Aust, May 1989; 14–18.
4. Rosenblatt J, Murtagh J. Hormone replacement therapy. Aust Fam Physician, 1995; 21:1345–1346.
5. Murkies AL. Common problems with hormone replacement therapy. Aust Fam Physician, 1992; 21:217–225.
6. Farrell E. Treatment options and menopause regimens. Aust Fam Physician, 1992; 21:240–246.
7. MacLennan A. Pill, patch, pellet or paste: what's new in HRT? Mod Med Aust, 1996; 39(12):40–46.
8. Murkies AL et al. Dietary flour supplementation decreases postmenopausal hot flushes: effect of soy and wheat. Maturitas, 1995; 21:189–195.
9. Seeman E, Young N. Osteoporosis. In: MIMS Disease Index (2nd edn). Sydney, IMS Publishing, 1996, 368–371.
10. Moulds RFW (Chairman). *Therapeutic guildelines: Endocrinology*. Melbourne: Therapeutic Guidelines Limited, 1997–98, 93–99.
11. Henderson BE, Paginini-Hill A, Ross RK. An epidemiological evaluation of the risks and benefits of hormone replacement therapy. 1989. Paper presented to Scientific Meeting, Australian Menopause Society, Brisbane. 23–24 September 1989.

87

Vaginal discharge

—

In all cases of abnormal vaginal discharge consider the possibility of the sexually transmitted diseases, gonorrhoea and non-specific urethritis.

Vaginal discharge is one of the commonest complaints seen by family physicians yet it is one of the most difficult to solve, especially if it is recurrent or persistent. It is present if the woman's underclothes are consistently stained or a pad is required. It is important to make a proper diagnosis, to differentiate between abnormal (physiological) and pathological discharge and to be aware of the considerable variation in secretion of vaginal fluid.

The differential diagnoses should include consideration of normal discharge; vaginitis, either infective or chemical; sexually transmitted diseases (STDs); and urinary tract infection.

Key facts and checkpoints

- A recent survey of a large family planning clinic found that 17% of women complained of vaginal discharge.[1]
- Vaginal discharge may present at any age but is very common in the reproductive years.
- Vaginal discharge is a common presentation of those STDs responsible for pelvic inflammatory disease.
- One of the simplest methods of making a proper diagnosis is a wet film examination. It saves expensive laboratory investigations.

A diagnostic approach

A summary of the safety diagnostic model is presented in Table 87.1.

Table 87.1   *Vaginal discharge: diagnostic strategy model*

Q. *Probability diagnosis*
A. Normal physiological discharge
    Vaginitis
    • bacterial vaginosis   40–50%
    • candidiasis   20–30%
    • trichomonas   10–20%

Q. *Serious disorders not to be missed*
A. Neoplasia
    • carcinoma
    • fistulas
    STDs/PID
    • gonorrhoea
    • chlamydia
    Sexual abuse, esp. children
    Tampon toxic shock syndrome (staphylococcal infection)

Q. *Pitfalls (often missed)*
A. Chemical vaginitis, e.g. perfumes
    Retained foreign objects, e.g. tampons, IUCD
    Endometriosis (brownish discharge)
    Ectopic pregnancy ('prune juice' discharge)
    Poor toilet hygiene
    Genital herpes (possible)
    Atrophic vaginitis

Q. *Seven masquerades checklist*
A. Depression   –
    Diabetes   √
    Drugs   √
    Anaemia   –
    Thyroid disease   –
    Spinal dysfunction   –
    UTI   √ (association)

Q. *Is the patient trying to tell me something?*
A. Needs careful consideration; possible sexual dysfunction.

Probability diagnoses

The two most common causes of vaginal discharge are physiological discharge and infective vaginitis.

Physiological discharge

Normal physiological discharge is usually milky-white or clear mucoid and originates from a combination of the following sources:

- cervical mucus (secretions from cervical glands)
- vaginal secretion (transudate through vaginal mucosa)
- vaginal squamous epithelial cells (desquamation)
- resident commensal bacteria
- cervical columnar epithelial cells

With physiological discharge there is usually no odour or pruritus.

In addition, the egg-white discharge accompanying ovulation may be noted. The discharge may be aggravated by the use of the pill. The normal discharge usually shows on underclothing by the end of the day. Clear or white, it oxidises to a yellow or brown on contact with air. It is increased by sexual stimulation.

Management:

- reassurance and explanation
- wear cotton underwear (not synthetic)
- bath instead of showering
- avoid douching and feminine deodorants
- use tampons instead of pads

Infective vaginitis

The commonest cause of infective vaginitis is bacterial vaginosis (formerly bacterial vaginitis, _Gardnerella vaginalis_ or _Haemophilus vaginalis_) which accounts for 40–50% of vaginitis.[2] _Candida albicans_ is the causative agent in 20–30% while _Trichomonas vaginalis_ causes about 20% in Australia. The comparable features are outlined in Table 87.2. Human papilloma virus infection of vaginal epithelium may cause excess discharge.

Serious disorders not to be missed

The 'not to be missed' group includes carcinoma of the vagina, cervix or uterus and sexually transmitted diseases, including pelvic inflammatory diseases caused by _Chlamydia trachomatis_ and _Neisseria gonorrhoeae_. Vaginal discharge is the most common presenting symptom of both of these serious STDs. Occasionally, infections of the endometrium and endosalpinx will produce a discharge that gravitates to the vagina.[1] Benign and malignant neoplasia anywhere in the genital tract may produce a discharge. Usually it is watery and pink or blood-stained.

Inspection should include vigilance for fistulas that may be associated with malignancy, inflammation or postirradiation.

Pitfalls

It is common to overlook the problem caused by hygienic preparations. Apart from the vaginal tampon, which may be retained (knowingly or otherwise), there is a variety of preparations that can induce a sensitivity reaction. These include deodorant soaps and sprays and contraceptive agents, especially spermicidal creams. Ironically, the various preparations used to treat the vaginitis may cause a chemical reaction.

Endometriosis of the cervix or vaginal vault may cause a bloody or brownish discharge.

Seven masquerades checklist

Of this group, diabetes mellitus leading to recurrent 'thrush', drugs causing a local sensitivity, and urinary tract infection have to be considered (Table 87.1).

Psychogenic considerations

This question needs to be answered, especially if the discharge is normal. The problem could

Table 87.2 _Characteristics of discharge for common causes of infective vaginitis (after Weisberg)_

Infective organism	Colour	Consistency	Odour	pH (normal 4–4.5)	Associated symptoms
Candida albicans	White	Thick (cream cheese)		4	Itch, soreness, redness
Trichomonas	Yellow/green	Bubbly, profuse (mucopurulent)	Malodorous, fishy	5–6	Soreness
Bacterial vaginosis	Grey	Watery, profuse, bubbly	Malodorous, fishy	5–6	—

be related to sexual dysfunction or it may reflect a problematic relationship, and the issue may need to be explored diplomatically. Vaginal discharge is an embarrassing problem for the patient and any discussion needs to be handled thoroughly and sensitively. A relevant sexual history may satisfactorily solve the problem.

The clinical approach

History

The history is important and should include:

- nature of discharge: colour, odour, quantity, relation to menstrual cycle, associated symptoms
- exact nature and location of irritation
- sexual history: arousal, previous STDs, number of partners and any presence of irritation or discharge in them
- use of chemicals such as soaps, deodorants, pessaries and douches
- pregnancy possibility
- drug therapy
- associated medical conditions, e.g. diabetes

Physical examination

Optimal facilities for the physical examination include an appropriate couch and good light, bivalve Sims' specula, sterile swabs (preferably with transport media), normal saline, 10% potassium hydroxide, slides and cover slips and microscope. Inspection in good light includes viewing the vulva, introitus, urethra, vagina and cervix. Look for the discharge and specific problems such as polyps, warts, prolapses or fistulas. To differentiate between vaginal and cervical discharge, wipe the cervix clear with a cotton ball and observe the cervix. Perform a pH test and a wet film.

Pitfalls to keep in mind include:

- The patient may have had a bath or a 'good wash' beforehand and may need to return when the discharge is obvious.
- A retained tampon may be missed in the posterior fornix, so the speculum should slide directly along the posterior wall of the vagina.
- Candida infection may not show the characteristic curds, 'the strawberry vagina' of trichomonas is uncommon and bubbles may not be seen.

Acetic acid 2% is useful in removing the discharge and mucus to enable a clearer view of the cervix and vaginal walls.

Investigations

- pH test with paper of range 4 to 6
- amine or 'whiff' test: add a drop of 10% KOH to vaginal secretions smeared on glass slide
- wet film microscopy of a drop of vaginal secretions

A culture is necessary if no diagnosis is made after this routine.

A full STD workup

- swabs from the cervix for chlamydia, *N. gonorrhoeae*
  — swab mucus from cervix first
  — swab endocervix
  — place in transport media
- Pap smear
- viral culture (herpes simplex)
  — scrape base of ulcer or, ideally, deroof a vesicle
  — immediately immerse in culture medium
  — transport rapidly to laboratory

Preparation of a wet film

To make a wet film preparation[2] (Fig. 87.1), place one drop of normal saline (preferably warm) on one end of an ordinary slide and one drop of 10% potassium hydroxide (KOH) on the other half of the slide. A sample of the discharge needs to be taken with a swab stick, either directly from the posterior fornix of the vagina or from discharge that has collected on the posterior blade of the speculum during the vaginal examination. A small amount of the discharge is mixed with both the normal saline drop and the KOH drop. A cover slip is placed over each preparation. The slide is examined under low power to get an overall impression, and under high power to determine the presence of lactobacilli, polymorphs, trichomonads, spores, clue cells and hyphae. A summary of various findings on

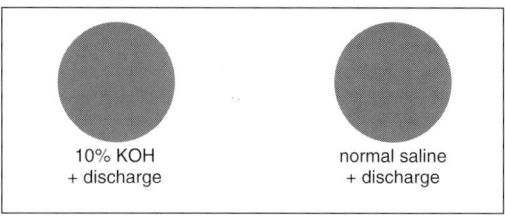

Examine for:
1. epithelial cells   4. trichomonads
2. polymorphs   5. clue cells
3. lactobacilli

Fig. 87.1 *Wet film method*

Table 87.3 *Wet film examination (after Weisberg)*

	Lactobacilli	Polymorphs	Epithelial cells	Clue cells	Other
Normal	+	None or occasional	+	–	
Candidiasis	+	None or occasional	+	–	Spores/hyphae
Trichomoniasis	Absent or scant	Numerous	+	–	Trichomonads
Bacterial vaginosis	Absent or scant	Numerous	+	2–50%	

wet film examination is presented in Table 87.3. Lactobacilli are long, thin Gram-positive rods; clue cells are vaginal epithelial cells that have bacteria attached so that the cytoplasm appears granular and often the entire border is obscured. They are a feature of bacterial vaginosis. Trichomonads are about the same size as polymorphs and to distinguish between the two one needs to see the movement of the trichomonad and the beating of its flagella under high power of the microscope. Warming the slide will often precipitate movement.

Refer to Figure 87.2.

Other investigations
Gram-stain smear and culture should be contemplated only if a diagnosis cannot be made on wet film.

Vaginal discharge in children
Staining on a child's underclothes may be due to excess physiological discharge, especially in the year before the menarche.[1] Vulvovaginitis is the most common gynaecological disorder of childhood, the most common cause being a non-specific bacterial infection.

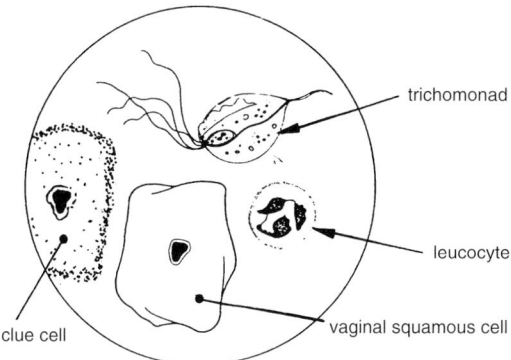

clue cell, trichomonad, leucocyte, vaginal squamous cell

Fig. 87.2 *Relative sizes of various cells or organisms as seen in a wet smear*

Important causes to consider
- poor hygiene—usually a non-specific bacterial vaginitis, e.g. coliforms
- 'sandbox' vaginitis: little girls sitting and playing in sand or dirt may develop irritation from particulate matter trapped in the vagina[3]
- foreign body: consider if a bloody malodorous vaginal discharge
- candidiasis (moniliasis)—uncommon but consider if antibiotic therapy or possibility of diabetes
- sexual abuse (must not be missed)
- pinworm infestation (Enterobius)
- sexually transmissible organisms—usually postpubertal

Symptoms
- itching or burning
- there may be a discharge that stains the underclothes
- ± dysuria

Examination
A careful general examination should be performed. In infants the best examination method is to place the child on her mother's lap with the legs held well abducted. Lateral traction applied to the labia allows the hymen orifice to be examined. Look for vulval or vaginal infection. Aspirate vaginal secretion with a medicine dropper for appropriate cultures. A Papanicolaou smear is advisable for a persistent problem since a sarcoma is a possibility.

An older child can be placed in one of two suitable positions:

1. Supine, legs apart in a frog-leg position, with bottom of feet touching (generally preferred).
2. Prone, knee/chest position. This allows a better view of the hymenal orifice but many children do not like this position.

A rectal examination is performed to try to feel for foreign bodies in the vagina and to assess the pelvic anatomy.

Vaginal discharge in the elderly

Vaginal discharge can occur in the elderly from a variety of causes including infective vaginitis, atrophic vaginitis, foreign bodies, poor hygiene and neoplasia. It is important to exclude malignancy of the uterus, cervix and vagina in the older patient.

Atrophic vaginitis

In the absence of oestrogen stimulation the vaginal and vulval tissues begin to shrink and become thin and dry. This renders the vagina more susceptible to bacterial attack because of the loss of vaginal acidity. Rarely, a severe attack can occur with a very haemorrhagic vagina and heavy discharge:

- yellowish non-offensive discharge
- tenderness and dyspareunia
- spotting or bleeding with coitus
- the vagina may be reddened with superficial haemorrhagic areas

Treatment
- Oral hormone replacement therapy.
- Local oestrogen cream or tablet, e.g. Vagifem. The tablet is preferred as it is less messy.

Vaginal candidiasis

Infection with the fungus *Candida albicans* is a common and important problem with a tendency to recurrence.

Clinical features
- intense vaginal and vulval pruritus
- vulval soreness
- vulvovaginal erythema (brick red)
- vaginal excoriation and oedema
- white curd-like discharge
- discomfort with coitus
- dysuria

Factors predisposing to vaginal candidiasis[1]

Endogenous: diabetes mellitus
                AIDS syndrome
                pregnancy
                debilitating diseases

Exogenous: oral contraceptives
               antibiotics
               immunosuppressants
               carbohydrate-rich diet
               orogenital/anogenital intercourse
               IUCD
               tight-fitting jeans
               nylon underwear
               humidity/wet bathing suit

Treatment

For the first attack of candidiasis it is appropriate to select one of the large range of vaginal imidazole therapies (clotrimazole, econazole, isoconazole, miconazole) for 1–7 days (Table 87.4). There appears to be no significant difference between imidazoles.[4] Nystatin is best reserved for recurrent cases or if there is local reaction to the imidazoles. Some therapists prefer creams to tablets and pessaries because cream can be applied to any tender vulval area, but a tablet and cream can be used simultaneously, especially for a heavy infection.

Gentian violet (0.5% aqueous solution) is useful for rapid relief, if available.

A recommended initial regimen is:
    clotrimazole 500 mg vaginal tablet as a single
    dose   ±
    clotrimazole 2% cream applied to vagina and
    vulva (for symptomatic relief)
An alternative regimen, especially for recurrent infections:
    nystatin pessaries once daily for 7 days
                and/or
    nystatin vaginal cream (100 000 U per 4 g)
    once daily for 7 days

Recalcitrant cases (proven by microscopy and if not pregnant)[5]
    fluconazole 150 mg (o) as a single dose
                or
    itraconazole 100 mg (o) once daily for 14 days
Note: A male sexual partner does not require
    treatment.[6]

Table 87.4   *Treatment of vaginal candidiasis*

| Length of treatment | Generic name | Vaginal therapy | |
		Tablets	Cream 5 g
Imidazoles			
1 day	clotrimazole	500 mg × 1	
(statim dose)	isoconazole	300 mg × 2	
3 days	clotrimazole	100 mg × 2	
	clotrimazole		2%
	econazole	150 mg	
	econazole		1.5%
	miconazole	200 mg	
6 days	clotrimazole	100 mg	
	clotrimazole		1%
7 days	miconazole	100 mg	2%
Nystatin			
7 days	nystatin	100 000 U	100 000 U
Oral therapy for recurrent recalcitrant infections		**Oral tablets**	
1 day	fluconazole	150 mg	
14 days	ketoconazole	200 mg daily	
14 days	nystatin	500 000 U tds	
14 days	fluconazole	50 mg	
14 days	itraconazole	100 mg	

Advice to the patient

- Bathe the genital area gently two or three times a day for symptomatic relief. In preparing for the antifungal preparation, use 1–3% acetic acid or sodium bicarbonate solution (1 tablespoon to 1 litre of water). Thoroughly cleanse the vagina, including recesses between rugae and the fornices and also the folds around the vulva.
- Dry the genital area thoroughly after showering or bathing.
- Wear loose-fitting cotton underwear.
- Avoid wearing pantyhose, tight jeans or tight underwear or using tampons.
- Avoid having intercourse or oral sex during the infected period.
- Do not use vaginal douches, powders or deodorants.

Trichomonas vaginalis

This flagellated protozoan, which is thought to originate in the bowel, infects the vagina, Skene's ducts and lower urinary tract in women and the lower genitourinary tract in men. It is transmitted through sexual intercourse and is relatively common in the female after the onset of sexual activity.

Clinical features

- profuse thin discharge (grey to yellow-green in colour)
- small bubbles may be seen in 20–30%
- pruritus
- malodorous discharge
- dyspareunia
- diffuse erythema of cervix and vaginal walls
- characteristic punctate appearance on cervix

Treatment[5]

- oral metronidazole 2 g as a single dose (preferable) *or* 400 mg bd for 7 days

or

tinidazole 2 g as a single dose (Table 87.5)

Table 87.5   *Oral treatment for bacterial vaginosis and trichomonas infections*

Length of treatment	Generic name	Oral dosage
1 day (statim dose)	tinidazole	500 mg × 4
	metronidazole	400 mg × 5
7 days (for recurrent)	tinidazole	500 mg daily
	metronidazole	400 mg bd

- use clotrimazole 100 mg vaginal tablet daily for 6 days during pregnancy
- attention to hygiene
- the sexual partner must be treated simultaneously
- the male partner should wear a condom during intercourse
- for resistant infections a 3–7 day course of either metronidazole or tinidazole may be necessary.

Bacterial vaginosis

Bacterial vaginosis is a clinical entity of mixed aetiology characterised by the replacement of the normal vaginal microflora (chiefly *Lactobacillus*) with a mixed flora consisting of *Gardnerella vaginalis*, other anaerobes such as *Mobiluncus* species, and *Mycoplasma hominis*.

Clinical features
- a grey, watery, profuse discharge
- malodorous
- no obvious vulvitis or vaginitis
- liberates an amine-like, fishy odour on admixture of 10% KOH
- ± dyspareunia and dysuria
- ± pruritus

Treatment
The same treatment (metronidazole or tinidazole) is used as for trichomonas vaginalis. Clindamycin 300 mg (o) bd for 7 days or 2% clindamycin cream can be used for resistant infections or during pregnancy. Normal vaginal pH can be restored using a variety of topical douches such as povidone iodine solution (1 tablespoon per litre of water), vinegar (3–4 tablespoons per litre of water), topical Acigel or a milky solution of yoghurt to restore *Lactobacillus* levels.

There is no evidence that treatment of the male sexual partner reduces the recurrence rate or provides any significant benefit.[7] The STD treatment guidelines of the US Centers for Disease Control state explicitly that such treatment is of no proven benefit.[8]

Retained vaginal tampon

A retained tampon, which may be impacted and cannot be removed by the patient, is usually associated with an extremely offensive vaginal discharge. Its removal can cause considerable embarrassment to both patient and doctor.

Method of removal
Using good vision the tampon is seized with a pair of sponge-holding forceps and quickly immersed under water without releasing the forceps. A bowl of water (an old plastic ice-cream container is suitable) is kept as close to the introitus as possible. This results in minimal malodour. The tampon and water are immediately flushed down the toilet if the toilet system can accommodate tampons (Fig. 87.3). An alternative method is to grasp the tampon with a gloved hand and quickly peel the glove over the tampon for disposal.

Tampon toxic shock syndrome
Staphylococcal infection
This rare dramatic condition is caused by the production of staphylococcal exotoxin associated with tampon use for menstrual protection. The syndrome usually begins within five days of the onset of the period.

(a)

(b)

Fig. 87.3 *Removal of an impacted vaginal tampon*

The *clinical features* include sudden onset fever, vomiting and diarrhoea, muscle aches and pains, skin erythema, hypotension progressing to confusion, stupor and sometimes death.

Management

Active treatment depends on the severity of the illness. Cultures should be taken from the vagina, cervix, perineum and nasopharynx. The patient should be referred to a major centre if 'shock' develops. Otherwise the vagina must be emptied, ensuring there is not a forgotten tampon, cleaned with a povidone iodine solution tds for 2 days, and flucloxacillin or vancomycin antibiotics administered.

- These women should not use tampons in the future.

Prevention

- Good general hygiene with care in handling and inserting the tampons.
- Change the tampon 3–4 times a day.
- Use an external pad at night during sleep.

When to refer

- evidence of sexual abuse to children to an experienced sexual assault centre
- recurrent, recalcitrant infections
- presence of carcinoma or fistula
- staphylococcal toxic shock syndrome

Practice tips

- Failure of treament may be due to diagnostic error, therapeutic error, sexual reinfection, chemical sensitivity to vaginal tablets, drug resistance or depressed host immunity.
- Patients with an infective cause appreciate the use of patient education material, especially that including preventive measures.

- Advise patients subject to vaginal infection about simple hygiene measures to keep the area dry and cool: avoid nylon underwear, pantyhose, tight jeans, wet swimsuits, perfumed soaps and vaginal deodorisers.
- A serious sequela is subsequent dyspareunia and vaginismus. The patient should be advised to have sufficient lubrication, such as KY jelly, to avoid distressing psychosexual problems.

References

1. Mackay EV et al. *Illustrated textbook of gynaecology* (2nd edn). Sydney: WB Saunders, Bailliere Tindall, 1992, 296–325.
2. Weisberg E. Wet film examination. Aust Fam Physician, 1991; 20:291–294.
3. Tunnessen WW Jr. *Signs and symptoms in paediatrics* (2nd edn). Philadelphia: Lippincott, 1988, 458–460.
4. O'Neill S, Howard S. Recurrent vulvovaginal candidiasis. Aust Fam Physician, 1989; 18:102.
5. Mashford ML (Chairman). *Antibiotic guidelines* (9th edn). Melbourne: Victorian Medical Postgraduate Foundation, 1996–97, 72–73.
6. Sobel JD. Vulvovaginal candidiasis. In: Holmes KK et al. (eds), *Sexually transmitted diseases*. New York: McGraw-Hill, 1990, 515–523.
7. Vejtorp M, Bollreup AC, Vejtory L et al. Bacterial vaginosis: a double-blind randomised trial of the effect of treatment of the sexual partner. Br J Obst Gynecol, 1988; 95:920–6.
8. US Department of Health and Human Services, Public Health Service, Centers for Disease Control. *Sexually transmitted diseases; treatment guidelines*. MMWR, 1989; 38:S–8.

88

Domestic violence and sexual assault

—

The root of Solomons seale when applied, taketh away in one or two nights, any bruise, blacke or blue spots gotton by falls or womens wilfulnesse, in stumbling upon their hasty husbands fists, or such like.

John Gerard 1545–1612

Domestic violence basically means the physical, sexual or emotional abuse of one partner by the other, almost invariably abuse of a female by a male. However, the abuse can be of an elderly parent by the children or from some other member of the household to another member. It usually results from abuse and/or imbalance of power in close relationships. One person in the relationship consistently dominates or threatens with power and the abused victim gradually gives over more power.

A major problem in dealing with domestic violence is that it is hidden and the victims are reluctant to divulge the cause of their injuries when visiting medical practitioners.

Key facts and checkpoints[1]

- Between one-quarter and one-third of relationships experience violence at some time.
- In 90–95% of cases the victims are women.
- 10% of women have been violently assaulted in the last year.
- 22% of homicides in Queensland in 1982–87 were spouse murders.
- In violent families with children, 90% of children witness the violence and 50% of children are victims of violence.

- 4% of relationships will experience chronic domestic violence (in 20% this occurs before marriage).
- Less than 20% of those who abuse their spouse abuse some other person.[2]
- Alcohol is a factor in 50% of domestic violence incidents (i.e. not the sole cause; it does make violence easier, and is used as an excuse). Other factors include work stress/pressure, financial stress and illness. However, there are no excuses for domestic violence.
- Pregnancy is a high-risk time for victims of domestic battering.
- 50% of people know someone affected by domestic violence, but one-third refuse to speak about it or get involved in any way because they regard it as a 'private matter'.
- One in five people think that domestic violence is acceptable in certain circumstances.

We usually think of domestic violence in terms of physical violence but it can take many forms.[3] These include:

- physical abuse
- psychological abuse
- economic abuse
- social abuse (e.g. isolation)
- sexual abuse

Possible presentations

- Physical injuries: usually bruising caused by punching, kicking or biting; also fractures, burns, genital trauma
- Physical symptoms, e.g. back pain, headache, depression, sexual dysfunction, anxiety

- Psychological problems (in both the woman and her children)

The physical injuries are rarely overlooked but the other symptoms are frequently overlooked.

A study by Stark et al[4] defines a three-stage sequence to the battering syndrome:

Stage 1: woman presents with injuries in the central anterior regions of the body (face, head and torso).

Stage 2: multiple visits to clinics, often with vague complaints.

Stage 3: development of psychological sequelae (alcohol, drug addiction, suicide attempts, depression).

Diagnosis

It is important to have a high index of suspicion and recognise and manage the problem to prevent further violence. If you suspect domestic violence—ASK! Talk to the woman alone:

- How are things at home?
- How are things with your spouse/children?
- Did anything unusual happen to bring about these injuries?
- Has there been any violence?
- You seem to be having a hard time.

It is vital to believe the woman's story. Women are most likely to seek help from their family doctor in preference to any other agency.[5] The doctor has to take the initiative because patients rarely complain about the violence.[3] They may present up to 30 times before they take action to end the violence.[3]

Assessment

- Delineate the problem — pattern of violence
  - effect on the woman and her children
  - resources available to women
  - social/cultural environment
- Examine and investigate presenting symptoms.
- Check for coexisting injuries (common target areas are breast, chest, abdomen and buttocks). Inspect the ears, teeth and jaw.
- Check the patient's general health status.
- Look for signs of alcohol or drug abuse.
- Keep accurate records and consider taking photographs.
- X-rays are helpful and may show old fractures.

Victims

The victims come from all socioeconomic and cultural groups. As a rule they enter the relationship as normal, independent, competent women but gradually lose their coping ability and self-esteem and may become compliant victims.[1] This has been demonstrated by Hazelwood and workers in their investigations of sexual sadists.[2] Unfortunately, many victims believe that somehow they deserve their punishment.

Many would like to leave home but the move is not so simple. Some do love their husbands and live in hope that the marriage will eventually work. They may feel that they cannot cope with living alone nor with the guilt and perceived failure of moving out.

Perpetrators

Perpetrators come from all walks of life and from all social and ethnic groups. They generally have inner drives to be strong, protective and powerful but can only achieve this at home through an inappropriate show of strength. However, they are basically insecure with poor self-esteem, poor communication skills, learned violence from family origins and an inability to express appropriate emotions which tend to manifest as anger and violence.[1]

Although they usually control their violence outside the home, there is evidence that some perpetrators are guilty of violent behaviour in the community.

Cycle of violence

A predictable pattern that is referred to as the 'cycle of violence' has been identified in many marriages. It is controlled by the perpetrator while the victim feels confused and helpless. The cycle repeats itself with a tendency for the violence to increase in severity (Fig. 88.1).

Management

The key to successful management is initial recognition of the problem and establishment of empathic caring and support for the victim and family. Do not try to fit the victims into the disease model. It must be emphasised that the perpetrators (as in most criminal activity) do not readily change their behavioural pattern and thus there is minimal prospect of the violence

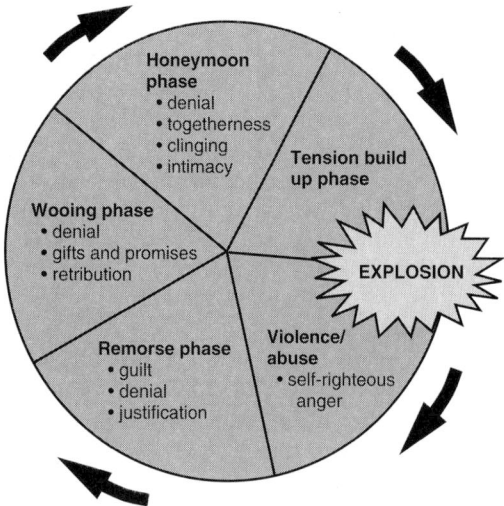

Fig. 88.1 *The cycle of domestic violence*

decreasing unless there is a dramatic reason to change. As with an alcohol problem, the person has to admit that he has a problem before effective counselling can begin. A management strategy is presented in Table 88.1. The safety of women and children is always the prime working rule.

Table 88.1 *Management strategy for domestic violence*

Treat the physical injury and
suspect domestic violence

↓

Establish the diagnosis

↓

Initiate crisis intervention
• organise admission to a refuge
• ensure informed consent for all actions
• consider notifying police

↓

Establish an empathic trusting relationship

↓

Build the victim's coping skills and self-esteem

↓

Make effective use of community resources
• support services
• women's support group
• domestic violence resource centre
• social services/police
• social workers

Useful strategies
Do believe her.

• Talk openly and explicitly about it.
• Express concern for her safety.
• Give information (i.e. about the course of action available to her, contacts for legal advice).
• Respect her right to make her own decisions.

Harmful strategies
Don't • deny domestic violence
• minimise the importance of domestic violence
• blame the victim
• treat with tranquillisers
• refer to a psychiatrist
• refer to marriage guidance if the husband isn't interested, but refer to specialist counsellors
• set explicit criteria/rules (takes away her power yet again)

It is uncommon to get the co-operation of the perpetrator in the management process. If they do seek help they require counselling by a skilled and experienced practitioner, as treatment will be prolonged and complex.

As a general rule the most effective intervention in arresting the violence is to arrest the violent person.[3]

Sexual assault

Medical practitioners dealing with the difficult and distressing problem of alleged sexual assault should be trained in the subject and familiar with the laws applicable to sexual assault in their own state. Rape involves considerable violence and physical injury in 5–10% of cases,[6] in which the victims fear for their lives. Apart from the inevitable psychological consequences, the possibility of pregnancy or acquired STD should be considered. The inexperienced practitioner should refer the patient to the nearest available resource but continue a caring involvement as the patient's GP. Survivors of sexual assault should be allowed to accept or decline various treatment options offered by the practitioner.

Management of the victim
What you should do for the patient first is to offer and provide privacy, safety, confidentiality and

emotional support. Believe them, listen to them and be non-judgmental.

Three important things to say initially to any victim:

- You are safe now.
- We are sorry this happened to you.
- It was not your fault.

Initial advice to the victim

If victim reporting to police:

1. Notify the police at once.
2. Take along a witness to the alleged assault (if there was a witness).
3. Do not wash or tidy yourself or change your clothing.
4. Do not take any alcohol or drugs.
5. Don't drink or wash out your mouth if there was oral assault.
6. Take a change of warm clothing.

If not reporting to police or unsure, contact any of the following:

1. a friend or other responsible person
2. Lifeline or Lifelink or a similar service
3. a doctor
4. a counselling service

Obtaining information

1. Obtain consent from the patient to record and release information.
2. Take a careful history and copious relevant notes.
3. Keep a record, have a protocol.
4. Obtain a kit for examination.
5. Have someone present during the examination (especially in the case of male doctors examining women).
6. Air-dry swabs (media destroy spermatozoa).
7. Hand specimens to police immediately.

Examination

If possible the patient should be clothed when seen. Have the patient undress while standing on a white sheet to collect debris, and note any injuries as each item is removed. Each part of the body should be examined, under good illumination, and all injuries measured and recorded carefully on a diagram.

Injuries should be photographed professionally. Examine the body and genital area with a

Wood's light to identify semen, which fluoresces. Palpate the scalp for hidden trauma. Collect appropriate swabs.

Making reports

Remember that as a doctor you are impartial. Never make inappropriate judgments to authorities (e.g. 'This patient was raped' or 'incest was committed'). Rather say: 'There is evidence (or no evidence) to support penetration of the vagina/anus' or 'There is evidence of trauma to _____'.

Postexamination

After the medical examination a discussion of medical problems should take place with the patient. This should be done in private and kept totally confidential. A management plan for physical injuries and emotional problems is discussed.

Consider the possibility of STD and possible referral. Consider also the possibility of pregnancy and the need for postcoital hormone tablets. Organise follow-up counselling and STD screening.

References

1. Kerr A. Domestic violence. Treat it seriously. Aust Fam Physician, 1989; 18:1362–1369.
2. Hazelwood R, Warren J, Dietz P. Compliant victims of the sexual sadist. Aust Fam Physician, 1993; 22:474–479.
3. Knowlden S, Helman T. How to treat domestic violence. Australian Dr Weekly, 21 April 1989; I–VIII.
4. Stark E. et al. *Wife abusing in the medical setting—an introduction to health personnel*. Rockville, Ma: National Clearing House for Domestic Violence, 1981, 7.
5. Western Australian Domestic Violence Task Force. *Break the silence*. Report to the Western Australian Government. Perth: Government Printer, 1986; 26–35, 162–163.
6. Tierney LM et al. *Current medical diagnosis and treatment* (35th edn). Stanford: Appleton & Lange, 1996, 667.

89

Basic antenatal care

—

An examiner, no lover of females, thrust a femur into her hand.
  'How many of these have you got?' he demanded.
  'Five.'
  'How do you come to that conclusion?' he asked contemptuously.
  'I have two of my own, the one in my hand, and the two of my unborn child.'

Anonymous anecdote

Pregnancy and childbirth are very important and emotional events in the lives of women and their families. Their care during and after pregnancy is one of the most satisfying aspects of the work of the family doctor, who generally chooses breadth of knowledge rather than depth of knowledge. The changing trend towards specialisation has meant a change of role for the city practitioner and now shared obstetric care is a commonly practised routine. The quality of care that can be given in family practice is often superior to that offered in the hospital antenatal clinic, partly because of the continuing personal care offered by the family doctor.[1]

Antenatal care presents preventive medicine opportunities *par excellence* and is the ideal time to develop an optimal therapeutic relationship with the expectant mother. The opportunities for anticipatory guidance should be seized and education about the multitude of possible sensations during pregnancy (such as heartburn, backache, leg cramps, various fears and anxieties) should be addressed. In other words, an optimal communication system should be established between the expectant couple and the health care system.

Early diagnosis of high-risk pregnancy is important but of little value unless followed by normal attendance for antenatal care.

The information presented here is a basis for the shared care strategy where family doctors share basic antenatal care with consultants and have a ready referral strategy for high-risk pregnancies.

The basic aim of antenatal care is to assess the risk of harm to mother and baby and apply the appropriate level of surveillance to minimise or eradicate harmful effects.

Preconceptual care

Preconceptual care is to be commended to the woman contemplating pregnancy and her family doctor is well placed to provide general health care and screening as well as genetic counselling.

General advice should include optimal nutrition and diet, weight control, regular exercise and discouragement of smoking, alcohol and drugs. Listeria infection is a problem if contracted, with foetal mortality being 30–50%. Protection is afforded by good personal and food hygiene. For those who ask, advise avoidance of unpasteurised dairy products, soft cheeses, cold meats and raw seafoods.

Folic acid is now generally recommended to commence 3–4 months prior to conception, continuing to 12 weeks post conception. Examination should include blood pressure, cardiac status, urinalysis and cervical smear.

Rubella serology should be estimated and, if required, immunisation 3 months prior to conception should be initiated. Test for seroconversion 3 months later. Vaccination should be avoided in early pregnancy.

Genetic counselling based on past obstetric or family history, advanced maternal age or other factors should be considered. This applies especially to Down syndrome, neural tube defect, congenital heart disease, cystic fibrosis and fragile X syndrome.

The initial visit

It is important to book the patient into hospital at the first visit and into the antenatal outpatient department if appropriate. It is mandatory to make an accurate estimation of the expected due date—the use of ultrasonography can help.

History checkpoints[2]
- Confirm the pregnancy by the menstrual history and by urine or serum human chorionic gonadotrophin if necessary.
- Previous obstetric history:
  — Gestation, length of labour, mode of delivery, birth weight of each baby.
  — Consider previous problems: foetal or neonatal abnormalities or deaths; preterm or growth-retarded infants.
  — Abortions: determine if there has been any termination of pregnancies or first or second trimester spontaneous abortions.
- Medical history:
  — Check for past evidence of diabetes, tuberculosis, anaemia, rubella, rheumatic fever, heart or renal disease, jaundice, depression, transfusions and rhesus status.
- Family history:
  — Features to consider are multiple pregnancies, hypertension and diabetes.
  — If any of these pertain to first-degree relatives, consider a glucose screening or tolerance test.
- Psychosocial history:
  — This is very important and includes an assessment of the emotional attitude.
- Drug history:
  — Includes intake of nicotine, alcohol, aspirin, illicit drugs, OTC drugs and prescribed drugs.
- Important points to consider:
  — Establish date of confinement (see obstetric calendar in Figure 89.1).
  — If maternal age > 37 years, consider feasibility of amniocentesis or chorionic villus sampling or other relevant tests (Down syndrome).
  — Consider unusual causes for severe nausea and vomiting, e.g. hydatidiform mole, cerebral tumour.

— Investigate possible exposure to rubella.
— If vaginal bleeding: if Rh negative, send blood sample for Rh antibodies—if absent, give one ampoule anti-D gammaglobulin within 72 hours of first bleed.

Physical examination
During the initial examination assess the patient's general physical and mental status. Examine the following:
- general fitness, colour (? anaemia)
- basic parameters: height, weight, blood pressure, pulse, urinalysis (protein and glucose)
- head and neck: teeth, gums, thyroid
- chest: including breasts/nipples
- abdomen: palpate for uterine size and listen to foetal heart (if indicated)

Perform the four classic techniques of palpation (applies to later visits):
1. Fundal palpation
2. Lateral abdominal palpation
3. Pawlik palpation
4. Deep pelvic palpation

- legs: note oedema or varicose veins

Speculum examination: perform a Pap smear and swab (if indicated by abnormal vaginal discharge).

Pelvic examination (optional): confirm uterus size and period of gestation by bimanual palpation.

Investigations
Standard antenatal investigations are outlined in Table 89.1 and a routine plan for antenatal care in Table 89.2.[3]

Visits during pregnancy

- initial in first trimester: 8–10 weeks
- up to 28 weeks: every 4–6 weeks
- up to 36 weeks: every 2 weeks
- 36 weeks–delivery: weekly

The average number of visits is twelve but the need for this number is being questioned, with some authorities recommending as few as six visits.

For each visit record:
- weight gain ✓
- blood pressure ✓
- urinalysis (protein and sugar); see Table 89.3

The calculation is made from the first day of the last menstrual period																															
January	1	2	3	4	5	6	7	8	9	10	11	12	13	14	15	16	17	18	19	20	21	22	23	24	25	26	27	28	29	30	31	January
October	8	9	10	11	12	13	14	15	16	17	18	19	20	21	22	23	24	25	26	27	28	29	30	31	1	2	3	4	5	6	7	*November*
February	1	2	3	4	5	6	7	8	9	10	11	12	13	14	15	16	17	18	19	20	21	22	23	24	25	26	27	28				February
November	8	9	10	11	12	13	14	15	16	17	18	19	20	21	22	23	24	25	26	27	28	29	30	1	2	3	4	5				*December*
March	1	2	3	4	5	6	7	8	9	10	11	12	13	14	15	16	17	18	19	20	21	22	23	24	25	26	27	28	29	30	31	March
December	6	7	8	9	10	11	12	13	14	15	16	17	18	19	20	21	22	23	24	25	26	27	28	29	30	31	1	2	3	4	5	*January*
April	1	2	3	4	5	6	7	8	9	10	11	12	13	14	15	16	17	18	19	20	21	22	23	24	25	26	27	28	29	30		April
January	6	7	8	9	10	11	12	13	14	15	16	17	18	19	20	21	22	23	24	25	26	27	28	29	30	31	1	2	3	4		*February*
May	1	2	3	4	5	6	7	8	9	10	11	12	13	14	15	16	17	18	19	20	21	22	23	24	25	26	27	28	29	30	31	May
February	5	6	7	8	9	10	11	12	13	14	15	16	17	18	19	20	21	22	23	24	25	26	27	28	1	2	3	4	5	6	7	*March*
June	1	2	3	4	5	6	7	8	9	10	11	12	13	14	15	16	17	18	19	20	21	22	23	24	25	26	27	28	29	30		June
March	8	9	10	11	12	13	14	15	16	17	18	19	20	21	22	23	24	25	26	27	28	29	30	31	1	2	3	4	5	6		*April*
July	1	2	3	4	5	6	7	8	9	10	11	12	13	14	15	16	17	18	19	20	21	22	23	24	25	26	27	28	29	30	31	July
April	7	8	9	10	11	12	13	14	15	16	17	18	19	20	21	22	23	24	25	26	27	28	29	30	1	2	3	4	5	6	7	*May*
August	1	2	3	4	5	6	7	8	9	10	11	12	13	14	15	16	17	18	19	20	21	22	23	24	25	26	27	28	29	30	31	August
May	8	9	10	11	12	13	14	15	16	17	18	19	20	21	22	23	24	25	26	27	28	29	30	31	1	2	3	4	5	6	7	*June*
September	1	2	3	4	5	6	7	8	9	10	11	12	13	14	15	16	17	18	19	20	21	22	23	24	25	26	27	28	29	30		September
June	8	9	10	11	12	13	14	15	16	17	18	19	20	21	22	23	24	25	26	27	28	29	30	1	2	3	4	5	6	7		*July*
October	1	2	3	4	5	6	7	8	9	10	11	12	13	14	15	16	17	18	19	20	21	22	23	24	25	26	27	28	29	30	31	October
July	8	9	10	11	12	13	14	15	16	17	18	19	20	21	22	23	24	25	26	27	28	29	30	31	1	2	3	4	5	6	7	*August*
November	1	2	3	4	5	6	7	8	9	10	11	12	13	14	15	16	17	18	19	20	21	22	23	24	25	26	27	28	29	30		November
August	8	9	10	11	12	13	14	15	16	17	18	19	20	21	22	23	24	25	26	27	28	29	30	31	1	2	3	4	5	6		*September*
December	1	2	3	4	5	6	7	8	9	10	11	12	13	14	15	16	17	18	19	20	21	22	23	24	25	26	27	28	29	30	31	December
September	7	8	9	10	11	12	13	14	15	16	17	18	19	20	21	22	23	24	25	26	27	28	29	30	1	2	3	4	5	6	7	*October*

Or: (approximately) subtract three from months and add seven to days
e.g. 19/8/89

$$\frac{+\ 7\ -\ 3}{26/5/90}$$ Or: Naegele's rule—add seven days, nine months

Fig. 89.1 *Obstetric calendar to determine expected due date*

Table 89.1 *Standard antenatal investigations*

Essential	Recommended or consider
First visit	*First visit*
• full blood examination	• HIV antibodies
• blood grouping and rhesus typing	• toxoplasmosis screen
• rubella antibodies	• hepatitis C screen
• cervical smear (if previous > 12 months)	
• midstream urine: microscopy and culture	
• HBs Ag (hepatitis surface antigen)	
• syphilis screen	
• haemoglobin electrophoresis (if indicated)	
Subsequent visits	*Subsequent visits*
• ultrasound 18–20 weeks (if doubt about foetal maturity)	• cervical swab (group B haemolytic streptococcus) 36 weeks
• glucose screening 28 weeks (diabetes exclusion test)	• test fetoplacental function (32–38 weeks)
• midstream urine (M&C), 28 weeks (if high risk)	• cardiotocographic monitoring
• haemoglobin 30 weeks	• rubella antibodies (? preferable to first visit)
• Rh antibodies (negative mother), 28 weeks and 36 weeks	

For prenatal diagnosis of genetic abnormalities:
• amniocentesis (14–16 weeks)
• chorionic villus sampling (10–11 weeks)
• alpha-fetoprotein
• consider triple test or quadruple test

Table 89.2 *A routine plan for antenatal care*

Week of preg-nancy	Date	Gestation (weeks)		BP	Weight (kg)	Urine		Foetus		Checklist of reminders
		date	size			protein	glucose	heart	position	
8–10										Confirm pregnancy and stage by examination Arrange basic investigations (Table 89.1) If Rh-negative arrange test for partner Consider psychosocial status Confirm hospital and medical arrangements Promote a healthy diet Discuss breast care
14										Discuss diet and general health Educate about recording first movements Arrange ultrasound 18 weeks to confirm dates, etc. Consider need for iron and folic acid
20										Record date of first movement Check that movements correspond with dates Confirm hospital booking Discuss coping abilities
26										Urinalysis, microscopy and culture Check foetal heart Reinforce value of breast-feeding Discuss antenatal classes and physiotherapy Check psychosocial issues Advise single mothers on available government benefits
28										Check haemoglobin and film Repeat antibody screen if Rh-negative Arrange glucose screening test
30										Check foetal position, presentation and heart Consider possibility of twins
32										Check breast care, diet, exercise program Consider special screening if necessary, e.g. repeated ultrasound
34										General check—health, breasts Check for signs of pre-eclampsia Check position ? breech
36										Check haemoglobin and film Arrange antibody test if Rh-negative Explain what to expect with onset of labour Check foetal position ? High vaginal swab for GBHS screen

(continues)

Table 89.2 *(continued)*

Week of pregnancy	Date	Gestation (weeks) date	Gestation (weeks) size	BP	Weight (kg)	Urine protein	Urine glucose	Foetus heart	Foetus position	Checklist of reminders
		Recorded observations								
37										Check breast care, diet, coping ability Explain hospital admission procedures Check foetal position (? engaged)
38										Check breast care, state of legs, coping ability Check foetal position (? engaged head) Reaffirm understanding of when to go to hospital
39										Check any special concerns Discuss future family planning

- uterine size/fundal height
- foetal heart (usually audible with stethoscope at 25 weeks and definitely by 28 weeks)
- foetal movements (if present)
- presentation and position of foetus (third trimester)
- presence of any oedema

Record day of first foetal movements (ask patient to write down the dates)

- primigravida: 17–20 weeks
- multigravida: 16–18 weeks

Fundal height

The relative heights of the uterus fundus are shown in Figure 89.2. The uterus is a pelvic organ until the twelfth week of pregnancy. After this time it can be palpated abdominally. At about 20–22 weeks it has reached the level of the umbilicus and reaches the xiphisternum between 36 and 40 weeks. Palpation of the fundal height is affected by obesity and tenseness of the abdominal wall.

Table 89.3 *Causes of proteinuria in pregnancy*

Urinary tract infection
Contamination from vaginal discharge
Pre-eclampsia toxaemia
Underlying chronic renal disease

Management of specific issues

Nutrition advice

A healthy diet is very important and should contain at least the following daily allowances:

Fig. 89.2 *Fundal height in normal pregnancy (in weeks); the height of the fundus is a guide to the period of gestation. Nulliparas experience lightening at about 36 weeks when the fundal height usually reverts to the 34 week level*

1. Eat most:
   - fruit and vegetables (at least 4 serves)
   - cereals and bread (4–6 serves)
2. Eat moderately:
   - dairy products—3 cups (600 mL) of milk or equivalent in yoghurt or cheese
   - lean meat, poultry or fish—1 or 2 serves (at least 2 serves of red meat per week)
3. Eat least:
   - sugar and refined carbohydrates (e.g. sweets, cakes, biscuits, soft drinks)
   - polyunsaturated margarine, butter, oil and cream

Bran with cereal helps prevent constipation of pregnancy.

If the ideal diet is followed, iron, vitamin and calcium supplements should not be necessary. Do not diet to lose weight. It is usual to gain about 12 kg during pregnancy.

Smoking, alcohol and other drugs[4]

Encourage patients to avoid all street drugs, alcohol, tobacco and caffeine (ideally). If they find this impossible, encourage the following daily limitations:

- 3–6 smokes
- 1 standard drink
- 1 cup of coffee or 2 cups of tea

Other household members should also stop smoking as passive smoking may be harmful to mother and child.

Breast-feeding

Mothers to be should be encouraged to breast-feed. Give advice and relevant literature. They can be directed to a local nursing mothers' group for support and guidance if necessary.

Antenatal classes

Referral to therapists conducting such classes can provide advice and supervision on antenatal exercises, back care, posture, relaxation skills, pain relief in labour, general exercises and swimming. Enrolment with the partner is recommended.

Normal activities

Mothers should be reassured that pregnancy is a normal event in the life cycle and that normal activities should be continued. Housework and other activities should be performed to just short of getting tired. The importance of getting sufficient rest and sleep should be emphasised.

Sex in pregnancy[5]

Coitus should be encouraged during pregnancy but with appropriate care, especially in the 4 weeks before delivery. Restriction would only seem necessary if there has been an adverse obstetric history and there are major complications in the current pregnancy.

The couple should be encouraged to be loving to each other and communicate their feelings freely, as the need for affection and physical contact is important. Coital techniques can be modified as the pregnancy progresses—posterior entry and the female superior position are quite suitable.

Travel

Pregnant women should avoid standing in trains. They should avoid international air travel after 28 weeks and travel after 36 weeks is usually not permitted. Patients should be counselled to wear a seat belt during car travel.

Psychosocial and emotional stress

Antenatal visits provide an ideal opportunity to become acquainted with the 'real' person and explore issues that help the patient. Provide whole person understanding with appropriate help and reassurance where necessary. Areas to be explored include support systems, attitudes of patient and partner to the pregnancy, sexuality, expectation of labour and delivery, financial issues, and attitudes of parents and in-laws.

Weight gain in pregnancy

Although a standard weight gain is given as 12 kg over 40 weeks of pregnancy, it is common for some women in Australia to gain up to 20 kg without adverse effects.[2]

Normal weight gain is minimal in the first 20 weeks, resulting in a 3 kg weight gain in the first half of pregnancy. From 20 weeks onwards there is an average weight gain of 0.5 kg per week. From 36 weeks the weight gain usually levels off.[2]

Foetal movement chart

If daily foetal movements exceed 10 and the regular pattern has not changed significantly, then usually the foetus is at no risk. However, if the movements drop to less than 10 per day, the patient should be referred to hospital for foetal monitoring.

Possible exposure to rubella

When contact with a possible case of rubella occurs during pregnancy it is essential to establish the immune status of the patient. If she is already immune no further action is necessary. If her immune status is unknown, perform a rubella Ig G titre and Ig M and repeat the Ig G and Ig M titres in 2–3 weeks.

Threatened miscarriage

If a threatened miscarriage occurs, check the blood group and test for rhesus antibodies in maternal serum. If the mother is Rh-negative and no antibodies are detected, give one ampoule of anti-D gammaglobulin intramuscularly. Assess her pelvis to rule out an ectopic pregnancy and, if indicated, perform pelvic scanning to confirm viability of the foetus or the presence of an extra-uterine gestation.

Pregnancy sickness[6]

- nausea and vomiting occur in more than 50% of women
- almost always disappears by the end of first trimester
- mild cases can be dealt with by explanation and reassurance; it is preferable to avoid drug therapy if possible
- simple measures:
  — small frequent meals
  — a fizzy soft drink may help
  — avoid stimuli such as cooking smells
  — take care with teeth cleaning
  — avoid oral iron
- medication (for severe cases):
  — pyridoxine 50–100 mg bd
  — if still ineffective add metoclopramide 10 mg tds

Heartburn[6]

Gastro-oesophageal reflux is a major source of discomfort to women in the latter half of pregnancy. Non-pharmacological treatment such as frequent small meals, avoidance of bending over and elevation of the head of the bed are the mainstays of treatment. Smoking, alcohol and caffeine (coffee, chocolate, tea) intake should be avoided. Regular use of antacids is effective, e.g. alginate/antacid liquid (Gaviscon, Mylanta Plus) 10–20 mL before meals and at bedtime. H_2-antagonists may be necessary.

Cramps

Pregnant women are more prone to cramp. If it develops they should be advised simply to place a pillow at the foot of the bed so that plantar flexion of the feet is avoided during sleep. Prolonged plantar flexion is the basis of the cramps. Tonic water prior to sleeping is helpful. There is no evidence that calcium supplements help cramps during pregnancy.[7]

Varicose veins

These can be troublesome as well as embarrassing. Wearing special supportive pantyhose (not elastic bandages) is the most comfortable and practical way to cope, in addition to adequate rest.

Haemorrhoids

Haemorrhoids in the later stages of pregnancy can be very troublesome. Emphasising the importance of a high-fibre diet to ensure regular bowel habit is the best management. Painful haemorrhoids may be eased by the application of packs soaked in warm saline or perhaps haemorrhoidal ointments containing local anaesthetic.

Dental hygiene

Dental problems can worsen during pregnancy so special care of teeth and gums, including a visit to the dentist, is appropriate. Continuation of cleaning with a softer brush is recommended.

Back pain

Back pain, especially low back pain, is common during pregnancy and special back care advice can help women cope with this problem, which can become debilitating. Advice with lifting, sitting, and resting, using a firm mattress and avoiding high-heeled shoes will help.

Physical therapy administered by a skilled therapist can be extremely effective for pregnant patients but certain safety rules should be followed:

- *First trimester:* use normal physical therapy and advise exercises.
- *Second trimester:* use supine side lying rotation and sitting techniques only; advise exercises.
- *Third trimester:* avoid physical therapy (if possible); encourage exercises.

Guidelines for treatment

- Keep mobilisation and manipulation to a minimum.
- Use mobilisation in preference to manipulation.
- Safeguard the sacroiliac joints in the last trimester.
- Encourage active exercises as much as possible.
- Avoid medications wherever possible.
- Give trigger point injections (8 mL 1% lignocaine) around the SIJs if necessary.

Exercise guidelines

Advise the patient that walking is an excellent exercise; for additional exercise activity:

- exercise at a mild to moderate level only
- avoid overheating
- allow for a long warm-up before exercise and a long cool-down
- choose low-impact or water exercise
- stop if there are adverse symptoms, e.g. any pain, bleeding, faintness, undue distress

Carpal tunnel syndrome

Splinting of the hand and forearm at night might be beneficial. If desperate, an injection of corticosteroid into the carpal tunnel can be very effective (check drug category for risk relative to dates). Sometimes operative division of the volar carpal ligament is necessary. Most problems subside following delivery.

Mineral supplements in pregnancy

Iron

Iron is not routinely recommended for pregnant women who are healthy, following an optimal diet and have a normal blood test. Those at risk, e.g. with poor nutrition, will require supplementation.

Folic acid

Folic acid is advised for *all* women contemplating pregnancy, starting 3–4 months prior to conception and continuing until 12 weeks after conception. Dose: 0.5 mg (o) daily.[8] In those at risk, e.g. previous neural tube defect, the dose is 5 mg per day.[9]

Advice on when to seek medical help

- if contractions, unusual pain or bleeding occur before term
- if the baby is less active than usual
- if the membranes rupture (with fluid loss)
- the onset of regular contractions 5–10 minutes apart

The heel-prick test

It is worth noting that the newborn infant has a routine heel-prick test to screen for phenylketonuria, hypothyroidism and cystic fibrosis.

References

1. Barker JH. *General practice medicine.* Edinburgh: Churchill Livingstone, 1984, 76–89.
2. Fung P, Morrison J. Obstetric share-care. Aust Fam Physician, 1989; 18:479–484.
3. Carson S, Gawthorn EC. A manual for primary health care. Sydney: Medical Observer, 1990; 3.1–3.20.
4. Smibert J. The principles of antenatal care. Aust Fam Physician, 1978; 9:1087–1094.
5. Beischer NA, Mackay EV. *Obstetrics and the newborn.* Sydney: Saunders, 1986.
6. Humphrey M. Common conditions in an otherwise normal pregnancy. In: MIMS Disease Index (2nd edn). Sydney: IMS Publishing, 1996, 116–120.
7. Hammer I et al. Calcium treatment of leg cramps in pregnancy. Acta Obstet Gynaecol Scand, 1981; 60:345–347.
8. Goh J, Erian M. An update on obstetric practice. Mod Med Aust, 1996; 8:20–25.
9. MRC Vitamin Study Research Group. Prevention of neural tube defects. Lancet, 1991; 338:131–137.

90

High-risk pregnancy

—

Grace the wyffe of William Baxter, beinge aboute three weeks before her tyme, was brought in bed the first day of December of two children, their bellies were growne and joyned together, from their breastes to their navells, and their faces were together.

John Richardson
Giving details of Siamese twins, born in 1655

Definition[1]

A high-risk pregnancy is one in which the foetus is at increased risk of stillbirth, neonatal morbidity or death, and/or the expectant mother is at increased risk for morbidity or mortality.

High-risk pregnancies may be predicted before conception in some women, especially those with serious medical problems and a poor obstetric history. Other high risks can be identified at the first antenatal visit and others develop during the course of pregnancy. The first antenatal visit is the most important visit and demands time and care to make an accurate assessment.

Accurate determination of EDD

It is vital to determine the expected due date of delivery (EDD) based on the exact time of the last normal menstrual period (sometimes misleading), the fundal height, the time of first foetal movements and, if in doubt, ultrasound assessment.

High-risk obstetric patients

Guidelines for high-risk pregnancy are presented in Table 90.1. Recognition of these high-risk pregnancies is important for the family doctor involved in shared care. Common categories that require special surveillance are:

- elderly primigravida
- grand multipara (fifth or greater pregnancy, especially if > 35 years)
- those with a poor obstetric history
- previous caesarean section
- severely disadvantaged social problem, e.g. sole teenage parent with drug problem
- hypertension
- obesity
- short stature
- diabetes mellitus
- prolonged infertility or essential drug or hormone treatment
- heavy smoking or alcohol intake

The onset during pregnancy of the following:

- little or no weight gain during the first half of the pregnancy
- complications such as pre-eclampsia, multiple pregnancies or antepartum haemorrhage
- abnormal presentation
- abnormal foetal growth

Urinary tract infection

Urinary tract infection includes pyelonephritis, cystitis and asymptomatic cases.

Acute pyelonephritis

This infection, usually due to *E. coli*, is one of the most common infective complications of pregnancy. Symptoms include fever, chills, vomiting and loin pain. Bladder symptoms such as frequency and dysuria are commonly absent. The patient should be hospitalised and usually requires intravenous antibiotic therapy and possibly rehydration.

Table 90.1 *Guidelines for specialist obstetric consultation*

	Major risk factors Obstetric consultation mandatory	Other risk factors Consultation should be considered

Past problematic obstetric history	• previous caesarean section
	• incompetent cervical os
	• 2nd trimester spontaneous abortion
	• rhesus/other blood group
	  incompatibility
	• thromboembolic disease
	• premature labour
		• multiple spontaneous or elective
		  abortions
		• premature delivery
		• previous stillbirth
		• neonatal death
		• grand multigravida

Problems related to pregnancy	• pre-eclampsia
	• rhesus/other blood group
	  incompatibility
	• significant vaginal bleeding
	• placenta praevia
	• postmaturity at 42 weeks
	• multiple pregnancy
	• polyhydramnios
	• need for amniocentesis
	  — genetic concerns
	  — abnormal AFP
	  — other
		• recurrent urinary infections
		• abnormal uterine growth
		• inadequate maternal weight gain
		• hypertension

General factors		• age > 35 : < 18 • obesity > 110 kg • prepregnancy weight < 45 kg • psychosocial problems • short stature < 152 cm • smoking > 10/day
Maternal disorders	• diabetes mellitus • systemic lupus erythematosus • sickle cell disease or other haemoglobinopathy	• anaemia: Hb < 10 g/dL • cardiovascular disease • chronic renal disease • alcohol or drug abuse • genital herpes
Perinatal problems	• premature labour • postmaturity (42 weeks) • disproportion • malpresentation • placental insufficiency	• non-vertex presentation (at term) • foetal arrhythmia • membranes ruptured > 18 hrs
Inadequate antenatal care		• late presentation (after 20 weeks) • no antenatal care • failed or poor attendance

Treatment of acute pyelonephritis

• amoxycillin 1 g IV 6 hourly for 48 hours, then 500 mg (o) 8 hourly (if bacteria sensitive) for 14 days[2,3]
• alternatives: cephalosporins, e.g. cephalothin IV and cephalexin 500 mg (o)

Acute cystitis

Patients with acute cystitis typically have dysuria and frequency. Treat for 10–14 days.

Treatment

• cephalexin 250 mg (o) 6 hourly[3]

or

• amoxycillin/potassium clavulanate (250/125 mg) (o) 8 hourly

or

• nitrofurantoin 50 mg (o) 6 hourly, if a beta-lactam antibiotic is contraindicated.

Note: Nitrofurantoin is contraindicated in the third[2] trimester of pregnancy as it may lead to haemolytic diseases in the newborn. Cotrimoxazole and sulphonamides should be avoided. Amoxycillin is recommended only if susceptibility of the organism is proven.

• a high fluid intake should be maintained during treatment.

Asymptomatic bacteriuria[2]

- 5–10% of pregnant asymptomatic women have positive cultures during pregnancy.
- Ideally all women should be screened for bacteriuria at their first visit.
- Less than 1% will subsequently develop bacteraemia.
- Approximately 5% of such women subsequently develop pyelonephritis during pregnancy with an increased risk of preterm labour, mid-trimester abortion and pregnancy-induced hypertension.

Treatment

Treatment is recommended according to culture sensitivities. It is preferable to delay it until the first trimester has passed.[2]

Hypertensive disorders in pregnancy[4]

Hypertensive disorders complicate about 10% of all pregnancies. Pregnancy may induce hypertension in previously normotensive women or may aggravate pre-existing hypertension.

A classification of hypertensive disorders in pregnancy:

- *Pregnancy-induced hypertension*
  Definition:
  SBP > 140 mmHg and DBP > 90 mmHg, occurring for first time after 20th week of pregnancy and regressing postpartum.
  or
  Rise in SBP > 25 mmHg or DBP > 15 mmHg from readings before pregnancy or in first trimester.

  Types:
  Hypertension without proteinuria
  Pre-eclampsia—hypertension + proteinuria
  Eclampsia—hypertension + convulsions

- *Essential (coincidental) hypertension*
  Chronic underlying hypertension occurring before the onset of pregnancy or persisting postpartum.

- *Pregnancy-aggravated hypertension*
  Underlying hypertension worsened by pregnancy.

Risk factors

The following are risk factors for pregnancy-induced hypertension:

- nulliparity
- family history of hypertension
- chronic hypertension
- diabetes complicating pregnancy
- multiple pregnancy
- hydatidiform mole
- hydrops fetalis
- hydramnios
- renal disease

Clinical features include hypertension, excessive weight gain, generalised oedema and proteinuria (urinary protein $> 0.3/24$ hours). Late symptoms include headache (related to severe hypertension), epigastric pain and visual disturbances.

Management

The optimal treatment is delivery, and induction of labour needs to be timed appropriately—based on parameters such as the blood pressure level and the development of proteinuria. The BP level must be kept below 160/100 mmHg, because at this level intrauterine death is likely to occur and there is a risk of stroke.

Antihypertensive drugs[4]

Contraindicated drugs are ACE inhibitors and diuretics. There is no place for the use of diuretics alone unless cardiac failure is present.
Commonly used medications:

- Beta-blockers, e.g. labetalol, oxprenolol and atenolol (used under close supervision and after 20 weeks gestation)
- Methyldopa: good for sustained BP control
- Nifedipine

Labetalol, hydralazine and diazoxide are useful for rapid control of BP in hypertensive crises.

Guidelines for referral/admission to hospital

- When BP reaches 140/90 mmHg
- Development of proteinuria

Anaemias[2]

During the course of a normal pregnancy the haemoglobin should remain above 11 g/dL. Levels below this, particularly less than 10 g/dL, require investigation. Iron demands during pregnancy are 725 mg, especially during the third trimester.

Types of anaemia in pregnancy:
- iron deficiency (approximately 50%)
- megaloblastic anaemia (usually due to folic acid deficiency)
- thalassaemia

Management
- If anaemia is found, measure serum ferritin, MCV, red cell folate and serum B12 as indicated
- Treatment is according to cause:
  — iron deficiency: ferrous sulphate 0.9 g (o) daily
  — megaloblastic anaemia: folic acid 5 mg (o) bd

Antepartum haemorrhage

If haemorrhage occurs under 24 weeks treat as for threatened miscarriage. If it occurs after 26 weeks admit to hospital for management. Remember to give anti-D if the mother is Rh-negative. Do not perform a vaginal examination.

Trauma: motor vehicle accidents

Abdominal trauma in pregnancy is usually associated with seat belt restraints during motor vehicle accidents. However, these injuries are far less severe than those that occur when people are not wearing seat belts. Women should be encouraged to wear seat belts and should not be given certificates stating that seat belts should not be worn in pregnancy.

The incidence of placental abruption following accidents is related to the severity of the accident and the extent of the external injuries. Injured patients should be admitted to a unit where cardiotocography can be performed regularly for 48 hours and perinatal intensive care can be provided if needed. Consider anti-D injection.

Consideration for induction

Possible indications for induction:
- post-term (41 weeks or over)

- maternal hypertension
- pre-eclamptic toxaemia
- intrauterine growth restriction
- diabetes mellitus

Drugs in pregnancy

Drugs have to be used with great care during pregnancy. An Australian categorisation of drug risk is presented in summary in Table 90.2. It is worth noting that β_2-agonists used to treat asthma have a Category A rating.

When to refer

If there is a possibility of cervical incompetence, refer for a specialist opinion before 14 weeks.

Referral to specialist centre[2]

The key to an optimal outcome is early identification of the high-risk pregnancy and early referral to a specialist team to supervise the management of the remainder of the pregnancy. This has been shown to improve neonatal morbidity and mortality significantly. It is important that family physicians, obstetricians, perinatologists and neonatalogists work as a harmonious team.

Table 90.3 *Common indications for a glucose screening test*

Diabetes in first-degree relatives
Advancing maternal age > 35
Gross maternal obesity
Polyhydramnios
Glycosuria
Signs and symptoms suggestive of diabetes
Poor obstetric history, e.g. stillborn, large babies
Early pre-eclamptic toxaemia

Table 90.2 *Examples of medicines in pregnancy: an Australian categorisation of risk (Australian Drug Evaluation Committee)*

	Category
Iron and haemopoietic agents	
• folic acid	A
• iron preparations (all types)	A
Antihistamines and antiemetics	
• phenothiazines, e.g. prochlorperazine	C
• meclozine, cyclizine	A
• other antihistamines	A or B2
Alimentary system agents	
• antacids	A
• H_2 receptor antagonists	B1
Cardiovascular	
• ACE inhibitor	D
• methyldopa	A
• calcium channel blockers	C
• beta-blockers	C
• digoxin	A
• diuretics (except spironalactone B3)	C
• glyceryl trinitrate	B2
Analgesics	
• aspirin	C
• paracetamol/acetaminophen	A
• codeine	A
• opioid analgesics	C
Hypnotics, sedatives, antipsychotic agents	
• barbiturates	C
• benzodiazepines	C
• chloral hydrate	A
• phenothiazines and butyrophenones	C
Antidepressants	
• tricyclics, e.g. amitriptyline	C
• tetracyclics, e.g. mianserin	B2
Anticonvulsants (all groups)	D
NSAIDs	C
Antimicrobials	
• penicillins	A
• cephalexin, cephalothin	A
• aminoglycosides	D
• nitrofurantoin	A
• tetracyclines	D
Corticosteroids	
• systemic	C
• inhalation	B3
Quinine	D

Code: Category A—no harmful foetal effect recorded.
  B—no harmful effects to date but limited experience (see ADEC guidelines for subgroups B1, B2, B3).
  C—have caused or suspected of causing harmful effects on foetus or neonates without causing malformations (reversible).
  D—have caused, are suspected to cause or may be expected to cause an increased incidence of foetal malformation or irreversible damage. Also may have adverse pharmacological effects.

References

1. Shires DB, Hennen BK, Rice DI. *Family Medicine.* New York: McGraw-Hill, 1987, 136–151.

2. Humphrey M. Common problems in an otherwise normal pregnancy. In: MIMS Disease Index (2nd edn). Sydney: IMS Publishing, 1996, 117–120.

3. Mashford ML. *Antibiotic guidelines* (9th edn). Melbourne: Victorian Medical Postgraduate Foundation, 1996, 168–170.

4. Michael CA. Hypertensive disease in pregnancy. In: MIMS Disease Index (2nd edn). Sydney: IMS Publishing, 1996, 260–263.

91

Postnatal care

—

As concerning the bringing up, nourishment and giving of suckle to the child, it shal be beste that the mother give her child sucke her selfe, for the mothers milk is more convenient and agreeable to the infant than any other woman's or other milke.

Thomas Raynalde 1540
The Byrthe of Mankynde

Education for the puerperium and caring for the baby should begin during pregnancy so that a new mother is familiar with the basic principles of motherhood, especially infant feeding.[1]

Postnatal care really begins with the birth of the baby. Once the airways are cleared the baby should be given to the mother as soon as possible and not taken from her except for essential management.

Mother should remain in the labour ward (if delivered in hospital) for at least an hour after her birth and until she has passed urine. She should be inspected frequently to exclude the possibility of a silent postpartum haemorrhage and vital signs checked before transferring to a lying-in ward.

Guidelines for the lying-in ward[1]

- Every mother needs rest but should have full toilet and shower facilities.
- The baby should be in a bassinet beside the mother and may be taken into bed any time mother likes.
- Room in: the baby should not go to the nursery unless it is sick or the mother requests it.
- There should be no visiting restrictions on close relatives but restrictions should be put on other visitors for the first 2–3 days.
- Demand feed to appetite.

- No test weighing.
- No complementary feeding unless mother is empty and baby screaming.
- A golden rule is that breast-feeding and the supply of mother's milk is a classic case of 'supply and demand'.
- The doctor should listen carefully to what the mother is saying (and not saying) during visits.

Postnatal consultations

The two-week consultation
Mother:
- Assess the coping ability of the new mother
- Look for signs/symptoms of postpartum depression
- Provide encouragement and advice
- Check breast-feeding

Baby:
- Routine examination
- Perform a Phenistix test on the baby's napkin (in case the Guthrie test has been missed in hospital)

The six-week consultation
This is basically a repeat of the previous consultation and a checklist is presented in Table 91.1.

Contraception

Breast-feeding, when it is truly on demand, is an extremely good contraceptive, but in reality some supplement is necessary for about three months in the average lactating woman.

Oral contraception
- The mini pill (progestogen only)
  — norethisterone 350 micrograms/day
                    or

— levonorgestrel 30 micrograms/day taken every night
- Transfer to combined OC when breast-feeding completed (oestrogens can suppress lactation).
- IUCD: If used, it should be fitted at or after 6 weeks.[2]

After-pains[1]

After-pains, which are more common and most intense after the second and subsequent pregnancies, are characterised by intermittent lower abdominal pains, like period pains, which are often worse during and after feeding. They are caused by oxytocin released from the posterior pituitary, which also causes the let-down reflex of nursing.

Treatment, after examination, is reassurance and analgesics in the form of paracetamol every 4 hours for 3 days or as long as necessary.

Breast-feeding

Insufficient milk supply

This is sometimes a problem in mothers who are under a lot of stress and find it hard to relax. A

Table 91.1 *Checklist for postnatal check at 4–6 weeks*

Mother
Pap smear (if not performed at first visit)
Check rubella status
Check for adequate contraception
Check if intercourse has been resumed and give advice (if appropriate)
Check bowel and urine control
Encourage abdominal and pelvic floor exercises
Check for back problems
Check weight, blood pressure and urine
Check breasts
Check perineum
Check psychological health, including coping ability
Check for postpartum thyroiditis
Discuss adequate diet, rest and personal care
Perform pelvic examination
Further follow-up if necessary
Give 'Personal Health Record' folder to mother
Baby
Routine examination
Check growth and feeding
Educate mother regarding immunisation schedule

---

let-down reflex is necessary to get the milk supply going, and sometimes this reflex is slow. If there is insufficient supply, the baby tends to demand frequent feeds, may continually suck its hand and will be slow in gaining weight.[1]

There are three important factors in establishing breast-feeding:

1. positioning the baby on the breast
2. the 'let-down'
3. supply and demand

The breasts produce milk on the principle of supply and demand. This means that the more the breasts are emptied, the more milk is produced.

Advice to mother
- Try to practise relaxation techniques.
- Put the baby to your breast as often as it demands, using the 'chest to chest, chin on breast' method.
- Express after feeds, because the emptier the breasts, the more milk will be produced.
- Make sure you get adequate rest, but if you feel tired go to your doctor for a check-up.

Engorged breasts

Engorgement occurs when the milk supply comes on so quickly that the breasts become swollen, hard and tender. There is an increased supply of blood and other fluids in the breast as well as milk. The breasts and nipples may be so swollen that the baby is unable to latch on and suckle.

Advice to mother
- Feed your baby on demand from day 1 until the baby has had enough.
- Finish the first breast completely; maybe use one side per feed rather than some from each breast. Offer the second breast if the baby appears hungry.
- Soften the breasts before feeds or express with a warm washer or shower, which will help to get the milk flowing.
- Avoid giving the baby other fluids.
- Express a little milk before putting the baby to your breast (a must if the baby has trouble latching on) and express a little after feeding from the other side if it is too uncomfortable.
- Massage any breast lumps gently towards the nipple while feeding.
- Apply cold packs after feeding and cool

washed cabbage leaves (left in the refrigerator) between feeds. Change the leaves every two hours.

- Wake your baby for a feed if your breasts are uncomfortable or if the baby is sleeping longer than 4 hours.
- Use a good, comfortable brassiere.
- Remove your bra completely before feeding.
- Take paracetamol regularly for severe discomfort.

Regular feeding and following demand feeding is the best treatment for engorged breasts.

Suppression of lactation[2]

Women may seek suppression of lactation for a variety of reasons such as weaning the baby, not wishing to breast-feed initially, or after stillbirth.

Mechanical suppression

The simplest way of suppressing lactation once it is established is to transfer the baby gradually to a bottle or a cup over a 3-week period. The decreased demand reduces milk supply, with minimal discomfort. If abrupt cessation is required, it is necessary to avoid nipple stimulation, refrain from expressing milk and use a well-fitting brassiere. Use cold packs and analgesics as necessary. Engorgement will gradually settle over a 2–3 week period.

Hormonal suppression

Hormonal suppression can be used for severe engorgement but only as a last resort. It is more effective if given at the time of delivery but may produce side effects. Avoid oestrogens.

- bromocriptine (Parlodel) 2.5 mg orally bd for 10–14 days[2] (nausea is a problem)

Drugs and lactation

Drugs that can affect lactation or a breast-fed infant are listed in Table 91.2.

Nipple problems with breast-feeding

Sore nipples

Sore nipples is a common problem, thought to be caused by the baby not taking the nipple into its mouth properly, often because of breast engorgement. The problem is preventable with careful attention to the feeding position of the baby.

Table 91.2 *Drugs taken by nursing mother that can affect breast-fed infant or lactation*

Contraindicated drugs

Antibiotics:
- aminoglycosides
- chloramphenicol
- nitrofurantoin
- metronidazole
- tetracycline
- sulphonamides

Antihistamines

Antineoplastics/cytotoxics

Benzodiazepines

Bromocriptine

Combined oral contraceptive /oestrogens

Ergotamine

Gold salts

H_2 antagonists, e.g. cimetidine, ranitidine

Illicit drugs, e.g. cocaine, cannabis, LSD

Lithium

Quinidine

Laxatives, e.g. senna

Alcohol (no harmful effects unless taken in excess)

Nicotine (increased respiratory distress in infants exposed)

Management advice to mother

It is important to be as relaxed and comfortable as possible (with your back well supported) and for your baby to suck gently, so:

- Try to use the 'chest to chest, chin on breast' feeding position.
- Vary the feeding positions (make sure each position is correct).
- Start feeding from the less painful side first if one nipple is very sore.
- Express some milk first to soften and 'lubricate' the nipple. (Avoid drying agents such as methylated spirits, soap and tincture of benzoin, and moisturising creams and ointments, which may contain unwanted chemicals and germs.)
- Gently break the suction with your finger before removing the baby from the breast. (Never pull the baby off the nipple.)
- Apply covered ice to the nipple to relieve pain.
- Keep the nipples dry by exposing the breasts to the air and/or using a hair dryer on a low setting.
- If wearing a bra, try Cannon breast shields inside the bra. Do not wear a bra at night.

Cracked nipples

Cracked nipples are usually caused by the baby clamping on the end of the nipple rather than applying the jaw behind the whole nipple. Not drying the nipples thoroughly after each feed and wearing soggy breast pads are other contributing factors. Untreated sore nipples may progress to painful cracks.

Symptoms

At first, the crack may be so small that it cannot be seen. The crack is either on the skin of the nipple or where it joins the areola. A sharp pain in the nipple with suckling probably means the crack has developed. Feeding is usually very painful, and bleeding can occur.

Management advice to mother[3]

Cracked nipples nearly always heal when you get the baby to latch onto the breast fully and properly. They usually take only 1–2 days to heal.

- Follow the same rules as for sore nipples.
- Do not feed from the affected breast—rest the nipple for 1–2 feeds.
- Express the milk from that breast by hand.
- Feed that expressed milk to the baby.
- Start feeding gradually with short feeds.
- A sympathetic expert such as an experienced nursing mother will be a great help if you are having trouble coping.
- Take paracetamol just before feeding to relieve pain.

Inverted nipples

An inverted nipple is one that inverts or moves into the breast instead of pointing outwards when the baby tries to suck from it. When the areola is squeezed, the nipple retracts inwards.

Treatment[3]

During pregnancy, rolling and stretching the nipple by hand can be helpful. The partner can assist with gentle oral and manual stimulation.

A simple treatment, which should start at the beginning of the seventh month of pregnancy, is the Hoffman technique:

1. Draw an imaginary cross on the breast with the vertical and horizontal lines crossing at the nipple.
2. Place the thumbs or the forefingers opposite each other at the edge of the areola on the imaginary horizontal line. Press in firmly and then pull the thumbs (or fingers) back and forth to stretch the areola.
3. In the vertical position, pull the thumbs or fingers upwards and downwards.

This procedure should be repeated about five times each morning. The nipple will become erect and is then easier to grasp, so that it can be slowly and gently drawn out.

Mastitis

Mastitis is basically cellulitis of the interlobular connective tissue of the breast. Usually restricted to lactating women it is caused mainly by a cracked nipple or poor milk drainage. The infecting organism is usually *Staphylococcus aureus* or more rarely *Escherichia coli* or *Candida albicans*. It is a serious problem and requires early treatment. Breast-feeding from the affected side can continue as the infection is confined to interstitial breast tissue and doesn't usually affect the milk supply.

Note: Mastitis must be treated vigorously—it is a serious condition.

Clinical features

- a lump and then soreness (at first)
- a red tender area
  possibly
- fever, tiredness, muscle aches and pains

Note: Candida infection usually causes severe breast pain—a feeling like a hot knife or shooting pains, especially during and after feeding. It may occur after a course of antibiotics.

Management

Prevention (in lactation)

- maintain free breast drainage
- attend to breast engorgement and cracked nipples

Treatment[4]

- antibiotics: resolution without progression to an abscess will usually be prevented by antibiotics:

    dicloxacillin 500 mg (o) qid for 10 days
      or
    flucloxacillin 500 mg (o) qid for 10 days
      or

cephalaxin 500 mg (o) qid for 10 days
If severe cellulitis:
flucloxacillin/dicloxacillin 2g IV 6 hourly
- therapeutic ultrasound ($2W/cm^2$ for 6 minutes) daily for 2–3 days
- aspirin or paracetamol for pain

Instructions to patients
- Keep the affected breast well drained.
- Continue breast-feeding: do it frequently and start with the sore side.
- Heat the sore breast before feeding, e.g. hot shower or hot face washer.
- Cool the breast after feeding: use a cold face washer from the freezer.
- Massage any breast lumps gently towards the nipple while feeding.
- Empty the breast well: hand express if necessary.
- Get sufficient rest.
- Keep to a nutritious diet and drink ample fluids.

Breast abscess

If tenderness and redness persist beyond 48 hours and an area of tense induration develops, then a breast abscess has formed. It requires surgical drainage under general anaesthesia, antibiotics, rest and complete emptying of the breast. Temporary weaning of breast-feeding from the affected side is necessary because of the surgical disruption.

For a description of surgical drainage refer to page 822.

Secondary postpartum haemorrhage[5]

Postpartum haemorrhage is any bright bleeding from the birth canal 24 hours or more after delivery. It may vary from very slight to torrential and may occur at any time up to 6 weeks postpartum.

Causes
- retained products of conception
- infection, especially at placental site
- laceration of any part of the birth canal

Treatment
- ergometrine 0.5 mg IM injection
- exploration under GA if blood loss > 250 mL

— gentle curettage required in the postpartum uterus
- antibiotics and blood as indicated

Note: Referral is necessary after the ergometrine injection. Occasionally a life-saving hysterectomy or ligation of the internal iliac arteries may be necessary.

Puerperal fever

The cause is genital infection in about 75% of patients. Other causes include urinary tract infection, mastitis and an intercurrent infection. Investigations include a vaginal swab for smear, culture and sensitivities (include anaerobic culture) and a midstream specimen of urine for microscopy and culture.

Treatment
- amoxycillin/potassium clavulanate plus metronidazole (while awaiting sensitivities)

Beware of severe puerperal sepsis such as Gram negative septicaemia or *Clostridium welchii* septicaemia.

Postnatal depressive disorders

It is quite common for women to feel emotional and flat after childbirth; this is apparently due to hormonal changes and to the anticlimax after the long-awaited event. There are three separate important problems:
1. postnatal blues
2. postnatal adjustment disorder
3. postnatal (or postpartum) depression

Postnatal blues
'The blues' is a very common problem (occurs in 80%) that arises in the first two weeks (usually days 3–10) after childbirth.

Clinical features
- feeling flat or depressed
- mood swings
- irritability
- feeling emotional (e.g. crying easily)
- tiredness
- insomnia
- lacking confidence (e.g. in bathing and feeding the baby)
- aches and pains (e.g. headache)

Fortunately 'the blues' is a passing phase and lasts only 4–14 days. Management is based on support, reassurance and basic counselling. Contact friends and relatives to help.

Advice to mother[2]

All you really need is encouragement and support from your partner, family and friends, so tell them how you feel.

- Avoid getting tired and rest as much as possible.
- Talk over your problems with a good listener (perhaps another mother with a baby).
- Accept help from others in the house.
- Allow your partner to take turns getting up to attend to the baby.

If 'the blues' lasts longer than four days, it is very important to contact your doctor.

Postnatal adjustment disorder

- occurs in first 6 months
- similar symptoms to 'the blues'
- anxiety with handling baby
- psychosomatic complaints
- fearful of criticism

Treatment

- support and reassurance
- cognitive therapy
- parentcraft support
- settles with time

Postnatal depression

Some women develop a very severe depression after childbirth. Always consider it in the frequent attender.

- occurs in 10–30% women
- in first 6–12 months (usually first 6)
- anxiety and agitation common
- marked mood swings
- poor memory and concentration
- typical depressive features

Treatment

- support, reassurance, counselling
- group psychotherapy
- couple therapy
- postnatal depression support group
- hospitalisation may be necessary, esp. if suicidal or infanticidal ideations
- medication, e.g. amitriptyline (esp. where anxiety is a major feature), dothiepin, sertraline

Note: Beware of puerperal psychosis with onset usually within first 2 weeks.

Sleep deprivation

Give advice and counselling. Use the 'sleep when baby sleeps' rule. Avoid sedatives.

Postpartum hypothyroidism

Postpartum hypothyroidism (postpartum thyroiditis) may be misdiagnosed as postpartum depression and should always be considered in the tired, apparently depressed woman in the first 6 months after delivery.

Sexual difficulties

Decreased libido is a common problem and often related to sleep deprivation. Only 50% of couples achieve intercourse by the 6 weeks check.[2] Decreased libido can also be due to one of the postnatal depressive disorders or to tension in adjusting to the new relationships.

Dyspareunia is common and should be treated symptomatically and with education. Simple lubrication or vaginal oestrogens can help until perineal healing is achieved.

Early intercourse is risky with deaths from air embolism reported in the first 2 weeks. Intercourse is not recommended in the first 6 weeks.

Elimination disorders[2]

Always enquire how the patient is coping with her bowels and urination. Simple advice such as stool softening and pelvic floor exercises will help. However, serious problems such as faecal incontinence secondary to a fistula from a third-degree tear, or urinary retention due to neuropraxia of the pelvic floor can develop and need urgent attention.

References

1. Smibert J. Practical postnatal care. Aust Fam Physician, 1989; 18:508–511.
2. McKenna M. Postnatal problems. In: MIMS Disease Index (2nd edn). Sydney: IMS Publishing, 1996, 423–425.
3. Murtagh J. *Patient education* (2nd edn). Sydney: McGraw-Hill, 1996, 6–10.
4. Mashford ML (Chairman). *Antibiotic guidelines* (9th edn). Melbourne: VMPF, 1996, 140.
5. Smibert J. Common puerperal complications. Aust Fam Physician, 18:824–827.

PART 6

MEN'S HEALTH

——

92
Scrotal pain

—

Acute scrotal pain in infancy and adolescence should be regarded as torsion of the testis until proved otherwise.

Scrotal pain in males can occur at all age groups but the child or adolescent with acute scrotal pain often poses a diagnostic challenge. Serious problems include testicular torsion, strangulation of an inguinoscrotal hernia, a testicular tumour and a haematocele, all of which require surgical intervention.

Key facts and checkpoints

- Torsion of the testis is the most common cause of acute scrotal pain in infancy and childhood.
- Torsion is also a feature of young men less than 25 years.
- Testicular pain can be referred to the abdomen.
- Torsion of the testis should form part of the differential diagnosis in a boy or young man who is vomiting and has intense pain in the inguinal region.
- The clinical picture of epididymo-orchitis can mimic torsion of the testis so closely that, in most children, the diagnosis should be made only at surgical exploration.[1]
- An abnormality predisposing to torsion of the testis is usually present bilaterally; the opposite testis should also be fixed to prevent torsion.
- Torsion must be corrected within four hours to prevent gangrene of the testis.

The clinical approach
History
It is important to determine whether there were any pre-existing predisposing factors or history of trauma.

Key questions
- Have you noticed any burning of urine or penile discharge?
- Have you had an injury to your scrotal region such as being struck by a baseball or falling astride something?
- Have you travelled overseas recently?
- Have you been aware of a lump in your testicle or groin?
- Have you had an illness lately and have you noticed swelling of the glands in your neck or near your ear?
- Do you have back pain or have you injured your back?

Examination
Both sides of the scrotum must be examined and contrasted. Inguinal and femoral hernial orifices, the spermatic cord, testis and epididymis must be checked on both sides. The patient should be examined standing and supine. The scrotum and its contents are examined systematically starting with the skin, which may include sebaceous cysts or rarely may exhibit thickening, sinuses or ulcers with inflammatory disorders such as filariasis and tuberculosis. A painful testis should be elevated gently to determine if the pain improves.

Investigations
Investigations that may help diagnose the painful testis in particular include:

- blood cell count
- urine analysis: micro and culture
- chlamydia antigen detection tests
- ultrasound
- technetium scan

Acute scrotal pain in children and adolescents

This problem is more likely to be encountered in the adolescent. A list of causes is presented in Table 92.1. Infants, however, can also have torsion of a testis or a testicular appendage, such as the hydatid of Morgagni.

Clinical problem

A 15 year old teenager presents with the relatively acute onset of pain in his lower right abdomen and scrotum. He has vomited several times. On examination the right testicle is tender, red and swollen.

Discussion

The two main differential diagnoses are acute epididymo-orchitis (which requires little more than conservative treatment) or torsion of the testis, which demands emergency surgical intervention (Fig. 92.1). Less commonly the problem would be a haematoma or an acute hydrocele mimicking testicular torsion. This patient, however, must be regarded as having torsion of the testis. Early operation with torsion is imperative because, if the testis is deprived of its blood supply for more than a few hours, infarction is inevitable and excision becomes necessary. Excluding mumps, no youth under the age of 18 years should be diagnosed as suffering from acute epididymo-orchitis until the testis has been exposed at operation and torsion excluded.

Table 92.1 *Causes of scrotal pain or swelling*

Torsion of the testis

Torsion of a testicular appendage

Epididymo-orchitis

Mumps orchitis

Acute hydrocele

Idiopathic scrotal oedema

Haematoma/haematocele

Neoplasm

Henoch-Schönlein purpura

Strangulated inguinoscrotal hernia

Referred pain

Scrotal skin conditions

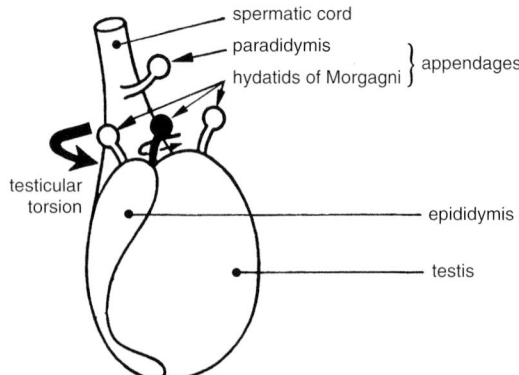

Fig. 92.1 *Torsion of the testis and an appendage: the 'black' hydatid of Morgagni is the one most likely to undergo torsion*

Torsion of the testis *v* epididymo-orchitis

With torsion of the testicle there is pain of sudden onset, described as a severe, aching, sickening pain in the groin that may be accompanied by nausea and vomiting. With epididymo-orchitis the attack usually begins with malaise and fever. The testicle soon becomes swollen and acutely tender; however, elevation of the scrotum usually relieves pain in this condition while tending to increase it with a torsion.

A comparison of the clinical presentations is given in Table 92.2.

Radiology as a diagnostic aid

Ultrasound is useful in distinguishing a cystic scrotal lump (such as a hydrocele) from a solid tumour. Its use to distinguish between a torsion and epididymo-orchitis is controversial as it cannot reliably detect changes that are diagnostic of early torsion. Since the investigation can involve unnecessary delay in treatment it is generally not recommended. A technetium scan can differentiate between the two conditions: in torsion the testis is avascular while it is hyperemic in epididymo-orchitis.

Time factor in surgical intervention

The optimal time to operate for torsion of the testis is within four (4) hours of onset of pain. About 85% of torsive testes are salvageable within six (6) hours but by ten (10) hours the salvage rate has dropped to 20%.[2]

At surgery the testicle is untwisted and if viable an orchidopexy is performed. A gangrenous testicle is removed. The opposite testis should be fixed by orchidopexy.

Table 92.2 *Clinical presentations of torsion of testis and acute epididymo-orchitis*

	Torsion of testis	Epididymo-orchitis
Typical age	Early teens, average range 5–15	Young adults Elderly
Onset	Usually sudden but can be gradual	Gradual
Severity of pain	Very severe	Moderate
Associated symptoms	Vomiting Groin pain Possibly abdominal pain	Fever
Examination of scrotum	Very tender and red Testis high and transverse Scrotal oedema	Swollen, tender and red; can be tender on rectal examination
	Possible an acute hydrocele	Possibly an acute hydrocele
Effect of gentle scrotal elevation	No change to pain or worse pain	Relief of pain
Investigations	Technetium scan (if available, time permits and diagnosis doubtful)	Leucocytosis Possibly pyobacteria of urine

Torsion of a testicular appendage

Vestigial remnants to the testis or the epididymis are present in 90% of the male population.[1] Torsion of the testicular appendage, the pedunculated hydatid of Morgagni, has a similar presentation to that of torsion of the testis but is less severe (see Fig. 92.1).

It can be diagnosed by the appearance of a dark blue nodule at the upper pole of the testis (provided that it is not masked by an associated hydrocele). Surgical exploration is advisable.

Scrotal pain at various ages
Acute epididymo-orchitis

Apart from mumps, acute epididymo-orchitis is usually caused by sexually transmitted pathogens in males 30–35 years and by urinary tract pathogens in patients over 35 years old. In older men it usually follows urinary tract obstruction and infection or instrumentation of the lower genitourinary tract.

Investigations

Blood cell count:	leukocytosis
Urine micro and culture:	pyuria, bacteria and possibly *E. coli.* A sterile culture suggests chlamydia infection[3]
Tests for chlamydia:	antigen detection kits
Ultrasound:	can differentiate a swollen epididymis from testicular tumour

Treatment
- bed rest
- elevation and support of the scrotum
- analgesics
- antibiotics (all doses 10–14 days)
  Sexually acquired
    amoxycillin/clavulanate 500/125 mg (o) 8 hourly for 10–14 days
                        plus
    doxycycline 100 mg (o) 12 hourly for 10–14 days
  Associated with urinary infection
    amoxycillin/clavulanate 500/125 mg (o) 8 hourly for 10–14 days
                        or
    trimethoprim 300 mg (o) daily for 10–14 days
                        or
    cephalexin 500 mg (o) 6 hourly for 10–14 days
                or (if resistance to above)
    norfloxacin 400 mg (o) 12 hourly for 10–14 days

Orchitis

Acute orchitis is invariably due to mumps and occurs during late adolescence. It is usually unilateral but may be bilateral.

Chronic orchitis may be due to syphilis, tuberculosis, leprosy or various helminthic infections such as filariasis. The majority are tuberculous in origin.

Testicular neoplasm

Testicular tumours can occur at all ages but are more common in young men aged 20–30 (teratoma) and 30–40 years (seminoma). Sometimes they can mimic an acute inflammatory swelling and present with acute pain.

Strangulated inguinoscrotal hernia

It is possible that a supposed testicular torsion is found to be a strangulated inguinoscrotal hernia, usually an indirect inguinal hernia extending into the scrotum. It can be detected by careful palpation of the base (neck) of the scrotum.

Trauma and haematoceles

A diffuse haematoma into the scrotum which causes no significant problems can follow surgery to the inguinal area, a blow to this area or a fracture of the pelvis. These conditions cause extravasation of blood distally. However, a haematocele of the tunica vaginalis can be either acute or an 'old clotted haematocele' following injury, such as a blow to the testis, or the drainage of a hydrocele.[5] Sometimes it can arise spontaneously. All types of haematoceles require surgical exploration to exclude testicular rupture or a tumour.

Trauma to the scrotum may produce urethral injury and extravasation of urine into the scrotum. This problem requires urgent surgery.

Problems of scrotal skin

Sebaceous cysts are common and may be infected and require drainage.

Fournier's gangrene (idiopathic gangrene of the scrotum) is an acute fulminating cellulitis affecting the scrotal skin. It usually develops suddenly and without any apparent cause. Gangrene of the scrotal skin appears early if the infection is not quickly checked with broad spectrum antibiotics. The end result is sloughing of the scrotal coverings, leaving the testes exposed.[5]

Referred pain

Pain can be referred to the scrotal region from ureteric colic and quite commonly from disorders of the thoracolumbar spine, notably a disc disruption at the T12–L1 level involving the L1 nerve root. The pain therefore may be referred or radicular.

When to refer

- Any suspicion of torsion of the testis.
- Sudden onset of acute scrotal pain at any age.
- A history of recurrent transient testicular pain in a young man.
- Presence of a tender testicular lump.
- Presence of a haematocele surrounding the testis.

Note: Referral should be most urgent, using the critical 4-hour guideline.

Practice tips

- Acute scrotal pain in infancy and adolescence should be regarded as torsion of the testis until proved otherwise.
- A history of recurrent transient pain (with or without swelling of the testis) in a young person means recurrent torsion. Urgent referral is essential.
- Although torsion usually occurs in the fully descended testis it can occur in an undescended testis.
- A pitfall is the phenomenon of 'testis redux' in which the descended testis undergoes torsion, is pulled into the superficial inguinal pouch by the cremasteric reflex and then becomes fixed by oedema.
- The development of acute hydrocele should be regarded with suspicion.
- Beware of the strangulated inguinoscrotal hernia presenting as a testicular torsion.
- Consider dissecting aneurysm in an older person presenting with testicular pain.

References

1. Jones PG. *Clinical paediatric surgery.* Sydney: Ure Smith, 1970, 231–236.
2. Gledhill T. Testicular torsion. Update, 1984; 2:136–140.
3. Berger RE. Urethritis and epididymitis. Semin Urol, 1983; 1:139.
4. Mashford L et al. *Antibiotic guidelines* (8th edn). Melbourne: Victorian Medical Postgraduate Foundation, 1996, 79–80.
5. Fry J, Berry H. *Surgical problems in clinical practice.* London: Edward Arnold, 1987, 87–88.

93

Inguinoscrotal lumps

—

He has a rupture, he has sprung a leake.

Ben Jonson (1573–1637)
The Staple of News

Lumps in the groin are common to both sexes but males are likely to have a greater variety of swellings in this area and several may be associated with scrotal lumps.

Lumps in the groin

The commonest swellings encountered in the groin or inguinal area are hernias (also known as 'ruptures') and enlarged lymph nodes. The diagnosis of a hernia is usually straightforward but it must be differentiated from other swellings, including Malgaigne's bulgings; these are not true hernias but diffuse swellings in both inguinal regions seen in people with poor lower abdominal musculature.[1] Table 93.1 lists the differential diagnoses of groin lumps.

Table 93.1 *Differential diagnoses of a groin mass*

Hernia—femoral, inguinal

Malgaigne's bulgings

Lipoma

Undescended testis

Spermatic cord swelling—encysted hydrocele, lipoma

Lymph node—localised, generalised

Haematoma (postfemoral artery puncture)

Neoplasm—lipoma, others

Psoas abscess

Vascular anomalies
• saphenous varix
• femoral aneurysm

Hernias

The commonest types of hernias in the groin are inguinal, femoral and a combination of the two. Rare hernias in the region are obturator, Spigelian (low abdominal), preperitoneal inguinal and prevascular femoral. The basic parts of a hernia are shown in Figure 93.1 and important anatomical landmarks in Figure 93.2. An indirect inguinal hernia is a hernia through the deep inguinal ring, originating lateral to the inferior epigastric vessels, following the path of the processus vaginalis, and can traverse the whole length of the inguinal canal (Fig. 93.3). In the male it closely approximates the spermatic cord and may enlarge as it passes through the superficial inguinal ring into the scrotum—an inguinoscrotal hernia.

Because of their narrow neck and oblique path in the inguinal canal such hernias are often irreducible and are prone to lead to strangulation of entrapped bowel.

A direct inguinal hernia originates medial to the inferior epigastric vessels and protrudes through the posterior wall of the inguinal canal,

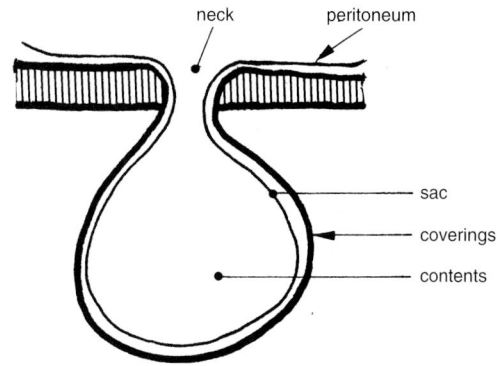

Fig. 93.1 *Basic components of a hernia*

Fig. 93.2 *Key landmarks in the left inguinal region: the deep inguinal ring lies above the mid-inguinal point (between the ASIS and the pubic tubercle); the femoral artery lies below this point*

Fig. 93.3 *Left indirect inguinal hernia: it emerges lateral to the inferior epigastric artery and passes into the scrotum medial to the pubic tubercle*

and is therefore separate from the spermatic cord (Fig. 93.4). It is almost always seen in men and rarely descends into the scrotum.[2] Due to a wider neck, strangulation and obstruction are most unusual. It must be emphasised that the distinction between a direct and an indirect inguinal hernia can be very difficult and the two may occur together.

A femoral hernia herniates through the femoral ring (also known as the femoral canal), which is the medial component of the femoral sheath. The hernia tends to bulge forwards and then upwards as it becomes larger. The neck is lateral to the pubic tubercle (Fig. 93.5).

Femoral hernias are often small, usually occur in females and may be unnoticed by the patient. They are particularly liable to produce bowel obstruction or strangulation.[2]

Guidelines with hernias

Acquired hernia
- always examine the scrotum
- frequently bilateral
- result from muscular weakness
- commonest—direct inguinal and femoral
- predisposing factors
  - age (more common with increasing age)
  - obesity
  - pregnancy
- precipitating factors (related to above factors)
  - increased intra-abdominal pressure
    - difficulty of micturition
    - straining at stool (constipation)
    - chronic cough, e.g. bronchitis
    - straining or lifting heavy objects
  - nerve damage, e.g. post appendicectomy
- complications
  - intestinal obstruction (Table 93.2)
  - incarceration
  - strangulation
  - sliding

Clinical features
The main symptoms and signs:[1]
- lump
- discomfort or pain
  - a dragging pain

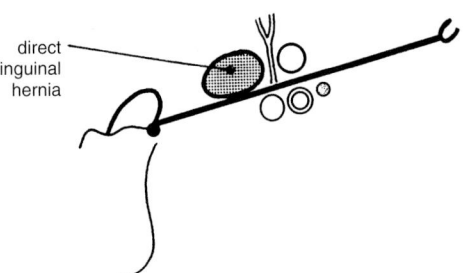

Fig. 93.4 *Left direct inguinal hernia: it emerges medial to the inferior epigastric artery and bulges forward*

Fig. 93.5 *Left femoral hernia: its neck is lateral to the pubic tubercle and it lies below the inguinal ligament*

Table 93.2 *Symptoms and signs of hernial obstruction*

Colicky abdominal pain

Nausea and vomiting

Constipation and failure to pass flatus

Abdominal distension

High-pitched tinkling bowel sounds

Local tenderness and swelling of the hernia

No expansile cough impulse

— worse after standing or walking
— referred to testicle (indirect inguinal)
• testicular pain—referred or with compression of the spermatic cord
• expansile impulse on coughing

Note: A femoral hernia is easily missed in obese patients.
Larger femoral hernia are often irreducible.
Always attempt reduction in the recumbent position (direct hernias usually reduce easily).
In over 50% of strangulated obturator hernias, pain is referred along the geniculate branch of the obturator nerve to the knee.[1]

Treatment of hernias

Surgery[3]

All symptomatic hernias require repair and all femoral hernias should be repaired. Obstructed and strangulated hernias require urgent surgery. The risk of strangulation is greatest with femoral hernias, moderate with indirect inguinal hernias and least with direct inguinal hernias.

Conservative

Asymptomatic inguinal hernias in patients with associated medical conditions, and who pose a significant operative risk, can be treated conservatively. A suitable truss to control a small inguinal hernia is a rat-tailed spring truss with a perineal band to prevent slipping.[1] Such a truss must be used with care and patients well instructed in its proper use. Trusses must always be applied over the inguinal canal with the patient lying flat and with the hernia reduced. Difficult reduction can be aided by a warm moist towelette.

Scrotal lumps

The scrotum contains the testes and distal parts of the spermatic cords, covered by layers of fascia and the dartos muscle. The testes are invested with tunica vaginalis derived from the peritoneal cavity during their descent.[1]

Disorders of the scrotum may be acute or chronic and bilateral or unilateral. Lumps may be cystic, solid or otherwise such as a varicocele, oedema and hernia. Solid lumps include a testicular tumour, epididymo-orchitis, and torsion of the testes. Cystic lumps include hydroceles, epididymal cysts and spermatoceles, and resolving extravasation. A comparison of scrotal lumps appears in Figure 93.6 and Table 93.3. Lumps in the scrotum usually develop from deeper structures, particularly the testes and their coverings, rather than scrotal skin.[1] Refer to Figure 93.6 for a comparison of scrotal lumps.

The cardinal sign of a true scrotal mass is that it is possible to get above it.

The patient usually presents with pain or a lump.

Examination of the scrotum

The scrotum should be examined with the patient supine and then standing. The left testis usually hangs lower than the right. On inspection note any sebaceous cysts in the scrotal skin (common), scabies if there are very pruritic nodules, and scrotal oedema which causes taut pitting skin. Careful palpation will elicit the relevant structures in the scrotum. Gently palpate each testis and epididymis between the thumb and the first two fingers. The spermatic cord is palpable as it enters the scrotum after passing through the superficial ring and the testis and epididymis are readily palpable.

After palpation test for translucency of any swelling in a darkened room by shining the beam of a strong torch from behind the scrotum through the swelling. Transilluminable swellings that light up with a red glow include hydroceles and cysts of the epididymis. Swellings that contain blood or other tissue, such as testicular tumours and most hernias, do not illuminate.

Unilateral scrotal swelling

It is important to determine whether the lump is inguinoscrotal or scrotal. It is scrotal if it is possible to get above the lump. If it is not possible to get above the lump then it is a large inguinal hernia or a combined hernia and hydrocele

Table 93.3 *Features of scrotal lumps*

	Possible clinical setting	Position	Palpation	Trans-illumination
Hydrocele	Any age Primary or secondary • tumour • infection • torsion	Confined to scrotum Anterior: surrounds testis except posteriorly	Smooth, pear-shaped Lax or tense Testis impalpable, non-tender	Yes
Cyst of epididymis *Epididymal cysts and spermatoceles clinically similar	Asymptomatic or dragging sensation	Behind and above testis	Smooth and tense Multilocular swelling Testis easily palpable Appears separate from testis	Yes
Chronic epididymo-orchitis	Non-specific Tuberculosis Chlamydia (Occasional associated small hydrocele)	Behind and above testis	Firm swelling Hard and craggy Normal testis	No
Varicocele	Dragging discomfort	Usually left-sided Along line of spermatic cord Above testis	Soft, like bunch of worms or grapes Collapses when patient supine and testis elevated Testis often smaller	No
Carcinoma	Young men 20–40 Painless lump Loss of testicular sensation	In body of testis Usually felt anteriorly May be hydrocele	Enlarged firm testis Feels heavy if large Normal epididymis (palpable)	No

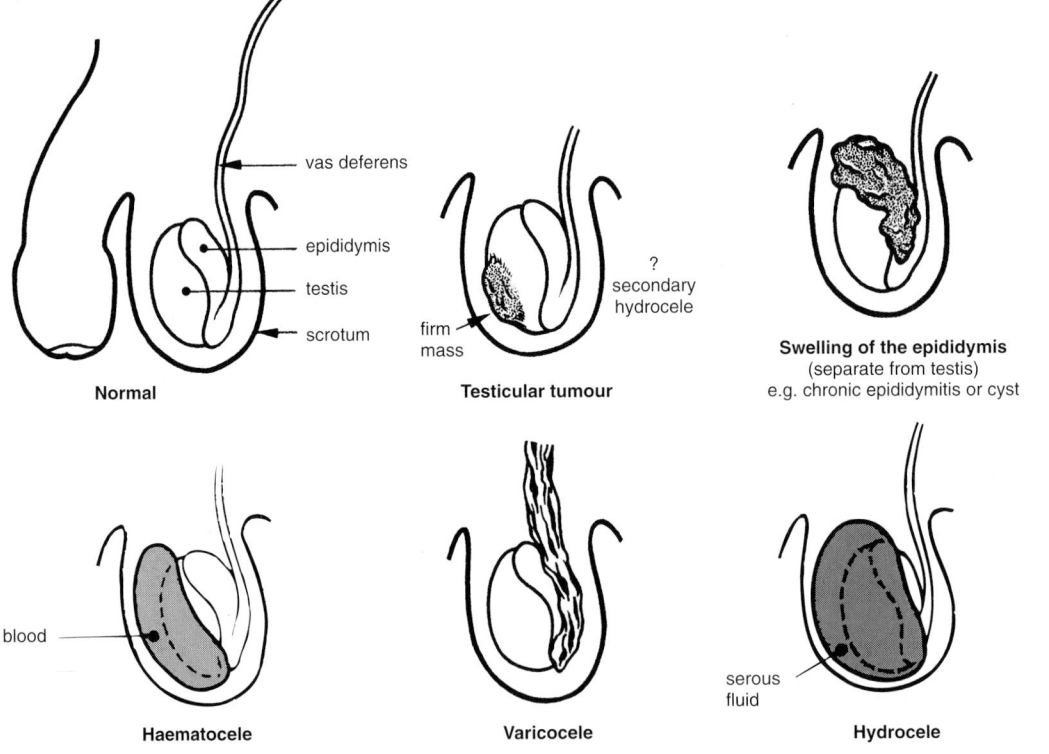

Fig. 93.6 *Basic comparison of scrotal lumps*

not possible
to palpate
above the
swelling

possible
to get
above the
swelling

Inguinoscrotal swelling
True scrotal swelling

Fig. 93.7 *Difference between a true scrotal swelling and an inguinoscrotal swelling*

(Fig. 93.7). The next feature to determine is whether the testis and/or epididymis can be palpated or whether they are obscured by a swelling such as a hydrocele.

Small testes

Testes are considered small in adults if less than 3.5 cm long. Small firm testes, 2 cm long or less, are a feature of Klinefelter's syndrome. Small soft testes indicate atrophy which may follow mumps orchitis, oestrogen therapy, hypopituitarism, cirrhosis and other related conditions.

Hydrocele

A hydrocele is a collection of clear amber fluid in the tunica vaginalis and can be primary or secondary. If a hydrocele develops it is important to rule out intrascrotal disease such as a tumour or infection. Ultrasound examination of the scrotum is helpful in assessing the state of the testis in the presence of a hydrocele. Hydroceles may be symptomless or cause dragging discomfort in the scrotum and groin.

Treatment of a primary hydrocele

Surgery is the most effective long-term treatment. A primary hydrocele can be treated by simple aspiration but the fluid usually reaccumulates and there is risk of bleeding or infection with repeated procedures.[4] However, aspiration followed by injection of a sclerosant agent (e.g. dilute aqueous phenol or STD) can prevent fluid accumulation and after two or three times can often cure the problem. This sclerotherapy may be complicated by pain and inflammatory reaction to the sclerosant.

Method
1. Inject LA into the scrotal skin down to the sac.
2. Insert an 18 or 19 gauge intravenous cannula through this site into the sac and remove the stilette, leaving the soft cannula in the sac (Fig. 93.8).
3. Remove the serous fluid initially by free drainage, possibly aided by manual compression on the sac and then by aspiration with a 20 mL syringe.
4. Record the volume.
5. Inject 2.5% sterile aqueous phenol or STD into the empty sac (10 mL for 200 mL of fluid removed, 15 mL for 200–400 mL and 20 mL for over 400 mL).

If the hydrocele re-forms (10% of cases) the procedure can be repeated after 6 weeks.

cannula

testis

hydrocele

Fig. 93.8 *Aspiration of hydrocele*

Encysted hydrocele of the cord

This is a localised fluid-filled segment of the processus vaginalis within the spermatic cord. It is palpable as a cystic lump in the upper scrotum.

It characteristically moves down with traction on the testis.

Epididymal cysts

The majority of epididymal cysts contain a clear colourless fluid. If the cysts communicate with the vasa efferentia a spermatocele filled with whitish fluid containing spermatazoa may form.

Epididymal cysts may be asymptomatic or they may cause discomfort and cosmetic embarrassment and should be excised. Fertility may be impaired in patients undergoing bilateral cyst excision.

Aspiration and injection of sclerosant agents can also be used for epididymal cysts.[4]

Varicoceles

A varicocele is a varicosity of the veins of the pampiniform plexus. It is seen in 8% of normal males and occurs on the left side in 98% of affected patients, due to a mechanical problem in drainage of the left renal vein. A relationship with infertility has been observed but its nature is controversial.

Most varicoceles are asymptomatic and incidental findings. They can cause a dragging discomfort in the scrotum. Treatment is indicated if it is symptomatic or for infertility. Firm-fitting underpants may relieve discomfort.[1] Surgical treatment is by venous ligation, above the deep inguinal ring. Ligation is indicated if there is any reduction in the size of the left testis.

Haematoceles

These can be either acute, resulting from trauma such as a fall astride, sports injury or tapping of a hydrocele, or chronic, where there is no obvious history of injury. Haematoceles are anterior to the testis and not transilluminable. Surgical drainage is required with acute injury where there is a possibility of testicular rupture (associated urethral injury has to be considered); and a tumour has to be excluded with the chronic type. Pressure atrophy of the testis can occur with injury and is much more common if early drainage is not instigated.

Testicular tumours

A mass that is part of the testis, and solid, is likely to be a tumour. Malignant testicular tumours account for about 2% of malignant tumours in men. They mainly affect fit young men and represent the commonest neoplasm in men aged 20–34 (Table 93.4).

Clinical features
- young men 20–40 years
- painless lump in body of testis (commonest feature)
- loss of testicular sensation
- associated presentations (may mask tumour)
  — hydrocele
  — varicocele
  — epididymo-orchitis
  — swollen testis with trivial injury
  — gynaecomastia (teratoma)

Golden rules
- All solid scrotal lumps are malignant until proved otherwise and must be surgically explored.
- Beware of hydroceles in young adults.
- Tumours can mimic acute epididymo-orchitis—the so-called 'inflammatory' or 'flash fire' presentation.[3]

Metastases
Testicular tumours spread by direct infiltration via the lymphatics and the bloodstream. Metastases typically occur in the para-aortic nodes so it is advisable to palpate carefully from the umbilical area upwards. Metastases also occur in the neck, liver and chest.

Investigations
Investigations to aid diagnosis include:[3]
- ultrasound of the testis: can detect and diagnose with considerable precision underlying

Table 93.4 *Testicular tumours*[1,4,5]

Tumour	Incidence (%)	Peak incidence (years)
Seminoma	40	25–40
Teratoma	32	20–35
Mixed seminoma/ teratoma	14	20–40
Lymphoma	7	60+
Other tumours e.g. interstitial (Leydig) gonadoblastoma	uncommon	variable

testicular lumps plus any invasion of the tunica
- tumour markers: alpha fetoprotein and human chorionic gonadotrophin

Investigations for staging include:

- chest X-ray
- CT scanning of abdomen, pelvis and chest for node involvement

Treatment

The initial treatment is orchidectomy with inguinal division of the spermatic cord. Specialised treatment that depends on the staging of the tumour gives good results for seminoma, which is very sensitive to radiotherapy. The results for teratoma are not as satisfactory as for seminoma.

Prognosis is good for most testicular tumours with 5 year cure rates of 85–90%.[3]

Early detection and testicular self-examination

Studies of testicular cancer have shown the benefits of early detection.[6] Common errors that caused a delay of diagnosis included incorrect diagnosis, neglecting to examine the testes, and failure to achieve a specific diagnosis to explain the symptoms. Delay on the part of the patient was the major determinant of total delay. It is important that we promote secondary preventive measures by encouraging testicular self-examination (TSE) as a simple procedure that all young men, especially those at risk, should learn to do.

Information for patients on TSE
- Examine the testicles yourself when warm and relaxed, e.g. after a warm bath or shower, when the scrotal skin is most relaxed, or in bed.
- Explore each testicle individually.
- Using both hands, gently roll the testicle between the thumb and the index and middle fingers (Fig. 93.9).

Fig. 93.9 *Testicular self-examination technique*

- If pain is experienced, too much pressure is being applied.
- The normal testicle is egg-shaped, firm to touch and should be smooth and free of lumps.
- Feel for any changes in size, shape or consistency.
- If you do find something abnormal, it is most likely it will be an area of firmness, or a small lump on the front or side of the testicle.
- If you find something you think is abnormal, you should see your doctor as soon as possible.
- Remember that not all lumps are due to cancer.

Undescended testes

A testis that is not in the scrotum may be ectopic, absent, retractile or truly undescended. The incidence is 2% in full-term males, 20% in premature male births and 1% at one year. More than two-thirds of undescended testes are located in the superficial inguinal pouch, that is, they are palpable in the groin.

Undescended testis

An undescended testis is one that cannot reach the bottom of the scrotum despite manual manipulation. After the indirect inguinal hernia it is the most common problem in paediatric surgery. The testis is usually normal but may become secondarily dysplastic if left outside the scrotum.

A truly undescended testis is one that has stopped in the normal path of descent and can occupy intra-abdominal, inguinal canal, emergent (just outside the external ring), high scrotal and mid-scrotal positions (Fig. 93.10a).[4] The cause of maldescent is probably mechanical.

Retractile testis

A retractile testis is one that can be manipulated into the scrotum irrespective of the position in which it is first located. It is a common condition. The testis can be present in the scrotum under circumstances such as a warm bath but retracted out of the scrotum when cold. Cremasteric contraction is absent in the first few months after birth and is maximal between 2 and 8 years.[1]

Ectopic testis

An ectopic testis is one that has left the normal path of descent and cannot be manipulated into the scrotum. It can be found in the perineum, upper thigh (femoral), base of the penis (prepubic), anterior abdominal wall or in the superficial inguinal pouch (Fig. 93.10a). True ectopic testes form only about 5% of all undescended testes (Fig. 93.10b).

Ascending testis

An 'ascending' testis is one that was in the scrotum in infancy but subsequently moved back to the groin because the spermatic cord failed to elongate at the same rate of body growth.

Examination[7]

The examination of the testes should take place in a warm room and relaxed environment. Begin by placing one finger on each side of the neck of the scrotum to prevent the testes from being retracted out of the scrotum by the other hand. The scrotum is then carefully palpated for a testis. If impalpable the fingertips of one hand are placed just medial to the anterior superior iliac spine and moved firmly towards the pubic tubercle where the other hand waits to entrap

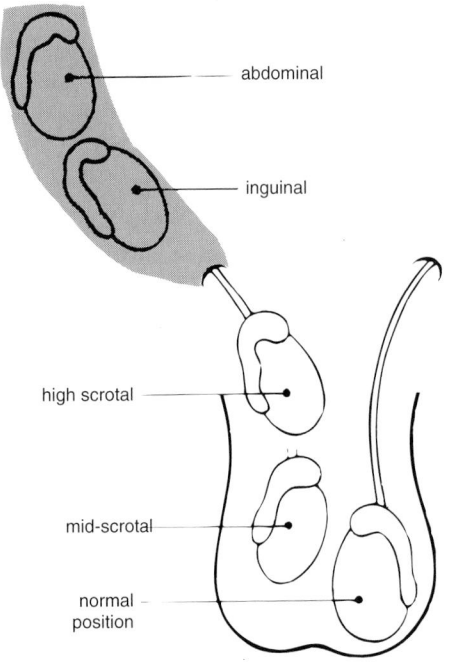

Fig. 93.10a *Undescended testis: arrested in the line of descent*

Fig. 93.10b *Undescended testis: ectopic*

the testis should it appear. The diagnosis then depends on carefully determining the range of movement.

The problem of non-descent

• testicular dysplasia
• susceptible to direct violence (if in inguinal region)
• risk of malignant change (seminoma) is 5–10 times greater than normal

Optimal time for surgery

The optimal time for orchidopexy is 12–18 months of age.[7] The production of spermatozoa is adversely affected in undescended testes from the age of 2 years onwards.[7] Exploration for the uncommon impalpable testis is worthwhile: 50% salvage rate, while in the other 50% either there is no testis or an abnormal and potentially neoplastic testis is removed.[7]

The advantages of early orchidopexy are summarised in Table 93.5.

Table 93.5 *Advantages of early orchidopexy (1 year)[4]*

Provides optimal chance of fertility
Corrects indirect inguinal hernias (coexists in 90%)
Reduces risk of trauma
Reduces risk of torsion
Reduces psychological consequences
Probably lessens the risk of malignancy (seminoma)

Hormone injections

Injections of chorionic gonadotrophic hormones are generally not recommended. They are ineffective except for borderline retractile testes.

Practice tip

Optimal times to operate in children
• Inguinal herniae—as soon as possible
• Umbilical herniae—wait until 4 years (most resolve by 2 years)
• Undescended testes—12–18 months

References

1. Fry J, Berry H. *Surgical problems in clinical practice*. London: Edward Arnold, 1987, 79–92.

2. Davis A, Bolin T, Ham J. *Symptom analysis and physical diagnosis* (2nd edn). Sydney: Pergamon Press, 1990, 212–220.

3. Hunt P, Marshall V. *Clinical problems in general surgery*. Sydney: Butterworths, 1991, 329–342.

4. Bullock N, Sibley G, Whitaker R. *Essential urology*. Edinburgh: Churchill Livingstone, 1989, 287–318.

5. Messing EM, Testicular seminoma. In: *Current therapy in genitourinary surgery* (2nd edn). New York: Resnick and Kursh, 1992, 168.

6. Bolse J, Vogelzang NJ, Goldman A et al. Impact of delay in diagnosis on clinical stage of testicular cancer. Lancet, 1981; 2:970–972.

7. Hutson J, Beasley S, Woodward A. *Jones clinical paediatric surgery*. Oxford: Blackwell Scientific Publications, 1992, 162–164.

94
Disorders of the penis

Ironically there is no organ about which more misinformation has been perpetuated than the penis.

William Masters & Virginia Johnson
Human Sexual Response

The most common penile disorders are those of psychosexual dysfunction and sexually transmissible diseases, but there are many other problems and these are most often related to the foreskin.

Disorders affecting the foreskin and glans
Phimosis
Phimosis is tightness of foreskin (prepuce), preventing its free retraction over the glans penis. The foreskin can be adherent to the glans penis even up to 5–6 years of age. It gradually separates until it becomes non-adherent usually by the age of six. Forcible retraction of the foreskin of any boy should be discouraged.

True congenital narrowing of the preputial orifice is rare. If the foreskin cannot be retracted by the age of 7 years and is causing symptoms such as balanitis then circumcision is recommended. Ballooning of the foreskin during micturition can be a feature.

Treatment
Inflammatory phimosis can be treated by local corticosteroid cream. True scarring requires circumcision.[1] Some patients with true phimosis may have problems once they start to have intercourse. They require circumcision.

Paraphimosis
In paraphimosis the foreskin is retracted, swollen and painful. This is because it has been pulled back over the glans and cannot be pulled forwards again. This problem occurs in older boys and the elderly, especially if a mild degree of phimosis is already present. Typically it occurs when the penis is erect or after catheterisation.

Management
Urgent manual reduction should be attempted first. It is usually performed without anaesthesia but a penile block (never use adrenaline in LA) may be appropriate.

Method 1
The glans penis and oedematous tissue distal to the constricting ring of foreskin are gently squeezed for several minutes to reduce the oedema. Manual reduction can then be performed by trying to advance the prepuce over the glans with the index fingers while gently compressing the glans with both thumbs (Fig. 94.1).

Fig. 94.1 *Acute paraphimosis: method of manual reduction*

Method 2

- Take hold of the oedematous part of the glans in the fist of one hand and squeeze firmly. A gauze swab or cool towelette will help to achieve a firm grip (Fig. 94.2).
- Exert continuous pressure until the oedema passes under the constricting collar to the shaft of the penis.
- The foreskin can then usually be pulled over the glans.

Fig. 94.2 *Acute paraphimosis: squeezing with a swab method*

Method 3

If manual reduction methods fail, a dorsal slit incision should be made in the constricting collar of skin under local or general anaesthetic (Fig. 94.3). The incision allows the foreskin to be advanced and reduces the swelling. Circumcision should be performed some days later when the inflammation has settled.[2]

Fig. 94.3 *Acute paraphimosis: dorsal slit incision in the constricting collar of skin*

Balanitis (balanoposthitis)

Balanitis is inflammation of the foreskin which usually affects the glans penis and tissues behind the foreskin (balanoposthitis). The inflammation may simply be redness or irritation of the glans and foreskin or bacterial infection. This quite common problem may be due to *Candida albicans* infection, but in infants may be caused by wet nappies and in the elderly by diabetes alone or with an associated organism.

Men presenting with balanitis should be screened for:

- diabetes
- Reiter's disease (especially if asymptomatic)

Treatment

- take swabs for culture
- careful washing behind foreskin

If yeasts present
— topical nystatin or miconazole or clotrimazole cream

If trichomonads present
— metronidazole or tinidazole (oral treatment)

If bacteria present
— appropriate antibiotic, e.g. chloramphenicol or chlortetracycline

Thickening of the foreskin with skin pallor suggests balanitis xerotica obliterans which responds to corticosteroid cream if it is mild. Circumcision is indicated for recurrent problems.

Foreskin hygiene

The normal foreskin in infants and children does not need special care and should not be retracted for cleaning from birth to 5 years of age. However, from the age of 6 or 7, males should practise proper hygiene by gently retracting the foreskin and washing the area as often as washing behind the ears.

Instructions to patients

- During a shower or bath slide the foreskin back towards your body (Fig. 94.4).
- Wash the end of the penis and foreskin with soap and water.
- After washing the area, dry the end of your penis and foreskin and then replace the foreskin.
- If the foreskin has a tendency to become irritated and smelly, slide the foreskin back sufficiently to allow free urination.

(a)   (b)   (c)

Fig. 94.4 *Foreskin hygiene: sliding foreskin back for washing*

Circumcision

Apart from abnormalities of the foreskin and religious reasons, circumcision for social reasons is generally discouraged. Arguments against circumcision are that it is not natural, it is unnecessary, it carries a small but significant risk of morbidity and mortality, and is associated with meatal stenosis. Circumcision is now performed less frequently and most practitioners do not appear to favour it for social reasons. Proponents, however, argue that it reduces the risk of periurethral bacterial colonisation, systemic infections such as septicaemia, carcinoma of the penis, and STDs. Indications for circumcision include phimosis, paraphimosis and recurrent balanitis. Boys with hypospadias should never be circumcised, since the foreskin may be a vital source of skin for subsequent repair.[2]

Using a dorsal slit of the foreskin as an alternative to routine circumcision produces a cosmetically unacceptable result and should only be used as an emergency measure.

Frenuloplasty

A congenitally tight frenulum may lead to a tear during intercourse. Repeated bleeding occurs. Division of the frenulum and suturing in the opposite direction is preferable to circumcision.

Disorders affecting the urethral meatus

Meatal stenosis

Meatal stenosis or stricture may be congenital or acquired. It may be acquired in the circumcised child, due to abrasion and ulceration of the tip of the glans. The incidence can be reduced by the application of Vaseline on the glans after circumcision.[1] Uncommon causes are direct trauma during circumcision and irritation from ammoniacal dermatitis. Meatal ulceration predisposes to meatal stenosis. It usually presents as pain during micturition or as slight bleeding on the napkin. In the child with mild meatal stenosis gentle dilation can be applied. Severe cases require surgical correction by meatotomy.

Catheter trauma is the usual cause in adults.

Hypospadias

Hypospadias is a condition where the urethra opens on the underside or ventral aspect of the penis. It occurs in 1 in 300 males.[1] Congenital hypospadias may be glandular (most common), coronal, penile or perineal.[3]

Hypospadias may cause the stream of urine to be deflected downwards or splash or drip back along the penile shaft. Unless it is glandular, surgical repair is usually advised, using the available foreskin. Chordee is corrected at the same time. These boys should not undergo routine circumcision.

Epispadias

Epispadias is where the urethra opens at the base of the penis, on its dorsal aspect. It occurs in 1 in 30 000 males.[1] Most patients are incontinent of urine because of a deficient bladder neck.

Penile warts

Penile warts are usually fleshy, papillomatous multiple outgrowths, commonly found around the coronal sulcus, the adjacent prepuce and the meatus. They are caused by human papilloma virus and usually transmitted sexually. Look for warts within the meatus by allowing dissecting forceps to spring open within the distal urethra. Treatment includes keeping the affected areas cool and dry and applying with extreme care 10–25% podophyllin solution or podophyllotoxin 0.5% paint to the warts (only) as directed. Alternative treatments include liquid nitrogen, 5-fluorouracil cream, diathermy or laser under general anaesthetic and repeated alpha interferon injections into the lesions. Ten per cent recur at 3 months.

Penile ulcers

A common cause related to sexual activity is trauma to the frenulum if it is congenitally tight. Such traumatic ulcers may be slow to heal and the frenulum may need surgical division. The ulcers may resemble a venereal ulcer, e.g. syphilitic chancre, herpes simplex or AIDS. Another important (although rare) cause is carcinoma of the penis. Various causes are listed in Table 94.1.

Carcinoma of the penis

Carcinoma of the penis is rare, occurring at a rate of 1 in 100 000 of the male population.[2] There is an association with the non-circumcised person, the theory being that smegma may be carcinogenic.

Carcinoma usually starts as a nodular warty growth (or ulcer) on the glans penis or in the coronal sulcus. Initially it may resemble a venereal wart. The presenting symptom may be a bloodstained or foul-smelling discharge as the lesion is usually hidden by the foreskin. It is

Table 94.1 *Causes of penile lesions*

Non-ulcerative
  Balanitis
  • *Candida albicans*
  • Reiter's syndrome
  • diabetes mellitus
  • poor hygiene

  Skin disease
  • psoriasis
  • lichen planus

  Venereal warts

Ulcerative
  Trauma (tender)
  Carcinoma (non-tender)
  Herpes simplex (tender)
  Syphilis (non-tender)
  Chancroid (tender)
  Behçet's syndrome

usually seen in elderly patients with poor hygiene.[3] Associated lymphadenopathy, which is present in 50% of patients on presentation, may be infective or neoplastic.

Priapism[4]

Priapism is a persistent painful erection not associated with appropriate sexual stimulation. The corpora cavernosa are engorged and painful, but the corpus spongiosum and glans remain flaccid.[2] The cause is usually poor venous drainage, but 10% reflect post-traumatic excess arterial inflow. Penile Doppler ultrasound distinguishes the differences. Venous priapism should be regarded as an emergency; if prolonged it may lead to venous thrombosis, resulting in impotence. Arterial priapism settles with rest.

Venous priapism is usually associated with intracavernosal injection for impotence with prostaglandin or papaverine. Haematological disorders such as sickle cell anaemia and leukaemia, metastatic malignant infiltration, spinal cord injuries and drugs such as anticoagulants, marijuana, phenothiazines and some antihypertensives are uncommon causes. Some cases are idiopathic.

Management[4] is an urgent blood film to exclude polycythemia and leukaemia; then, under local anaesthesia, repeated saline flushing and aspiration of thick blood from the ipsilateral corpora cavernosa with a 16g needle through the glans penis. If resolution is incomplete, use a very slow injection of 10 mL of saline containing aramine 1 mg into the corpus cavernosum, followed by massage. A poor response at one hour may require a second aramine injection, carefully monitoring for hypertension. Venous bypass surgery is rare if drainage can be established.

Peyronie's disease

Peyronie's disease is a fibrotic process, sometimes associated with Dupuytren's contracture, that affects the shaft of the penis and results in discomfort and deformity on erection. Typically, the patient presents with painful 'crooked' erections. There is abnormal curvature of the erect penis. The penile deformity may prevent satisfactory vaginal penetration. On examination a nontender hard plaque may be palpable in the shaft of the penis. Mild cases require reassurance and daily vitamin E tablets for 6 months to reduce discomfort.[4] The problem may increase, remain static or spontaneously lessen over 1–2 years. Occasionally, surgical treatment by penile tuck is indicated if the patient's erection is so deformed that sexual intercourse is difficult, or rarely by penile implant if the patient is impotent.[2]

Haematospermia

Haematospermia, which is blood in the semen, presents as a somewhat alarming symptom. It is sometimes encountered in young adults and middle-aged men. The initial step is to determine that the blood is actually in the semen and not arising from warts inside the urethral meatus or from the partner.

It usually occurs as an isolated event but can be secondary to urethral warts or prostatitis, or with prostatomegaly or prostatic tumour (especially in elderly patients). If a micro-urine shows no accompanying haematuria, and prostatic specific antigen and blood pressure are normal, reassurance and a 6 week review is appropriate as spontaneous cessation of haematospermia is the rule.

References

1. Hutson J, Beasley S, Woodward A. *Jones clinical paediatric surgery*. Oxford: Blackwell Scientific Publications, 1992, 175–179.

2. Bullock N, Sibley G, Whitaker R. *Essential urology*. Edinburgh: Churchill Livingstone, 1989, 287–299.

3. Hunt P, Marshall V. *Clinical problems in general surgery*. Sydney: Butterworths, 1991, 365–368.

4. Lawson P. Difficult male urological problems. Urology Seminar Proceedings. Box Hill Hospital, 1977; 2–4.

95
Disorders of the prostate

—

Mind and body, like man and wife, do not always agree to die together.

Charles Colton 1780–1832

The main function of the prostate gland is to aid in the nutrition of sperm and keep the sperm active. It does not produce any hormones so there is usually no alteration in sexual drive following prostatectomy.

Prostatitis

Prostatitis embraces a group of conditions with voiding discomfort and pain in the prostate referred to the perineum, low back, urethra and testes. It typically affects men aged 25–50. Prostatitis usually occurs in the absence of identifiable bacterial growth, when it is termed non-bacterial prostatitis. The prostate may develop acute or chronic bacterial infection.

Bacterial prostatitis is usually caused by *E.coli* (commonest), *Streptococcus faecalis*, *Pseudomonas* or *Staphylococcus*. Some chronic infections have been shown to be associated with *Chlamydia trachomatis*.[1]

Prostatodynia means the presence of symptoms typical of prostatitis but without objective evidence of inflammation or infection (Table 95.1).

It is preferable to use the term 'prostatitis syndromes' to embrace the four terms used in Table 95.1.

Clinical features of acute bacterial prostatitis
Symptoms
• fever, sweating, rigors
• pain in perineum (mainly), back and suprapubic area

• urinary frequency, urgency and dysuria
• variable degrees of bladder outlet obstruction
• ± haematuria

Signs
• fever
• rectal examination: prostate exquisitely tender, swollen, firm, warm, indurated

Complications
• abscess
• recurrence
• epididymo-orchitis
• acute retention
• bacteraemia/septicaemia

Chronic bacterial prostatitis
Chronic bacterial prostatitis is diagnosed by a history of mild irritative voiding with perineal, scrotal and suprapubic pain. Ejaculatory pain can occur. The gland may be normal on clinical examination or tender and boggy. It should be suspected in men with recurrent UTI (refer Table 95.2).

Investigations
• Fractional urine specimens and expressed prostatic secretions (EPS) obtained after prostatic massage can show excess white cells.
• Culture of the urine or ejaculate may be negative or give low counts.
• Prostatic stones (demonstrated by plain X-ray or transrectal ultrasound) may prevent successful treatment.
• Prostatic specific antigen (PSA): elevation occurs with inflammation and may cause confusion with cancer.

Table 95.1 *Classification of prostatitis syndromes*

	Prostatic pain	Prostatic rectal examination	Positive bladder culture	Positive prostatic secretion culture
Acute bacterial prostatitis	Yes	Very tender swollen	Yes	Yes
Chronic bacterial prostatitis	Often	Normal or indurated	Occasionally	Low counts
Non-bacterial prostatitis	Often	Normal	Occasionally	No
Prostatodynia	Often	Normal	No	No

Table 95.2 *Features of chronic bacterial prostatitis*

Difficult to treat

Relapsing infection

Perineal pain

Some leucocytes in expressed prostatic secretion

Treatment

Acute bacterial prostatitis[2]

amoxycillin (or ampicillin) 1 g IV 6 hourly

+

gentamicin 5 mg/kg/day as a single daily dose

until there is substantial improvement, when therapy may be changed to an appropriate oral agent, based on the sensitivity of the pathogen(s) isolated, for the remainder of 14 days.[2]

For milder infection, oral treatment with amoxycillin/potassium clavulanate, trimethoprim or norfloxacin is suitable. Urinary retention or abscess formation almost always requires endoscopic deroofing for drainage.

Chronic bacterial prostatitis

Treatment of this condition is made difficult by uncertainty in differentiating it from non-bacterial prostatitis as cultures may grow low counts of what may be normal flora. Avoid over-treatment with antibiotics. Reassurance is important and it is worth suggesting frequent ejaculation and hot baths. Massage only for recalcitrant cases.

doxycycline 100 mg (o) daily for 1 month

or

trimethoprim 300 mg (o) daily for 1 month

or

norfloxacin 400 mg (o) 12 hourly for 1 month

or

ciprofloxacin 500 mg (o) 12 hourly for 1 month[2]

Non-bacterial prostatitis

This is the commonest by far. It is often recurrent and each episode can last several months. Antibiotic therapy is inappropriate. The symptoms may reflect retrograde passage of urine into prostatic tissue with urate crystallisation. Emphasise good voiding habits.[2] Avoid straining at the end of micturition. Encourage normal sexual activity and use stress management. Prescribe allopurinol 300 mg daily for at least 3 months for each episode as it reduces prostatic urate deposition and relieves symptoms.[3]

Prostatodynia

Perform a thorough genitourinary tract investigation. Some patients have urethral sphincter spasm and may respond to diazepam or the alpha-blocking agent minipress 0.5 mg bd. Psychological counselling may be appropriate. Occasionally alcohol and caffeine induce flares of prostatodynia which may often be regarded as synonymous with non-bacterial prostatitis.

Very rare causes of prostatitis include tuberculosis, gonorrhoea, parasites and fungi.

Lower urinary tract symptoms (LUTS)

These symptoms can be grouped as voiding symptoms (obstructive) or storage symptoms (irritative). Irritative symptoms may be caused by a bladder problem only. Obstructive symptoms are usually caused by the prostate (which can also cause irritative symptoms). The old term 'prostatism' is ill defined and best dropped.

Voiding (obstructive) symptoms:

- hesitancy
- weak stream
- postmicturition dribble
- urinary retention

Storage (irritative) symptoms:

- urgency
- urge incontinence
- frequency
- nocturia
- dysuria
- suprapubic pain

Bladder outlet obstruction

Symptoms of bladder outlet obstruction (BOO) are present in most men after the age of 60. The commonest cause is benign prostatic obstruction. Benign prostatic hypertrophy is a histological diagnosis which, strictly, should not be used for symptoms. Only 10–15% require surgery for relief of obstructive symptoms.[1] Bladder outlet obstruction can also be caused by bladder neck obstruction and urethral sphincter spasm.

Clinical features of BOO:
- hesitancy
- frequency of micturition
- urgency
- nocturia
- slow interrupted flow
- terminal dribbling
- acute retention (the presenting problem in 15% of patients)
- retention with overflow incontinence (less common)

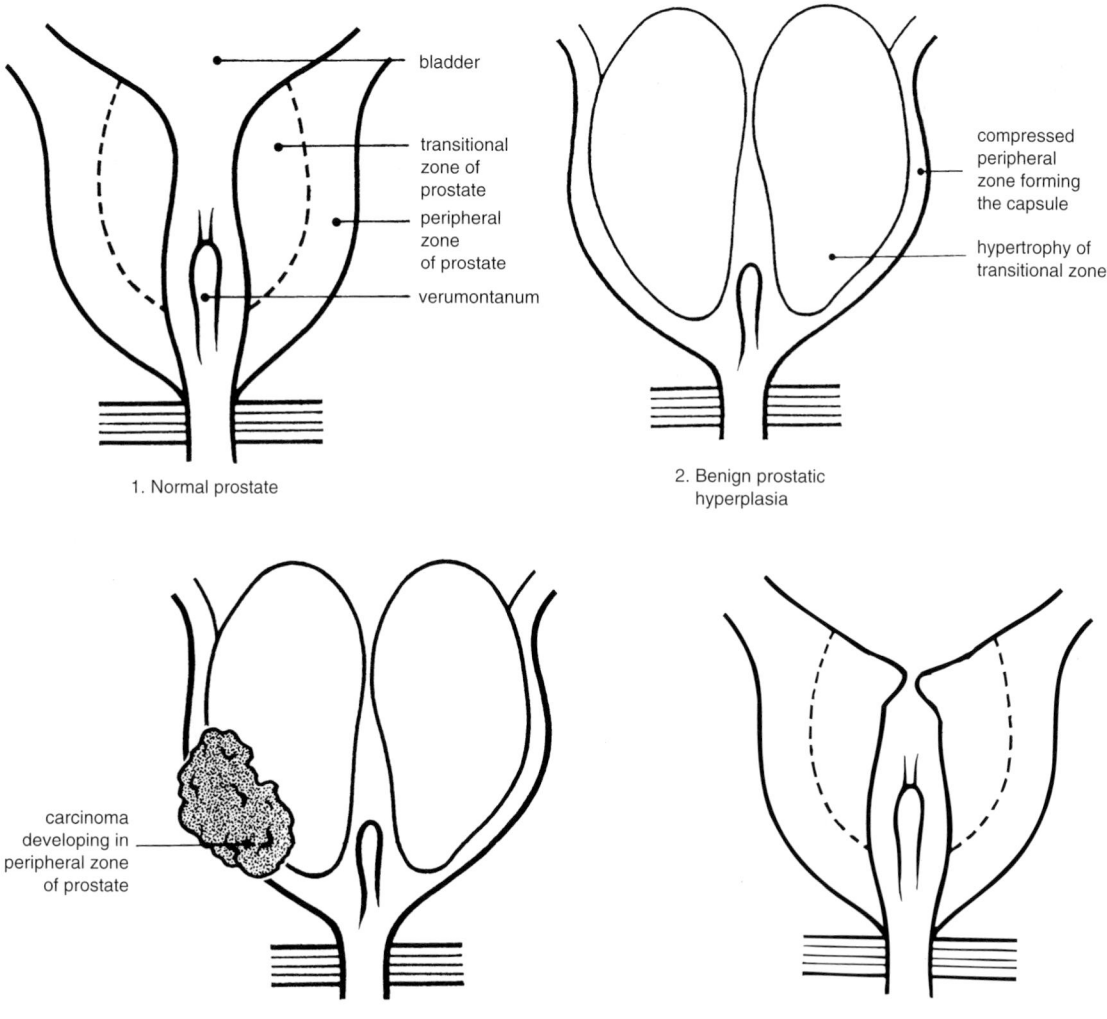

1. Normal prostate

bladder

transitional zone of prostate

peripheral zone of prostate

verumontanum

2. Benign prostatic hyperplasia

compressed peripheral zone forming the capsule

hypertrophy of transitional zone

3. Carcinoma of prostate

carcinoma developing in peripheral zone of prostate

4. Bladder neck obstruction

Fig. 95.1 *Diagrammatic comparison of bladder outlet obstruction*

- haematuria from ruptured submucosal prostatic veins can occur
- rectal examination usually detects an enlarged prostate

Note: Small glands can also cause outlet obstruction.

Investigations

These include

- urine culture
- renal function
- prostate specific antigen
- prostatic needle biopsy (with or without transrectal ultrasound) if carcinoma suspected
- voiding flow rate of <10 mL/sec tends to confirm that the symptoms reflect obstruction and not bladder irritability

Complications of prostatic obstruction

- retention
- urinary infection
- bladder calculus formation
- uraemia

Self-help advice for patients with mild symptoms (after cancer excluded)

- Avoid certain drugs, especially OTC cough and cold preparations.
- Reduce caffeine.
- Avoid fluids before bedtime.
- Urinate when you need to (do not hang on).
- Wait 30 seconds after voiding and try to void again.

Medical treatment

Patients with mild symptoms may be helped with alpha-adrenergic blocking drugs such as phenoxybenzamine, tamsulosin, terazosin and prazosin to inhibit contraction of the muscle in the bladder neck and urethra.[1] A typical dose is prazosin 0.5 mg bd, or 1 mg nocte after commencing with 0.5 mg nocte. It can be increased to a maximum of 2 mg bd. Symptoms are not improved by increasing beyond this dose. The 5 alpha reductase inhibitors (e.g. finasteride) reduce prostatic volume. Urine flow improves by 3 months, plateauing at 6 months, but not to the same degree as with surgery. It is not very effective for symptomatic control. Both drugs are used long-term. They do not summate.

Surgical management

The most effective treatment for obstruction is transurethral resection of the prostate (TURP), or laser ablation (Fig. 95.2). Transurethral incision of the prostate (TUIP) gives identical results with small glands. Open prostatectomy accounts for less than 1% of benign prostatic surgery today.

Permanent springs (stents) placed in the prostatic urethra under local anaesthesia are an option for the very frail patient. Microwave and heat treatment are new methods but less effective.

Absolute indications for prostatectomy include deterioration in renal function, the development of upper tract dilatation, retention (following drainage and assessment) and

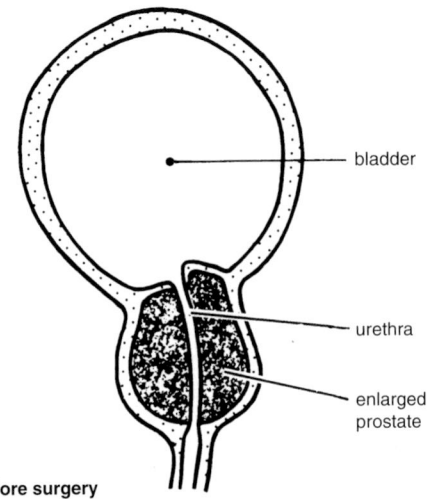

Before surgery

bladder

urethra

enlarged prostate

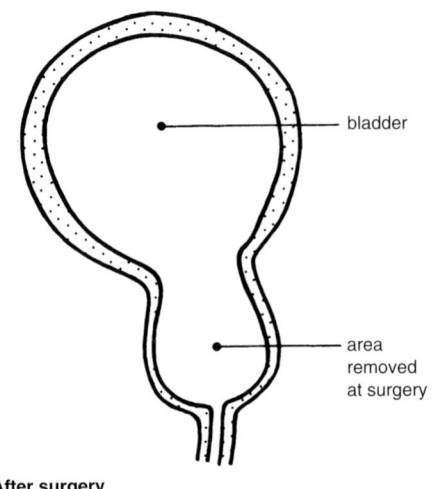

After surgery

bladder

area removed at surgery

Fig. 95.2 *The process of prostatectomy*

bladder stones. Eighty per cent of patients have surgery for bothersome symptoms.

Postoperative guidelines for the patient
- There may be urgency even to the point of incontinence for a few days.
- Bleeding can occur intermittently for three weeks, so increase fluid intake.
- Erectile function is usually unchanged (neither better nor worse) but loss of erection probably occurs in 5% of patients.
- Avoid intercourse for three weeks.
- Orgasms continue but there is usually no emission with ejaculation. The semen is ejaculated back into the bladder.
- If obstructive problems recur early there may be a stricture.

Note: • Persisting postoperative frequency bothers about 15% of patients.
  • 10–15% reveal unsuspected carcinoma.

Drugs and LUTS

Certain drugs can cause LUTS due to the effect of the drug on the bladder. It is very important for the family doctor to enquire about these drugs when evaluating such a patient. The problem is mainly an adverse effect of drugs with anticholinergic activity.

Anticholinergics
- atropine and hyoscine compounds
  e.g. disopyramide
    mazindol
    phenothiazines
    dicyclomine
    propantheline
    other belladonna alkaloids
- antidepressants
    especially tricyclic compounds
- antiParkinson agents
  e.g. amantadine
    benzhexol
    benztropine
    biperiden
    orphenadrine
    procyclidine

Beta-adrenoceptor agonists
- ephedrine
- salbutamol
- terbutaline

- OTC preparations (mainly for coughs and colds)
  e.g. sympathomimetics including ephedrine

Carcinoma of the prostate

Prostate carcinoma is the commonest malignancy in men and the third commonest cause of death from malignant disease in Australia. It is rare before the age of 50. By the age of 80 years 80% of men have histologic carcinoma within the gland but most are dormant.[4] Prostatic carcinoma may be asymptomatic, even when it has extended beyond the prostate. It usually commences in the peripheral part of the gland. There are dramatic racial differences in the frequency that tend to change with migration, indicating that prostate cancer reflects environmental influences (and possibly dietary fat).

Clinical features

Unsuspected carcinomas are often detected by prostate specific antigen (PSA) or histologically after TURP. Clinical prostatic carcinoma presents typically with rapidly progressive symptoms of lower urinary tract obstruction or of metastatic spread, especially to bone (pelvis and vertebrae).[4] Symptoms include bladder outflow obstruction 70%, acute retention 25%, back pain 15%, haematuria 5% and uraemia 5%.[1] Other symptoms include tiredness, weight loss and perineal pain.

Digital rectal examination (DRE) may reveal a nodule (50% are not carcinoma). Locally advanced cancer typically reveals a hard, nodular and irregular gland. The tumour may be large enough to obliterate the median sulcus. The borders may lack definition. On the other hand, with cancer, the prostate may feel normal.

Investigations to detect carcinoma
Blood analysis
- prostate specific antigen (PSA)
  — normal level less than 4 ng/mL
  — can be elevated without cancer
  — is prostate specific, not prostate cancer specific
  — can be 'normal' in 5% of cancers[5]
  — levels between 4 and 10 are equivocal
  — levels > 10 are only suggestive of cancer

Biopsy[5]

Consider biopsy (with or without transrectal ultrasound) if the DRE is positive or if the PSA is elevated.

Correlations:

PSA 4–10 with abnormal DRE—38% have cancer

PSA > 10 with normal DRE—30% have cancer

PSA > 10 with abnormal DRE—65% have cancer

Investigations to stage disease

• radionuclide bone scan (not necessary if PSA < 20)

Screening

The value of screening asymptomatic men is debatable. If it has a place it would consist of a PSA and DRE annually from 55–70 years if life expectancy exceeds 10 years.[5]

Treatment of prostate cancer[5]

Patients over 70 with no symptoms require no treatment. The treatment depends on the age of the patient and the stage of the disease. Repeating the PSA in three months is a useful strategy.

For tumours that are potentially curable, radical prostatectomy or local radiotherapy are the options.

Radiotherapy

The cure rate is 10% less than with surgery but the difference does not become apparent for 10 years. The main adverse reactions are faecal urgency and diarrhoea together with urine frequency. Impotence is common two years after radiotherapy.

Radical prostatectomy

• Should be reserved for patients under 70 with PSA < 30.
• Long-term cure rates of 80% must be balanced with urine incontinence rates (sufficient to need a pad) of 10–20% and frequently impotence.

Hormone manipulation

For metastatic or locally advanced disease, androgen deprivation is the cornerstone of treatment, the options being:

• bilateral orchidectomy

or

• daily antiandrogenic tablets
    e.g. cyproterone acetate (Androcur)
         flutamide (Eulexin)

or

• LHRH agonists: depot injections of luteinising hormone releasing hormone (LHRH) analogues
    e.g. goserelin (Zoladex)
         leuprorelin acetate (Lucrin)

Treatment combinations for small volume metastatic prostate carcinoma *may* prolong life:

e.g. • orchidectomy plus flutamide
     • LHRH agonists plus flutamide—LHRH agonists cause an initial surge of testosterone so a preliminary antiandrogenic agent is necessary to prevent a flare in the cancer.

References

1. Bullock N, Sibley G, Whitaker Q. *Essential urology*. Edinburgh: Churchill Livingstone, 1989, 287–299.

2. Mashford ML. *Antibiotic guidelines* (7th edn). Melbourne: Victorian Medical Postgraduate Foundation, 1996, 78–79.

3. Persson BE, Ronquist G, Ekblom M. Ameliorative effect of allopurinol on nonbacterial prostatitis: a parallel double-blind controlled study. J of Urology (American Urology Ass.), 1996; 155:961–964.

4. Kumar PJ, Clark ML. *Clinical medicine* (2nd edn). London: Bailliere Tindall, 1990, 486–488.

5. Lawson P. *Disorders of the prostate*. Seminar proceedings notes (adapted from the Australian Prostate Health Council's information notes). Box Hill Hospital, Melbourne, 1993.

PART 7

SEXUALLY RELATED PROBLEMS

——

96
The infertile couple

—

You notice that the tabetic has the power of holding
water for an indefinite period. He is also impotent—in
fact, two excellent properties to possess for a quiet
day on the river.

Dr Dunlop 1913
Teaching at Charing Cross Hospital

Definition

Infertility is defined as the absence of conception after a period of 12 months of normal unprotected sexual intercourse.[1] It can be a very
distressing and emotional problem for the
couple who need considerable care, empathy
and relatively rapid investigation of their
problem. In assessing a couple with the problem
of subfertility (this term is a preferable way of
describing the condition to the patients), it is
appropriate to involve both partners in the consultation. In determining the cause of the subfertility, three basic fertility parameters should be
investigated.[2]

1. The right number of sperm have to be placed
   in the right place at the right time.
2. The woman must be ovulating.
3. The tubes must be patent and the pelvis sufficiently healthy to enable fertilisation and
   implantation.

Key facts and checkpoints

- Infertility affects 10–15% of all cohabitating
  couples.[3]
- This incidence increases with age.
- After the age of 32 fertility decreases by 1.5%
  per year.

- About 15% of couples who do not use contraception fail to achieve a pregnancy within
  12 months.[4]
- More than 10% remain unsuccessful after
  2 years.[4]
- About 50% of couples will seek medical
  assistance.[3]
- The main factors to be assessed are ovulation,
  tubal patency and semen analysis.
- About 30% of couples have an identifiable
  male factor. Male infertility affects 5% of men.
- Female factors account for about 45%: tubal
  problems account for about 20% and ovulatory
  disorders about 20%. Polycystic ovary syndrome is a common factor.
- The initial investigation for the man is semen
  analysis on two occasions. The initial investigation for the woman is a basal body temperature chart followed by midluteal progesterone
  measurement.
- About 15–18% of cases have no apparent
  explanation.
- A significant number (25%) have combined
  male and female problems.
- Current specialised treatment helps the majority of subfertile couples to achieve pregnancy.[5]

Physiological factors[5,6]
Male fertility
Fertility in the male requires:

- normal hypothalamic function producing
  gonadotrophin-releasing hormone (GnRH)
- normal pituitary function producing the gonadotrophic hormones follicle stimulating hormone (FSH) and luteinising hormone (LH)
- normal seminiferous tubule and Leydig cell
  function
- normal sperm transport and delivery

Facts about sperm viability
- The maximum number of viable sperm is found in the ejaculate after a 48 hour abstinence.
- After entering receptive cervical mucus, sperm are capable of fertilising an egg for at least 48 hours.
- sperm survive for less than 30 minutes in the vagina.

Female fertility
Fertility in the female requires:
- normal function of the ovulatory cycle, which requires:
  — normal hypothalamic-pituitary function producing the hormones GnRH, FSH and LH
  — normal ovarian function with follicular response to FSH and LH (Fig. 96.1)
  — appropriate prolactin levels (which are normally low); excessive prolactin secretion (hyperprolactinaemia) causes anovulation
- normal tubal transport and access of the ovum to incoming sperm
- receptive cervical mucus
- normal uterus to permit implantation of the fertilised ovum

Probabilities of pregnancy
About 50% of normal couples, having unprotected intercourse at least twice a week, will probably achieve pregnancy in 6 months, 80% in 1 year and 90% in 2 years.[5]

Causes of infertility
Significant causes of infertility are summarised in Table 96.1 and illustrated in Figure 96.2.

A diagnostic approach
It is important to see both partners, not just the woman.

History
The following basic facts should be ascertained.

The man
- sexual function
- previous testicular problems/injury, e.g. orchitis, trauma, undescended testes
- medical problems: diabetes, epilepsy, tuberculosis, renal disorders
- past history (PH) of sexually transmitted diseases
- PH of mumps
- PH of urethral problems
- genitourinary surgery, e.g. hernia
- recent severe febrile illness
- occupational history (exposure to heat, pesticides, herbicides)

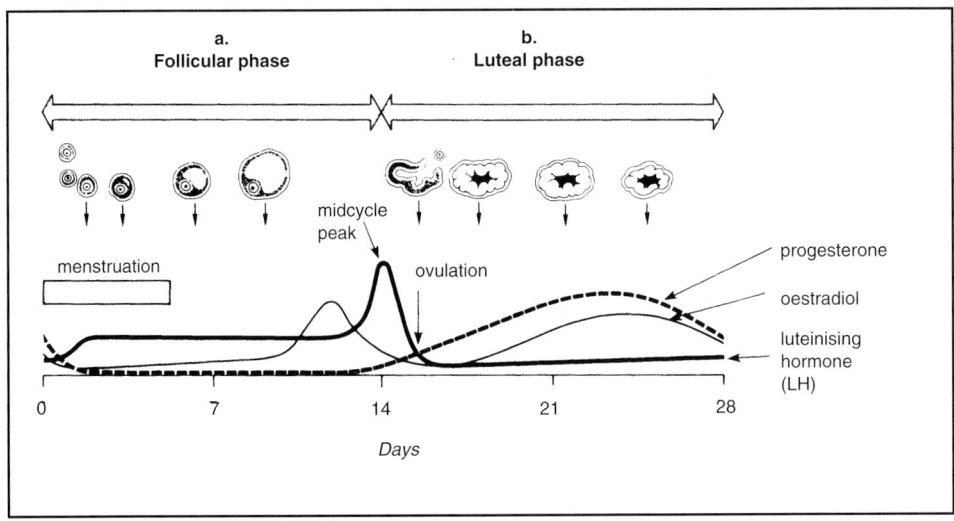

Fig. 96.1 *The normal ovulatory cycle: the midcycle peak of LH and FSH is at 14 days and ovulation occurs shortly afterwards*

Table 96.1 *Significant causes of infertility*

Female factors

Ovulation disorders
- ovarian failure
- stress
- polycystic ovary syndrome
- weight-related ovulation disorders
- hyperprolactinaemia
- other endocrine disorders
- idiopathic eugonadotropic anovulation

Tubal disease
- pelvic inflammatory disease
- endometriosis
- previous ectopic pregnancy
- previous tubal ligation
- previous peritonitis

Uterine and cervical abnormalities
- congenital
- acquired

Endometriosis

Male factors

Reduced sperm production
- congenital cryptorchidism (maldescent)
- inflammation, e.g. mumps orchitis
- antispermatogenic agents
  - chemotherapy
  - drugs
  - irradiation
  - heat
- idiopathic
- Klinefelter's syndrome (46 XXY)

Hypothalamic pituitary disease
- hypogonadotropic disorder

Disorders of coitus
- erectile dysfunction
- psychosexual ejaculatory failure
- retrograde ejaculation
  - genitourinary surgery
  - autonomic disorders, e.g. diabetes
  - congenital abnormalities

Ductal obstruction

Couple factors

Joint subfertility
Psychosexual dysfunction

- drug intake (possible adverse effects from)
  - alcohol
  - chemotherapy
  - anabolic steroids
  - aminoglycoside antibiotics
  - sulphasalazine
  - cimetidine/ranitidine
  - colchicine
  - spironolactone
  - antihypertensive agents
  - narcotics
  - phenytoin
  - nitrofurantoin
  - nicotine
  - marijuana

The woman
- evidence of previous fertility
- onset of menarche
- menstrual history
- symptoms of ovulation
- symptoms of endometriosis
- PH of sexually transmitted disease and pelvic infection
- previous IUCD
- PH of intra-abdominal surgery, e.g. appendicitis, ovarian cyst
- PH of genitourinary surgery, including abortions
- obstetric history
- body weight: eating disorders (anorexia, obesity)
- drug intake
  - alcohol
  - smoking, especially > 20/day
  - oral contraception
  - anabolic steroids
  - major tranquillisers

Combined history
- frequency and timing of intercourse
- adequate penetration with intercourse, and ejaculation
- use of lubricants
- attitudes to pregnancy and subfertility
- expectations for the future

Physical examination
A general assessment of body habitus, general health including diabetes mellitus, and secondary sexual characteristics should be noted in both man and woman. Urinalysis should be performed on both partners.

The man
- secondary sexual characteristics; note any gynaecomastia
- genitalia
  - size and consistency of the testes
    - normal size 3.5 to 5.5 cm long; 2 to 3.5 cm wide
    - small testes < 3.5 cm long
    - Klinefelter's 2 (or less) cm long (typical)
  - palpate epididymis and vas (present and non-tender is normal)

GnRH

hypothalamus

anterior
pituitary

FSH

LH

prolactin

FSH

LH

FSH   LH

excess
prolactin
inhibits
ovulation

ovum

oestrogens
progesterone

testosterone

| ovulation | tubal disorders | uterine disorders | cervical-vaginal factors | potency-sperm dysfunction | vas blockage | testicular dysfunction | ? adequate coitus |

Female factors   **Male factors**   **Combined factors**

X indicates possible disorder causing infertility

Fig. 96.2 *The major factors involved in subfertility*   ADAPTED FROM KUMAR AND CLARKE

— evidence of varicocele
— PR: check prostate
— note penis and location of urethra

The woman
• secondary sexual characteristics
• thyroid status
• genitalia and breasts
• vaginal and pelvic examination
  — assess uterus and ovaries (normal—present, mobile and non-tender)
  — the adnexae (any masses)

Investigations
These are usually performed after referral but the family doctor should organise initial investigations to assess where to refer, e.g. andrologist, endocrinologist, gynaecologist.

Initial investigations

Male—semen analysis

It is advisable to obtain two samples at least 2–3 weeks apart. It requires a complete ejaculation, preferably by masturbation, after at least 3 days sexual abstinence. Use a clean, dry wide-mouthed bottle; condoms should not be used. Semen should be kept warm and examined within 1 hour of collection.[6]

Normal values: volume > 3 mL
                 concentration > 20 million sperm/mL
                 motility > 60% after 2 hours
                 normal forms > 60%

Female—ovulation status

• educate about temperature chart and cervical mucus diary, noting time of intercourse (take

temperature with thermometer under tongue before getting out of bed in the morning)
- midluteal hormone assessment (21st day of cycle), i.e. serum progesterone and prolactin

Subsequent investigations
Diagnostic laparoscopy—direct visualisation corpus luteum, tubes; check tubal patency by insulfating blue dye from the cervix through tubes to peritoneal cavity.

Further investigations (if necessary)

Male

If azoospermia or severe oligospermia:
- serum FSH (if 2.5 times normal, indicates irreversible testicular failure)—this is the most important endocrine test in the assessment of male infertility
- antisperm antibodies (in semen or serum)

Female

(other investigations may be necessary)
- thyroid function tests: ? hypothyroidism
- hysterosalpingogram (rarely used now)
- endometrial biopsy
- ultrasound of pelvis
- computerised tomography of the pituitary fossa
- chlamydia (cervical culture)

Note: Ovulation or its absence is best demonstrated by luteal progesterone.

Essential investigations are outlined in Table 96.2.

Management principles[3]
- Both partners should be involved in management decisions since fertility is a couple's problem.
- Infertility can cause considerable emotional stress, including the taking or placing of blame by one partner or the other, and subsequent guilt feelings; hence sensitive and empathetic

Table 96.2 *Essential investigations of the subfertile couple*

Basal body temperature chart and cervical mucus diary
Semen analysis
Serum progesterone and prolactin (day 21) in female
Laparoscopy and/or ultrasound of ovaries
Rubella immune status (female)

support is essential. This may include marital counselling.
- Since recent advances have helped this problem so much, there is no place for guesswork or for empirical therapy and early referral is necessary.

Polycystic ovary syndrome (PCOS)
PCOS is a common chronic anovulatory disorder affecting 2–5% of women of reproductive age. It should not be confused with the common ultrasonographic diagnosis of cystic ovaries with no clinical features.

Clinical features of PCOS:
- oligo- or amenorrhoea
- hirsutism (70%)
- obesity (50%)

PCOS has a strong hereditary basis and can begin in the pubertal years. There are variations of the syndrome including normal menstruation (20%) and abnormal uterine bleeding (50%).

Two important consequences are infertility and an increased risk of endometrial cancer (if anovulatory).

Investigations show raised serum testosterone, raised LH level and reversed FSH/LH ratio. Transvaginal ultrasound aids diagnosis. Early consultant referral is important. Current treatment is multiple incisions via laparoscopy.

Counselling the subfertile couple[7]
The counselling of subfertile couples has to be adapted to the level reached by the couple along the infertility pathway. The needs of each couple may be very different depending on their emotional nature, their lifestyle, moral, religious and ethical beliefs. However, their suffering can run very deep and deserves attention, time and opportunities for free expression of feelings and concerns.

The medical counselling model developed by Craig and Colagiuri[7] (Fig. 5.1) is very useful as it empowers patients to make their own decision through facilitation as opposed to the directive and advisory medical model.

The couple are provided initially with accurate and appropriate information. Anxiety is alleviated by reassurance and by dispelling myths such as their problem being caused by an unfavourable position for intercourse, leakage of excess semen from the vagina or previous use of the pill.

The facilitation process enables the couple to ventilate any feelings of guilt, anxiety, fear, anger and sexuality. The style of questioning should aim to explore the influence that the problem has had on the couple and then the influence they have over it. These processes then lead to decision making by the couple about further management strategies.

A graph of emotional responses to the infertility (Fig. 96.3) can be used to help the couple explore their current and past emotional responses to their problem. Apart from helping them realise that their problem is not unique, it provides opportunities for ventilation of important feelings that can act as a basis for counselling.

Treatment

If the problem has been identified, specific treatment needs to be prescribed by the consultant, e.g.

- Anovulation can be treated with ovulation induction drugs such as clomiphene, bromocriptine, gonadotrophins or GnRH.

- Endometriosis can be treated medically or surgically (peritubal adhesions).
- Male problems—little can be done (including testosterone and vitamins) to enhance semen quality. Corticosteroids may help if sperm antibodies are present. Consider IVF and related technology for male factor infertility.
- Severe tubal disease—use in-vitro fertilisation and embryo transfer (IVF-ET).
- Unexplained subfertility—consider gamete intrafallopian transfer (GIFT), a modification of IVF. This method, in which eggs and sperm are placed into the Fallopian tubes, is best used in the treatment of infertility of unknown aetiology and carries a pregnancy rate of about 30% per couple.[2]

When to refer

A family doctor should perform the initial investigations of a couple with infertility, including temperature chart, semen analysis and hormone levels, to determine whether it is a male or female problem and then organise the appropriate referral.

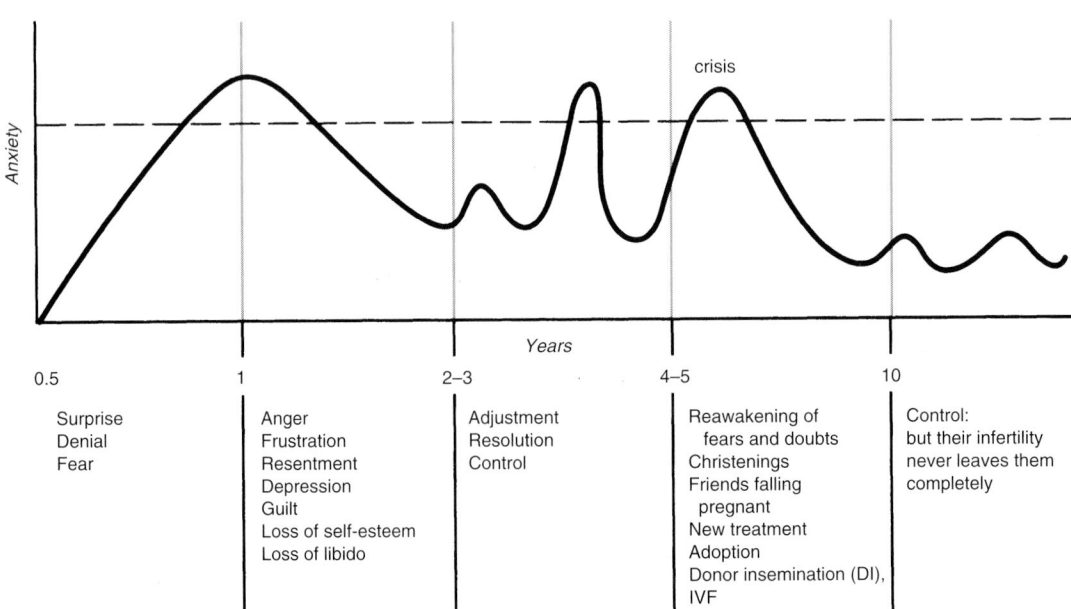

Fig. 96.3 *Emotional responses to infertility*   COLAGIURI AND CRAIG[7] REPRINTED WITH PERMISSION

References

1. Kumer PJ, Clark ML. *Clinical medicine* (2nd edn). London: Bailliere Tindall, 1990, 792–794.

2. Wood C, Kovacs G. *Infertility: all your questions answered.* Melbourne: Hill of Content, 1996.

3. Jequier AM. Infertility. In: MIMS Disease Index (2nd edn). Sydney: IMS Publishing, 1996, 273–278.

4. Smith H. Female infertility. Mod Med Aust, August 1990; 98–106.

5. Knowlden S, Helman T. How to treat infertility. Australian Dr Weekly, 25 August 1989; I–VII.

6. DeKrester D. Female infertility. Mod Med Aust, July 1990; 98–109.

7. Craig S. A medical model for infertility counselling. Aust Fam Physician, 1990; 19:491–500.

97
Sexual dysfunction

The functional form of impotence fills the coffers of the quacks, and swells the list of suicides.

Rutherford Morrison (1853–1939)

Family doctors are often asked to provide advice and help for sexual concerns and are continually challenged to detect such problems presenting in some other guise. Since we deal with so much illness, including debilitating problems, and prescribe so many drugs we must be aware and sensitive to the possible implications of their various effects on sexual health.

Sexual disorders can be considered in three major groups: sexual dysfunction, sexual deviation and gender role disorders. This chapter will confine itself to a discussion of sexual dysfunction.

Sexual dysfunction

Sexual dysfunction in men refers to persistent inability to achieve normal sexual intercourse while in women it refers to a persistent lack of sexual satisfaction.[1]

Several studies have demonstrated that sexual concerns and problems are common with a prevalence ranging from 10–70% of the population.[2] Difficult problems are summarised in Table 97.1. These studies have also indicated that patients are certainly willing to discuss their sexuality and wish their family doctors to become involved in counselling and management of their problems. Between 25% and 30% of sexual difficulties have an organic cause, while the remainder are emotional or psychogenic in origin.[3] The unique place of general practice and the family doctor provides ideal opportunities to address the sexual concerns of patients.

Table 97.1 *Sexual dysfunction: difficult problems*

Sexual desire
• low libido

Sexual arousal
• erectile impotence
• failure of arousal in women

Sexual orientation/activity
• homosexuality
• fetishism

Orgasm
• premature ejaculation
• retarded ejaculation
• orgasmic dysfunction in women

Male problems
• low libido
• erectile difficulties
• premature ejaculation
• failure to ejaculate, or retarded ejaculation

Female problems
• low libido
• failure of arousal
• vaginismus
• orgasmic difficulties
• dyspareunia

The most common problem influencing an effective outcome is difficulty in communication between doctor and patient, which prejudices effective history taking and counselling. The problem is not content-related, much of which is based on common sense, but the ubiquitous problem of communication.

If, as a practitioner, you counsel on the assumption that astounding ignorance about sexuality still exists in our society, you will be amazed at the results and at how relatively simple it is to help so many confused people who often have unrealistic expectations of their partners and themselves.

Opportunistic sexuality education

The family doctor has many opportunities to provide education in sexuality throughout the lifelong care of the patient and it is wise to have a strategy that matter of factly incorporates enquiries and information about sexual health.

Examples include:

- antenatal and postnatal care
- contraceptive requests
- parents concerned about their children's sex play
- serious illness—medical and surgical
- adolescent problems
- menopause problems

Presentation of sexual concerns

Although some patients may present directly with a complaint of sexual dysfunction, many will be less direct and use some other pretext or complaint as a 'ticket of entry' for their sexual concerns. Despite a seemingly terse approach the issue must be recognised and treated with considerable importance. This may mean scheduling an appropriate time to discuss the concerns.

Sometimes patients are unaware of an association between their medical problem and underlying sexual issues.[2] Doctors may recognise such an association and initiate a tactful psychosocial history that includes questions about sexuality. Examples are chronic backache, pelvic pain, vaginal discharge, tiredness, insomnia and tension headache (see Table 97.2).

The effect of illness on sexual function

Doctors seldom enquire about the impact of an illness on the sexual function of patients and their partners and tend to be unaware of the sexual needs of elderly people (Table 97.3). It is most appropriate to enquire about these issues in our patients, e.g. the postmyocardial infarction patient, the postprostatectomy patient, the patient taking antihypertensives or other drugs, and the postmastectomy or posthysterectomy patient (Table 97.4). Diabetes deserves special attention as 27–55% of diabetic men reported some erectile difficulties.[2]

Table 97.2 *How sexual issues may present in family practice*[2]

Minor non-sexual complaint—'entry ticket'

Specific sexual concern

Marital or relationship problem

Non-sexual problem (as perceived by the patient)

Sexual enquiry and counselling as part of illness management

Sexual enquiry as part of total health check-up

Infertility

Menopausal problems

Table 97.3 *Medical conditions affecting sexual performance*

Cardiovascular
- previous myocardial infarction
- angina pectoris
- peripheral vascular disease
- hypertension and its treatment

Respiratory
- asthma
- chronic obstructive airways disease

Endocrine
- diabetes mellitus
- hypothyroidism
- hyperthyroidism
- Cushing's syndrome

Neurological
- multiple sclerosis
- neuropathy
- spinal cord lesions
- Parkinson's disease

Musculoskeletal
- arthritis

Depression

Renal
- renal failure

Urological problems
- prostatectomy
- phimosis
- Peyronie's disease
- priapism

Hepatobiliary
- cirrhosis

Surgical
- vaginal repair
- hysterectomy
- others

Trauma
- motor vehicle accidents

Cancer

Other
- Klinefelter's syndrome

Table 97.4 *Drugs affecting sexual arousal and function*

Male	Female
Alcohol	Alcohol
Narcotics	Narcotics
Marijuana	Marijuana
Anticholinergics	Combined oral contraceptive
Antiepileptics	
Antihypertensives	CNS depressants
Antihistamines	Antihypertensives (selected)
Benzodiazepines	Antiepileptics
Disulfiram	
Psychotherapeutic drugs	
Oestrogens	
Cytotoxic drugs	

Taking a sexual history

It is important to be alert for psychiatric disorders and situational factors and not to predict a person's sexual disposition. Avoid being too formal or too familiar but aim to display a wise, matter-of-fact, empathic, common-sense rapport. Tactfully explore the patient's attitude to sexuality and examine the relationship. Ideally, it is best to see a couple together if the problem is occurring within a steady relationship. As a practitioner, you have to be comfortable with your own sexuality and learn to be relaxed, confident and understanding when dealing with sexual concerns.

Enquiry about possible child sexual abuse is an important part of the history.

Probing questions for a suspected sexual problem

- Do you have any trouble passing urine or any vaginal discharge (women)?
- Are you sexually active?
- What is the physical side of your marriage/relationship like?
- Do you have any pain or discomfort during intercourse?
- Is your relationship good?
- Do you communicate well? Generally? Sexually?
- Do you have any difficulties in your sexual relationships?
- What is your sexual preference?
- Are you attracted to men, women or both?
- Have you experienced the 'coming out' process?

- What drugs are you taking?
- Do you take recreational drugs, e.g. alcohol, marijuana, nicotine?

Specific questions about sexuality

- Do you get aroused/turned on? What turns you on?
- Do you look forward to making love?
- Do you spend much time on love play?
- Does lovemaking make you feel happy and relaxed?
- Do you worry about getting pregnant (women)?
- What do you do about contraception?
- Do you worry about getting an STD?
- Do you worry about getting AIDS?
- How often do you reach a climax during lovemaking?
- How often do you have intercourse, or sexual activity without intercourse?
- Do you 'come' together?

Female

- Do you have enough lubrication? Are you wet enough?
- Do you find intercourse uncomfortable or painful?

Male

- Do you have trouble getting a full erection?
- How long does it take you to 'come' after you insert your penis?
- Do you 'come' too quickly?

Background history for an admitted problem

- Can you think of any reasons why you have this problem?
- What sex education did you have as a child? At home or at school?
- Were your parents happily married?
- Were sexual matters something that could be discussed in the home?
- Did you come from a religious family?
- Did you receive warnings or prohibitions as a child?
- What was the family attitude to masturbation, extramarital sex, menstruation, contraception, etc.?
- What is your attitude to masturbation?
- Were you fondled or sexually abused by an adult, especially a member of the family?
- Were there healthy shows of affection such as touching or hugging between family members?

- Did you have any upsetting sexual experiences during childhood and adolescence?
- What was your first sexual experience like?

Examination

The routine medical examination should include the basics such as urinalysis, BP measurement, genital examination and a neurological where indicated. A careful vaginal and pelvic examination should be an opportune educational experience for the patient and an exercise in preventive medicine.

Investigations

No particular routine tests are recommended. Tests for male impotence are outlined on page 928. Tests that may help exclude significant causes of low libido are those for diabetes, liver dysfunction, thyroid dysfunction and endocrine dysfunction. Endocrine dysfunction tests include prolactin, free testosterone, FSH, LH and oestradiol estimations. Other investigations may include pelvic ultrasonography, colposcopy or laparoscopy.

Exploring sexual myths

The acceptance in part or in total of many sexual myths that have prevailed in our society may have affected the relationship of a couple, especially in the context of the modern trend towards openness in discussing sexuality. It is worthwhile to help patients identify whether any of these myths have influenced their concerns by exploring common myths and their significant consequences to the individual or couple.

Sexual myths that could be explored include:[2]

- men need sex, women need love
- men need more sex than women
- men must be the instigators
- men know all about it
- sex = intercourse
- in this enlightened age everyone understands sexual issues

Sexual myths in the male[4]

- A hard erection is essential for good sex.
- A man should not show his feelings.
- A real man is always horny and ready for sex.
- As a person gets older there is no change in sexual interest, response or performance.
- As a person gets older there is a loss of interest in sex.

- Sexual performance is what really counts.
- Men are responsible for their partner's sexual pleasure.
- Sex must lead to orgasm.
- A man and his partner must reach orgasm simultaneously.

Basic sexual counselling

The family doctor can learn to be an effective sex counsellor. Sex counselling can be emotionally demanding and, while good interviewing skills, interest, support and basic advice are important, additional skills are needed to be an effective counsellor.

The fundamental methods involve:

- good communication and allowing a 'comfortable' exchange of information
- giving the patient 'permission' to talk openly about sexual matters
- providing basic 'facts of life' information
- dispelling sexual myths, correcting other misunderstandings
- gentle guidance for appropriate insight
- de-emphasising the modern-day obsession with performance and orgasm and emphasising the value of alternate forms of sexual expression, e.g. caressing, kissing, and manual and oral stimulation
- reducing the patient's anxiety
- bolstering self-images affected by feelings of rejection, avoidance, guilt, resentment or incompetence
- reassuring the patient that he or she is normal (where appropriate)

Inappropriate doctor behaviour is presented in Table 97.5.

Table 97.5 *Sexual counselling: inappropriate doctor behaviour*

Overfamiliarity
Being too formal
Being too talkative
Blunt questioning
Being judgmental
Making assumptions about the other's sexuality
Imposing one's own beliefs and standards
Dogmatism
Tackling problems beyond one's experience

An interesting realisation after counselling families in sexuality is that most of the problems are not difficult and often spring from basic ignorance of normal sexual function; it's simply a matter of setting the record straight. The greatest hurdle is 'getting started' with delineating the problem. Once that barrier is crossed, satisfactory results appear to follow.

Another significant realisation is that sexual problems can be grossly underestimated. Human beings generally have a basic craving for intimacy, touching, stroking and loving sex. Apparently 'good' harmonious relationships can lack this type of intimacy, which may lead to various psychosomatic manifestations.

Ideally the family doctor should undertake a course in sexual counselling to promote confidence in the counselling process. Patients can be taught basic methods (where appropriate) such as sensate focus, squeeze or stop–start techniques for premature ejaculation, self-exploration using Kegel's exercises, fantasy conditioning with videos, and behaviour modification. Complex problems, especially those involving impotence, infertility and sexual deviations or perversions, demand referral to an expert.

The PLISSIT counselling model

The PLISSIT counselling model developed by Annon[5] can be used to build the skills needed to deal with sexual problems, especially if there is a psychological element.[3]

The mnemonic PLISSIT stands for:

- P is for permission giving
- LI is for limited information
- SS is for specific suggestion
- IT is for intensive therapy

'Permission giving' allows patients to talk about sex, ask questions, feel guilty and so on. Their problems are shared with a reflective listening confidant.

Most medically trained people can probably provide the limited information required about sexual physiology and behavioural patterns.[3] 'Specific suggestion' provides ideas for self-help and may include key reference books, and relevant audiotapes or videotapes (Table 97.6). Videos can certainly arouse interest, ideas and motivation for a renewal of sexual activity. With a little support and permission, the patient can take simple action to remedy or improve a problem.

Table 97.6 *Educational aids for sexual dysfunction*

Recommended books
- Comfort A. *The joy of sex.* London: Mitchell Beazley, 1987.
- Zilbergeld B. *Men and sex. A guide to sexual fulfilment.* Medindie SA: Souvenir Press, 1979.
- Castleman M. *Making love* (mainly for men.) Penguin.
- Crooks R, Baur K. *Our sexuality.* Menlo Park, Ca: Benjamin/Cummings Publishing Co. 1984.
- Williams W. *It's up to you—a self-help book for the treatment of erectile problems.* Sydney: Williams & Wilkins, 1989.
- Rickard-Bell R. *Loving sex: happiness in mateship.* Brighton Le Sands: Wypikaninkie Publications, 1992.
- Gochros, Fischer. *Treat yourself to a better sex life.* Simon & Schuster.
- Kitzinger S. *Women's experience of sex.* Penguin.
- Phelps K. *Confronting sexuality.* Sydney: Harper Collins, 1993.
- Heiman J, Lo Piccolo J. *Becoming orgasmic: a sexual growth program for women.* Sydney: Simon & Schuster, 1988.

Recommended videos
- The lovers' guide I and II. Andrew Stanway.
- The language of love.

Intensive therapy, whether psychiatric or emotional, calls for deeper involvement and can be a dangerous area for the inexperienced. Referral to the appropriate practitioner is usually advisable.[3]

Analogous roles of the penis and clitoris

An explanation of the analogous roles of the penis and clitoris (proposed by Cohen and Cohen) is a very useful strategy for educating patients and helping them to understand the relationship of intercourse and penile and clitoris stimulation with orgasm. The simple model (Fig. 97.1) can be shown to patients to explain, for example, why some women are unable to achieve orgasm by intercourse alone, especially using the conventional missionary position.[2,6] It can readily be explained that clitoral stimulation in women is analogous to penile stimulation in men. Such information is very helpful for women and also to men who may perceive themselves as inadequate lovers. The use of such explanatory aids greatly facilitates the educational process and makes it more 'comfortable' for all concerned.

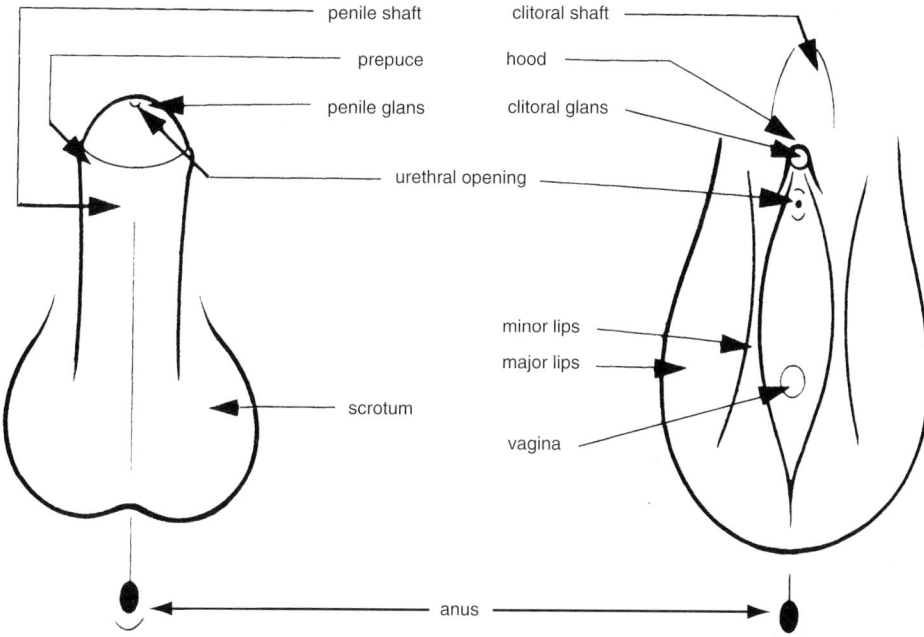

Fig. 97.1 *Analogous structures in male and female genitalia*   REPRODUCED WITH PERMISSION FROM G. AND M. COHEN,
CANADIAN FAMILY PHYSICIAN, 852, 31:767–71

Erectile dysfunction

Erectile dysfunction (impotence) is the inability to achieve or maintain an erection of sufficient quality for satisfactory intercourse. It doesn't refer to ejaculation, fertility or libido. Patients often use the term to refer to a problem of premature ejaculation, hence careful questioning is important.

Erectile dysfunction is a common problem, affecting 2% of males at 45 years and 25% of males aged 65.[7]

The most effective and practical approach to the man with erectile dysfunction is to determine the response to an intrapenile injection where prostaglandin E_1 is preferred to papaverine.

Causes of erectile dysfunction

- Psychogenic: related to stress, interpersonal or intrapsychic factors, e.g. depression, marital disharmony
- Neurogenic: disorders affecting the parasympathetic sacral spinal cord, e.g. multiple sclerosis; it usually develops gradually
- Vascular
- Diabetes
- Hormone disorder
  — androgen deficiency, e.g. testicular disease

  — hypothyroidism
  — hyperprolactinaemia (rare) → impotence and loss of libido due to secondary testosterone deficiency
- Drug-induced
  — alcohol
  — nicotine (four times the risk by age 50)
  — pharmaceutical preparations
- Unknown

History

The nature of the onset of erectile dysfunction is very important and this includes the nature of the relationship. Of particular importance is a drug history including alcohol, nicotine, street drugs and pharmaceutical agents, particularly antihypertensives (beta-blockers and thiazide diuretics), antidepressants, antipsychotics and H_2-receptor antagonists. Ask about nocturnal and early morning erections.

Examination

This should include a rectal examination and examination of the vascular and neurological status of the lower limbs and the genitalia, especially the testicles and penis. Check the cremaster and bulbocavernosus reflexes.

Investigations

First-line blood tests:

- free testosterone   ? androgen deficiency
- thyroxine   ? hypothyroidism
- prolactin   ? hyperprolactinaemia
- luteinising hormone
- glucose

Other blood tests to consider:

- LFTs, especially GGT (alcohol effect)

Nocturnal penile tumescence

This is an electronic computerised test used to detect and measure penile erections during REM sleep. Normally, there are 3–5 spontaneous erections lasting 20–35 minutes. The test helps to differentiate between psychogenic (normal studies) and organic (poor function). A very simple screening test is to use the snap gauge device.

Dynamic tests of penile function[7]

These tests include injections of drugs into the corpus cavernosum (which is the simplest method) to assess function. If the patient does not have overt psychogenic impotence and the diagnosis is uncertain, the response to intracavernosal injections of prostaglandin E (PGE) can be tested. A good response to PGE indicates that the patient has psychogenic or neurogenic impotence (e.g. due to pelvic nerve division during colon resection). Responses at higher doses indicate an incomplete organic disorder, e.g. partial arterial occlusion, venous leak, or diabetic neuropathy (early). Total failure to respond suggests arterial occlusion or an idiopathic disorder of the corpora cavernosa.

Management

This should comprise appropriate patient education including a videotape of the specific recommended treatment and technique. The partner should be included in the discussions and general management process with an emphasis on bolstering the couple's self-image which may have been affected by feelings of rejection or avoidance.

Psychogenic disorders

These will involve psychotherapy and sex behavioural modification as outlined under sexual counselling. Referral to a consultant may be appropriate.

Hormonal disorders

- testosterone for androgen deficiency: primary testicular disease (e.g. Klinefelter's syndrome) or gonadotrophin deficiency

> *Stepwise trial*

1. Oral: testosterone undecanoate (Andriol)
2. IM: testosterone enanthate (Primoteston Depot) or testosterone esters (Sustanon)
3. Subcutaneous implantation: testosterone implants (last 5–6 months)

- thyroxine for hypothyroidism
- bromocriptine for hyperprolactinaemia

Oral medication

- sildenafil (Viagra) 50 mg (o) 1 hour before sex Avoid it in those on nitrates for angina.

Intrapenile injection

- Alprostadil intracavernosal injections (Fig. 97.2)
  — self-administered after supervised teaching (use a penile model if available)
  — start with a lower dose
  — maximum of three a week
  — if prolonged erection > 2 hours take 2 pseudoephedrine tablets—repeat at 3½ hours if necessary (provided not hypertensive)

The co-operation of the partner is essential and urological backup must be arranged.

Transurethral alprostadil (Muse)

Urethral pellet: initial dose 250 mcg

Vacuum constriction

Vacuum constriction devices may have a place in management.

Surgery

- malleable penile prosthesis
- inflatable penile prosthesis (Fig. 97.3)
- vascular surgery where appropriate

Female orgasmic difficulties

It is necessary to determine whether the woman has been anorgasmic or can experience orgasms from other activities such as masturbation, manual or oral stimulation, even though she is non-orgasmic during intercourse.

The use of the Cohen model (Fig. 97.1) is very helpful in emphasising the importance of clitoral stimulation.

Therapy includes:

- sensate focus exercises[8]
- advice on the most appropriate positions for intercourse

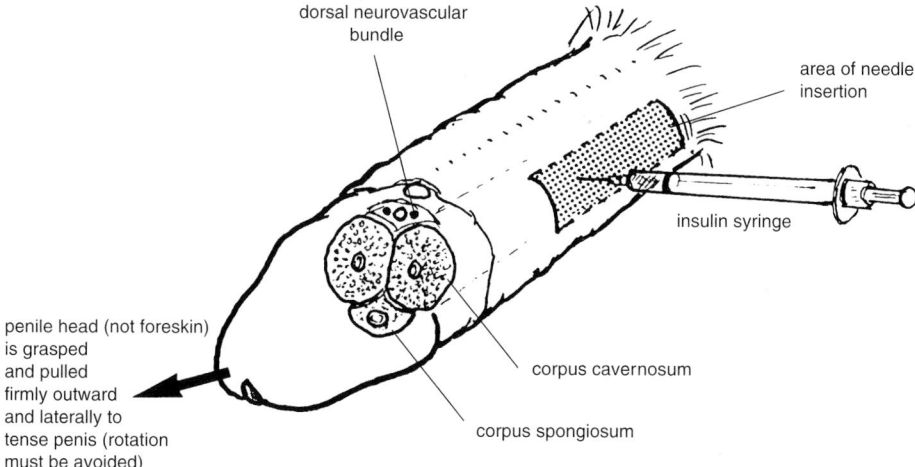

dorsal neurovascular bundle

area of needle insertion

insulin syringe

penile head (not foreskin) is grasped and pulled firmly outward and laterally to tense penis (rotation must be avoided)

corpus cavernosum

corpus spongiosum

Fig. 97.2 *Penile self-injection technique. The needle insertion is at 90° to the penis into the corpus cavernosum laterally at 1–3 o'clock (shown here) and 9–11 o'clock close to the penile base. It should avoid the midline neurovascular bundle and the ventral corpus spongiosum.*

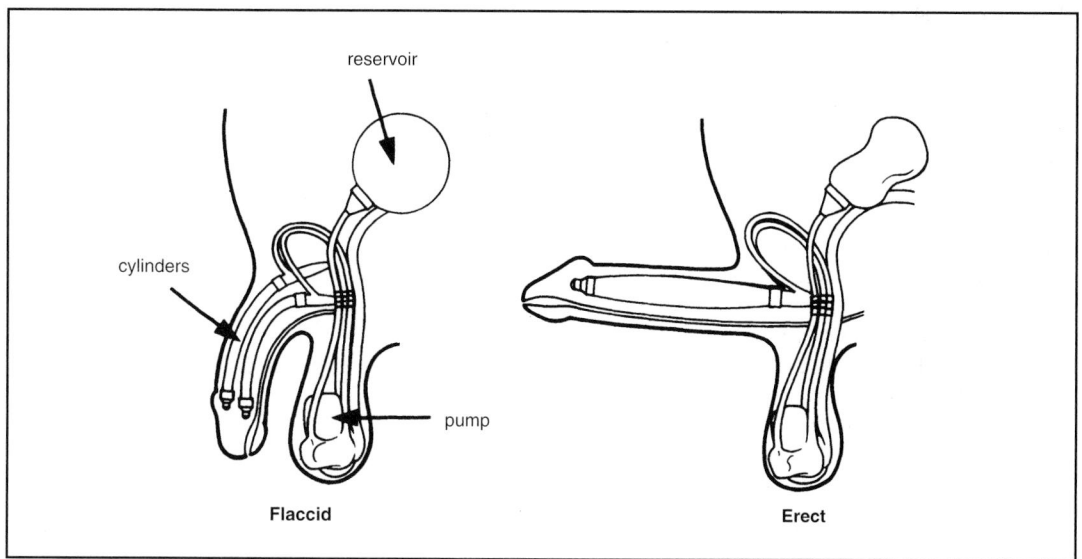

reservoir

cylinders

pump

Flaccid

Erect

Fig. 97.3 *An inflatable prosthesis, showing positioning of the components*

- permission to use
  — sexual aids: books, magazines
  — visual tapes
  — self-stimulation

Premature ejaculation

Premature ejaculation is a common problem that may not be clearly described by the patient so a careful history is necessary to define the problem. Both patient and partner may complain about the problem.

There are many approaches to treatment but they are aimed either at prolonged ejaculatory control or at satisfactory sexual activity without preoccupation with ejaculation and anticipation of better control with time and experience.

The standard management strategies to enhance ejaculatory control include a combination of three techniques:[8]

- graded sensate focus
- Masters' and Johnson's squeeze technique[9]
- Semans' 'stop–start' technique[10]

The tricyclic antidepressant, clomipramine, has been reported to be very effective, e.g. 25–50 mg/day.[11]

The small penis syndrome

In general practice it is not uncommon to counsel men and adolescent males for anxiety, sometimes pathological, about the relatively small size of their penis and its possible impact on sexual adequacy. Some males appear to be preoccupied with the size of their penis, especially when reaching the sexually active phase of their life. It is a manifestation of abnormal body image perception.

This attitude is related to the myth that a man's sexual performance depends on the size of his penis. The patient may present with minor (often trivial) non-sexual complaints as a 'ticket of entry' into the consulting room or perhaps as a manifestation of anxiety or depression related to preoccupation with penile size.

Measurement

Irrespective of physique or facial configuration most men are concerned about penile size.[12] However, as for all parts of the body, there is considerable variation in size and shape of the penis.

The average adult penis, when measured from the symphysis pubis to the meatus, is 3–4 inches (7.5–10.5 cm) long when flaccid (Table 97.7).[12,13] The erect penis has an average length of 6 inches (15 cm) with a range of slightly more than one inch (2.5 cm).[12,13] This increase in size is not necessarily related to the original flaccid state.

Masters and Johnson[14] point out that a penis that is larger in its flaccid state does not increase in length proportionately during erection.

Table 97.7 *Average penile size*

		Flaccid	*Erect*
Length	inches	3–4	5–7
	centimetres	7.5–10.5	12–18
Circumference	inches	2.5–4	4–6
	centimetres	6–10	8–12

Psychological factors

Virility and performance are not related to the size of the penis.[12] Orgasm in the female does not depend on deep vaginal penetration. Penile size was found to have little relationship to a partner's satisfaction from sexual intercourse. The vagina, which is 4 inches (10 cm) long in the unstretched state, tended to accommodate itself to the size of the penis.

Counselling

Counselling the male with fears about sexual inadequacy related to penile size is based on providing reassuring information about the preceding anatomical and physiological facts. The reasons for the patient's concerns should be explored. It should be pointed out that the feeling of inadequacy often follows comparisons with unreal images of macho men portrayed in the media.

If a potential problem is suspected, a useful strategy is to raise the issue subtly by using the third person; in a casual matter-of-fact manner, say something like 'It's interesting how many men worry about such things as their performance and the size of their penis'.

It is important to emphasise that there is no way of physically enlarging a penis, and this includes regular masturbation and coitus. Furthermore, it should be explained that size has absolutely no relationship with physical serviceability or with the capacity to satisfy a partner.

Sexuality in the elderly

The sexual needs of the elderly in our society tend to be ignored or misunderstood. While sexual activity and sexual interest generally decline with age, our elderly are not asexual and their sexuality has to be recognised and understood. They have the same needs as younger people—namely, the need for closeness, intimacy and body contact.[15] The same studies have shown that significant numbers of elderly people continue to enjoy both sexual interest and activity throughout their lives. Their activity is determined by factors such as marital status, knowledge about sexuality, prior patterns of sexual expression, privacy and physical health.

A common problem is that termination of sexual activity stems from the belief that people feel they are 'over the hill' and have a performance anxiety. This applies particularly to people who have invariably experienced orgasm with intercourse and then start failing to maintain this pattern.

Many women require additional lubrication and need advice about the use of oestrogen cream or lubricating jelly.

The application of the PLISSIT model applies to the elderly with an emphasis initially on permission.

References

1. Kumar PJ, Clark ML. *Clinical medicine* (2nd edn). London: Bailliere Tindall, 1990, 997–998.
2. Cohen M, Cohen G. The general practitioner as an effective sex counsellor. Aust Fam Physician, 1989; 18:207–212.
3. Richardson JD. Sexual difficulties: a general practice speciality. Aust Fam Physician, 1989; 18:200–204.
4. Williams W. *It's up to you—a self-help book for the treatment of erectile problems*. Sydney: Williams & Wilkins, 1985, 16–34.
5. Annon JS. *Behavioural treatment of sexual problems. Brief therapy.*
Hagerstown, Maryland: Harper & Rowe, 1976, 45–119.
6. Hite S. *The Hite report: a nationwide study of human sexuality*. New York: Dell Publishing Co, 1976, 229.
7. Keogh EJ. Medical management of impotence. Mod Mend Aust, Feb. 1991; 52–65.
8. Ross MW, Channon-Little LD. *Discussing sexuality*. Sydney: MacLennan & Petty, 1991, 42–66.
9. Masters WH, Johnson VE. *Human sexual inadequacy*. Boston: Little, Brown and Company, 1970.
10. Semans JH. Premature ejaculation. A new approach. South Med J, 1956; 49: 353.
11. McMahon CG. Ejaculatory dysfunction. Current Therapeutics, 1996; 37(3):49–73.
12. Green R. *Human sexuality*. Baltimore: Williams & Wilkins, 1975, 22–23.
13. Katchadourian HA, Lunde DT. *Fundamentals of human sexuality*. New York: Holt, Rinehart & Winston, 1975, 44.
14. Masters WH, Johnson VE. *Human sexual response*. Boston: Little, Brown, 1966, 191–193.
15. Cohen M. Sex after sixty. Can Fam Physician, 1984; 30:619–624.

98

Sexually transmitted diseases

He who immerses himself in sexual intercourse will be assailed by premature ageing, his strength will wane, his eyes will weaken, and a bad odour will emit from his mouth and his armpits, his teeth will fall out and many other maladies will afflict him.

Moses ben Maimon (1135–1204)
Mishneh Torah

Sexually transmitted diseases (STDs) are a group of communicable diseases, usually transmitted by sexual contact. Their incidence has been of widespread significance during the past 30 years and they are a major public health problem in all countries.

The STDs have developed a high profile in modern society with the advent of HIV infection, hepatitis B, *Chlamydia trachomatis* as a major cause of pelvic inflammatory disease, the emergence of penicillin-resistant gonorrhoea and the increasing frequency of the human papilloma (wart) virus infection with its association with carcinoma of the cervix. STDs are summarised in Table 98.1.

Key facts and guidelines

- In western society most patients with STDs are in the 15–30 year age group.[1]
- Gonorrhoea and syphilis are no longer the commonest STDs.
- Chlamydial infection, hepatitis B, human papilloma virus and genital herpes are now common infections.
- Not all STDs are manifest on the genitals.
- Not all genital lesions are STDs.
- The 5% rule[2]
  — 5% of urethritis (STD) in males is lower UTI

  — 5% of lower UTI in females is urethritis (STD)
- *Chlamydia trachomatis* is now the commonest cause of urethritis.
- NSU typically causes dysuria in men but may be asymptomatic. It usually causes no symptoms in women.
- Gonorrhoea may cause no symptoms, especially in women.
- STDs such as donovanosis, lymphogranuloma venereum and chancroid occur mainly in tropical countries. Donovanosis is common in Australian Aborigines.
- The presentation of STD in children, especially vaginitis, should alert practitioners to consider sexual abuse.
- HIV infection, which is predominantly sexually transmitted, should be considered in any person at risk of STD as well as IV drug users. It must be appreciated that it can present as an acute febrile illness (similar to Epstein-Barr mononucleosis) before going into a long asymptomatic 'carrier' phase.

Collection of specimens

It is mandatory to collect the appropriate specimens before treatment, because of the epidemiological implications.

Material requirements (obtainable from laboratories):

- standard swabs
- stiff wire swabs
- glass slides
- teflon-coated slides for viral or chlamydial microscopy
- transport media (three types)
  — Stuart's (or Amies or similar)

Table 98.1 *Sexually transmitted diseases: causative organisms and treatment*

STD	Causative organism/s	Treatment
Bacterial		
Gonorrhoea	*Neisseria gonorrhoeae*	Ciprofloxacin (o) or ceftriaxone IM or spectinomycin IM + doxycycline or azithromycin
Chlamydia urethritis Non-specific urethritis	*Chlamydia trachomatis* *Ureaplasma urealyticum* *Mycoplasma hominis*	Doxycycline (o) or azithromycin (o) as above
Cervicitis and PID	*Neisseria gonorrhoeae* *Chlamydia trachomatis* mixed 'vaginal' flora	Mild: doxycycline + metronidazole or tinidazole add amoxycillin + probenecid (if *N. gonorrhoeae*) Severe: add cephalosporins (IV use in hospital)
Syphilis	*Treponema pallidum*	Benzathine penicillin: best to refer
Bacterial vaginosis	*Gardnerella vaginalis* other anaerobes	Tinidazole or metronidazole + clindamycin 2% cream
Granuloma inguinale (Donovanosis)	*Calymmatobacterium granulomatis*	Doxycycline or azithromycin
Chancroid	*Haemophilus ducreyi*	Erythromycin or azithromycin: best to refer
Lymphogranuloma venerum	*Chlamydia trachomatis*	Doxycycline: best to refer
Viral		
AIDS	HIV_1, HIV_2	AZT/DDI/nevirapine
Genital herpes	Herpes simplex virus	Aciclovir
Genital warts	Papilloma virus	Podophyllotoxin paint or imiquimod cream
Hepatitis	HBV, HCV	Immunoglobulin/interferon
Molluscum contagiosum	Pox virus	Various simple methods, e.g. deroofing with needle
Fungal		
Vaginal thrush (possible) Balanoposthitis	*Candida albicans*	Any antifungal preparation
Protozoal		
Vaginitis, urethritis Balanoposthitis	*Trichomonas vaginalis*	Tinidazole or metronidazole
Arthropods		
Genital scabies	*Sarcoptes scabiei*	Permethrin 5% cream
Pediculosis pubis	*Phthirus pubis*	Permethrin 1% lotion

— chlamydial
— viral

Your laboratory will advise on the most appropriate test kits and methods of collection.

Presenting conditions[2]

Most STDs fit into one (or sometimes more) of the easily definable categories of clinical presentation:

• urethritis—discharge and/or dysuria

• vaginitis—discharge + irritation + odour + dyspareunia
• cervicitis/pelvic inflammatory disease (PID) (possible symptoms)
— pelvic pain/lower abdominal pain (PID)
— backache (PID)
— mild discharge
— mucopurulent cervical discharge
— dyspareunia (PID)
— dysuria
• ulcer

- lump
- pruritus
- rash with   — secondary syphilis
                  — HIV infection
                  — hepatitis B

Vaginitis

Vaginitis is presented in more detail in Chapter 87. The common pathogens are:

- *Candida albicans* → vaginal thrush
- *Trichomonas vaginalis*
- *Gardnerella vaginalis* → bacterial vaginosis

Of the three common pathogens, only *Trichomonas* is considered to be sexually transmitted and the only vaginitis requiring routine treatment of partners.

    Gardnerella is more a marker of the condition than a true pathogen. Bacterial vaginosis (also termed anaerobic vaginosis) is really an altered physiological state rather than an infection or inflammation. The hallmark of the condition is the absence of lactobacilli. It is important to note that anaerobic vaginosis is frequently asymptomatic and found by accident when vaginal swabs are made for other purposes. In these circumstances treatment is not warranted.

Collection of specimens

Make two slides:

- one smear for air-drying and Gram stain
- one wet film preparation, under a cover slip, for direct inspection for the
    — pseudohyphae of *Candida*
    — 'clue cells' of *Gardnerella*
    — motile *Trichomonas*

Treatment (in summary)[1,2]

- *Candida* on Gram stain: any antifungal preparation
    e.g. clotrimazole 500 mg vaginal tablets statim and clotrimazole 1% cream daily (or nystatin) for symptomatic relief
- *Gardnerella* on Gram stain:
    e.g. metronidazole 400 mg (o) bd for 7 days or clindamycin 2% cream
    Aci-jel topically bd
- *Trichomonas* on wet film:
    e.g. tinidazole or metronidazole 2 g (o) statim and treat partner

Urethritis

The important STDs that cause urethritis are gonorrhoea and non-specific urethritis (NSU: also termed non-gonococcal urethritis), which is three times more common than gonorrhoea.[2] NSU is commonly due to *Chlamydia trachomatis* but may also be caused by *Ureaplasma* and other unknown organisms.

Symptoms of urethritis

In males

The main symptoms (if present) are:

- a burning sensation when passing urine (dysuria)
- a penile discharge or leakage (clear, white or yellow)

Sometimes there is no discharge, just pain. Sometimes the infection is asymptomatic. Most often the symptoms are trivial with NSU. Although a creamy pus-like discharge is typical of gonorrhoea, and a less obvious milky-white or clear discharge typical of NSU, it is often difficult to differentiate the causes from the discharge. In some males the only complaint is spots on the underpants or dampness under the foreskin. Epididymo-orchitis in the young male should be presumed to be a complication of an STD urethritis.

In females

Gonorrhoea often causes no symptoms but can produce vaginal discharge or dysuria or pelvic inflammatory disease (PID). NSU usually causes no symptoms but may cause vaginal discharge, dysuria or PID. NSU is the commonest form of PID, which can result in infertility.

Gonococcal infection of anus and throat

In both sexes, gonorrhoea may infect the anus or oropharynx. Anorectal gonorrhoea may be asymptomatic or may present as a mucopurulent anal discharge (a feeling of dampness) and anal discomfort.

    Oropharangeal gonorrhoea may be asymptomatic or present as a sore throat or dysphagia.

Collection of specimens

Take two swabs:

- standard swab for *Gonococcus* (into the urethral meatus): place into Stuart's transport medium

- wire swab for *Chlamydia* (2–4 cm into the urethra and twist around), after wiping away frank pus and exudate (Fig. 98.1). Place into *Chlamydia* transport medium.

Note: A wire swab and dedicated chlamydia transport medium are essential for *Chlamydia* diagnosis, as sap from wooden swabs and chemicals from some plastics kill *Chlamydia*. But culture now less important.

In males direct immunofluorescence or ELISA will usually provide the diagnosis of chlamydial infection. The PCR chlamydia urine test (95% specific) is the preferred test.

Special notes
- Take an MSU in males who have dysuria but no discharge.

or

Take urethral swabs from females who have dysuria but not frequency. The presence of large numbers of coliform in a urethral swab culture is suggestive of bacterial cystourethritis (lower UTI).

- If there are gonococci on Gram stain, treat with ciprofloxacin and doxycycline; if no gonococci on Gram stain, treat with tetracycline; and if microscopy unavailable give both antibiotics.

Chlamydia urethritis

Incubation period
Symptoms appear 1–2 weeks after intercourse, although the incubation period can be as long as 12 weeks or as short as 5 days (compare with IP of gonorrhoea—about 2–3 days).

Treatment
doxycycline 100 mg (o) 12 hourly for 10 days [3]

or

azithromycin 1g (o) single dose (preferred)

A second course may be required if the symptoms persist or recur (about one in five cases).

urethra with urethritis

Fig. 98.1 *Taking a urethral swab*

Second-line treatment is erythromycin 500 mg qid for 7 days. All sexual partners, even if asymptomatic, need to be treated in the same way. If a female partner has proven cervicitis the treatment must be as for PID. Sexual intercourse must be avoided until the infection has cleared up in both partners. The importance of compliance must be stressed.

Prevention
Using condoms for vaginal and anal sex provides some protection.

Gonorrhoea

Incubation period
Gonorrhoea has a short incubation period of 2–3 days and symptoms usually appear 2–7 days after vaginal, anal or oral sex. The incubation period can be as long as 3 weeks.

Other manifestations of gonorrhoea
- Epididymo-orchitis and prostatitis (males)
- Urethral stricture is not uncommon in males

Treatment
If there is infection with penicillin-resistant gonococci (PPNG) due to β-lactamase (penicillinase) production (a problem prevalent in South-East Asia and eastern Australia), the following should be used:[3]

ciprofloxacin 500 mg (o) as a single dose

or

ceftriaxone 250 mg IM (with lignocaine 1%) as a single dose

or

spectinomycin 2 g IM as a single dose

plus

doxycycline 100 mg (o) bd for 10 days

or

azithromycin 1 g (o) as a single dose

Where PPNG prevalence is low:

amoxycillin 3 g (o) as a single dose + probenecid 1 g (o)

plus

doxycycline or azithromycin 1 g (o) as a single dose

If the above antibiotics are inappropriate, e.g. pregnancy:

erythromycin 500 mg (o) bd for 10 days

or

roxithromycin 300 mg (o) daily for 10 days

Sexual partners must be examined and treated

and sexual intercourse must be avoided until the infection has cleared. Follow-up culture is advisable, especially in females.

Prevention

Using condoms for vaginal, anal and oral sex provides good protection. Sexually active men and women (especially those at risk) need at least annual checks.

Cervicitis

Cervicitis is often a forerunner to pelvic inflammatory disease. If there is cervicitis only (mucopus at the cervix without uterine pain or tenderness) treat as for urethritis (the likely organisms are *Chlamydia trachomatis* or *Neisseria gonorrhoeae*) e.g. ciprofloxacin plus doxycycline.

Pelvic inflammatory disease

Pelvic inflammatory disease (PID) is covered in more detail in Chapter 84. It is not always an STD. The intrauterine device is also a common cause. Often multiple pathogens are involved in the infection.

Common pathogens are *Neisseria gonorrhoeae* and *Chlamydia trachomatis*. Swabs from the cervical os frequently underestimate the organisms involved and thus treatment needs to be directed to all possible pathogens.

Mucopurulent cervicitis is now known to be an early sign of PID, usually due to *Chlamydia*.[2]

Specimen collection

Cervical and urethral swabs for urethritis for *N. gonorrhoeae* and *C.trachomatis*.

Treatment

Therapy for PID is deliberately vigorous because the major aim is to prevent infertility and the consequent need for IVF in the long term. The detailed treatment is outlined on page 850.

Summary[2,3]

Mild infection:
a 14 day course of doxycycline 100 mg bd
and
metronidazole 400 mg bd or tinidazole 500 mg (o) daily (clindamycin if pregnant)
Add Sultrin vaginal cream if heavy discharge

If gonorrhoea: add amoxycillin 3 g (o) statim + probenecid 1 g (o)
Severe PID: hospitalise for IV therapy

Ulcers

STD causes of genital ulcers are presented in Table 98.2. Most genital ulcers are herpes—any small genital ulcer which is superficially ulcerated, scabbed, red-edged, multiple and painful is invariably herpes.

Syphilis is uncommon and may get overlooked, especially with anal chancres.

Chancroid is almost always an imported disease.

Table 98.2 *STD causes of anogenital ulcers*

	Pain	Specimen collection
Common		
Herpes simplex virus	Yes	Scraping for direct immunofluorescence Swab for antigen detection and culture into viral transport medium
Uncommon		
Treponema pallidum (primary chancre)	No	Exudate for dark ground microscopy and serum for leutic screen (reagin or treponemal tests)
Haemophilus ducreyi	Yes	Scraping for Gram stain and special culture
Calymmatobacterium granulomatis (granuloma inguinale)	No	Scraping for special stains

Genital herpes

The incubation period is usually 3–6 days but can be longer. A firm microbiological diagnosis is recommended. Swab for culture.

Symptoms

With the first attack there is a tingling or burning feeling in the genital area. A crop of small vesicles then appears; these burst after 24 hours to leave small, red, painful ulcers. The ulcers form scabs and heal after a few days. The glands in the groin can become swollen and tender, and the patient might feel unwell and have a fever.

The first attack lasts about 2 weeks.

Males

The virus usually affects the shaft of the penis, but can involve the glans and coronal sulcus, and the anus (Fig. 98.2).

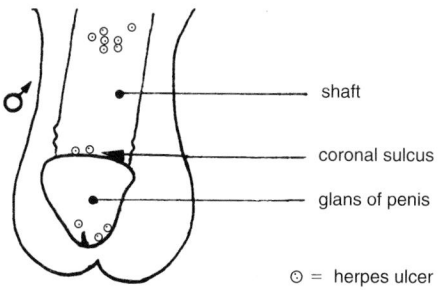

shaft

coronal sulcus

glans of penis

☉ = herpes ulcer

Fig. 98.2 *Usual sites of vesicles/ulcers in males*

Females
Vesicles develop around the opening of, and just inside, the vagina and can involve the cervix and anus (Fig. 98.3). Passing urine might be difficult, and there can be a vaginal discharge. In about 25%, the cervix is the only site of lesions and these cases may be asymptomatic.

In both sexes, it can affect the buttocks and thighs. A serious but uncommon complication, especially in females, is the inability to pass urine.

Transmission
It can be caught by direct contact through vaginal, anal or oral sex. Rarely is it transferred to the genitals from other areas of the body by the fingers. Sometimes it appears spontaneously in stable relationships.

Recurrence
Half of those who have the first episode have recurrent attacks; the others have no recurrence. Fortunately, attacks gradually become milder and less frequent, last 5–7 days and usually stop eventually. Recurrences after many months or years can be precipitated by menstruation, sexual intercourse, masturbation, skin irritation and emotional stress. Condom use reduces the risk by about 50%.

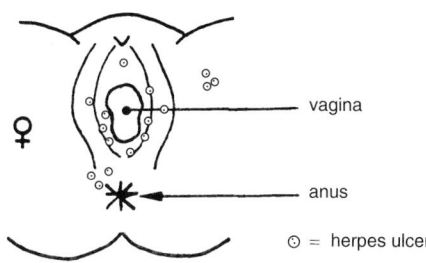

vagina

anus

☉ = herpes ulcer

Fig. 98.3 *Usual sites of vesicles/ulcers in females*

Treatment of genital herpes
Antimicrobial therapy

Topical treatment

The proven most effective topical therapy is topical aciclovir (not the ophthalmic preparation). Other topical preparations provide relief but do not alter significantly the course of the infection; they should be applied as soon as the symptoms start.

Alternatives:
10% silver nitrate solution applied with a cotton bud to the raw base of the lesions, rotating the bud over them to provide gentle debridement. Repeat once or twice. This promotes healing and spreading.

or

10% povidone-iodine (Betadine) cold sore paint on swab sticks for several days.
Pain relief can be provided in some patients with topical lignocaine.

Oral treatment

For the first episode of primary genital herpes (preferably within 24 hours of onset):
> aciclovir 200 mg 5 times a day for 7–10 days
> or until resolution of infection[2]
>> or
> famciclovir 250 mg (o) tds for 7–10 days
>> or
> valaciclovir 500 mg (o) bd for 7–10 days

This appears to reduce the duration of the lesions from 14 days to 5–7 days.[2] The drugs are not usually used for recurrent episodes, which last only 5–7 days. A 5 day course of any of the drugs can be used for a rather severe recurrence. Very frequent recurrences (six or more attacks in 6 months) benefit from continuous low-dose therapy (as above) for 6 months (e.g. valaciclovir 500 mg (o) once daily).

Supportive treatment (advice to the patient)
• Rest and relax as much as possible. Warm salt baths can be soothing.
• Icepacks or hot compresses can help.
• Painkillers such as aspirin or paracetamol give some relief.
• If urination is painful, pass urine under water in a warm bath.
• Keep the sores dry; dabbing with alcohol or using warm air from hairdryer can help.
• Leave the rash alone after cleaning and drying; do not poke or prod the sores.

• Wear loose clothing and cotton underwear. Avoid tight jeans.

Counselling

Since genital herpes is distressing and recurrent, patients are prone to feel stressed and depressed and can be assisted by appropriate counselling and support. Sexual abstinence should be practised while lesions are active. Consider referral to a self-help/support group.

Prevention

Spread of the disease can be prevented by avoiding sexual contact during activity of the lesions. Condoms offer some protection (not absolute) and patients should wash their genitals with soap and water immediately after sex. Condoms should always be used where a partner has a history of this infection.

Syphilis

In Australia syphilis usually presents either as a primary lesion or through chance finding on positive serology testing (latent syphilis).

It is important to be alert to the various manifestations of secondary syphilis. The classification and clinical features of syphilis are presented in Table 98.3 (see also Chap. 26).

Transmission

• sexual intercourse (usual common mode)
• transplacental to foetus
• blood contamination: IV drug users
• direct contact with open lesions

Management

The management of syphilis has become quite complex and referral of the patient to a specialist

Table 98.3 *Classification and clinical features of syphilis*

Type	Time period	Infectivity	Clinical features
Acquired Early (within first 2 years of infection)			
Primary	10–90 days, average 21	Infectious	Hard chancre Painless Regional lymphadenopathy
Secondary	6–8 weeks after chancre	Infectious	Coarse non-itchy maculopapular rash Constitutional symptoms (may be mild) Condylomata lata Mucous membrane lesions
Early latent	months to 2 years	Infectious	No clinical features but positive serology
Late (after the 2nd year of infection)			
Late latent	2 years plus	Non-infectious	
Tertiary (now rare)		Non-infectious	Late benign: gummas or Cardiovascular or Neurosyphilis
Congenital			
Early	within first 2 years of life	Infectious	Stillbirth or failure to thrive Nasal infection: 'snuffles' Skin and mucous membrane lesions
Late	after second year of life	Non-infectious	Stigmata, e.g. Hutchinson's teeth Eye disease CNS disease Gummas

facility for diagnosis, treatment and follow-up is recommended.

Recommended antimicrobial therapy

Early syphilis (primary, secondary or latent) of not more than one year's duration:[3]

benzathine penicillin 1.8 g IM as a single dose

or

procaine penicillin 1 g IM daily for 10 days

For patients hypersensitive to penicillin:

doxycycline 100 mg (o) 12 hourly for 14 days

or

erythromycin 500 mg (o) 6 hourly for 14 days

Note: Sex should be avoided until ulcers healed. Sexual contacts in the past 3 months should have treatment.

Late latent syphilis: more than one year or indeterminate duration:

benzathine penicillin 1.8 g IM once weekly for 3 doses, or procaine penicillin

Cardiovascular and neurosyphilis and congenital syphilis are also treated with penicillin but require special regimens.

Lump

Common pathogens:

- wart (papilloma) virus—condylomata acuminata, venereal 'warts'
- molluscum contagiosum (pox) virus

Uncommon:

- *Treponema pallidum*—condylomata lata

Diagnosis

Warts and molluscum contagiosum have a distinctive appearance and are readily diagnosed by inspection. Removal for diagnosis is usually not required. Condylomata acuminata are multiple lesions that resemble warts superficially but are covered by abundant exudate. They occur in secondary syphilis and luetic screen is positive.

Treatment of warts

Counselling and support are necessary. Not all genital warts are sexually transmitted.

Warts may be removed by chemical or physical means, or by surgery. Treatment needs to be individualised. For small numbers of readily accessible warts the simplest treatment is:[3]

- podophyllin 25% solution in tinct. benz. co.

— apply with a cotton wool swab to each wart

— wash off in 4 hours, then dust with talcum powder

— repeat twice weekly until warts disappear

or

- podophyllotoxin 0.5% paint (a more stable preparation)

— apply bd with plastic applicator for 3 days

— repeat in 4 days and then weekly for 4–6 cycles if necessary

Note: The normal surrounding skin should be spared as much as possible.

Avoid this treatment in pregnancy on cervical, meatal or anorectal warts.

Cryotherapy (liquid nitrogen) or laser or diathermy under general anaesthetic can be used for multiple lesions. Intralesional injection of alpha interferon is yet another treatment. However, the most promising treatment is topical imiquimod (Aldara) cream applied tds to each wart for 4–12 weeks.

All females (including partners of males with warts) should be referred to a specialised clinic where colposcopy is available, because of the causal link of warts to cervical cancer.

Treatment of molluscum contagiosum

These lesions often resolve spontaneously. There are many treatment choices to provoke resolution. These include:

- deroofing aseptically with a needle or sharp-pointed stick and expressing the contents (recommended)
- lifting open the tip with a sterile needle inserted from the side and applying 10% povidone-iodine (Betadine) solution
- liquid nitrogen (for a few seconds)
- application of 25% podophyllin in tinct. benzoin co.
- application of 30% trichloroacetic acid
- destruction with electrocautery or diathermy

Itch

Common pathogens:

Sarcoptes scabiei (scabies)

Phthirus pubis (pubic lice)

Candida albicans

- vulvovaginitis—females
- balanitis—males

Non-STD itchy rashes on genitals include dermatitis and psoriasis.

Diagnosis

Scabies: inspection on scraping and microscopy.

- Inspection: scabies is diagnosed by a very itchy, lumpy rash. It is rare to find the tiny mites, but it may be possible to find them in the burrows, which look like small wavy lines.

Pubic lice: inspection for moving lice and nits (eggs) on hair shaft.

Candida albicans: swab for Gram stain and *Candida* culture.

Treatment

Scabies[3]

Permethrin 5% cream if > 2 months of age. Apply to whole body from jawline down (include every flexure and area), leave overnight, then wash off. Wash clothing and linen after treatment and hang them in sun.

or

Benzyl benzoate 25%, left for 24 hours before washing off.

The whole family and close contacts must be treated regardless of symptoms which can take weeks to develop. One treatment is usually sufficient. It can be repeated in a week if necessary.

Note: Persistence of the itch after treatment is common. If the itch has not abated after 7 days, re-treat. After this, reassurance is usually all that is required. Also prescribe a topical antipruritic, e.g. crotamiton cream for 3–5 days and an oral antihistamine for the itch.

Pubic lice

Permethrin 1% lotion: apply to pubic hair and surrounding area, leave for 10 minutes and then wash off.

or

Pyrethrins 0.165% with piperonyl butoxide 2% in foam base; apply as above.

Shaving pubic hair is also effective. Bed clothes and underwear should be washed normally in hot water after treatment and hung in the sun to dry. Repeat the treatment after 7 days. Sometimes a third treatment is necessary. Sexual contacts and the family must be treated (young children can be infested from heavily infested parents). Where the lice or the nits are attached to eyelashes, insecticides should not be used: apply Vaseline liberally to the lashes.

Candidiasis

Topical imidazole, e.g. clotrimazole 1% applied 2-3 times daily

Extragenital STDs
Viral hepatitis

Sexual activity is a factor in the transmission of hepatitis B (in particular), hepatitis A (where faecal-oral contact is involved), hepatitis C (probably) and hepatitis D.[1]

Hepatitis B[1]

In western societies, sexual transmission of HBV is a common mode of spread and there is a higher prevalence in homosexual men and prostitutes. HBV prevalence in homosexual men is correlated with insertive and receptive anogenital contact and oroanal contact.

There is no specific therapy for hepatitis B, so prevention is important. Interferon α-2 can be used for complications such as chronic active hepatitis.

Prevention[1]

Several prevention strategies are available; they include:

- immunisation
- prevention of infection in health care establishments
- management of exposure (needlestick injuries, etc)
- management of infants of mothers who are hepatitis B carriers
- condoms, which offer some reduction of risk of sexual transmission
- personal hygiene

Immunisation

Immunisation should be encouraged in hepatitis B marker-free people at risk of acquiring this infection. At-risk groups include sexual partners of carriers, institutional individuals, all homosexuals, prostitutes and drug addicts. Some health workers are exposed to risk.

Management of exposure

Sexual partners of acute cases and chronic carriers who are negative for surface antigen (HBsAg) and antibody can be offered hepatitis B immunoglobin, and routine hepatitis B immunisation should be commenced.

Hepatitis C

Although there have been doubts about the potential for sexual transmission of hepatitis C, Tedder et al. in 1991[4] have demonstrated strong evidence for the sexual transmission of HCV. Interferon can be used for complications.

Human immunodeficiency virus infection

HIV infection (colloquially called AIDS, although this represents only the severe end of the disease spectrum) is predominantly sexually transmitted in the community. In Australia about 95% of current AIDS cases are sexually transmitted, 80–90% in homosexual or bisexual men.[1] The important risk factors in these men are receptive anal intercourse and multiple sexual partners.

Sexual transmission to women[1]

Although the heterosexual partners of infected men are at risk of infection, spread to and from women has been relatively uncommon in developed countries, but now appears to be increasing significantly. In central Africa, heterosexual spread appears to be an important means of transmission. Genital ulcerative diseases such as syphilis and genital herpes may be associated with an increased risk of heterosexual transmission.

HIV infection is considered in more detail in Chapter 24.

The full STD check-up[5]

Family doctors may be consulted by a prostitute or other sexually active female requesting a thorough check-up. Such people require certificates from time to time and may not have access to a public STD clinic. The visit should provide an opportunity for counselling and education about her health risks.

The screening program includes:

- Full sexual history.
- Physical examination: genital appearance, skin, breasts, oropharynx, lymph nodes, abdomen, careful anogenital examination.
- Investigations (guide only):
  1. Pap smear: 6–12 monthly.
  2. Endocervical swabs for chlamydia and gonorrhoea 1–3 monthly (depending on risk).

3. High vaginal swab and 'wet film prep' for vaginal pathogens 1–3 monthly.
4. HIV antibody test (with informed consent)—not ordered more often than every 3 months.
5. Syphilis screening test: RPR/VDRL (as for 4).
6. Hepatitis B screening: if negative, organise hepatitis B vaccination.
7. Rubella IgG as base-line test: if negative, advise rubella vaccination.

Consider

8. Throat swabs for gonorrhoea (if oral sex without condoms).
9. Urethral swab for gonorrhoea and chlamydia if urinary symptoms.
10. Anorectal swab for gonorrhoea if sexual history indicates need.

When to refer

Syphilis

- probably all suspected or confirmed cases but certainly for suspected tertiary syphilis
- HIV-positive patients, and
- suspected treatment failure

Pubic lice and scabies

- unresolved rash or itch despite apparently appropriate treatment

Genital warts

- urethral or cervical warts
- associated cervical HPV changes on cytology
- refractory warts

Gonorrhoea or non-specific urethritis

- if complications, pelvic spread or extragenital problems develop, or symptoms persist after two courses of antibiotics.

Practice tips

- Do not presume that the patient or his/her partner has acquired an STD outside their relationship.
- The itch of scabies or pubic lice can be distressing: prescribe the topical antipruritic (crotamiton cream) and/or an oral antihistamine.
- Reassure the patient that the itch will gradually subside over a few weeks (especially with scabies). This allays anxiety that may lead to overzealous self-medication.

- Make every attempt to confirm or exclude genital herpes, using the appropriate investigations.
- Use aciclovir or similar antivirals for first episodes of genital herpes and when recurrences are either frequent or painful.

Table 98.4 *STDs: Twelve golden rules of management (Venereology Society of Victoria)*

1. An STD can only be diagnosed if the possibility is considered.
2. An adequate sexual history is paramount.
3. A proper history and careful examination must precede laboratory investigations.
4. Remember the sexual partner(s)!
5. Treatment consists of the appropriate antibiotic in correct dosage for an adequate period of time.
6. A patient concerned about STDs is probably an 'at risk' patient.
7. Counselling and education are fundamental to STD management.
8. Penicillin will not cure NSU.
9. *Not* all vaginal discharges are thrush.
10. Multiple, painful genital ulcers are most often due to herpes simplex.
11. Prompt, accurate treatment of PID is necessary to preserve fertility.
12. Remember the three Cs—Consent, Confidentiality and Counselling—of HIV antibody testing.

- Twelve golden rules of management are presented in Table 98.4.

Acknowledgment

Part of this text, on hepatitis B, is reproduced from the *Handbook on sexually transmitted diseases*. 'Commonwealth of Australia copyright, reproduced by permission'. Professor John Turnidge has given permission to adopt his categories of presenting conditions.

References

1. NH&MRC Handbook on sexually transmitted diseases. Canberra: Department of Community Services and Health, 1990, 1–55.
2. Turnidge J. Sexually transmitted diseases. CHECK Programme. Melbourne: RACGP, 1989, Unit 210/211.
3. Mashford ML. *Antibiotic guidelines* (9th edn). Melbourne: Victorian Medical Postgraduate Foundation, 1996, 66–78.
4. Tedder RS, Gilson RJC, Briggs M et al. Hepatitis C virus: evidence for sexual transmission. BMJ, 1991; 302:1299–1302.
5. Bradford D. Sexually transmitted disease. CHECK Programme. Melbourne: RACGP, 1993; Unit 252/253, 7–8.

PART 8

PROBLEMS OF THE SKIN

99

A diagnostic and management approach to skin problems

The skilful doctor knows by observation, the mediocre doctor by interrogation, the ordinary doctor by palpation.

Chang Chung-ching (c. AD 170–196)

The diagnosis of skin problems depends on astute clinical skills based on a systematic history and examination and, of course, experience. If the diagnosis is in doubt it is appropriate to refer the patient to a skilled co-operative consultant, as the referral process is an excellent educational opportunity for the GP. Another opinion from a colleague/s in a group practice is also very educative. At least, cross-referencing the skin lesion with a colour atlas facilitates the learning process.

Terminology of skin lesions
Primary lesions
- *Macule.* Circumscribed area of altered skin colour < 1 cm diameter (Fig. 99.1).
- *Patch.* Macule of > 1 cm diameter (Fig. 99.1).
- *Papule.* Palpable mass on skin surface < 1 cm diameter (Fig. 99.2).
- *Maculopapule.* A raised and discoloured circumscribed lesion.
- *Nodule.* Circumscribed palpable mass > 1 cm diameter (Fig. 99.2)
- *Plaque.* A flat-topped palpable mass > 1 cm diameter.
- *Wheal.* An area of dermal oedema (can be any size).

- *Angio-oedema.* A diffuse area of oedema extending into subcutaneous tissue.
- *Vesicle.* A fluid-filled blister < 1 cm in diameter (Fig. 99.3).

Fig. 99.1 *Macule and patch*

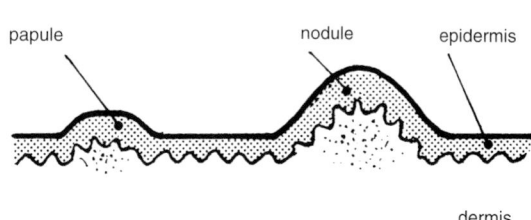

Fig. 99.2 *Papule and nodule*

Fig. 99.3 *Vesicle and bulla*

- *Bulla.* A vesicle > 1 cm diameter (Fig. 99.3).
- *Pustule.* A visible collection of pus in the skin < 1 cm diameter.
- *Abscess.* A localised collection of pus in a cavity > 1 cm diameter.
- *Furuncle.* A purulent infected hair follicle; includes:
  — folliculitis (small furuncles)
  — boils (larger furuncles)
- *Carbuncle.* A cluster of boils discharging through several openings.
- *Purpura.* Bleeding into the skin appearing as multiple haemorrhages.
- *Petechiae.* Purpuric lesions 2 mm or less in diameter.
- *Ecchymosis.* Larger purpuric lesion.
- *Haematoma.* A swelling from gross bleeding.
- *Telangiectasia.* Visible dilatation of small cutaneous blood vessels.
- *Comedo.* A plug of keratin and sebum in a dilated sebaceous gland.
- *'Blackhead'.* An open comedo.
- *'Whitehead'.* A closed comedo.

Secondary lesions

- *Scales.* An accumulation of excess keratin that presents as flaking.
- *Crust.* Superficial dried secretions (serum and exudate).
- *Ulcer.* A circumscribed deep defect with loss of all the epidermis and part or all of the dermis (Fig. 99.4); they usually heal with scarring.
- *Erosion.* A skin defect with complete or partial loss of the epidermis; they heal without scarring (Fig. 99.4).
- *Fissure.* A linear split in the epidermis and dermis (Fig. 99.4).
- *Atrophy.* Thinning or loss of epidermis and/or dermis with loss of normal skin markings.
- *Sclerosis.* Thickening of the dermis with induration of subcutaneous tissue; resembles a scar but may arise spontaneously, e.g. scleroderma.
- *Scar.* A healed dermal lesion where normal structures are replaced by fibrous tissue.

Fig. 99.4 *Ulcer, erosion and fissure*

- *Hypertrophic scar.* Rises above the skin surface.
- *Atrophic scar.* Settles below the skin surface.
- *Keloid.* Overgrowth of dense fibrous tissue extending beyond the original wound.
- *Excoriation.* Scratch marks causing an erosion or an ulcer (loss of epidermis).
- *Lichenification.* Thickening secondary to chronic scratching or rubbing (in dermatitis).

Defining terms

Terms that are continually referred to in skin disease include:

nummular	= coin-like	interchangeable
discoid	= disc-like	
annular	= ring-like	
circinate	= circular	
arcuate	= curved	
reticulate	= net-like	
pityriasis	= (pityron = bran): fine bran-like scaly desquamation	
guttate	= 'dew drop'	
rosea	= rose-coloured	
morbilliform	= like measles	
morphoea	= circumscribed scleroderma or skin infiltrate	

A diagnostic approach

The diagnostic approach of Robin Marks[1] presented here helps to achieve order in the midst of confusion. He describes the importance of simplifying the diagnostic process by being a 'lumper' rather than a 'splitter'. Most common dermatological problems fall into one of seven categories (Table 99.1). A problem that does not fit into one of these seven groups is either an unusual condition or an unusual presentation of a common condition and probably merits a consultant's opinion.

History

The three basic questions are:[1]

1. Where is the rash and where did it start?
2. How long have you had the rash?
   The split into three time zone groups (Table 99.2) is very useful. This question leads on to the next question regarding itch, as the patient is unlikely to tolerate an itchy eruption.
3. Is the rash itchy?
   If so, is it mild, moderate or severe? The nature of the itch is very helpful diagnostically. A severe itch is one that wakes the

Table 99.1 *Common dermatological conditions*

Infections
   bacterial • impetigo
   viral   • warts
                • herpes simplex, herpes zoster
                • exanthemata
   fungal   • tinea
                • candidiasis

Acne

Psoriasis

Atopic dermatitis (eczema)

Urticaria
   acute and chronic
   papular • pediculosis
              • scabies
              • insect bites

Sun-related skin cancer

Drug-related eruptions

Table 99.2 *How long has the rash been present?*

Acute (hours–days)	urticaria
	atopic dermatitis (allergic contact dermatitis particularly)
	insect bites
	drugs
	herpes
	viral exanthemata
Acute → chronic (days–weeks)	atopic dermatitis
	impetigo
	scabies
	pediculosis
	drugs
	pityriasis rosea
	psoriasis
	tinea
	candida
Chronic (weeks–months)	psoriasis
	atopic dermatitis
	tinea
	warts
	cancers
	skin infiltrations (such as granulomata, xanthomata)

patient at night and leads to marked excoriation of the skin, while a mild itch is one that is only slightly upsetting for the patient and may not be noticeable for significant periods during the day.

Three questions the doctor must consider
1. Could this be a drug rash?
2. Has this rash been modified by treatment?
3. Do any contacts have a similar rash?

Further questions for the patient
- Do you have contact with a person with a similar eruption?
- What medicines are you taking or have taken recently?
- Have you worn any new clothing recently?
- Have you been exposed to anything different recently?
- Do you have a past history of a similar rash or eczema or an allergic tendency, e.g. asthma?
- Is there a family history of skin problems?

The nature of itching[1]
The characteristics of the itch are very useful in dividing up the diagnoses: an eruption that is not itchy is unlikely to be scabies and one that is very itchy is unlikely to be a skin tumour (Table 99.3).

However, nothing is absolute and variations to the rule will occur; e.g. tinea, psoriasis and pityriasis versicolor are sometimes itchy and sometimes not. Chickenpox can vary from being intensely itchy, especially in adults, to virtually no itching.

Relieving or aggravating factors of the itch provide useful diagnostic guidelines; e.g. Whitfield's ointment applied to an itchy eruption for a provisional diagnosis of ringworm would make the itch worse if it were due to eczema.

Physical examination[1]
Examine the skin in good light, preferably natural light, and ensure that any make-up is removed.

Table 99.3 *Is the rash itchy?*

Very	urticaria
	atopic dermatitis
	scabies, pediculosis
	insect bites
	chickenpox (adults)
	dermatitis herpetiformis
	Grover's disease
Mild to moderate	tinea
	psoriasis
	drugs
	pityriasis rosea
	candida
	stress itching/lichen simplex
Often not	warts, tinea
	impetigo, psoriasis
	cancers
	viral exanthemata
	seborrhoeic dermatitis

There are two basic stages in the physical examination of a rash. The first is an assessment of the characteristics of the individual lesion and the second is the distribution or pattern of the lesions.

Characteristics of the individual lesion

The single most important discriminating feature is whether it involves the dermis alone or the epidermis as well (Table 99.4). If the lesion involves the epidermis there will be scaling, crusting, weeping, vesiculation or a combination of these (Fig. 99.5). If the dermis alone is involved the lesion is by definition a lump, a papule or a nodule (Fig. 99.6). No lesion ever involves the epidermis without involving the dermis as well.

Other characteristics of individual lesions which must be sought are the colour, the shape and the size. It is important to feel the skin during the physical examination and to note the consistency of the lesion (Is it firm or soft?). The activity of the lesion may also be useful: does it have a clearing centre and an active edge?

Distribution of the lesions

The clinician must decide whether the lesions are localised or widespread. If they are widespread, are they distributed centrally, peripherally, or both? (Table 99.5). Diagnosis is often helped when the skin lesions are in a specific area (Table 99.6 and Figs 99.7 and 99.8). Itchy papules on the penis associated with a widespread pruritus is likely to be scabies. However, care has to be taken because many misdiagnoses are made instinctively on the distribution, e.g. anything in the flexures is dermatitis or anything on the feet is tinea.

Another feature of an eruption which should

Fig. 99.5 *Epidermal skin lesion*

Fig. 99.6 *Dermal skin lesion*

be sought on examination is whether the lesions are all at the same stage of evolution.

It is necessary to perform a complete physical examination as well. There is, after all, no such thing as a skin disease but rather disease affecting the skin. The clinician must always bear this in mind when managing patients complaining of a skin eruption. Disease does not affect the skin in isolation and it is unforgivable to look only at the skin and ignore the patient as a whole.

Note: In every case examine the mouth, scalp, nails, hands and feet.

Diagnostic tools

Appropriate diagnostic tools include:
- a magnifying lens
- a diascope, which is a glass slide or clear plastic spoon that is used to blanch vascular

Table 99.4 *Appearance of individual lesions*

Epidermal	atopic dermatitis
	psoriasis
	tinea
	pityriasis rosea
	impetigo, herpes, warts
	cancers
	scabies
	solar keratoses
Dermal	urticaria
	insect bites, pediculosis, scabies
	drugs
	skin infiltrations
	viral exanthemata

Table 99.5 *Distribution of the rash*

Widespread	atopic dermatitis
	psoriasis
	scabies
	drugs
	urticaria
Central trunk	tinea versicolor
	pityriasis rosea
	viral exanthemata
Peripheral	atopic dermatitis
	herpes zoster
	tinea
	psoriasis
	warts
	insect bites

Table 99.6 *Specific areas affected*

Face	rosacea
	impetigo
	atopic dermatitis
	psoriasis
	photosensitive, e.g. drugs
	herpes simplex
	acne
	cancers
	viral exanthemata
Scalp	psoriasis
	seborrhoeic dermatitis
	pediculosis
	tinea
	chickenpox
Flexures	atopic dermatitis
	psoriasis
	seborrhoeic dermatitis
	tinea
	candida
	pediculosis
Mouth	aphthous ulcers
	herpes simplex
	candida
	measles
Nails	psoriasis
	tinea
Penis	scabies

Tables 99.1 to 99.6 have been prepared by Dr Robin Marks[1] and are reproduced with his permission.

lesions in order to determine their true colour
- a 'maggylamp', which is a hand-held fluorescent light with an incorporated magnifier; the device allows shadow-free lighting and magnification

- a dermatoscope—very valuable in the diagnosis of pigmented tumours but it does require skill and familiarity to achieve effective use
- Wood's light
- swabs for culture
- skin biopsy (even with psoriasis, etc.)

Office tests and diagnostic aids
Wood's light

Wood's light examination is an important diagnostic aid for skin problems in general practice. It has other uses, such as examination of the eye after fluorescein staining. (A new, low-cost, small ultraviolet light unit called 'the black light' is available.)

Method
Simply hold the ultraviolet light unit above the area for investigation in a dark room.

Limitations of Wood's light in diagnosis
Not all cases of tinea capitis fluoresce, because some species that cause the condition do not produce porphyrins as a by-product. See Table 99.7 for a list of the skin conditions that do fluoresce. Wood's light is really only useful for hair-bearing areas.

Porphyrins wash off with soap and water, and a negative result may occur in a patient who has shampooed the hair within 20 hours of presentation. Consequently, a negative Wood's light reading may be misleading. The appropriate way of confirming the clinical diagnosis is to send specimens of hair and skin for microscopy and culture.

Eyelids
seborrhoeic dermatitis/blepharitis
xanthelasma
allergic contact dermatitis

Face
cancers
acne
rosacea
systemic lupus erythematosus
atopic dermatitis
pityriasis alba
impetigo
keratoacanthoma

Lips
herpes simplex
Candida chelitis
leukoplakia

Scalp
tinea capitis
psoriasis
seborrhoeic dermatitis
pediculosis

Ears
seborrhoeic dermatitis
allergic contact dermatitis
solar keratosis

Nasolabial folds
perioral dermatitis
seborrhoeic dermatitis

Folliculitis
sycosis barbae (*Staph. aureus*)
tinea barbae

Chin
perioral dermatitis
seborrhoeic dermatitis
rosacea

Fig. 99.7 *Typical sites on the face affected by the skin conditions indicated*

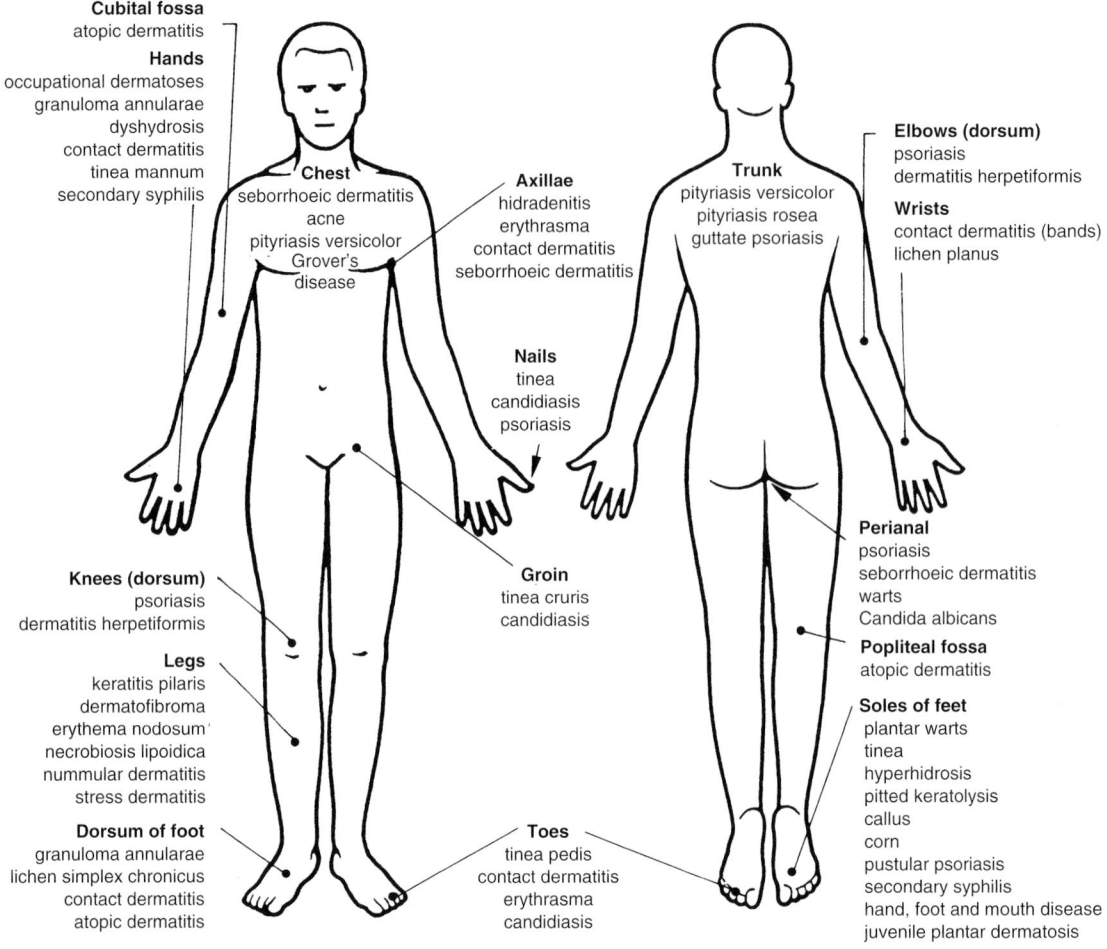

Cubital fossa
atopic dermatitis
Hands
occupational dermatoses
granuloma annularae
dyshydrosis
contact dermatitis
tinea mannum
secondary syphilis

Chest
seborrhoeic dermatitis
acne
pityriasis versicolor
Grover's
disease

Axillae
hidradenitis
erythrasma
contact dermatitis
seborrhoeic dermatitis

Trunk
pityriasis versicolor
pityriasis rosea
guttate psoriasis

Elbows (dorsum)
psoriasis
dermatitis herpetiformis

Wrists
contact dermatitis (bands)
lichen planus

Nails
tinea
candidiasis
psoriasis

Knees (dorsum)
psoriasis
dermatitis herpetiformis

Legs
keratitis pilaris
dermatofibroma
erythema nodosum
necrobiosis lipoidica
nummular dermatitis
stress dermatitis

Dorsum of foot
granuloma annularae
lichen simplex chronicus
contact dermatitis
atopic dermatitis

Groin
tinea cruris
candidiasis

Toes
tinea pedis
contact dermatitis
erythrasma
candidiasis

Perianal
psoriasis
seborrhoeic dermatitis
warts
Candida albicans

Popliteal fossa
atopic dermatitis

Soles of feet
plantar warts
tinea
hyperhidrosis
pitted keratolysis
callus
corn
pustular psoriasis
secondary syphilis
hand, foot and mouth disease
juvenile plantar dermatosis

Fig. 99.8 *Typical regional location of various skin conditions*

Skin scrapings for dermatophyte diagnosis

Skin scrapings is an excellent adjunct to diagnosis of fungal infections. Requirements are a scalpel blade, glass slide and cover slip, 20% potassium hydroxide (preferably in dimethylsulfoxide) and a microscope.

Table 99.7 *Skin conditions that produce fluorescence in Wood's light*

Tinea capitis	green
Erythrasma	coral pink
Pityriasis versicolor	pink-gold
Pseudomonas pyocyanea	yellowish-green
Porphyria cutanea tarda	red (urine)
Squamous cell carcinoma	bright red

Method
• Scrape skin from the active edge.
• Scoop the scrapings onto the glass microscope slide.
• Cover the sample with a drop of potassium hydroxide.
• Cover this with a cover slip and press down gently.
• Warm the slide and wait at least 5 minutes for 'clearing'.

Microscopic examination
• Examine at first under low power with reduced light.
• When fungal hyphae are located, change to high power.
• Use the fine focus to highlight the hyphae (Fig. 99.9).

epidermal cells

fungal hyphae

Fig. 99.9 *Diagrammatic representation of microscopic appearance of fungal hyphae*

Note: Some practice is necessary to recognise hyphae.

Other uses of microscopy
Detection of the scabies mite: the burrow of the scabies mite is found (can be difficult!) and the epidermis is decisively scraped with a No. 15 scalpel blade, and transferred to a slide after adding a drop of liquid paraffin. The mite is very distinctive.

Patch testing
Patch testing is used to determine allergens in allergic contact dermatitis. Read in 48 hours.

Biopsies
Punch or shave biopsies can be useful (see Figs 104.10 and 104.11).

Hair
Send hair samples for microscopy and root analysis.

Terminology of topical skin preparations
Bases or vehicles are a mixture of powders, water and greases (usually obtained from petroleum). The relative blending of these compounds determines the nature of the base, e.g. lotion, cream, ointment, gel or paste.

An *emollient* is a topical agent that is softening or soothing to the skin. It also acts as a skin moisturiser and is therefore used on dry skin or dermatoses related to dry skin, e.g. atopic dermatitis. Examples are:
- mineral or vegetable oil
- white petrolatum (Vaseline)
- aqueous cream

An *astringent* is a topical agent that has styptic or binding properties with an ability to stop secretions from skin or tissues. An example is aluminium acetate solution (Burow's solution); the aluminium acetate acts as a protein precipitator and is a very effective soothing agent and antipruritic.

A *keratolytic* is an agent that softens or breaks up keratin. Examples are:
- urea 10%: for xerosis or keratosis pilaris
- urea 20%: cracked palms and soles
- salicylic acid 4–10%

An *antipruritic* agent is one that relieves itching. Examples are:
- menthol (0.25%)
- phenol (0.5%)
- coal tar solution (2–10%)
- camphor (1 or 2%).

A *lotion* is a suspension of an insoluble powder in water. Modern lotions use an emulsifying agent, which eliminates the need to shake the lotion. An example is calamine lotion (zinc oxide 5, calamine 15, glycerine 5, water to 100).

Paints and *tinctures* are rapidly drying liquid preparations which are very useful for intertriginous areas, especially between the toes and natal cleft. 'Tincture' is the preparation when alcohol is the vehicle. Example: podophyllin in tinct. benz. co. (for genital warts).

Cream is a suspension of a powder in an emulsion of oil and water with the addition of an emulsifying agent.

Ointment is a suspension of a substance in an oily vehicle.

Gels are substances with a greaseless, water-miscible base.

Pastes are similar to ointments in composition but are more viscid. They consist of an ointment to which another agent such as starch has been added.

Emulsions are mixtures of two immiscible liquids, one being dispersed throughout the other in small droplets.

Table 99.8 gives guidelines for choosing a topical vehicle.

Traditional chemicals used in extemporaneous preparations[2]

Salicylic acid: produces painless destruction of epithelium, thereby facilitating absorption. Consider its use for psoriasis, neurodermatitis, tinea of palms and feet, seborrhoeic dermatitis.

Resorcinol: a topical keratolytic with bactericidal and fungicidal properties. Consider its use for psoriasis, acne, rosacea, seborrhoeic dermatitis.

Tar: the two commonly found tar preparations are used for their anti-inflammatory, soothing and antimitotic properties. Consider their use for psoriasis, atopic dermatitis, seborrhoeic dermatitis and neurodermatitis.

Menthol and *phenol:* added to various preparations for their soothing and cooling effects. Consider for use in pruritic problems such as varicella, urticaria and atopic dermatitis.

Sulphur: of benefit in dermatoses, due mainly to its keratolytic properties. The other actions of sulphur are scabicidal, parasiticidal and fungicidal. Consider its use for acne, rosacea, seborrhoeic dermatitis, psoriasis and tinea.

Dithranol: for psoriasis.

Table 99.8 *Guidelines for choosing a topical vehicle*

Disorder	Topical vehicle
Acute inflammation: erythema, weeping	wet dressing solution lotions
Subacute inflammation: erythema, scaling	creams gels (for hairy areas)
Chronic inflammation: scaling, dryness, thickening	ointments impregnated tapes

Selection of corticosteroid preparations

- Class I and class II preparations are appropriate for most problems.
- Creams or lotions are used for 'weeping' lesions, the face, flexures and hair-bearing areas.
- Use ointments for dry and scaly skin.
- Use ointments and occlusive vehicles for dry and chronic skin surfaces.
- Ointments should not be used on weeping surfaces.
- Stubborn dermatoses such as psoriasis respond better to preparations under occlusion, such as plastic wrap applied overnight with appropriate securing in place.
- Use a gel or lotion for the scalp.
- For *Candida* infection, e.g. complicating seborrhoeic napkin dermatitis, mix 1% hydrocortisone in equal quantities with an antifungal preparation such as nystatin.
- Use the weakest strength for chronic dermatoses but treat severe acute dermatoses aggressively.
- Steroids not needed if no inflammation present.

Cautions

- Avoid high-potency preparations on the face, in flexures and on infants.
- Corticosteroids can mask or prolong an infection.
- Long-term use can cause striae and skin atrophy, perioral dermatitis, 'steroid acne' and rosacea.
- Excessive use of more potent preparations can cause adrenal suppression; predispositions include use > 2 weeks, and use on thinner skin such as face, genitalia and intertriginous areas.
- Avoid sudden cessation: alternate with an emollient or a milder preparation.

The relative clinical potency of topical corticosteroids is given in Table 99.9.

Skin tips

- Do no harm. Introduce the mildest possible preparation to alleviate the problem.
- Creams tend to be drying.
- Ointments tend to reduce dryness and have greater skin penetration. If wet—use a wet

Table 99.9 *Potency ranking of the most commonly used topical corticosteroid preparations in Australia and New Zealand*

Generic name	Formulation
Group I Mild	
Hydrocortisone 0.5%	Cream
Hydrocortisone acetate 0.5%	Cream
Hydrocortisone 1%	Cream
Hydrocortisone acetate 1%	Cream, ointment
Group II Moderately potent	
Alclometasone diproprionate 0.05%	Cream, ointment
Betamethasone valerate 0.02%	Cream, ointment
Betamethasone valerate 0.05%	Cream, ointment, gel
Clobetasone butyrate 0.05%	Cream, ointment
Triamcinolone acetonide 0.02%	Cream, ointment
Triamcinolone acetonide 0.05%	Cream, ointment
Group III Potent	
Betamethasone valerate 0.1%	Cream, ointment, scalp lotion
Betamethasone diproprionate 0.05%	Cream, ointment, lotion
Diflucortolone valerate 0.1%	Cream, ointment, fatty ointment
Fluocinolone acetonide 0.025%	Cream, gel, ointment
Fluclorolone acetonide 0.025%	Cream
Fluorcortolone hexanoate 0.25%	Cream
Halcinonide 0.1%	Cream
Hydrocortisone butyrate 0.1%	Cream, lipocream
Methylprednisolone aceponate 0.1%	Cream, ointment
Mometasone furoate 0.1%	Cream, ointment, lotion
Group IV Super-potent	
Betamethasone diproprionate 0.05% (enhanced)	Cream, ointment
Clobetasol propionate 0.05%	Cream, ointment, scalp application
Preparations containing other agents	
Triamcinolone acetonide 0.01% +	
neomycin, gramicidin, nystatin	Cream, ointment
Betamethasone valerate 0.1% + gentamicin	Cream, ointment
Hydrocortisone 1% + clioquinol 1%	Cream
Hydrocortisone 1% + clioquinol 3%	Cream
Hydrocortisone 1% + clotrimazole	Cream

dressing (wet soaks and a lotion). If dry—use an ointment (salve).

- Occlusive dressings with plastic wraps permit more rapid resolution of stubborn dermatoses.
- Most toilet soaps use alkaline and are very drying; they should not be used on dry skin or dermatitis with dry skin. Soap substitutes include neutral soaps (Dove, Neutrogena), superfatted soaps (Oilatum) and non-soap cleanser (Cetaphil).
- Bath additives can be useful for dermatoses such as psoriasis, atopic dermatitis and for pruritus. For some people it may be better not to add it to the bath (diluting effect; accident from slipping) but to massage the oil into the dry itchy skin after the bath.
- Always give careful instructions to the patient regarding application of preparations: use a prepared handout if available.

- Alter the treatment according to the response.
- Explain the costs involved, especially where a preparation is expensive.
- Avoid combination creams unless clear evidence of secondary infection proven by culture and sensitivity.

Rules for prescribing creams and ointments

How much cream?[3]

On average, 30 g of cream will cover the body surface area of an adult. Ointments, despite being of thicker consistency, do not penetrate into the deeper skin layers so readily, and the requirements are slightly less. Pastes are applied thickly, and the requirements are at least 3–4 times as great as for creams.

Table 99.10 *Suitable quantities of skin preparations for specific body areas*[4] (twice daily application for 1 week)

| | Creams and ointments | | Lotions |
	Corticosteroids	Others	
Face and neck	15–30 g	15–30 g	100 mL
Both hands	15–30 g	25–50 g	200 mL
Scalp	15–30 g	50–100 g	200 mL
Both arms	30–60 g	100 g	200 mL
Both legs	100 g	100–200 g	200 mL
Trunk	100 g	400 g	500 mL
Groins and genitalia	15–30 g	15–25 g	100 mL

The 'rule of nines', used routinely to determine the percentage of body surface area affected by burns (Fig. 99.10), may also be used to calculate the amount of a topical preparation that needs to be prescribed.

For example:

- if 9% of the body surface area is affected by eczema, approximately 3 g of cream is required to cover it
- 9 g of cream is used per day if prescribed three times daily
- a 50 g tube will last 5–6 days

One gram of cream will cover an area approximately 10 cm × 10 cm (4 square inches), and this formula may be used for smaller lesions.

Table 99.10 provides guidelines for approximate weekly quantities of skin preparations required to cover specific areas of the body.

Some general rules

Remember:

- to use cream or lotions for acute rashes
- to use ointments for chronic scaling rashes
- that a thin smear only is necessary
- that 30 g
  - will cover the adult body once
  - will cover hands twice daily for 2 weeks
  - will cover a patchy rash twice daily for 1 week
- that 200 g will cover a quite severe rash twice daily for 2 weeks

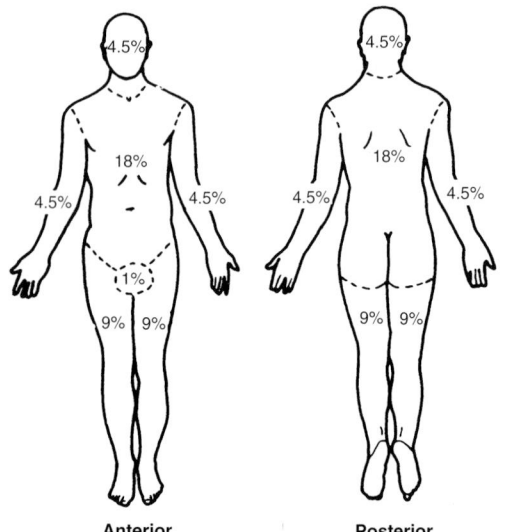

Anterior   Posterior

Fig. 99.10 *'Rule of nines' for body surface area*

References

1. Marks R. A diagnostic approach to common dermatological problems. Aust Fam Physician, 1982; 11:696–702.
2. Kelly B. Extemporaneous preparations. Aust Fam Physician, 1993; 22:842–844.
3. Gambrill J. How much cream? Aust Fam Physician, 1982; 11:350.
4. George CF et al. London: British National Formulary, Number 31, 1996; 451–456.

100

Pruritus

—

Pruritus (the Latin word for itch) is defined simply as the desire to scratch.

It is one of the most important dermatological symptoms and is usually a symptom of primary skin disease with a visible rash. However, it is a subjective symptom and diagnostic difficulties arise when pruritus is the presenting symptom of a systemic disease with or without a rash. An associated rash may also be a manifestation of the underlying disease.

The broad differential diagnoses of pruritus are:

- skin disease
- systemic disease
- psychological and emotional disorders

Physiology[1]

Itch arises from the same nerve pathway as pain, but pain and itch are distinct sensations. The difference is in the intensity of the stimulus. Unrelieved chronic itch, like unrelieved pain, can be intolerable and cause suicide. There are many similarities: both are abolished by analgesia and anaesthesia; subdued by counter-irritation, cold, heat and vibration; and referred itch occurs just like referred pain. Antihistamines which act on the HI receptor are often ineffective, suggesting that histamine is not the only mediator of itch.[1]

Localised pruritus

Pruritus may be either localised or generalised. Localised itching is generally caused by common skin conditions such as atopic dermatitis (Table 100.1). Scratch marks are generally presented. Pruritus is a feature of dry skin. An intense localised itch is suggestive of scabies, also known as 'the itch'.

Itching of the anal and vulval areas is a common presentation in general practice.

A careful examination is necessary to exclude primary skin disease; a detailed history and examination should be undertaken to determine if one of the various systemic diseases is responsible.

The history may provide a lead to the diagnosis; e.g. the itching of polycythaemia may be triggered by a hot bath which can cause an unusual prickling quality that lasts for about an hour.[2] On the other hand the itching may be caused by a primary irritant such as a 'bubble bath' preparation.

Table 100.1 *Primary skin disorders causing significant pruritus*

Atopic dermatitis (eczema)
Urticaria
Dermatitis herpetiformis
Grover's disease
Scabies
Pediculosis
Asteatosis (dry skin)
Lichen planus
Chickenpox
Contact dermatitis
Insect bites

Generalised pruritus

Pruritus may be a manifestation of systemic disease. It can accompany pregnancy, especially towards the end of the third trimester (beware of cholestasis), and disappear after childbirth. These women are then prone to pruritus if they take the contraceptive pill.[3]

Systemic causes are summarised in Table 100.2 and a summary of the diagnostic strategy model is given in Table 100.3.

Table 100.2 *Systemic conditions that can cause pruritus*

Pregnancy

Chronic renal failure

Liver disorders:
- cholestatic jaundice, e.g. carcinoma of head of pancreas
  primary biliary cirrhosis
  drugs: chlorpromazine, antibiotics
- hepatic failure

Malignancy
- lymphoma: Hodgkin's disease
- leukaemia, esp. chronic lymphatic leukaemia
- disseminated carcinoma

Haematological disorders
- polycythaemia rubra vera
- iron deficiency anaemia
- pernicious anaemia (rare)
- macroglobulinaemia

Endocrine disorders
- diabetes mellitus
- hypothyroidism
- hyperthyroidism
- carcinoid syndrome
- hyperparathyroidism

Malabsorption syndrome
- gluten sensitivity (rare)

Tropical infection/intestinal parasites
- filariasis
- hookworm

Drugs
- alkaloids
- opiates, cocaine
- quinidine
- chloroquine
- CNS stimulants

Senile pruritus

Polyarteritis nodosa

Irritants
- fibreglass
- others

Psychological and emotional causes
- anxiety/depression
- psychosis
- parasitophobia

Table 100.3 *Generalised pruritus: diagnostic strategy model*

Q. *Probability diagnosis*
A. Psychological/emotional[3]
   Old dry skin (senile pruritus)

Q. *Serious disorders not to be missed*
A. Neoplasia
   - lymphoma/Hodgkin's
   - leukaemia: CLL
   - other carcinoma
   Chronic renal failure
   Primary biliary cirrhosis

Q. *Pitfalls*
A. Pregnancy
   Tropical infection/infestation
   Polycythaemia
   Generalised sensitivity, e.g. fibreglass, bubble bath

Q. *Seven masquerades checklist*
A. Depression   √
   Diabetes   √
   Drugs   √
   Anaemia   √ iron deficiency
   Thyroid   √ hyper and hypo
   Spinal dysfunction −
   UTI   −

Q. *Is the patient trying to tell me something?*
A. Quite likely: consider anxiety, parasitophobia.

Guidelines

- The prevalence of itching in Hodgkin's disease is about 30%. The skin often looks normal but the patient will claim that the itch is unbearable.[2]
- Pruritus can be the presenting symptoms of primary biliary cirrhosis and may precede other symptoms by 1–2 years.[3] The itch is usually most marked on the palms and soles.
- Pruritus can occur in both hyperthyroidism and hypothyroidism, especially in hypothyroidism where it is associated with the dry skin.

Investigations to consider

- urinalysis
- pregnancy test
- FBE and ESR
- renal function tests
- liver function tests
- thryoid function tests
- random blood sugar
- stool examination (ova and cysts)
- chest X-ray
- lymph node biopsy (if present)
- immunological tests for primary biliary cirrhosis

Treatment

The basic principle of treatment is to determine the cause of the itch and treat it accordingly. Itch of psychogenic origin responds to appropriate therapy, such as amitriptyline for depression.[1]

If no cause is found:

- apply cooling measures, e.g. air-conditioning, cool swims
- avoid rough clothes; wear light clothing
- avoid known irritants
- avoid overheating
- avoid vasodilatation, e.g. alcohol, hot baths/ showers (keep showers short and not too hot)
- treat dry skin with appropriate moisturisers, e.g. propylene glycol in aqueous cream
- topical treatment
  - emollients to lubricate skin
  - local soothing lotion such as calamine, including menthol or phenol (avoid topical antihistamines)
  - pine tar preparations, e.g. Pinetarsol
  - crotamiton cream
- sedative antihistamines (not very effective for systemic pruritus)
- non-sedating antihistamines during day
- antidepressants or tranquillisers (if psychological cause and counselling ineffective)

Pruritic skin conditions

Scabies

Scabies is a highly infectious skin infestation caused by a tiny mite called *Sarcoptes scabiei*. The female mite burrows just beneath the skin in order to lay her eggs. She then dies. The eggs hatch into tiny mites, which spread out over the skin and live for only about 30 days. The excreta of the mites cause an allergic rash. Diagnosis is by microscopic examination of skin scrapings.

Clinical features

- intense itching (worse with warmth and at night)
- erythematous papular rash
- usually on hands and wrists
- common on male genitalia (see Chap. 98)
- also occurs on elbows, axillae, feet and ankles, nipples of females (Fig. 100.1)

Spread

The mites are spread from person to person through close personal contact (skin to skin), including sexual contact. They may also be spread through contact with infested clothes or

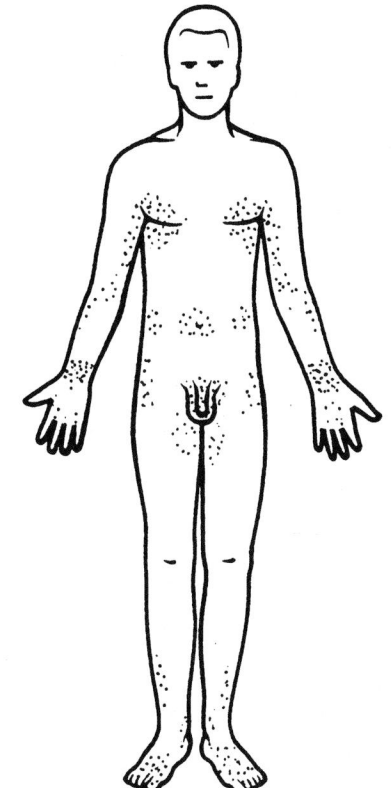

Fig. 100.1 *Typical distribution of the scabies rash*

bedding, although this is uncommon. Sometimes the whole family can get scabies. The spread is more likely with overcrowding and sexual promiscuity.

Treatment

For all ages (except children under 2 months)
   permethrin 5% cream (preferable)
            or
  benzyl benzoate 25% emulsion
  (dilute with water if under 10 years)

- apply to entire body from jawline down (including under nails, in flexures and genitals)
- leave permethrin overnight, then wash off thoroughly
- leave benzyl benzoate for 24 hours
- avoid hot baths or scrubbing before application
- treat the whole family at the same time even if they do not have the itch
- wash clothing and bedclothes as usual in hot water and hang in sun
- one treatment is usually sufficient but repeat

scabicide treatment in one week for moderate and severe infections
- for children under 2 months use sulphur 5% cream daily for 2–3 days or crotamiton 10% cream daily for 3–5 days

Dermatitis herpetiformis

This extremely itchy condition is a chronic subepidermal vesicular condition in which the herpes simplex-like vesicles erupt at the dermo-epidermal junction. The vesicles are so pruritic that it is unusual to see an intact one on presentation.

Some consider that it is always caused by a gluten-sensitive enteropathy. Most patients do have clinical coeliac disease.

Clinical features
- most common in young adults
- vesicles mainly over elbows and knees (extensor surfaces)
- also occurs on trunk, especially buttocks and shoulders (Fig. 100.2)
- vesicles rarely seen by doctors
- presents as excoriation with eczematous changes
- masquerades as scabies, excoriated eczema or insect bites
- typically lasts for decades
- associated with gluten-sensitive enteropathy
- skin biopsy shows diagnostic features

Treatment
- gluten-free diet
- dapsone (usually dramatic response)

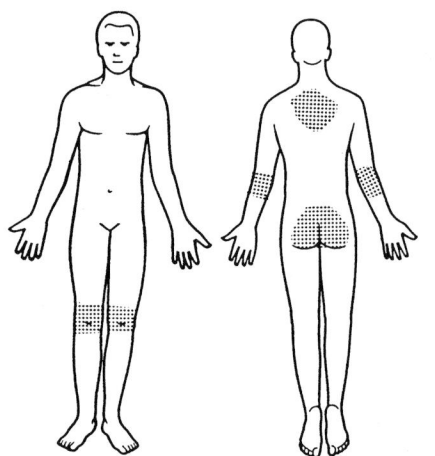

Fig. 100.2 *Typical distribution of dermatitis herpetiformis*

Lichen planus

Lichen planus is an epidermal inflammatory disorder of unknown aetiology characterised by pruritic violaceous flat-tipped papules, mainly on the wrists and legs.

Clinical features
- young and middle-aged adults
- small, shiny, lichenified plaques
- symmetrical and flat-tipped
- violaceous
- flexor surfaces: wrists, forearms, ankles
- can affect oral mucosa—white streaks or papules or ulcers
- can affect nails and scalp

Management
- explanation and reassurance
- usually resolves over months, leaving discoloured marks without scarring
- recurrence rare
- asymptomatic lesions require no treatment
- topical moderately potent corticosteroids (may use occlusive dressing)
- intralesional corticosteroids for hypertrophic lesions

Pruritus ani

The generalised disorders causing pruritus may cause pruritus ani. However, various primary skin disorders such as psoriasis, dermatitis, contact dermatitis and lichen planus may also cause it, in addition to local anal conditions. It is covered in more detail in Chapter 32.

Pruritus vulvae

Causes of an itchy vulva to consider are:
- candidiasis (rash, cottage cheese discharge)
  — broad spectrum antibiotics
  — diabetes mellitus
  — contraceptive pill
- poor hygiene and excessive sweating
- tight clothing
- sensitivity to soaps, cosmetics and contraceptive agents
- overzealous washing
- local skin conditions
  — psoriasis
  — dermatitis/eczema (uncommon cause)
- post anal conditions, e.g. haemorrhoids
- infestations
  — threadworms (children)
  — scabies
  — pediculosis pubis

- infections
  - — trichomonas
  - — urinary tract infection
  - — genital herpes
- menopause: due to oestrogen deficiency
- topical antihistamines
- vulval carcinoma
- psychological disorder, e.g. psychosexual problem, STD phobia

Treatment is according to the causation.

Jock itch

Jock itch is a term used to describe a common infection of the groin area in young men, usually athletes, that is commonly caused by a tinea infection, although there are other causes of a groin rash (Table 100.4). The dermatophytes responsible for tinea cruris (Dhobie itch) are *Trichophyton rubrum* (60%), *Epidermophyton floccosum* (30%) and *Trichophyton mentagrophytes*.[4] The organisms thrive in damp, warm, dark sites. The feet should be inspected for evidence of tinea pedis. It is transmitted by towels and other objects, particularly in locker rooms, saunas and communal showers.

Clinical features of tinea cruris
- itchy rash
- more common in young males
- strong association with tinea pedis (athlete's foot)
- usually acute onset
- more common in hot months—a summer disease
- more common in physically active people
- related to chafing in groin, e.g. tight pants, and especially nylon 'jock straps'
- scaling, especially at margin
- well-defined border (Fig. 100.3)

Table 100.4 *Common causes of a groin rash (intertrigo)*

Simple intertrigo

Skin disorders
- psoriasis
- seborrhoeic dermatitis
- dermatitis/eczema

Fungal
- candida
- tinea

Erythrasma

Contact dermatitis

definite erythematous border

Fig. 100.3 *Dermogram for tinea cruris*

If left untreated the rash may spread, especially to the inner upper thighs, while the scrotum is usually spared. Spread to the buttocks indicates *T. rubrum* infection.

Diagnostic aids
- Skin scrapings should be taken from the scaly area for preparation for microscopy (see p. 960).
- Wood's light may help the diagnosis, particularly if erythrasma is suspected.

Management of tinea cruris
- Soak the area in a warm bath and dry thoroughly.
- Apply an imidazole topical preparation, e.g. miconazole or clotrimazole cream; rub in a thin layer bd for 3–4 weeks.
- Apply tolnaftate dusting powder bd when almost healed to prevent recurrence.
- If itch is severe, a mild topical hydrocortisone preparation (additional) can be used.[4]
- If weeping: Burow's solution compresses dry the area.
- For persistent or recurrent eruption, use oral griseofulvin for 6–8 weeks, or terbinafine for 2–4 weeks.

Candida intertrigo

Candida albicans superinfects a simple intertrigo and tends to affect obese or bedridden patients, especially if incontinent.[5]

Clinical features
- occurs equally in men and women
- erythematous scaly rash in groin
- less well-defined margin than tinea (Fig. 100.4)
- associated satellite lesions
- yeast may be seen on microscopy

indefinite border with satellite macular lesions
at the edge

Fig. 100.4 *Dermogram for candidiasis of crural area*

Treatment
- Treat underlying problem.
- Apply an imidazole preparation such as miconazole 2% or clotrimazole 1%.
- Continue treatment for 2 weeks after symptoms resolve.
- Use Burow's solution compresses to dry a weeping area.
- Use short-term hydrocortisone cream for itch or inflammation (long-term aggravates the problem).

Erythrasma
Erythrasma, a common and widespread chronic superficial skin infection, is caused by the bacterium *Corynebacterium minutissimum*, which can be diagnosed by coral pink fluorescence on Wood's light examination. Itch is not a feature.

Clinical features
- superficial reddish-brown scaly patches
- enlarges peripherally
- mild infection but tends to chronicity if untreated
- coral pink fluorescence with Wood's light
- common sites: groin, axillae, submammary, toe webs (Fig. 100.5)

Treatment
- erythromycin or tetracycline (oral)
- topical imidazole

Asteatotic eczema (winter itch)
This often unrecognised problem, which can be very itchy, is a disorder of the elderly. It is a form of eczema that typically occurs on the legs of the elderly, especially if they are subjected to considerable scrubbing and bathing. Other predisposing factors include low humidity (winter, central heating) and diuretics. The problem may be part of a malabsorption state.

Clinical features
- dry skin
- fine scaling and red superficial cracking
- 'crazy paving' appearance
- occurs on legs, especially shins
- also occurs on thighs, arms and trunk

Treatment
- avoid scrubbing with soaps
- use aqueous cream and a soap substitute
- apply topical steroid diluted in white soft paraffin

Grover's disease
Also known as transient acantholytic dermatosis, Grover's disease produces small, firm, intensely pruritic, reddish-brown papules with minimal scale, mainly on the upper trunk. It usually occurs in middle-aged to elderly men (typically 70–80 years). Diagnosis is by biopsy. Treatment is to relieve the itch until spontaneous resolution occurs. Effective treatments include oral corticosteroids and ultraviolet light.

Lichen simplex
Lichenification is a form of dermatitis caused by repeated scratching or rubbing, which results in epidermal thickening. Lichen simplex is the term

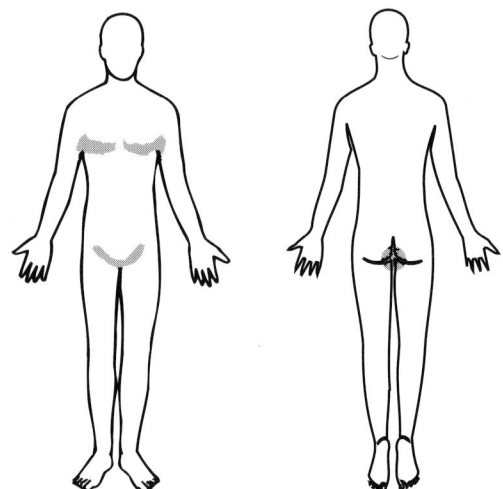

Fig. 100.5 *Typical sites of erythrasma*

used when no primary dermatological cause can be found.

Urticaria

Urticaria is a common condition that mainly affects the dermis. It can be classified as acute (minutes to weeks) or chronic (lasting more than two months).

The three characteristic features are:

• transient erythema
• transient oedema
• transient itch

Classification according to site

1. *Superficial*: affecting superficial dermis = urticaria; occurs anywhere on body, especially the limbs and trunk.
2. *Deep*: affecting subcutaneous tissue = angiooedema; occurs anywhere but especially periorbital region, lips and neck.

Checklist of causes[3]

• Allergies (acute allergic urticaria is dramatic and potentially very serious)
  — azo dyes
  — drugs: penicillin and other antibiotics
  — foods: eggs, fish, cheese, tomatoes, others
  — infections: bacteria, parasites, protozoa, yeasts
• Pharmacological
  — drugs: penicillin, aspirin, codeine
  — foods: fish, shellfish, nuts, strawberries, chocolate, artificial food colourings, wheat, soybeans
  — plants: nettles, others
• Systemic lupus erythematosus
• Physical
  — cholinergic: response to sweating induced by exercise and heat, e.g. young athletes
  — heat, cold, sunlight
• Pregnancy (last trimester)
• Unknown (idiopathic)—80%; possible psychological factors

Investigations

• full blood examination—look for eosinophilia of parasites
• ANF and DNA binding—consider SLE
• challenge tests

Treatment

• Avoid any identifiable causes.
• Avoid salicylates and related food preparations, e.g. tartrazine.
• Consider elimination diets.
• Use oral antihistamines e.g. cyproheptadine, or a non-sedating one, e.g. astemizole or terfenadine.
• Give short course of systemic corticosteroids if severe. e.g. prednisolone 50 mg once daily for 10–14 days.[6]
• Use topical soothing preparation if relatively localised, e.g. crotamiton 10%, or phenol 1% in oily calamine.
• Lukewarm baths with Pinetarsol or similar soothing bath oil.

References

1. Walsh TD. *Symptom control.* Oxford: Blackwell Scientific Publications, 1989, 286–294.
2. Hunter JAA, Savin JA, Dahl MV. *Clinical dermatology.* Oxford: Blackwell Scientific Publications, 1989, 216.
3. Fry L et al. *Illustrated encyclopedia of dermatology.* Lancaster: MTP Press, 1981, 313–315 and 485–488.
4. Gin D. Tinea infection. In: MIMS Disease Index (2nd edn). Sydney: IMS Publishing, 1996, 512.
5. Cowen P. Candidiasis, cutaneous. In: MIMS Disease Index (2nd edn). Sydney: IMS Publishing, 1996, 89–91.
6. Levine M, Lexchin J, Pellizzari R. *Drugs of choice: a formulary for general practice.* Ottawa: Canadian Medical Association, 1995, 15–33.

<h1>101</h1>

<h1>Common skin problems</h1>

The power of making a correct diagnosis is the key to all success in the treatment of skin diseases; without this faculty, the physician can never be a thorough dermatologist, and therapeutics at once cease to hold their proper position, and become empirical.

Louis A. Duhring (1845–1913)

Skin disorders are very common in general practice. According to Fry, 13% of the population (UK)[1] will be treated for skin disorders each year with the most common conditions being acute infections, dermatitis (eczema), warts, urticaria, pruritus, acne and psoriasis. According to Bridges-Webb et al,[2] 13% of the problems managed in Australian general practice will be skin problems with the most common problems (in order of frequency) being dermatitis/eczema, solar/hyper keratosis, laceration, malignant neoplasm, bruise, skin ulcer, dermatophytosis, boil/carbuncle, naevi and warts.

This chapter will focus on the common dermatoses.

Dermatitis/eczema

The terms 'dermatitis' and 'eczema' are synonymous and denote an inflammatory epidermal rash, acute or chronic, characterised by vesicles (acute stage), redness, weeping, oozing, crusting, scaling and itch.

Dermatitis can be divided into *exogenous* causes (allergic contact and primary irritant) and *endogenous*, which implies all forms of dermatitis not directly related to external causative factors. Endogenous types are atopic, nummular (discoid), dyshydrotic, pityriasis alba, lichen simplex chronicus, seborrhoeic.

The meaning of atopy

The term 'atopic' refers to a hereditary background or tendency to develop one or more of a group of conditions such as allergic rhinitis, asthma, eczema, skin sensitivities and urticaria. It is not synonymous with allergy.

An estimated 10% of the population are atopics with allergic rhinitis being the most common manifestation.[3]

Atopic dermatitis

Features of classical atopic dermatitis:[4]
- itch
- usually a family history of atopy
- about 3% of infants are affected, signs appearing between 3 months and 2 years and manifest by 5 years
- often known trigger factors (Table 101.1) are evident
- dust mite allergy is not always obvious especially for periorbital rash
- lichenification may occur with chronic atopic dermatitis
- flexures usually involved
- dryness is usually a feature

> ### Criteria for diagnosis
> - itch
> - typical morphology and distribution
> - dry skin
> - history of atopy
> - chronic relapsing dermatitis

Distribution

The typical distribution of atopic dermatitis changes as the patient grows older. In infants the rash appears typically on the cheeks of the face, the folds of the neck and scalp. It may then

Table 101.1 *Trigger factors for atopic dermatitis*

Dust mite (common)

Sweating

Sand, e.g. in sandpits

Extremes of hot and cold

Rapid temperature changes

Soap and water/frequent washing, especially in winter

Chlorinated water

Bubble baths

Infection (viral, bacterial, fungal)

Allergy

Stress/emotional factors

Skin irritants

• wool, e.g. sheepskin covers
• brushed nylon or silk clothing
• chemical disinfectants
• detergents
• petrochemical products
• pollens

Scratching and rubbing

Perfumes

Poor general health

Foodstuffs (consider)
• cow's milk
• beef
• chicken
• nuts
• eggs
• food colourants
• oranges   .
• wheat

Note: The relationship to food is controversial and uncertain. Rash testing is misleading. Consider eliminating the foodstuffs and reintroducing one at a time. If sensitive, the children go bright red a few minutes after feeding.

spread to the limbs and groins. The change from infancy through to adulthood is presented in Figures 101.1a, b, c.

During childhood a drier and thicker rash tends to develop in the cubital and popliteal fossae and on the hands and feet, which may be dry, itchy, fissured and painful.

Prognosis

It is generally correct that children tend to 'grow out of' the problem as the function of their oil and sweat glands matures. The skin becomes less dry, less overheated and irritable.[5] About 60% of patients have virtually normal skin by 6 years and 90% by puberty.[5]

Treatment

Advice to parents of affected children:

• Avoid soap and perfumed products. Use a bland bath oil in the bath and aqueous cream as a soap substitute.
• Older children should have short, tepid showers.
• Avoid rubbing and scratching—use gauze bandages with hand splints for infants.
• Avoid overheating, particularly at night.
• Avoid sudden changes of temperature, especially those that cause sweating.

Fig. 101.1a *Relative distribution of atopic dermatitis in infants*

Fig. 101.1b *Atopic dermatitis in children*

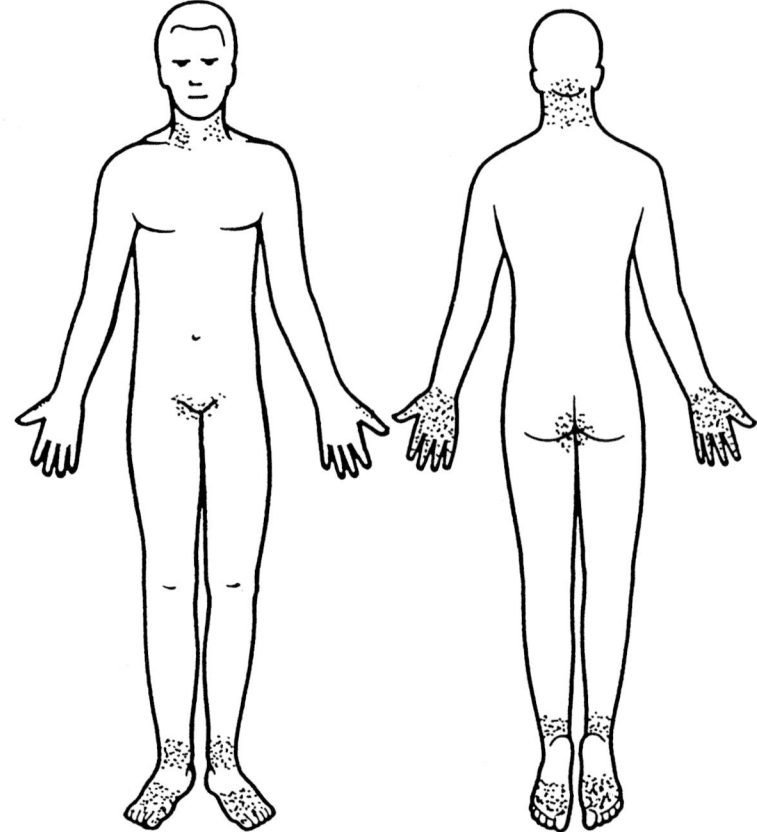

Fig. 101.1c *Typical distribution of atopic dermatitis in adults*

- Wear light, soft, loose clothes, preferably made of cotton. Cotton clothing should be worn next to the skin.
- Avoid wool next to the skin.
- Avoid dusty conditions and sand, especially sandpits.
- Avoid contact with people with 'sores', especially herpes.
- Keep the skin moist.

Consider dust mite strategies:

- dust mite covers (premium grade) for bedding
- wash linen in hot water >55°C
- consider replacing fabric on chairs and carpet

Education and reassurance

Explanation, reassurance and support are very important. Emphasise that atopic dermatitis is a superficial disorder and will not scar or disfigure under normal circumstances. The child should be treated normally in every respect. Counselling is indicated where family stress and psychological factors are contributing to the problem.

Medication

Note: Corticosteroid creams (for acute phase) and ointments (for chronic phase) are the basis of treatment.

Mild atopic dermatitis

- soap substitutes, such as aqueous cream
- emollients (choose from)
  - aqueous cream
  - sorbolene with 10% glycerol
  - bath oils, e.g. Alpha-Keri
- 1% hydrocortisone ointment (if not responding to above)

Moderate atopic dermatitis

- as for mild
- topical corticosteroids (twice daily)
  - vital for active areas
  - moderate strength, e.g. fluorinated, to trunk and limbs

— weaker strength, e.g. 1% hydrocortisone, to face and flexures
— use in cyclic fashion for chronic cases, e.g. 10 days on, 4 days off
• oral antihistamines at night for itch

Severe dermatitis
• as for mild and moderate eczema
• potent topical corticosteroids to worse areas (consider occlusive dressings)
• consider hospitalisation
• systemic corticosteroids (rarely used)
• allergy assessment if unresponsive

Weeping dermatitis (an acute phase)
This often has crusts due to exudate. Burow's solution diluted to 1 in 20 or 1 in 10 can be used to soak affected areas. Saline (1 teaspoon to 500 mL water) dressings can also be used: soak old sheets till damp and lay on the areas.

General points of dermatitis management
Acute weeping → wet dressings (saline or Burow's)
Acute → creams
Chronic → ointments, with or without occlusion
Lichenified → ointments under occlusion
Infection → antibiotics

Other types of atopic dermatitis

Nummular (discoid) eczema
• chronic, red, coin-shaped plaques
• crusted, scaling and itchy
• mainly on the legs, also buttocks and trunk
• often symmetrical
• common in middle-aged patients
• may be related to stress
• tends to persist for months

Treatment as for classical atopic dermatitis.

Pityriasis alba
• these are white patches on the face of children and adolescents
• very common mild condition
• more common around the mouth and on cheeks
• can occur on the neck and upper limbs, occasionally on trunk
• it is a subacute form of atopic dermatitis
• full repigmentation occurs eventually

Treatment
• reassurance
• simple emollients
• restrict use of soap and washing
• may prescribe hydrocortisone ointment (rarely necessary)

Lichen simplex chronicus
• circumscribed thick plaques of lichenification
• often a feature of atopic dermatitis
• caused by repeated rubbing and scratching of previously normal skin
• due to chronic itch of unknown cause
• at sites within reach of fingers, e.g. neck, forearms, thighs, vulva, heels, fingers
• may arise from habit

Treatment
• explanation
• refrain from scratching
• fluorinated corticosteroid ointment with plastic occlusion

Dyshydrotic dermatitis (pompholyx)
• typically aged 20–40
• itching vesicles on fingers
• may be larger vesicles on palms and soles
• commonly affects sides of digits and palms
• lasts a few weeks
• tends to recur
• possibly related to stress

Treatment
• as for atopic dermatitis
• potent fluorinated corticosteroids topically
• oral corticosteroids may be necessary

Asteatotic dermatitis
This is the common very itchy dermatitis that occurs in the elderly, with a dry 'crazy paving' pattern, especially on the legs (see page 970). 'Asteatotic' means without moisture.

Cracked (fissured) hands/fingers
This common cause of disability is usually due to dermatitis of the hands, or a very dry skin. It is usually part of the atopic dermatitis problem and it is important to consider allergic contact dermatitis.

Management of hand dermatitis
Hand protection:
• Avoid domestic or occupational duties that involve contact with irritants and detergents.

- Wear protective work gloves; cotton-lined PVC gloves.
- Avoid toilet soaps—use a substitute, e.g. Dove, Neutrogena.
- Cetaphil lotion is a useful soap substitute.
- Apply emollients, e.g. 2% salicylic acid in white soft paraffin (at night).
  If necessary:
  — hydrocortisone 1% ointment (not cream), or
  — stronger fluorinated preparation, or
  — tar preparation (at night).

Cracked heels

Cracked painful heels are a common problem, especially in adult women. It is a manifestation of very dry skin.

Treatment

- Soak the feet for 30 minutes in warm water containing an oil such as Alpha-Keri or Derma oil.
- Pat dry, then apply an emollient foot cream, e.g. Nutraplus (10% urea).

Contact dermatitis

Acute contact (exogenous) dermatitis can be either *irritant* or *allergic*.

Features

- itchy, inflamed skin
- red and swollen
- papulovesicular
- may be dry and fissured

Irritant contact dermatitis

Caused by primary irritants, e.g. acids, alkalis, detergents, soaps, oils, solvents. This is irritation, not allergy.

Allergic contact dermatitis

Caused by allergens that provoke an allergic reaction in some individuals only—most people can handle the chemicals without undue effect. This allergic group also includes photo-contact allergens. Contact dermatitis is due to delayed hypersensitivity, sometimes with a long time of days to years. It is common in industrial or occupational situations where it usually affects the hands and forearms.

Common allergens

- ingredients in cosmetics, e.g. perfumes, preservatives
- topical antibiotics, e.g. neomycin
- topical anaesthetics, e.g. benzocaine
- topical antihistamines
- plants: rhus, grevillea, primula, poison ivy
- metal salts, e.g. nickel sulphate, chromate
- dyes
- perfumes
- rubber/latex
- resins and glues
- coral

Note: The skin of mangoes cross-reacts with rhus and grevillea.

Clinical features[4]

- dermatitis ranges from faint erythema to 'water melon' face oedema
- worse in periorbital region, genitalia and hairy skin; least in glabrous skin, e.g. palms and soles

Note: can be delayed onset.

- think of rhus, grevillea or poison ivy allergy if puffy eyes

Diagnostic hallmarks[4]

- site and shape of lesions suggest contact
- linear lesions a feature
- allergic causes may be found by patch testing
- improvement when off work or on holiday

Diagnosis

- careful history and examination
- consider occupation; family history; vacation or travel history; clothes, e.g. wetsuits, new clothes, Lycra bras; topical applications, e.g. medicines, cosmetics
- refer to a dermatologist for patch testing

Management

- determine cause and remove it
- wash with water (only) and pat dry (avoid soap)
- if acute with blistering, apply Burow's compresses
- oral prednisolone for severe cases (start with 60 mg for adults)
- topical corticosteroid cream
- oral antibiotics for secondary infection

Seborrhoeic dermatitis

Seborrhoeic dermatitis is a very common skin inflammation that usually affects areas abundant in sebaceous glands or intertriginous areas. It is therefore common in hair-bearing areas of the body, especially the scalp and eyebrows. It can also affect the face, neck, axillae and groins, eyelids (blepharitis), external auditory meatus and nasolabial folds. The presternal area is often involved.

There are two distinct clinical forms: seborrhoeic dermatitis of infancy; and the adult form, which mainly affects young adults.

Studies have indicated that it may be caused by a reaction to the yeast *Pityrosporum ovale*. It is also associated with HIV infection and Parkinson's disease.

Principles of treatment

- Topical sulphur, salicylic acid and tar preparations are first-line treatment: they kill the yeast.
- Ketoconazole cream is most effective.
- Ketoconazole shampoo for scalp twice weekly for 4 weeks.
- Topical corticosteroids are useful for inflammation and pruritus and best used in combination. Avoid corticosteroids if possible.

Seborrhoeic dermatitis of infancy

This rash may be known as 'cradle cap' if it affects the scalp, or nappy rash/diaper dermatitis if it involves the napkin area.

It can be difficult to differentiate the rash from that of atopic dermatitis but seborrhoeic dermatitis tends to appear very early (before atopic dermatitis), even in the first month of life and mostly within the first 3 months, when androgen activity is most prevalent. The different features

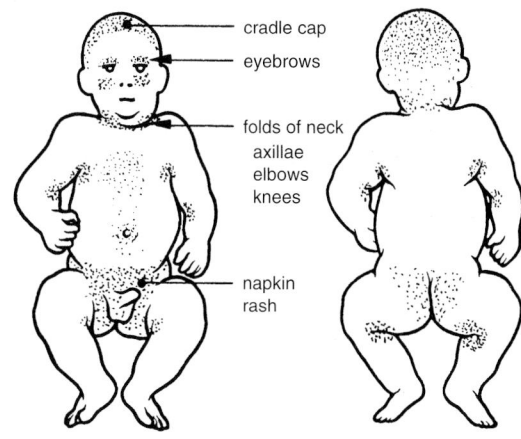

Fig. 101.2 *Seborrhoeic dermatitis: typical distribution in infants*

are summarised in Table 101.2 and the distribution is presented in Figure 101.2.

Seborrhoeic dermatitis usually appears as red patches or blotches with areas of scaling. This becomes redder when the baby cries or gets hot. Cradle cap may appear in the scalp. A flaky, scurf-like dandruff appears first, and then a yellowish, greasy, scaly crust forms. This scurf is usually associated with reddening of the skin.

The dermatitis can become infected, especially in the napkin area, and this may be difficult to treat. If untreated, it often spreads to many areas of the body. It is said that cradle cap and nappy rash 'may meet in the middle'.

Treatment

Simple basic methods:

- Keep areas dry and clean.
- Bathe in warm water, pat areas dry with a soft cloth.

Table 101.2 *Differential diagnosis of seborrhoeic dermatitis and atopic dermatitis in infancy*

	Seborrhoeic dermatitis	Atopic dermatitis (eczema)
Age of onset	mainly within first 3 months	usually after 2 months
Itchiness	nil or mild	usually severe
Distribution	scalp, cheeks, folds of neck, axillae, folds of elbows and knees	starts on face elbow and knee flexures
Typical features	cradle cap red and yellow greasy scale	vesicular and weeping becomes dry and cracked
Napkin rash	common prone to infection with *Candida*	less common
Other features	may become generalised	may become generalised

- Keep skin exposed to air and sun as much as possible.
- Avoid toilet soaps for washing (use emulsifying ointment or Cetaphil lotion).
- Rub scales of cradle cap gently with baby oil, then wash away loose scales.
- Change wet or soiled nappies often.
- For mild areas on body, apply a thin smear of zinc cream.

Medication
Scalp

- 1% sulphur and 1% salicylic acid in sorbolene cream
- apply overnight to scalp, shampoo off next day with a mild shampoo
- use 3 times a week

Face, flexures and trunk

- 2% sulphur and salicylic acid in aqueous or sorbolene cream
- hydrocortisone 1% (irritation on face and flexures)
- betamethasone 0.02–0.05% (if severe irritation on trunk)

Napkin area

- mix equal parts 1% hydrocortisone with nystatin or ketoconazole 2% or clotrimazole 1% cream

Prognosis
Most children are clear by 18 months (rare after 2 years).

Adult seborrhoeic dermatitis

Clinical features:

- any age from teenage onwards
- the head is a common area: scalp and ears, face, eyebrows, eyelids (blepharitis), nasolabial folds (Fig. 101.3)
- other areas: centre of chest, centre of back, scapular area, intertriginous areas, especially perianal (Fig. 101.4)
- red rash with yellow greasy scale
- secondary monilial infection common in flexures
- dandruff a feature of scalp area
- worse with stress and fatigue

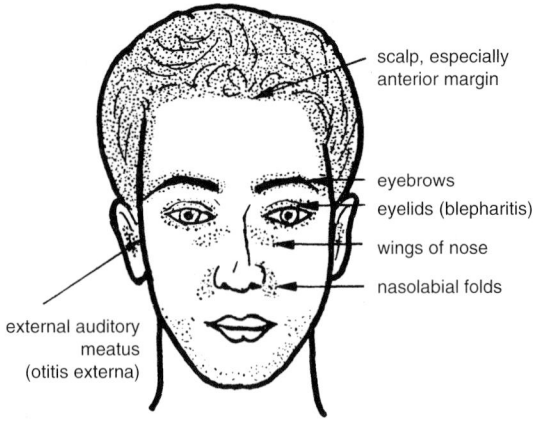

Fig. 101.3 *Seborrhoeic dermatitis: facial distribution in adults*

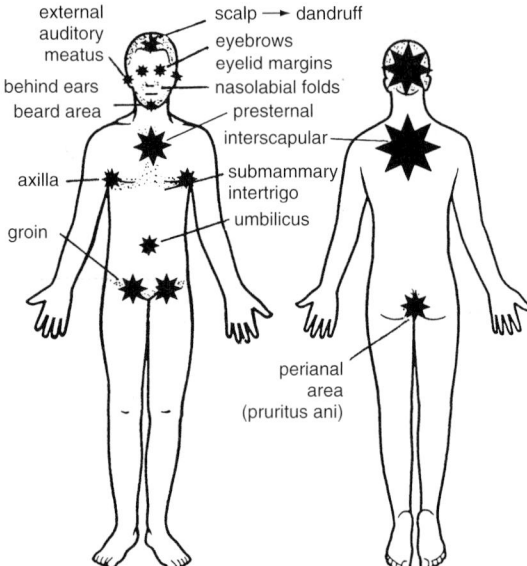

Fig. 101.4 *Seborrhoeic dermatitis: possible distribution in adults*

Treatment

Scalp

Options

1. salicylic acid 2% + sulphur 2% in aqueous cream overnight—shampoo off next day using selenium sulphide or zinc pyrithione shampoo (apply 3 times a week)
2. ketoconazole shampoo; immediately after using medicated shampoo (leave 5 minutes), twice weekly
3. betamethasone gel to scalp (if very itchy)

Face and body
- wash regularly using bland soap
- salicylic acid 2% + sulphur 2% (± tar) in aqueous cream

or

ketoconazole 2% cream (very effective); apply once daily for 4 weeks
- hydrocortisone 1% bd (if inflamed and pruritic)

Psoriasis

Psoriasis is a chronic skin disorder of unknown aetiology which affects 2–4% of the population. It appears most often between the ages of 10 and 30, although its onset can occur any time from infancy to old age. It has a familial predisposition although its mode of inheritance is debatable. If one parent is affected there is a 25% chance of developing it; this rises to 65% if both parents are affected.[3]

The feature of psoriasis is the increased frequency of mitosis and synthesis of DNA (suppressed by tar and dithranol) combined with enzyme and immune abnormalities. The result is overproduction of skin cells leading to thickening of the skin and overscaling.

Capillary dilatation explains the redness.

Types of psoriasis	Differential diagnosis
infantile	seborrhoeic dermatitis, atopic dermatitis
plaque (commonest)	seborrhoeic dermatitis, discoid eczema, solar keratoses, Bowen's disease
guttate	pityriasis rosea, secondary syphilis, drug eruption
flexural	tinea, candida intertrigo, seborrhoeic dermatitis
scalp (sebopsoriasis)	seborrhoeic dermatitis, tinea capitis
nail	tinea, idiopathic onycholysis
pustular (palmoplantar)	tinea, infected eczema
exfoliative	severe seborrhoeic dermatitis

Factors that may worsen or precipitate psoriasis
- infection, especially Group A streptococcus
- trauma or other physical stress
- emotional stress

- sunburn
- puberty/menopause
- drugs
  - antimalarials, e.g. chloroquine
  - beta-blockers
  - lithium
  - NSAIDs
  - oral contraceptives

The typical patient
- older teenager or young adult
- possible family history
- onset may follow stress, illness or injury
- rash may appear on areas of minor trauma—the Kobner phenomenon
- rash improves on exposure to sun but worse with sunburn
- worse in winter
- itching not a feature
- lesions are most unlikely to appear on the face

Arthropathy
About 5% can develop a painful arthropathy (fingers, toes or a large joint) or a spondyloarthropathy (sacroiliitis).[6]

The rash
The appearance depends on the site affected. The commonest form is plaque psoriasis which begins with red lesions that enlarge and develop silvery scaling. The commonest sites are the extensor surfaces of the elbows and knees; then the scalp, sacral areas, genitals and nails are affected (Fig. 101.5).

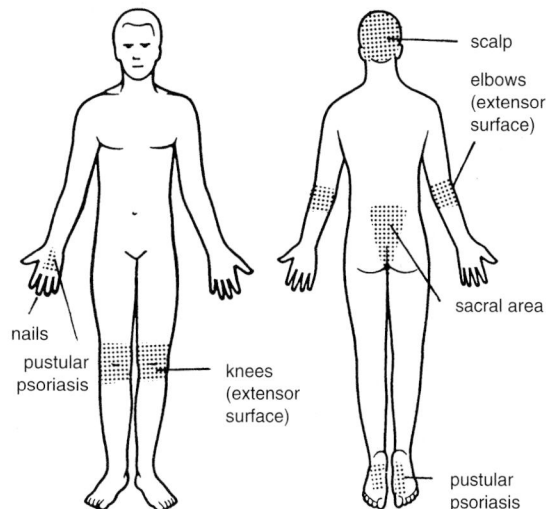

Fig. 101.5 *Psoriasis: typical skin distribution*

Diagnosis

Psoriasis is a clinical diagnosis but biopsy may be needed for confirmation. No laboratory test (including blood testing) is available.

Principles of management

While realising there is no cure for psoriasis the aim of treatment is to relieve discomfort, slow down the rapid skin cell division and work in consultation with a specialist to achieve these aims.[6]

- Provide education, reassurance and support.
- Promote general measures such as rest, and holidays preferably in the sun.
- Advise prevention, including avoidance of skin damage and stress if possible.
- Tailor treatment (including referral) according to the degree of severity and extent of the disease.

Treatment options

1. Topical therapy
   - dithranol (anthralin): concentrations range from 0.05 to 2% (maximum)
     — effective on difficult thick patches

   Note: Facts about dithranol
     — Stains light-coloured hair purple so don't use on scalp.
     — Start in low concentration and build up according to tolerance and response.
     — Use in strengths 0.05% (children), 0.1%, 0.25%, 0.5% and 2.0% (max.).
     — Can use a higher strength of 0.25% to start but only for short contact therapy (30 minutes before shower).
     — Irritates skin, causing a burning sensation.
     — Don't use it on face, genitalia or flexures.
   - tar preparations: effective but also messy to use
   - corticosteroids: the mainstay of therapy for small plaques; use 1% hydrocortisone on more sensitive areas (genitals, groin, axillae, face) but use stronger types elsewhere, e.g. betamethasone dipropionate
   - calcipotriol ointment
     — easy to use but expensive
     — apply twice daily for a minimum of 6 weeks
     — tends to irritate face and flexures

- wash hands after use
- used for chronic stable plaques (not for severe extensive rash)
- bland preparations and emollients: these can be used for dryness, scaling and itching, e.g. liquor picis carbonis (LPC) and menthol (or salicylic acid) in sorbolene base

---

Recommended topical regimens

Combined method for mild to moderate psoriasis (a good starting method)
— Dithranol 0.1%, salicylic acid 3%, LPC (tar) 10% in white soft paraffin (preferable) or sorbolene cream.
— Leave overnight (warn about dithranol stains—use old pyjamas and sheets).
— Review in 3 weeks then gradually increase strength of dithranol to 0.25%, then 0.5% then 1%. Can cut down frequency to 2–3 times per week.
— Shower in the morning and then apply a topical fluorinated corticosteroid.

Short contact anthralin therapy (SCAT method)
— apply dithranol 2% in sorbolene cream
— wash off in shower after 10–15 minutes

General adjunctive therapy
— tar baths, e.g. Pinetarsol or Polytar
— tar shampoo, e.g. Polytar, Ionil-T
— sunlight (in moderation)

2. Systemic therapy
   - methotrexate: can have dramatic results in severe cases
   - cyclosporin (hospital use only)
   - corticosteroids (for erythrodermic psoriasis only)
   - acitretin—a vitamin A derivative effective in severe intractable psoriasis (never used in females of child-bearing age)
3. Physical therapy
   - phototherapy (UVB ultraviolet light): needs careful supervision
   - UVB plus coal tar (Goeckerman regimen): reserved for severe psoriasis;
     a. tar bath
     b. UVB
     c. 2–5% crude coal tar
   - Ingram regime: also for severe psoriasis (best as inpatient)
     a. tar bath
     b. UVB
     c. 0.1%–0.5% dithranol in Lassar's paste

- photochemotherapy (PUVA = psoralen + UVA)—reserved for non-responders to UVB treatment or other therapies. A variation is REPUVA = retinoid + psoralen + UVA
- intralesional corticosteroids—an excellent and effective treatment for isolated small or moderate-sized plaques that can be readily given by the family doctor

Method of injection

Mix equal parts of triamcinolone acetonide 10 mg/mL, or similar corticosteroid, and plain local anaesthetic or normal saline and, using a 25 g or 23 g needle, infiltrate the psoriatic plaque intradermally to cover virtually all the plaque. A small plaque can be covered by a single insertion while a larger plaque may require separate insertions (Fig. 101.6)

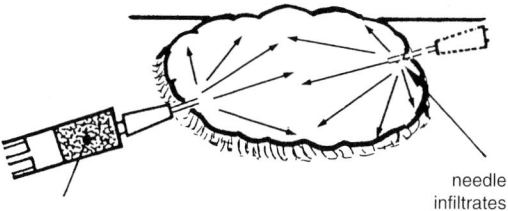

long-acting corticosteroid   needle infiltrates all areas of plaque

Fig. 101.6 *Intralesional corticosteroid injection technique for psoriatic plaque (requiring double injection—small plaques need only one infiltration)*

Other practice tips

Chronic stable plaque psoriasis
- apply stronger fluorinated corticosteroid (II–III class) cover with Duoderm Thin and leave for 7 days (other occlusive dressings can be used)

or

- tar (as an alternative to dithranol), e.g. crude coal tar 1–4% plus salicylic acid 3–5% in sorbolene cream. It can be left on overnight and washed off in the morning.

or

- calcipotriol ointment, apply bd

Resistant localised plaque
Intralesional injection with corticosteroid diluted 50:50 with N saline or local anaesthetic

Maintenance for milder stabilised plaque psoriasis
Salicyclic acid 3%, LPC 8% in sorbolene

Scalp psoriasis
- apply 20% urea cream for 4 days, then
- tar preparations for the scalp

Genital psoriasis
Apply corticosteroids

Flexural psoriasis
Note that fissuring, e.g. inframammary, natal cleft, is a feature.
- apply topical steroids—fluorinated if possible.

Nappy rash

Nappy rash (or diaper dermatitis) is an inflammatory contact dermatitis occurring in the napkin area and can be a common presentation of mild or moderate underlying skin disease. It is found in children up to 2 years old and has a peak incidence from 9–12 months.[8]

Most children will develop nappy rash at some stage of infancy with an estimated 50% having it to a significant extent. The commonest type is *irritant dermatitis*, but consider also

- *candida albicans* (invariably present although often not obvious)
- seborrhoeic dermatitis
- atopic dermatitis
- psoriasis

Causes of nappy rash
The main predisposing factor in all types is dampness due to urine and faeces. Other causes or aggravating factors are:

- a tendency of the baby to eczema
- a tendency of the baby to seborrhoeic dermatitis
- infection, especially monilia (thrush)
- rough-textured nappies
- detergents and other chemicals in nappies
- plastic pants (aggravates wetness)
- excessive washing of the skin with soap
- too much powder over the nappy area (avoid talcum powders)
- teething aggravates (punched out lesions)

Irritant dermatitis
This is a type of contact dermatitis with the erythema and scaling conforming to the napkin area. The flexures are usually spared. It is related to the activity of faecal proteases and lipases and probably not to the activity of ammonia (from urea) as previously promoted. The problem can

vary from mild erythema to a severe blistering eruption with ulceration. Ultrabsorbent disposable nappies appear to be better than cloth nappies.[9] Diarrhoea is a causative factor of irritant dermatitis. If the eruption extends further than the points of contact with the nappy an underlying skin disease such as seborrhoeic or atopic dermatitis must be suspected. Psoriasis always involves the skin folds.

Seborrhoeic dermatitis (SD)

This affects mainly the flexures of the natal cleft and groin. It is important to look for evidence of SD elsewhere, such as cradle cap and lesions on the face and axillae.

Atopic dermatitis

Atopic dermatitis can involve the napkin area. Pruritus is a feature and the child may be observed scratching the area. There may be evidence of atopic dermatitis elsewhere, such as the face.

Candidiasis (monilia nappy rash)

Superinfection of intertrigo or napkin dermatitis will result in a diffuse, red, raw, shiny rash that will involve the flexures and extend beyond the napkin area as 'satellite lesions'. *Candida* tends to invade the skin folds and the foreskin of male babies.

Uncommon causes

Psoriatic nappy rash

This presents as a dry scaling eruption, primarily on the napkin area, but can extend to the flexures, trunk and limbs. The edge of the rash is sharply demarcated. The typical psoriatic scale is absent. It tends to occur in the first weeks of life. There is usually a family history.

Infections

Bacterial infections to consider include staphylococcal folliculitis, impetigo and perianal streptococcal dermatitis. Culture of the lesion will reveal the cause.

Impetigo

If there is staphylococcus superinfection, bullae and pus-filled blisters will be present.

Histiocytosis X (Letterer-Siwe disease)

There is a similar rash to seborrhoeic dermatitis but the lesions are purpuric. In this serious disease the child is very ill and usually lymphadenopathy and hepatosplenomegaly may be found.

Zinc deficiency

May be more common than realised.

Management of nappy rash

Basic care (instructions to patients):

1. Keep the area dry. Change wet or soiled nappies frequently and as soon as you notice them. Disposable nappies are helpful.
2. After changing, gently remove any urine or moisture with diluted sorbolene cream or warm water.
3. Wash gently with warm water, pat dry (do not rub) and then apply any prescribed cream or ointment to help heal and protect the area. Vaseline or zinc cream applied lightly will do. Stoma adhesive powder is an excellent protector.
4. Expose the bare skin to fresh air wherever possible. Leave the nappy off several times a day, especially if the rash is severe.
5. Do not wash in soap or bath too often—once or twice a week is enough.
6. Avoid powder and plastic pants.
7. Use special soft nappy liners that help protect the sensitive skin.
8. Thoroughly rinse out any bleach or disinfectants.

Medical treatment

Some principles:

- The cornerstone of treatment is prevention.
- Emollients should be used to keep skin lubricated, e.g. mixture of zinc oxide and castor oil or Vaseline.
- A mild topical corticosteroid is the treatment of choice.
- It is usual to add an antifungal agent.
- Be careful of excessive use of corticosteroids, especially fluorinated steroids.
- If infection is suspected, confirm by swab or skin scraping.

Treatment

Atopic dermatitis	1% hydrocortisone
Seborrhoeic dermatitis	1% hydrocortisone + ketoconazole cream
Candida	topical nystatin at each nappy change
Widespread (candida present)	1% hydrocortisone cream mixed in equal quantities with nystatin or clotrimazole cream (apply qid after changes)

| Psoriatic dermatitis | tar preparation, or 1% hydrocortisone |
| Impetigo | topical mupirocin; oral antibiotics if severe |

Facial rashes

Common facial skin disorders include acne, rosacea, perioral dermatitis and seborrhoeic dermatitis. These conditions must be distinguished from SLE.

Acne

Acne is inflammation of the sebaceous (oil) glands of the skin. At first there is excessive sebum production due to the action of androgen. These glands become blocked (blackheads and whiteheads) due to increased keratinisation of the sebaceous duct. The bacteria in the sebum produce lipases with the resultant free fatty acids, provoking inflammation.

Types of acne[10]
- *Infantile.* Occurs in the first few months of life, mainly on the face. Affects mainly boys and is a self-limiting minor problem. Reassurance only is required in most cases. Some are severe and may scar.
- *Adolescent.* The most common type, occurring around puberty. Acne is rare under 10 years; ages 13–16 are commonest and it is worse in males aged 18–19. It is slightly less common in girls and worse around 14 years with premenstrual exacerbations.
- *Cosmetica.* In females, associated with the prolonged use of skin care products, e.g. moisturiser, foundation cream and heavy make-up.
- *Oil.* Occurs mainly on the legs of workers exposed to petroleum products.

Taking a history
Enquire about use of skin preparations—therapeutic or cosmetic; exposure to oils; possible diet relationships and drug intake.

Drugs that aggravate acne:[10]

- corticosteroids
- chloral hydrate
- iodides or bromides
- lithium
- phenytoin
- quinine
- oral contraceptives

Management
Support and counselling
Adolescents hate acne; they find it embarrassing and require the sympathetic care and support not only of their doctor but also of their family. It should not be dismissed as a minor problem.

Education
People with acne should understand its pathogenesis and be given leaflets with appropriate explanations. Myths must be dispelled:

- It is not a dietary or infectious disorder.
- It is not caused by oily hair or hair touching the forehead.
- Ordinary chemicals (including chlorine in pools) do not make it worse.
- Blackheads are not dirt, and will not dissolve in hot, soapy water.

Reassure the patient that acne usually settles by the age of 20.

General factors
- Diet is considered not to be a factor but if there is a causal relationship with any foods, e.g. chocolate, avoid them.
- Special soaps and overscrubbing are unhelpful. Use a normal soap and wash gently.
- Avoid oily or creamy cosmetics and all moisturisers. Use cosmetics sparingly.
- Avoid picking and squeezing blackheads.
- Exercise, hair washing and shampoos are not of proven value.
- Ultraviolet light such as sunlight may help improve acne.

Principles of treatment
1. Unblock the pores (follicular ducts) with keratolytics such as sulphur compounds, salicylic acid (5–10%); with benzoyl peroxide (2.5%, 5% or 10%) or retinoic acid (tretinoin) 0.01% gel, cream (0.025%, 0.05% or 0.1%), lotion or liquid.
2. Decrease bacteria in the sebum with systemic antibiotics—tetracyclines or erythromycin— or with topical antibiotics such as clindamycin.
3. Decrease sebaceous gland activity with oestrogens, spironolactone, cyproterone acetate, or isotretinoin

Note: Oral isotretinoin is teratogenic.

Recommended treatment regimes

Topical regimens

Suitable for mild to moderate acne

> *Basic starting regimen (benzoyl peroxide and tretinoin)*

- Use tretinoin 0.01% gel or 0.05% cream or iso-tretinoin 0.05% gel: apply each night (photo-sensitive).
- After 2 weeks, add benzoyl peroxide 2.5% or 5% gel once daily (in the morning). That is, maintenance treatment is:
  — tretinoin or isotretinoin at night
  — benzoyl peroxide gel mane.
- Maintain for 3 months and review.

> *Alternative regimens, if recalcitrant*

- Clindamycin HCl 600 mg in 60 mL of 70% iso-propyl alcohol, e.g. Clindatech. Apply with fin-gertips twice daily.
  Alternative bases for clindamycin, especially if the alcohol is too drying or irritating:
  — Cetaphil lotion (Alcon) 100 mL, or
  — Dermatech liquid 100 mL
  Clindamycin is particularly useful for preg-nant women and those who cannot tolerate antibiotics or exfoliants.[10]
- Erythromycin 2% gel
- Azelaic acid, apply bd

Oral antibiotics

Use for inflammatory acne:

- tetracycline 1 g per day or doxycycline 100 mg per day or minocycline 100 mg per day
- use half this dose if mild
- reduce dosage according to response
  e.g. tetracycline 250 mg per day or every second day
  or
  doxycycline 50 mg per day
  or
  minocycline 50 mg nocte
- reserve minocycline for resistant cases
- erythromycin or cotrimoxazole are alternatives
- give a minimum 12 week trial

Other therapies

Severe cystic or recalcitrant acne (specialist care)

- isotretinoin (Roaccutane)
- dapsone

Females not responding to first-line treatment

- combined oral contraceptive pill, e.g. ethinyl-oestradiol/cyproterone acetate (Diane-35 ED)

Note: Response to any acne treatment occurs in 6–8 weeks.

Rosacea

Rosacea is a common persistent eruption of unknown aetiology. It is typically chronic and persistent with a fluctuant course.

Clinical features

- mainly 30–50 years
- on forehead, cheeks, nose and chin (Fig. 101.7)
- periorbital and perioral areas spared
- vascular changes—erythema and telangiec-tasia
- inflammation—papules and pustules

Complications

- blepharitis
- conjunctivitis, rarely keratitis and corneal ulcer
- associated rhinophyma in some cases

Management

- Apply cool packs if severe.
- Avoid factors that cause facial flushings, e.g. excessive sun exposure, heat, alcohol, spicy foods, hot drinks.

Systemic antibiotics

- tetracycline (first choice)
  erythromycin (second choice)
  e.g. 500–1000 mg daily, then 250 mg daily

Fig. 101.7 *Rosacea: typical facial distribution*

when controlled, for a total of 8–10 weeks. Repeated for recurrences: avoid maintenance. If using doxycycline, start with 100 mg then 50 mg daily.

• metronidazole 200 mg bd for 10 days for resistant cases

Topical agents

• 2% sulphur in aqueous cream tds (milder cases)

or

metronidazole gel bd (more severe cases)

Note: Hydrocortisone 1% cream is effective, but steroids are best avoided and strong topical steroids should not be used because of severe rebound vascular changes.

Perioral dermatitis

Clinical features:

• acne-like dermatitis of lower face
• usually young women
• around mouth and on chin, sparing adjacent perioral area (Fig. 101.8)
• frequently begins at the nasolabial folds
• multiple small red pustules and papules
• on a background of erythema and scaling
• may be related to pregnancy and oral contraception
• may be related to repeated topical corticosteroid (especially fluorinated) use

Treatment

• Tetracycline 250 mg bd for 6–8 weeks.
• Discontinue any topical corticosteroid therapy.

Fig. 101.8 *Perioral dermatitis: typical distribution*

Tinea

Tinea, or ringworm infections, are caused mainly by three major classes of dermatophytic organisms that have the ability to invade and proliferate in keratin of the skin, nails and hair. It is most useful to perform skin scrapings and microscopy to look for encroaching septate hyphae.[11] Confirm the diagnosis by fungal culture. Tinea cruris is presented on page 969.

Tinea pedis (athlete's foot)

Tinea pedis is usually caused by *Trichophyton rubrum* and is the commonest type of fungal infection in humans. Candida intertrigo and erythrasma are important differential diagnoses.

Symptoms

The commonest symptoms are itchiness and foot odour. Sweat and water make the top layer of skin white and soggy. There is scaling, maceration and fissuring of the skin between the fourth and fifth toes and also third and fourth toes.

Management

Advice to the patient:

• Keep your feet as clean and dry as possible.
• Carefully dry your feet after bathing and showering.
• After drying your feet, use an antifungal powder, especially between the toes.
• Remove flaky skin from beneath the toes each day with dry tissue paper or gauze.
• Wear light socks made of natural absorbent fibres, such as cotton and wool, to allow better circulation of air and to reduce sweating. Avoid synthetic socks.
• Change your shoes and socks daily.
• If possible, wear open sandals or shoes with porous soles and uppers.
• Go barefoot whenever possible.
• Use thongs in public showers such as at swimming pools (rather than bare feet).

Medication

Clotrimazole 1%, ketoconazole 2% or miconazole 2% cream or lotion, applied after drying, bd or tds for 2–3 weeks. If severe and spreading, prescribe oral griseofulvin or terbinafine after confirming the diagnosis by fungal culture (see p. 986).

Tinea corporis

Tinea corporis (ringworm infection of the body) is usually caused by *Trichophyton rubrum* (60%) or *Microsporum canis*.[11] A potent source of facial tinea is the guinea pig (can present as pustular folliculitis).

Clinical features

- spreading circular erythematous lesions
- slight scaling or vesicles at the advancing edge
- central areas usually normal
- mild itch
- may involve hair, feet and nails

Management

- clotrimazole 1% or miconazole 2% cream or ketoconazole 2% cream, applied bd for 3–4 weeks
- oral terbinafine or griseofulvin if no response

Tinea manuum

Tinea manuum is ringworm infection of the hand, usually presenting with scaling of the palms and plantar aspects of the fingers. The differential diagnoses are atopic dermatitis and contact dermatitis of the hands.

Clinical features

- usually unilateral
- spreading edge
- erythematous; fine scaling
- may be associated with tinea pedis

Treatment

- topical clotrimazole 1%, ketoconazole 2% or miconazole 2% cream for 6 weeks or, if resistant, terbinafine 250 mg or griseofulvin 500 mg daily for 6 weeks.

Tinea capitis

In Australia tinea capitis is usually due to *Microsporum canis* acquired from cats and dogs.

Clinical features

- usually in children (rare after puberty)
- patches of partial alopecia
- scaly patches
- small broken-off hair shafts
- hairs fluoresce yellow-green with Wood's light (not invariably, e.g. with *T. tonsurans* infection)

Treatment

- griseofulvin (o)   Adults: 500–1000 mg daily
                      Children: 10 mg/kg/day
                      (max. 250 mg)

  6 week course

Kerion

Kerion of the scalp and beard area may present like an abscess—tender and fluctuant. Usually occurs on the scalp, face or limbs. A fungal cause is possible if the hairs are plucked out easily and without pain (if painful and stuck, bacterial infection is likely).

Tinea incognito

This is the term used for unrecognised tinea infection due to modification with corticosteroid treatment. The lesions are enlarging and persistent, especially on the groins, hands and face.

The sequence is initial symptomatic relief of itching, stopping the ointment or cream and then relapse.

Tinea unguium (toenails and finernails)

These onychomycosis problems are chronic and very resistant to treatment:

- usually associated with tinea pedis
- nails may show white spots
- may be yellow-brown and crumbling
- may start from edge (periphery) and spread towards base

Treatment[11,12]

Fingernails: terbinafine 250 mg (o) daily for 6 weeks, or griseofulvin 500 mg daily (o) for 6 months

Toenails: terbinafine 250 mg (o) daily for 12 weeks, or griseofulvin for 12–18 months

New treatments: amorolfine nail lacquer 1–2 times weekly (fingernails: 6 months; toenails: 6 or more months)

> **Topical tip**

Cut affected nail well back, elevate the nail slightly at the edges and apply tincture of Daktarin to and under nail bd for several weeks.

Griseofulvin treatment: significant side effects include headaches and (long-term) bone marrow suppression or liver toxicity. Regular screening with FBE and LFTs advisable.

Pityriasis versicolor (tinea versicolor)

Pityriasis versicolor is a superficial yeast infection of the skin (usually on the trunk) caused by *Pityrosporum orbiculare* (*Malassezia furfur*). The old name, tinea versicolor, is inappropriate because the problem is not a dermatophyte infection. It occurs worldwide but is more common in tropical and subtropical climates. There are two distinct presentations:

1. reddish brown, slightly scaly patches on upper trunk
2. hypopigmented area that will not tan, especially in suntanned skin

The term 'versicolor' means variable colours.

Clinical features

- mainly young and middle-aged adults
- brown on pale skin or white on tanned skin
- trunk distribution (Fig. 101.9)
- patches may coalesce
- may involve neck, upper arms, face and groin
- scales removed by scraping show characteristic short stunted hyphae with spores on microscopy

Differential diagnosis

Seborrhoeic dermatitis of trunk (more erythematous), pityriasis rosea, vitiligo, pityriasis alba (affects face).

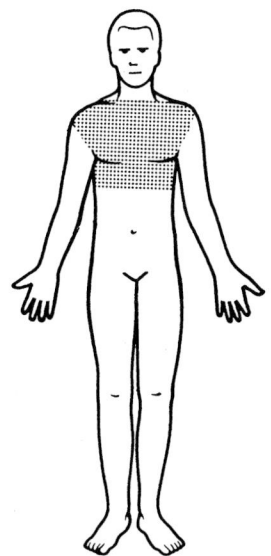

Fig. 101.9 *Pityriasis versicolor: typical truncal distribution (corresponding area on back)*

Treatment

- Selenium sulfide (Selsun yellow shampoo). Wash area, leaving on for 5–10 minutes, then wash off. Do this daily for 2 weeks (at night), then every second day for 2 weeks, then monthly for 12 months. Shampoo scalp twice weekly.

    and/or

- Clotrimazole, miconazole or ketaconazole cream/lotion nocte for 2–4 weeks

    or

- Terbinafine 1% cream twice daily[12] for 2 weeks

    or

- Sodium thiosulphate 25% solution bd for 4 weeks (wash off after 10 minutes)

    or

    (for persistent or recurrent problems)

- Ketoconazole 200 mg daily for 7–10 days or 400 mg single dose[13]

Note: Ketoconazole may be hepatotoxic. Always perform LFTs first (do not use long-term). Griseofulvin is inappropriate because the rash is not a fungal infection.

Warn patients that the white patches will take a long time to disappear and that cure does not equate with disappearance.

Dry skin

Disorders associated with scaling and roughness of the skin include:

- atopic dermatitis—all types, e.g. pityriasis alba, nummular eczema, asteatotic dermatitis
- ageing skin
- psoriasis
- ichthyotic disorders
- keratosis pilaris

Itching may be a feature of dry skin (but is not inevitable).

Aggravating factors:

- low humidity, e.g. heaters, air-conditioners
- frequent immersion in water
- heat/hot water
- toilet soaps

Management

- Ensure humidification if there is central heating.
- Reduce bathing.
- Bathe or shower in tepid water.
- Use a soap substitute, e.g. Dove or Neutrogena/ Cetaphil lotion.

- Pat dry—avoid vigorous towelling.
- Rub in baby oil after bathing (better than adding oil to the bath
- Avoid wool next to the skin (wear cotton).
- Use emollients, e.g. Alpha-Keri lotion, QV skin lotion.
- Use moisturisers, e.g. Nutraplus, Calmurid.

Sunburn

Sunburn is normally caused by ultraviolet B (UV-B) radiation which penetrates the epidermis and superficial dermis, releasing substances such as leukotrienes and histamines which cause redness and pain. Severe sunburn may develop on relatively dull days because thin clouds filter UV-B poorly.

Clinical presentations:

Minor sunburn	Mild erythema with minimal discomfort for about 3 days.
Moderate	Moderate to severe erythema within a few hours; worse the following day—red, hot and moderately painful. Settles in 3–4 days with some desquamation.
Severe	Classic signs of inflammation—redness, heat, pain and swelling. Skin develops vesicles and bullae. Systemic features develop with very severe burns, e.g. fever, headache, nausea, delirium, hypotension. May require IV fluids.

Differential diagnosis

- general photosensitivity: consider drugs, e.g. thiazide diuretics, tetracyclines, sulphonamides, phenothiazines, griseofulvin, NSAIDs
- acute systemic lupus erythematosus may present as unexpectedly severe sunburn
- photocontact dermatitis

Treatment

Hydrocortisone 1% ointment or cream for severe sunburn, early. Repeat in 2–3 hours and then the next day. Hydrocortisone is not useful after 24 hours and should be used for unblistered erythematous skin, not on broken skin.

Oral aspirin eases pain. Oil in water baths or bicarbonate of soda paste may help and wet applications such as oily calamine lotions may give relief.

Prevention

Avoid exposure to summer sunlight 10 am to 3 pm (or 11 am to 4 pm summer time saving). Use natural shade—beware of reflected light from sand or water and light cloud. Use a sunscreen with a minimum of SPF 15+. Wear broad-brimmed hats and protective clothing.

References

1. Fry J. *Common diseases* (4th edn). Lancaster: MTP Press Limited, 1985, 337–339.
2. Bridges-Webb C. Morbidity and treatment in general practice. Med J Aust: Supplement, 19 October 1992, 26–27.
3. Berger P. *Skin secrets*. Sydney: Allen & Unwin, 1991, 93–170.
4. Brown P. Dermatitis/eczema. In: MIMS Disease Index (2nd edn). Sydney: IMS Publishing, 1996, 142–144.
5. Millard LG. Irritable papular rashes. Medicine International,1988; 49:2007–2011.
6. Brown M. Psoriasis. In: MIMS Disease Index (2nd edn). Sydney: IMS Publishing, 1996, 430–432.
7. Buxton PK. *ABC of dermatology*. London: British Medical Association, 1989, 40.
8. Gallachio V. Nappy rash. Aust Fam Physician, 1988; 17:971–972.
9. Aldridge S. Nappy rash. Aust Paed Review, 1991; 2(1):2.
10. Berger P. Acne—pathogenesis and treatment. Mod Med Aust, September 1990; 83–89.
11. Gin D. Tinea infections. In: MIMS Disease Index (2nd edn). Sydney: IMS Publishing, 1996, 511–513.
12. Levine M, Lexchin J, Pelizzzari R. *Drugs of choice: a formulary for general practice.* Ottawa: Canadian Medical Association, 1995, 15–33.
13. Hunter JAA, Savin JA, Dahl MV. *Clinical dermatology.* Oxford: Blackwell Scientific Publications, 1989, 162–163.

102

Acute skin eruptions

—

They say love's like the measles—all the worse when it comes late in life.

Douglas Jerrold (1803–57)

The sudden appearance of a rash which is a common presentation in children (Chap. 74), usually provokes patients and doctors alike to consider an infectious aetiology, commonly of viral origin. However, an important cause to consider is a reaction to a drug.

A knowledge of the relative distribution of the various causes of rashes helps with the diagnostic methodology. Many of the eruptions are relatively benign and undergo spontaneous remission. Fortunately, the potentially deadly rash of smallpox is no longer encountered.

Serious eruptions that demand accurate diagnosis and management include:

- primary HIV infection
- secondary syphilis
- Stevens-Johnson syndrome
- purpuric eruption of meningococcal septicaemia, typhoid, measles, other septicaemia

A list of important causes of acute skin eruptions is presented in Table 102.1.

The diagnostic approach

The diagnostic approach to skin eruptions presupposes a basic knowledge of the causes, and then a careful history and physical examination should logically follow.

The history should include:

- site and mode of onset of the rash
- mode of progression
- drug history
- constitutional disturbance, e.g. pyrexia, pruritus
- respiratory symptoms

Table 102.1 *Important causes of acute skin eruptions*

Maculopapular
- measles
- rubella
- scarlet fever
- viral exanthem (fourth disease)
- erythema infectiosum (slapped face syndrome or fifth disease)
- roseola infantum (sixth disease)
- Epstein-Barr mononucleosis (primary or secondary to drugs)
- primary HIV infection
- secondary syphilis
- pityriasis rosea
- guttate psoriasis
- urticaria
- erythema multiforme (may be vesicular)
- drug reaction
- scabies
- Ross River and Barmah Forest infection

Maculopapular vesicular
- varicella
- herpes zoster
- herpes simplex
- eczema herpeticum
- impetigo
- hand, foot and mouth disease
- drug reaction

Maculopapular pustular
- pseudomonas folliculitis
- staphylococcus aureus folliculitis
- impetigo

Purpuric (haemorrhagic) eruption
- purpura, e.g. drug-induced purpura, severe infection
- vasculitis (vascular purpura)
  — Henoch-Schönlein purpura
  — polyarteritis nodosa

- herald patch?
- diet—unaccustomed food
- exposure to irritants
- contacts with infectious disease

• bleeding or bruising tendency.

The examination should include:

• skin of whole body
• nature and distribution of rash
• soles of feet
• mucous membranes
• oropharynx
• conjunctivae and the lymphopoietic system (? lymphadenopathy ? splenomegaly).

Laboratory investigations may include:

• a full blood examination
• syphilis serology
• Epstein-Barr mononucleosis test
• HIV test
• rubella haemagglutination tests ($\times$ 2)
• viral and bacterial cultures

Acute skin eruptions in children

The following skin eruptions (some of which may also occur in adults) are outlined in childhood infectious diseases (Chap. 74).

• measles (p. 761)
• rubella (p. 761)
• viral exanthem (fourth disease) (p. 763)
• erythema infectiosum (fifth disease) (p. 763)
• roseola infantum (sixth disease) (p. 763)
• Kawasaki's disease (p. 764)
• varicella (p. 758)
• impetigo (p. 767)

Pityriasis rosea

Pityriasis rosea is a common but mild acute inflammatory skin disorder. Although a viral agent is suspected to be the cause, no infective agent has been demonstrated.

Clinical features

• any age, mainly young adults (aged 15–30)
• preceding herald patch (1–2 weeks); can have 2–3, but none in 20%
• oval, salmon-pink or copper-coloured eruption
• coin-shaped patches with scaly margins
• follows cleavage lines of skin (Fig. 102.1)
• on trunk ('T-shirt' distribution)
• occurs also on upper arms, upper legs, neck, face (rare) and axillae
• patients not ill
• itch varies from nil to severe (typically minor itching)
• scale is on inner aspect of active border

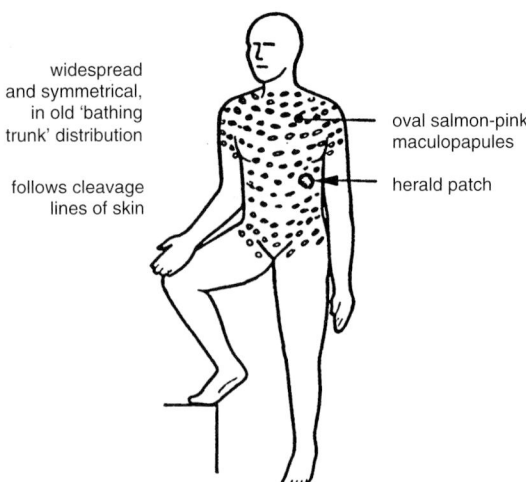

widespread and symmetrical, in old 'bathing trunk' distribution

follows cleavage lines of skin

oval salmon-pink maculopapules

herald patch

Fig. 102.1 *Pityriasis rosea: typical distribution*

Differential diagnosis

Herald patch — tinea corporis
Generalised rash — seborrhoeic dermatitis (slower onset), guttate psoriasis, drug eruption (Table 102.2), secondary syphilis

Prognosis

A mild self-limiting disorder with spontaneous remission in 2–10 weeks (average 2–5). It does not appear to be contagious.

Management

• Explain and reassure with patient education handout.[1]
• Bathe and shower as usual, using a neutral soap, e.g. Neutrogena.
• Use a soothing bath oil, e.g. QV bath oil.
• For bothersome itch: apply mild topical corticosteroid ointment or calamine lotion with 1% phenol or urea cream.

Table 102.2 *Drugs that cause eruptions suggestive of pityriasis rosea*[2]

Main drugs
• gold salts
• penicillamine
• captopril

Others
• arsenicals
• barbiturates
• bismuth
• clonidine
• metoprolol
• metronidazole

- Ultraviolet therapy is good but, like psoriasis, sunburn must be avoided. Expose rash to sunlight or UV therapy (if florid) three times a week.

Secondary syphilis

The generalised skin eruption of secondary syphilis varies and may resemble any type of eruption from psoriasiform to rubelliform to roseoliform. The rash usually appears 6–8 weeks after the primary chancre.

Features of the rash
- initially faint pink macules
- then becomes maculopapular
- can involve whole of body (Fig. 102.2)
- palms and soles involved
- dull red in colour and round
- more prolific on flexor surfaces
- symmetrical and relatively coarse
- asymptomatic

Associations (possible)
- mucosal ulcers: 'snail track'
- lymphadenopathy
- patchy hair loss
- condylomata lata

Treatment
- as for primary syphilis (Chap. 98)

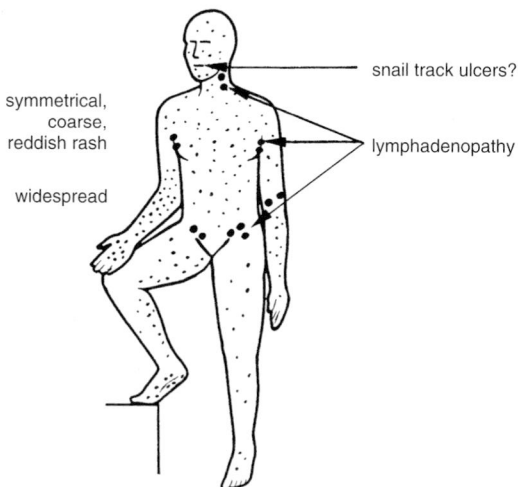

symmetrical, coarse, reddish rash

widespread

snail track ulcers?

lymphadenopathy

Fig. 102.2 *Secondary syphilis: typical features*

Primary HIV infection

A common manifestation of the primary HIV infection is an erythematous, maculopapular rash, although other skin manifestations such as a roseola-like rash and urticaria can occur.

Clinical features
- symmetrical
- may be generalised
- lesions 5–10 mm in diameter
- common on face and/or trunk
- can occur on extremities including palms and soles (Fig. 102.3)
- non-pruritic

If such a rash accompanied by an illness like glandular fever occurs, HIV infection should be suspected and specific tests ordered.

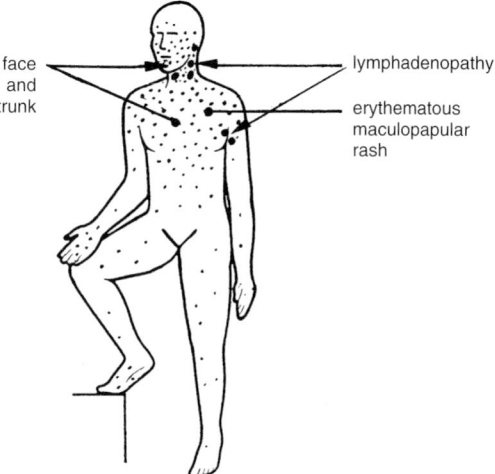

face and trunk

lymphadenopathy

erythematous maculopapular rash

Note: mimics glandular fever

Fig. 102.3 *Primary HIV infection: typical features*

Guttate psoriasis

Guttate psoriasis is the sudden eruption of small (less than 5 mm), very dense, round red papules of psoriasis on the trunk (Fig. 102.4). The rash may extend to the limbs.

It is usually seen in children and adolescents and often precipitated by a streptococcal throat infection. The rash soon develops a white silvery scale. It can persist for up to 6 months. It may undergo spontaneous resolution or enlarge to form plaques.

Treatment includes ultraviolet light and tar preparations.

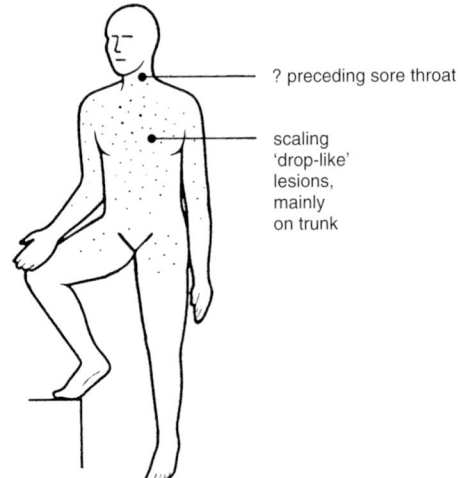

Fig. 102.4 *Guttate psoriasis: small, drop-like lesions, mainly on trunk*

? preceding sore throat

scaling 'drop-like' lesions, mainly on trunk

Epstein-Barr mononucleosis

The rash of Epstein-Barr mononucleosis is almost always related to antibiotics given for tonsillitis. The primary rash, most often non-specific, pinkish and maculopapular (similar to that of rubella), occurs in about 5% of cases only. The secondary rash, which can be extensive and sometimes has a purplish-brown tinge, is most often precipitated by one of the penicillins (Fig. 102.5).

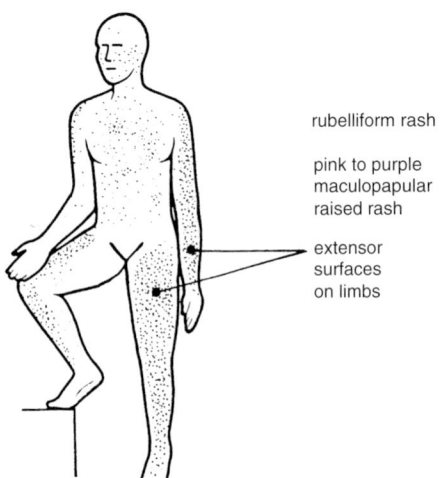

Fig. 102.5 *Epstein-Barr mononucleosis: typical rash induced by penicillin, amoxycillin or ampicillin*

rubelliform rash

pink to purple maculopapular raised rash

extensor surfaces on limbs

- ampicillin ⎫ 90–100%
- amoxycillin ⎭ association
- penicillin   up to 50%

Drug eruptions

A rash is one the most common side effects of drug therapy, which can precipitate many different types of rash; the most common is toxic erythema (Table 102.3). Most drug-evoked dermatoses have an allergic basis with the eruption appearing approximately 10 days after administration, though much sooner if previously sensitised.[3] The most common drugs that cause skin eruptions are summarised in Table 102.4.

The most important fact to realise about drug reactions is that their appearances are so variable—they may mimic almost any cutaneous disease and, in addition, create unique appearances of their own.

When taking a history it is appropriate to enquire about medications or chemicals that may be overlooked such as aspirin, vitamins, toxins, laxatives and medicated toothpaste.

Toxic erythema

The maculopapular erythematous eruption is either morbilliform or scarlatiniform. It is more pronounced on the trunk than on the limbs and face but may become confluent over the whole body.

Table 102.3 *Most common types of drug eruptions (after Thomas)*[3]

	Relative frequency %
Toxic erythema	45
Urticaria	25
Erythema multiforme	7
Eczematous dermatitis	5
Fixed drug reaction	3
Photosensitivity	3
Others • acne form • psoriasiform • pigmentation • erythema nodosum • toxic epidermal necrolysis • purpuric • pigmentary • exfoliative	

Table 102.4 *Most common drugs that cause skin eruptions*

Antimicrobials	• penicillin/cephalosporins • sulphonamides • tetracyclines • nitrofurantoin • streptomycin • griseofulvin • metronidazole
Diuretics	• thiazides • frusemide
Anticonvulsants	• carbamazepine • phenytoin
Tranquillisers	• phenothiazines • barbiturates • chlordiazepoxide
Anti-inflammatory and analgesics	• gold salts • aspirin/salicylates • codeine/morphine • pyrazolones, e.g. BTZ • other NSAIDs
Hormones	• combined oral contraceptive • stilboesterol • testosterone
Others	• phenolphthalein • serum • amiodarone • cytotoxic drugs • quinidine/quinine • bromides and iodides • sulphonylureas • allopurinol • warfarin • amphetamines

Drugs that typically cause toxic erythema include:
• antibiotics — penicillin/cephalosporins
          — sulphonamides
• thiazides
• carbamazepine
• barbiturates
• allopurinol
• gold salts

Photosensitivity
Several antibiotics increase the sensitivity of the skin to ultraviolet light and may lead to a rash with a distribution according to sunlight exposure. The photosensitive rash may be erythematous, resembling sunburn; eczematous; or vesicular.

Typical drugs: tetracyclines
    sulphonamides/
      sulphonylureas
    thiazides and frusemide

phenothiazines
retinoids
amiodarone
griseofulvin
antihistamines, esp.
  promethazine
antimalarials
psoralens

Fixed drug eruption
The mechanism of fixed drug eruption is unknown. The most commonly affected areas are the face, hands and genitalia. The lesions, which are usually bright red but can have other characteristics, are fixed in site and appearance within hours of the drug's administration.

Typical drugs: phenolphthalein
    tetracyclines
    penicillins
    sulphonamides
    salicylates
    the oral contraceptive pill
    barbiturates
    chlordiazepoxide
    quinine

Treatment of any drug reaction
The important aspect of management is to recognise the offending agent and withdraw it. The rash should be treated according to its nature.

There is a therapeutic impulse to prescribe antihistamines but they should be reserved for the treatment of urticarial drug eruptions. They may actually delay healing in purpuric, erythematous and vesiculobullous reactions. Antihistamines may act as allergens and show cross-sensitivity with phenothiazines, sulphonamides and topical antihistamines.

Table 102.5 lists drugs with the highest skin reaction rates.

Table 102.5 *Drugs with the highest skin reaction rates*

• penicillin and derivatives
• sulphonamides
• thiazide diuretics
• barbiturates
• quinidine
• anticonvulsants
• blood products
• gold salts

Erythema multiforme

Erythema multiforme is an acute eruption affecting the skin and mucosal surfaces.

Clinical features:

- mainly in children, adolescents, young adults
- symmetric
- erythematous papules
- mainly backs of hands, palms and forearms (Fig. 102.6)
- also on feet and toes, mouth
- occasionally on trunk and genitalia
- polymorphic
- vesicles and bullae may develop
- self-limiting (up to 2 weeks)

Stevens-Johnson syndrome

A very severe and often fatal variant. Sudden onset with fever and constitutional symptoms.

Causes and associations

Erythema multiforme is a vasculitis affecting the skin and mucosa. Herpes simplex virus (usually type I) is the commonest known association.

Associations include:

- unknown 50%
- herpes simplex virus 33%
- other infections, e.g.
  - mycoplasma pneumonia
  - tuberculosis
  - streptococcus
- connective tissue disorders, e.g. SLE
- neoplasia
  - Hodgkin's disease
  - myeloma
  - carcinoma
- deep X-ray therapy
- drugs
  - barbiturates
  - penicillin
  - sulphonamides
  - phenothiazines
  - phenytoin

Treatment

Identify and remove cause, e.g. withdraw drugs.

Symptomatic treatment, e.g. antihistamines for itching.

Refer severe cases.

Erythema nodosum

Erythema nodosum is characterised by the onset of bright red, raised, tender nodules on the shins. It is an acute, inflammatory, immunological reaction in the subcutaneous fat. The nodules may appear on the thighs and the arms. Adult females are typically affected. An arthritic reaction can affect the ankles and knees.

Causes/associations

- Sarcoidosis (commonest known cause)
- Infections
  - Streptococcal infections
  - viral infections
  - tuberculosis
  - leprosy
  - fungal infections
- Inflammatory bowel disorders
- Drugs
  - sulphonamides
  - tetracyclines
  - oral contraceptives
  - bromides and iodides
- Unknown (about 40%)

Investigations

Tests include FBE, ESR, chest X-ray (the most important), Mantoux test.

Treatment

Identify the cause if possible. Rest and analgesics for the acute stage. Systemic corticosteroids speed resolution if severe episodes.

Prognosis

There is a tendency to settle spontaneously over 3–8 weeks. The lesions may recur.

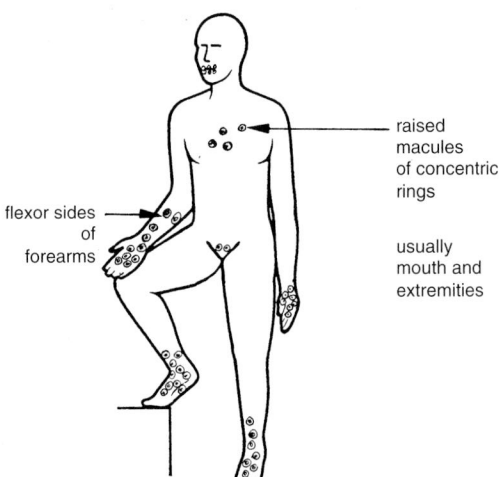

flexor sides of forearms

raised macules of concentric rings

usually mouth and extremities

Fig. 102.6 *Erythema multiforme: typical distribution*

Herpes zoster

Herpes zoster (shingles) is caused by re-activation of varicella zoster virus (acquired from the primary infection of chickenpox) in the dorsal root ganglion. The term comes from the Greek *herpes* (to creep) and *zoster* (a belt or girdle). Shingles is from the Latin *cingere* (to gird) or *cingulum* (a belt). In most instances the reason for reactivation is unknown, but occasionally it is related to an underlying malignancy, usually leukaemia or a lymphoma, to immunosuppression, or to a local disease or disturbance of the spine or spinal cord, such as a tumour or radiotherapy.

The incidence is 3.4 cases per 1000 population per year. A person of any age can get herpes zoster but it is more common in people over 50 years.

Clinical features

The main features are:

- the condition is preceded by several days of radicular pain with hyperaesthesia
- unilateral patchy rash in one or two contiguous dermatomes
- intense erythema with papules in affected skin
- later crusting and separation of scabs after 10–14 days, often with depigmentation, and
- regional lymphadenopathy

Distribution

Any part of the body may be affected, but thoracic and trigeminal dermatomes are the most common. It follows the distribution of the original varicella rash (worse on the face and trunk).

Cranial nerve involvement

The trigeminal nerve: 15% of all cases.

- ophthalmic branch—50% affects nasociliary branch with lesions on tip of nose and eyes (conjunctivae and cornea)
- maxillary and mandibular—oral, palatal and pharyngeal lesions

The facial nerve: lower motor neurone facial nerve palsy with vesicles in and around external auditory meatus (notably posterior wall)—the Ramsay Hunt syndrome.

Complications

Rare: meningoencephalitis
Uncommon: motor paralysis

Common:

- postherpetic neuralgia; increased incidence with age and debility, with duration greater than 6 months:

less than 50 years	1%
50–59 years	7%
60–69 years	21%
70–79 years	30–50%

- the neuralgia resolves within one year in 70–80% of these patients but in others it may persist for years
- eye complications of ophthalmic zoster including keratitis, uveitis and eyelid damage

Management

- Appropriate detailed explanation and reassurance. Dispel myths: namely, that it is not a dangerous disease, the patient will not go insane nor die if the rash spreads from both sides and meets in the middle.
- Explain that herpes zoster is only mildly contagious but children can acquire chickenpox after exposure to a person with the disorder. It is advisable to avoid contact with infants and young children who have never had chickenpox and avoid contact with the immunocompromised and those undergoing chemotherapy. Consider giving varicella zoster immunoglobulin to those immunocompromised contacts who have no history of varicella.
- Treating the rash: Instruct the patient to avoid overtreating the rash, which may become infected. Calamine lotion may be soothing but removal of the calamine can be painful. For a hot painful rash tepid water compresses are soothing and a drying lotion, e.g. menthol in flexible collodion, is most suitable. Aciclovir ointment can be used, although some authorities do not favour its use because of stinging.[4]
- Oral medication[6]
  — Analgesics such as aspirin or paracetamol with or without codeine should be first-line therapy.
  — Antiviral therapy may reduce the duration of the disease and the infectivity of the rash. It should be used in all immunocompromised patients, those with ophthalmic zoster and also in any patient where the rash has been present for less than 72 hours.[5]
  Dose:[6] aciclovir 800 mg 5 times daily for 7 days.
  or

doppler. Measure ankle and brachial systolic pressures and then determine the ankle brachial index (ABI), which is the ankle pressure divided by the brachial pressure. Typical levels are:

normal   > 0.9 (venous ulcer)
ischaemic   < 0.5 (arterial ulcer)
claudicant 0.5–0.9 (mixed arterial-venous ulcer, significant ischaemia if < 0.7)

The ability to determine the cause of the ulceration and thus treat accordingly, especially with pressure dressings, has been a major advance in management. An ABI < 0.8 warrants caution in applying any compression.

Venous ulceration

Venous ulceration (synonyms: 'varicose', 'stasis' and 'gravitational' ulcers) accounts for the majority of leg ulcers. Chronic venous insufficiency is one of the most common medical problems in the elderly, with an estimated incidence of 5.9%.[4]

The problem is invariably secondary to deep venous thrombophlebitis. The subsequent chronic venous hypertension produces trophic changes such as hyperpigmentation, fibrotic thickening, induration and oedema. The end point of this process is ulceration, which affects 3% of those with varicose veins and 30% of those with trophic changes.[5]

Clinical features of venous ulcers[6]
- occur in same area as venous eczema
- shallow (but can reach periosteum)
- more common medial than lateral
- sometimes circumferential
- granulating floor sometimes with surrounding cellulitis
- notoriously slow in healing
- generally not tender but can be painful
- associated pain is usually relieved by raising the leg

On examination, superficial varicosities are usually but not invariably present. Pitting oedema may be present early but with time fibrosis and firm induration develop. Other clinical features include dermatitis (eczema), punctuate capillary proliferation, haemosiderin, hyperpigmentation and 'atrophie blanche'.[7]

Arterial (ischaemic) ulcers

Ischaemic ulcers are generally localised to the most peripheral areas below the ankle joint, such as the tips of the toes and the point of the heel, or to pressure points such as the heels, malleoli or head of the first metatarsal.
  Clinical features:
- painful
- punched out
- minimal granulation tissue

Management is directed towards reperfusion.

Management of venous leg ulcers

A major advance in the management of venous ulcers has been the finding that wounds heal better in an occluded or semi-occluded state.[7] A moist environment also aids healing.

Principles of optimal management
- explanation about the cause, and promotion of patient compliance
- promoting clean granulation tissue to permit healing
- meticulous cleansing and dressing (avoid sensitising preparations)
- prevention and control of infection—antibiotics if cellulitis (cephalexin or erythromycin)
- firm elastic compression bandage—use a minimal stretch bandage from base toes to just below the knee. The degree of compression depends on the blood flow and is proportional to it
- bed rest with elevation (if severe, 45–60 minutes twice a day and at night): ensure legs are elevated higher than the heart
- encourage early ambulation
- appropriate modification of lifestyle including weight reduction
- good nutrition includes a healthy balanced diet with ample protein and complex carbohydrates

Note: Firm compression is the single most important factor in the healing of venous ulcers.[5] Options include elastic stockings, elastic bandages, Unna's boots and legging orthoses.[8]

Cleansing/debridement agents
There are many cleansing agents, including:
  N saline, benzoyl peroxide and Intra Site Gel. As a rule, avoid antiseptics.

A good combination is N saline cleansing followed by Intra Site Gel for debridement. Hydrogels such as Intra Site Gel, which have been found to be effective at debridement (including black necrotic areas), have generally replaced enzyme dressings.

Medicated occlusive bandages

There are several suitable occlusive paste bandages for ambulant patients which ideally should be left on for 7–14 days. All contain zinc oxide with the indicated additives, e.g. Calaband (calamine), Ichthaband (ichthammol), Quinaband (clioquinol + calamine), Tarband (coal tar), Viscopaste and Zincaband (zinc oxide only).

Patch testing for an allergic response should be performed for a few days beforehand.

Pitfalls and other factors to be considered

- Treat the primary cause by surgery or other means, e.g. varicose veins, vascular insufficiency.
- If oedema, elevate legs and prescribe diuretics. An ulcer will not heal in the presence of significant ankle oedema.
- Be careful of allergy to local applications, e.g. zinc.
- Be careful of irritation from local applications, e.g. antibiotics. Antibiotic-impregnated dressings are not generally recommended.
- Never apply corticosteroid preparations directly to ulcers.
- Avoid heavy packing of the wound.
- Consider grafting (pinch skin or split thickness).
- Consider oxpentifylline 400 (Trental) for chronic occlusive arterial disease.

Post-healing and prevention of ulcers

- Encourage preventive measures such as regular walking, good nutrition, no smoking, elevation of leg when resting, great care to avoid trauma.
- Apply emollients for varicose eczema.
- Wear a compression grade elastic stocking for varicose ulcers, e.g. Jobst Fast-Fit, Tensor Press.

A recommended treatment routine for a leg ulcer is presented in Table 103.4. It is desirable (for the outpatient) to leave the dressings and bandages in place for one week, perhaps two weeks, depending on the state of the dressing.

Table 103.4 *A recommended leg ulcer treatment method*

Clean with normal saline
- If slough, apply Intra Site Gel
- Dressing: non-adherent paraffin gauze
- Padding bandage, e.g. Velband
- Occlusive paste bandage, e.g. Icthaband or Viscopaste (7–14 days), from base of toe to just below knee, plus compression bandage
  or
  Compression bandage, e.g Elastocrepe or Eloflex, to just below knee
- Consider Tubigrip stockinette cover

Unna's boots

Unna's boots have an important place in the management of severe ulceration despite the discomfort and inconvenience for the patient. They appear to provide excellent fixed compression and to encourage healing, and one particular study showed their superiority to elastic stockings (7.3 weeks compared to 18.4 weeks).[9]

Principles of management for chronic ulcers are summarised in Table 103.5.

Table 103.5 *Principles of management of chronic ulcers[11]*

Ulcer type	Major management principles
Venous	Control venous insufficiency • compression bandage • improve calf muscle pump action (ambulation, exercises) • vertical leg drainage
Arterial	Vascular assessment for surgical intervention
Mixed venous/ arterial	Vascular assessment for surgical intervention
Pressure	Eliminate or reduce pressure

Decubitus ulcers (pressure sores)

Pressure sores tend to occur in elderly immobile patients, especially those who are unconscious, paralysed or debilitated. The cause is skin ischaemia from sustained pressure over a bony area, particularly the heels, sacrum, hips and buttocks. Poor general health, including anaemia, is a predisposing factor.

Clinical features:

- preliminary area of fixed erythema at pressure site
- relatively sudden onset of necrosis and ulceration
- ulcer undermined at edges

- possible rapid extension of ulcers
- necrotic slough in base

Management

Prevention

- Good nursing care including turning patient every 2 hours.
- Regular skin examinations by the nursing and medical staff.
- Special care of pressure areas, including gentle handling.
- Special beds, mattresses (e.g. air-filled ripple) and sheepskin to relieve pressure areas.
- Good nutrition and hygiene.
- Control of urinary and faecal incontinence.
- Avoid the donut cushion.

Treatment of ulcer

Use above measures, plus:

- Clean base with saline solution (applied gently via a syringe) or Intra Site Gel.
- General guidelines for dressings:
  — deep ulcers: alginates, e.g. Tegagel, Kaltostat
  — shallow ulcers: hydrocolloids, e.g. Duo-derm, CGF, Cutinova Hydro
  — dry or necrotic ulcers: hydrogels, e.g. Intra-site, Solosite
  — heavy exudative ulcers: foams, e.g. Lyofoam.
- Give vitamin C, 500 mg bd.
- Give antibiotics for spreading cellulitis (other-wise of little use).
- Healing is usually satisfactory but, if not, sur-gical intervention with debridement of necrotic tissue and skin grafting may be nec-essary. This is very effective if the patient can cope.

Undressing wounds

Removal of dressings from ulcerated wounds is very important. The contact layer should be removed slowly to prevent detachment of fragile epithelial surface cells and trauma to healthy granulation tissue.[10]

Trophic ulcers

Trophic ulcers are due to neuropathy causing loss of sensation (invariably diabetic) and usually follow an injury of which the patient was unaware.

A feature is a deep punched-out lesion (similar to ischaemic ulcers) over pressure points. A common site is the ball of the foot under the first metatarsal head, but the heel or a bunion may also be affected.

The ulcers may extend to the bone and into joints. They are prone to secondary infection.

Treatment is based on controlling the diabetes and clearing infection with appropriate antibi-otics, but referral for surgical management is usually essential.

Dermatitis artefacta and neurotic excoriations

These self-inflicted ulcerated or erosive skin lesions have a psychological basis.

Dermatitis artefacta

In this condition, patients deny self-trauma and may have deep-seated psychological problems; or they may be malingering or manipulative for secondary gain.

Neurotic excoriations

These lesions, which are usually identical to the artefactual lesions, are caused by patients who admit to scratching, picking or digging at their skin. It occurs at times of stress and treatment is seldom successful. Treatment consists of coun-selling and topical antipruritics such as:

- coal tar solution (liquor picis carbonis) and menthol in sorbolene cream
                                  or
- menthol (0.5%) or phenol (1.0%) in aqueous cream.

References

1. Cormack J, Marinker M, Morrel D. In: *Practice. A handbook of primary health care*. London: Kluwer-Harrap Handbooks, 1980; 3:01–09.

2. Davis A, Bolin T, Ham J. *Symptom analysis and physical diagnosis* (2nd edn). Sydney: Pergamon Press, 1990, 380–389.

3. Stacey MC. Chronic venous ulcers. Sydney: Medical Observer, 29 March 1991; 31–32.

4. Beauregard S, Gilchrest BA. A survey of skin problems and skin care regimens in the elderly. Arch Dermatol, 1987; 123:1638–1643.

5. Fry J, Berry HE. *Surgical problems in clinical practice*. London: Edward Arnold, 1987, 115–117.

6. Buxton P. *ABC of dermatology*. London: BMJ, 1989, 34–39.

7. Fitzpatrick JE. Stasis ulcers: update on a common geriatric problem. Mod Med Aust, June 1990; 81–88.

8. Vernick SH, Shapiro D, Shaw FD. Legging orthosis for venous and lymphatic insufficiency. Arch Phys Med Rehab, 1987; 68:459–461.

9. Hendricks WM, Swallows RT. Management of stasis leg ulcers with Unna's boots versus elastic support stockings. J Amer Acad Dermatol, 1985; 12:90–98.

10. Rowland J. Pressure ulcers: a literature review and a treatment scheme. Aust Fam Physician, 1993; 22:1819–1827.

11. Findlay D. Wound management and healing in general practice. Annual Update Course notes, Monash University, 1996; 13–16.

104

Common lumps and bumps

—

It will never get well if you pick it.

American proverb

Lumps and bumps are very common presentations and the skin a very common site for neoplastic lesions. Most of these lesions only invade locally, with the notable exception of malignant melanoma. Pigmented skin tumours thus demand very careful consideration, although only a very few are neoplastic. The optimum time to deal with the problem and cure any skin cancer is at its first presentation. The family doctor thus has an important responsibility to screen these tumours and is faced with two basic decisions: the diagnosis and whether to treat or refer.

Most skin lumps are benign and can be left *in situ*, but the family doctor should be able to remove most of these lumps if appropriate and submit them for histological verification. The main treatment options available in family practice are: biopsy, cryotherapy, curette and cautery, excision or intralesional injections of corticosteroid.[1] A list of common and important lumps is presented in Table 104.1.

Skin cancer

The three main skin cancers are the non-melanocyctic skin cancers—basal cell carcinoma (BCC) and squamous cell carcinoma (SCC)—and melanoma. The approximate relative incidence is BCCs 80%, SCCs 15–20%, and melanomas less than 5%.[2] The incidence of non-melanotic skin cancer is approximately 800 new cases per 100 000 population per year, and 25 per 100 000 for melanoma. About 80% of skin

Table 104.1 *Important lumps and their tissue of origin*[3]

Skin and mucous membranes
- fibroepithelial polyp (skin tag)
- sebaceous cyst
- implantation cyst
- mucocele
- hypertrophic scar and keloid
- warts and papillomas
- pox virus lumps
  - — molluscum contagiosum
  - — orf
  - — milker's nodules
- seborrhoeic keratoses
- granuloma annularae
- dermatofibroma
- solar keratoses
- keratoacanthoma

malignant tumours
- *basal cell carcinoma (BCC)*
- *squamous cell carcinoma (SCC)*
- *Bowen's disease*
- *malignant melanoma*
- *Kaposi's sarcoma*
- *secondary tumour*

Subcutaneous and deeper structures
- lipoma
- neurofibroma
- soft fibroma
- lymph node

musculoskeletal
- ganglion

cancer deaths are due to melanoma and the rest mainly due to SCC.[2]

A diagnostic approach to the lump

As with any examination, the routine of *look, feel, move, measure, auscultate* and *transilluminate* should be followed.

1006

The lump or lumps can be described thus:

- number
- shape: regular or irregular
- size (in metric units)
- position
- consistency (very soft, soft, firm, hard or stony hard)
- mobility
- surface or contour
- special features
  - exact anatomical site
  - relation to anatomical structures
  - colour
  - temperature (of skin over lump)
  - tenderness
  - pulsation (transmitted or direct)
  - impulse
  - reducibility
  - percussion
  - fluctuation (? contains fluid)
  - bruit
  - transilluminability
  - special signs
    - slipping sign
    - emptying sign of cavernous haemangioma
  - regional lymph nodes
  - ? malignancy (is it 1° or 2° ?)

Relation of the lump to anatomical structures[3]

The question 'In what tissue layer is the lump situated?' needs to be addressed.

- Is it in the skin? The lump moves when the skin is moved, e.g. sebaceous cyst.
- Is it in subcutaneous tissue? The skin can be moved over the lump. The slipping sign: if the edge of the lump is pushed, the swelling slips from beneath the finger, e.g. lipoma.
- Is it in muscle? The lump is movable when the muscle is relaxed but on contraction of the muscle this movement becomes limited.
- Is it arising from a tendon or joint? Movement of these structures may cause a change in the mobility or shape of the tumour.
- Is it in bone? The lump is immobile and best outlined with the muscles relaxed.

Fibroepithelial polyps

Synonyms: skin tags, acrochordon, benign squamous papilloma.

Clinical features:

- benign skin overgrowth

- increased incidence with age
- commonest on neck, axillae, trunk, groins
- no malignant potential
- can be irritating or unsightly to patient

Management

- can leave or remove
- snip off with scissors or bone forceps (Figs 104.1a,b)

or

- tie base with fine cotton or suture material

or

- diathermy base

or

- apply liquid nitrogen (Fig. 104.2)

These methods do not require local anaesthetic.

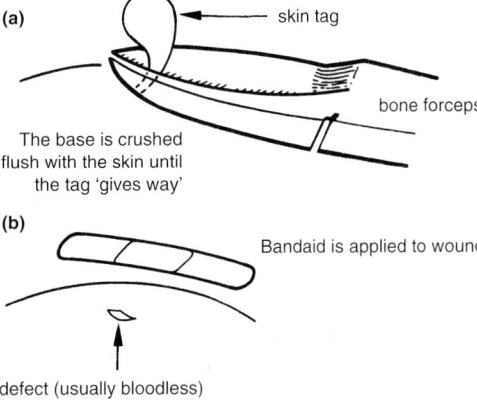

Fig. 104.1 *Removal of skin tag using bone forceps*

Fig. 104.2 *Removal of skin tag by liquid nitrogen: a cotton bud soaked in liquid nitrogen is applied to the forceps, which grasp the tag firmly*

Sebaceous cyst

Synonyms: 'pilar' cysts, wens, epidermoid cysts (similar in appearance)
Clinical features:

- firm to soft regular lump
- fixed to skin but not to other structures (Fig. 104.3a)
- found mainly on scalp—then face, neck, trunk, scrotum
- contains sebaceous material
- may be a central punctum containing keratin
- tendency to inflammation

Management

Can leave if small and not bothersome.

Surgical removal methods

There are several methods of removing sebaceous cysts after infiltrating local anaesthetic over and around the cyst. These include:

Method 1. Incision into cyst

Make an incision into the cyst to bisect it, squeeze the contents out with a gauze swab and then avulse the lining of the cyst with a pair of artery forceps or remove with a small curette.

Method 2. Incision over cyst and blunt dissection

Make a careful skin incision over the cyst, taking care not to puncture its wall. Free the skin carefully from the cyst by blunt dissection. When it is free from adherent subcutaneous tissue, digital pressure will cause the cyst to 'pop out'.

Method 3. Standard dissection

Incise a small ellipse of skin to include the central punctum over the cyst (Fig. 104.3b). Apply forceps to this skin to provide traction for dissection of the cyst from the adherent dermis and subcutaneous tissue. Ideally, forceps should

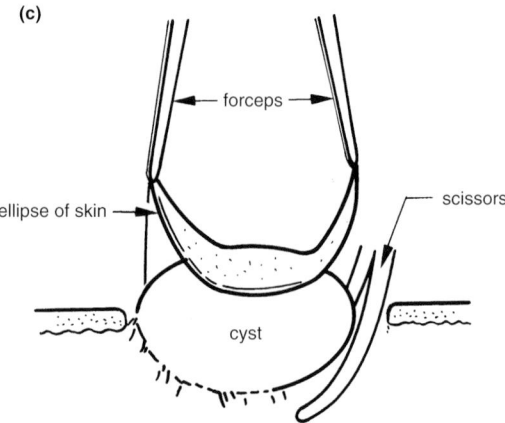

Fig. 104.3b,c *Standard dissection of a sebaceous cyst*

be applied at either end. The objective is to avoid rupture of the cyst. Inserting curved scissors (e.g. McIndoe's scissors), free the cyst by gently opening and closing the blades (Fig. 104.3c). Bleeding is not usually a problem. When the cyst is removed, obliterate the space with subcutaneous catgut. The skin is sutured with a vertical mattress suture to avoid a tendency to inversion of the skin edges into the slack wound. Send the cyst for histopathology.

Treatment of infected cysts

Incise the cyst to drain purulent material. When the inflammation has resolved completely the cyst should be removed by Method 1 or Method 3 (above).

Implantation cyst

Synonym: implantation dermoid
Clinical features:

- small cystic swelling
- may be tender
- usually follows puncture wounds
- especially on finger pulp, e.g. hairdressers, sewers
- contains mucus

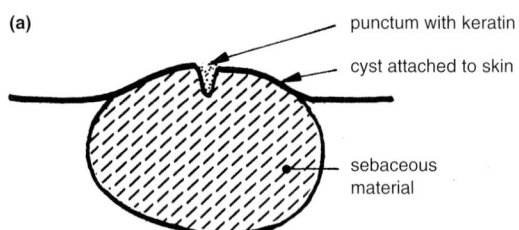

Fig. 104.3a *Configuration of a sebaceous cyst*

Management
- incision removal (similar to sebaceous cyst)

Mucocele

A mucous retention cyst.
  Clinical features:

- a benign tumour
- cyst containing mucus
- appears spontaneously
- common on lips and buccal mucosa
- smooth and round
- yellow or blue colour

Management
- incision removal

Hypertrophic scar

A hypertrophic scar is simply a lumpy scar caused by a nodular accumulation of thickened collagen fibres. It does not extend beyond the margins of the wound and regresses within a year.

Keloid

A keloid is a special type of hypertrophic scar that extends beyond the margins of the wound.
  Clinical features:

- firm, raised, red-purple, skin overgrowth
- common on ear lobes, chin, neck, shoulder, upper trunk
- hereditary predisposition
- follows trauma, even minor, e.g. ear piercing
- may be burning or itchy and tender

Management
- prevention (avoid procedures in keloid-prone individuals)
- intradermal injection of corticosteroids in early stages (2–3 months) or X-ray treatment of surgical wounds within 2 weeks of operation.[4]

Warts and papillomas

Warts are skin tumours caused by the human papilloma virus (HPV). The virus invades the skin, usually through a small abrasion, causing abnormal skin growth. Warts are transmitted by direct or fomite contact and may be autoinoculated from one area to another.[5]
  Clinical features:

- average incubation period—4 months

- increased incidence in children and adolescents
- peak incidence around adolescence
- occurs in all races at all ages
- about 25% resolve spontaneously in 6 months[5] and 70% in 2 years
- present as various types

Types of warts

These include common warts, plane warts, filiform warts (fine elongated growths, usually on the face and neck), digitate warts (finger-like projections, usually on scalp), genital and plantar (Fig. 104.4).

Common warts

Skin-coloured tumours with a rough surface, found mainly on the fingers, elbows and knees.

Plane warts

Skin-coloured, small and flat, occurring in linear clusters along scratch lines. Mainly occur on the face and limbs. Difficult to treat because they contain very few virus particles. Prone to Koebner's phenomenon, which is seeding when a scratch passes through a plane wart.

Treatment options for warts

Topical applications:[5]

- salicylic acid, e.g. 5–20% in flexible collodion (apply daily or bd)
- formaldehyde 2–4% alone or in combination
- podophyllin 10–25% in tinct. benz. co. *or* podophyllotoxin 0.5% (better) for anogenital warts—it is good on mucosal surfaces but does not penetrate normal keratin
- cytotoxic agents, e.g. 5-fluorouracil: very good for resistant warts such as plane warts and periungual warts

Cryotherapy

Carbon dioxide (−56.5°C) or liquid nitrogen (−195.8°C) destroys the host cell and stimulates an immune reaction.

Note: Excessive keratin must be pared before freezing.
      Results often disappointing.

Curettage

A most common treatment; some plantar warts can be removed under LA with a sharp spoon curette. The problem is a tendency to scar so

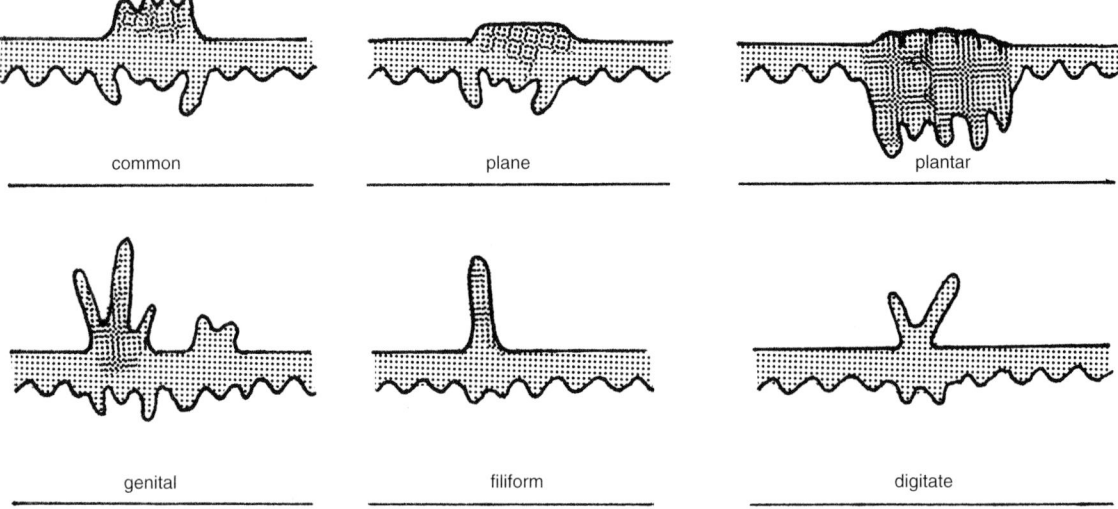

common	plane	plantar

genital	filiform	digitate

Fig. 104.4 *Configuration of various types of warts*

avoid over a pressure area such as the sole of the foot.

Electrodissection
A high-frequency spark under LA is useful for small, filiform or digitate warts. A combination of curettage and electrodissection is suitable for large and persistent warts.

Vitamin A and the retinoids
- topical retinoic acid, e.g. tretinoin 0.1% cream (Retin-A) is effective on plane warts
- systemic oral retinoid, acitretin (Neotigason) for recalcitrant warts (with care)

Specific wart treatment
The method chosen depends on the type of wart, its site and the patient's age.

Plantar warts: refer Chapter 62.

Genital warts: podophyllotoxin 0.5% paint (see Chap. 98).

Filiform and digitate warts: liquid nitrogen or electrodissection.

Plane warts: liquid nitrogen; salicylic acid 20% Co, e.g. Wartkil; consider 5-fluorouracil cream or Retin-A.

Common warts: a recommended method:
1. Soak the wart/s in warm soapy water.

2. Rub back the wart surface with a pumice stone.
3. Apply the paint (only to the wart; protect the surrounding skin with Vaseline). The paint: formalin 5%, salicylic acid 12%, acetone 25%, collodion to 100%.[4]

Do this daily or every second day. Carefully remove dead skin between applications.

Periungual warts (fingernails): consider 5-fluoro-uracil or liquid nitrogen. Always use a paint rather than ointment or paste on fingers.

Pox virus lumps

Skin tumours can be caused by pox viruses, some of which result from handling infected sheep, cows and monkeys and other animals such as deer. Hence they are usually found in sheep shearers, farmers and zookeepers.

Molluscum contagiosum
This common pox virus infection can be spread readily by direct contact, including sexual contact (p. 949).
  Clinical features:

- common in school-age children
- single or multiple (more common)
- shiny, round, pink-white papule
- hemispherical up to 5 mm
- central punctum gives umbilical look

- can be spread by scratching and use of steroids

Treatment options
- liquid nitrogen (a few seconds)
- pricking the lesion with a pointed stick soaked in 1% or 2.5% phenol
- application of 15% podophyllin in friar's balsam (compound benzoin tincture)
- application of 30% trichloracetic acid
- destruction by electrocautery or diathermy
- ether soap and friction method
- lifting open the tip with a sterile needle inserted from the side (parallel to the skin) and applying 10% povidone-iodine (Betadine) solution (parents can be shown this method and continue to use it at home for multiple tumours)
- covering with a piece of Micropore tape—change every day (may take a few months)

Orf
Orf is due to a pox virus and presents as a single papule or group of papules on the hands of sheep-handlers after handling lambs with contagious pustular dermatitis. The papules change into pustular-like nodules or bullae with a violaceous erythematous margin. It clears up spontaneously in about 3–4 weeks without scarring and usually no treatment is necessary.

Practice tip. Rapid resolution (days) can be obtained by an intralesional injection of triamcinolone diluted 50:50 in normal saline.[6]

Milker's nodules
In humans 2–5 papules appear on the hands about one week after handling cows' udders or calves' mouths. The papules enlarge to become tender grey nodules with a necrotic centre and surrounding inflammation. The patient can be reassured that the nodules are a self-limiting infection and spontaneous remission will occur in 5–6 weeks without residual scarring. One infection gives lifelong immunity.

Practice tip: Intralesional corticosteroid injection (as for orf).

Seborrhoeic keratoses
Synonyms: seborrhoeic wart, senile wart, senile keratoses (avoid these terms).

Clinical features:
- very common
- increasing number and pigmentation with age > 40 years
- sits on skin, appears in some like a 'sultana' pressed into the skin, i.e. well-defined border
- has a 'pitted' surface
- may be solitary but usually multiple
- common on face and trunk, but occurs anywhere
- usually asymptomatic
- usually causes patients some alarm (confused with melanoma)

Management
- usually nil apart from reassurance
- does not undergo malignant change
- can be removed for cosmetic reasons
- light cautery to small facial lesions
- freezing liquid nitrogen (especially if thin) decolours the tumour
- 10% (or stronger) phenol solution applied carefully—repeat in 3 weeks
- apply trichloroacetic acid to surface: instil gently by multiple pricks with a fine-gauge needle, twice weekly for 2 weeks
- may drop off spontaneously
- if diagnosis uncertain, remove for histopathology

Granuloma annularae
Granuloma annularae are a common benign group of papules arranged in an annular fashion.
Clinical features:
- most common among children and young adults
- firm papules grouped in a 'string of pearls' pattern
- dermal nodules
- may be associated with minor trauma
- associated with diabetes
- usually on dorsum or sides of fingers (knuckle area), backs of hands, the elbows and knees

Management
- check urine/blood for sugar
- give reassurance (they usually subside in a year or so)
- cosmetic reasons: intradermal injection of triamcinolone 10% or similar corticosteroid (dilute equal volume with N saline)

Dermatofibroma

Synonyms: sclerosing haemangioma; histio-cytoma.

This is a common pigmented nodule arising in the dermis due to a proliferation of fibroblasts, believed to develop as an abnormal response to minor trauma. The nodule gives a characteristic button-like feel and dimpling when laterally compressed (pinched) from the side with the fingers.

Clinical features:

- usually multiple
- firm, well-circumscribed nodules
- oval, 0.5–1.5 cm in diameter
- freely mobile over deeper structures
- slightly raised in relation to skin
- mainly on limbs, especially legs
- may itch
- mainly in women
- variable colour, pink or brown, tan or grey or violaceous
- characteristic 'dimple' sign on pinching margins

Treatment

- reassurance
- simple excision if requested

Solar keratosis

Solar keratoses are reddened, adherent, scaly thickenings occurring on light-exposed areas, with a potential for malignant change, especially on the ears.

Clinical features:

- sun-exposed fair skin
- mainly on face, ears, scalp (if balding), forearms, dorsum of hands (especially) and feet
- dry, rough, adherent scale
- discomfort on rubbing with towel
- scale can separate to leave oozing surface
- a small proportion undergo malignant change

Management

- reduced exposure to sunlight
- can disappear spontaneously
- liquid nitrogen if superficial
  or
  5-fluorouracil 5% cream daily for 3–4 weeks
- surgical excision for suspicious and ulcerating lesions
- biopsy if doubtful

Keratoacanthoma

Keratoacanthomas (KA) occur singly on light-exposed areas. The major problem is differentiation from squamous cell carcinoma (SCC), especially if on the lip or ear. The relative growth rates of three types of skin tumours are shown in Figure 104.5.

Fig. 104.5 *Relative growth rates of three types of skin tumours: keratoacanthoma, squamous cell carcinoma and basal cell carcinoma*

Clinical features:

- rapidly growing lesion on sun-exposed skin
- raised crater with central keratin plug (Fig. 104.6)
- grows to 2 cm or more
- arises over a few weeks, remains static, then spontaneously disappears after about 6 months; can leave a big scar
- can be confused with SCC

Management

- remove by excision—perform biopsy
- if clinically certain—curettage/diathermy
- treat as SCC (by excision) if on lip/ear

The recommended treatment is surgical excision and histological examination. Ensure a 2–3 mm margin for excision. Most patients will not tolerate a tumour for 6 months on an exposed area such as the face while waiting for a spontaneous

Fig. 104.6 *A typical keratoacanthoma*

remission. Also, if it is an SCC, a potentially lethal cancer has remained *in situ* for an unnecessarily long period.

Basal cell carcinoma (BCC)

Clinical features:

- most common skin cancer (80%)
- age: usually > 35 years
- more frequent in males
- mostly on sun-exposed areas: face (mainly), neck, upper trunk, limbs (10%)
- may ulcerate easily = 'rodent ulcer'
- slow-growing over years
- has various forms: nodular, pigmented, ulcerated, etc.
- stretching the skin demarcates the lesion, highlights pearliness and distinct margin
- does not metastasise via lymph nodes or bloodstream
- local spread is a problem
- can spread deeply if around nose, eye or ear

Clinical types

1. cystic nodular
2. ulcerated
3. pigmented
4. superficial
5. morphoeic (fibrotic)
6. common: pearly edge, telangiectasia, ulcerated

Management

- excision (3 mm margin) is best
- if not excision, do biopsy before other treatment
- radiotherapy is an option
- Moh's chemotherapy—a new form of treatment where the tumour removal is microscopically controlled.

Squamous cell carcinoma (SCC)

SCC is an important malignant tumour of the epidermis; it is also found on sun-exposed areas, especially in fair-skinned people. It tends to arise in premalignant areas such as solar keratoses, burns, chronic ulcers, leukoplakia and Bowen's disease, or it can arise *de novo*.

Clinical features:

- usually > 50 years
- initially firm thickening of skin, especially in solar keratosis
- surrounding erythema

- the hard nodules soon ulcerate
- occurs on the hands and forearms and the head and neck
- ulcers have a characteristic everted edge
- capable of metastases and may involve regional nodes
- SCCs of ear, lip, oral cavity, tongue and genitalia are serious and need special management

Management

- Early excision of tumours < 1 cm with 3 mm margin, to deep fat level.
- Referral for specialised surgery and/or radiotherapy if large, in difficult site or lymphadenopathy.
- SCCs of the ear and lip, which have considerably more malignant potential, can be excised by wedge excision.

Bowen's disease

Bowen's disease begins as a slowly enlarging, sharply demarcated, thickened red plaque, especially on the lower legs of females. It may resemble solar keratosis or a patch of psoriasis. It remains virtually unchanged for months or years. It may become very crusty, ulcerate or bleed. It has a great potential for malignant change since it is a full thickness squamous cell carcinoma *in situ*.

Management

- biopsy first for diagnosis
- wide surgical excision if small
- skin grafting may be required
- cryotherapy or radiotherapy

Note: Biopsy a single patch of suspected psoriasis or dermatitis not responding to topical steroids.

Malignant melanoma

These are usually enlarging pigmented lesions with an irregular notched border. Refer to Chapter 105, on pigmented skin lesions.

Secondary tumour

These complex tumours may metastasise from the lung, melanoma or bowel and may arise in surgical scars, e.g. for carcinoma of the breast.

Kaposi's sarcoma

Kaposi's sarcoma presents as brownish-purple papules on the skin and mucosa. Apart from the well known presentation in immunocompromised individuals, it is seen as a primary tumour mostly in elderly men of central or eastern European origin.

Lipoma

Lipomas are common benign tumours of mature fat cells situated in subcutaneous tissue.
  Clinical features:

• soft and may be fluctuant
• well defined; lobulated
• rubbery consistency
• may be one or many
• painless
• most common on limbs (especially arms) and trunk
• can occur at any site

Management

• reassurance about benign nature
• removal for cosmetic reasons or to relieve discomfort from pressure

Surgical excision

Many lipomas can be enucleated using a gloved finger, but there are a few traps: some are deeper than anticipated, and some are adjacent to important structures such as large nerves and blood vessels. Others are tethered by fibrous bands, and can recur. Recurrence is also possible if excision is incomplete.

Method

1. Outline the extent of the lipoma and note its anatomical relationships.
2. Infiltrate the area with 1% lignocaine with adrenaline (include the deepest part of the lipoma).
3. Make a linear incision (Fig. 104.7a) in the overlying skin, preferably in a natural crease line for about two-thirds of its length. The lipoma should bulge through the wound. For large lipomas, incise an ellipse of skin (Fig. 104.7b).
4. Insert a gloved finger between the skin and fatty tumour to determine whether it will shell out. It is important to seek the outer edge of each lobule, dissect it and bring it to the surface (Fig. 104.7c).

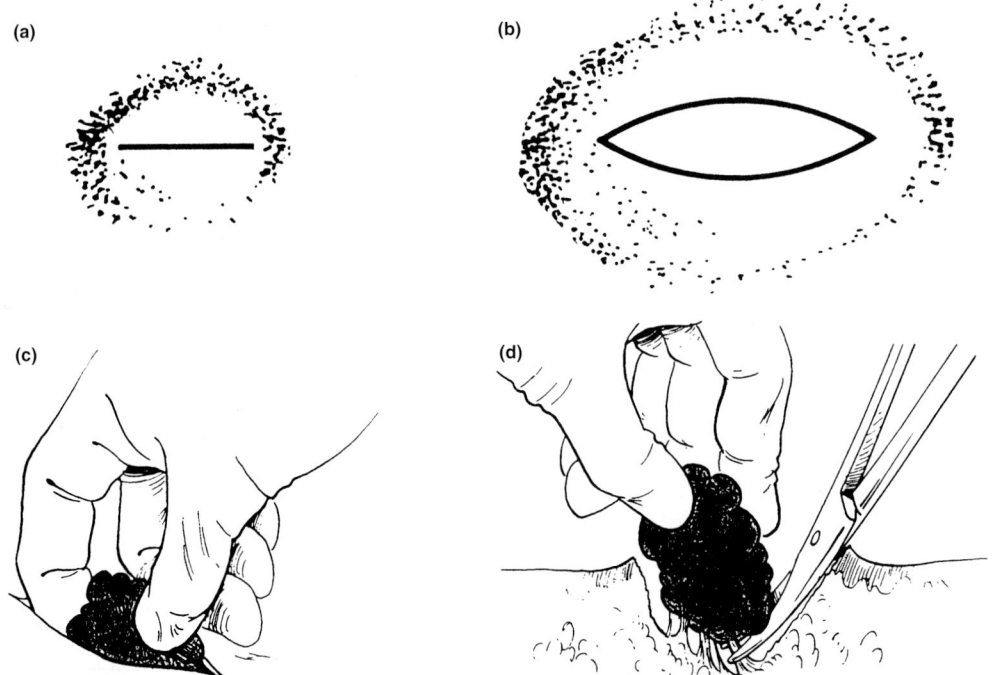

Fig. 104.7 (a) *Linear incision for small lipomas;* **(b)** *elliptical incision for large lipomas;* **(c)** *gloved-finger dissection to bring the lipoma to the surface;* **(d)** *blunt scissors dissection to free the lipoma from tethering fibrous bands*

5. If necessary, insert curved scissors and use a blunt opening action to free any fibrous bands tethering the lipoma (Fig. 104.7d).
6. Ensure that all the fatty tissue is removed. Send it for histological examination.
7. Use a gauze swab to control bleeding and remove debris from the dead space.
8. Close the dead space with interrupted catgut sutures.
9. Close the skin with interrupted or subcuticular sutures.

Neurofibroma

These benign tumours are firm (sometimes soft) painless subcutaneous lumps aligned lengthwise in the long axis of the limb in relation to peripheral nerves. The lumps are more mobile from side to side than along the long axis. Some are tender to pressure with associated pain and paraesthesia on the nerve distribution.

Ganglion

Ganglia are firm cystic lumps associated with joints or tendon sheaths.
  Clinical features:
• deep subcutaneous lumps
• around joints or tendon sheaths
• mostly around wrists, fingers, dorsum of feet
• immobile, fixed to deep tissues
• translucent
• contain viscid gelatinous fluid
• associated with arthritis and synovitis
• may disappear spontaneously
• recurrences common

Management
• can be left—wait and see
• do not 'bang with a Bible'
• needle aspiration and steroid injection
                  or
  surgical excision (can be difficult)

Injection treatment of ganglia

Ganglia have a high recurrence rate after treatment, with a relapse of 30% after surgery. A simple, relatively painless and more effective method is to use intralesional injections of long-acting corticosteroid, such as methylprednisolone acetate.[7]

Method
1. Insert a 21 gauge needle attached to a 2 mL or 5 mL syringe into the cavity of the ganglion.

2. Aspirate some (not all) of its jelly-like contents, mainly to ensure the needle is *in situ*.
3. Keeping the needle exactly in place, swap the syringe for an insulin syringe containing up to 0.5 mL of steroid.
4. Inject 0.25–0.5 mL (Fig. 104.8).
5. Rapidly withdraw the needle, pinch the overlying skin for several seconds and then apply a light dressing.
6. Review in 7 days and, if still present, repeat the injection using 0.25 mL of steroid.

Up to six injections can be given over a period of time, but 70% of ganglia will disperse with only one or two injections.[7]

Fig. 104.8 *Injection treatment of ganglion*

Some preferred therapeutic options
Liquid nitrogen therapy

Ideally, liquid nitrogen is stored in a special, large container and decanted when required into a small thermos flask or spray device.
  The easiest method of application to superficial skin tumours (Table 104.2) is via a ball of cotton wool rolled rather loosely on the tip of a wooden applicator stick. The ball of cotton wool should be slightly smaller than the lesion, to prevent freezing of the surrounding skin.

Method (basic steps)
1. Inform the patient what to expect.
2. Pare excess keratin with a scalpel.
3. Use a cotton wool applicator slightly smaller (not larger—see Fig. 104.9a) than the lesion.
4. Immerse it in nitrogen until bubbling ceases.
5. Gently tap it on the side of the container to remove excess liquid.

Table 104.2 *Superficial skin tumours suitable for cryotherapy*

Warts (plane, periungual, plantar, anogenital)

Skin tags

Seborrhoeic keratoses

Molluscum contagiosum

Solar keratoses

6. Hold the lesion firmly between thumb and forefinger.
7. Place applicator vertically (Fig. 104.9b) on tumour surface.
8. Apply with firm pressure: do not dab.
9. Freeze until a 2 mm white halo appears around the lesion.

Explain likely reaction to patient, such as the appearance of blisters (possibly blood blisters). The optimal time for retreatment of warts is in 2–3 weeks (not longer than 3 weeks).

Biopsies

There are various methods for taking biopsies from skin lesions. These include scraping, shaving and punch biopsies, all of which are useful but not as effective or safe as excisional biopsies.

Shave biopsies

This simple technique is generally used for the tissue diagnosis of premalignant lesions and some malignant tumours, but not melanoma.

| Method |

1. Infiltrate with LA.
2. Holding a number 10 or 15 scalpel blade horizontally, shave off the tumour just into the dermis (Fig. 104.10).
3. Diathermy may be required for haemostasis.

The biopsy site usually heals with minimal scarring.

Punch biopsy

This biopsy has considerable use in general practice, where full-thickness skin specimens are required for histological diagnosis. (Good quality disposable biopsy punches are available from Derma Tech Laboratories.)

| Method |

1. Clean the skin.
2. Infiltrate with LA.

(a)

(b)

(c)

Fig. 104.9 *Application of liquid nitrogen:* **(a)** *applicator too large;* **(b)** *correct size and approach of applicator;* **(c)** *correct size but wrong position of applicator*

3. Gently stretch the skin between the finger and thumb to limit rotational movement.
4. Select the punch (4 mm is the most useful size) and hold it vertically to the skin.
5. Rotate (in a clockwise, screwing motion) with firm pressure to cut a plug about 3 mm in depth (Fig. 104.11). Remove the punch.

Fig. 104.10 *Shave biopsy*

excision
scalpel held
horizontally

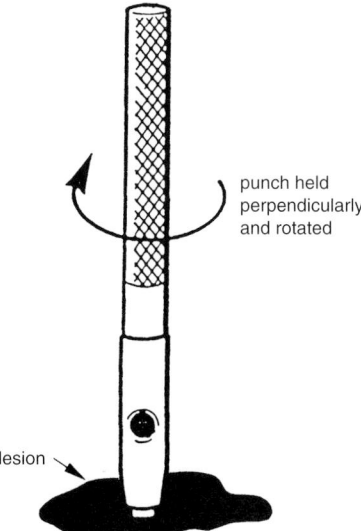

Fig. 104.11 *Punch biopsy*

punch held
perpendicularly
and rotated

lesion

- necrobiosis lipoidica
- hypertrophic lichen planus

Triamcinolone is the appropriate long-acting corticosteroid (10 mg/mL). It may be diluted in equal quantities with saline.

Method

1. The steroid should be injected into the lesion (not below it).
2. Insert a 25 or (preferably) 27 gauge needle, firmly locked to a small insulin-type 1 mL syringe, into the lesion at the level of the middle of the dermis (Fig. 104.12).
3. High pressure is required with some lesions (e.g. keloid).
4. Inject sufficient steroid to make the lesion blanch.
5. Several sites will be needed for larger lesions, so preceding LA may be required in some instances. Avoid infiltration of steroid in larger lesions: use multiple injections.

6. Use fine-toothed forceps or a tissue hook to grip the outer rim of the plug.
7. Exert gentle traction and undercut the base of the plug parallel to the skin surface, using fine-pointed scissors or a scalpel.
8. Place the specimen in fixative.
9. Secure haemostasis by firm pressure or by diathermy.
10. Apply a dry dressing or a single suture to the defect.

Steroid injections into skin lesions

Suitable lesions for steroid injections are:

- plaque psoriasis
- granuloma annulare
- hypertrophic scars (early development)
- keloid scars (early development)
- alopecia areata
- lichen simplex chronicus

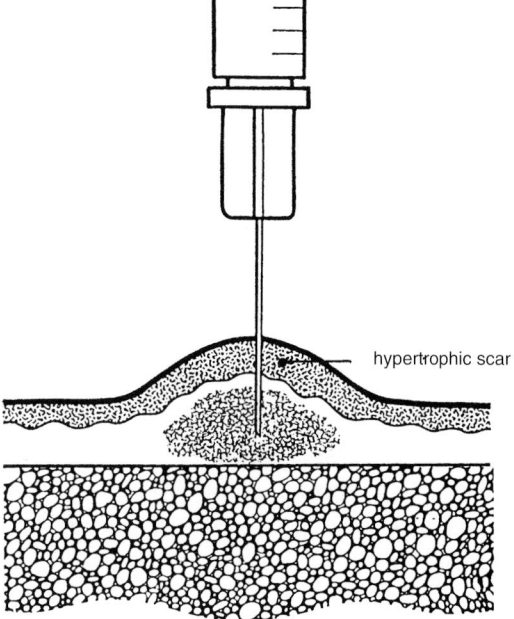

hypertrophic scar

Fig. 104.12 *Injection of corticosteroid into mid-dermis*

Elliptical excisions

Small lesions are best excised as an ellipse. Generally, the long axis of the ellipse should be along the skin tension lines identified by natural wrinkles.

The intended ellipse should be drawn on the skin (Fig. 104.13). The placement will depend on

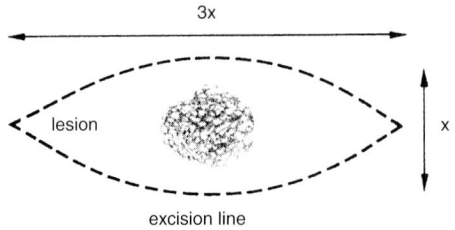

Fig. 104.13· *Ellipse excision*

such factors as the size and shape of the lesion, the margin required (usually 2–3 mm) and the skin tension lines.

General points
- The length of the ellipse should be three times the width.
- This length should be increased (say, to four times) in areas with little subcutaneous tissue (dorsum of hand) and high skin tension (upper back).
- A good rule is to obtain an angle at each end of the excision of 30° or less.
- These rules should achieve closure without 'dog ears'.

Excisions on the face
It is important to select optimal sites for elliptical excisions of tumours of the face. As a rule it is best for incisions to follow wrinkle lines and the direction of hair follicles in the beard area. Therefore, follow the natural wrinkles in the glabella area, the 'crow's feet' around the eye, and the nasolabial folds (Fig. 104.14). To determine non-obvious wrinkles, gently compress the relaxed skin in different directions to demonstrate the lines.

For tumours of the forehead make horizontal incisions, although vertical incisions may be used for large tumours of the forehead. Ensure that you keep your incisions in the temporal area quite superficial, as the frontal branch of the facial nerve is easily cut.

When to refer

Referral should be considered for:
- suspicion of melanoma
- tumours larger than 1 cm
- recurrent tumours, despite treatment
- incompletely excised tumours, especially with poor healing
- doubts about appropriate treatment
- recommended treatment beyond skills of practitioner

Fig. 104.14 *Recommended lines for excisions on face*
ADAPTED FROM J.S. BROWN, *MINOR SURGERY: A TEXT AND ATLAS*, CHAPMAN AND HALL, LONDON, 1986

References

1. Paver R. The surgical management of cutaneous tumours in general practice. Mod Med Aust, March 1991; 43–51.
2. Marks R. Skin cancer. In: MIMS Disease Index. (2nd edn). Sydney: IMS Publishing, 1996, 469–472.
3. Davis A, Bolin T, Ham J. *Symptom analysis and physical diagnosis* (2nd edn). Sydney: Pergamon Press, 1990, 302–306.
4. de Launey WE, Land WA. *Principles and practice of dermatology* (2nd edn). Sydney: Butterworths, 1984, 280–281.
5. Berger P. Warts: how to treat them successfully. Mod Med Aust, August 1990, 28–32.
6. Reddy J. Intralesional injection for orf: a practice tip. Aust Fam Physician, 1993; 22:65.
7. La Villa G. Methylprednisolone acetate in local therapy of ganglion. Clinical Therapeutics, 1986; 47:455–457.

105

Pigmented skin lesions

The management of pimented skin lesions is a constant concern for all practitioners and requires careful evaluation based on the natural history of these lesions and the increasing incidence of malignant melanoma in particular.

Most pigmented lesions are benign and include simple moles or melanocytic naevi, seborrhoeic keratoses, freckles and lentigines. Reassurance is all that is necessary in the management of these problems.

However, one-third of all melanomas arise in pre-existing naevi, many of which are dysplastic, and it is the recognition and removal of such naevi that is so important in the prevention of melanoma.[1]

Malignant melanoma is doubling in incidence each decade, which is an alarming statistic considering the public education programs about the hazards of sun exposure. Of equal interest is the fact that the cure rate for melanoma is also increasing, reflecting earlier diagnosis and treatment.[2]

A classification of pigmented skin lesions is given in Table 105.1.

Key facts and checkpoints

- The incidence of melanoma is greatest in white caucasians and increases with proximity to the equator.

Table 105.1 *Classification of pigmented skin lesions*

Non-melanocytic
- pigmented basal cell carcinoma
- seborrhoeic keratoses (page 1011)
- solar keratoses (page 1012)
- dermatofibroma (page 1012)
- pyogenic granuloma
- foreign body granuloma
- talon noir (black heel)
- tinea nigra
- Becker's naevus

Melanocytic
Non-melanoma:
- freckles
- lentigines
- naevi
  1. congenital
  2. acquired
     — junctional → compound → intradermal
     — dysplastic
     — halo
     — blue
     — Spitz

Melanoma:
1. lentigo maligna (Hutchinson's melanotic freckle)
2. superficial spreading melanoma
3. nodular melanoma
4. acral lentiginous melanoma

- The early diagnosis and treatment of melanoma profoundly affects the prognosis.
- Melanoma is extremely rare before puberty, but 70% generate before the age of 21.
- Most people have 5–10 melanocytic naevi on average.
- Multiple dysplastic naevi carry a higher risk of malignant change, which may occur in young adults. Such patients require regular observation (with photography).

Pyogenic granuloma

Synonyms: granuloma, granuloma telangiectaticum, acquired haemangioma

A pyogenic granuloma is a vascular lesion (without pus) due to a proliferation of capillary vessels. It is considered to be an abnormal reaction to minor trauma.

Clinical features:

- common in children and young adults
- usually on hands and face
- bright red 'raspberry'-like lesion
- raised, sometimes pedunculated
- friable—bleeds easily

Management

It must be distinguished from amelanotic melanoma or anaplastic SCC. Shave biopsy with electrocautery of base. The specimen must be sent for histological examination. They are prone to recur.

Talon noir ('black heel')

Talon noir is a black spotted appearance on the heel and is common in sportspeople. A similar lesion (probably smaller) is often found on the other heel.

'Black heel' is formed by small petechiae caused by the trauma of the sharp turns required in sport: shearing stress on the skin of the heel produces superficial bleeding. The diagnosis can be confirmed by gentle paring of the callus to reveal the multiple small petechial spots in the epidermis; these are then pared away. If there is doubt about the diagnosis (malignant melanoma is the main differential diagnosis), the lesion should be excised.

Tinea nigra

Tinea nigra is characterised by solitary black macular lesions on the palm or sole. The simple technique of taking skin scrapings to reveal fungal elements will allow easy differentiation from malignant melanoma.

Becker's naevus

Becker's naevus is a faint, brown, diffuse pigmented area with a component of coarse hairs and is usually found on the shoulder and upper trunk. It occurs mainly in boys around puberty.

It is not a birthmark, it is benign and reassurance is appropriate.

Freckles

Freckles are small brown macules (usually < 0.5 cm), coloured by excessive epidermal melanin without any increase in the number of naevus cells (melanocytes). They occur mainly on light-coloured skin and tend to darken in summer and fade in winter. Cosmetic improvement can be achieved through the use of sunscreens.

Lentigines

Lentigines are small rounded, brown to black macular areas ranging from 1 mm to 1 cm or more across. They are very common and may appear in childhood as a few scattered lesions, often on areas not exposed to the sun. They may erupt during pregnancy. In the elderly, lentigines often develop on sun-damaged skin, usually on the backs of the hands (so-called 'liver spots') and on the face.

Unlike freckles they have increased numbers of melanocytes.

Management

Treatment is usually unnecessary. Liquid nitrogen or excision can be used for cosmetically unacceptable lesions. Sunscreens are needed to prevent further darkening of existing lesions.

Congenital melanocytic naevi

These moles are present at birth and are sometimes large.

Clinical features:

- variable colour: brown to black
- sometimes hairy and protruding
- increased risk of malignant change (especially in larger ones)

Common acquired naevi

These are the common moles for which an opinion is so often sought. The moles are localised benign proliferation of naevus cells. There may be a sharp increase in numbers during pregnancy. New lesions appear less frequently after the age of 20. The types are junctional, compound and intradermal. Naevi in children are usually the junctional type with proliferating naevus cells clumped at the dermoepidermal junction. With time the naevus cells 'move' into the dermis. A compound naevus has both junctional and dermal elements. With maturation all the naevus cells move into the dermis. Refer to Figure 105.1.

Clinical features

Junctional

- usually < 5 mm
- circular-shaped macules
- may be slightly elevated
- colour usually brown to black
- may be 'fuzzy' border with brownish halo

Most naevi of the palms, soles and genitals are junctional but there is no evidence to support the traditional view that naevi in these sites have more malignant potential.[2]

Compound

- dome-shaped, slightly raised pigmented nodules
- up to 1 cm in diameter
- colour varies from light to dark brown/black, but lighter than junctional naevi
- most are smooth but surface can be rough or verrucoid
- larger ones may be hairy, especially after puberty
- become 'flesh'-coloured in time

Intradermal

- look like compound but less pigmented

- often skin-coloured
- may evolve to pink or brown senile nodules or to soft pedunculated tags

Malignant potential of common acquired melanocytic naevi

Junctional: have significant potential to undergo malignant change (as long as junctional activity is present)

Compound: very rarely undergo malignant change

Intradermal: these are totally benign lesions

Management
- Provide appropriate reassurance.
- Observe.
- If lesion is changing or there is uncertainty, perform surgical excision (2–3 mm margin) for histopathology.

Halo naevus

A halo naevus consists of a depigmented halo around a central melanocytic naevus. It is the result of an autoimmune reaction. The central naevus gradually involutes. It tends to occur around puberty.

Caution: A halo can occur around a melanoma.

Management
Measure the lesion. Reassure and do nothing, as it usually disappears over the next few years; if

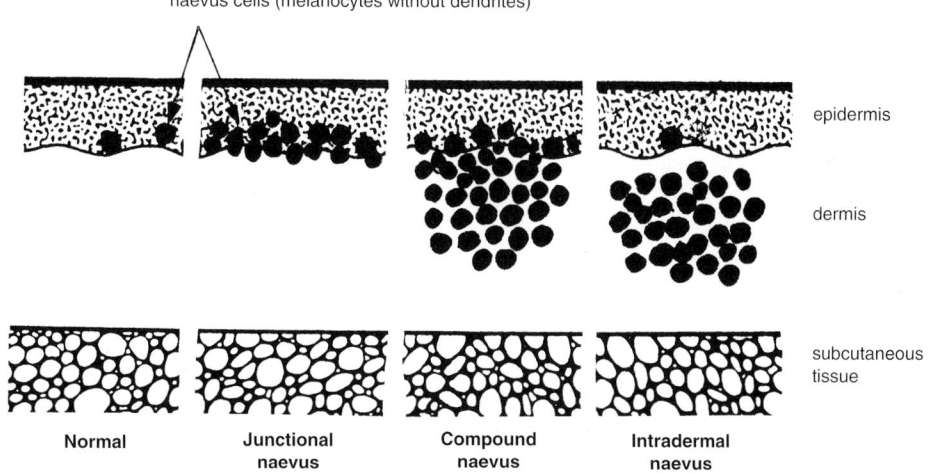

naevus cells (melanocytes without dendrites)

epidermis

dermis

subcutaneous tissue

Normal   Junctional naevus   Compound naevus   Intradermal naevus

Fig. 105.1 *Comparison of melanocyte (naevus cell) distribution in various common acquired naevi*

doubtful at all, remove and obtain histological diagnosis.

Blue naevus

A blue naevus presents as a solitary slate-grey-blue dermal lesion. Blue naevi usually present in childhood and adolescence on the lower back and buttocks and the limbs, especially dorsa of the hands and feet. Malignant change is rare. Often excised for cosmetic reasons.

Spitz naevus (benign juvenile melanoma)

Spitz naevi are also called benign juvenile melanomas or spindle cell naevi.
  Clinical features:

- solitary pigmented or erythematous nodules
- often appear in children, usually 4–8 years
- develop over 1–3 months
- well circumscribed, dome-shaped lesions

Management

Surgical excision is treatment of choice (because of rapid growth and best 'reassurance' policy).

Dysplastic melanocytic naevi

These are large irregular moles which appear predominantly on the trunk in young adults. They can be familial or sporadic and are markers of an increased risk of melanoma, rather than necessarily being premalignant lesions. Even so, melanoma may arise within these lesions more frequently than would be expected by random chance.[3]
  They are considered to be intermediate between benign naevi and melanoma.
  Clinical features:

- age: adolescence onwards
- large > 5 mm (variable size)
- most common on trunk
- irregular and ill-defined border
- irregular pigmentation
- background redness
- variable colours: brown, tan, black, pink
- variation of colours within the naevus
- most are stable and do not progress to melanoma

Dysplastic naevus syndrome

The presence of multiple, large, irregular pigmented naevi, mainly on the trunk, presents a difficult management problem, especially if there is a family history of melanoma. The lifetime risk of melanoma may approach 100% for such patients.

Management

Use a follow-up program (similar to excised early melanoma) of 6 monthly review for 2 years (3 monthly if family history of melanoma) and yearly thereafter, provided no lesions become malignant during the first 2 years. During this time the patient and family should become well versed in surveillance. Apart from measurement, good professional quality photographs of areas of the body or specific lesions of concern may also be helpful.
  Any suspicious lesions should be excised for histological examination.

Advice to patients

To decrease your chances of getting a melanoma, you should protect yourself from the sun. These rules should be followed:

- Try to avoid direct sunlight when the sun is at its strongest (from 10 am to 3 pm).
- Always wear a broad-brimmed hat and T-shirt in the sun.
- Use a factor 15+ sunscreen on exposed skin and renew the sunscreen regularly.
- Sunbaking might give you a good tan but it is also going to increase your chances of getting a melanoma, so you should avoid it.

Melanoma

The early diagnosis of melanoma is vital to outcome. Thickness of a melanoma when it is removed is the major factor determining prognosis: it is vital to detect melanomas when they are in the thin stage and look like an unusual freckle.
  In Australia, only about 30% of melanomas develop in pre-existing melanocytic naevi (moles).[2,3] The majority arise in apparently normal skin. Initially the tumour tends to spread laterally in many cases and it should be removed at this stage when it is easily cured. An irregular border or margin is suggestive of the tumour.

Clinical features
- typical age range 30–50 years (average 40)
- can occur anywhere on the body
  - more common — lower limbs in women
  - — upper back in men
- often asymptomatic
- can bleed or itch

Change
The sign of major importance is a recent change in a 'freckle' or mole:
- change in size: at edge or thickening
- change in shape
- change in colour: brown, blue, black, red, white, including combinations
- change in surface
- change in the border
- bleeding or ulceration
- other symptoms, e.g. itching
- development of satellite nodules
- lymph node involvement

Types of melanoma

Lentigo maligna[3]
Lentigo maligna (Hutchinson's melanotic freckle) is a slow-growing form of intraepidermal melanoma which occurs on areas exposed to light (usually the face), predominantly in the elderly. If allowed to remain it may become invasive and the prognosis will be similar to that for other invasive melanomas. These lesions have all the variations in size, shape and colour of superficial melanomas.

Superficial spreading melanoma
Like lentigo maligna, the initial growth is in a lateral or radial intraepidermal manner, rather than in an invasive downward or vertical manner. It exhibits a striking colour variation. It accounts for 70% of melanomas.

Nodular melanoma
Nodular melanoma, which accounts for 20% of melanomas, has no radial growth phase. It is typically found on the trunk and limbs of young to middle-aged individuals. It may have a 'blueberry'-like nodule. Prognosis is determined by thickness at the time of excision.

Acral lentiginous melanoma
These typically occur on palms, soles and distal phalanges. They have a poorer prognosis than other types. They occur mainly in dark-skinned races.

Variations
Amelanotic melanomas are flesh-coloured papules that increase in size or change shape. These lesions can be extremely difficult to diagnose and the poor prognosis associated with them is due to late diagnosis rather than an increased malignancy.

The features and associations of melanoma subtypes are presented in Table 105.2.

Prognosis
Determinants of prognosis include:[3]
- thickness (Breslow classification)
- level or depth (worse in level 4 or 5) (Fig. 105.2)
- site (worse on head and neck, trunk)
- sex (worse for men)
- age (worse > 50 years)
- amelanotic melanoma
- ulceration

Vertical growth is associated with invasion and the prognosis worsens with depth. The chance of cure is greater than 90% if a melanoma is removed when it is less than 0.75 mm thick.[3] If the lesion is allowed to invade to a thickness of

Table 105.2 *Features and associations of melanoma subtypes (after Kelly)*[4]

Melanoma subtype	Frequency %	Radial growth phase	Location	Average age	Occupation profile
Superficial spreading	70	+	Trunk (back), limbs (legs)	Middle-aged	Indoor worker
Nodular	20	−	Trunk, limbs	Middle-aged	Indoor worker
Lentigo maligna	7.5	+	Head, neck	Elderly	Outdoor worker
Acral lentiginous	2.5	+	Palms, soles mucosae	Not known	Not known

Reproduced with permission of J. Kelly[4]

Fig. 105.2 *Assessment of tumour level: the levels of melanoma invasion*   PRODUCED BY PERMISSION J. KELLY[4]

4 mm or more, the likelihood of a cure is reduced to less than 30%.[3]

The influence of tumour thickness on 5 year survival rates is shown in Table 105.3.

Staging is based on the tumour level (depth) shown in Figure 105.2:

Level 1—confined to the epidermis (*in situ*)
Level 2—tumour cells extend into the superficial (papillary) dermis
Level 3—tumour cells fill up the superficial dermis
Level 4—tumour cells extend into the deeper (reticular) layer
Level 5—invasion of subcutaneous tissue

Differential diagnosis

There are several common skin lesions that may be mistaken for melanoma.[1] They are:

1. Haemangioma (thrombosed)
2. Dermatofibroma (sclerosing haemangioma)
3. Pigmented seborrhoeic keratosis
4. Pigmented basal cell carcinoma
5. Junctional and compound naevi
6. Blue naevi
7. Dysplastic naevi
8. Lentigines

Facilitating early diagnosis of melanoma

An adequate light source without shadows is essential. Refer to page 959 for use of the 'maggy-lamp' and the dermatoscope.

Table 105.3   *The influence of tumour thickness on 5 year survival rates (after Kelly)*[4]

Range of tumour thickness (mm)	5 year survival rates %
< 0.76	95–100
0.76–1.5	70–98
1.51–4.0	55–85
> 4.0	30–60

Reproduced with permission of J. Kelly[4]

Clinical examination of the skin[1]

It is important to examine the entire skin and not just the lesion presented by the patient. Comparison of pigmented skin lesions is very helpful in differentiating between benign and malignant. One satisfactory routine is:

• Starting at the head, examine the hairline, backs of ears, neck, back, and backs of the arms. Pull down the underwear to expose the buttocks; examine the backs of the legs.
• With the patient facing you, examine the anterior hairline, the front of the ears, the forehead, cheeks and neck, moving downwards to the anterior chest. Move bra straps as required to achieve complete coverage. Then examine the abdomen, pulling down the underwear to examine as far as the pubic hairs.
• Then examine the anterior surfaces of the legs. The 'maggylamp' is very useful for this examination.

After scanning the entire skin surface and comparing and contrasting naevi, specific lesions may be examined with the dermatoscope.

Compare suspicious lesions with similar lesions elsewhere on the patient's skin.

Applying the ABCDE system[1]

A = **A**symmetry
Melanoma is almost always asymmetrical. Most non-melanoma lesions are symmetrical, oval or round.

B = **B**order
The border of the melanoma is usually well defined, especially in the more malignant, compared with the dysplastic naevus which is almost always indistinct with a fading out 'shoulder' effect. The border of the melanoma is irregular while most benign lesions have a regular edge.

C = **C**olour
The classic blue-black colour is helpful but the *variety* of colours present in most melanomas is the most helpful. Magnification usually visualises greys, whites, violets, reds, oranges and shades of brown interspersed in the darker blue-black pigmentation. Early melanomas developing in dysplastic naevi tend not to have this deep pigmentation.

D = **D**iameter
The majority of melanomas when first seen are at least 7 mm in diameter, especially if arising from a pre-existing naevus. However, it is possible to diagnose small nodular melanomas < 5 mm.

E = **E**levation
Elevation indicates invasion and is a sign of more advanced disease.

Diagnosis by exclusion

In the diagnostic process consider the lesions outlined in the differential diagnosis and check out the various characteristics. Haemangiomas may have an emptying sign when pressed with a finger. Pigmented BCCs can be difficult if they are fully pigmented but this is uncommon. The characteristic pearly-grey look and the telangiectasia are usually still visible on magnification with the 'maggylamp'. The most useful feature of dysplastic naevi is that they are usually multiple and lesions for comparison can generally be found elsewhere. Dysplastic naevi also have greater breadth and height and often a darker nodule in the centre—the 'target' sign.

Management points for naevi and melanomas

- Do not inject local anaesthetic directly into the lesion.
- Incisional biopsy of a melanoma or suspicious mole is best avoided.
- Accurate clinical diagnosis, with the definitive treatment performed in one stage, is optimal, rather than excision biopsy with follow-up surgery.

Management tips[1]

- The solitary dysplastic naevus has no significant malignant potential.
- Multiple excision of naevi is not justified.
- If in doubt, perform excision biopsy with a margin of 2–3 mm. Refer to Figure 105.3 for the protocol for a suspicious lesion.

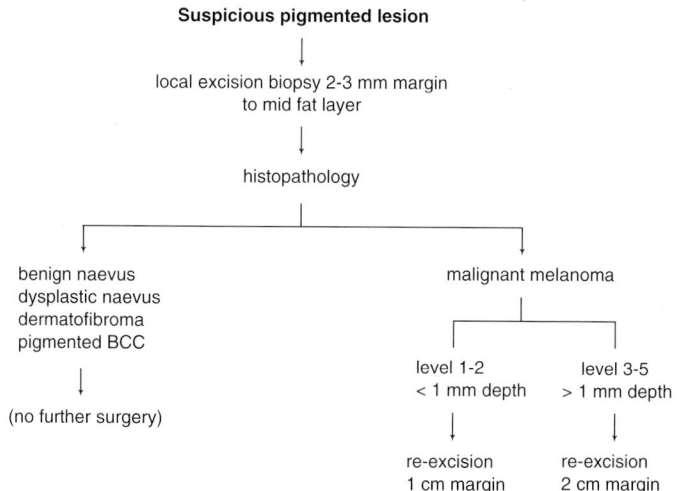

Fig. 105.3 *Plan for management of a suspicious pigmented lesion*   AFTER PETER SINCLAIR[5]

- If melanoma is strongly suspected, referral to a consultant is necessary.
- Beware of the pigmented BCC—it is easily missed but it usually has a shiny surface.
- Do not freeze a pigmented lesion—take a biopsy.

Counselling

An encouragingly positive and supportive approach can realistically be taken for most patients, as the overall survival for melanoma in Australia is more than 80%.[1]

Even with tumours greater than 4 mm thickness, 50% of patients will survive.

Follow-up

Follow-up tends to be based on the tumour thickness:[1]

1 mm	6 monthly review for 2 years
1–2 mm	4 monthly for 2 years, 6 monthly for next 2 years, then yearly for 10 years
> 2 mm	review by both specialist and GP, regularly, for 10 years

The first sign of metastasis is usually to the lungs so a yearly chest X-ray is advisable.

References

1. McCarthy W. The management of melanoma. Aust Fam Physician, 1993; 22:1177–1186.
2. Lauritz B. Pigmented skin lesions. In: Monash University Medical School's Annual Update Course for GPs. Course Proceedings, 1992, 33–34.
3. Marks R. Skin cancer. In: MIMS Disease Index (2nd edn). Sydney: IMS Publishing, 1996, 469–472.
4. Kelly J. The management of early skin cancer in the 1990s. Aust Fam Physician, 1990; 19:1714–1729.
5. Sinclair P. Whitehorse Division of GP refresher course. Marysville, 1997, 4.

PART 9

COMMON CONTINUING MANAGEMENT PROBLEMS

106

Alcohol problems

If you want to keep a dead man, put him in whisky;
if you want to kill a live man put whisky in him.

Thomas Guthrie (1803–73)

Excessive drinking of alcohol is one of the most common and socially destructive problems in Australia. One survey found that 5% of Australian men and 1% of women were alcohol-dependent. It also showed that 84% of men and 80% of women drink alcohol, with 22% of the population drinking alcohol every day.[1]

Skinner refers to the prevalence of 'alcoholism' in North America as about 5–7% of the adult group, with a much larger group (20–30%) of individuals having drinking problems without major symptoms of alcoholism.[2] Abstainers represent 10–20% of populations.

Excessive and harmful drinking

People are said to be dependent on alcohol when it is affecting their physical health and social life yet they do not seem to be prepared to stop drinking to solve their problems.

For men, excessive drinking is more than four standard drinks of alcohol a day. For women, drinking becomes a serious problem at lesser amounts—two standard drinks a day. This level can also affect the foetus of the pregnant woman. High-risk or harmful drinking occurs at

Table 106.1 *NH&MRC guidelines: number of standard drinks each day*

	Low risk	Hazardous	Harmful
Men	0–4	5–6	> 6
Women	0–2	3–4	> 4

more than six drinks a day for men and four drinks a day for women. The NH&MRC's guidelines for drinking are summarised in Table 106.1.

Extent of the problem

- Alcohol is estimated to have a harmful effect on about 1 in 10 people.
- At least 15% of all patients admitted to hospital have an alcohol-related illness.
- About 50% of fatal traffic accidents involve alcohol.
- The author's study[3] identified alcohol dependence in 9.7% of the population studied and a further group of problem drinkers that included the 'explosive' or binge drinker (Fig. 106.1) Problem drinkers represent about 15–20% of the population.

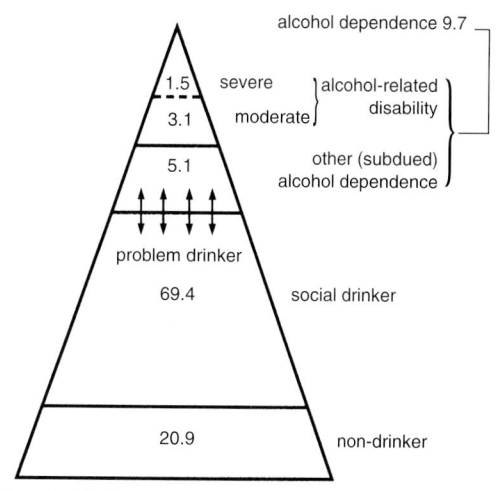

Fig. 106.1 *Prevalence of alcohol drinking patterns in the adult population (figures expressed as a percentage)*

Identifying the problem

As a profession we generally seem to be very slow in recognising the problem drinker; we need to train ourselves to have a sixth sense in early detection of the heavy or problem drinker.

Clinical pointers

Alcohol abuse should be suspected in any patient presenting with one or more of the physical or psychosocial problems presented in Table 106.2. Target areas for clinical scrutiny are outlined in Table 106.3. The facial features of the patient can be a helpful pointer, albeit of the more advanced drinker. These include:

- plethoric facies
- puffy 'greasy' facies
- telangiectasia
- rosacea + rhinophyma
- suffused ('bloodshot') conjunctivae
- prominent lower lip with chelitis of corners of mouth
- smell of stale alcohol or very 'minty' sweet breath (masking effect)

Table 106.3 *Target areas for clinical scrutiny*

Young and middle-aged bachelors
Divorced or separated individuals
Alcoholic beverage trade: bar trade, hotel staff
Professionals: politicians, doctors and others
Travelling professions, e.g. seamen, salesmen, truck drivers
Armed forces, especially returned servicemen
Authors, journalists and related workers
Social club patrons, e.g. sporting clubs

Taking a drinking history

This requires tact and skill and it must be noted that many problem drinkers considerably understate the level of their intake.

Useful strategies
- Ask questions as part of a matter-of-fact enquiry into health risk factors such as smoking and diet.

Table 106.2 *Adverse clinical effects of alcohol*

Psychological and social effects	Physical effects
• loss of self-esteem	• brain damage (if severe)
• irritability	• depression
• devious behaviour	• epilepsy
• anxiety and phobias	• Wernicke-Korsakoff syndrome
• depression	• insomnia—nightmares
• paranoia	• hypertension
• stress	• heart disease
• relationship breakdown	— arrhythmias
• child abuse	— cardiomyopathy
• poor work performance	— beri-beri heart disease
• memory disturbances	• liver disease
• financial problems	• pancreatic disease
• accidents	• dyspepsia (indigestion)
• driving offences	• acute gastritis
• crime–violence	• stomach ulcers
• personal neglect	• sexual dysfunction
• attempted suicide	• hand tremor
• pathological jealousy	• peripheral neuropathy
	• myopathy
	• gout
	• obesity
	• other metabolic/endocrine effects
	— hyperlipidaemia
	— pseudo-Cushing's syndrome
	— osteoporosis
	— osteomalacia
	• haemopoiesis
	— macrocytosis
	— leucopenia
	— thrombocytopenia

- Place the onus of denial on the patient by asking questions such as 'When did you last drink alcohol?' rather than 'Do you ever drink alcohol?'
- Record your patient's intake quantitatively in terms of standard drinks or grams of alcohol.
- Confirm the history by enquiring about the time spent drinking per day and expenditure on alcohol.

Useful questions
- When did you last drink alcohol?
- Do you like alcohol?
- What is your usual intake each day? Each week?
- What type of alcohol do you prefer to drink?
- Do you take a drink in the morning?
- Do you eat breakfast?
- When was the last time you felt nauseated or 'off-colour' in the morning?
- When do you get heartburn?
- Do you drink with your mates or family or at the club?
- How long do you usually go without alcohol?
- When was the last time you were drunk?
- When was the last time you cannot remember a drinking session?
- About how much alcohol can you take before it affects you?
- Has alcohol had any effects on you?
- Does it give you the shakes?
- Do you ever need to take alcohol to help you get to sleep?
- Do you need it to steady your nerves?

Questionnaires
There are several questionnaires that can be most helpful, assuming the patient is fully co-operative. Two or more positive replies for the CAGE questionnaire[4] are suggestive of a problem drinker.

1. Have you ever felt you should CUT down on your drinking?
2. Have people ANNOYED you by criticising your drinking?
3. Have you ever felt bad or GUILTY about your drinking?
4. Have you ever had a drink first thing in the morning to steady your nerves or get rid of a hangover? (an EYE-OPENER)

Another very practical questionnaire is AUDIT (The Alcohol Use Disorders Identification Test) developed by the WHO to facilitate the early detection of problem drinkers.

Laboratory investigations

The following blood tests may be helpful in the identification of excessive chronic alcohol intake.

- blood alcohol
- serum gamma glutamyl transferase (GGT): elevated in chronic drinkers (returns to normal with cessation of intake)
- mean corpuscular volume (MCV) : > 96fl

Other changes:

- abnormal liver function tests (other than GGT)
- high-density lipoproteins elevated
- low-density lipoproteins lowered
- serum uric acid elevated

Measuring alcohol intake

One standard drink contains 10 g of alcohol, which is the amount in one middy (or pot) of standard beer (285 mL), two middies of low-alcohol beer or five middies of super-light beer. These are equal in alcohol content to one small glass of table wine (120 mL), one glass of sherry or port (60 mL) or one nip of spirits (30 mL) (Fig. 106.2)

| 1 middy of standard beer (285 mL or 10 oz) | 1 glass of wine (120 mL or 4 oz) | 1 glass of sherry or port (60 mL or 2 oz) | 1 nip of spirits (30 mL or 1 oz) |

Fig. 106.2 *Standard drinks*

1 stubby or can of beer   = 1.3 standard
                                              drinks
1 × 750 mL bottle of beer = 2.6 standard
                                              drinks
1 × 750 mL bottle of wine = 6 standard
                                              drinks

The 0.05 level

To keep below the 0.05 blood alcohol level
drinking and driving limit, a 70 kg man or
woman should not exceed:

2 standard drinks in 1 hour
3 standard drinks in 2 hours
4 standard drinks in 3 hours

The rule is that one standard drink is eliminated
per hour so it is important to spread drinking time.

Approach to management

The challenge to the family doctor is early recognition of the problem. There are specific target
areas which should be considered carefully by
the general practitioner (Table 106.3). Several
studies have shown that early intervention and
brief counselling by the doctor are effective in
leading to rehabilitation.[5] Some of the results are
very revealing:

- Patients expect their family doctor to advise on
  safe drinking levels.[6]
- They will listen and act on our advice.[7]
- Treatment is more effective if offered before
  dependence   or   chronic   disease   has
  developed.[7,8]

Of prime concern to the GP is the assessment
of whether the patient is interested in changing
his or her excessive drinking behaviour. The proposed model of change by Prochaska and Di
Clemente helps identify the stage reached by the
patient (Fig. 106.3).[9]

Precontemplators are satisfied users who are
either unconcerned about their drinking or have
no desire to change. However, if there is any
evidence of ambivalence or concern about
drinking then the opportunity exists for motivational interviewing techniques.

Patients tend to have little insight into their
problem and often need the development of
unpleasant sequelae to make them aware of
their alcohol-related problem. Furthermore,
patients are not likely to offer concern about
their drinking problem spontaneously but are
often receptive to the initiative coming from their
doctor.

The family doctor is ideally placed to identify
and treat the problem of alcohol because the
individual who abuses alcohol will tend to
surface at some point in the provision of primary
health care.

Of particular concern are teenage and early
adult drinking patterns, often influenced by environmental factors including the home and sporting clubs. Fortunately, many young people are
able to control their drinking as they mature, provided they survive the risk-taking behaviour
period. However, those who remain single tend
to adopt drinking as part of their lifestyle. When
the duration of excessive drinking increases to
10 or 15 years, patients tend to present with
classic alcohol-related diseases.[2] According to
Skinner, alcohol dependency usually develops
in individuals in their early twenties, yet most
patients admitted to alcohol treatment programs
have a history of heavy drinking of 10–20 years
with associated alcohol-related morbidity.

Alcohol-sensitising drugs

Drugs that cause a most unpleasant reaction
when taken with alcohol include disulfiram and
calcium carbimide. Their role is controversial
and they should be restricted to a co-operative
and highly motivated patient who gives informed
consent.

The reaction causes nausea, vomiting, flushing, dizziness and dyspnoea.

Management

The best results are obtained with early recognition of the problem and prompt intervention
to resolve it; the patient's admission of the
problem and a resolve to face it; firm support
and interest by the medical team and appropriate support from family and friends. The patient
should set their own goals and develop a contract with their GP.

A brief practical management plan[10]

Giving patients feedback about their level of
alcohol consumption, presenting objective
evidence of harm and setting realistic goals for
reducing alcohol intake induces many to change
their drinking behaviour.

A six-step management plan, which has been
employed in a general-practice early intervention program, is as follows:

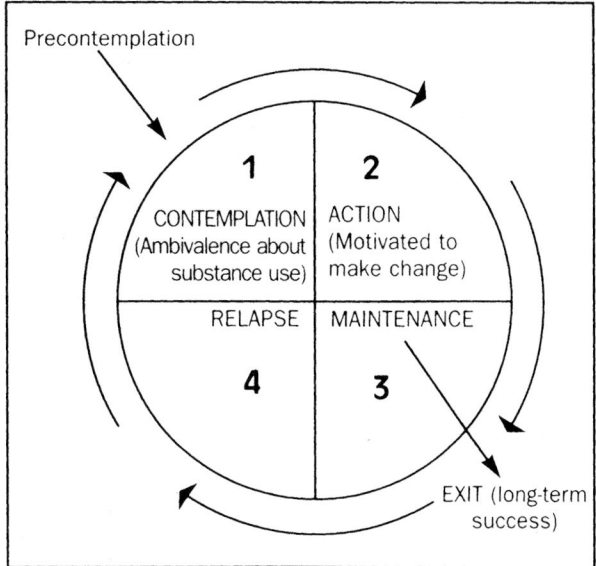

Fig. 106.3 *Prochaska's and Di Clemente's proposed model of change to facilitate the identification of behavioural stages and the provision of counselling for treating dependence on alcohol, tobacco and other drugs*

1. *Feed back* the results of your assessment and specifically the degree of risk associated with their daily alcohol intake and bout drinking. Emphasise any damage that has already occurred.
2. *Listen* carefully to their reaction. They will need to ventilate their feelings and may respond defensively.
3. *Outline the benefits* of reducing drinking:
   - save money
   - less hassles from family
   - sleep better
   - have more energy
   - be less depressed
   - lose weight
   - better physical shape
   - lessen the risk of:
     — hypertension
     — liver disease
     — brain disease
     — cancer
     — accidents
4. *Set goals* for alcohol consumption which you both agree are feasible. In most cases this will involve reduction to below certain 'safe limits'.
   - For men: *no more than* 3–4 drinks 3–4 times per week (aim for less than 12 per week).
   - For women: *no more than* 2–3 drinks 2–3 times per week (aim for less than 8 per

week). Pregnant women should not have more than 1 drink 2–3 times per week. Some authorities recommend total abstinence.

These are the *upper safe limits* and are *not* amounts that patients should be recommended to drink if their intake is normally lower.

For patients who have already experienced some physical damage or substantial psychosocial problems, it is best to advise a period of total abstinence. For patients who are physically dependent on alcohol, long-term abstinence is advisable.

5. *Set strategies* to keep below the upper safe limits:
   - Quench thirst with non-alcoholic drinks before having an alcoholic one.
   - Have the first alcoholic drink *after* starting to eat (avoid drinking on an empty stomach).
   - Switch to low-alcohol beer.
   - Take care which parties you go to: avoid constant parties and other high-risk situations.
   - Think of a good explanation for cutting down on your drinking.
   - Have a physical workout when bored or stressed.
   - Explore new interests—fishing, cinema, social club, sporting activity.

6. *Evaluate* progress by having patients monitor their drinking by using a diary; check that any abnormal blood test results are returning to normal. Make a definite appointment for follow-up and give appropriate literature such as *Alcohol and health*. Obtain consent for a telephone follow-up. A useful minimum intervention plan is presented in Table 106.4.

The use of disulfiram[11]

In compliant patients, disulfiram 250–500 mg (o) daily can be used—such treatment has hazards and the patient requires intensive supportive therapy.

Follow-up (long consultation one week later)

Review the patient's drinking diary. Explore any problems, summarise, listen and provide support and encouragement. If appointment is not kept, contact the patient.

Specialist services

According to progress and the patient's wishes and consent, specialist treatment units, group therapy and attendance at meetings of Alanon or Alcoholics Anonymous are potential sources of help to keep the alcohol-dependent person abstinent and coping.

Withdrawal symptoms

Symptoms of a 'hangover' include headache, nausea, irritability, malaise and a mild tremor. Withdrawal from alcohol in a chronic problem drinker includes:

- agitation
- prominent tremor
- sweating
- insomnia
- seizures
- delirium tremens

Table 106.4 *Minimum intervention technique plan (5–10 minutes)*

1. Advise reduction to safe levels
2. Outline the benefits
3. Provide a self-help pamphlet
4. Organise a diary or other feedback system
5. Obtain consent for a telephone follow-up
6. Offer additional help, e.g. referral to an alcohol and drug unit or to a support group

---

Treatment for moderate symptoms is based on diazepam. The aim is to prevent development of delirium tremens. Maintain fluid, electrolytes and nutrition. Add vitamin B complex including thiamine because the patients are invariably thiamine deficient.

Recommended treatment for acute withdrawal symptoms[11]

- diazepam 10–20 mg (o) every 2 hours (up to 120 mg (o) daily) titrated against clinical response (taper off after 2 days)
- thiamine 100 mg IM or IV daily for 3–5 days, then 100 mg (o) daily
- vitamin B group supplement (o) or IM daily.

Delirium tremens

DTs is a serious life-threatening withdrawal state. It has a high mortality rate if inadequately treated and hospitalisation is always necessary.

Clinical features:

- may be precipitated by intercurrent infection or trauma
- 1–5 days after withdrawal (usually 3–4 days)
- disorientation, agitation
- clouding of consciousness
- marked tremor
- visual hallucinations, e.g. spiders, pink elephants
- sweating, tachycardia, pyrexia
- signs of dehydration

Treatment[11]

- hospitalisation
- correct fluid and electrolyte imbalance with IV therapy
- treat any systemic infection
- thiamine (vitamin B_1) 100 mg IM or IV daily for 3–5 days, then thiamine 100 mg (o) daily
- diazepam 5 mg by slow IV injection (over several minutes) every half hour until symptoms subside

or

diazepam 10–20 mg (o) every 2 hours (up to max. 120 mg daily) until symptoms subside

This dose is usually required for 2–3 days, then should be gradually reduced till finished. If psychotic features, e.g. hallucinations and delusions, add

haloperidol 2.5–5 mg (o) bd.

Note: Chlormethiazole is not recommended because of its potential to produce excessive CNS depression and dependency.[11]

References

1. Rankin JS. The size and nature of the misuse of alcohol and drugs in Australia. Proceedings of 29th International Congress of Alcoholism and Drug Dependence, Sydney, February 1970, 10–20.

2. Skinner HA. Early detection and basic management of alcohol and drug problems. Australian Alcohol and Drug Review, 1985; 4:243–249.

3. Murtagh JE. Stigmata of alcohol dependence. Aust Fam Physician, 1985; 14:204–205.

4. Mayfield D, McLeod G, Hall P. The CAGE questionnaire. Am J Psych, 1974; 131:1121–1123.

5. Skinner HA. Early intervention for alcohol and drug problems: core issues for medical education. Australian Alcohol and Drug Review, 1986; 5:69–74.

6. Cockburn J, Killer D, Campbell E, Sanson-Fisher RW. Measuring general practitioners' attitudes towards medical care. Family Practice, 1987; 3:192–199.

7. Wallace P, Cutler S, Haines A. Randomised controlled trial of general practitioner intervention in patients with excessive alcohol consumption. BMJ, 1988; 297:663–668.

8. Saunders JB. The WHO project on early detection and treatment of harmful alcohol consumption. Australian Drug and Alcohol Review, 1987; 6:303–308.

9. Prochaska JO, Di Clemente CC. Towards a comprehensive model of change. In: Miller WRJ, Heath N eds, *Treating addictive behavior*. New York: Plenum, 1986, 3–27.

10. Saunders JB, Roche AM. One in six patients in your practice. NSW medical education project on alcohol and other drugs. Sydney: A drug offensive pamphlet 1989, 1–6.

11. Moulds RFW. *Psychotropic drug guidelines* (3rd edn). Victorian Medical Postgraduate Foundation, 1995, 80–83.

107

Allergic disorders including hay fever

—

The nostril membrane is so irritable that light dust, contradiction, an absurd remark—anything—sets me sneezing and I can be heard in Taunton with a favourable wind, a distance of six miles. Turn your mind to this little curse. If consumption is too powerful for physicians, at least they should not suffer themselves to be outwitted by such little upstart disorders as the hay fever.

Sydney Smith 1835
Letter to Dr Holland

Allergic disorders affect approximately 20% of the population. The most common allergies are those associated with IgE mediated (immediate, or Type 1) hypersensitivity such as allergic rhinoconjunctivitis (hay fever), atopic dermatitis (eczema) and allergic asthma.[1]

Less commonly encountered but of increasing clinical importance in the community are IgE mediated allergies to foods such as peanuts and/or other nuts and seafoods (crustaceans or molluscs) which may cause urticaria, angioedema, anaphylaxis and even death. Peanuts are one of the most common causes of food-induced anaphylaxis in adults. A clinically significant cross-reactivity between peanuts and other legumes is uncommon, but allergy to tree nuts such as almonds and walnuts may occur in up to 50% of those with peanut allergy.[2] Another special case is the oral allergy syndrome in which people with some degree of seasonal allergy to grass pollens or birch pollen suffer oral itch and swelling when they come into contact with certain fruits. This problem may be alleviated by desensitisation to pollens.[2]

Natural rubber latex allergy, associated with the introduction of universal precautions to decrease transmissible diseases, is an increasingly important cause of Type 1 hypersensitivity, affecting particularly medical and paramedical personnel. Patients who have had multiple operations or procedures are another high-risk group. Diagnosis is suggested by history and confirmed by specific skin tests or the detection of serum specific IgE. The development of urticaria on contact with latex is highly suggestive of underlying Type 1 hypersensitivity. An interesting association between latex allergy and sensitivity to fruit is recognised, most commonly banana, kiwifruit or avocado.[2]

Atopy

Atopy refers to those 40% of people who have an inherited tendency for an exaggerated IgE antibody response to common environmental antigens.[1] There will be a positive response to one or more allergen skin-prick tests, and usually a family history of allergic disorders. Of those who are atopic, one-half to one-third manifest an allergic disorder, most commonly allergic rhinitis, asthma, atopic dermatitis or allergic gastroenteropathy.

Common allergens causing immediate hypersensitivity

It is helpful to consider important allergen exposure during history taking. Table 107.1 lists sources of common allergens.

Table 107.1 *Sources of common allergens*[1]

Inhalants
Pollens, domestic animals, house dust mites, mould spores, cockroaches
Foods
Peanuts, fish, shellfish, milk, eggs, wheat
Other
Drugs, latex, insect venoms, occupational

Inhalant allergies

Allergic rhinoconjunctivitis and asthma are the main manifestations. The history provides a strong pointer to the causative allergen. If symptoms are seasonal, pollen allergy is most likely; perennial symptoms indicate an allergy to dust mites, household pets or moulds. Certain activities which precipitate symptoms may also provide a clue—these include mowing lawns, dusting and vacuuming.

Food allergy and intolerance

IgE mediated food allergy usually manifests in infancy and childhood with gastrointestinal symptoms such as anorexia, nausea, vomiting and spitting up of food, colic, diarrhoea and failure to thrive.

Foods that commonly cause allergic reactions include milk and other dairy products, eggs and peanuts. Other foods implicated include oranges, soya beans, nuts, chocolate, fish, shellfish and wheat.

The allergic reactions are not to be confused with non-immunological food intolerance such as lactose intolerance.

Peanut allergy

Peanuts are one of the most common causes of food-induced anaphylaxis in adults. The diagnosis is confirmed by demonstration of peanut-specific IgE by either skin-prick tests with peanut extract or RAST testing. Reaction to peanuts usually begins within minutes of ingestion, the first symptoms being oropharyngeal itching or burning. Flushing, urticaria, wheeze, stridor, angioedema and collapse may follow.[3] The combination of peanut allergy and asthma is dangerous, as evidenced by fatal or near fatal reactions in young children.[4] The key to management is avoidance of peanut-containing foods. Desensitisation is currently not recommended. Those at risk should carry an anaphylaxis kit (Table 107.2).

Latex allergy

The clinical manifestations of Type 1 hypersensitivity reactions to latex protein are wide-ranging, from urticaria to life-threatening anaphylaxis and death. It is believed that some episodes of intraoperative anaphylaxis are due to the patient—who has been sensitised to latex—reacting after mucosal contact with

Table 107.2   *Adult anaphylaxis kit*[3]

Epi Pen (0.3 mg adrenaline 1:1000 IM injection)
  Inject into outer thigh muscle at first sign of swelling of throat or tongue, or other reaction, e.g. breathlessness

Medihaler Epi MDI (adrenaline metered aerosol spray)
  Spray 10–20 times in milder reactions only, e.g. local lip tingling or swelling

Oral antihistamines
  e.g. 10 mg loratadine tablets (x2)
  Take 1 tablet after adrenaline injection

Prednisolone 25 mg tablets (x2)
  Take immediately after adrenaline

gloves worn by operating staff. Some institutions now provide latex-free operating suites in response to this serious problem.[5]

Latex allergy is thus a significant problem for at-risk people, including health care workers, patients with spina bifida or other spinal cord abnormalities, and those who have had multiple operations.

Symptoms

Contact dermatitis (Type 4 hypersensitivity), urticaria, worsening atopic dermatitis, allergic rhinoconjunctivitis, asthma, allergy to multiple fruits and possibly anaphylaxis.

Diagnosis

Skin-prick tests (dangerous and best left to experts) are more sensitive than blood tests at this stage but carry a risk of anaphylaxis. Measurement of serum specific IgE is safe although less sensitive. Contact allergy (Type 4) is identified by patch testing.

Management

Total avoidance. Health care workers who are allergic can never again wear latex gloves.[6]

Tests for specific IgE
Skin-prick tests

This is the preferred method as results can be read at the first consultation, provided the high-quality allergen preparations are used. A positive test alone may be of no diagnostic significance if the patient is asymptomatic to the specific allergens. A negative test is very useful for excluding IgE mediated allergy.

Detection of serum specific IgE

A number of tests including radioallergosorbent (RAST) tests[1] and enzyme linked immunosorbent tests (ELISA) measure allergen-specific IgE in the serum. They are no more accurate than skin testing, are expensive and do not provide an immediate result.

Indications include: history and skin tests not matching, extensive eczema, dermographism, infants and very young children, immunotherapy work-up, antihistamine use in past 48 hours.

Management principles[1]

Allergen avoidance

If relevant from history and skin-prick testing, special attention should be paid to reducing exposure to house dust mites and mould, to pet selection and specific food avoidance. Change of occupation and environment may be necessary for some people.

Pharmacotherapy

Drugs are used to alleviate symptoms where avoidance methods have failed or are impractical. Examples include antihistamines (H_1-receptor and H_2-receptor antagonists), adrenaline (emergency use), sodium cromoglycate, corticosteroids, some anticholinergics and sympathomimetics.

Immunotherapy (desensitisation)

This involves repeated administration of small increasing doses of allergen by subcutaneous injection. This is the treatment of choice for severe wasp or bee venom allergy and for resistant allergic rhinoconjunctivitis where a single causative allergen can be identified. Patients should be observed for at least 45 minutes and adequate resuscitation facilities are essential.

Management of specific allergic disorders

- asthma: see Chapter 109, p. 1051
- atopic dermatitis: see Chapter 101, p. 972
- urticaria: see Chapter 100, p. 965
- anaphylaxis and angioedema: see Chapter 114, p. 1111

Rhinitis/hay fever

Rhinitis is inflammation of the nose causing sneezing, nasal discharge or blockage for more than an hour during the day. Rhinitis is subdivided into various types:

- According to time span:
  - seasonal rhinitis: occurs only during a limited period, usually springtime
  - perennial rhinitis: present throughout the year
- According to pathophysiology:
  - allergic rhinitis: an IgE mediated atopic disorder
  - vasomotor rhinitis: due to parasympathetic overactivity

Both allergic and vasomotor rhinitis have a strong association with asthma.

The classification can be summarised as:

- seasonal allergic rhinoconjunctivitis = hay fever
- perennial rhinitis
  - allergic (usually due to house dust mites)
  - non-allergic= vasomotor
    - eosinophilic
    - non-eosinophilic

Clinical features of rhinitis

Nasal symptoms:

- sneezing
- nasal obstruction and congestion
- hypersecretion: watery rhinorrhoea, postnasal drip
- reduced sense of smell
- itching nose (usually allergic)

Throat symptoms:

- dry and sore throat
- itching throat

Irritated eyes (allergic)

Abnormal nasal mucous membrane—pale, boggy, mucoid discharge. A transverse nasal crease indicates nasal allergy, especially in a child.

Allergens

- pollens from trees (spring) and grass (in summer)
- moulds
- house dust mites (perennial rhinitis)
- hair, fur, feathers (from cats, dogs, horses, birds)
- some foods, e.g. cow's milk, eggs, peanuts, peanut butter

Diagnosis

Allergic rhinitis—nasal allergy:

- detection of allergen-specific IgE antibodies (not specific)

- RAST test or skin testing for specific allergens (can get false negatives)

Vasomotor rhinitis—a diagnosis of exclusion.

Other causes of rhinitis

- Chronic infection (viral, bacterial, fungal)
- Rhinitis of pregnancy
- Rhinitis medicamentosa—following overuse of OTC decongestant nasal drops or sprays
- Drug-induced rhinitis
  - various antihypertensives
  - aspirin
  - phenothiazines
  - oral contraceptives
  - cocaine, marijuana
- Chemical or environmental irritants (vasomotor rhinitis)
  - smoke and other noxious fumes
  - paints and sprays
  - cosmetics

Factors aggravating rhinitis (vasomotor)

- emotional upsets
- fatigue
- alcohol
- chilly damp weather
- air-conditioning
- sudden changes in temperature and humidity

Allergic rhinitis

Allergic rhinitis may be seasonal or perennial. Its prevalence varies from 5–20% with a peak prevalence in children and young adults up to 20%.[7] The symptoms are caused by release of powerful chemical mediators such as histamine, serotonin, prostaglandins and leukotrienes from sensitised mast cells.[7]

Seasonal allergic rhinoconjunctivitis (hay fever)

This is the most common type of allergic rhinitis and is due to a specific allergic reaction of the nasal mucosa, principally to pollens. The allergens responsible for perennial allergic rhinitis include inhaled dust, dust mite, animal dander and fungal spores.

Most cases of hay fever begin in childhood with one half having the problem by the age of 15 and 90% of eventual cases by the age of 30.[8] Approximately 20% suffer from attacks of asthma.

While patients with hay fever tend to have widespread itching (nose, throat and eyes), those with perennial rhinitis rarely have eye or throat symptoms but mainly sneezing and watery rhinorrhoea.

Nasal polyps

Nasal polyps are round, soft, pale pedunculated outgrowths arising from the nasal or sinus mucosa. They occur in patients with all types of rhinitis, especially allergic rhinitis. Symptoms include nasal obstruction and loss of smell.

Simple polyps can be readily snared and removed, but referral to a specialised surgeon is advisable since the aim is to remove the polyp with the mucosa of the sinuses (often ethmoid cells) from which it arises. This reduces the incidence of recurrence.

Management

Management consists of four main areas:

1. appropriate explanation and reassurance
2. allergen avoidance
3. pharmacological treatment
4. immunotherapy

Advice to the patient

- Keep healthy, eat a well-balanced diet, avoid 'junk food' and live sensibly with balanced exercise, rest and recreation. If your eyes give you problems, try not to rub them, avoid contact lenses and wear sunglasses.
- Avoid using decongestant nose drops and sprays: although they soothe at first, a worse effect occurs on the rebound.
- Avoidance therapy: avoid the allergen, if you know what it is (consider pets, feather pillows and eiderdowns).
- Sources of the house dust mite are bedding, upholstered furniture, fluffy toys and carpets. Seek advice about keeping your bedroom or home dust-free, especially if you have perennial rhinitis.
- Pets, especially cats, should be kept outside.
- Avoid chemical irritants such as aspirin, smoke, cosmetics, paints and sprays.

Allergen avoidance

This is difficult during the spring pollen season, particularly where patients are living in high-pollen (e.g. country farming) areas, or spending considerable time outdoors in the course of work or sporting and recreational activities.

Pharmacological therapy[9]

Therapy can be chosen from:
1. antihistamines
   - oral (not so effective for vasomotor rhinitis)
   - intranasal spray (rapid action)
   - ophthalmic drops
2. decongestants (oral or topical)
3. sodium cromoglycate
   - intranasal: powder insufflation or spray
   - ophthalmic drops for associated conjunctivitis
4. corticosteroids
   - intranasal (not so effective for non-eosinophilic vasomotor rhinitis)
   - oral (very effective if other methods fail)
   - ophthalmic drops for allergic conjunctivitis

Immunotherapy

Consider hyposensitisation/immunotherapy when specific allergens are known and conventional response is inadequate. Immunotherapy to grass pollen is generally very effective and should be considered in moderate to severe springtime hay fever.

Antihistamines

Oral antihistamines are the first line of treatment for seasonal hay fever and are generally effective where symptoms are intermittent, or when they can be used prophylactically before periods of high pollen exposure. The newer generation, so-called 'non-sedating' antihistamines that do not cross the blood-brain barrier are used in preference to the first-generation drugs, although some degree of sedation may occur even with these. Terfenadine is best avoided in the elderly. A list of non-sedating antihistamines is presented in Table 107.3. It is claimed by some that the new topical preparation, levocabastine, as an intranasal spray, is rapidly effective for an exacerbation of symptoms.

Oral decongestants

Oral sympathomimetics, either used alone or in combination with antihistamines (where they may help reduce drowsiness), may be of value particularly where nasal discharge and stuffiness are major symptoms. Side effects include nervousness and insomnia. They should be used cautiously in patients with hypertension, heart disease, hyperthyroidism, glaucoma and prostatic hypertrophy.

Intranasal therapy[9]

Intranasal decongestants should be used for limited periods only (i.e. less than a week) or intermittently (3–4 doses per week) because of the potential problems with rebound congestion and rhinitis medicamentosa. They are often of particular value during the first week of treatment with intranasal corticosteroids (where the onset of action is delayed several days), improving nasal patency and allowing more complete insufflation of the corticosteroids. Adverse reactions similar to those of oral decongestants may occur.

Intranasal sodium cromoglycate acts by preventing mast cell degranulation and is effective without serious side effects. The capsule variety must be used (the spray form requires 1–2 hourly dosage to be effective); it is useful in perennial allergic rhinitis but is not as effective as intranasal corticosteroids for springtime hay fever.

Intranasal corticosteroid sprays are the most effective agents for treating seasonal allergic rhinitis. Side effects are minimal and adrenal suppression is not a problem with normal usage. Patients should be informed that these medications will not give immediate relief (often taking 10–14 days to have peak effect) and must be used continuously throughout the hay fever season.

Table 107.3 *Non-sedating antihistamines (oral regimens)*

Generic name	Onset	Dosage
Astemizole	Relatively slow	10 mg daily
Cetirizine	Rapid	10 mg daily or bd
Fexofenadine	Rapid	60 mg bd
Loratadine	Very rapid	10 mg daily
Terfenadine	Rapid	60 mg bd

Table 107.4 *Intranasal preparations for rhinitis*

	Brand name	Dosage	Comments
Sodium cromoglycate	Rynacrom powder (capsules)	Insufflate 1 capsule, qid	Compliance a problem
	Rynacrom nasal spray	Spray 4–6 times daily	
Beclomethasone dipropionate	Aldecin nasal Beconase nasal	100 μg spray each nostril bd or tds	
Budesonide	Rhinocort nasal	100–200 μg each nostril daily	
Ipratropium bromide	Atrovent	1–2 sprays per nostril tds prn	Useful for vasomotor rhinitis and profuse rhinorrhoea Care needed with elderly
Various sympathomimetics e.g. phenylephrine		2, 3 or 4 times daily (max. 7 days)	Short-term use only Care with elderly, prostatic hypertrophy

Intranasal levocabastine—this antihistamine preparation usually involves 2 sprays per nostril bd to qid.

Table 107.4 lists intranasal preparations for rhinitis.

Ophthalmic preparations

Sodium cromoglycate eyedrops are usually very effective for springtime conjunctivitis. They can be used as necessary (there is no dosage limit) and are most helpful when used prophylactically before periods of high pollen exposure. Decongestant eyedrops may also be helpful (care with narrow angle glaucoma), while corticosteroid eyedrops are reserved for resistant allergic conjunctivitis and should be used with care to exclude infection and glaucoma. Antihistamine eyedrops (levocabastine) are yet another option.

Other treatments

Corticosteroids (oral)

These can be very effective where other treatments or methods have failed. A 6–10 day short course can be used. An example of a 6 day 'rescue course' is prednisolone 25, 25, 20, 15, 10, 5 mg daily doses.

Ipratropium bromide (Atrovent)[9]

The nasal preparation of this topical anticholinergic is often very effective when rhinorrhoea is the major problem.

Table 107.5 summarises recommended steps in management.

When to refer

- Where surgical intervention is required, such as with nasal obstruction from polyps, bulky nasal turbinates and deviated septum.
- For immunotherapy.

Practice tips

- Avoid long-term use of topical decongestant nasal drops.
- Avoid topical antihistamine preparations.
- Prescribe sodium cromoglycate eyedrops for the hay fever patient with itchy eyes.
- Be careful of severe systemic reactions that can occur with intradermal skin testing and with immunotherapy. Resuscitation facilities should be available.

Table 107.5 *Summary of recommended treatment steps for rhinitis*

Allergic rhinitis
- patient education
- allergen avoidance (if possible)
- non-sedating antihistamines

  or

- inhaled corticosteroids (the most effective)
- sodium cromoglycate (Opticrom) eye drops
- oral corticosteroids (if topicals ineffective)
- immunotherapy if applicable

Vasomotor rhinitis
- patient education
- trigger avoidance (if possible)
- inhaled corticosteroids
- anticholinergics, e.g. ipratropium bromide
- nasal surgery if necessary

References

1. Loblay RH. Allergies (Type 1). In: MIMS Disease Index (2nd edn). Sydney: IMS Publishing, 1996, 12–15.

2. O'Hehir R. Update in allergic diseases. Update Course for GPs handbook. Monash University, 1996, 19–20.

3. Douglas R, O'Hehir R. Peanut allergy. Med J Aust, 1997; 166:63–64.

4. Sampson HA, Mendleson L, Rosen JP. Fatal and near fatal anaphylactic reactions to food in children and adolescents. N Eng J Med, 1992; 327:380–384.

5. Katelaris CH et al. Prevalence of latex allergy in a dental school. Med J. Aust, 1996; 164:711–714.

6. Walls RS. Latex allergy: a real problem. Med J Aust, 1996; 164:707.

7. Scoppa J. Rhinitis (allergic and vasomotor). In: MIMS Disease Index (2nd edn). Sydney: IMS Publishing, 1996, 450–451.

8. Fry J. *Common diseases* (4th edn). Lancaster: MTP Press, 1985, 134–138.

9. Sharp A, Murtagh J. Hay fever (seasonal allergic rhinitis). Aust Fam Physician, 1995; 24:1899–1900.

108

Anxiety

—

Anxiety is an uncomfortable inner feeling of fear or imminent disaster. The criterion for anxiety disorder as defined at the International Classification of Health Problems in Primary Care (ICHPPC-2-Defined) (WONCA, 1985)[1] is:

generalised and persistent anxiety or anxious mood, which cannot be associated with, or is disproportionately large in response to a specific psychosocial stressor, stimulus or event.

Anxiety is a normal human emotion and most of us experience some temporary degree of anxiety in our lives as a normal reaction to stress and misfortune. Table 108.1 presents the scale formulated by psychologists to quantify life's main stresses. However, some people are constantly anxious to the extent that it is abnormal and interferes with their lives. They suffer from an anxiety disorder, a problem that affects 5–10% of the population.

The symptoms of anxiety, which are psychological or physical in manifestation, can vary enormously from feeling tense or tired to panic attacks.

Classification of anxiety

The following list represents approximately the categories of anxiety disorders recognised by the DSM-III-R:[2,3]

- generalised anxiety disorder
- panic disorder, with or without agoraphobia

Table 108.1 *Life change and stress survey of recent experiences*

Life event	Life change units
Death of spouse	100
Divorce	73
Marital separation	65
Jail term	63
Death of close family member	63
Personal injury or illness	53
Marriage	50
Fired at work	47
Marital reconciliation	45
Retirement	45
Change in health of family member	44
Pregnancy	40
Sex difficulties	39
Business readjustment	39
Death of close friend	37
Change to different line of work	36
Mortgage (large)	31
Change in responsibility at work	29
Son or daughter leaving home	29
Outstanding personal achievement	28
Spouse begins or stops work	26
Begin or end school	26
Trouble with boss	23
Change in work hours or conditions	20
Change in residence	20
Change in schools	20
Mortgage or loan (modest)	17
Change in sleeping habits	16
Vacation	13
Christmas	12

Adapted from the Journal of Psychomatic Research, 1967: Vol 11; 216.

- phobic disorder, including social phobia
- obsessive compulsive disorder
- post-traumatic stress disorder

Generalised anxiety disorder

Generalised anxiety comprises excessive anxiety and worry about various life circumstances and is not related to a specific activity, time or event such as trauma, obsessions or phobias.

General features:

- persistent unrealistic and excessive anxiety
- worry about two or more life circumstances for 6 months or longer
- about one-third present with mainly neurological symptoms, one-third with cardiovascular symptoms and one-third with mainly gastrointestinal symptoms[2]

Diagnostic criteria for generalised anxiety disorder

Three or more of:

- irritability
- restless, 'keyed up' or 'on edge'
- easily fatigued
- difficulty concentrating or 'mind going blank'
- muscle tension
- sleep disturbance

Clinical features

Psychological

- apprehension/fearful anticipation
- irritability
- exaggerated startle response
- sleep disturbance and nightmares
- impatience
- panic
- sensitivity to noise
- difficulty concentrating or 'mind going blank'

Physical

- Motor tension
  - muscle tension/aching
  - tension headache
  - trembling/shaky/twitching
  - restlessness
  - tiredness/fatigue
- Autonomic overactivity
  - dry mouth
  - palpitations/tachycardia
  - sweating/cold clammy hands
  - flushes/chills
  - difficulty swallowing or 'lump in throat'
  - diarrhoea/abdominal distress

- frequency of micturition
- difficulty breathing/smothering feeling
- dizziness or lightheadedness

Note: Psychological disturbances are also referred to as disturbances of vigilance and scanning.

Symptoms and signs according to systems

Neurological	dizziness, headache, trembling, twitching, shaking, paraesthesia
Cardiovascular	palpitations, tachycardia, flushing, chest discomfort
Gastrointestinal	nausea, indigestion, diarrhoea, abdominal distress
Respiratory	hyperventilation, breathing difficulty, air hunger
Cognitive	fear of dying, difficulty concentrating, 'mind going blank', hypervigilance

Diagnosis of anxiety

The diagnosis is based on:

- the history: it is vital to listen carefully to what the patient is saying
- exclusion of organic disorders simulating anxiety by history, examination and appropriate investigation
- exclusion of other psychiatric disorders, especially depression

Main differential diagnoses

Note that this conforms to the seven masquerades list. Refer to Table 108.2.

- depression
- drug and alcohol dependence/withdrawal
- benzodiazepine dependence/withdrawal
- hyperthyroidism
- angina and cardiac arrhythmias
- iatrogenic drugs
- caffeine intoxication

Important checkpoints

Five self-posed questions should be considered by the family doctor before treating an anxious patient:[1]

- Is this hyperthyroidism?
- Is this depression?
- Is this normal anxiety?
- Is this mild anxiety or simple phobia?
- Is this moderate or severe anxiety?

Table 108.2 *Significant differential diagnoses of anxiety*

Psychiatric disorders
- depression
- drug and alcohol dependence/withdrawal
- benzodiazepine dependence/withdrawal
- schizophrenia
- acute or chronic organic brain disorder
- presenile dementia

Organic disorders
- drug-related
  — amphetamines
  — bronchodilators
  — caffeine excess
  — ephedrine
  — levodopa
  — thyroxine
- cardiovascular
  — angina
  — cardiac arrhythmias
  — mitral valve prolapse
- endocrine
  — hyperthyroidism
  — phaeochromocytoma
  — carcinoid syndrome
  — hypoglycaemia
  — insulinoma
- neurological
  — epilepsy, especially complex partial seizures
  — acute brain syndrome
- respiratory
  — asthma
  — acute respiratory distress
  — pulmonary embolism

Management of anxiety

The management applies mainly to generalised anxiety as specific psychotherapy is required in other types of anxiety. Much of the management can be carried out successfully by the family doctor using brief counselling and support.[2]

Management principles

- The aim is to use non-pharmacological methods and avoid the use of drugs if possible.
- Give careful explanation and reassurance
  — explain the reasons for the symptoms
  — reassure the patient about the absence of organic disease (can only be based on a thorough examination and appropriate investigations)
  — direct the patient to appropriate literature to give insight and support (Table 108.3).
- Provide practical advice on ways of dealing with the problems.
- Advise on the avoidance of aggravating substances such as caffeine, nicotine and other drugs.

Table 108.3 *Recommended reading for the anxious patient*

Herbert Benson	*The Relaxation Response*, Collins, London, 1984.
Dale Carnegie	*How to Stop Worrying and Start Living*, rev. edn, ed. Dorothy Carnegie, Angus and Robertson, Sydney, 1985.
Ainslie Mears	*Relief without Drugs*, Fontana, Glasgow, 1983.
Norman Peale	*The Power of Positive Thinking*, Cedar, London, 1982.
Claire Weekes	*Peace from Nervous Suffering*, Angus and Robertson, London, 1972.
Claire Weekes	*Self-help for your Nerves*, Angus and Robertson, London, 1976.

- Advise on general measures such as stress management techniques, relaxation programs and regular exercise and organise these for the patient (don't leave it to the patient).
- Advise on coping skills, including personal and interpersonal strategies, to manage difficult circumstances and people (in relation to that patient).

Patient education material

The author has found the following handout material to be invaluable in helping to manage less severe cases of generalised anxiety.[4]

Self-help

It is best to avoid drugs if you can; instead look at factors in your lifestyle that cause you stress and anxiety and modify or remove them (if possible). Be on the lookout for solutions. Examples are changing jobs and keeping away from people or situations that upset you. Sometimes confronting people and talking things over will help.

Special advice

Be less of a perfectionist: do not be a slave to the clock; do not bottle things up; stop feeling guilty; approve of yourself and others; express yourself and your anger. Resolve all personal conflicts. Make friends and be happy. Keep a positive outlook on life, and be moderate and less intense in your activities.

Seek a balance of activities, such as recreation, meditation, reading, rest, exercise and family/social activities.

Relaxation

Learn to relax your mind and body: seek out special relaxation programs such as yoga and meditation.

Make a commitment to yourself to spend some time every day practising relaxation. About 20 minutes twice a day is ideal, but you might want to start with only 10 minutes.[5]

- Sit in a quiet place with your eyes closed, but remain alert and awake if you can. Focus your mind on the different muscle groups in your body, starting at the forehead and slowly going down to the toes. Relax the muscles as much as you can.
- Pay attention to your breathing: listen to the sound of your breath for the next few minutes. Breathe in and out slowly and deeply.
- Next, begin to repeat the word 'relax' silently in your mind at your own pace. When other thoughts distract, calmly return to the word 'relax'.
- Just 'let go': this is a quiet time for yourself, in which the stresses in body and mind are balanced or reduced.

Medication

Doctors tend to recommend tranquillisers only as a last resort or to help you cope with a very stressful temporary period when your anxiety is severe and you cannot cope without extra help. Tranquillisers can be very effective if used sensibly and for short periods.

Pharmacological treatment

Acute episodes

The following drugs are recommended for patients who have intermittent transient exacerbations not responding to other measures.[6]

diazepam 2–5 mg(o) as a single dose
repeated bd as required
or
diazepam 5–10 mg (o) nocte
or
oxazepam 15–30 mg (o) as a single dose
repeated bd as required

Special notes:
- Recommended (if necessary) for up to 2 weeks, then taper off to zero over next 4 weeks.
- Reassess in 7 days.
- Oxazepam is preferred in women patients; middle-aged men generally respond well to short-term diazepam.

- Be wary of drug-seeking behaviour, e.g. unfamiliar patients, especially if they request a specific benzodiazepine.
- Consider beta-blockers in patients with sympathetic activation such as palpitations, tremor or excessive sweating, e.g. propranolol 10–40 mg (o) tds.[6] They do not relieve the mental symptoms of anxiety, however.

Long-term treatment

If non-pharmacological treatment is ineffective for persisting disabling anxiety, the drugs of choice are:

diazepam 2–5 mg (o) bd or tds (or 5–10 mg nocte)
or
oxazepam 15–30 mg (o) bd

Try to wean the patient off medication each 6–12 months.

An alternative to benzodiazepines is:
buspirone 5 mg (o) tds[6]
- increase if necessary to 20 mg (o) tds
- continue for several weeks after symptoms subside
- mean effective dose is 20–25 mg daily
- response takes 7–10 days
- does not appear to cause sedation

Panic disorder

Patients with panic disorder experience sudden, unexpected, short-lived episodes of intense anxiety. These tend to be recurrent and occur most often in young females.

The DSM-III-R diagnostic criteria for panic disorder with or without agoraphobia include:

- the attack was unexpected and not triggered by the person being the focus of attention
- four attacks within a 4 week period
or
one or more attacks followed by at least one month of persistent fear of having another attack
- at least four of the following symptoms during at least one of the attacks:
  — shortness of breath (dyspnoea) or smothering sensations
  — dizziness, unsteady feelings or faintness
  — palpitations or accelerated heart rate (tachycardia)
  — trembling or shaking
  — sweating
  — choking

— nausea or abdominal distress
— depersonalisation or derealisation
— numbness or tingling sensations (paraesthesias)
— flushes (hot flashes) or chills
— chest pain or discomfort
— fear of dying
— fear of going crazy or of doing something uncontrolled

Organic disorders that simulate a panic attack are hyperthyroidism, phaeochromocytoma and hypoglycaemia.

Management

Reassurance, explanation and support (as for generalised anxiety). This is the mainstay of treatment.

If hyperventilating, breathe in and out of a paper bag.

Cognitive behaviour therapy

This aims to reduce anxiety by teaching patients how to identify, evaluate, control and modify their negative, fearful thoughts and behaviour. If simple psychotherapy and stress management fails then patients should be referred for this therapy.

Patients' fears, especially if irrational, need to be clearly explained by the therapist, examined rationally and challenged, then replaced by positive calming thoughts.[2]

Pharmacological treatment[6]

Acute episodes, i.e the panic attack:

diazepam 5 mg (o)
or
oxazepam 15–30 mg (o)
or
alprazolam 0.25–0.5 mg (o)

Prophylaxis[6]

imipramine 50–75 mg (o) nocte
increasing every 2–3 days to 150 mg nocte by day 7
dosage can be increased further depending on response and/or adverse effects
or
benzodiazepines
alprazolam 0.25–6 mg (o) daily in divided doses

Alternatives: the newer generation antidepressants can be used if the above are ineffective.

Note: Medication should be withdrawn slowly.

Medication for panic disorder may need to be continued for 6–12 months.

Phobic disorders

In phobic states the anxiety is related to specific situations or objects. Patients avoid these situations and become anxious when they anticipate having to meet them. A list of phobias is presented in Table 108.4.

The three main types of phobic states are:

• specific phobias
• agoraphobia
• social phobias

Table 108.4 *Phobias*

Name of phobia	Fear or aversion of
Acrophobia	heights
Aerophobia	draughts
Agoraphobia	open spaces
Aichmophobia	sharp objects
Ailurophobia	cats
Algophobia	pain
Androphobia	men
Anthophobia	flowers
Anthropophobia	people
Arachnophobia	spiders
Aquaphobia	water
Astraphobia	lightning
Aviatophobia	flying
Bacteriophobia	bacteria
Bathophobia	depth
Brontophobia	thunder
Cancerophobia	cancer
Cardiophobia	heart disease
Claustrophobia	closed spaces
Cynophobia	dogs
Demonophobia	demons
Dromophobia	crossing streets
Equinophobia	horses
Genophobia	sex
Gynophobia	women
Haptephobia	being touched
Herpetophobia	creeping, crawling things
Homophobia	homosexuals
Hypsophobia	falling
Hypnophobia	going to sleep
Mysophobia	dirt, germs, contamination
Necrophobia	death
Neophobia	anything new
Numerophobia	numbers
Nyctophobia	darkness
Ochlophobia	crowds
Pyrophobia	fire
Taphophobia	being buried alive
Scotophobia	blindness
Sociophobia	social situations
Theophobia	God
Xenophobia	strangers
Zoophobia	animals

The ten most common phobias (in order) are spiders, people and social situations, flying, open spaces, confined spaces, heights, cancer, thunderstorms, death and heart disease.[7]

Specific phobias

These are common among normal children and include fear of specific things such as snakes, spiders, thunder, darkness, dogs and heights. The problem is seldom encountered in practice and there is usually no call for drug therapy.

Agoraphobia

Avoidance includes the many situations involving the issues of distance from home, crowding or confinement. Typical examples are travel on public transport, crowded shops and confined places. The patients fear they may lose control, faint and suffer embarrassment.

The condition is commonly associated with depression, obsessions, marital and family disharmony, or drug and alcohol abuse.[8]

Social phobias

Social phobias include anxiety-provoking social gatherings when the person feels subject to critical public scrutiny, e.g. canteens, restaurants, staff meetings, speaking engagements. The sufferer may be a shy, self-conscious, premorbid personality.[2] Social phobias, including performance anxiety and symptoms, are often related to sympathetic overactivity.

Management

The basis of treatment for all phobic disorders is psychotherapy that involves behaviour therapy and cognitive therapy.

Pharmacological treatment[6]

This should be used only if non-pharmacological measures fail.

Agoraphobia with panic: use medications as for panic attacks.

Social phobia: if problematic, a trial of a newer antidepressant agent, e.g. fluoxetine, is recommended.[6]

Social phobia with performance anxiety: propranolol 10–40 mg (o) 30–60 minutes before the social event or performance.

Specific phobia: pharmacotherapy is not recommended.

Obsessive compulsive disorder

Anxiety is associated with obsessive thoughts and compulsive rituals.

The obsessions are recurrent and persistent intrusive ideas, thoughts, impulses or images that are usually resisted by the patient, e.g. a religious person having recurrent blasphemous thoughts.

Compulsions are repetitive, purposeful and intentional behaviours conducted in response to an obsession to prevent a bad outcome for the person, e.g. excessive washing of the genitals.

Mild obsessional or compulsive behaviour can be regarded as normal in response to stress.

Management

Optimal management is a combination of psychotherapeutic and pharmacological treatment, namely:

- cognitive behaviour therapy for obsessions
- exposure and response prevention for compulsions
- clomipramine 50–75 mg (o) nocte increasing gradually to 150–250 mg (o) nocte[6]

An alternative agent to clomipramine (if not tolerated or ineffective) is fluoxetine 10–80 mg (o) daily after breakfast.[6]

Post-traumatic stress disorder

This term describes the various symptoms and behaviour that follow a psychologically distressing event or experience outside the range of usual human experience, e.g. violent crime such as an armed hold-up, warfare, or natural disasters such as bushfires. The symptoms usually develop immediately after the event but can be delayed for months or years.

Typical symptoms and features:

- recurrent and intrusive distressing recollections
- recurrent distressing dreams of the event
- acting or feeling as if the event were recurring
- intense distress on exposure to resembling events
- persistent avoidance of events that symbolise or resemble the trauma
- increased arousal symptoms, e.g. insomnia, hypervigilance, exaggerated startle response, poor concentration, moodiness

Treatment

This is difficult and involves counselling, the basis of which is facilitating abreaction of the experience by individual or group therapy.[6] The aim is to allow the patient to face up openly to memories. Persistent symptoms are an indication for referral.

Pharmacological treatment

There is no specific indication for drugs but medication can have benefit in the treatment of panic attacks, generalised anxiety or depression.[6] Long-term use of benzodiazepines is not recommended but short-term use for their anti-anxiety and hypnotic effects may be appropriate for the very anxious patient.

Hyperventilation

Hyperventilation syndrome can be a manifestation of anxiety. The main symptoms are:

- lightheadedness, faintness or dizziness
- breathlessness
- palpitations
- sweating
- dry mouth with aerophagy
- agitation
- fatigue and malaise

Other symptoms include paraesthesia of the extremities, perioral paraesthesia and carpopedal spasm.

Management

- reassurance
- encourage patients to identify the cause and then control their rate and depth of breathing
- first aid management is to raise the carbon dioxide level by rebreathing from a paper (not plastic) bag or from cupped hands (if a bag is unavailable)

Adjustment disorder with anxious mood

This term is reserved for patients who present with anxiety symptoms within 3 months of response to an identifiable psychosocial stressor. It is the most common presentation of anxiety symptoms and should be regarded as a separate entity to a generalised anxiety disorder.[6]

The symptoms are in excess of the normal expected reaction to the stressor but have persisted for less than 6 months following the removal of the stressor.

The basic treatment is non-pharmacological—counselling, relaxation and stress management.

A short-term course of drug treatment can be used in severe or persisting cases, e.g.

diazepam 2–5 mg (o) daily or bd[6]
or
oxazepam 15–30 mg (o) daily or bd (up to 14 days)

Anxiety in children

Anxiety disorders can occur in childhood. Panic attacks are not uncommon. Children are generally more responsive to non-pharmacological approaches. Separation anxiety disorders for real, threatened or imagined separation can occur; if severe and persistent, treatment (with care) with imipramine is recommended.[6]

Benzodiazepine usage

The use of benzodiazepines as anxiolytics should be restricted and they should be used discretely. Markus et al[9] recommend reserving benzodiazepines to the following clinical situations.

1. Self-perpetuating anxiety following a precipitating event and not responding to non-pharmacological management. Give a short course for 2 weeks.
2. Situational anxiety affecting lifestyle, e.g. plane travel, dental appointments. Intermittent use only.
3. Emergency short-term use for agoraphobia or panic attacks.

They should not be used to treat depression, obsessional neuroses or chronic psychoses and should be used with caution in bereavement and crisis situations.

Problems associated with benzodiazepine use include:[1]

- impaired alertness, oversedation
- dependence
- increased risk of accidents
- adverse effects on mood and behaviour
- interaction with alcohol and other drugs
- potential for abuse and overdose
- risks during pregnancy and lactation
- muscle weakness
- sexual dysfunction
- diminished motivation
- lowered sense of competency
- lower self-esteem

Benzodiazepine withdrawal syndrome

This syndrome is usually relatively delayed in its onset and may continue for weeks or months.[1] Withdrawal features include:

- anxiety (rebound)
- depression
- insomnia
- nausea
- loss of appetite
- tremor
- confusion
- intolerance of loud noise, bright light or touch
- visual hallucinations
- epileptic seizures

There are several strategies to help the consenting patient to stop benzodiazepines, ranging from stopping completely to very gradual withdrawal. An effective method is to withdraw the drug very slowly while providing counselling and support, including referral to a self-help group. Antidepressants can be substituted if there is evidence of depression, while beta-blockers may help the withdrawal syndrome if other measures have failed.

When to refer

- if the diagnosis is doubtful
- if drug and alcohol dependence or withdrawal complicate the management
- if depression or a psychosis appears to be involved
- failure of response to basic treatment

Practice tips

- Be careful not to confuse depression with anxiety.
- A depressive disorder can be the cause of anxiety symptoms.
- For anxiety, especially with cardiovascular symptoms (palpitations and/or flushing), always consider the possibility of hyperthyroidism and order thyroid function tests.

- Always try non-pharmacological measures to manage anxiety whenever possible.
- Be careful with use of benzodiazepines: aim at short-term treatment only.
- Tips to beat stress
  — listen to music
  — do things that you enjoy
  — look at positives
  — develop strategies to laugh
  — go to the movies or a show weekly
  — consider a pet
  — your job is what you do (not who you are)
  — regular chats with close friends
  — exercise 30 minutes, 4 to 5 times a week
  — learn to meditate

References

1. Wilkinson G. *Anxiety: recognition and treatment in general practice*. Oxford: Radcliffe Medical Press, 1992, 5–62.

2. Vine RG, Judd FK. Anxiety disorders and panic states. In: MIMS Disease Index (2nd edn). Sydney: IMS Publishing, 1996, 43–45.

3. Gelder M. Diagnosis and management of anxiety and phobic states. Medicine International, 1988; 45:1857–1861.

4. Murtagh J. *Patient education* (2nd edn). Sydney: McGraw-Hill, 1996, 127.

5. Beattie R. Anxiety: patient education. Aust Fam Physician, 1985; 14:901.

6. Moulds RFW. *Psychotropic drug guidelines* (3rd edn). Melbourne: Victorian Medical Postgraduate Foundation, 1996–97, 124–139.

7. Anonymous author. Making it to the top ten. Melbourne: The *Sun*, 3 March 1990, 67.

8. Fryer AJ. Agoraphobia. Modern problems in pharmacopsychiatry, 1987; 22:91–126.

9. Markus AC, Murray Parker C, Tomson P et al. *Psychological problems in general practice*. Oxford: Oxford University Press, 1989, 12–43.

109
Asthma

—

After I'd written to you yesterday I had an attack of asthma and an incessantly running nose, which forced me to tramp about, lighting cigarettes at every tobacconist etc. And worse was to come: I went to bed about midnight, feeling all right after spending a long time inhaling smoke, but 3 or 4 hours later came the real attack of the summer.

Marcel Proust 1901
Letter to his mother

Asthma is defined as 'a chronic inflammatory disorder of the airways in which many cells play a role. In susceptible individuals this inflammation causes symptoms which are usually associated with widespread but variable airflow obstruction that is often reversible either spontaneously or with treatment, and it also causes an associated increase in airway responsiveness to a variety of stimuli'.[1] It can also be defined as a cough or wheeze associated with heightened airway responsiveness to inhaled histamine.[2] Asthma is a common and potentially fatal disorder; it is now regarded as an inflammatory disorder of the airways, which are hyperactive in the asthmatic patient.

Chronic asthma is an inflammatory disease with the following pathological characteristics:

- infiltration of the mucosa with inflammatory cells (especially eosinophils)
- oedema of the mucosa
- damaged mucosal epithelium
- hypertrophy of mucus glands with increased mucus secretion
- smooth muscle constriction (Fig. 109.1)

Key facts and checkpoints

- Asthma continues to be underdiagnosed and undertreated.[3] It is increasing worldwide.
- It has an unacceptable mortality rate of approximately 5 per 100 000 of the population.
- About one child in four or five has asthma (usually in a mild form).
- It tends to develop between the ages of two and seven.
- Most children present with a cough.

(a)

lining (mucosa)   muscle wall

(b)

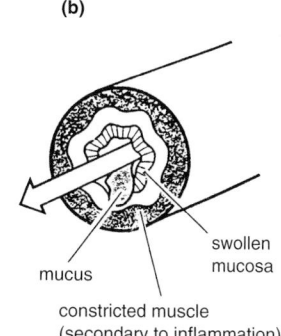

mucus

swollen mucosa

constricted muscle (secondary to inflammation)

Fig. 109.1 *Airway changes in asthma:* **(a)** *normal airway;* **(b)** *airway in asthma*

- Most children are free from it by puberty.
- At least 1 in 7 adolescents has asthma.
- About one adult in ten has asthma.
- All family doctors should keep abreast of developments in asthma management to achieve best possible control at all times in their patients.
- Three valuable home 'gadgets' to help the asthmatic are the mini peak flow meter, the large volume spacing device and the pump with nebuliser.
- The focus of management should be on prevention; an acute asthmatic attack represents failed treatment.
- Measurement of function is vital as 'objective measurement is superior to subjective measurement'.
- Spirometry is the key investigation.
- Doubling the radius of the airway increases the flow rate 16 times.
- The earlier steroid therapy is introduced, the better the outcome.
- Avoid concomitant medication that exacerbates asthma, e.g. beta-blockers, aspirin, NSAIDs.
- Future aerosols will have non-CFC propellants leading to increased lung deposition and thus lower dosage.

Causes of asthma

No single cause for asthma has been found, but a variety of factors may trigger an attack. These include specific factors such as viruses and allergens and non-specific factors such as weather changes and exercise. A checklist of trigger factors is:

- infections, especially colds
- allergies, e.g. to animal fur, feathers, grass pollens, mould
- allergy to house dust, especially the dust mites
- cigarette smoke, other smoke and fumes
- sudden changes in weather or temperature
- occupational irritants, e.g. wood dust, synthetic sprays, chemicals
- drugs, e.g. aspirin, NSAIDs, beta-blockers (oral, parenteral or topical)
- certain foods and food additives may trigger asthma
  e.g. monosodium glutamate
    metabisulphites/sulphite preservatives/
    food colouring agents
    seafood
    nuts
- exercise, especially in a cold atmosphere
- emotional upsets or stress

Additional points
- Patients with asthma should not smoke.
- Atopic patients should avoid exposure to furred or feathered domestic animals if they have problems.
- About 90% of children with atopic symptoms and asthma demonstrate positive skin-prick responses to dust mite extract. Total eradication of house dust mite from the home is difficult.

Clinical features
The classic symptoms are:

- wheezing
- coughing (especially at night)
- tightness in the chest
- breathlessness

Note: Asthma should be suspected in children with recurrent nocturnal cough and in people with intermittent dyspnoea or chest tightness, especially after exercise.

Severe symptoms and signs are presented under the section on dangerous asthma later in this chapter.

Examination[4]
Physical signs may be present if the patient has symptoms at the time of examination.

The absence of physical signs does not exclude a diagnosis of asthma. If wheeze is not present during normal tidal breathing it may become apparent during a forced expiration. Wheeze does not necessarily indicate asthma.

Investigations
- Measurement of peak expiratory flow rate (PEFR): demonstrates variation in values over a period of time.
- Spirometry: a value of $< 75\%$ for FEV_1/VC ratio indicates obstruction. It is the more accurate test and recommended for those who can perform it, i.e. most adults and children > 6 years.
- Measurement of PEFR or spirometry before and after bronchodilator: has a characteristic $> 20\%$ improvement for PEFR and $> 15\%$ in FEV_1.
- Inhalation challenge tests: airway reactivity is tested in a respiratory laboratory to inhaled histamine, methacholine and hypertonic saline. Sometimes useful to confirm diagnosis.
- An exercise challenge may also be helpful.
- Allergy testing may be appropriate.

- Chest X-ray: not routine but useful if complications suspected or symptoms not explained by asthma.
- Mannitol inhalation test (coming).

Four big advances in the management of asthma

1. The realisation that asthma is an inflammatory disease. Therefore the appropriate first or second line treatment in moderate to severe asthma is inhaled sodium cromoglycate or corticosteroids.
2. The regular use of the mini peak flow meter.
3. The use of spacers attached to inhalers/puffers.
4. Improved and more efficient inhalers.

Reasons for suboptimal asthma control are presented in Table 109.1.

Treating inflammatory airways disease

If inflammatory airways disease is undertreated there is the risk of irreversible airways obstruction from submucosal fibrosis. One of the most common mistakes in medical practice is to fail to introduce inhaled corticosteroids for the management of patients with moderately severe asthma.

Table 109.1 *Reasons for suboptimal asthma control*[1,3]

Poor compliance

Inefficient use of inhaler devices

Procrastination in introducing optimal therapy

Failure to prescribe preventive medications, particularly inhaled corticosteroids for chronic asthma

Using bronchodilators alone and repeating these drugs without proper evaluation

Patient fears
- inhaled or oral corticosteroids
- concern about aerosols and the ozone layer
- overdosage
- developing tolerance
- embarrassment
- peer group condemnation

Doctor's reluctance to
- use corticosteroids
- recommend obtaining a mini peak flow meter
- recommend obtaining a compressed air-driven nebuliser unit

Measurement of peak expiratory flow (PEF)

Patients with moderate to severe chronic asthma should be encouraged to obtain a PEF meter and measure their PEFR. PEF meter objective readings are more useful than subjective symptoms in assessing asthma control. They allow the establishment of a base-line of the 'patient's best'; they monitor changes; they allow the assessment of asthma severity and response to treatment.

Anyone older than 6–7 years can usually test PEFR accurately. The PEFR should be measured in the morning and at night before inhaling the bronchodilator and then 10 minutes later. Ideally it should be performed three times for each test and the best reading recorded. The predicted normal values are a most useful guide. At some stage the patient's best PEFR should be compared with the gold standard, namely FEV_1.

Warning signs when using PEF are:

- falling of PEFR and poor control
- readings less than 70% of normal best
- more morning dipping than normal
- erratic readings
- less response to bronchodilator than normal

Figure 109.2 shows a typical PEF recording of worsening asthma.

Large volume spacers[2]

Some people who have trouble using metered dose inhalers (MDIs) can have a special 'spacer' fitted onto the mouthpiece of the inhaler. One puff of the MDI is put in the spacer. The patient breathes in from its mouthpiece, taking one deep inhalation, then 1–2 very deep breaths, or 4–6 normal breaths. This method is useful for adults having trouble with the MDI and for younger children (older than 3 years). Spacers are very efficient, overcome poor technique and cause less irritation of the mouth and throat (Fig. 109.3). They allow increased airway deposition of inhalant and less oropharyngeal deposition.

Note: It is recommended to wash spacers with detergent and dry in sunlight every 10 days.

Small volume spacers

Children under 4 years can use an MDI and a small volume valved spacer (Aero Chamber, Breath-A-Tech) with a face mask.

Fig. 109.2 *Typical peak expiratory flow record showing signs of worsening asthma*

Management principles

Aims of management:

- Abolish symptoms and restore normal airway function.[2]
- Maintain best possible lung function at all times—keep asthma under control.
- Reduce morbidity.
- Control asthma with the use of regular anti-inflammatory medication and relieving doses of beta$_2$ agonist when necessary.

Long-term goals:

- Achieve use of the least drugs, least doses and least side effects.
- Reduce risk of fatal attacks.

Fig. 109.3 *Using a spacer device. Rules: children—all puffs in at once, then inhale; adults—single puff, single breath*

- Reduce risk of developing irreversible abnormal lung function.

Definition of control of asthma

- no cough, wheeze or breathlessness most of the time
- no nocturnal waking due to asthma
- no limitation of normal activity
- no overuse of beta$_2$ agonists
- no severe attacks
- no side effects of medication

The six step asthma management plan

The National Asthma Campaign of Australia has developed this plan, which can be summarised for both patient and doctor in the following point form. An important underlying theme for the plan is careful attention to educating the patient and family.

1. *Assess the severity of the asthma* (Table 109.2)
   - Establish the peak expiratory flow rate (PEFR).
   - Both doctor and patient should agree on severity and common goals of treatment.
   - Consider symptoms and effect on living.
   - Consider medication requirements.

Table 109.2 *Assessment of asthma severity*[1,2]

Grade	History	Medication use (bronchodilator	Lung function		
			Best PEFR (% predicted)	PEFR % variability (over 2 weeks)	FEV₁ (% predicted)
Mild	Episodic Mild occasional symptoms with exercise	Occasional use of bronchodilator for symptoms	Normal 100%	6–10%	> 75%
Moderate	Symptoms most days Virtually asymptomatic on effective treatment Several known triggers apart from exercise	Needed most days	70–100%	11–25%	50–75%
Severe	Symptoms most days Wakes at night with cough/wheeze Chest tightness on waking Hospital admission or emergency department attendance in past 12 months Previous life-threatening episodes	Needed more than 3 times a day or High dose inhaled steroids > 800–1200 μg daily or Oral steroids in past 12 months	≤ 70%	> 25%	<50%

2. *Achieve best lung function*
   - Prescribe drug therapy to keep PEFR at best and to minimise symptoms.
   - Maintain the 'best' PEFR.
   - If PEF remains below predicted PEF level, treatment with high-dose inhaled steroids achieves optimal lung function in about 66% of patients.[5] (Appendix V).
3. *Avoid trigger factors*
   - Note any domestic or occupational triggers.
   - Triggers can be inhaled or ingested.
   - If an allergen is clearly identified, avoid it, e.g. get rid of the cat, don't smoke, house dust mite avoidance strategies.
4. *Maintain best lung function with optimal medication*
   - Organise an optimal medication program.
   - Consider inhaled medications, monitored with PEF, with as few drugs, doses and side effects as possible.
   - Ensure the patient understands the difference between 'preventer' and 'reliever' medications.

5. *Know your action plan*
   (prepare an easy-to-follow action plan)
   - This must cover three points:
     — recognition that asthma is deteriorating
     — patient initiates own extra medication
     — getting access to medical attention
6. *Check your asthma regularly*
   Review and educate the patient regularly and provide continuing care, even when the asthma is mild.

Patient (and family) education

This aspect is vital and patients can be referred to an asthma education resource centre. However, the family doctor should be continually educating and encouraging the patient to follow the six step asthma management plan.

Asthmatics tend to use 'denial' as a coping mechanism and are generally 'non-attenders' when well.

Prevention of attacks is the best treatment, and all asthmatics and their families should aim to know the disorder very well and become expert in managing it.

Know your asthma (advice for patients)

- Read all about it.
- Get to know how severe your asthma is.
- Try to identify trigger factors such as tobacco smoke and avoid them. There is an 80% increase in asthma incidence in children whose parents smoke.
- Become expert at using your medication and inhalers. A big problem is incorrect inhaler technique (35% of patients).
- Use your inhalers correctly and use a spacer if necessary.
- Know and recognise the danger signs and act promptly.
- Have regular checks with your doctor.
- Have physiotherapy: learn breathing exercises.
- Keep fit and take regular exercise.
- Keep to ideal weight.
- Work out a clear management plan and an action plan for when trouble strikes.
- Get urgent help when danger signs appear.
- Learn the value of a peak expiratory flow meter (for anyone over 6 years old).
- Get a peak flow meter to help assess severity and work out your best lung function.
- Keep at your best with suitable medications.
- Always carry your bronchodilator inhaler and check that it is not empty (learn about the water flotation test).

Pharmacological agents to treat asthma

It is useful to teach patients the concept of the 'preventer' and the 'reliever' for their asthma treatment. The pharmacological treatment of asthma is summarised in Table 109.3.

Table 109.3 *Pharmacological treatment of bronchial asthma*

	Generic types	Examples	Nebulising solution	Oral	Aerosol (metered dose inhalation)	Dry powder (inhalation)	Injection
Bronchodilators							
1. β₂-adrenoceptor agonists	Salbutamol	Ventolin	✓	✓	✓	✓	✓
	Salmeterol	Serevent			✓	✓	
	Terbutaline	Bricanyl	✓	✓	✓	✓	✓
	Eformoterol	Foradile				✓	
	Fenoterol	Berotec	✓		✓		
	Adrenaline				✓		✓
2. Anticholinergics	Ipratropium bromide	Atrovent	✓		✓		
3. Methylxanthines	Theophylline	Brondecon		✓			
		Nuelin		✓			
		Theo-dur		✓			
	Aminophylline						✓
Mast cell stabilisers	Sodium cromoglycate }	Intal	✓		✓	✓	
		Intal forte			✓		
	Nedocromil sodium	Tilade			✓		
Corticosteroids	Beclomethasone	Becotide (50, 100)			✓	✓	
		Becloforte (250)			✓	✓	
	Budesonide	Pulmicort (various strengths)	✓		✓	✓	
	Fluticasone	Flixotide			✓	✓	
	Prednisolone			✓			
	Hydrocortisone	Solu-cortef					✓
Leucotriene antagonists	Montelukast	Singulair		✓			
	Zafirlukast	Accolate		✓			

'Preventer' drugs or anti-inflammatory agents

These medications are directed towards the underlying abnormalities—bronchial hyper-reactivity and associated airway inflammation.

Corticosteroids

Inhaled

Types	beclomethasone
	budesonide
	fluticasone
Dose range	400–2000 μg (adults); aim to keep below 1600 μg (if possible)
Availability	• metered dose inhaler
	• Turbuhaler
	• Rotacaps
	• Disks
Frequency	twice daily (helps compliance)
Side effects	• oropharyngeal candidiasis, dysphonia (hoarse voice)
	• bronchial irritation: cough
	• adrenal suppression (doses of 2000 μg/daily; sometimes as low as 800 μg)

Note: Rinse mouth out with water and spit out after using inhaled steroids.

Oral

Prednisolone is used mainly for exacerbations. It is given with the usual inhaled corticosteroids and bronchodilators.

Dose	up to 1 mg/kg/day for 1–2 weeks
Side effects	these are minimal if drug is used for short periods

Long-term use: osteoporosis, glucose intolerance, adrenal suppression, thinning of skin and easy bruising.
Oral corticosteroids can be ceased abruptly.

Cromolyns

These are sodium cromoglycate (SCG) and nedocromil sodium. SCG is available as dry capsules for inhalation, metered dose aerosols and a nebuliser solution. The availability of the metered aerosol and spacer has helped the use of SCG in the management of asthma in children. Adverse effects are uncommon; local irritation may be caused by the dry powder. Systemic effects do not occur.

Nedocromil is used for the treatment of mild–moderate persistent asthma in adults, for frequent episodic asthma in children over 2 years of age and for the prevention of exercise-induced asthma. The initial dose is 2 inhalations qid. Adverse effects are uncommon.

Leukotriene antagonists

These new drugs which include montelukast and zafirlukast are very useful for seasonal asthma, aspirin sensitive asthma and reduce the need for inhaled steroids. Montelukast is taken as a 5 or 10 mg chewable tablet once daily.

'Reliever' drugs or bronchodilators

The three groups of bronchodilators are:

- the β_2-adrenoceptor agonists (β-agonists)
- methylxanthines—theophylline derivatives
- anticholinergics

β_2-agonists

The inhaled route of delivery is the preferred route and the vehicles of administration include metered dose inhalation, a dry powder, and nebulisation where the solution is converted to a mist of small droplets by a flow of oxygen or air through the solution (Fig. 109.4).

Oral administration of β_2-agonists is rarely required. The inhaled drugs produce measurable bronchodilation in 1–2 minutes and peak effects by 10–20 minutes. The traditional agents such as salbutamol and terbutaline are short-acting preparations. The new longer-acting agents include salmeterol and formoterol.

Fig. 109.4 *Demonstration of the mechanism of the jet nebuliser*

Theophylline derivatives

These oral drugs may have complementary value to the inhaled agents but tend to be limited by side effects and efficacy.

Indications for preventive therapy[4]

Guidelines for introducing preventive asthma therapy in adults and children include any of the following:

- requirement of β_2–agonist > 3–4 times each week or > 1 canister every 3 months (excluding pre exercise)
- symptoms (non-exercise) > 3–4 times per week between attacks
- spirometry showing reversible airflow obstruction during asymptomatic phases
- asthma significantly interfering with physical activity despite appropriate pre-treatment
- asthma attacks > every 6–8 weeks
- infrequent asthma attacks but severe or life-threatening

Prophylactic agents

This term is reserved for those medications that are taken prior to known trigger factors, particularly for exercise-induced asthma.

Exercise-induced asthma

- β_2-agonist inhaler (puffer); two puffs immediately before exercise last 1–2 hours. New longer-acting agents such as salmeterol are more effective.
- Sodium cromoglycate or nedocromil, two puffs.
- Combination β_2-agonist + sodium cromoglycate.
- Paediatricians often recommend a non-drug warm-up program as an alternative to medication.

A general management plan for chronic asthma is summarised in Figure 109.5.

Correct use of the asthma metered dose inhaler (MDI) (puffer)

Did you know that . . . ?

- faulty inhaler technique occurs in at least one-third of users
- 90% of the medication sticks to the mouth and does not reach the lungs
- it is the inhalation effort—not the pressure from the aerosol—that gets the medication to the lungs

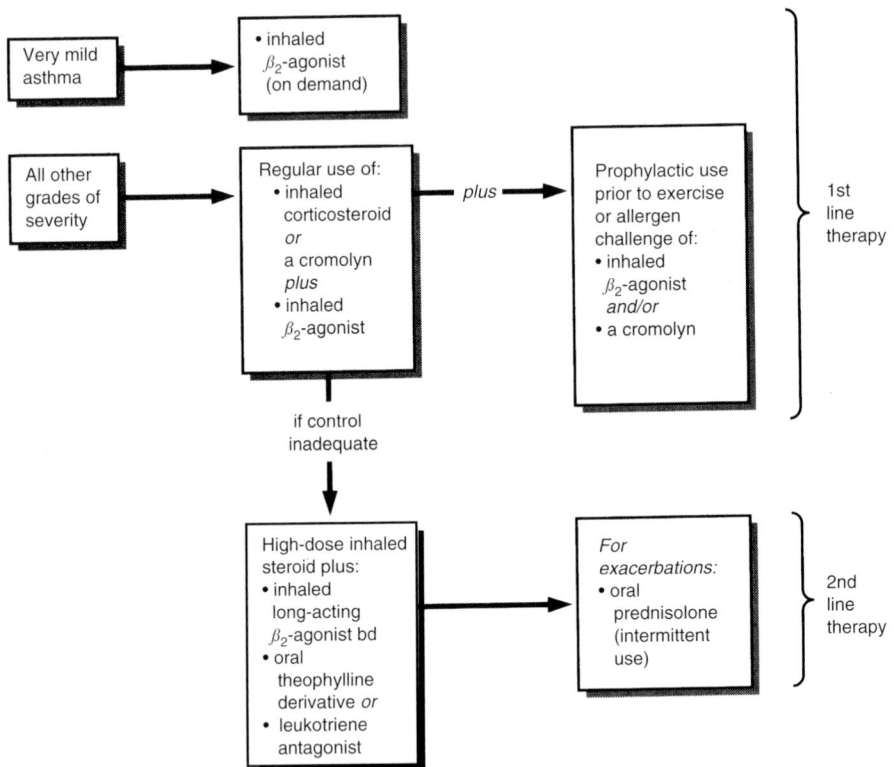

Fig. 109.5 *Management plan for chronic asthma*   ADAPTED FROM SEALE JP, *ASTHMA*[2] WITH PERMISSION OF *MIMS AUSTRALIA,* A DIVISION OF MEDIMEDIA AUSTRALIA PTY LIMITED

- it is important to instruct patients properly and check their technique regularly

The two main techniques

The open-mouth technique and the closed-mouth technique are the main methods, and both are effective. The patient and doctor should choose the technique that suits them best. Both techniques are suitable for most adults. Most children from the age of 7 can learn to use puffers quite well.

Instructions for patients

| The open-mouth technique | (Fig. 109.6)

1. Remove the cap. Shake the puffer vigorously for 1–2 seconds. Hold it upright (canister on top) to use it (as shown).
2. Hold the mouthpiece of the puffer 4–5 cm (about three finger-breadths) away from your mouth.
3. Tilt your head back slightly with your chin up. Open your mouth and keep it open.
4. Slowly blow out to a comfortable level.
5. Just as you start to breathe in (slowly) through your mouth, press the puffer firmly, once. Breathe in as far as you can over 3–5 seconds. (Do not breathe in through your nose.)
6. Close your mouth and hold your breath for about 10 seconds; then breathe out gently.
7. Breathe normally for about one minute, then repeat the inhalation.

| The closed-mouth technique | (Fig. 109.7)

The method is basically identical to the open-mouth technique except that you close your lips around the mouthpiece.

Common mistakes

- holding the puffer upside down
- holding the puffer too far away
- pressing the puffer too early and not inhaling the spray deeply
- pressing the puffer too late and not getting enough spray
- doing it all too quickly: not breathing in slowly and holding the breath
- squeezing the puffer more than once
- not breathing in deeply

Extra points

1. The usual dose of standard MDI is one or two puffs every 3–4 hours for an attack.
2. If you do not get adequate relief from your normal dose, you should contact your doctor.
3. It is quite safe to increase the dose, such as to 4–6 puffs.
4. If you are using your inhaler very often, it usually means your other asthma medication is not being used properly. Discuss this with your doctor.

Autohaler

The Autohaler is a breath-activated MDI which can improve lung deposition in patients with poor inhaler technique.

Fig. 109.6 *Using the metered dose inhaler: the open-mouth technique*

Fig. 109.7 *Using the metered dose inhaler: the closed-mouth technique*

The Turbuhaler

The Turbuhaler is a dry powder delivery system that is widely used as an alternative to the metered dose inhaler. It is a breath-activated device.

Other dry powder devices are the Accuhaler, Diskhaler and Rotahaler.

Dangerous asthma

Failure to recognise the development of a severe attack has cost the lives of many asthmatics. The severe attacks can start suddenly (even in mild asthmatics) and catch people by surprise.

High-risk patients

People who have experienced one or more of the following are more likely to have severe attacks:

- a previous severe asthma attack
- previous hospital admission, especially if to intensive care
- hospital attendance in the past 12 months
- long-term oral steroid treatment
- carelessness with taking medication
- night-time attacks, especially with severe chest tightness
- recent emotional problems

Early warning signs of severe asthma or an asthma atack:

- symptoms persisting or getting worse despite adequate medication
- increased coughing and chest tightness
- poor response to two inhalations
- benefit from inhalations not lasting 2 hours
- increasing medication requirements
- sleep being disturbed by coughing, wheezing or breathlessness
- chest tightness on waking in the morning
- low peak expiratory flow readings

Dangerous signs

- marked breathlessness, especially at rest
- sleep being greatly disturbed by asthma
- asthma getting worse quickly rather than slowly, despite medication
- feeling frightened
- difficulty in speaking; unable to say more than a few words
- exhaustion
- drowsiness or confusion
- chest becoming 'silent' with a quiet wheeze, yet breathing still laboured

- cyanosis
- chest retraction
- respiratory rate greater than 25 (adults) or 50 (children)
- pulse rate > 120
- peak flow < 100 L/min or < 40% predicted FEV_1
- oximetry on presentation (SaO_2) < 90%

Asthma action plans

Examples of action plans for patients are presented below.

Action plan

If you are distressed with severe asthma:

- Call an ambulance and say 'severe asthma attack' (best option)
  or
- Call your doctor
  or
- If you are having trouble finding medical help, get someone to drive you to the nearest hospital

Keep using your bronchodilator inhaler continuously if you are distressed.

The following is an example of an asthma action plan that the patient keeps on a card for easy reference.

Asthma Action Plan

Name ....

Contact Dr .... Tel. ....

Hospital tel. ....

Measure peak flow before reliever

Best peak flow: 600 (example) ....

Peak flow	*Treatment*
1. Below 480 (or 80% of best)	Double dose of preventer
2. Below 360 (or 60% of best)	Start prednisolone and contact doctor
3. Below 240 (or 40% of best)	Continue reliever and dial 000 for ambulance

The acute asthma attack

Summary (adult dosage)[4,5]

- continuous nebulised salbutamol (or terbutaline) if nebuliser available (if not: 6–10 puffs of β_2-agonist inhaler, preferably with spacer, using two loading puffs at a time followed by 4–6 breaths)

    Ipratropium bromide may be mixed with β_2-agonist for concurrent nebulisation.
- parenteral β_2-agonist, e.g. salbutamol 500 μg IM, SC
- corticosteroids, e.g. prednisolone 50 mg (o) statim then daily

    or

    hydrocortisone 250 mg IV or IM, 6 hourly
- oxygen 8L/min by face mask
- monitor PEF

The management of status asthmaticus is presented on page 1114.

Asthma in children

The prevalence of asthma is increasing in childhood and the management (especially in infants) is always a concern for the family doctor.

Key checkpoints

- Bronchodilators, inhaled or oral, are ineffective under 12 months.
- The delivery method is a problem in children and Table 109.4 gives an indication of what systems can be used at various levels.
- In the very young, e.g. 1–2 years old, a spacer with a face mask such as Aero Chamber or Breath-A-Tech can deliver the aerosol medication.
- The PEF rate should be measured in all asthmatic children older than 6 years. Children under 6 years generally cannot cope with the meters and those with mild asthma don't usually need PEF measurement.
- The Turbuhaler is usually not practical under 7–8 years.

Prophylaxis in children

The non-steroidal medications, sodium cromoglycate (SCG) and/or nedocromil sodium by inhalation, are the prophylactic drugs of choice in childhood chronic asthama of mild to moderate severity.

- They have no significant side effects. Avoid nedocromil in children > 2 years.
- A symptomatic response occurs in about 1–2 weeks (can take up to 4–6 weeks).
- SCG (Forte) is an alternative to low-dose inhaled corticosteroids once the asthma is stable, especially if there are steroid side effects.

If there is no clinical response to these agents in 4 weeks, consider use of inhaled corticosteroids, but the risks versus benefits must always be considered. Any dose equal to or greater than 400 μg in children can have side effects, including growth suppression and adrenal suppression. Aim for a maintenance of 100–400 μg, which keeps the child symptom-free. Once this stage is reached, consider stopping treatment or changing to SCG or nedocromil sodium.

Leukotriene antagonists taken orally aged 6 years and above is another option.

Guidelines for the management of asthma in children (1–4 years) are summarised in Table 109.5. Delivery systems for children are presented in Table 109.4.

When to refer

- If you are doubtful about the diagnosis.
- For problematic children.
- For advice on management when asthmatic control has failed or is difficult to achieve.

Practice tips

- Reassure the patient that 6–10 inhaled doses of a β_2-agonist is safe and appropriate for a severe attack of asthma.

Table 109.4 *Delivery systems for asthma in children*

Vehicle of administration	Age in years			
	Less than 2	2–4	5–7	8 and over
Inhaler alone			*	√
Inhaler + small volume spacer + face mask	√	√		
Inhaler + large volume spacer		√	√	√
Nebuliser/air compressor/face mask	√	√	√	√
Dry powder inhalers, e.g. Turbuhaler, Rotahaler			*	√

* possible in some individual children

Table 109.5 *Management plan for children 1–4 years*

Grade of asthma	Agent	Vehicle
Mild	β_2-agonist	Inhaler + spacer Nebuliser
Moderate	β_2-agonist	Inhaler + spacer or Nebuliser
	sodium cromoglycate ↓ if unresponsive corticosteroid	Inhaler + spacer or Nebuliser
Severe	β_2-agonist ↓	Inhaler + spacer or Nebuliser
	corticosteroid theophylline ipratropium bromide prednisolone	Sprinklers (oral) Nebuliser Oral

Note: Improvised 'spacer' with paper cup or plastic soft-drink bottle: an aerosol may be administered to children by plunging the mouthpiece of the inhaler through the base of the cup and then holding the open end of the cup over the child's mouth, or by cutting out the base of a plastic soft-drink bottle and holding this over the mouth while the inhaler is inserted into the open top of the bottle.

- It is important to achieve a balance between undertreatment and overtreatment.
- Beware of patients, especially children, manipulating their peak flow.
- Get patients to rinse out their mouth with water and spit it out after inhaling corticosteroids.
- Patients who are sensitive to aspirin/salicylates need to be reminded that salicylates are present in common cold cure preparations and agents such as Alka-Seltzer.[3]
- Possible side effects of inhaled drugs can be reduced by always using a spacer with the inhaler, using the medication qid rather than bd, rinsing the mouth, gargling and spitting out after use, and using corticosteroid sparing medications.

References

1. International Consensus Report on Diagnosis and Treatment of Asthma. National Heart, Lung and Blood Institute. Bethesda, Maryland, 1992; 1–2.

2. Seale JP. Asthma. In: MIMS Disease Index. Sydney: IMS Publishing, 1991–92, 59–65.

3. Rees J, Price J. *ABC of asthma* (2nd edn). London: BMJ, 1989, 1–34.

4. Asthma management handbook 1996. National Asthma Campaign. Melbourne, 1996; 8–75.

5. Rubinfeld AR. How to treat asthma. Aust Dr Weekly, 1 February 1991, I–VIII.

110

Epilepsy

—

The fit makes the patient fall down senseless; and without his will or consciousness presently every muscle is put in action; as if all the powers of the body were exerted to free itself from some great violence. In these strong and universal convulsions, the urine, excrements and seed, are sometimes forced away, and the mouth is covered with foam, which will be bloody, when the tongue is bit, as it often is in the agony.

William Heberden (1718–1801)

Epilepsy is defined as a 'tendency to recurrence of seizures'. It is a symptom, not a disease. A person should not be labelled 'epileptic' until at least two attacks have occurred.[1] Epilepsy is common and affects about one person in 50. Both sexes are about equally involved, and it seems to run in some families. Famous people who have had epilepsy include Julius Caesar, Thomas Edison and Handel.

The most important factors in the management of epilepsy are the accurate diagnosis of the type of seizures; identification of the cause and appropriate investigation; the use of first-line drugs as the sole therapy of some weeks; and adjustment of the dose, according to clinical experience and plasma levels, to give maximum benefit.

To be accurate in diagnosing seizures the diagnosis must be based on:

- the observation of a witness to the seizures
- a general and neurological examination
- an electroencephalogram (EEG), although this has considerable limitations
- a computerised tomography (CT) scan or preferably MRI (especially if the EEG is focal and a tumour is suspected)

Long-term ambulatory EEG recording now provides more information and, coupled with video monitoring, it will make a permanent record of the seizure which can be reviewed at will. The CT scan or MRI scan is necessary to exclude a focal cause (such as a cyst, tumour, malformation or abscess) which might be treatable by surgery. The MRI scan now shows developmental migration disorders.

The scans will identify mesotemporal sclerosis (an abnormality in the hippocampus due to birth hypoxia), thereby making some 'idiopathic' seizures into secondary seizures from a known cause.

Epilepsy usually starts in early childhood.

An underlying organic lesion becomes more common in epilepsy presented for the first time in patients over the age of 25 and thus more detailed investigation is required.[1]

Optimal management includes adequate psychosocial support with education, counselling, advocacy and appropriate referral.

Types of epileptic seizures/ syndromes

Epileptic seizures are classified in general terms as generalised and partial (Table 110.1). Partial seizures are about twice as common as generalised seizures and usually due to acquired pathology.[2]

Generalised seizures

The epileptic discharge affects both cerebral hemispheres simultaneously from the outset. The seizure may be primary (no focus) or secondary due to acquired cerebral pathology.

Table 110.1 *Classification of epileptic seizures*

1. Generalised seizures
Convulsive
tonic clonic (previously called grand mal)
clonic
Non-convulsive
tonic ⎫ drop
atonic ⎭ attacks
absence (petit mal)
atypical absence
myoclonic

2. Partial seizures (non-convulsive)
Simple partial (consciousness retained)
with motor signs (Jacksonian)
with somatosensory symptoms
with psychic symptoms
Complex partial (consciousness impaired)

3. Secondary generalised seizures (convulsive)
Simple partial seizures evolving to tonic clonic seizures
Complex partial seizures evolving to tonic clonic seizures
Simple partial seizures evolving to complex partial seizures and then to tonic clonic seizures

The main features are:
- abrupt impairment or loss of consciousness
- possible bilateral symmetrical motor events

Types

- Tonic-clonic (formerly called grand mal) seizure: this is the classic convulsive seizure with muscle jerking (pp. 699–700)
- Tonic seizure: stiffness only, often with a 'drop' (hallmark of Lennox Gastaut syndrome)
- Clonic seizure: jerks only
- Atonic seizure: loss of tone, and 'drops'
- Absence seizure (formerly called petit mal): involves loss of consciousness with no or only very minor bilateral muscle jerking, mainly of the face[2] (p. 510)
- Myoclonic seizure: bilateral discrete muscle jerks, which may be very severe, and loss of consciousness

Partial seizures

In partial seizures the epileptic discharge begins in a localised focus of the brain and then spreads out from this focus. The clinical pattern depends on the part of the brain affected.

- simple partial seizures: consciousness is retained (pp. 509–510)
- complex partial seizures: consciousness is clouded so that the patient does not recall the complete seizure (p. 509).

Both these types of partial seizure can evolve into a bilateral tonic clonic seizure; this is termed a secondary generalised seizure and is usually due to diffuse brain pathology.[1]

Investigations

Standard minimum investigations are:

- serum calcium and electrolytes
- fasting glucose
- EEG (usually with sleep deprivation)
- syphilis serology

Other tests may include:

- chest X-ray
- brain scan
- video EEG (limited mainly to frequent seizures or to diagnostic dilemmas)
- magnetic resonance imaging (MRI)
- CT scanning (if MRI unavailable)

A patient presenting with the first seizure after the age of 25 years will require more detailed investigation.

Approaches to management

- An accurate diagnosis of the seizure type is essential.
- An underlying brain disease has to be investigated and treated.
- A decision has to be made about whether drug therapy is appropriate. Most seizures require long-term antiepileptic (anticonvulsant) drug therapy aimed at suppressing the underlying seizure activity in the hope that it may subside, so that 'cure' ultimately occurs and treatment may be ceased. A summary of antiepileptic drugs is presented in Table 110.2.
- The choice of drug depends on the seizure type, on consideration of the age and sex of the patient and on efficacy in relation to toxicity.
- Treatment should be initiated with one drug and pushed until it controls the events or causes side effects, irrespective of the medication blood level. The disorder can usually be controlled by one drug provided adequate serum or plasma concentrations are reached.[3]
- If a maximum tolerated dosage of this single drug fails to control the seizures, replace it with an alternative agent. Add the second drug and obtain a therapeutic effect before removing the first drug.

Table 110.2 *Antiepileptic drugs*

The following antiepileptic drugs are used

Benzodiazepines
  clonazepam
  diazepam
Carbamazepine
Corticotrophin
Phenobarbitone and related drugs
  methylphenobarbitone
  primidone
Phenytoin
Sodium valproate
Succinimides
  ethosuximide

New drugs (mainly as 'added on' therapy)

Lamotrigine
Vigabatrin
Gabapentin
Felbamate
Clobazam
Topiramate
Tiagabine

- It is important to review the need for anticonvulsants every 12 months. Consider drug withdrawal if the patient has been free of seizures for several years (best under specialist supervision). Up to 60% of children have a mild self-limiting condition and can settle after medication is withdrawn.

- Special attention should be given to the adverse psychological and social effects of epilepsy. Emotional and social suport is important and advice about epilepsy support groups is appropriate.

Drug therapy

The following are important specific considerations:

- It is best to select the most effective recommended drug for a specific seizure type (Table 110.3).
- Young women prefer carbamazepine to phenytoin because of the adverse effects of gingival hypertrophy and hirsutism of phenytoin.
- Each drug has specific adverse effects (Table 110.4) while all drugs tend to be sedating, especially phenobarbitone and its derivatives.
- Twice daily dosage is usually practical.
- Phenytoin should be increased in small increments (25–50 mg) above a dose of 300 mg daily.
- Phenytoin or carbamazepine will bring about control in at least 80% of patients with tonic clonic seizures.[1] Do not use these drugs together as they have a similar action.

Adverse drug reactions

Patients should be warned about significant side effects:

Table 110.3 *Recommended selection of antiepileptics in epilepsy*

Type of seizure	First-line therapy	Second-line therapy (select from)
Tonic/clonic	Sodium valproate In young women (still reproductive) use carbamazepine	Phenytoin Vigabatrin Carbamazepine Lamotrigine Gabapentin Tiagabine Topiramate Phenobarbitone
Absence (petit mal)	Ethosuximide	Sodium valproate (first line if associated with other seizure type) Clonazepam Lamotrigine
Myoclonic	Sodium valproate	Clonazepam Lamotrigine
Simple partial (Jacksonian) and Complex partial	Carbamazepine	Phenytoin Sodium valproate Topiramate Gabapentin Lamotrigine Tiagabine Vigabatrin

Table 110.4 *Commonly used antiepileptics: usual dose and adverse reactions*

	Usual starting adult dose	Average satisfactory adult dose (mg/kg/day)	Therapeutic plasma concentration range (μmol/L)	Significant adverse reactions
Carbamazepine	100–200 mg daily or bd, increasing gradually to control (max. 2 g/day)	30	25–50 free level 6–13	Anorexia, nausea, vomiting, dizziness, drowsiness, skin rashes, tinnitus, ataxia, diplopia Small risk of spina bifida in foetus Drug interactions, e.g. COC, warfarin, other anticonvulsants
Clonazepam	0.25 mg bd increasing to control	0.1–0.2	0.08–0.24	Drowsiness, fatigue, muscle weakness, ataxia, dizziness Respiratory problems Interacts with alcohol
Ethosuximide (used only in absence seizures)	20–30 mg/kg/day in 2 divided doses	30	300–700 (all free)	Anorexia, nausea, vomiting Diarrhoea Drowsiness, ataxia, headache
Lamotrigine	25 mg/day increasing to 100–200 mg/day	1.5–5	–	Beware of blood dyscrasias Drowsiness, skin rashes, nausea, headache, dizziness, ataxia Beware of severe rashes: introduce slowly
Phenobarbitone	30–90 mg bd	2–4	45–130	Drowsiness Dizziness, ataxia Skin rashes Mood changes, e.g. excitable Interacts with warfarin, COC, other anticonvulsants
Phenytoin	5 mg/kg/day in 2 divided doses	5–6	40–80 free level 4–8	Drowsiness, fatigue, mental confusion, ataxia, nystagmus, slurred speech, anorexia, dizziness, nausea, vomiting Skin reactions Gum hypertrophy, hirsutism Foetal malformations, e.g. cleft lip and palate, congenital heart disorders
Sodium valproate	500 mg bd, increasing to achieve control (up to 2–3 g/day)	20–30 Standard dose: 500 mg mane 1000 mg nocte	300–750 free level 30–75	Drowsiness, tremor, hair loss Platelet effect Risk of neural tube defects in foetus Hepatic failure Interacts with other anticonvulsants To be avoided in pregnancy
Vigabatrin	500 mg bd increasing to 2g bd	30–40	Not relevant	Drowsiness Behavioural disturbances Dizziness

- Nausea, dizziness, ataxia, visual disturbance or excessive tiredness/fatigue indicate excessive dosage of carbamazepine or phenytoin.
- Most drugs can cause a rash.
- Gingival hyperplasia is a classic effect of phenytoin.
- Hirsutism can occur with phenytoin while hair loss can occur with sodium valproate.
- Sodium valproate has rare but potentially serious toxic effects
  — liver toxicity
  — dysmorphogenic effects (specifically spina bifida) on foetus during pregnancy (therefore it is a risk in women of child-bearing age, especially if inadvertent pregnancy occurs due to pill failure related to antiepileptic interaction).
- LFTs should be performed every two months for six months after starting sodium valproate.[1] Liver toxicity is much more common in the under 2 years old age group.

Patient education

Points worth emphasising:
- Most patients can achieve complete control of seizures.
- Most people lead a normal life—they can expect to marry, have a normal sexual life and have normal children.
- Patients need good dental care, especially if they are taking phenytoin.
- A seizure in itself will not usually cause death or brain damage unless in a risk situation such as swimming, or prolonged.
- Patients cannot swallow their tongue during a seizure.
- Take special care with open fires.
- Encourage patients to cease intake of alcohol.
- Adequate sleep is important.

Driving
One has to be very careful about driving. Most people with epilepsy can drive but each case has to be considered individually. Applicants for learner's licence need to be seizure-free for 2 years, with an annual medical review for 5 years following receipt of the licence. Restrictions range from 1 month to 2 years, depending on the circumstances of the seizures.

Employment
People with epilepsy can hold down most jobs, but if liable to seizures they should not work close to heavy machinery, in dangerous surroundings, at heights (such as climbing ladders) or near deep water. Careers are not available in some services, such as the police, military, aviation (pilot, traffic controller) or public transport (e.g. bus driver).

Sport and leisure activities
Most activities are fine, but epileptics should avoid dangerous sports such as scuba diving, hang-gliding, parachuting, rock climbing, car racing and swimming alone, especially surfing.

Table 110.5 outlines contraindications for sporting activities. These apply to patients who suffer from very frequent seizures, especially the complex partial seizures with prolonged postictal states.[4]

Avoid trigger factors
- fatigue
- lack of sleep
- physical exhaustion
- stress
- excess alcohol
- prolonged flashing lights if photosensitive, e.g. video games (this applies to those with a proven response to a proper EEG with photic stimulation)

Table 110.5 *Sporting activities: contraindications*[4]

Absolute contraindications
- flying and parachuting
- motor racing
- mountain and rock climbing
- high diving
- scuba diving
- underwater swimming, especially competitive
- hang-gliding
- abseiling

Relative contraindications
- aiming sports such as archery and pistol shooting
- contact sports such as boxing, rugby, football, including soccer, where heading the ball is involved
- competitive cycling for children with absence epilepsy
- bathing and swimming
- gymnastics, especially activities such as trampolining and climbing on bars
- ice skating and skiing
- javelin throwing

Epilepsy in children
Refer to Chapter 50, on faints, fits and funny turns (p. 505).

Photosensitive epilepsy in children

Some children suffer from photosensitive epilepsy related to exposure to computer and video games. There is some evidence that such children may not have seizures if they keep one eye covered. If television provokes seizures, strategies such as watching it with ambient lighting and using the remote control rather than approaching the set will minimise the problem.

Epilepsy in the elderly

The elderly require the same diagnostic approach as any other age group. However, they are sensitive to side effects of drugs and may require a lower dose than younger patients. It must be remembered that antidepressant or major tranquilliser drugs can precipitate a generalised seizure.

Pregnancy and epilepsy[5]

Although the outcome is successful for more than 90% of epileptic women, there is a slightly increased risk of prematurity, low birth weight, mortality, defects and intervention. About 45% of women have an increased number of seizures, due mainly to a fall in antiepileptic drug levels.

All antiepileptic drugs are potentially teratogenic, with different drugs being related to different defects: phenytoin has been related to cleft lip and palate and congenital heart disease, while sodium valproate (in particular) and carbamazepine have been associated with spina bifida. All antiepileptic drugs are expressed in breast milk but in such reduced concentrations as not to preclude breast-feeding.

Pitfalls in management of epilepsy[3]

Misdiagnosis

The main pitfall associated with seizure disorders and epilepsy is misdiagnosis. It should be realised that not all seizures are generalised tonic clonic in type. The most common misdiagnosed seizure disorder is that of complex partial seizures (an underdiagnosed disorder) or the tonic or atonic seizures.

The diagnosis of epilepsy is made on the history rather than the EEG so a very detailed description of the events from eye witnesses is important.

The features of complex partial seizure (described on p. 509) have many variations, the commonest being a slight disturbance of perception or consciousness. The complex partial seizure may evolve to a generalised tonic clonic seizure. A simple partial seizure may also do this.

In tonic clonic seizures the patient may become momentarily rigid or fall to the ground and perhaps have one or two jerks only.

Misdiagnosing behavioural disorders

It is important to differentiate between a fit and a behavioural disorder, but it can be difficult. About 20% of apparently intractable 'seizures' are considered to be non-epileptic (pseudoseizures), i.e. emotionally based.[6] Ancillary testing, especially with video EEG recording, can help overcome these diagnostic problems but the differentiation may be difficult as the most common situation for pseudoseizures is in the person who has real fits.

Overtreatment

Polypharmacy

Polypharmacy may be counterproductive for the patient and the seizure disorder. This is especially applicable to drugs with a high incidence of side effects. If a patient is taking several medications, management of the case needs questioning and perhaps reconsidering with a consultant's help.

Seizure control may be improved by reducing polypharmacy. When initiating treatment it is best to select one drug and increase its dose until its maximum recommended level, the onset of side effects or appropriate control. If control is not obtained, the drug should be replaced with an alternative agent but a crossover period is essential. Monotherapy is preferred but combination therapy is often acceptable.

Prolonged treatment

The question should be asked at some stage 'Does this patient really need medication?' Some patients are kept on antiepileptics for too long without any attempt being made to wean them off medication or to transfer them onto antiepileptics less prone to side effects. Patients should not be left on inappropriate drugs especially if side effects and drug interactions are a problem.

Drug interactions

Drug interactions with antiepileptics should always be kept in mind. The most serious of all is the interaction with the oral contraceptive pill, because pregnancy can occur. Erythromycin and carbamazepine interact.

Management of status epilepticus

Definition

Status epilepticus is the situation in which a patient suffers from two or more generalised seizures without regaining consciousness between seizures, or suffers from continuous partial seizures.[7]

Focal status

- a high index of suspicion is needed to diagnose
- oral medication usually adequate
- avoid overtreatment

Generalised status

Absence attack (petit mal)

- hospitalisation
- IV diazepam

Tonic-clonic (dangerous!)[7]

- ensure adequate oxygenation: attend to airway (e.g. Guedel tube); give oxygen
- diazepam 0.05 mg/kg/minute IV until the seizures cease or respiratory depression begins (beware of respiratory depression and other vital parameters)

or

- clonazepam 1 mg IV statim then 0.5–1 mg/min IV until seizures cease or respiratory depression begins

or

- phenytoin 1000 mg IV over 20–30 minutes

or

- midazolam 0.05–0.1 mg/kg IV (max. 10–15 mg) or 0.15 mg/kg IM

Other drugs to consider:

- phenobarbitone; thiopentone; paraldehyde; valproate (can use rectally)

Note: Midazolam is suitable for all types of seizures.

Diazepam can be given rectally. In an adult, 10 mg is diluted in 5 mL of isotonic saline and introduced via the nozzle of the syringe into the rectum. The dose in children is 0.5 mg/kg.

DOs and DON'Ts for the onlookers of a seizure

- Don't move the person (unless necessary for safety).
- Don't force anything into the person's mouth.
- Don't try to stop the fit.
- Do roll the person on to his or her side with the head turned to one side and chin up.
- Do call for medical help if the seizure lasts longer than 10 minutes or starts again.
- Do remove false teeth and help clear the airway once the fit is over.

When to refer[2]

Specialist referral is advisable under the following circumstances:

- uncertainty of diagnosis
- at onset of seizure disorder to help obtain a precise diagnosis
- when seizures are not controlled by apparent suitable therapy ? wrong drug ? suboptimal dose ? progressive underlying disorder
- when the patient is unwell, irrespective of laboratory investigation
- when a woman is considering pregnancy (preferable) or has become pregnant: to obtain therapeutic guidance during a difficult phase of management
- for assessment of the prospects for withdrawing treatment after some years of absolute seizure control

Practice tips

- The EEG has considerable limitations in diagnosis. It is diagnostic in less than 50%,[1] although more diagnostic if conducted under sleep deprivation. An accurate eye witness account of the seizure is the most reliable diagnostic aid.
- During evaluation look for evidence of neurofibromatosis.
- Beware of interactions between antiepileptics and the oral contraceptive pill.
- Interactions between erythromycin and carbamazepine can cause toxicity.
- Always aim to achieve monotherapy.
- An important toxic reaction can occur with combined phenytoin and carbamazepine.
- Patients should not drive while medication is being adjusted, particularly if weaning is being attempted.

• The development of sophisticated surgical techniques means that surgery can be used in selected patients with poor control. Evaluation for surgery is a very specialised area.

References

1. Scott AK. Management of epilepsy. In: *Central nervous system*. London: BMJ, 1989, 1–2.

2. Eadie MJ. Epilepsy. In: MIMS Disease Index (2nd edn). Sydney: IMS Publishing, 1996, 175–178.

3. Ianseck R. *Pitfalls in neurology*. Proceedings Handbook: Annual Update Course for General Practitioners. Monash University Medical School, 1992, 1–4.

4. Cordova F. Epilepsy and sport. Aust Fam Physician, 1993; 22:558–562.

5. Kilpatrick C. Epilepsy poses special problems. Aust Dr Weekly, 19 February 1993, 48.

6. Theodore HR. Neurotrek. A PC based system for automated recording of epileptic seizures and similar events. Patient Management, 1992; 16:15–16.

7. Moulds RFW (Chairman). *Therapeutic Guidelines: Neurology*, Therapeutic Guidelines Limited, 1997, 100–101.

111

Hypertension

Hypertension is a serious community disorder and the most common condition requiring long-term drug therapy in Australia. It is a silent killer because most people with hypertension are asymptomatic and unaware of their problem. Epidemiological studies have demonstrated the association between hypertension and stroke, coronary heart disease, renal disease, heart failure and atrial fibrillation. Treatment is life-long, hence the need for careful workup.

Definitions and classification

- The various categories of blood pressure are arbitrarily defined according to blood pressure values for both diastolic and systolic readings (Table 111.1).[1,2]

> For adults aged 18 years and older hypertension is:
> diastolic pressure > 90 mmHg
> systolic pressure > 140 mmHg

- Isolated systolic hypertension is that ≥ 140 mmHg in the presence of a diastolic pressure < 90 mmHg.
- Hypertension is either essential or secondary (Table 111.2).
- Essential hypertension is the presence of sustained hypertension in the absence of underlying, potentially correctable renal, adrenal or other factors.
- Malignant hypertension is that with a diastolic pressure > 120 mmHg and exudative

Table 111.1 *Classification of blood pressure in adults aged 18 years and older measured as sitting blood pressure (mmHg)[1,2]*

Range (mmHg)	Category
Diastolic	
< 85	Normal blood pressure
85–89	High normal blood pressure
90–99	Mild hypertension
100–109	Moderate hypertension
> 110	Severe hypertension
Systolic (assumes 'normal' or 'high normal' diastolic blood pressure)	
< 130	'Normal' systolic blood pressure
140–149	Borderline isolated systolic hypertension
≥ 140	Isolated systolic hypertension

- Adapted from the 1988 Report of the Joint National Committee on Detection, Evaluation and Treatment of High Blood Pressure.
- The classification is based on the average of two or more readings on at least three or more occasions.
- In subjects aged 50 or less the diastolic level always takes precedence over the systolic level.
- Before diagnosis is made the variation between readings should not exceed 10 mm of mercury for systolic blood pressure or 6 mm of mercury for diastolic blood pressure.

vasculopathy in the retinal and renal circulations.
- Refractory hypertension is BP > 140/90 despite maximum dosage of two drugs for 3–4 months.
- Since cardiovascular risk is increased when there has been hypertensive end organ damage, and the presence of such organ damage will influence the approach to treatment, it is appropriate to classify hypertension into stages as outlined in the 1978 WHO Expert Report and reconfirmed in the 1993 Guidelines (Table 111.3).

Table 111.2 *Classification of hypertension*

Essential (90–95%)

Secondary (approximately 5–10%)

Renal (3–4%)
- glomerulonephritis
- reflux nephropathy
- renal artery stenosis
- other renovascular disease

Endocrine
- primary aldosteronism (Conn's syndrome)
- Cushing's syndrome
- phaeochromocytoma
- oral contraceptives
- other endocrine factors

Coarctation of the aorta

Immune disease, e.g. polyarteritis nodosa

Drugs

Pregnancy

Table 111.3 *Classification of hypertension by extent of organ damage (WHO guidelines)*

Stage I	No objective signs of organic changes
Stage II	At least one of the following signs of organ involvement:
	• left ventricular hypertrophy (X-ray, etc.)
	• generalised and focal narrowing of the retinal arteries
	• proteinuria and/or slight elevation of plasma creatinine concentration (1.2–2.0 mg/dL)
	• ultrasound or radiological evidence of atherosclerotic plaque
Stage III	Both symptoms and signs have appeared as a result of organ damage. These include:
	• Heart: angina pectoris myocardial infarction heart failure
	• Brain: TIA, stroke hypertensive encephalopathy
	• Optic fundi: retinal haemorrhages and exudates ± papilloedema
	• Kidney: plasma creatinine concentration > 2.0 mg/dL, renal failure
	• Vessels: dissecting aneurysm, symptomatic arterial occlusive disease

Key facts and checkpoints

- In the United States, 15% of 18–24 year olds and 60% of 65–74 years olds have hypertension.[3]

- In the US, studies show that only 54% of all hypertensives are aware of their disease and only 11% are being treated adequately. Similar figures have been shown in the UK.[4]
- The risk of cardiovascular disease rises significantly with increasing blood pressure.
- If both parents have hypertension there is a 50% chance of the offspring developing hypertension and if one parent has HT there is a 25% chance.
- Headache may occur in hypertensive patients (most are asymptomatic): it is typically early morning, occipital and throbbing: it appears to be related to severity of blood pressure.
- Any dizziness in hypertensive patients is usually due to postural hypertension from treatment.
- An analysis of the results available from 17 randomised controlled trials involving 47 653 subjects followed for an average of 5 years showed that an average fall in blood pressure of 11/5 mmHg conferred a 38% reduction in stroke, and a 16% fall in the incidence of coronary heart disease.
- Target organs (including some specific examples) that can be damaged by hypertension include the heart (failure, LVH, ischaemic disease), the kidney (renal insufficiency), the retina (retinopathy), the blood vessels (peripheral vascular disease, dissecting aortic aneurysm) and the brain (cerebrovascular disease).
- Deaths in hypertensive patients have been shown to be due to stroke 45%, heart failure 35%, renal failure 3% and others 17%.[4]
- Factors increasing chances of dying in hypertensive patients are: male patient; young patient; family history; increasing diastolic pressure.[4]

Secondary hypertension

Secondary hypertension may be suggested in patients below 40 by the history (Table 111.4), physical examination, severity of hypertension or the initial laboratory findings. It is also more likely in patients whose blood pressure is responding poorly to drug therapy, patients with well-controlled hypertension whose blood pressure begins to increase, and patients with accelerated or malignant hypertension.[2]

The most common causes of secondary hypertension are various renal diseases, such as renovascular disease, chronic glomerulonephritis, chronic pyelonephritis (often associated with

Table 111.4   *Clinical features suggesting secondary hypertension*[5]

Clinical features	Likely cause
Abdominal systolic bruit	Renal artery stenosis
Proteinuria, haematuria, casts	Glomerulonephritis
Bilateral renal masses with or without haematuria	Polycystic disease
History of claudication and delayed femoral pulse	Coarctation of the aorta
Progressive nocturia, weakness	Primary aldosteronism (check serum potassium)
Paroxysmal hypertension with headache, pallor, sweating, palpitations	Phaeochromocytoma

reflux nephropathy) and analgesic nephropathy.[1] There will often be no physical findings to suggest the existence of such renal diseases, but an indication will generally be obtained by the presence of one or more abnormalities when the urine is examined. Clinical pointers include proteinuria, an abnormal urine sediment, general atheroma, smokers and abdominal bruit.

Physical findings that may suggest secondary hypertension include epigastric bruits (indicating possible renal artery stenosis) and abdominal aortic aneurysm. Less common findings include abdominal flank masses (polycystic kidneys), delayed or absent femoral pulses (coarctation of the aorta), truncal obesity with pigmented striae (Cushing's syndrome), and tachycardia, sweating and pallor (phaeochromocytoma).

Further investigation will be required to confirm or reveal secondary hypertension.

Conn's syndrome: clinical features
- weakness due to hypokalaemia
- polyuria and polydypsia
- Na $\uparrow$, K $\downarrow$, alkalosis
- aldosterone $\uparrow$ (serum and urine)
- plasma renin $\downarrow$

Phaeochromocytoma: clinical features
Paroxysms or spells of

- hypertension
- headache (throbbing)
- sweating
- palpitations
- pallor/skin blanching
- rising sensation of tightness in upper chest and throat (angina can occur)

24 hour urinary free catecholamines $\uparrow$ (VMA)

Detection of hypertension[1]
Hypertension can only be detected when blood pressure is measured. Therefore every reasonable opportunity should be taken to measure blood pressure.

Diagnosis should not be made on the basis of a single visit. Initial raised blood pressure readings should be confirmed on at least two other visits within the space of 3 months; average levels of 90 mmHg diastolic or more, or 140 mmHg systolic or more, are needed before hypertension can be diagnosed. This will avoid the possibility of an incorrect diagnosis, committing an asymptomatic normotensive individual to unjustified, lifelong treatment.

Measurement[1]
Blood pressure varies continuously and can be affected by many outside factors. Care should therefore be taken to ensure that readings accurately represent the patient's usual pressure. The essential steps in this process are outlined below.

Position
Patients should be seated with their bare arm supported and positioned at heart level. Any sleeve should be loose above the sphygmomanometer cuff.

Cuff size and placement
A cuff size that will completely occlude the brachial artery is essential for accurate measurement. Cuffs that are too short or too narrow may give falsely high readings. The cuff's rubber bladder should have a width of at least 40% of the circumference of the patient's arm and a length at least double that. The commonly used

cuffs are often shorter than this recommendation. Suitable cuffs are made by Trimline (PyMaH) and Accosan. Several sizes, including cuffs for children and the obese, should be available. The bladder of the cuff deteriorates over about two years and should be replaced at intervals.[6]

A preferable cuff placement is to have the tubes emerging from the bladder point proximally (Figure 111.1) thus leaving the cubital fossa free.[6]

Equipment
Ideally, measurement should be taken with a reliable and properly maintained sphygmomanometer. Otherwise, a recently calibrated aneroid manometer or a calibrated electronic instrument can be used. It is essential that all equipment is maintained regularly. All tubing connections should be airtight.

Palpation
Initially, systolic blood pressure should be recorded by the palpatory method at the radial or brachial artery (the brachial artery is felt just medial to the biceps tendon in the cubital fossa). This will prevent low auscultatory systolic pressures caused by a 'silent gap'.

Note this reading and add 30 mmHg to it as the upper level to which to inflate the cuff, while accurately measuring the BP with the bell of the stethoscope over the brachial artery.

Taking the reading
While the BP is being measured, the cuff should be deflated at a rate no greater than 2mm of mercury for each beat. One of the commonest

Fig 111.1 *Correct placement of the cuff*

errors is to allow the column of mercury to fall too rapidly.

Pressure should be recorded to the nearest 2 mm of mercury (it should not end in 5). Parallax errors should be avoided when reading levels (Figure 111.2).[6,7] Wait 60 seconds and repeat the BP measurement.

Recording
On each occasion when BP is taken, two or more readings should be averaged. Wait at least 30 seconds before repeating the procedure. If the first two readings differ by more than 6 mmHg systolic or 4 mmHg diastolic, more readings should be taken.

Both systolic and diastolic levels should be recorded. For the diastolic reading the disappearance of sound (Phase 5)—that is, the pressure when the last sound is heard and after which all sound disappears—should be used.[8] This is more accurate than the muffling of sounds (Phase 4) (Fig. 111.3), which should only be used if the sound continues to zero.

Heart rate and pulse
At the same time the BP is measured, the heart rate and rhythm should be measured and recorded. A high heart rate may indicate undue stress that is causing the associated elevated BP reading. An irregular heart rhythm may cause difficulty in obtaining an accurate BP reading.

BP modifying factors
Apprehension: Patient should be rested for at least 5 minutes and made as relaxed as possible.

Caffeine: Patients should not take caffeine for 4–6 hours before measurement.

Smoking: Patients should also avoid smoking for 2 hours before measurement.

Eating: Patients should not have eaten for 30 minutes.

Strategies for high initial readings
If the initial reading is high (DBP > 90, SBP > 140) repeat the measures after 5 minutes of quiet rest. The 'white coat' influence in the medical practitioner's office may cause higher readings so measurement in other settings such as the home or the workplace should be managed whenever possible.

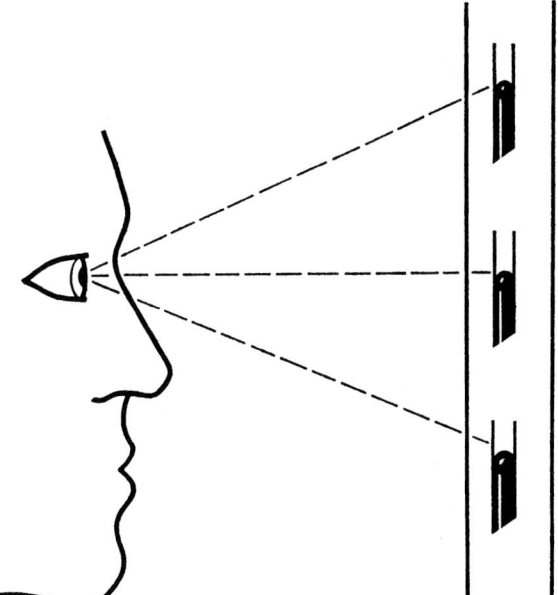

Fig 111.2 *Correct eye level: the observer should be within 1 metre of the manometer, so the scale can be easily read to avoid a parallax error—the eye should be on the same horizontal level as the mercury meniscus*

Confirmation and follow-up[1]

Repeated blood pressure readings will determine whether initial high levels are confirmed and need attention, or whether they return to normal and need only periodic checking. Particular attention should be paid to younger patients to ensure that they are regularly followed up.

Initial diastolic blood pressure readings of 115 mmHg or more, particularly for patients with target organ damage, may need immediate drug therapy.

Once an elevated level has been detected, the timing of subsequent readings should be based on the initial pressure level, as shown in Table 111.5.

If mild hypertension is found, observation with repeated measurement over 3–6 months should be followed before beginning therapy. This is because levels often return to normal.

Ambulatory 24 hour monitoring

This is not required for the diagnosis and follow-up of most hypertensive patients but in some patients with fluctuating levels, borderline hypertension or refractory hypertension (especially where the 'white coat' effect may be significant) ambulatory monitoring has a place in management. Studies have shown that this method provides a more precise estimate of blood pressure variability than casual recordings. This has implications for the timing of drug therapy in individual patients.

'White coat' hypertension

This group may comprise up to 25% of patients presenting with hypertension. These people have a type of conditioned response to the clinic or office setting and their home BP and ambulatory BP profiles are normal. They appear to be at low risk of cardiovascular disease but may progress to sustained hypertension.

Evaluation

As well as defining the blood pressure problem, the clinical evaluation for suspected hypertension should also determine

- whether the patient has potentially reversible secondary hypertension
- whether target organ damage is present
- whether there are other potentially modifiable cardiovascular risk factors present and
- what co-morbid factors exist.

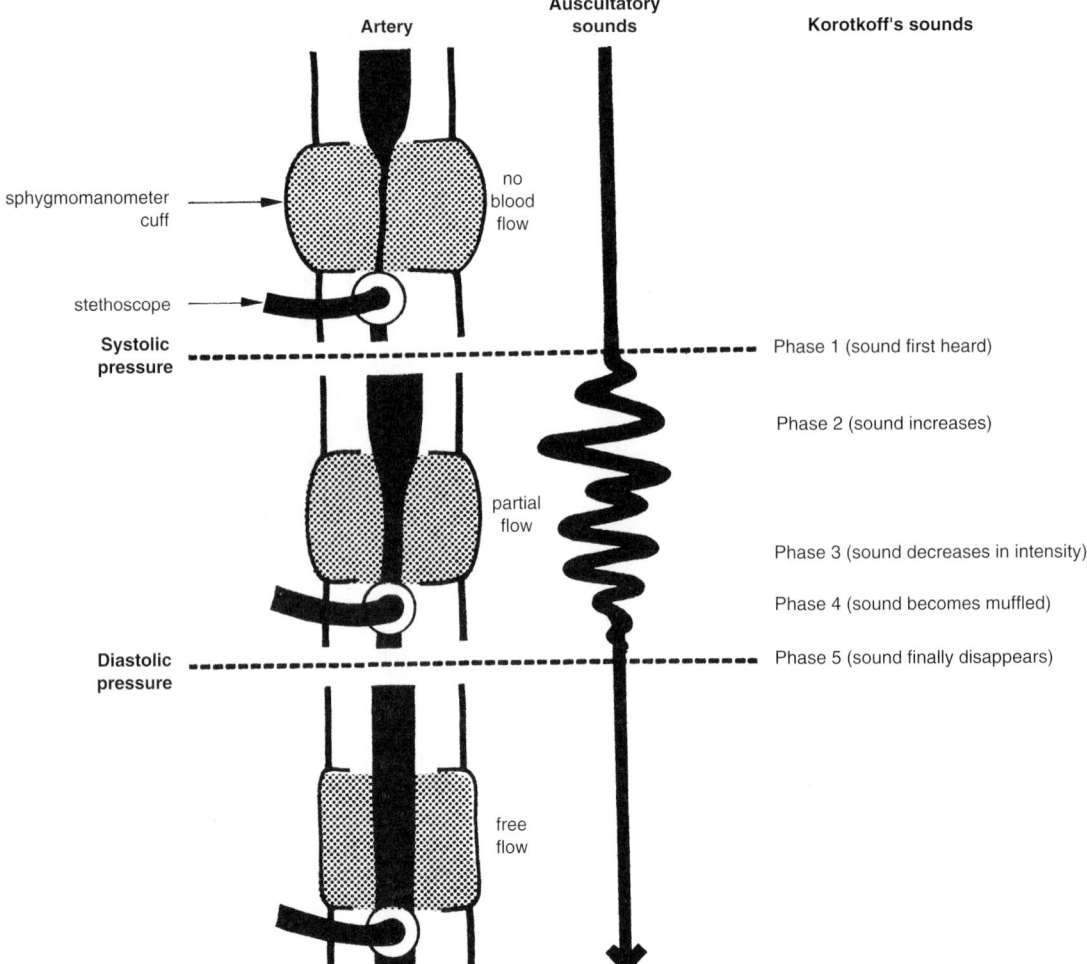

Fig 111.3 *Illustration of blood pressure measurement in relation to arterial blood flow, cuff pressure and auscultation*

Table 111.5 *Follow-up criteria for initial blood pressure measurement for adults 18 years and older[1,2]*

Range (mmHg)	Recommended follow-up*
Diastolic	
< 85	Recheck within 2 years
85–89	Recheck within 1 year
90–99	Confirm within 2 months
100–109	Evaluate or refer within 4 weeks
> 110	Evaluate or refer immediately or within 1 week
Systolic, when diastolic is < 90	
< 130	Recheck within 2 years
130–139	Recheck in 1 year
140–159	Confirm within 2 months
> 180	Evaluate or refer within 1 week

* If recommendations for follow-up of diastolic and systolic blood pressure are different the shorter recommended time for recheck and referral should take precedence.[2]

Medical history

The following should be included in the medical history of the patient:

History of hypertension

- method and date of initial diagnosis
- known duration and levels of elevated blood pressure
- symptoms that may indicate the effects of high blood pressure on target organ damage, such as headache, dyspnoea, chest pain, claudication, ankle oedema and haematuria
- symptoms suggesting secondary hypertension (Table 111.4)
- the results and side effects of all previous antihypertensive treatment

Presence of other diseases and risk factors

- a history of cardiovascular, cerebrovascular or peripheral vascular disease, renal disease, diabetes mellitus or recent weight gain
- other cardiovascular risk factors, including obesity, hyperlipidaemia, carbohydrate intolerance, smoking, salt intake, alcohol consumption, exercise levels and analgesic intake
- other relevant conditions, such as asthma or psychiatric illness (particularly depressive illness)

Family history

Particular attention should be paid to the family history of hypertension, cardiovascular or cerebrovascular disease, hyperlipidaemia, obesity, diabetes mellitus, renal disease, alcohol abuse and premature sudden death.

Medication history

A history of all medications, including over-the-counter products, should be obtained because some can raise blood pressure or interfere with antihypertensive therapy. These include:

- oral contraceptives
- hormone replacement therapy
- steroids
- non-steroidal anti-inflammatory agents (NSAIDs)
- nasal decongestants and other cold remedies
- appetite suppressants
- amphetamines
- monoamine oxidase inhibitors
- analgesics
- ergotamine
- cyclosporin
- carbenoxolone and licorice

Caffeine intake[1]

Caffeine has an acute dose-related pressor effect. People who have recently ingested significant amounts will have a blood pressure reading which is elevated above their usual level. The amount of caffeine in a cup (225 ml) in common dietary sources is as follows:

Instant coffee	90 mg
Brewed coffee	125 mg
Decaffeinated coffee	4.5mg
Tea	60 mg
Chocolate drinks (e.g. hot chocolate)	5 mg
Cola drinks	25 mg

Alcohol intake[1]

Alcohol has a direct pressor effect that is dose-related. An assessment of the average daily number of standard drinks is important—more than two standard drinks (20 g alcohol) a day is significant.

Physical examination

The approach to the physical examination is to examine possible target organ damage and possible causes of secondary hypertension. The main features to consider in the physical examination are illustrated in Figure 111.4.

The four grades of hypertensive retinopathy are illustrated in Figure 111.5.

Leg pulses and pressure

To assess the remote possibility of coarctation of the aorta in the hypertensive patient, perform at least one observation comparing:

1. the volume and timing of the radial and femoral pulses
2. the blood pressure in the arm and leg

Blood pressure measurement in the leg

- Place the patient prone.
- Use a wide, long cuff at mid-thigh level.
- Position the bladder over the posterior surface and fix it firmly.
- Auscultate over the popliteal artery.

Investigations

The following are the basic screening tests recommended for all patients:

- Urine tests
  — urinalysis (for protein and glucose)
  — micro-urine (casts, red and white cells)
  — urine culture (only if urinalysis abnormal)
- Biochemical tests
  — potassium and sodium
  — creatinine and urea
  — glucose
  — uric acid
  — cholesterol (total, HDL, LDL ratios)
- ECG

Other investigations, such as echocardiography, renal imaging studies (especially renal ultrasound), 24 hour urinary catecholamines, aldosterone and plasma renin, are not routine and should be done only if specifically indicated. A chest X-ray may serve as a base-line against

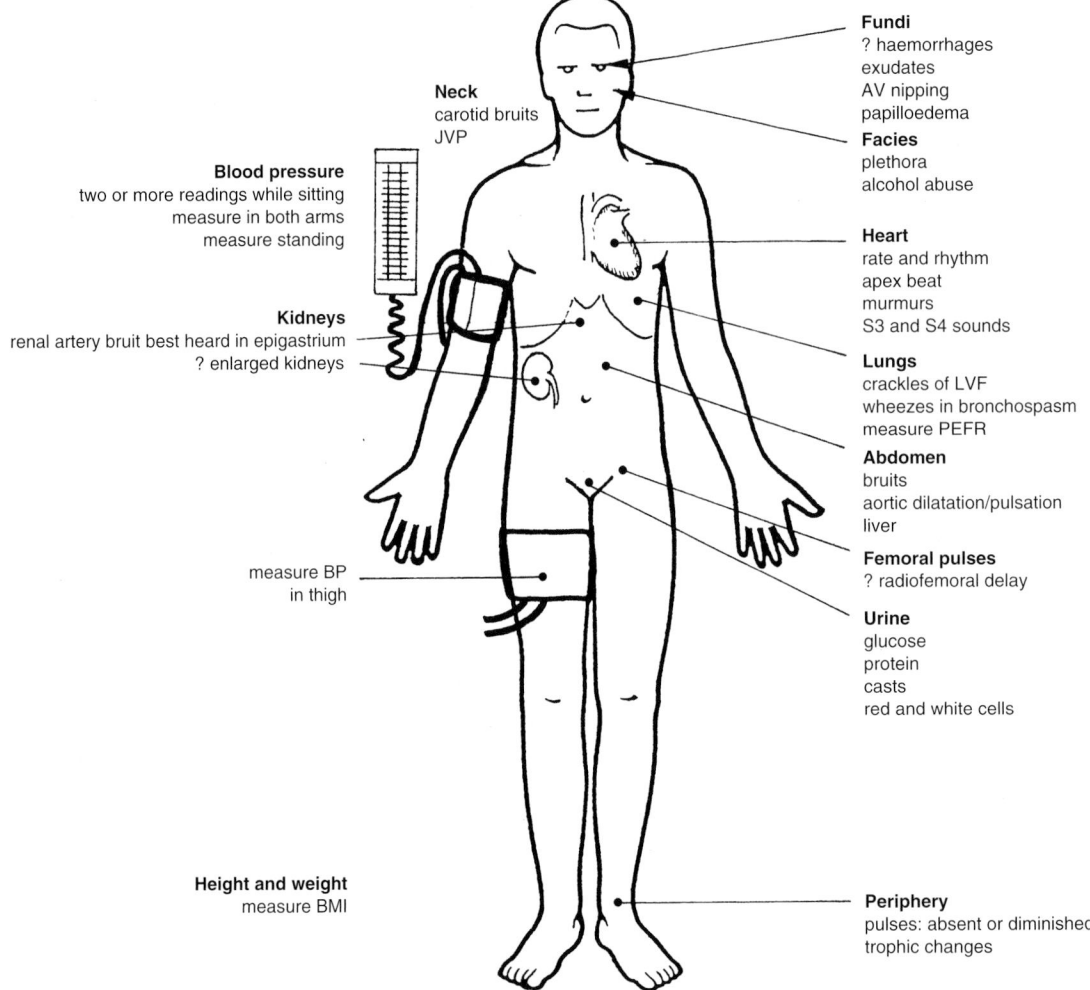

Fig 111.4 *Physical examination of patient with hypertension: what to look for*

which to measure future changes. However, if a chest X-ray shows the heart is enlarged, it is more likely to represent chamber dilatation than increased ventricular wall thickness.[1] Specific renal studies now favoured include isotope scans, doppler studies of renal arteries and renal arteriography.

Treatment

A correct diagnosis is the basis of management. Assuming that the uncommon secondary causes are identified and treated, treatment will focus on essential hypertension.

Management principles

- The overall goal is to improve the long-term survival and quality of life.
- Promote an effective physician–patient working relationship.
- Aim to reduce the levels to $^{140}\!/_{90}$ mmHg or less (ideal).
- Undertake a thorough assessment of all cardiovascular risk factors.
- Instruct all patients in the use of non-drug treatment strategies and their potential benefits.
- In patients with mild to moderate hypertension and no target organ damage, consider ambulatory or home BP monitoring.

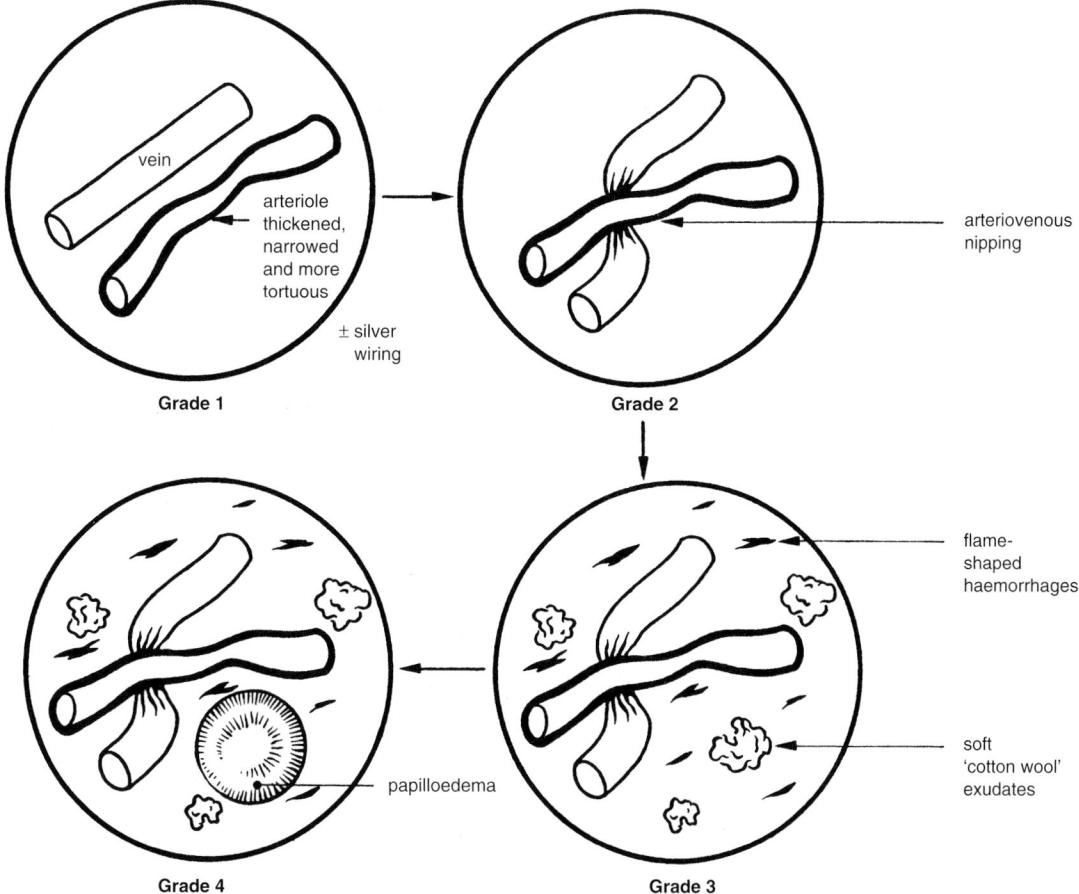

Fig 111.5 *The four grades of hypertensive retinopathy*

- Drug therapy should be given to those with:
  — sustained high initial readings
  — target organ damage
  — failed non-drug measures.
- Make a careful selection of an antihypertensive drug and an appraisal of the side effects against the benefits of treatment.
- Avoid drug-related problems such as postural hypotension.
- Avoid excessive lowering of blood pressure.
- Aim to counter the problem of patient non-compliance.
- Be aware of factors that may contribute to drug resistance.

Patient education

Patient education should include appropriate reassurances, clear information and easy-to-follow instructions. It is important to establish

patients' understanding of the concept of hypertension and its consequences by quizzing them about their knowledge and feelings.

Correction of patients' misconceptions[1]
Patients are likely to have several misconceptions about hypertension which may adversely affect their treatment.

For example, they might believe that:

- hypertension can be cured
- they do not need to continue treatment once their BP is controlled
- they do not have a problem because they do not have symptoms
- they need to take additional pills, or stop treatment in response to symptoms they believe are caused by high or low blood pressure levels
- they need not take prescribed pills if they attend to lifestyle factors such as exercise and diet

- they can gauge their blood pressure by how they feel

Tips for optimal compliance
- Establish a good caring rapport.
- Give patients a card of their history with BP readings.
- Give advice about pill-taking times.
- Set therapeutic goals.
- Establish a recall system.
- Provide patient education material.

On review:
- Ask if any pills were missed by accident.
- Attempt to reduce waiting time to a minimum, e.g. direct a patient to a spare room upon arrival.
- Review all cardiovascular risk factors.
- Enquire about any side effects.

Non-pharmacological treatment modalities

If the average diastolic BP at the initial visit is 90–100 mmHg, and there is no evidence of end-organ damage, non-pharmacological therapy is indicated for a 3 month period without use of antihypertensive drugs. Remember to remove, revise or substitute drugs which may be causing hypertension, e.g. NSAIDs, corticosteroids, oral contraceptives, hormone replacement therapy.

Behaviour intervention measures include:

- *Weight reduction*
There is considerable evidence that weight loss and gain are linked to a corresponding fall and rise in BP. Hovell has estimated that for every 1 kg of weight lost, blood pressure dropped by 2.5 mmHg systolic and 1.5 mmHg diastolic.[9] The BMI should be calculated for all patients and where required a weight loss program organised to reduce the BMI to between 20 and 25.
- *Reduction of alcohol intake*[1]
The direct pressor of alcohol is reversible. Drinking more than 20 g of alcohol a day raises blood pressure and makes treatment of established hypertension more difficult. People with hypertension should limit their alcohol intake to one or two standard drinks (10 g) per day. Reduction or withdrawal of regular alcohol intake reduces BP by 5–10 mmHg.
- *Reduction of sodium intake*
Some individuals seem to be more sensitive to salt restriction. Advise patients to put away the salt shaker and use only a little salt with their food. Reduction of sodium intake to less than 100 mmol sodium per day is advised.
- *Increased exercise*
Regular aerobic or isotonic exercise helps to reduce BP.[10] Hypertensive patients beginning an exercise program should do so gradually. Walking is an appropriate exercise. Weights and other forms of isometric exercises should be avoided because they will significantly elevate blood pressure in the hypertensive subject.
- *Reduction of particular stress*
If avoiding stress or overwork is difficult, recommend relaxation and/or meditation therapy.
- *Other dietary factors*
There is evidence that lactovegetarian diets and magnesium supplementation can reduce BP.[11,12] A diet high in calcium, and low in fat and caffeine, may also be beneficial. Avoid licorice and licorice-containing substances.
- *Smoking*
Smoking causes acute rises in blood pressure but does not appear to cause sustained hypertension. However, the elimination of smoking is important as it is a strong risk factor for cardiovascular disease and continuing to smoke may negate any benefits of antihypertensive therapy.[1]
- *Management of sleep apnoea*

Pharmacological therapy

The benefits of drug therapy appear to outweigh any known risks to individuals with a persistently raised diastolic pressure > 95 mmHg. Although the ideal antihypertensive drug has yet to be discovered there are many effective antihypertensive drugs available.[13] Deciding which one to use first involves an assessment of the patient's general health, the medication's known side effects, the simplicity of its administration and its cost. A useful plan is outlined in Figure 111.6.

Various disorders such as diabetes, asthma, chronic obstructive airways disease, Raynaud's phenomenon, heart failure, and elevated serum urate and/or lipid levels may restrict the use of some classes of drugs.

When to treat
- failed genuine non-pharmacological trial
- all SBP 140–180 or DBP 90–110

Goals of treatment
- <130/85: Adults < 65 years
Diabetes; Renal Disease
- <140/90: Adults > 65 years

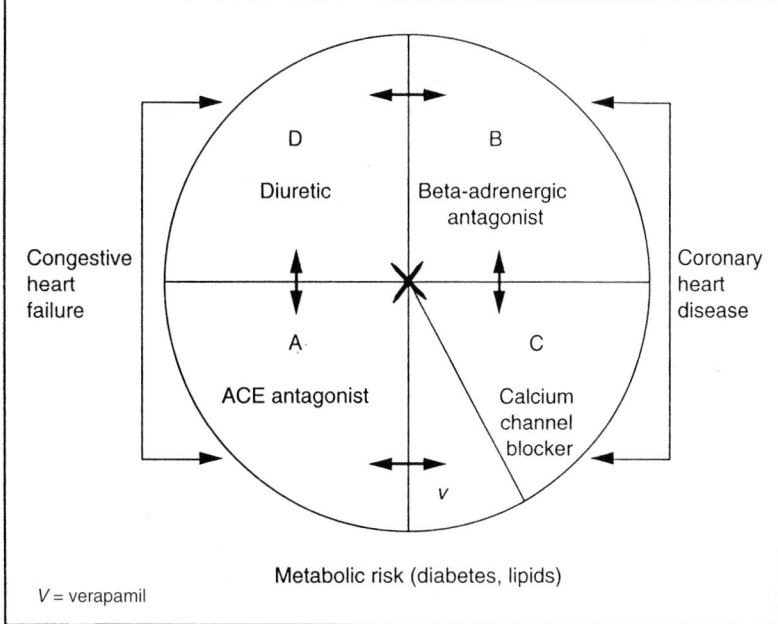

Fig 111.6 *Common combinations of the therapeutic drug classes used for first-line therapy of hypertension*

- *Adjacent drug classes are useful combinations in that effects on blood pressure are additive and adverse effects are no more likely than with either drug used alone.*
- *Verapamil (V) generally should not be used with β-antagonists.*
- *Drug groups that are diametrically located on the diagram may be used together, but may not have fully additive effects.*
- *Drugs on the left side should be combined in patients with hypertension and heart failure, and those on the right side are useful in patients with hypertension and coexisting coronary heart disease.*
- *Drug groups on the lower panel lack metabolic effects and may be preferred combinations in the presence of diabetes or lipid abnormalities as well as hypertension.*
- *Prazosin and other α-antagonists are also often used as monotherapy and may be combined with any of the above drug groups.*
- *Small doses of centrally acting anti-adrenergic drugs (e.g. methyldopa, clonidine) can probably also be used with any of the other agents although data on their use in combination are scarce with the newer drug groups.*

ADAPTED FROM MANAGEMENT OF HYPERTENSION: A CONSENSUS STATEMENT, MED J AUST, 1994, 160: SUPPLEMENT 21 MARCH. © COPYRIGHT 1994. *THE MEDICAL JOURNAL OF AUSTRALIA.* REPRODUCED WITH PERMISSION

Guidelines

- Start with a single drug.
- A period of 4–6 weeks is needed for the effect to become fully apparent.
- If ineffective, consider increasing the drug to its maximum recommended dose, or add an agent from another compatible class, or substitute with a drug from another class.
- Use only one drug from any one class at the same time.
- A summary of first-line therapy options and the uses of the various pharmacological agents is shown in Table 111.6.
- Measure the BP at the same time each day.
- A good strategy is to get patients to self-measure.

Starting regimens

The traditional method has been to use stepwise therapy until ideal control has been reached, commencing with:

1. thiazide or thiazide-like diuretic or β-blocker (cardioselective)
2. combination of diuretic and β-blocker
3. add a vasodilator

However, the newer classes of drugs can be used as first-line agents.

The following are useful combinations:[1,5]

Initial agent	Additional drugs
diuretic	β-blocker
	ACE inhibitor
	or
	α-blocker

Table 111.6 *First-line pharmacological options for the management of hypertension[7]*

Drug class					
Diuretic	*Beta-blocker*	*Calcium channel antagonist*	*ACE inhibitor*	*Central-acting agent*	*Alpha-blocker*
Typical examples and starting dose (oral therapy)					
chlorothiazide 250 mg daily	atenolol 25–50 mg daily	verapamil SR 160 mg daily	captopril 6.25 mg bd	methyldopa 125 mg bd	prazosin 0.5 mg nocte
hydrochloro-thiazide 12.5 mg daily	metoprolol 50 mg daily	felodipine SR 2.5 mg daily	enalapril 5 mg daily	clonidine 50 μg, bd	terazosin 0.5 mg nocte
	pindolol 5 mg daily	amlodipine 2.5 mg daily	lisinopril 5 mg daily		
indapamide 2.5 mg daily	propranolol 40 mg daily	nifedipine 10 mg bd	ramipril 2.5 mg daily		*Note*: labetalol (100 mg bd) is a combined α and β blocker
		diltiazem 180 mg daily	perindopril 2 mg daily		
			Angiotensin II receptor antagonist		
			losarten 50 mg daily		
			irbesartan 150 mg daily		
Recommended in					
Heart failure (mild) Older patients	Anxious patient Young patients Angina Postmyocardial infarction Migraine	Asthma Angina PVD Raynaud's phenomenon	Heart failure PVD Diabetes Raynaud's	Asthma Pregnancy	Asthma PVD Heart failure LUTS (prostatism)
Contraindications					
Maturity onset diabetics Hyperuricaemia	Asthma COAD History of wheeze Heart failure Heart block (2°,3°) PVD Brittle IDDM	Heart block 2nd & 3rd degree (verapamil, diltiazem)	Bilateral renal artery stenosis	Liver disease (methyldopa)	Heart failure (mechanical obstruction)
Precautions					
Hypokalaemia Thiazides + ACE inhibitors Renal failure	Avoid abrupt cessation with angina Use with verapamil Use with NSAIDs Use in smokers	With β-blockers and digoxin CCF	Chronic renal disease Avoid K sparing diuretics and NSAIDs	Depression	Elderly patients
Important side effects					
Rashes Sexual dysfunction Weakness Blood dyscrasias Muscular cramps Hypokalaemia Hyponatraemia Hyperuricaemia Hyperglycaemia Lipid metabol-ism effect	Fatigue Insomnia Vivid dreams Bronchospasm Cold extremities Sexual dysfunction Lipid metabolism effect	Headache Flushing Ankle oedema Palpitations Dizziness Nausea Constipation (verapamil) Nocturia, urinary frequency	Cough Weakness Rash Dysgeusia (taste) Hyperkalaemia First dose hypotension Angioedema	Sedation Dry mouth Bowel disturbances Fatigue Orthostatic hypotension Sexual dysfunction Haemolytic anaemia (methyldopa)	First dose syncope Orthostatic hypotension Weakness Palpitations Sedation Headache

β-blocker	Diuretic
	Calcium antagonist
	(except verapamil and
	diltiazem)
α-blocker	Diuretic
	β-blocker
ACE inhibitor	Diuretic
	Calcium antagonist
Calcium	β-blocker
antagonist	ACE inhibitor
Diuretic	Central acting agent
	ACE inhibitor
Author's	
preference	
Diuretic	ACE inhibitor
	or
	β-blocker

Relatively ineffective combinations[1]
Diuretic and calcium antagonist
Beta-blockers and ACE inhibitors

Undesirable combinations[1]
More than one drug from a particular pharmacological group: beta-blockers and verapamil (heart block, heart failure); potassium-sparing diuretics and ACE inhibitors (hyperkalaemia).

Diuretics[1,5]
- Thiazides are good first-line therapy for hypertension.
- Hypokalaemia can be corrected with potassium-sparing diuretics or changing to another first-line drug.
- Loop diuretics are less potent as antihypertensive agents but are indicated where there is concomitant cardiac or renal failure and in resistant hypertension.
- Thiazides are less effective where there is renal impairment.
- Thiazides may precipitate acute gout.
- NSAIDs may antagonise the antihypertensive and natriuretic effectiveness of diuretics.
- A diet high in potassium and magnesium should accompany diuretic therapy, e.g. lentils, nuts, high fibre.
- Avoid use if significant dyslipidaemia.
- Indapamide has different properties to the thiazide and loop diuretics and has less effect on serum lipids.

Beta-blockers
- NSAIDs may interfere with the hypotensive effect of beta-blockers.

- If blood pressure is not reduced by one beta-blocker it is unlikely to be reduced by changing to another.
- Verapamil plus a beta-blocker may unmask conduction abnormalities causing heart block.
- In patients with ischaemic heart disease, or susceptibility to it, treatment must not be stopped suddenly—this can precipitate angina at rest.

Calcium antagonists
- These drugs reduce blood pressure by vasodilatation.
- The properties of individual drugs vary, especially their effects on cardiac function.
- The dihydropyridine compounds (nifedipine and felodipine) tend to produce more vasodilatation and thus related side effects.
- Unlike verapamil or diltiazem (which slow the heart), dihydropyridine drugs can be used safely with a beta-blocker.
- Verapamil is contraindicated in second and third degree heart block.
- Verapamil and diltiazem should be used with caution in patients with heart failure.
- These drugs are efficacious with ACE inhibitors, beta-blockers, prazosin and methyldopa.

ACE inhibitors
Angiotensin-converting enzyme is responsible for converting angiotensin I to angiotensin II (a potent vasoconstrictor and stimulator of aldosterone secretion) and for the breakdown of bradykinin (a vasodilator). ACE inhibitors are effective in the elderly; improve survival and performance status in cardiac failure; are protective of renal function in diabetes; and cardioprotective in postmyocardial infarction. For patients with normal renal function, the dose should not exceed 150 mg daily for captopril, 40 mg daily for enalapril or lisinopril, 10 mg daily for ramipril, and 8 mg daily for perindopril.

Disturbance in taste is usually transitory and may resolve with continued treatment. Cough, which occurs in about 15% of patients, may disappear with time or a reduction in dose but it often persists and requires a change in drug in some patients. Angioedema, a potentially life-threatening condition, may occur in 0.1–0.2% of subjects. Like cough, it is a class effect and will mitigate against use of any ACE inhibitor.

Angiotensin II receptor antagonists

Irbesartan and losarten are not ACE inhibitors but are angiotensin II receptor blocking drugs used for mild to moderate hypertension alone or with other antihypertensive agents. Cough does not appear to be a significant adverse effect; otherwise, the adverse effects are similar to ACE inhibitors.

Prazosin

A specific problem is the 'first dose phenomenon'; this involves acute syncope about 90 minutes after the first dose, hence treatment is best initiated at bedtime. Prazosin potentiates beta-blockers and works best if used with them. It is a useful first-line therapy in patients who are unsuitable for diuretic or beta-blocker therapy, e.g. those with diabetes, asthma or hyperlipidaemia.

Vascular smooth muscle relaxants

(other than calcium channel antagonists)

These include hydralazine, minoxidil and diazoxide, which are not used for first-line therapy but for refractory hypertensive states and hypertensive emergencies.

Mild hypertension[1]

Mild hypertension in adults is defined as a diastolic pressure (Phase 5) persistently between 90 and 99 mmHg, without target organ damage.[14] This group includes those with 'white coat' hypertension.

Mildly hypertensive people have almost twice the risk of vascular disease compared with normotensive people, and evidence shows that morbidity and mortality rise with an increase in blood pressure.[1] The long-term risk in patients with 'white coat' hypertension has yet to be defined.

Patients treated appropriately have fewer strokes and pressure-related cardiovascular complications than those not treated. Drug treatment has potential side effects which cannot be ignored; sometimes the risks from this form of treatment could exceed those if the patient remains untreated.[14] Therefore, the initial approach to the management of mild hypertension should be based on non-drug measures and should focus on behaviour change. In this way, overt side effects are avoided and risk prevention measures enhanced.

Often the success of this approach is improved by using people with particular skills, such as

dietitians. If after 6 months or more these methods have not succeeded, then drug therapy may be necessary.[14]

Practical guidelines for patients with persistent diastolic blood pressure between 90 and 99 mmHg are shown in Figure 111.7.

Moderate hypertension[1]

If diastolic pressure is 100–109 mmHg then a more aggressive approach is necessary, particularly for patients with target organ damage. Appropriate non-pharmacological measures should be tried in all subjects, especially where success is possible, e.g. obesity, high alcohol intake. This will fail in the majority, who will require drug therapy. If there is poor response to initial therapy a second drug may be prescribed after a short time. The interval between the changes in treatment may also be reduced. Combination therapy may be more effective than maximum doses of any single agent.

Severe hypertension[5]

The blood pressure of those with severe hypertension may be life-threatening. Patients with an average diastolic ﹒ pressure of more than 110 mmHg should be checked immediately for hypertensive complications, particularly marked fundoscopic changes, proteinuria or cardiac failure. They are more likely to have an underlying cause, e.g. renovascular disease. Hospitalisation may be necessary for these patients.

In such cases the opinion of a specialist is important, because of the likely risk of serious illness or death. A dihydropyridine calcium channel blocker (e.g. nifedipine, amlodipine, felodipine) with early addition of a beta-blocker or ACE inhibitor is suitable for urgent lowering of blood pressure.

Hypertensive emergencies

A hypertensive emergency occurs when high blood pressure causes the presenting cardiovascular problem. Typical presentations of hypertensive emergencies (which are rare) include hypertensive encephalopathy, acute stroke, heart failure, dissecting aortic aneurysm and eclampsia.

In all such cases referral to a specialist is essential and the patient should be hospitalised

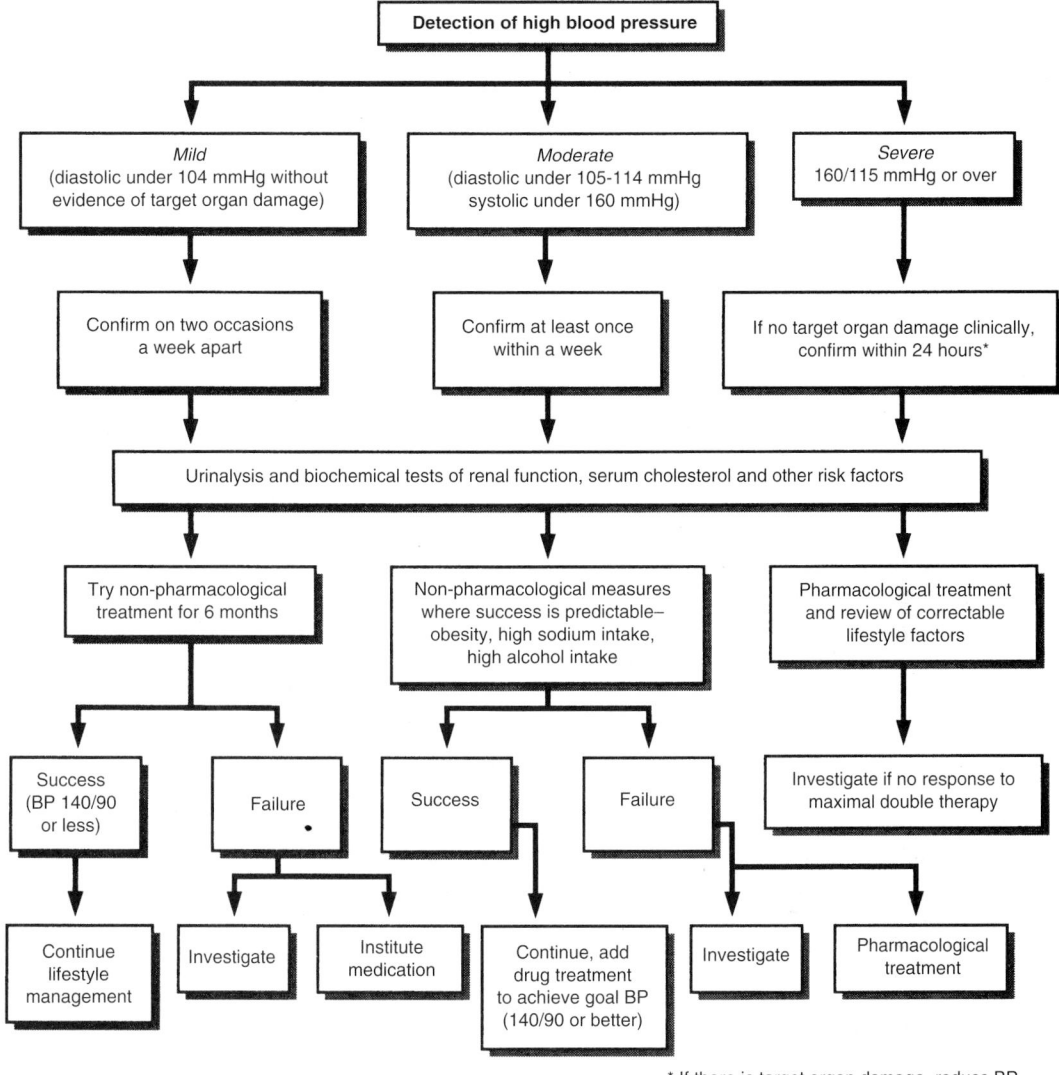

Fig 111.7 *Decision tree for managing hypertension* AS RECOMMENDED BY THE NATIONAL HEART FOUNDATION

immediately for monitoring and treatment. Treatment must be individualised, mindful of the nature of the underlying problem and associated disorders.

Such treatment is the same as for severe hypertension. Otherwise, sodium nitroprusside IV in an intensive care setting is the optimal treatment.

Isolated systolic hypertension[1]

Isolated systolic hypertension is most frequently seen in elderly people.

Definition: systolic BP $\geq$ 140 mmHg with a DBP < 90 mmHg

Patients with isolated systolic hypertension should be treated in the same way as those with classic systolic/diastolic hypertension. Evidence that reducing isolated systolic blood pressure decreases the mortality and morbidity risk has been demonstrated by the SHEP (systolic hypertension in the elderly) study.[16]

Non-pharmacological therapy should be commenced as is relevant to the patient. If drugs are used the SBP should be cautiously lowered to between 140 and 160 mmHg. The drugs of choice are diuretics, calcium channel-blocking agents and ACE inhibitors.

Refractory hypertension

Refractory hypertension exists where control has not been achieved despite reasonable treatment for 3–4 months. A review of a possible secondary cause is appropriate.

Checklist of possible reasons[1]

- drug-related causes: doses too low; inappropriate combinations; effects of other drugs, e.g. antidepressants, adrenal steroids, NSAIDs, sympathomimetics, nasal decongestants, ergotamine, oral contraceptives, psychotropics
- poor compliance with therapy
- renovascular hypertension
- nicotine; licorice; caffeine (strong coffee)
- obesity
- excessive alcohol intake
- excessive salt intake
- renal insufficiency and other undiagnosed causes of secondary hypertension
- illicit substances, e.g. amphetamines, cocaine, anabolic steroids

When adequate control is not possible and the cause is not obvious, the patient should be referred to a specialist. Measurement outside the clinic may help in the assessment of such people, as may 24 hour ambulatory monitoring.

Hypertension in children and adolescents

The recording of blood pressure should be part of the normal examination in children and used in their continuing care. Blood pressure should be measured in all children who are unwell. Blood pressure is less frequently measured in children for a number of reasons, such as the unavailability of an appropriately sized cuff or difficulty in measuring BP in the infant or toddler.

The children of parents with hypertension should be closely watched. Those at risk of secondary hypertension, e.g. renal or cardiovascular disease, urological abnormalities and diabetes mellitus, should have routine measurements. Those children with visual changes, headache or recurrent abdominal pain or seizures, and those

on drugs such as corticosteroids or the pill, should have their blood pressure checked regularly.

Although secondary causes of hypertension are more common in children than in adults, young people are still more prone to developing essential rather than secondary hypertension. Renal parenchymal disease and renal artery stenosis are the major secondary causes.

The upper limits of normal BP for children in different age groups are:[1]

Age (in years)	Arterial pressure (mmHg)
14–18	135/90
10–13	125/85
6–9	120/80
5 or less	110/75

The proper cuff size is very important to avoid inaccurate readings and a larger rather than a smaller cuff is recommended. The width of the bladder should cover 75% of the upper arm. In infants and toddlers use of an electronic unit may be necessary. Although cessation of sound (Phase 5) is the better reflection of true diastolic pressure, there is often no disappearance of sound in children and so estimation of the point of muffling has to be recorded.

Diagnostic evaluation and drug treatment for children are similar to those for adults. When a child is obese, reduction in weight may adequately lower BP. ACE inhibitors or calcium channel-blocking agents are preferable in the young hypertensive, with diuretics a second agent. ACE inhibitors should be avoided in postpubertal girls.

Hypertension in the elderly

Blood pressure shows a gradual increasing linear relationship with age.

Guidelines for treatment

- Isolated systolic hypertension is worth treating.[16]
- Older patients may respond to non-pharmacological treatment.
- Reducing dietary sodium is more beneficial than with younger patients.
- If drug treatment is necessary, commence with half the normal recommended adult dosage. 'Start low and go slow.'
- Patients over 70 and in good health should be treated the same as younger patients.

- A gradual reduction in blood pressure is recommended.
- Drug reactions are a limiting factor.
- Drug interactions are also a problem: these include NSAIDs, antiParkinson drugs and phenothiazines.

Specific treatment

1st line choice: indapamide (preferred) or thiazide diuretic (low dose)[1]; check electrolytes in 2–4 weeks: if hypokalaemia develops add a K-sparing diuretic rather than K supplements. Use a combination thiazide and K-sparing diuretic. Diuretics may aggravate bladder difficulties, e.g. incontinence.

2nd line choice: beta-blockers (low dose) where diuretic cannot be prescribed or if angina.

Other effective drugs (especially for isolated systolic hypertension):
- ACE inhibitors (especially with heart failure)
- calcium channel antagonists

Both these groups are generally well tolerated but constipation may be a problem with verapamil.

Renal function and electrolytes should be monitored when ACE inhibitors are started.

Special management problems

These conditions are summarised in Table 111.7.

Diabetes mellitus

Factors contributing to hypertension may be the same in Type II (NIDDM) diabetes and non-diabetic hypertensive patients. In both Type I and Type II diabetes, nephropathy can be a significant contributor. The monitoring of patients for early signs of nephropathy with measurements of microalbumin excretion is helpful. Microalbuminuria can also be detected in non-diabetic hypertensives where it appears to be a marker of cardiovascular disease. Diabetic autonomic neuropathy can cause orthostatic hypotension. Diabetics with persistent or sustained DBP > 90 mmHg and proteinuria need treatment. The threshold for treatment of hypertension in the diabetic is lower than in the non-diabetic. Control of hypertension is an important factor in limiting progression of diabetic renal disease.

Treatment

- Use basic non-pharmacological treatments, especially weight reduction, if applicable.
- ACE inhibitors and calcium channel blockers are useful first-line drugs because they do not affect insulin and diabetes control.
- Other suitable drugs are prazosin, hydralazine and methyldopa.
- Diuretics added to an ACE inhibitor are effective but caution is required because they can aggravate glucose intolerance.
- Proteinuria and renal function need to be monitored.

Pregnancy

Hypertension in pregnancy can be either pre-eclampsia (pregnancy-induced hypertension) or essential hypertension. Blood pressure levels normally drop during the second trimester and rise in the third. A DBP > 80 mmHg in late pregnancy is considered unacceptable. Preferred drugs to use are methydopa, labetalol and beta blockers. Diuretics and ACE inhibitors should not be used. Hypertensive pregnant women should be supervised in association with a specialist unit.

Surgical patients

Patients whose BP is under control before surgery should continue the same treatment. If oral medication is affected by the surgery, parenteral treatment may be needed to avoid rebound hypertension. This is a particular problem with clonidine and possibly methyldopa. Withdrawal of other drugs, such as beta-blockers, may have adverse consequences.

Renal disease

Renal function is not adversely affected by the treatment of severe or malignant hypertension. Use a loop diuretic, e.g. frusemide, initially. Beta-blockers, calcium antagonists, prazosin and methyldopa can be used, while caution is needed with ACE inhibitors, particularly if there is underlying renovascular disease.

Heart failure

First-line treatment for associated hypertension includes ACE inhibitors and diuretics. Other suitable drugs are a hydralazine-nitrate combination and methyldopa. Calcium antagonists should be used with care and verapamil and beta-blockers should be avoided.

Ischaemic heart disease

Recommended drugs are beta-blockers and calcium antagonists.[7] The non-dihydropyridine agents should be used with care with a beta-blocker but the dihydropyridine agents are quite safe.

Obstructive airways disease

Apart from beta-blockers, all other routine antihypertensives can be used.

Impotence

It is prudent to avoid antihypertensives that are possibly associated with impotence, e.g. thiazide diuretics, methyldopa, resperine and beta-blockers. Suitable agents to use are ACE inhibitors and calcium blockers.

Can hypertension be overtreated?[17]

Yes. Excessive blood pressure reduction, particularly if acute, can seriously compromise perfusion in vital organs, especially if blood flow is already impaired by vascular disease. Careful monitoring of the patient, including standing BP measurement, is important.

One should avoid excessive blood pressure reduction in the setting of acute stroke, where there is a tight carotid artery stenosis (particularly if symptomatic) and in the elderly subject (especially if there is postural hypotension).

It has been suggested that lowering DBP < 85 mmHg in particular subgroups (e.g. those with ischaemic heart disease) may raise the cardiovascular risk above that associated with a lesser reduction in blood pressure.[18] However, the relationship between cardiovascular risk and blood pressure is a continuous one. Moreover, the SHEP Study did not show any adverse effects of lowering DBP in patients with pre-existing coronary heart disease. The safety of lowering DBP to levels below 85 mmHg has been demonstrated in the Hypertension Optimal Treatment (HOT) Study.[19]

Step-down treatment of mild hypertension[17]

This is an important concept that recognises that drug treatment need not necessarily be lifelong. If blood pressure has been well controlled for several months to years it is often worth reducing the dosage or the number of drugs.

A 'drug holiday' (cessation of treatment) can be hazardous, however, because satisfactory control is usually temporary and hypertension will re-emerge. Careful monitoring under such circumstances is mandatory.

When to refer[5]

- Refractory hypertension—adequate control not possible and cause not obvious.
- Suspected 'white coat' hypertension—for ambulatory blood pressure monitoring.

Table 111.7 *Choice of drugs in patients with coexisting conditions*

	Diuretic	ACE inhibitors	Calcium antagonists	β-blockers
Asthma/COAD	✓	✓	✓	✗
Bowel disease/constipation	✗	✓	✗	✓
Bradycardia/heart block	✓	✓	care	✗
Cardiac failure	✓*	✓*	care	✗
Depression	✓	✓	✓	✗
Diabetes	✗	✓*	✓	✗
Dyslipidaemia	✗	✓	✓	✗
Hyperuricaemia/gout	✗	✓*	✓*	✗
Impotence	✗	✓	✓	✗
Ischaemic heart disease	✓	✓	✓*	✓*
Peripheral vascular disease	✓	✓	✓*	✗
Pregnancy	✗	✗	✓	✓
Raynaud's phenomenon	✓	✓	✓*	✗
Renal artery stenosis	✓	✗*	✓*	✓*
Renal failure	✓	care	✓	✓
Tachycardia (resting)	✗	✗	care	✓*

* drug/s of choice. Calcium antagonists need to be selected with care—some are suitable, others not

- Severe hypertension—diastolic BP > 115 mmHg.
- Hypertensive emergency.
- If there is evidence of ongoing target organ impairment.
- If there is significant renal impairment (serum creatinine > 0.1 mmol/L).
- If a treatable cause of secondary hypertension is found.

Practice tips

- Hypertension should not be diagnosed on a single reading.
- At least two follow-up measurements with average systolic pressure > 140 mmHg or diastolic pressures > 90 mmHg are required for the diagnosis.
- Beware of using beta-blockers in a patient with a history of wheezing.
- Add only one agent at a time and wait about 4 weeks between dosage adjustments.
- Excessive intake of alcohol can cause hypertension and hypertension refractory to treatment.
- If hypertension fails to respond to therapy, an underlying renal or adrenal lesion may have been missed.
- The low-pitched bruits of renal artery stenosis are best heard by placing the diaphragm of the stethoscope firmly in the epigastric area.
- Older patients may respond better to diuretics, calcium antagonists and ACE inhibitors.
- Younger patients may respond better to beta-blockers or ACE inhibitors.

References

1. Hypertension Guideline Committee, 1991 report. *Hypertension: diagnosis, treatment and maintenance.* Adelaide: Research Unit RACGP (South Australian Faculty), 1991.
2. The 1988 Report of the Joint National Committee on Detection, Evaluation and Treatment of High Blood Pressure. National High Blood Pressure Education Program. Bethesda, Maryland: National Heart, Lung and Blood Institute, National Institute of Health, May 1988. NIH Publication No. 88–1088.
3. Sloane PD, Slatt PD, Baker RM. *Essentials of family medicine.* Baltimore: Williams and Wilkins, 1988, 149–153.
4. Sandler G. High blood pressure. In: *Common medical problems.* London: Adis Press, 1984, 61–106.
5. Stokes G. Essential hypertension. In: MIMS Disease Index. Sydney: IMS Publishing, 1991–92, 265–271.
6. Fraser A. Measurement of blood pressure. Aust Fam Physician, 1989; 18:355–359.
7. *ABC of hpertension.* London: British Medical Association. 1989, 1–50.
8. Bates B. *A guide to physical examination and history taking* (5th edn). Philadelphia: Lippincott, 1991, 284.
9. Hovell MF. The experimental evidence for weight loss treatment of essential hypertension. A critical review. Am J Public Health, April 1982; 72(4):359–368.
10. Blair SN, Goodyear NN, Gibbons LW, Cooper KH. Physical fitness and incidence of hypertension in healthy normotensive men and women. JAMA, 1984; 252(4):487–490.
11. Rouse IL, Beilin LJ. Vegetarian diet and blood pressure. Editorial review. J Hypertension, 1984; 2:231–240.
12. Kestlefoot H. Urinary cations and blood pressure—population studies. Ann Clin Research, 1984; 16 Supp (43):72–80.
13. Jennings G, Sudhir K. Initial therapy of primary hypertension. Med J Aust, 1990; 152:198–202.
14. Guidelines for the treatment of mild hypertension. Memorandum from a WHO/ISH meeting. Endorsed by Participants at the Fourth Mild Hypertension Conference. Bulletin of the World Health Organisation, 1986; 64(1):31–35.
15. Mashford ML (Chairman). *Cardiovascular drug guidelines* (2nd edn). Melbourne: Victorian Medical Postgraduate Foundation, 1995–96, 59–68.
16. SHEP Co-operative research group. Prevention of stroke by antihypertensive drug treatment in older persons with isolated systolic hypertension. J Amer Med Assn, 1991; 265:3255–3264.
17. Vandongen R. Drug treatment of hypertension. Aust Fam Physician, 1989; 18:345–348.
18. Cruickshank JM, Thorp JM, Zacharias FJ. Benefits and potential harm of lowering high blood pressure. Lancet, 1987; 1:581–584.
19. The HOT study group. The Hypertension Optimal Treatment Study. Blood Pressure, 1993; 2:6.

112

Dyslipidaemia

The landmark Scandinavian Simvastatin Survival Study (4S) published in 1994, may well be remembered as the study that finally put to rest many of the apprehensions and misconceptions regarding lipid-lowering therapy.

Duffy and Meredith 1996[1]

Dyslipidaemia is the presence of an abnormal lipid/lipoprotein profile in the serum and can be classified as:

- predominant hyperglyceridaemia
- predominant hypercholesterolaemia
- mixed pattern with elevation of both cholesterol and triglyceride (TG)

Modern epidemiological studies have established the facts that elevated plasma cholesterol causes pathological changes in the arterial wall leading to coronary artery disease (CAD), and that lipid-lowering therapy results in reduction of coronary and cerebrovascular events with improved survival.

These studies which can be summarised by their acronyms—4S,[2] PLAC I,[3] PLAC II,[4] ACAPS,[5] KAPS,[6] REGRESS[7] and WOSCOPS[8]—all reinforce the benefits of lipid-lowering therapy for dyslipidaemia and the primary prevention of coronary heart disease.

Established facts[9,10,11]

- Major risk factors for CAD include:
  — increased LDL cholesterol + reduced HDL cholesterol
  — ratio LDLC/HDLC > 4
- Risk increases with increasing cholesterol levels (90% if > 7.8 mmol/L)

- Levels TG > 10 mmol/L increases risk of pancreatitis
- Management should be correlated with risk factors
- 10% reduction of total cholesterol gives 20% reduction in CAD after 3 years

Investigations[9]

The following fasting tests are recommended in all adult patients 18 years and over:
- serum triglyceride
- serum cholesterol and HDLC & LDLC if ≥ 5.5 mmol/L
- TFTs if overweight elderly female

Confirm an initial high result with a second test at 6–8 weeks. Patients requiring treatment are summarised in Table 112.1. Testing should occur at least every 5 years.

Appropriate treatment goals[11]

- Total cholesterol < 5.0 mmol/L
- LDLC < 3.5 mmol/L
- HDLC > 1.0 mmol/L
- triglycerides < 2.0 mmol/L (4.0 for category V)

Treat all risk factors.

Non-pharmacological measures

- Dietary measures
  — keep to ideal weight
  — reduce fat intake, esp. dairy products and meat
  — avoid 'fast' foods and deep fried foods
  — replace saturated fats with mono or polyunsaturated fats
  — limit high-cholesterol foods, e.g. egg yolk, offal, fish roe

Table 112.1 *Patients requiring treatment (National Heart Foundation)*

Risk category		Initiate drug therapy if lipid level (mmol/L) is	Target
1.	Highest risk Existing CHD or other vascular diseases	TC > 5.0 or LDLC > 3.0 or TG > 2.0	< 4.5 < 2.5 < 2.0
2.	High risk (one or more of) • diabetes • positive family history CHD • hypertension • smoking • familial hypercholesterolaemia • HDLC < 1.0	TC > 6.0 or LDLC > 4.0 or TG > 4.0	< 5.0 < 3.0 < 2.0
3.	Lower risk (others)	TC > 7.0 or LDLC > 5.0 or TG > 8.0	< 6.0 < 4.0 < 4.0

— always trim fat off meat, remove skin from chicken
— avoid biscuits and cakes between meals
— eat fish at least twice a week
— high-fibre diet, esp. fruit and vegetables
— increase complex carbohydrates
— alcohol intake 0–2 standard drinks/day
— drink more water
• Regular exercise
• Cessation of smoking
• Co-operation of family is essential
• Exclude secondary causes, e.g. hypothyroidism, obesity, alcohol excess (especially ↑ TG), specific diuretics

Checkpoints
• diet therapy effective (TG↓, LDLC↓) within 6–8 weeks
• continue at least 6 months before considering drug therapy in all but the highest-risk category

Pharmacological measures

The choice of the lipid-lowering agent depends on the pattern of the lipid disorder.[10,11] See Table 112.2. Use the following agents in addition to diet.

Moderate LDLC elevation
Choose one of the following:

First-line agents
1. Bile acid sequestrating resins
   • e.g. cholestyramine 4 g daily in fruit juice increasing to maximum tolerated dose
   • adverse effects: GIT side effects, e.g. constipation, offensive wind

2. HMG-CoA reductase inhibitors ('statins')
   • e.g. atorvastatin 10 mg (o) nocte, increase to max. 40 mg/day
       or
     cervistatin 0.2 mg (o) nocte, increase to 0.3 mg
       or
     fluvastatin 20 mg (o) nocte, increase to max. 80 mg/day
       or
     simvastatin 10 mg (o) nocte, increase to max. 40 mg/day
       or
     pravastatin 10 mg (o) nocte, increase to max. 40 mg/day
   • adverse effects: GIT side effects, myalgia, abnormal liver function
   • monitor: measure LFTs (ALT and CPK) and CK as base-line
       repeat LFTs after 4–8 weeks, then every 6 weeks for 6 months

Second-line agents
3. Nicotinic acid
   • nicotinic acid 250 mg (o) with food daily, increase to max. 500 mg tds
   • adverse effects: flushing, gastric irritation, gout
   • minimise side effects with gradual introduction; take with food and aspirin cover
4. Probucol
   • probucol 500 mg (o) bd
   • problems: slow response, care with hepatic disease

Table 112.2 *Lipid-lowering drugs*

Drug	Dose	Usage	Adverse effects	Safety monitoring
The statins	**Night dose**			
Atorvastatin				
Pravastatin	10–40 mg	↑ cholesterol		
Simvastatin				
Fluvastatin	20–80 mg		muscle pains;	creatine kinase
Cervistatin	0.2–0.3 mg		raised liver enzymes	liver enzymes
Resins				
Cholestyramine	8g bd	↑ cholesterol	GIT dysfunction;	
Colestipol	10g bd		drug interactions	
Gemfibrozil	600 mg bd	↑ triglycerides	GIT dysfunction; myositis; interaction with statins and warfarin	liver enzymes coagulation
Nicotinic acid	100 mg tds to 500 mg tds	↑ cholesterol and triglycerides	flushing; raised glucose, urate and liver enzymes	glucose urate liver enzymes
Probucol	500 mg bd	↑ cholesterol	GIT dysfunction; arrhythmias	liver enzymes ECG
Fish oils n-3 fatty acids	2 g daily	↑ triglycerides	minimal	bleeding time

5. Oestrogen[11]
   • oestradiol valerate 2 mg (o) mane
     ± medroxyprogesterone acetate
   This hormone replacement therapy can reduce LDLC and is a physiological intervention in postmenopausal females, especially after hysterectomy. It has limited efficacy.

Severe LDLC elevation
Combined 'statin' and resin
    cholesteramine 4–8 g (o) mane
            plus
  a 'statin' (p. 1091)

Moderate to severe (isolated) TG elevation
    gemfibrozil 600 mg (o) bd

Note: Slow response; monitor LFTs; predisposes to gallstones and myopathy.

Alternatives
    nicotinic acid
            or
    n-3 fish oil concentrate 6 g (o) daily in divided doses to max. 15 g/day

Note: Reduction in alcohol intake is essential.

Mixed hyperlipidaemia (↑ TG + ↑ LDLC)
    If TG < 4: a 'statin'
    If TG > 4: gemfibrozil
Consider combination therapy,

e.g. fish oil + 'statin'
    gemfibrozil + resin

Note: Statin + gemfibrozil increases risk of myopathy and requires specialised supervision.

Special considerations
The decision to commence drug therapy should be based on at least two separate measurements at an accredited laboratory.

Be careful with β-blockers and diuretics affecting lipid levels.

Length of treatment
Possibly lifelong (up to 75 years)

Follow-up investigations
• serum lipids
• LFTs (ALT and CPK)
• possibly creatinine kinase

Special groups
Children
In general there is little justification for using lipid-regulating drugs in children, especially as the drugs have been shown to reduce heart disease within 2–5 years in adults.[10] Initial dietary

advice and avoidance of smoking is recommended. Bile acid sequestrating resins are safe to use.

The elderly[10]

The role of lipid therapy remains unclear. Generally, elderly patients with established CHD should receive standard lipid management unless their general medical status is poor.

Pregnancy[11]

As a general rule the increase in cholesterol level associated with pregnancy subsides after delivery. Systematically absorbed lipid-lowering agents may be unsafe during pregnancy and should be avoided.

References

1. Duffy SJ, Meredith IJ. Treating mildly elevated lipids. Current Therapeutics, 1996; 37(4):49–58.

2. Scandinavian Simvastatin Survival Study Group. Randomised trial of cholesterol lowering in 4444 patients with coronary heart disease: the Scandinavian Simvastatin Survival Study (4S). Lancet, 1994; 344:1383–1389.

3. Pitt B, Mancini BJ, Ellis SG et al. Pravastatin limitation of atherosclerosis in the coronary arteries (PLAC I): reduction in atherosclerosis progression and clinical events. J Am Coll Cardiol, 1995; 26:1133–1139.

4. Byington RP, Furberg CD, Crouse JR et al. Pravastatin, lipids and atherosclerosis in the carotid arteries (PLAC II). Am J Cardiol, 1995; 76:54C–59C.

5. Furberg CD, Adams HP, Applegate WB et al. for the Asymptomatic Carotid Plaque Study (ACAPS) Research Group. Effect of lovastatin and warfarin on early carotid atherosclerosis and cardiovascular events. Circulation, 1994; 90:1679–1687.

6. Salonen R, Nyyssonen K, Porkkala-Sarataho E, Salonen JT. The Kuopio Atherosclerosis Prevention Study (KAPS): effect of pravastatin treatment on lipids, oxidation resistance of lipoproteins, and atherosclerosis progression. Am J Cardiol, 1995; 76:34C–39C.

7. Jukema JW, Bruschke AVG, van Boven A et al. Effects of lipid lowering by pravastatin on progression and regression of coronary artery disease in symptomatic men with normal to moderately elevated serum cholesterol levels. The Regression Growth Evaluation Statin Study (REGRESS). Circulation, 1995; 91:2528–2540.

8. Shepherd J, Cobbe SM, Ford I et al. Prevention of coronary heart disease with pravastatin in men with hypercholesterolaemia. N Eng J Med, 1995; 333:1301–1307.

9. Department Human Services and Health. Schedule Benefits. Canberra: Commonwealth of Australia, November 1996, 25–28.

10. National Heart Foundation (Australia). Guide to plasma lipids for doctors, 1996.

11. Mashford ML et al. *Cardiovascular drug guidelines* (2nd edn). Victorian Medical Postgraduate Foundation Inc., 1995–96; 41–45.

113

Rational prescribing

—

Even in medicine; though it is easy to know what honey, wine and hellebore, cautery and surgery are, to know how and to whom and when to apply them so as to effect a cure is no less an undertaking than to be a physician.

Aristotle (384–322 BC)

As most patient encounters with general practitioners result in a prescription[1] the importance of rational prescribing assumes great significance in primary health care delivery. Prescribing is one of the special skills of our discipline. The prescribing doctor has a great responsibility to keep up to date in the principles and practice of therapeutics.

In the first instance, the prescriber should consider the question 'is this drug really necessary?' before prescribing it. Alternatively, non-pharmacological measures should be considered including nutritional advice, relaxation techniques, exercise programs and other appropriate natural modalities.

An issue that is often not appreciated by critics of drug prescribing is that much of it is patient-driven; some patients believe that there should be a biochemical solution to every discomfort. Haslock describes this as a 'sociological trend in patients, and in the population as a whole, for increasing demand for treatment'.[2] This demand should not lead us to prescribe drugs in a cavalier fashion nor should concerns about side effects prevent us writing a prescription where indicated.

Special attention should be given to the issue of compliance, especially in children, the elderly and the handicapped. Examples of significant areas include the management of asthma, where delivery systems are significant, and in insulin dependent diabetes. The top 10 drugs used in Australia in terms of daily dose used, prescription counts and costs are presented in Table 113.1

Table 113.1   *The top 10 drugs in Australia 1997*[3]

	Daily dose used	Prescription counts	Cost
1.	salbutamol	amoxycillin	simvastatin
2.	frusemide	paracetamol	omeprazole
3.	enalapril	salbutamol	ranitidine
4.	simvastatin	simvastatin	enalapril
5.	ranitidine	codeine 30 mg with paracetamol	ipratropium bromide
6.	ipratropium bromide	ranitidine	amlodipine
7.	amlodipine	temazepam	captopril
8.	budesonide	enalapril	salbutamol
9.	felodipine	atenolol	famotidine
10.	hydrochlorothiazide with amiloride	cefaclor	pravastatin

Guidelines for the optimal use of medication [4]

- an awareness of the part drugs play in treating illness and maintaining health
- knowledge sufficient to choose the most effective medication/s for the patients concerned, taking into account their clinical condition, risk, benefit, dosage, length of treatment, cost, monitoring of effect and consideration of alternatives
- information which enables patients to use drugs correctly and safely [4]

Key facts and checkpoints

- Any drug, prescribed or non-prescribed, has the potential to cause adverse effects which should always be kept in mind by the doctor. The importance of taking a drug history can never be underestimated.
- Adverse drug reactions are more probable in elderly patients; as they are the main consumers of drugs, often taking several (sometimes potent) different drugs simultaneously, special care should be taken, including regular reviews.
- Prescribing of the following groups of drugs requires special care and attention, particularly in the elderly:
  — antibiotics
  — analgesics, especially opioid analgesics
  — anticoagulants
  — non-steroidal anti-inflammatory drugs
  — antihypertensives and other cardiac drugs
  — anxiolytic and hypnotic drugs, especially the benzodiazepines
- Prescribing should ideally be accompanied by patient education information about the drug/s, including written instructions.
- It is important for the prescribing doctor to consider possible drug interactions and contraindications (absolute and relative) before writing the prescription.
- The patient should be invited to contact the prescriber with any concerns about the effects of any drug/s.
- A good professional relationship between patient, pharmacist and doctor should be encouraged and developed. The future use of computer-generated prescriptions and computer programs covering patient drug information, interactions and contraindications will assist rational prescribing.

- As a rule, practitioners should aim for monotherapy for a specific condition and keep polypharmacy to a minimum, especially when treating a number of different conditions.
- Antibiotic resistance is a problem in Australian medical practice and likely to worsen if the current high level of antibiotic use is maintained. [5]

Prescribing in the elderly

Some of the problems associated with prescribing and adverse drug reactions in the elderly have been discussed in Chapter 8 (pp. 63–64). Adverse drug reactions are three times more common in patients aged over 65 than in those aged under 50 years. [6] Approximately 15% of elderly patients admitted to hospital are suffering adverse drug reactions. [7]

One study showed that the drugs mainly responsible for these admissions were antihypertensives (including beta-blockers), analgesics and NSAIDs, digoxin, diuretics, psychotropics and hypnotics. [8] Most adverse reactions are type A (dose-related) rather than type B (idiosyncratic). [6]

The elderly are very prone to adverse effects to most of the more potent drugs, especially those for cardiac dysfunction and hypertension (Table 113.2). Both ACE inhibitors and calcium channel blockers have been shown to produce a greater fall in blood pressure in elderly compared with younger subjects, presumably related also to a reduced homeostatic response. [9]

In view of the increased susceptibility of the elderly to adverse drug reactions and their multiple disease states a very conservative and critical approach to prescribing is necessary. The starting dose of a drug in the elderly should be at the lower end of the recommended range. Further dosage increments should be gradual and reviewed regularly. It is important to individualise doses for the elderly, being mindful of the potential for reduced renal clearance and other physiological factors.

Anticoagulant prescribing

The important and responsible task of rational prescribing of anticoagulants is presented in Chapter 36 (pp. 355–357).

Table 113.2 *Drug side effects in the elderly: common presentations*[6]

Drug	Side effects
Benzodiazepines	Confusion, falls, psychomotor impairment
Beta-blockers	Confusion, falls, asthma, insomnia
Cimetidine	Confusion
Digoxin	Nausea, confusion
Diuretics	Incontinence, falls, hyponatraemia, hypokalaemia
Levodopa	Confusion, falls, dystonia, hallucinations, agitation, postural hypotension
Metoclopramide	Confusion, extrapyramidal symptoms
Narcotic analgesics	Constipation, confusion
NSAIDs	Confusion, GIT bleeding, oedema, renal dysfunction, headache
Phenothiazines	Confusion, postural hypotension, falls, constipation
Phenytoin	Confusion, falls, ataxia, parkinsonism, urinary problems
Prazosin	Postural hypotension, incontinence
SSRI antidepressants	Nausea, agitation, insomnia
Theophylline	Nausea, tremor, confusion
Tricyclic antidepressants	Confusion, falls, postural hypotension, constipation, urinary problems, eye problems
Verapamil	Constipation

Antibiotic prescribing

Antibiotics are substances produced by micro-organisms that suppress the growth of other micro-organisms. Apart from these natural substances, agents are produced synthetically in the laboratory to achieve the same purpose. The term 'antimicrobial agent' encompasses all agents that attack micro-organisms.

Antimicrobial agents can be classified as bactericidal (kills organisms) or bacteriostatic (prevents growth of organisms). Both types are effective therapeutically although both also rely on natural host defences to eradicate the pathogenic micro-organisms. A particular agent may exhibit both bactericidal and bacteriostatic properties, depending on the conditions of activity.

Beta-lactams, such as penicillins and cephalosporins, and aminoglycosides, such as gentamicin and streptomycin, are the typical examples of bacteriocidal agents while the macrolides, such as erythromycin and roxithromycin, and the tetracyclines are examples of bacteriostatic drugs.

Antimicrobial agents are classified into five major groups according to the site on the cellular biochemical pathway where the drug is primarily active[10] (Fig. 113.1).
1. inhibition of synthesis and damage to cell wall
2. inhibition of synthesis or damage to cytoplasmic membrane
3. inhibition of synthesis of nucleic acid
4. inhibition of protein synthesis
5. modification of folic acid metabolism, affecting energy metabolism

Beta-lactams

The beta-lactams include a diverse group of agents which are structurally related and exhibit bactericidal activity directed at the bacterial cell wall (Fig. 113.1). They include the penicillins, cephalosporins, monolactams, e.g. aztreonam, and carbapenems, e.g. imipenem.

The penicillins can be subclassified as follows:[11]

- narrow spectrum—benzylpenicillin (penicillin G), procaine penicillin, benzathine penicillin and phenoxymethylpenicillin
- broad spectrum—ampicillin, amoxycillin
- antistaphylococcal—methicillin, cloxacillin, dicloxacillin, flucloxacillin
- antipseudomonal—piperacillin and ticarcillin

The cephalosporins are subdivided into three classes or 'generations':
- first generation
  — oral: cefaclor, cephalexin
  — parenteral: cephalothin, cephazolin
- second generation (all parenteral): cephamandole, cefoxitin, cefotetan (these agents have a limited place in clinical medicine)
- third generation (all parenteral): cefotaxime, ceftriaxone, ceftazidime, cefpirome
  These have an extended spectrum of activity covering most enteric Gram-negative rods but limited activity against enterococci and MRSA

Practice points
- The development of beta-lactamase enzyme in resistant micro-organisms has been a major problem, e.g. methicillin-resistant *Staphylococcus aureus* (MSRA). This has led to the development of beta-lactamase inhibitors such as clavulanic acid and sublactam which inhibit

Cell wall synthesis

beta-lactams
• penicillins
• cephalosporins
• monolactams
• carbapenems
glycopeptides
• vancomycin
• teicoplanin
beta-lactamase inhibitors
bacitracin (topical)

Nucleic acid synthesis
quinolones, e.g.
 • norfloxacin
 • ciprofloxacin
rifampicin
nitrofurantoin
nitroimidazoles

Protein synthesis
aminoglycosides, e.g.
 • gentamicin
 • streptomycin
tetracyclines
chloramphenicol
clindamycin
macrolides, e.g.
 • erythromycin
 • roxithromycin

**Cell wall
(cytoplasmic)
membrane**
 polymyxins
 polyene antifungals

Folic acid metabolism
 sulphonamides
 trimethoprim
 isoniazid

Fig. 113.1 *The bacterial cell, showing the five main antimicrobial sites or mechanisms of inhibition of micro-organisms*

the organisms when used in combination with penicillins such as amoxycillin and ticarcillin.
• The antistaphylococcal penicillins are stable to beta-lactamase produced by staphylococci.
• Flucloxacillin is generally well tolerated but can cause cholestatic jaundice. The problem is largely restricted to older patients (>55 years), especially with renal impairment, and also longer courses. There is evidence that the related dicloxacillin is less hepatotoxic but probably less effective for serious infections.
• Penicillin hypersensitivity (anaphylaxis, angioedema and urticaria) is due to an IgE antibody reaction against penicillin antigens. The reaction can be delayed for up to 72 hours. Unless the rashes are urticarial they may not represent an acute hypersensitivity reaction.
• Maculopapular rashes associated with

(amoxy) ampicillin may not be hypersensitivity (allergic) reactions.[11] The same may apply to the symptom of diarrhoea.
• Cross-reactivity between the groups can occur so a history of an immediate reaction is a contraindication to giving penicillin and most other beta-lactam drugs.[11]

Aminoglycosides
The aminoglycosides include gentamicin, tobramycin, netilmicin, amikacin and streptomycin. They are basically bactericidal and are effective against Gram-positive and Gram-negative organisms. Their toxicity and potential for developing resistance are limiting factors. They are all potentially ototoxic and nephrotoxic and should be reserved for serious infections such as hospital-acquired sepsis.

Sulphonamides and trimethoprim

Sulphonamides have limited use because of serious side effects, especially in the elderly.

The combination of the sulphonamide, sulphamethoxazole, with trimethoprim enjoyed widespread usage as a broad spectrum agent against urinary tract and respiratory tract infections.[11] However, the development of resistance and adverse effects has limited its use.

Tetracyclines

Tetracyclines are broad spectrum agents that inhibit a wide variety of Gram-positive and Gram-negative organisms and other micro-organisms such as rickettsiae, chlamydia and mycoplasmas. They have many clinical uses, including antimalarial, but increasing bacterial resistance and the development of other agents have restricted their use. Tetracyclines should not be prescribed for pregnant women, children younger than 8 years, or anyone with renal impairment or severe liver disease.

Quinolones[11]

Nalidixic acid is an original member of this group. Norfloxacin, ciprofloxacin, enoxacin and fleroxacin are newer members with a broad spectrum of activity. They generally have poor activity against streptococci, are expensive and should be reserved for the treatment of infections resistant to less expensive agents or where the oral agent is essential.

Quinolones damage the joints of immature animals and are therefore not recommended in children less than 14 years old.

Macrolides

Macrolides include erythromycin, roxithromycin, clarithomycin and azithromycin. They have a wide spectrum of activity against Gram-positive and Gram-negative cocci and anaerobes, Mycoplasma, Chlamydia, Legionella, Bordatella and Corynebacteria, but not against Gram-negative rods.

Ansamycins

These include rifampicin and rifabutin which are active against Gram-positive organisms and the mycobacterial species. Rifampicin is used mainly in the treatment of tuberculosis and MRSA but the emergence of resistance has led to its use in combination with other quite different agents.

Lincosamides

The main agent is clindamycin which is active against Gram-positive aerobes and most anaerobes. The problem of serious diarrhoea (pseudomembranous colitis) has limited its use.

Antibiotic resistance

The continual emergence of resistant strains of organisms remains a serious problem. Bacterial resistance was initially thought to be caused entirely by chromosomal change but has been shown to arise also from a transmissible, extrachromosomal segment of DNA referred to as a plasmid. Resistance-conferring plasmids have been identified in virtually all bacteria. A classic example is the production of β-lactamase enzyme by several organisms, particularly *Staph. aureus*, which inactivate β-lactam antimicrobials. Most resistances emerging in our community are due to the high levels of antibiotic prescribing for patients in Australia.[5]

Predictable examples of almost 100% resistance include *Staph. aureus* to penicillin and amoxycillin, streptococci to aminoglycosides, Enterococci to cephalosporins, *Klebsiella* to amoxycillin, and *Pseudomonas aeruginosa* to amoxycillin ± clavulanate and most cephalosporins.[12]

Organisms that are developing increased resistance to co-trimoxazole include *E. coli*, *Proteus mirabilis* and *Streptococcus pneumoniae*. Emerging resistances in respiratory pathogens are found in β-lactamase producing *Haemophilus influenzae* and *Moxarella catarrhalis*. *Streptococcus pneumoniae* is becoming resistant to co-trimoxazole and penicillin. Almost half of *E. coli* strains are now resistant to amoxycillin while 15% are resistant to trimethoprim. Strains resistant to amoxycillin-clavulanate are now being encountered.[5]

Other significant resistances include:

- Methicillin-resistant *Staph. aureus* (MRSA): this is an ongoing problem in nursing homes and hospitals. Resistance to fluoroquinolones such as ciprofloxacin has increased dramatically. Vancomycin remains the mainstay of therapy.
- Vancomycin-resistant enterococci (VRE) (a major nosocomial problem) especially in the US.
- Multidrug-resistant tuberculosis (MDR-TB) is also an emerging problem especially in HIV

patients and some South-East Asian immi-grants, especially with isoniazid resistance.

- Penicillin-resistant *Neisseria gonorrhoea* is a continuing emerging problem in South-East Asia and other developing countries.
- Resistance to quinolones is now being seen at a low level in many Gram-negative pathogens.[5]

General guidelines for antibiotic prescribing[12]

Rules of thumb

Choose the agent with the
- narrowest spectrum that will cover the likely pathogens
- lowest cost if efficacy and safety are otherwise equal
- fewest serious side effects

Avoid whenever possible
- topical antibiotics, as resistance is much more likely to develop (exceptions include eye infections and vaginitis)
- antibiotic combinations, except in proven clinical circumstances or when coverage is difficult with a single drug
- prophylactic antibiotics, unless they are of proven benefit (in general only in *some* elective surgery)

Value of microscopy in directing therapy

Remember the power of the microscope in making rapid diagnoses (Table 113.3). Always read test results from *top down* (microscopy first) as valuable information is given there.

Table 113.3 *Relative value of microscopy in rapid diagnosis of microbiological specimens*

Specimen		Value of microscopy
Vaginal swab	++++	Diagnostic
Urethral swab	++++	Diagnostic
CSF	++++	Diagnostic
Wound/pus swab	+++	Very useful
Micro-urine*	++	Usually helpful
Sputum*	++	Usually helpful
Faeces	+	Occasionally helpful
Throat swab	–	Rarely useful
Blood culture	–	Rarely useful

* Poor specimen collection reduces value

Infections requiring more than 7 days treatment

Treatment should be given for 5–7 days. Table 113.4 gives important exceptions.

Table 113.4 *Important infections requiring more than 7 days' treatment*

Infection	Minimum
Streptococcus pyogenes pharyngitis	10 days
Pelvic inflammatory disease	2 weeks
Chlamydial infection	10 days
Deep-seated staphylococcal infection	2–6 weeks
Deep-seated anaerobic infection	6 weeks
Osteomyelitis	2–26 weeks
Endocarditis	4–6 weeks
Tuberculosis	9 months
Syphilis	10 days

Single-dose treatment

Single-dose therapy has good efficacy in the following circumstances:
- uncomplicated urinary tract infection
- uncomplicated gonorrhoea
- candida vaginitis
- *Trichomonas* vaginitis
- giardiasis
- intestinal helminth infestations

Guidelines for antibacterial drug selection

The choice of antibiotic for a particular infection is based on knowledge of common pathogens, prevailing resistances of importance, simple pharmacology and host modifying factors.[12,13] See Table 113.5.

Psychotropic and nervous system medication prescribing

Considerable skill is required for the rational prescribing of these agents, especially antipsychotic agents, antidepressants and the anxiolytic and hypnotic agents.

Benzodiazepines are of particular concern because of dependency with all ages. They are especially of concern in the elderly, who are the main long-term users of benzodiazepines.

Benzodiazepines

The use of benzodiazepines as anxiolytics should be restricted and they should be used discretely. Markus et al.[14] recommend reserving

Those who stop medication have an equal obligation to:

- ascertain whether there is still a need for its therapeutic action
- take the necessary steps, if the need exists, to provide an alternative

There is evidence that peptic ulcers that develop in patients taking NSAIDs heal faster if the NSAID is dropped.[21]

There is no evidence that using an enteric-coated NSAID preparation or using the rectal route for administration reduces gastric damage as it is mediated almost entirely systemically after the NSAID has been absorbed.[19] Furthermore, trials have indicated that the efficacy of using H_2-receptor antagonists for preventing NSAID gastrointestinal complications is low to absent.

NSAIDs and the elderly

NSAIDs with short half-lives, e.g. ibuprofen and diclofenac, may be safer in the elderly and all NSAIDs should be used in reduced dosage. Patients should be monitored for fluid retention and hypertensive control.[6,18]

Prescribing recommendations

- Recommend intermittent use of NSAIDs based on appropriate patient education. Intermittent courses for 14 days can work well in chronic conditions, remembering that it takes about 10 days for NSAIDs to achieve maximal effectiveness.
- Use paracetamol as an alternative, especially for osteoarthritis conditions.
- Consider protective combinations e.g. diclofenac + misoprostol.

Analgesic prescribing

The general practitioner has an important responsibility not only to relieve patients' pain skilfully and completely (if possible) but to ensure that the appropriate drugs are prescribed without leading to dependence.

Pain can be divided into three categories: nociceptive pain, neurogenic pain and muscle pain, each requiring different therapeutic agents.[18] For nociceptive pain the traditional analgesics are used: paracetamol, aspirin, other NSAIDs and opioids. Neurogenic pain is treated with antidepressants, antiepileptics and membrane stabilisers. Agents used to treat muscle pain are muscle relaxants and baclofen.

Chronic pain such as chronic low back pain represents a challenge but the challenge is to manage acute pain skilfully and prevent chronicity. O'Reilly[22] has provided some useful guidelines for the role of the general practitioner in the management of chronic pain:

- Emphasise that cure is unlikely.
- Encourage the patient to accept responsibility for pain management.
- Provide ongoing support and interest.
- Promote activity rather than rest.
- Educate patients about their condition: review X-rays and discuss drugs, especially the long-term disadvantages of narcotics and sedatives.
- Encourage time-contingent vs pain-contingent use of medication.
- Withdraw unsuitable drugs, e.g. narcotics and sedatives.
- Consider use of undiagnosed depression or anxiety as amplifiers of pain perception and treat where necessary.
- Promote the use of relaxation, distraction and heat or ice packs rather than increased medication.
- Discuss strategy for management of flare-ups in advance.
- Refer for psychological support: cognitive behavioural psychologist or psychiatrist recommended.

Analgesics in common use[18]

Paracetamol

Paracetamol has minimal anti-inflammatory activity but moderate analgesic (equipotent with aspirin) and antipyretic properties. It is metabolised by the liver and has an excretion half-life of approximately 4 hours. Adverse effects are uncommon but gastrointestinal discomfort such as dyspepsia and nausea can occur occasionally. It is well tolerated by patients with peptic ulcers and has no effect on platelet function. Use of 4 g or more per day over 12 months has been associated with chronic liver disease.

Usual dosage: 1 g (o) 4 hourly (max. 4 g/day)

Aspirin

Aspirin has both analgesic and anti-inflammatory activity and is a very effective drug in adults for mild to moderate acute pain. It has an extremely short half-life and is metabolised to salicylic acid which shares the above properties. The major problems with aspirin are gastrointestinal discomfort, ulceration and bleeding.

Usual dosage: 600 mg (o) 4 hourly (max. 4 g/day)

Opioid analgesics

These agents are usually reserved for the treatment of severe pain. Commonly used agents are the weaker opioids—codeine, oxycodone, dextropropoxyphene—and the stronger ones—morphine, pethidine and methadone. Other types are dextromoramide, pentazocine, paraveretum and fentanyl.

Adverse effects, which are common, dose-dependent and quite variable, include nausea and vomiting, constipation, respiratory depression and dysphoria.

Codeine

Codeine, which is methymorphine, is metabolised to morphine. Controlled trials have shown codeine 32 mg to be no more effective than aspirin 600 mg.[23] Disturbing side effects include nausea and constipation.

Usual dosage: 30–60 mg (o) 4 hourly (max. 180 mg/day)

Oxycodone

Oxycodone is a synthetic opioid that is very effective orally. It is useful for moderate pain in bridging the gap between the simple analgesics and strong opioids.[23] The oral form has a duration of action of 4 hours. It is well absorbed through the rectal mucosa and is useful as a night-time suppository with a duration of 7–8 hours.[18]

Adverse side effects include nausea, constipation, confusion and itch.

Usual dosage: 10 mg (o) 4 hourly (max. 60 mg/day)
30 mg rectally 12 hours

Dextropropoxyphene

This controversial drug is structurally related to methadone.

Adverse effects include dysphoria, confusion, lightheadedness and constipation. It has been associated with relatively sudden death when taken in overdose, especially with alcohol.[18] Continuous use should be discouraged, particularly in elderly patients and those with cardiac disease.[18]

Morphine

Morphine is the most effective opioid for the relief of cancer pain (see Chap. 7). It is worth noting that injections are not more effective than oral administration in achieving pain relief. It should be titrated according to patients' needs. Dose reduction may need to be made in patients with impaired liver or renal function and in elderly or debilitated patients.

Note: Dose requirements vary considerably and patient response should be monitored frequently. There may be no upper limit to dosage in cancer patients.

Usual dosage:[18]
10 mg (o) 4 times daily
IM or SC injection: 7.5–15 mg
intravenous:
bolus—2.5–5 mg followed by 1–2 mg increments at 5 minute intervals
slow—2.5–5 mg over 5–10 minutes, then increments
infusion—2–5 mg per hour

Methadone

Methadone is an effective oral analgesic with a long but variable half-life; it is given, preferably, once or at most twice a day. Unsuitable for acute pain, it is valuable for chronic pain, although long-acting morphine preparations have displaced it. It should not be used in elderly patients or those with renal dysfunction. Its place is in management of narcotic dependency but it needs to be used with care because of the risk of respiratory depression and accumulation.

Pethidine

Pethidine is a synthetic opioid with a short duration of action. A problematic adverse effect is accumulation of its toxic metabolite (norpethidine) which can cause myoclonic and general seizures.[23] It has no place in the management of chronic pain whether cancer or non-cancer.

Combined analgesics

Combined analgesics are freely available both as prescribed and over-the-counter (OTC) preparations for moderately severe pain. They usually consist of a simple analgesic such as paracetamol or aspirin combined with an opioid analgesic (usually codeine). The analgesics have an additive effect because they act at different receptor sites. The use of such preparations is generally not recommended but if both agents are needed it is advisable to prescribe them separately thus enabling individual dose adjustments.[18]

Analgesics in the elderly

As a general rule, most elderly patients are more sensitive to opioid analgesics and to aspirin and other NSAIDs but there may be considerable individual differences in tolerance between patients. Patients over 65 years should receive lower initial doses of opioid analgesics with subsequent doses being titrated according to the patient's needs.[18]

Some general rules and tips[18]

- Give analgesics at fixed times by the clock rather than 'prn' for ongoing pain.
- Regularly monitor your patient's analgesic requirements and modify according to needs and adverse effects.
- Start with a dose towards the lower end of the dose range and then titrate upwards depending on response.
- Provide ongoing interest and support. This will magnify any placebo effect.
- Avoid using compound analgesics and prescribe simple and opioid analgesics separately.
- Never cut suppositories in half with the intention of halving the dose.
- Reserve the use of antiemetics for the development of nausea and vomiting with opioids. Extrapyramidal reactions (dystonia and oculogyric crises) can be a problem with antiemetics.
- Advise patients about the benefits of high-fibre foods if on analgesics. Prescribe a bulking agent or lactulose if necessary.

Therapeutic drug monitoring

Drug monitoring by measuring the serum or plasma concentration of prescribed drugs provides an objective basis for adjusting dosage in individual patients, especially where the more toxic drugs are involved.

Drugs with the following characteristics are those that are commonly monitored:[24]

- drugs with a definable relationship between plasma concentration and clinical effects, e.g. theophylline
- drugs with well defined 'therapeutic' and 'toxic' levels for plasma drug concentrations, e.g. phenytoin

- drugs with a narrow 'therapeutic index' where toxic and therapeutic levels are close, e.g. digoxin
- drugs where there is no easily measured therapeutic response, e.g. antiarrhythmic drugs
- drugs for which plasma concentration has prognostic significance in overdosage, e.g. paracetamol

Commonly monitored drugs include:

- *aminoglycosides*: gentamicin, tobramycin, amikacin
- *antiepileptics*: carbamazepine, clonazepam, ethosuximide, phenobarbitone, phenytoin, valproate
- *antiarrhythmias*: amiodarone, disopyramide, flecainide, lignocaine, procainamide, quinidine, sotalol
- *antidepressants*: amitriptyline, imipramine, nortriptyline
- cyclosporin
- digoxin
- lithium
- salicylate
- theophylline

As a general rule, most samples are taken just before a dose.

Prescription writing

The official guideline for prescribing in Australian general practice is the Pharmaceutical Benefits Scheme (PBS) which provides a Schedule of Pharmaceutical Benefits for all practitioners.

The essential legal requirements of a prescription are:[25]

- doctor's name
- address and telephone number
- date on which the prescription is written
- patient's name and address
- entitlement number (for patients holding Health Benefits Card)
- the prescribed item:
  — generic or proprietary name or formula
  — form of the preparation (tablet, mixture, etc.)
  — strength in metric
  — quantity to be dispensed
  — repeats to be issued (if any)
  — dosage in metric
  — directions to the patient

The prescription should be regarded as a

Table 113.8 *Prescription writing: abbreviations acceptable by common usage*

Abbreviation	Derivation	Meaning
NP	Nomen propem	Label the container with the name of its contents
R$_x$	Recipe	Take (to the pharmacist)
Ft	Fiat	Make up
m	Misce	Mix
M	Mitte	Send (to the patient)
Sig	Signa	Label, let it be labelled
Tab	Tabella	Tablet
Cap	Capsula	Capsule
Mist	Mistura	Mixture
Elix	Elixir	Elixir
Garg	Gargarisma	Gargle
Collut	Collutorium	Mouthwash
Syr	Syrupus	Syrup
Lot	Lotio	Lotion
Emuls	Emulsio	Emulsion
Ung	Unguentum	Ointment
Crem	Cremor	Cream
Applic	Applicatio	Application
Past	Pasta	Paste
Pig	Pigmentum	Paint
Tr	Tinctura	Tincture
Pulv	Pulvis	Powder
Gutt	Guttae	Drops
Narist	Naristillae	Nose drops
Aurist	Auristillae	Ear drops
Occulent	Occulentum	Eye ointment
Amp	Ampulla	Ampoule
ex aq	ex aqua	In water
Lin	Linimentum	Liniment

Instructions to the patient

stat	statim	immediately (for the first dose)
prn	pro re nate	when required or occasionally
md	more dicto	as directed
bd	bis diem	twice daily
tds	ter die sumendum	to be taken three times daily
tid	ter in die	three times a day
in	imni nocte	every night
qid	quater in die	four times daily
qqh	quarta quaque hora	every fourth hour
ac	ante cibum	before meals
cc	cum cibum	with meals
pc	post cibum	after meals
m	mane	in the morning
n	nocte	at night
n et m	nocte et mane	night and morning
hs	hora somni	at bedtime

'sacred' legal document and not subject to misinterpretation. Legibility is very important to enable accurate dispensing by the pharmacist who has an invaluable role to play in reinforcing the patient's drug education and compliance and acting as a watchdog for possible prescribing errors.

The traditional abbreviated terminology used for prescription writing is summarised in Table 113.8. An example of a prescription item is given in Figure 113.2 on page 1106.

References

1. Bridges-Webb C, Britt H, Miles DA et al. Morbidity and treatment in general practice in Australia 1990–1991. Med J Aust (Supplement) 1992; 157:51–57.

2. Haslock I. Should we use non-steroidal anti-inflammatory drugs? Aliment Pharmacol Therap, 1988; 25:1–8.

3. Top 10 drugs. Australian Prescriber, 1997; 20(1):17.

4. Pharmaceutical Health and the Rational Use of Medicines (PHARM) Working Party. *A policy on the quality use of medicines*. Canberra: Commonwealth Dept of Health, Housing and Community Services, 1992.

5. Turnidge J, Bell J. Antibiotic resistance: the Australian situation. Current Therapeutics, 1996; 37:59–64.

6. Scharf S, Christophidis N. Drug treatment in the elderly. In: MIMS Disease Index (2nd edn). Sydney: IMS Publishing, 1996,159–160.

7. Williamson J. Chopin JM. Adverse reactions to prescribed drugs in the elderly: a multicentre investigation. Age and Ageing, 1980; 9:73–80.

8. Brian RH. Medication problems in old age. Patient Management, 1988; 5:27–31.

9. Swift CG. Pharmcodynamics, changes in homeostatic mechanisms, receptor and target organ sensitivity in the elderly. British Medical Bulletin, 1990; 46:36–52.

10. Brody TM et al. *Human Pharmacology*. St Louis: Mosby, 617–632.

11. Mashford ML (Chairman). *Antibiotic guidelines* (9th edn). Melbourne: Victorian Medical Postgraduate Foundation, 1996–97: 7–17.

12. Turnidge J. *ABC of antibiotics*. Sydney: Pfizer, 1990.

Dr A B CEED
M.B., B.S.
WHITEBURN CLINIC
17 MEDIBANK CRESCENT
MEDICARE VIC
Ph: 9999 9000

6 8 3 7 9 4 0

Pharmaceutical Benefits Entitlement Number

| S | M | | 6 | 7 | 0 | | 2 | 6 | 3 | | H | A |

☐ SAFETY NET ENTITLEMENT CARD HOLDER

☑ CONCESSIONAL OR DEPENDANT, RPBS BENEFICIARY OR SAFETY NET CONCESSION CARD HOLDER.
(Cross Relevant Box)

PATIENT'S NAME _____ *Jack Citizen*

ADDRESS _____ *8 / 1296 Circuit St, Glendale*

DATE *14 , 4 , 1997* _____ POST CODE *9926*

☑ PBS   ☐ RPBS   ☐ BRAND SUBSTITUTION NOT PERMITTED

(tick appropriate box)

℞ *doxycycline 100 mg tabs*

Sig. T̄ daily pc

Mitte.   7   1 rpt

Cease:

DOCTOR'S SIGNATURE - - - - - *A G Practitioner* - - - - - - - -

I certify that I have received this medication and the information relating to any entitlement to free or concessional pharmaceutical benefits is not false or misleading

___ / ___ / ___   _____

Date of Supply   Patient's or Agent's Signature

P.B. 35 (10/96)   Agent's Address

Fig. 113.2 *Example of a prescription item*

13. Chambers I, Munro R. Antibacterial drug selection in common infections In: MIMS Disease Index (2nd edn). Sydney: IMS Publishing, 1996; 39–41.

14. Markus AC et al. *Psychological problems in general practice*. Oxford: Oxford University Press, 1989, 12–43.

15. Moulds RFW (Chairman). *Psychotropic drug guidelines* (3rd edn). Melbourne: Victorian Medical Postgraduate Foundation, 1996–97, 129–147.

16. Khalig N, Wood PNH. *Arthritis and rheumatism in the eighties*. London: Arthritis and Rheumatism Council, 1986.

17. Baum C, Kennedy DL, Forbes MB. Utilisation of NSAIDs. Arthritis Rheum, 1985; 28:686–692.

18. Moulds RFW (Chairman). *Analgesic guidelines* (3rd edn). Melbourne: Victorian Medical Postgraduate Foundation, 1997–98.

19. Ryan P. Pharmacology of musculoskeletal treatment agents. Monash Distance Education: Graduate Diploma in Family Medicine Notes 1995; 6(1):8–15.

20. Brooks PM, Yeomans ND. NSAIDs gastropathy: is it preventable? Aust NZ Med, 1992; 22:685–691.

21. Lancaster–Smith MJ, Jaderberg ME, Jackson DA. Ranitidine in the treatment of NSAIDs—associated gastric and duodenal ulcers. GUT, 1991; 32:252–255.

22. O'Reilly S. Treatment of chronic non-malignant pain in general practice. Aust Fam Physician, 1994; 23:2281.

23. Crammond T. Pain relief. In: MIMS Disease Index (2nd edn). Sydney: IMS Publishing, 1996, 380–385.

24. Shenfield GM. Therapeutic drug monitoring: when is it of value? In: MIMS Disease Index (2nd edn). Sydney: IMS Publishing, 1996, 502–505.

25. Liddell M. Prescription writing. In: Department of Community Medicine & General Practice, Monash University, Final Year Handbook 1997; 2:C:2–4.

PART 10

ACCIDENT AND EMERGENCY MEDICINE

114
Emergency care

—

When Elisha arrived, he went alone into the room and saw the boy lying dead on the bed. He closed the door and prayed to the Lord. Then he lay down on the boy, placing his mouth, eyes and hands on the boy's mouth, eyes and hands. As he lay stretched out over the boy, the boy's body started to get warm—the boy sneezed seven times and then opened his eyes.

II Kings 4: 32–5
(A miracle or successful artificial resuscitation?)

Definition of the emergency

'An event demanding immediate medical attention.'

The demand is determined by patients, relatives, neighbours, nurses, police and others, but is sometimes modified by the doctor or his or her staff.

The common concept of emergencies is an organic one, but the cause is often emotional, or of social origin. The general practitioner has to learn to understand the patient's feeling of urgency and the cure by reassurance may not be simple at all, but can require great skill and understanding. Despite this, the general practitioner must be available and organised to cope with the medically defined emergency when it comes. Emergency care outside the hospital represents one of the most interesting and rewarding areas of medical practice. City doctors will have to modify their degree of availability, equipment and skills according to paramedical emergency services, while others, especially remote doctors, will need total expertise and equipment to provide optimal circumstances to save their patients' lives.

In dealing with a specific emergency, the doctor adopts a different approach. Instead of taking a history and performing an examination in the usual way, he or she replaces this with a technique of rapid assessment and immediate management. In fact, the diagnosis may be possible on the information available over the telephone.

Time criticality

An important yet obvious concept is that of 'time criticality' which implies that certain patients are at high risk of a critical outcome of deterioration if there is significant delay in appropriate management.

Key facts and figures

- The commonest emergency calls in a survey of a typical community were[1] accidents and violence (50.7%), abdominal pain (9.9%), dyspnoea (7.2%), chest pain (5.8%), syncope/blackout (5.2%), other acute pain (5.0%).
- The prevalence of emergency calls was 2.6 per 1000 population per week.
- The commonest specific conditions in this study were lacerations 19%, fractures 11%, injuries from transport accidents 11%, bronchial asthma 4%, ischaemic heart pain 3.5%, appendicitis 3%.
- The commonest causes of sudden death were myocardial infarction 67%, accidents 10%, cerebrovascular accidents 7%, pulmonary embolism 6%, suicide 4%.
- The main vital emergency procedures were cardiopulmonary resuscitation, intubation and ventilation, intravenous access including cutdown, intravenous (or rectal) dextrose and arrest of haemorrhage.

Principles of management

The important principles of management of the emergency call can be summarised as follows:

1. The practitioner must be aware of life-threatening conditions.
2. It is important to 'get up and go' when the call signals danger.
3. The provisional diagnosis should follow the telephone call.
4. The practitioner should be prepared mentally and physically:
   PLAN, EQUIP and PRACTISE
5. Chest pain/collapse/myocardial infarction (collectively) represents *the* premium emergency call.
6. Beware of children with respiratory distress and traumatic injuries.
7. The most savable patients are those with blood loss. Hence IV fluids for intravascular volume expansion and blood availability are essential.
8. The necessary basic skills to cope with most emergencies involve ABC—airway, breathing, circulation.
9. Have the equipment and the skills to handle potentially HIV-contaminated body fluids.[2]
10. Carrying a defibrillator is ideal for the doctor attending emergencies: 70% of cardiac arrests occur in the home.

Vital basic skills

1. Rapid intravenous access: direct or cutdown (including 50% Dextrose).
2. Cardiopulmonary resuscitation including upper airway relief, intubation and ventilation, treatment of cardiac arrhythmias and defibrillation.
3. Cricothyroidotomy.
4. Arrest of haemorrhage.
5. Knowledge of usage of common emergency drugs.

When to get up and go

The following symptoms and signs make attendance at the emergency mandatory:

- unconsciousness
- convulsions
- chest pain in an adult, especially associated with pallor and sweating
- pallor and sweating in any patient with pain, collapse or injury
- collapse, especially at toilet

- significant haemorrhage
- breathlessness, including bronchial asthma
- the agitated patient threatening homicide or suicide (take a policeman for company)
- serious accidents
- asthmatic patients

Don't forget the value of oxygen

Ideally, the doctor who attends emergency calls should carry an oxygen delivery unit or at least rely on the simultaneous arrival of an ambulance with resuscitation equipment. Most cases require a high flow rate of 8–10 L/minute.

Typical medical emergencies requiring oxygen:

- bronchial asthma
- acute pulmonary oedema
- acute anaphylaxis
- myocardial infarction
- cardiopulmonary arrest
- collapse

Twelve golden rules

Here are twelve important rules for the diagnostic approach to the emergency call.

1. Always consider the possibility of hypoglycaemia and opioid overdosage in the unconscious patient.
2. Consider intra-abdominal bleeding first and foremost in a patient with abdominal pain who collapses at toilet.
3. Acute chest pain represents myocardial infarction until proved otherwise.
4. Exclude acute epiglottitis in a child with a sudden onset of respiratory distress and pallor.
5. Consider the possibility of a ruptured intra-abdominal viscus in any person, especially a child, with persistent post-traumatic abdominal pain.
6. Always consider the possibility of acute anaphylaxis in patients with a past history of allergies.
7. Always consider the possibility of depression in a postpartum woman presenting with undifferentiated illness or problems in coping with the baby.
8. Always consider ectopic pregnancy in any woman of child-bearing age presenting with acute abdominal pain.
9. If a patient is found cyanosed always consider upper airway obstruction first.

10. Beware of the asthmatic who is cyanosed with a 'silent chest' and tachycardia.
11. Consider ventricular fibrillation or other arrhythmia foremost in an adult with sudden collapse or dizziness.
12. The sudden onset of severe headache adds up to subarachnoid haemorrhage.

Emergencies in the elderly

Elderly patients suffer from their own spectrum of emergency problems. The commonest problems encountered in the author's study[1] were:

- chest pain, especially ischaemic heart disease
- syncope/blackout, e.g. arrhythmias, sudden death, TIAs, CVAs.
- dizziness/giddiness, e.g. arrhythmias, postural hypotension
- dyspnoea, e.g. acute cardiac failure, asthma
- abdominal pain, e.g. biliary colic, bowel obstruction

Special problems in the elderly include:

- fractures from falls, e.g. neck of femur, radius, humerus
- cerebrovascular accidents
- ruptured aneurysms
- problems of dementia and delirium
- abdominal colic syndromes, e.g. renal colic, biliary colic

Important medical emergencies in adults

This section includes summarised protocols for management of emergencies.

Acute anaphylaxis and anaphylactic reactions

Common causes: bee stings, wasp stings, other bites, parenteral antibiotics especially penicillin

Other causes: allergic extracts, blood products, antivenom, radiological contact materials, anaesthetic agents

Note: The early danger symptom is itching of the palms of hands and soles of the feet.

Differential diagnosis: syncope
  Refer to the adult anaphylaxis kit on page 1037.

First-line treatment

- oxygen 6–8 L/min (by face mask)
- adrenaline 0.3–0.5 mg (1:1000) SC or IM (if more severe) best given in upper body, e.g. deltoid (mg = mL of 1:1000 adrenaline)

If no rapid improvement
  adrenaline 1 in 10 000: (dilute 1 mL 1:1000 in 9 mL saline)
  5–10 mL IV over 2–5 minutes

Repeat adrenaline every 10 minutes as necessary (IM or IV)

- insert IV line and infuse
  colloid solution, e.g. Haemaccel (500 mL → 1 L)
      or
  crystalloid solution, e.g. N saline (1.5 L → 3 L)
  1 part colloid = 3 parts crystalloid (by volume)
- salbutamol aerosol inhalation (or nebulisation if severe)
- promethazine 10 mg IV slowly (or 25 mg IM)
      or
  diphenydramine 10 mg IV (or 25 mg IM)
- admit to hospital (observe at least 4 hours)

> **If not responding**

Continue adrenaline every 10 minutes:

- hydrocortisone 500 mg IV (takes 3 hours to be effective)
- establish airway (oral airway or endotracheal intubation) if required

Angioedema and acute urticaria

Acute uticaria and angioedema are essentially anaphylaxis limited to the skin, subcutaneous tissues and other specific organs. They can occur together.

Treatment

Uncomplicated cutaneous swelling—antihistamines
  e.g. diphenhydramine or promethazine 50 mg (o) or 25 mg IM if more severe
Upper respiratory involvement
  — adrenaline 0.3 mg SC
  — antihistamine IM

Acute pulmonary oedema

- keep the patient propped up in bed
- oxygen by mask or intranasally (6 L/min)
- insert IV line
- morphine 1 mg/min IV (slowly up to 5–10 mg) + metoclopramide 10 mg IV
- frusemide 20 mg IV, increasing to 80 mg IV as necessary
- glyceryl trinitrate (nitroglycerin) 300–600 μg sublingual. Can use IV nitrates in preference to morphine
- venesection (if desperate)

Give digoxin if rapid atrial fibrillation and patient not already taking it.

An intravenous infusion of glyceryl trinitrate is superceding morphine use.

Note: keep in mind underlying cause
e.g. myocardial infarction (? silent)
arrhythmia
cardiomyopathy
anaemia

Status asthmaticus

Status asthmaticus is a life-threatening condition that is resistant to standard treatment. It requires intensive medication because of marked obstruction to the air passages, due to severe smooth muscle spasm and inflammation, producing mucosal oedema and mucous impaction.

Initial treatment

• oxygen 8 L/min by mask
• continuous nebulised 0.5% salbutamol (or terbutaline) by face mask, using compressed (8 L/min) oxygen for nebulisation

Note: can use salbutamol with ipratropium (0.025%)—2 mL of each with 4 mL saline, usually for second nebulisation

• insert IV line
• hydrocortisone 4 mg/kg (e.g. 200–250 mg) IV statim

If no response in 30 minutes (or deterioration):
• chest X-ray to exclude complications
• arterial blood gases/pulse oximetry
• IV administration of
salbutamol 200–400 μg (over 2 min) statim

or

adrenaline 1:10 000 IV (1 mL over 30 seconds)   if on monitor
then
IV infusion of
salbutamol 7.5 μg/kg/hr
hydrocortisone

Note: Aminophylline 250 mg over 5 minutes can be given as a loading dose (if patient not taking prior oral theophylline, if failing to respond and on a cardiac monitor).

If not responding, exhausted and moribund:
• intubation with IPPV
• hydration with IV fluids

Consider isoflurane or halothane inhalation to 'break' bronchospasm.

Hypoglycaemia

• 50% dextrose 20–50 mL IV
(if IV line difficult, administer rectally by pressing the nozzle of a large syringe into the anus and injecting slowly)
or
glucagon 1 mL IM
then oral glucose

Myocardial infarction

Refer to page 352.
First-line management:
• arrange ambulance and hospitalisation
• oxygen (face mask) 6 L/min
• insert IV line
• glyceryl trinitrate (nitroglycerin) 300 μg (½ tab) SL, or spray
• aspirin 300 mg (1 tab)
• morphine 1 mg per minute IV
until pain relief (up to 15 mg)
± metoclopramide 10 mg IV for vomiting

Note: Avoid IM injections.

Hyperventilation

Rebreathe slowly from a paper (not plastic) bag
or
Into cupped hands

Status epilepticus and serial seizures

Status epilepticus = repeated convulsions
without regaining
consciousness after
initial tonic-clonic seizure
Serial seizures = repeated convulsions
after regaining
consciousness

Management

• ensure adequate oxygenation: attend to airway (e.g. Guedel tube); give oxygen 8 L/min
• diazepam 0.05 mg/kg/minute IV until the seizures cease or respiratory depression begins (beware of respiratory depression and other vital parameters)

or

• clonazepam 1 mg IV statim then 0.5–1 mg/min IV until seizures cease or respiratory depression begins

or

• phenytoin 1000 mg IV over 20–30 min

or

• midazolam 0.05–0.1 mg/kg IV (max. 10–15 mg)
or 0.15 mg/kg IM

Other drugs to consider:
• phenobarbitone; thiopentone; paraldehyde; valproate (can use rectally)

Bites and stings

Bites and stings from animals, spiders and insects are commonplace in Australia and the United States but fatal bites are uncommon.

Snake bites

Snake bites are more common and severe in those handling snakes and in those trying to kill the snake. Snakes are more aggressive when mating or sloughing their skin (about four times a year). They strike for one-third of their length at 3.5 metres/second. Over 70% of bites are on the legs.

First aid

1. Keep the patient as still as possible.
2. Do not wash, cut, manipulate the wound, apply ice or use a tourniquet.
3. Immediately bandage the bite site very firmly (not too tight). A 15 cm crepe bandage is ideal: it should extend above the bite site for 15 cm, e.g. if bitten around the ankle the bandage should cover the leg to the knee.
4. Splint the limb to immobilise it: a firm stick or slab of wood would be ideal.
5. Transport to a medical facility for definitive treatment. Do not give alcoholic beverages or stimulants.
6. If possible, the dead snake should be brought along.

Note: A venom detection kit is used to examine a swab of the bitten area or a fresh urine specimen (the best) or blood.

The bandage can be removed when the patient is safely under medical observation. Observe for symptoms and signs of envenomation.

Envenomation

Not all patients become envenomated and the antivenom should not be given unless there is evidence of this. Envenomation is more likely when the snake has a clear bite, such as in snake handlers or barefooted people or hands placed in burrows.

Important early symptoms of snake bite envenomation include:
• nausea and vomiting (a reliable early symptom)
• abdominal pain

• excessive perspiration
• severe headache
• blurred vision
• difficulty speaking or swallowing
• coagulation defects, e.g. haematuria
• tender lymphadenopathy

Refer to Figure 114.1 for detailed effects.

Investigations and observation
• venom detection kit: wound site (best) or urine
• careful observations, e.g. vital signs, conscious state
• test all urine for blood and protein
• watch for coagulopathy, e.g. spitting and coughing blood, bleeding from wounds/IV site, haematuria
• serial whole blood clotting time (a plain glass tube): normal < 5–8 min, > 15 min significant
• coagulation screen

Treatment of envenomation
• reassure patient at all times
• set up a slow IV infusion of N saline
• give IV antihistamine cover (15 min beforehand) and 0.3 mL adrenaline 1:1000 SC (0.1 mL for a child)
• dilute the specific antivenom (1 in 10 in N saline) and infuse slowly over 30 min via the tubing of the saline solution
• have adrenaline, oxygen and steroids on standby
• monitor vital signs
• provide basic life support as necessary

Note 1: The use of prophylactic adrenaline is controversial and some authorities reserve it for a reaction to the antivenom. It is best avoided with brown snake envenomation and with coagulopathy.

Note 2: Do not give antivenom unless clinical signs of envenomation or biochemical signs, e.g. positive urine, or abnormal clotting profile.

Note 3: 1 ampoule may be sufficient but 3 or more may be needed, especially if coagulopathy

Spider bites

The toxin of most species of spider causes only localised pain, redness and swelling, but the toxin of some, notably the deadly Sydney funnel-web spider (*Atrax robustus*), can be rapidly fatal.

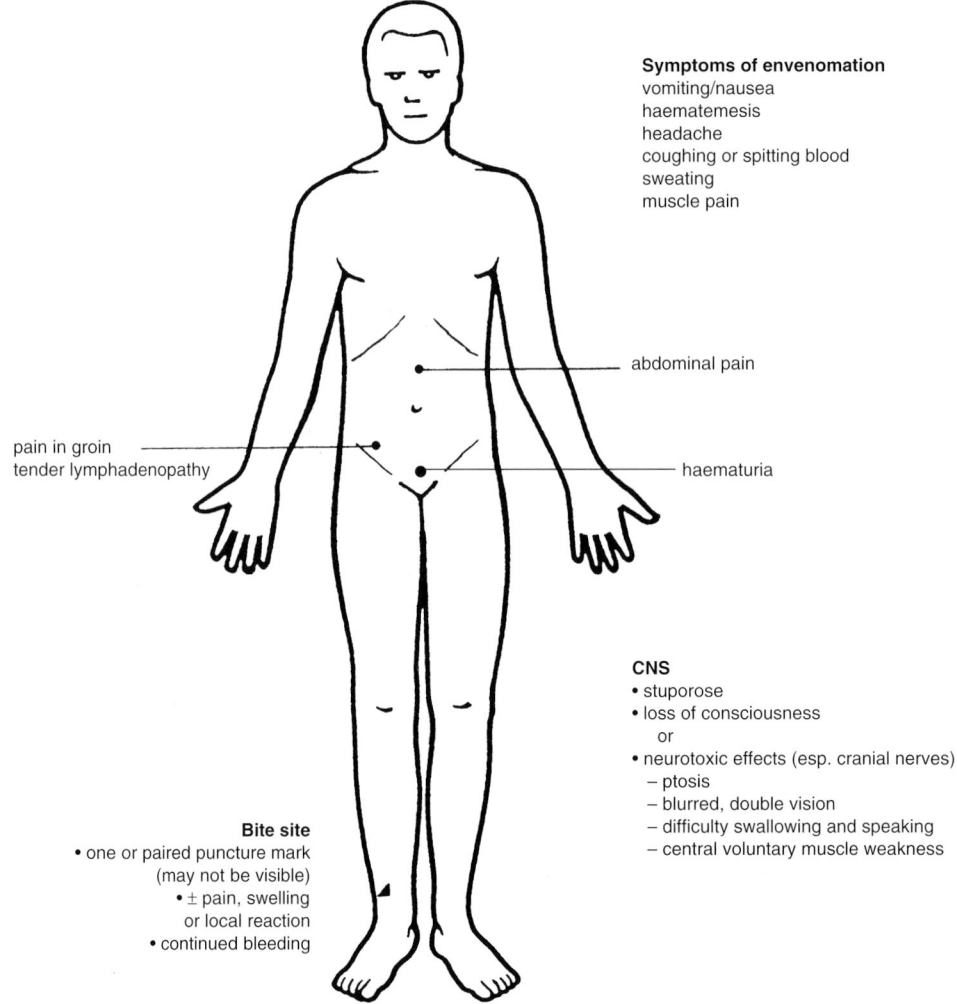

Symptoms of envenomation
vomiting/nausea
haematemesis
headache
coughing or spitting blood
sweating
muscle pain

abdominal pain

pain in groin
tender lymphadenopathy

haematuria

CNS
• stuporose
• loss of consciousness
  or
• neurotoxic effects (esp. cranial nerves)
  – ptosis
  – blurred, double vision
  – difficulty swallowing and speaking
  – central voluntary muscle weakness

Bite site
• one or paired puncture mark
  (may not be visible)
• ± pain, swelling
  or local reaction
• continued bleeding

NB: The greatest danger is respiratory obstruction and failure

Fig. 114.1 *How to recognise snake bite envenomation*

First aid
Sydney funnel-web: as for snake bites.
Other spiders: apply an ice pack, do not bandage.

Treatment

1. | *Sydney funnel-web* |

   Signs of envenomation (in order):
   • muscle fasciculation—limb → tongue/lip
   • marked salivation or lacrimation
   • piloerection
   • dyspnoea
   • neurological symptoms, e.g. disorientation, coma

Treatment — specific antivenom
    — resuscitation and other supportive measures

2. | *Other spider bites* |

   The toxins of most species of spiders cause only localised symptoms but the venom of a selected few, namely the red-back spider of Australia (*Latrodectus mactans hasseltii*) and its related black widow spider (*Latrodectus mactus*), can cause envenomation. This is rarely fatal but is more serious in the young, the frail and the elderly. The clinical features of envenomation are presented in Figure 114.2.

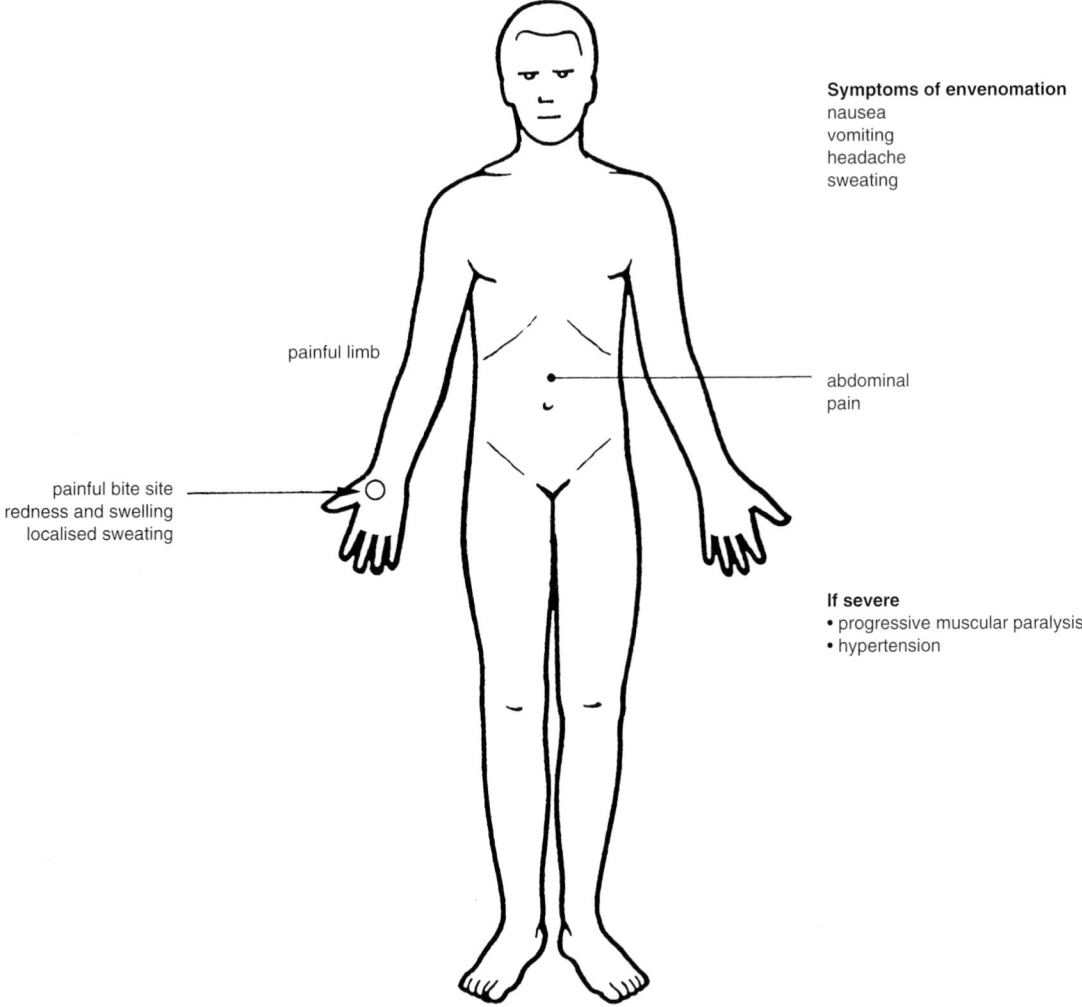

Symptoms of envenomation
nausea
vomiting
headache
sweating

painful limb

abdominal
pain

painful bite site
redness and swelling
localised sweating

If severe
• progressive muscular paralysis
• hypertension

Fig. 114.2 *How to recognise* Latrodectus mactus *envenomation*

Treatment of envenomation (rarely needed)
— give antihistamine, e.g. IM
— antivenom IM injection 15 min later

Bee stings

First aid

1. Scrape the sting off sideways with a fingernail or knife blade. Do not squeeze it with the fingertips.
2. Apply 20% aluminium sulphate solution (Stingose) or methylated spirits.
3. Apply ice to the site.
4. Rest and elevate the limb that has been stung.

If anaphylaxis, treat as outlined earlier.

Preventive measures (if hypersensitive)

• Avoid bees (and wasps) if possible.
• Immunotherapy to honey bee (or wasp venom). There is no cross-allergy between the honey bee, the 'yellow jacket wasp' and the paper wasp. Specific hyposensitisation against the Vespula species is required. For the bee use pure venom antigen.
• Immunotherapy should be offered to those:
— with a history of asthma who have had a single severe reaction to a bee sting
— who have had a minimum of three stings with serial crescendo reactions
— occupationally exposed who manifest severe reactions

— with elevated venom-specific IgE (RAST) antibodies, or positive venom prick tests

Centipede and scorpion bites

The main symptom is pain, which can be very severe and prolonged.

First aid

1. Apply local heat, e.g. hot water with ammonia (household bleach)
2. Clean site.
3. Local anaesthetic, e.g. 1–2 mL of 1% lignocaine infiltrated around the site.
4. Check tetanus immunisation status.

Box jellyfish or sea wasp (Chironex fleckeri)

This is the most dangerous jellyfish in Australian waters and has been responsible for at least 80 extremely painful and sudden deaths.[3] Death can occur in minutes due to cardiopulmonary failure. The jellyfish is limited to tropical waters north of the Tropic of Capricorn and is found in coastal waters during the summer.

Prevention

• Avoid swimming, paddling and wading in 'jellyfish alert' areas in unsafe months.
• Otherwise, use a 'stinger suit'.

Treatment

• The victim should be removed from the water to prevent drowning.
• Inactivate the tentacles by pouring vinegar over them for 30 seconds (do not use alcohol)—use up to 2 litres of vinegar at a time.
• Check respiration and the pulse.
• Start immediate cardiopulmonary resuscitation.
• Give box jellyfish antivenom IM or by IV injection.
• Provide pain relief if required (ice, lignocaine and analgesics).

Stinging fish

The sharp spines of the stinging fish have venom glands which can produce severe pain if they spike or even graze the skin. The best known of these is the stonefish. The toxin is usually heat-sensitive.

Envenomation

• intense pain
• localised swelling
• bluish discolouration

Treatment

• Clean the wound.
• Bathe or immerse the affected part in very warm to hot (not scalding) water—this may give instant relief.[3]
• Give simple analgesics.
• If pain persists, give a local injection/infiltration of lignocaine 1% or even a regional block. If still persisting, try pyridoxine 50 mg intralesional injection.
• A specific antivenom is available for the sting of the stonefish. Can be given IM or IV.

Mollusc bite (blue-ringed octopus, cone shell)

Mollusc venoms can be rapidly fatal because of prolonged muscular weakness leading to respiratory paralysis.

Treatment

• compression bandage to bite site (usually hand/arm)
• immobilise the limb
• arrange transport (preferably by ambulance) to a medical facility
• observe (and manage) for respiratory paralysis—ensure adequate ABC

Sandfly bites

For some reason, possibly the nature of body odour, the use of oral thiamine may prevent sandfly bites.

Dose: thiamine 100 mg orally, daily

Other bites and stings

This includes bites from ants, wasps and some jellyfish.

First aid

1. Wash the site with large quantities of cool water.
2. Apply vinegar (liberal amount) or aluminium sulfate 20% solution (Stingose) to the wound for about 30 seconds.
3. Apply ice for several minutes.
4. Use soothing anti-itch cream or 5% lignocaine cream or ointment if very painful.

Medication is not usually necessary unless an acute allergic reaction develops.

The embedded tick

Some species of ticks can be very dangerous to human beings, especially to children. If they attach themselves to the head or neck, usually behind the ear, a serious problem exists. As it is impossible to distinguish between dangerous and non-dangerous ticks, early removal is mandatory. The tick should be totally removed—and the mouth-parts of the tick must not be left behind. Do not attempt to grab the tick by its body and tug. This is rarely successful in dislodging the tick, and more toxin is thereby injected into the host.

As an office procedure, many practitioners grasp the tick's head as close to the skin as possible with fine forceps or tweezers, and pull the tick out sideways with a sharp rotatory action. This is acceptable, but not as effective as the methods described here.

First aid outdoor removal method
- Saturate the tick with petrol or kerosene and leave for 3 minutes.
- Loop a strong thin thread around the tick's head as close to the skin as possible, and pull sharply with a twisting motion.

Office procedure
- Infiltrate a small amount of LA into the skin around the site of embedment.
- With a number 11 or 15 scalpel blade, make the necessary very small excision, including the mouth-parts of the tick, to ensure total removal (Fig. 114.3).
- The small defect an usually be closed with a bandaid (or Steri-strips).

Human bites and animal bites

These bites can cause problems of suppurative infection and management in general. They are outlined in Chapter 116.

A pot pourri of emergency calls
Electric shock

Useful facts:
- Direct current (DC) from welding machines or lightning produces more electrolyte tissue damage and burns than AC (domestic supply).
- Injuries occur at sites distant from entry or exit.
- Severe muscle contractions can cause bone fracture.
- Household shocks tend to cause cardiac arrest (ventricular fibrillation) and myocardial damage is common.
- Ischaemic necrosis of a limb is a common effect.
- Apparently minor initial injuries may be very misleading (Fig. 114.4).
- Neurological deficits and psychoneurotic sequelae are common in survivors.

Principles of management
- Make the site safe: switch off the electricity. Use dry wool to insulate rescuers.
- 'Treat the clinically dead.'
- Attend to ABC.
- Give a precordial thump in a witnessed arrest.
- Consider a cervical collar (? cervical fracture).

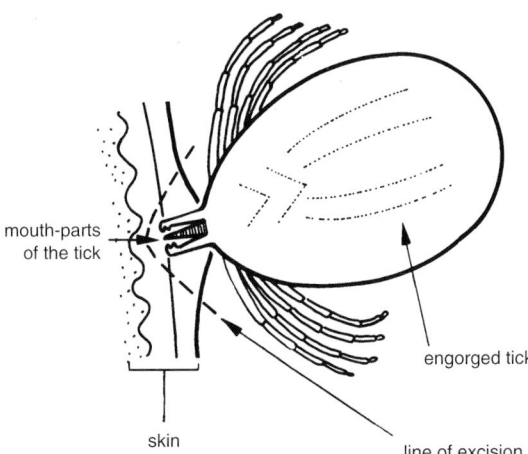

Fig. 114.3 *Removing the embedded tick*

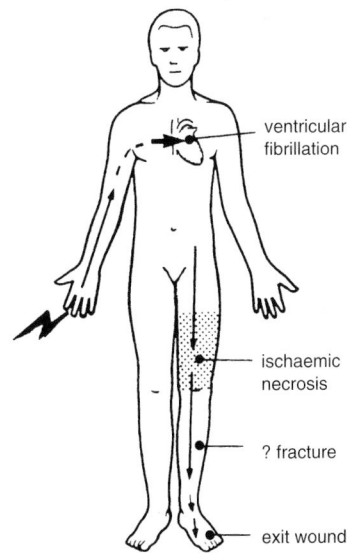

Fig. 114.4 *Effect of electric shock passing through the body*

- Provide basic cardiopulmonary resuscitation, including defibrillation (as required).
- Give a lignocaine infusion (100 mg IV) after cardiac arrest.[4]
- Investigate and consider
  — careful examination of all limbs
  — X-ray of limbs or spine as appropriate
  — check for myoglobinuria and renal failure
  — give tetanus and clostridial prophylaxis
- Get expert help—intensive care unit, burns unit.

Lightning strike

Prevention (during an electrical storm):

- Don't shelter under trees (splash phenomenon—Fig. 114.5).[5]
- Avoid using telephone.
- Avoid holding metal objects, e.g. golf clubs.
- Keep as low to ground as possible.

Clinical effects:

- Burn injury (90%): the 'flashover' phenomenon—clothing disintegrates
- Blast injury, e.g. ruptured spleen, subdural, ruptured eardrum
- Electrical injury as for houshold shock (uncommon)

Fig. 114.5 *'Splash effect' where current is reflected from tree*

Diagnosing the hysterical 'unconscious' patient

One of the most puzzling problems in emergency medicine is how to diagnose the unconscious patient caused by a conversion reaction. These patients really experience their symptoms (as opposed to the pretending patient) and resist most normal stimuli, including painful stimuli.

Method

1. Hold the patient's eye or eyes open with your fingers and note the reaction to light. Now hold a mirror over the eye and watch closely for pupillary reaction. The pupil should constrict with accommodation from the patient looking at his or her own image.

or

2. Hold the patient's fist above the nose and drop it. The 'hysterical' patient will usually just miss hitting the nose.

Petrol sniffing

The three main acute problems:

1. Fitting: give diazepam IV (as for convulsions). May require paraldehyde IM.
2. Agitation/aggressive behaviour: try to calm patient in a well lit room. Give sedation with diazepam. Give haloperidol for hallucinations or delusions.
3. General debilitation: this may include acute infections, e.g. chest infection or anaemia. Investigation and referral for breaking the habit is necessary.

Near drowning

The rule to remember is that victims can respond to resuscitation after considerable immersion time (up to 30 minutes) and that mouth-to-mouth resuscitation should always be attempted even if pulseless or with fixed dilated pupils. The usual routine of basic life support and CPR apply.

Artificial surfactant given via an endotracheal tube has been used successfully in the UK.

There is no significant difference in outcome and management between salt water and fresh water drowning.

Opioid (heroin) overdose

Refer to page 702.

Migraine

Refer to pages 523–524.

Vital emergency skills

Cardiopulmonary resuscitation (CPR)

Cardiopulmonary arrest (CPA). It is essential that all doctors are familiar with the protocol for instituting basic life support in such an eventuality. Sick patients do visit our offices daily and the potential for sudden collapse including a cardiac arrest is ever present. About 75% of arrests are due to ventricular fibrillation and more than 75% of victims have severe coronary artery disease.[6] After three (3) minutes of CPA (unconsciousness, no pulse, no respiration) there is an increasing risk of permanent cerebral dysfunction.

Important causes of sudden death are outlined in Table 114.1.[7]

The ABC basic life support for cardiac arrest should be followed, but ideally DABC is best (defibrillation first if a defibrillator is available—the outcome appears to be directly related to the speed of defibrillation).

Basic life support

The following represents a logical ABC plan for the adult patient who collapses or is found apparently unconscious.

1. Shake and shout at the patient.
2. Check breathing.
3. Check pulse (feel carotid adjacent to thyroid cartilage).
4. Call for help (if no pulse).
5. Finger sweep oropharynx (clear it).

Table 114.1 *Causes of sudden death*

Cardiac arrhythmias
  ventricular fibrillation (75%)
  ventricular tachycardia
  torsade de pointes VT (? drugs)
  sick sinus syndrome
  severe bradycardia

Sudden pump failure
  acute myocardial infarction
  cardiomyopathy

Cardiovascular rupture
  myocardial rupture
  dissecting aneurysm aorta
  subarachnoid haemorrhage

Acute circulatory obstruction
  pulmonary embolism

Others include
  pulmonary hypertension
  mitral valve prolapse
  electrolyte abnormalities
  glue sniffing

6. Place victim on back on firm surface.
7. Thump precordium (if arrest witnessed).
8. Tilt head back (to maximum).
9. Lift chin (use airway if available).
10. Commence basic life support:
    - expired air resuscitation (EAR)—5 quick breaths
    - external chest compression
    - one rescuer: 15 : 2 (compressions/breaths)
                      80 beats/min
    - two rescuers: 5 : 1
                      60 beats/min

The basic schedule for cardiopulmonary resuscitation is presented in Table 114.2 and a flow chart for basic life support in Figure 114.6.

Fig. 114.6 *Algorithm for basic life support: CPR in the collapsed patient*

Table 114.2 *Basic schedule for CPR*

	Infant < 1 year	Child	Adult
Compression (rate per min)	100	80	60
Depth of compression (cm)	1–2	3	4–5
Position of compression	centre sternum	centre sternum	4 cm above xiphisternum
Method	2 fingers	1 hand	2 hands
Ventilation (rate per minute)	20	16	12
Head tilt	Nil	Mid	Full

For optimal airway patency:
1. Clear foreign matter
   • from mouth: use finger sweep
   • from airway: blow between shoulder blades
   • consider a Heimlich manoeuvre
2. Lay patient supine on flat, firm surface (A). Note how the soft tissue of the pharynx can obstruct the airway by falling backwards.

(A)

3. In order to overcome this, apply a heat tilt (B) plus a chin lift (C) or jaw thrust manoeuvre.
   (*Note:* avoid excessive movement of the neck if spinal injury is suspected, but clearing the airway has first priority.)

Slight flexion of the neck with small cushion

Fig. 114.7 *Basic life support: A = Airway*

Method of expired air resuscitation

With the victim's head in the 'sniffing the morning air' position (head totally tilted back and chin pulled forward) the rescuer takes a deep breath and seals his or her lips around the mouth or nose of the victim. Pinch the victim's nose if using mouth-to-mouth resuscitation. Four or five quick full puffs are given within 10 seconds (Figs 114.7 and 114.8). EAR is the only method of artificial respiration that successfully ventilates the patient.[6] If the chest does not move easily, obstruction is present. If available a sucker should be used to clear the oropharynx. Firmly fitting dentures should be left in place as they make artificial respiration easier. A resuscitube or Laerdal pocket mask (which should be in the doctor's bag) is ideal for EAR and saves mouth-to-mouth contact.

External chest compression

Compressions are safely performed by finding the xiphisternal notch then placing the broad heel of one hand over the lower half of the sternum (in adults) with the heel of the second hand placed over the first with the fingers interlocked. Remember to keep the arms and elbows straight as the sternum is rhythmically depressed for 4–5 cm. Try to keep to this position as

Expired air resuscitation:
1. Five full breaths within 10 seconds.
2. Observe rise of chest, not of abdomen.
3. Look, listen and feel for exhalation.
4. Check the carotid pulse.
5. If no pulse, commence full cardiopulmonary resuscitation.

In a two-operator CPR, the person ventilating is best situated on the opposite side of the patient from the person performing chest compression.

Fig. 114.8 *Basic life support: B = Breathing*

1. If carotid or femoral pulse is absent, immediately commence external cardiac compression.
2. See page 1121 for rhythm

(A)

(B)

External cardiac compression with fingers locked (A), and with fingers extended (B). Heel of one hand placed on lower sternum 2 finger-breadths above the xiphoid sternal junction. Heel of second hand placed on first. Ensure fingers don't exert pressure. The patient should be lying on a firm surface, the operator level with shoulder.

Fig. 114.9 Basic life support: C = Circulation

'wandering' causes fractured ribs or worse. The fingers must be kept off the chest.

Maintain the compression for 0.5 second, then relax—compressions should be smooth, regular and uninterrupted.

Check pupil size and reaction to light and the carotid or femoral pulse. The compressions should ideally produce an impulse in the femoral pulse. Another person can check for carotid or femoral pulsation during CPR (Fig. 114.9).

Maintenance of CPR

Consider ceasing CPR if there is no improvement in 30 minutes. Exceptions where prolonged CPR can be successful are cold water drowning, marine envenomation, snake bite, and certain poisonings, e.g. cyanide and organophosphate.

Note: Ventilation of the patient in the first minutes is the key to success especially if a bag and mask are available to perform this. It must not be neglected during basic or advanced cardiorespiratory life support.

Advanced cardiac life support

Advanced life support depends on the availability of skilled personnel and appropriate equipment.

Optimal initial support involves:

• endotracheal intubation (otherwise bag and oxygen)

• ECG monitoring
• intravenous access (large peripheral or central vein)

Optimal initial therapy involves:

• defibrillation
• oxygen
• cardioactive drugs, especially adrenaline

If an ECG recording is unavailable the best course of action is:

• defibrillation
      if unsuccessful
• adrenaline IV

Fig. 114.10 *Standard position of two paddles for defibrillation*

Fig. 114.11 *Protocol for advanced cardiac life support*

Defibrillation

The ideal defibrillator is an automatic machine, e.g. Heartstart, which automatically delivers regulated shocks, e.g. 200J → 200J → 360J over about 1 minute.

For defibrillation, two paddles should be placed correctly on the chest wall, using one of two positions:

- one to right of upper sternum and the other over the apex of the heart (Fig. 114.10 on p. 1123)
- one over anterior wall of chest and the other under tip of left scapula

Hairs on the chest should be shaved to accommodate the paddles.

A protocol for advanced cardiac life support is presented in Fig. 114.11.[8]

Urgent intravenous access

It is preferable to aim for transcutaneous cannulation of veins initially so a peripheral line should be introduced into a vein in the cubital fossa. Several lines may be required with massive blood loss.

Alternative routes:

- central venous cannulation: most doctors should be able to cannulate the external jugular vein with a standard cannula
- peripheral venous cutdown
- intraosseous infusion (see p. 792)

Urgent intravenous cutdown

In emergencies, especially those due to acute blood loss, transcutaneous cannulation for the infusion of fluids or transfusion of blood can be difficult. For the short-term situation, a surgical cutdown into the long saphenous vein at the ankle or the cephalic vein at the wrist is lifesaving. Ideally, the long saphenous vein should be used in children.

Surface anatomy

Long saphenous vein. The vein lies at the anterior tip of the medial malleolus. The best site for incision is centred about 2 cm above and 2 cm anterior to the most prominent medial bony eminence (Fig. 114.12a).

Cephalic vein. The cephalic vein 'bisects' the bony eminences of the distal end of the radius as it winds around the radius from the dorsum of the hand to the anterior surface of the

(a)

(b)

(c)

Fig. 114.12 *Urgent intravenous cutdown:* **(a)** *site of incision over long saphenous vein (medial perspective);* **(b)** *site of incision over cephalic vein at wrist (radial or lateral perspective);* **(c)** *method of introduction of catheter into vein*

forearm. The incision site is 2–3 cm above the tip of the radial styloid (Fig. 114.12b).

Method of cutdown

After fitting gloves and using a skin preparation:

1. Make a 1.5–2 cm transverse skin incision over the vein.

2. Locate the vein by blunt dissection (do not confuse the vein with the pearly white tendons).

3. Loop an aneurysm needle or fine curved artery forceps under and around the vein.

4. Place the ligature around the distal vein and use this to steady the vein.

5. Place a loose knotted ligature over the proximal end of the vein.

6. Incise the vein transversely with a small lancet or scissors or by a carefully controlled stab with a scalpel.

7. Use a vein elevator (if available) for the best possible access to the vein.

8. Insert a catheter (Fig. 114.12c); use 14 or 16 g.

9. Gently tie the proximal vein to the catheter.

10. After connecting to the intravenous set and checking the flow of fluid, close the wound with a suitable suture material.

References

1. Murtagh J. The anatomy of a rural practice. Aust Fam Physician, 1981; 10:564–567.

2. Hogan C. The management of emergencies in general practice. Aust Fam Physician, 1989; 19:1211–1219.

3. Sutherland SK. Venomous bites and stings. In: MIMS Disease Index (2nd edn). Sydney: IMS Publishing, 1996, 563–567.

4. Walpole BG. Electric shock. Aust Fam Physician, 1989; 18:1252–1258.

5. Crocker B, Thomson S. Lightning injuries. Patient Management, Nov. 1991; 51–55.

6. Kumer PJ, Clarke MC. *Clinical medicine* (2nd edn). London: Bailliere Tindall, 1990, 541.

7. Schroeder SA. *Current medical diagnosis and treatment*. East Norwalk: Appleton & Lange, 1990, 280.

8. Young S. Cardiopulmonary resuscitation in VMPF. Emergency management—in the first hour, Course Proceedings, 1991, 8–9.

115

Stroke and transient ischaemic attacks

—

A mild attack of apoplexy may be called death's retaining fee.

Giles Menage (1613–92)

Definitions

A *stroke* is a focal neurological deficit lasting longer than 24 hours and is caused by intra-cerebral haemorrhage or infarction.

A *transient cerebral ischaemic attack (TIA)* is a focal neurological deficit due to cerebral ischae-mia, lasting less than 24 hours.

A *stroke in evolution* is an enlarging neurolog-ical deficit, presumably due to infarction, which increases over 24–48 hours.

Key checkpoints

- A stroke or TIA must be considered a medical emergency.
- Clinical assessment, investigations and treat-ment should be commenced quickly.
- The best approach to stroke management is aggressive attention to primary and secondary prevention.
- The main risk factors for stroke are atrial fibril-lation, hypertension, smoking, age and diabetes.
- Cardiac disease is now a more recognised source of emboli.
- Consider the possibility of a patent foramen ovale (in 20% population) in relatively young people presenting with a stroke: this leads to paradoxical emboli (from veins to the brain).
- Consider the possibility of endocarditis if there is a heart murmur.
- Order a CT scan on all patients with suspected TIAs and strokes (if not referring to a stroke

unit): if normal repeat in 7–10 days. (MRI may replace the CT scan.)
- Keep in mind athersclerotic disease of aortic arch as a source of cerebral embolism.

Modifiable risk factors for cerebrovascular disease[1]

Major: hypertension, smoking, cardiovascu-lar disease, atrial fibrillation (esp. valvular AF), diabetes

Others: cardiac failure, dyslipidaemia, obesity, alcohol excess, oral contra-ception, migraine, stress

Control of risk factors is the key approach to management. Control of hypertension, including systolic hypertension in the elderly, and smoking cessation are vital factors for reduction of the incidence of stroke. Studies have shown that a reduction of blood pressure of 14/8 mmHg is associated with about 50% reduction in stroke incidence.[1]

Stroke

Interesting facts[2]

- Stroke is the third most common cause of death in Australia.
- About one-third of victims will die within one month.
- About 50% of ischaemic strokes are preceded by TIAs.
- Thromboembolism from vascular disease outside the brain causes 70% of strokes and 90% of TIAs.
- Such sources are atheromatous plaques within the carotid or vertebral systems or cardiac causes, e.g. postmyocardial infarction.

- Echocardiography is an important investigation with TIAs since LV dysfunction and the size of the left atrium are the strongest independent predictors of thromboembolism.

Pathophysiological groups of cerebral infarction

The three main groups are:
- single penetrator or small vessel disease (lacunar syndrome)—probably due to *in situ* small vessel disease
- cardioemboli
- large vessel artery to artery embolic infarcts (Table 115.1)

Diagnostic guidelines

- Sudden stroke is typical of embolism.
- The clinical picture depends on the vessel involved.
- In young people <50 years consider patent foramen ovale.
- With cerebral haemorrhage the stroke evolves steadily, often over hours: the putamen (50%) is the commonest site.
- Lacunar CVAs — small deep infarcts
  - pure motor hemiplegia most common effect
  - lack of cortical signs
  - the neurological deficit may progress over 24–36 hours
  - outcome usually good
- Investigate all, including subarachnoid haemorrhage (SAH), with CT scans (may need a lumbar puncture for SAH diagnosis).
- Carotid duplex scan can accurately determine atherosclerotic narrowing of the extracranial carotid circulation.

Pitfalls

- mistaking visual or sensory migraine equivalents in young adults for TIAs

Table 115.1 *Types and incidence of stroke*[2]

Stroke subtype		Frequency (%)
Haemorrhage		
• primary intracerebral		10
• subarachnoid		5
Cerebral infarction		85
• single penetrator (lacunar)	20%	
• cardioembolic	40%	
• large vessel (artery to artery)	40%	
	Total	100

- mistaking a CVA for labyrinthitis (rare over 50 years)
- failure to perform carotid duplex scan before starting aspirin for TIA or small stroke (because of missing small haemorrhage, unsuspected tumour or a subdural)
- diagnosing small stroke as a lacune (may be a stroke in evolution)

Management

Immediate

- Stabilise ventilation—consider intubation and oxygen.
- Exclude head trauma.
- Obtain urgent CT or MRI scan.
- Treat any seizures.
- Treat any hypoglycaemia.

General

- Carry out investigations, including carotid duplex scan.
- Treat hypertension (if appropriate) and other risk factors.
- Give IV fluid, electrolyte and nutritional support (nil orally until swallowing has been assessed).
- Good nursing care is the cornerstone of management.
- Physiotherapy and speech therapy.
- Vigorous rehabilitation.
- Intracerebral haemorrhage: consider urgent surgical evacuation for haematomas of the posterior fossa (cerebellum) and cerebral white matter. Shunt insertion may be needed. No medical therapy is of proven value.
- SAH: requires urgent referral (vasospasm and rebleeding are the main causes of morbidity and mortality):
  nimodipine ± surgery
- Infarction: early intervention within 3 (ideally) to 6 hours of onset with tissue plasminogen activator (rtPA) is currently under investigation, as are cytoprotective agents. Recent trials indicate improved outcomes with rtPA (but not with streptokinase). However, there appears to be a 5–7% risk of intracerebral haemorrhage.[1]

Transient ischaemic attacks
Features

- sudden onset
- complete clinical recovery in less than 24 hours

- average duration is 5 minutes
- consciousness usually preserved
- 90% usually in anterior circulation
- carotid TIAs—unilateral features
- vertebrobasilar TIAs—often have bilateral or crossed features

A comparison of the main clinical features of carotid (anterior circulation) ischaemia and vertebrobasilar (posterior circulation) ischaemia is presented in Figure 115.1. The carotid circulation accounts for 80% of TIAs.

Differential diagnoses of TIAs are presented in Table 115.2.

Some ischaemic syndromes
- transient monocular blindness (amaurosis fugax)
- transient hemisphere attacks
- the 'locked in' syndrome
- vertebrobasilar, e.g.
  — bilateral motor loss
  — crossed sensory and motor loss
  — diplopia
  — bilateral blurring or blindness

Amaurosis fugax
This is the sudden transient loss of vision in one eye (like a 'curtain or shade' coming from above or below) due to the passage of an embolus through the retinal vessels. It is a feature of a TIA in the carotid artery circulation and is often the first clinical evidence of carotid stenosis.[3] About 20%

Table 115.2 *Differential diagnosis of TIAs*

- Classic migraine (with aura)
- Unusual migraine variants
  - e.g.   hemiplegic
          ophthalmoplegic
          retinal
- Focal epileptic seizures
  - e.g.   complex partial
          simple partial
- Multiple sclerosis
- Transient global amnesia
- Intracranial structural lesions
  - e.g.   anteriovenous malformation
          tumour
- Vestibular disorders
  - e.g.   acute labyrinthitis
- Benign paroxysmal positional vertigo
- Ménière's syndrome
- Adverse drug reactions
- Toxic reactions
- Peripheral nerve lesions
  - e.g.   carpal tunnel syndrome
          Bell's palsy

of all TIAs present as amaurosis fugax.[4] Amaurosis fugax may forewarn of the development of hemiparesis or blindness and should be considered a matter for urgent attention and rectification.

Transient hemisphere attack (usually middle cerebral artery)
- affects motor or sensory or both
- usually face and arm (more than leg)
- dysphasia common

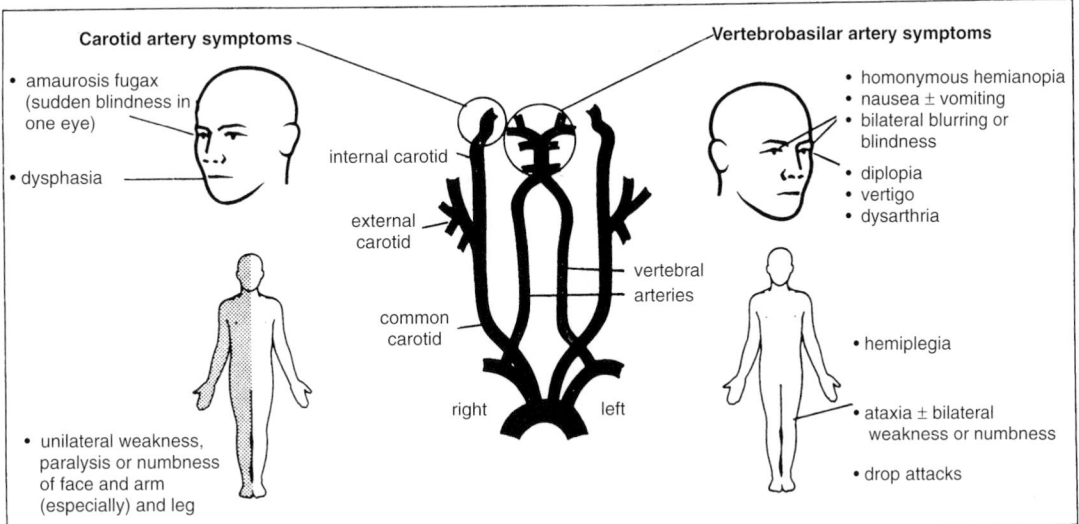

Fig. 115.1 *Cerebral arterial circulation with some important clinical features of carotid and vertebrobasilar ischaemia*
REPRODUCED FROM C. KENNA AND J. MURTAGH, *BACK PAIN AND SPINAL MANIPULATION*, BUTTERWORTHS, SYDNEY, 1989, WITH PERMISSION

The 'locked in' syndrome

In this syndrome, which may be transient or persistent, patients remain conscious and aware of their dilemma but are unable to speak or move the limbs, particularly the arms. It may be possible to communicate with patients using eye responses to commands. The cause is invariably a lesion in the brainstem.

Significance of TIAs

- Five years after a TIA, 22–51% (average 1 in 3) patients (without treatment) will have a stroke.[3,5] This figure may be higher for those with ipsilateral high-grade (70% or more) carotid stenosis.
- The highest risk is in the first 6 months.
- A carotid artery TIA has more serious prognostic significance. Such patients are at high risk of developing a stroke that is potentially preventable.
- Referral for investigation is appropriate.
- All patients should have a carotid duplex and CT scan at presentation.
- Cardiac status should be addressed because of an association with myocardial infarction.

Investigations

- full blood count
- blood glucose, creatinine and cholesterol
- thyroid function tests
- carotid duplex doppler (the investigation of choice)
- ECG
- transoesophageal echocardiography
- CT scan (with contrast)

Treatment

- Aim to minimise the risk of a major stroke.
- Determine cause and correct (if possible).
- Advise cessation of smoking and treat hypertension (if applicable).
- Anti-platelet therapy (especially for carotid ischaemia):

    aspirin 100–300 mg (o) daily (gives 30% protection from stroke or death after TIA)[6]

    or

    ticlopidine 250 mg (o) bd after food if aspirin contraindicated (concern about neutropenia so monitor blood)
- Anticoagulation therapy:

    warfarin — for vertebrobasilar ischaemia (with increasing frequency of TIAs)

    — for failed anti-platelet therapy

    — atrial fibrillation (selected cases) >65 years of age
- Carotid endarterectomy has been proven to have a place in the management of carotid artery stenosis and the decision depends on the expertise of the unit.[7] There is no evidence that surgery is appropriate for the asymptomatic patient with a stenosis <60% or the symptomatic patient with a stenosis less than 30%, but there is a significant benefit for a stenosis greater than 70% (and possibly >60% in asymptomatic patients). If the stenosis is >90% refer immediately.

Atrial fibrillation[1,2]

- the main source of cardioembolic infarction
- increased with risk factors—hypertension, previous embolism and recent CHF (previous 3 months)
- with non-valvular AF, annual risk of CVA is 2.5% (no risk factors) to 17.6% (2+ risk factors)

Management

- valvular disease: warfarin—target INR 2–3
- non-valvular AF — no risk factors: aspirin 100–300 mg/day

    — risk factors: warfarin: INR 2–3

    — if warfarin contraindicated: aspirin

Indications for carotid duplex studies

- bruit in neck
- TIAs
- crescendo TIAs (more frequent and longer lasting)
- vertebrobasilar insufficiency symptoms
- hemispheric stroke
- prior to major vascular surgery, e.g. CABG

When to refer

- consider referral most cases
- suspicion of SAH
- carotid artery stenosis on carotid duplex scan
- cerebellar haemorrhage on CT scan

• stroke in a young patient < 50 years (consider patent foramen ovale and other less common causes)

References

1. Moulds RFW (Chairman). *Therapeutic Guidelines: Neurology*. Melbourne: Therapeutic Guidelines, 1997, 79–85.

2. Donnan G. How to treat: TIA and stroke. Australian Doctor, 16 Sept. 1994; 1–4.

3. Kumar PJ, Clark ML. *Clinical Medicine* (2nd edn). London: Bailliere Tindall, 1990, 907–913.

4. Crimmins DS. How to investigate the patient with TIA. Mod Med Aust, 1995; 38(12):71–74.

5. Joff R. Diagnosis and treatment of transient ischaemic attacks. Mod Med Aust, 1994; 37(8):18–23.

6. Leicester J. Stroke and transient cerebral ischaemic attacks. In: MIMS Disease Index (2nd edn). Sydney: IMS Publishing, 1996, 87–489.

7. Donnan G (Chair). NH&MRC Working Party. Clinical practice guidelines: Prevention of stroke—the role of anticoagulants, antiplatelets and carotid endarterectomy. Consultation document draft 1996.

116

Common skin wounds and foreign bodies

—

The variety of foreign bodies which have found their way into the rectum is hardly less remarkable than the ingenuity displayed in their removal.

A turnip has been delivered PR by the use of obstetric forceps.

A stick firmly impacted has been withdrawn by inserting a gimlet into its lower end.

A tumbler, mouth downwards, has several times been extracted by filling the interior with a wet plaster of Paris bandage, leaving the end of the bandage extruding, and allowing the plaster to set.

Bailey and Love 1943
A short practice of surgery

Injuries to the skin, including simple lacerations, abrasions, contusions and foreign bodies, are among the commonest problems encountered in general practice. To manage these cosmetically important injuries well is one of the really basic and enjoyable skills of our profession.

Key guidelines

- A well-prepared treatment room with good sterilisation facilities, instruments, sterile dressings and an assistant facilitates management.
- With lacerations check carefully for nerve damage, tendon damage and arterial damage.
- Beware of slivers of glass in wounds caused by glass—explore carefully and X-ray (especially with high-resolution ultrasound) if in doubt.
- Beware of electrical or thermal wounds because marked tissue necrosis can be hidden by slightly injured skin.
- Beware also of roller injuries such as car wheels.

- Beware of pressure gun injuries such as oil and paint. The consequences can be disastrous.
- Avoid suturing the tongue, and animal and human bites, unless absolutely necessary.
- Keep drawings or photographs of wounds in your medical records.
- Have a management plan for puncture wounds, including medical needlestick injuries.
- Gravel rash wounds are a special problem because retained fragments of dirt and metal can leave a 'dirty' tattoo-like effect in the healed wound.

Contusions and haematomas

A contusion (bruise or ecchymosis) is the consequence of injury causing bleeding in subcutaneous or deeper tissue while leaving the skin basically intact. It might take weeks to resolve, especially if extensive.

A haematoma is a large collection of extravasated blood that produces an obvious and tender swelling or deformity. The blood usually clots and becomes firm, warm and red; later (about 10 days) it begins to liquify and becomes fluctuant.

Principles of management
- Explanation and reassurance
- RICE (for larger bruises/haematomas) for 48 hours
  R: rest
  I: ice (for 20 minutes every 2 waking hours)
  C: compression (firm elastic bandage)
  E: elevation (if a limb)
- Analgesics: paracetamol/acetaminophen

- Avoid aspiration (some exceptions)
- Avoid massage
- Heat may be applied after 72 hours as local heat or whirlpool baths
- Consider possibility of bleeding disorder if bleeding out of proportion to injury

Problematic haematomas

Some haematoma in certain locations can cause deformity and other problems.

Haematoma of nasal septum[1]

Septal haematoma following injury to the nose can cause total nasal obstruction. It is easily diagnosed as a marked swelling on both sides of the septum when inspected through the nose (Fig. 116.1). It results from haemorrhage between the two sheets of mucoperiosteum covering the septum. It may be associated with a fracture of the nasal septum.

Note: This is a most serious problem as it can develop into a septal abscess. The infection can pass readily to the orbit or the cavernous sinus through thrombosing veins and may prove fatal, especially in children. Otherwise it may lead to necrosis of nasal septal cartilage followed by collapse and nasal deformity.

Treatment
- Remove blood clot through an incision, under local anaesthetic.
- Prescribe systemic (oral) antibiotics, e.g. penicillin or erythromycin.
- Treat as a compound fracture if X-ray reveals a fracture.

Haematoma of the pinna[1]

When trauma to the pinna causes a haematoma between the epidermis and the cartilage, a permanent deformity known as 'cauliflower ear' may result. The haematoma, if left, becomes organised and the normal contour of the ear is lost.

The aim is to evacuate the haematoma as soon as practical and then to prevent it reforming. One can achieve a fair degree of success even on haematomas that have been present for several days.

Method

Under aseptic conditions insert a 25 g needle into the haematoma at its lowest point and aspirate the extravasated blood (Fig. 116.2a). Apply a padded test tube clamp to the haematoma site and leave on for 30–40 minutes (Fig. 116.2b). Generally, daily aspiration and clamping are sufficient to eradicate the haematoma completely.

(a)

(b)

Fig. 116.2 *Treatment of haematoma of the pinna*

Fig. 116.1 *Inferior view of nasal cavity showing bilateral swelling of septal haematoma*

Pretibial haematoma

A haematoma over the tibia (shin bone) can be persistently painful and slow to resolve. An efficient method is, under very strict asepsis, to inject 1 mL lignocaine 1% and 1 mL hyaluronidase and follow with immediate ultrasound. This may disperse or require drainage.

Abrasions

Abrasions vary considerably in degree and potential contamination. They are common with bicycle or motorcycle accidents and skateboard accidents. Special care is needed over joints such as the knee or elbow.

Rules of management

- Clean meticulously, remove all ground-in dirt, metal, clothing and other material.
- Scrub out dirt with sterile normal saline under anaesthesia (local infiltration or general anaesthesia for deep wounds).
- Treat the injury as a burn.
- When clean, apply a protective dressing (some wounds may be left open).
- Use paraffin gauze and non-adhesive absorbent pads such as Melolin.
- Ensure adequate follow-up.
- Immobilise a joint that may be affected by a deep wound.

Lacerations

Lacerations vary enormously in complexity and repairability. Very complex lacerations and those involving nerves or other structures should be referred to an expert.

Principles of repair

- Good approximation of wound edges minimises scar formation and healing time.
- Pay special attention to debridement.
- Avoid deep layers of suture material in a contaminated wound—consider drainage.
- Inspect all wounds carefully for damage to major structures such as nerves and tendons and for foreign material:
  — shattered glass wounds require careful inspection and perhaps X-ray.
  — high-energy wounds, e.g. motor mowers, are prone to have metallic foreign bodies and associated fractures.

- Be ready to take X-rays of wounds to look for foreign objects or fractures (compound fractures).
- Trim jagged or crushed wound edges, especially on the face.
- All wounds should be closed in layers.
- Avoid leaving dead space.
- Do not suture an 'old' wound (greater than 8 hours) if it is contaminated with primary closure: leave 4 days before suturing if not infected.
- Take care in poor healing areas such as backs, necks, calves and knees; and in areas prone to hypertrophic scarring such as over the sternum of the chest and the shoulder.
- Use atraumatic tissue-handling techniques.
- Everted edges heal better than inverted edges.
- Practise minimal handling of wound edges.
- A suture is too tight when it blanches the skin between the thread—it should be loosened.
- Avoid tension on the wound, especially in fingers, lower leg, foot or palm.
- The finest scar and best result is obtained by using a large number of fine sutures rather than a fewer thicker sutures more widely spread.
- Avoid haematoma.
- Apply a firm pressure dressing when appropriate, especially with swollen skin flaps.
- Consider appropriate immobilisation for wounds. Many wound failures are due to lack of immobilisation from a volar slab on the hand or a back slab on the leg.

Practical aspects

Suture material (Table 116.1)
- Monofilament nylon sutures are generally preferred for skin repair.
- Use the smallest calibre compatible with required strains.

Table 116.1 *Selection of suture material (guidelines)*

Skin	nylon 6/0	face
	nylon 3/0	back, scalp
	nylon 5/0	elsewhere
Deeper tissue (dead space)	catgut 4/0	face
	Dexon/Vicryl 3/0 or 4/0	elsewhere
Subcuticular	catgut 4/0	
Small vessel ties	plain catgut 4/0	
Large vessel ties	chromic catgut 4/0	

- The synthetic, absorbable polyglycolic acid or polyglactin sutures (Dexon, Vicryl) are stronger than catgut of the same gauge, but do not use these (use catgut instead) on the face or subcuticularly.

Instruments
Examples of good quality instruments:
- locking needle holder (e.g. Crile-Wood 12 cm)
- skin hooks
- iris scissors

Holding the needle
The needle should be held in its middle; this will help to avoid breakage and distortion, which tend to occur if the needle is held near its end (Fig. 116.3).

Dead space
Dead space should be eliminated to reduce tension on skin sutures. Use buried absorbable sutures to approximate underlying tissue. This is done by starting suture insertion from the fat to pick up the fat/dermis interface so as to bury the knot (Fig. 116.4).

Everted wounds
Eversion is achieved by making the 'bite' in the dermis wider than the bite in the epidermis (skin surface) and making the suture deeper than it is wide. Shown are:
- simple suture (Fig. 116.5a)
- vertical mattress suture (Fig. 116.5b)

The mattress suture is the ideal way to evert a wound.

Number of sutures
One should aim to use a minimum number of sutures to achieve closure without gaps but sufficient sutures to avoid tension. Place the sutures as close to the wound edge as possible.

Special techniques for various wounds
The three-point suture
In wounds with a triangular flap component, it is often difficult to place the apex of the flap accurately. The three-point suture is the best way to achieve this while minimising the chance of strangulation necrosis at the tip of the flap.

Fig. 116.3 *Correct and incorrect methods of holding the needle*

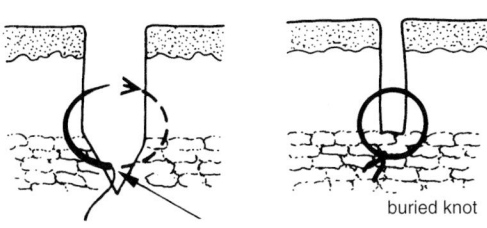

Introduce needle here

Fig. 116.4 *Eliminating dead space*

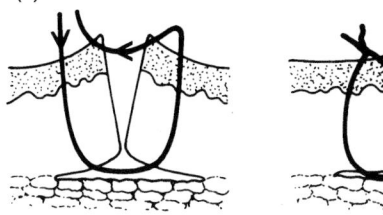

Fig. 116.5 *Everted wounds:* **(a)** *correct and incorrect methods of making a simple suture;* **(b)** *making a vertical mattress suture*

Method

1. Pass the needle through the skin of the non-flap side of the wound.
2. Pass it then through the subcuticular layer of the flap tip at exactly the same level as the reception side.
3. Finally, pass the needle back through the reception side so that it emerges well back from the V flap (Fig. 116.6).

Triangular flap wounds on the lower leg

Triangular flap wounds below the knee are a common injury and are often treated incorrectly. Similar wounds in the upper limb heal rapidly when sutured properly, but lower limb injury will not usually heal at first intention unless the apex of the flap is given special attention.

Proximally based flap

A fall through a gap in flooring boards will produce a proximally based flap; a heavy object (such as the tailboard of a trailer) striking the shin will result in a distally based flap.

Often the apex of the flap is crushed and poorly vascularised; it will not survive to heal after suture.

Treatment methods (under infiltration with LA)

1. Preferred method: To attempt to salvage the distal flap, scrape away the subcutaneous tissue on the flap and use it as a full-thickness graft.
2. An alternative is to excise the apex of the flap, loosely suture the remaining flap and place a small split-thickness graft on the raw area (Fig. 116.7).

For both methods apply a suitable dressing and strap firmly with a crepe bandage. The patient should rest with the leg elevated for three days.

Distally based flap (Fig. 116.8)

This flap, which is quite avascular, has a poorer prognosis. The same methods as for the proximally based flap can be used. Trimming the flap and using it as a full thickness graft has a good chance of repair in a younger person but a poor chance in the elderly.

Repair of cut lip

While small lacerations of the buccal mucosa of the lip can be left safely, more extensive cuts require careful repair. Local anaesthetic infiltration may be adequate, although a mental nerve block is ideal for larger lacerations of the lower lip.

For wounds that cross the vermilion border, meticulous alignment is essential. It may be advisable to premark the vermilion border with gentian violet or a marker pen. It is desirable to have an assistant.

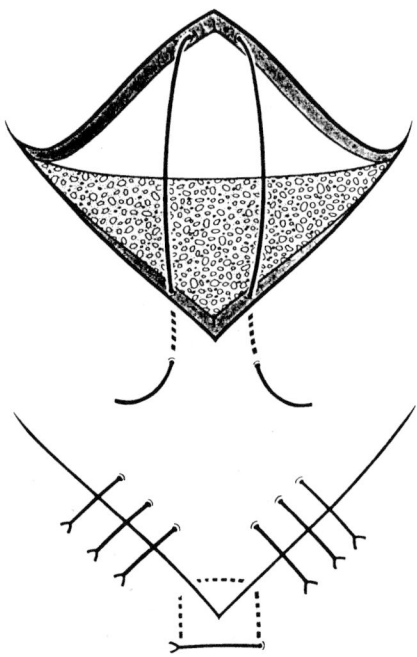

Fig. 116.6 *The three-point suture*

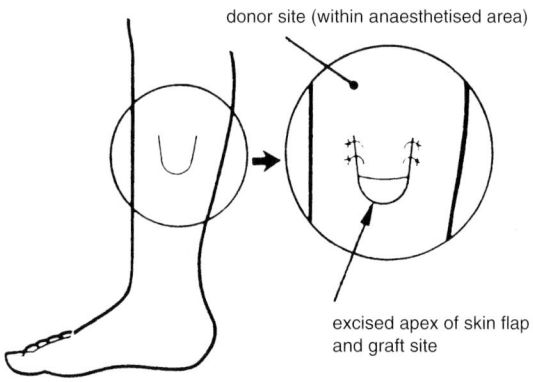

donor site (within anaesthetised area)

excised apex of skin flap and graft site

Fig. 116.7 *Triangular flap wound repair: proximally based flap*

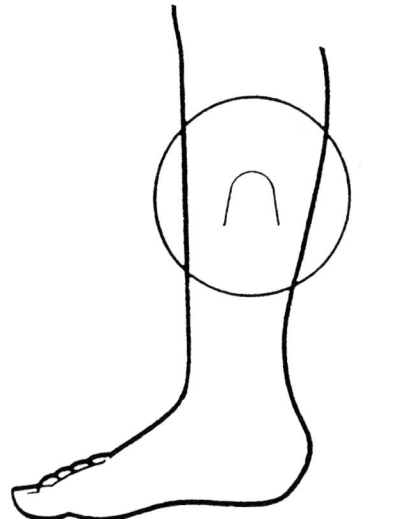

Fig. 116.8 *Triangular flap wound repair: distally based flap*

Method

1. Close the deeper muscular layer of the wound using 4/0 CCG. The first suture should carefully appose the mucosal area of the lip, followed by one or two sutures in the remaining layer.
2. Next, insert a 6/0 monofilament nylon suture to bring both ends of the vermilion border together. The slightest step is unacceptable (Fig. 116.9). This is the key to the procedure.
3. Close the inner buccal mucosa with interrupted 4/0 plain catgut sutures.
4. The outer skin of the lip (above and below the vermilion border) is closed with interrupted nylon sutures.

Post repair

1. Apply a moisturising lotion along the lines of the wound.
2. Remove nylon sutures in 3–4 days (in a young person) and 5–6 days (in an older person).

Repair of lacerated eyelid

General points:

- Preserve as much tissue as possible.
- Do not shave the eyebrow.
- Do not invert hair-bearing skin into the wound.
- Ensure precise alignment of wound margins.
- Tie suture knots away from the eyeball.

Method

1. Place an intermarginal suture behind the eyelashes if the margin is involved.
2. Repair conjunctiva and tarsus with 6/0 catgut.
3. Then repair skin and muscle (orbicularis oculi) with 6/0 nylon (Fig. 116.10).

Repair of tongue wound

Wherever possible, it is best to avoid repair to wounds of the tongue because these heal rapidly. However, large flap wounds to the tongue on the dorsum or the lateral border may require suturing. The best method is to use buried catgut sutures.

Method

1. Get patient to suck ice for a few minutes, then infiltrate with 1% lignocaine LA and leave 5–10 minutes.
2. Use 4/0 or 3/0 catgut sutures to suture the flap to its bed, and bury the sutures (Fig. 116.11).

Fig. 116.9 *The lacerated lip: ensuring meticulous suture of the vermilion border*

Fig. 116.10 *The lacerated eyelid*

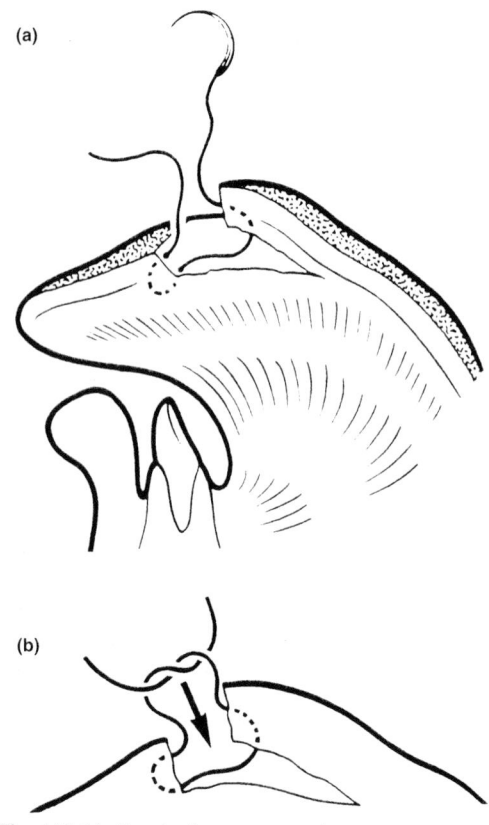

(a)

(b)

Fig. 116.11 *Repair of tongue wound*

It should not be necessary to use surface sutures. If it is, 4/0 silk sutures will suffice.

The patient should be instructed to rinse the mouth regularly with salt water until healing is satisfactory.

The amputated finger

In this emergency situation, instruct the patient to place the severed finger directly into a fluid-tight sterile container, such as a plastic bag or sterile specimen jar. Then place this 'unit' in a bag containing iced water with crushed ice.

Note: Never place the amputated finger directly in ice or in fluid such as saline. Fluid makes the tissue soggy, rendering micro-surgical repair difficult.

Care of the finger stump

Apply a simple, sterile, loose, non-sticky dressing and keep the hand elevated.

Bite wounds

Human bites

Human bites and clenched fist injuries can present a serious problem of infection. Anaerobic organisms in the oral cavity, e.g. Vincent's, can penetrate the damaged tissue and form a deep-seated infection. Streptococcal and staphylococcal organisms are common pathogens. Complications of the infected wounds include cellulitis, wound abscess and lymphangitis.

Principles of treatment
- Clean and debride the wound carefully, e.g. aqueous antiseptic solution or hydrogen peroxide.
- Give prophylactic penicillin if a severe or deep bite.
- Avoid suturing if possible.
- Tetanus toxoid (although minimum risk).
- Consider rare possibility of HIV and hepatitis B or C infections.
- If infected, take a swab, give procaine penicillin 1 g IM and amoxycillin/clavulanate, tds for 5 days.[2]

Dog bites

Non-rabid

Dog bites typically have poor healing and carry a risk of infection with anaerobic organisms, including tetanus, staphylococci and streptococci. Puncture wounds are more prone to infection than laceration.

Principles of treatment
- Clean and debride the wound with aqueous antiseptic, allowing it to soak for 10–20 minutes.
- Aim for open healing—avoid suturing if possible (except in 'privileged' sites with an excellent blood supply such as the face and scalp).
- Apply non-adherent, absorbent dressings (paraffin gauze and Melolin) to absorb the discharge from the wound.
- Tetanus prophylaxis: immunoglobulin or tetanus toxoid.
- Give prophylactic penicillin for a severe or deep bite: 1.5 million units procaine penicillin IM statim, then orally for 5–10 days. Tetracycline or amoxycillin/clavulanate are alternatives.

- Inform the patient that slow healing and scarring are likely.

Rabid or possibly rabid dog (or other animal)

(not currently applicable in Australia)
- Wash the site immediately with detergent or saline (preferable) or hydrogen peroxide or soap (if no other option).
- Do not suture.
- If rabid: human rabies immune globin (passive)
  antirabies vaccine (active)
- Uncertain: capture and observe animal consider vaccination

Cat bites
Cat bites have the greatest potential for suppurative infection. The same principles apply as for the management of human or dog bites, but use erythromycin or doxycycline or cephelexin.[2] It is important to clean a deep and penetrating wound. Another problem is cat-scratch disease, presumably caused by a Gram-negative bacterium, *Bartonella henselae.*

Clinical features of cat-scratch disease
- an infected ulcer or papule pustule at bite site (30% of cases) after three days or so[3]
- 1–3 weeks later: fever, headache, malaise
  regional lymphadenopathy (may suppurate)
- intradermal skin test positive
- benign self-limiting course
- sometimes severe symptoms for weeks, especially in immunocompromised
- treat with erythromycin or roxithromycin[2]

Coral cuts
Wounds from coral cuts are at risk of serious infection with vibrio organisms (marine pathogens) or *Streptococcus pyogenes.* Such wounds require cleaning with antiseptics, debridement, dressing and antibiotic cover with doxycycline 100 mg bd for 7 days.

Scalp lacerations in children
If lacerations are small but gaping use the child's hair for the suture, provided it is long enough.

Method
Make a twisted bunch of the child's own hair on each side of the wound. Tie a reef knot and then an extra holding knot to minimise slipping. Ask an assistant to drop compound benzoin tincture solution (Friar's balsam) on the hair knot. Leave the hair suture long and get the parent to cut the knot in five days.

Forehead and other lacerations in children
Despite the temptation, avoid using reinforced paper adhesive strips (Steri-strips) for children with open wounds. They will merely close the dermis and cause a thin, stretched scar. They can be used only for very superficial epidermal wounds in conjunction with sutures.

Adhesive glue for wound adhesion
A tissue adhesive glue can be used successfully to close superficial smooth and clean skin wounds, particularly in children. An expensive commercial preparation Histoacryl (active ingredient enbucrilate) is available, but Superglue also serves the purpose although sterility and toxicity have to be considered. The glue should be used only for superficial, dry, clean and fresh wounds. No gaps are permissible with this method.

Wound anaesthesia in children
New topical preparations which provide surface anaesthesia are being used for wound repair in children. They include lignocaine and prilocaine mixture (EMLA cream) and adrenaline and cocaine (AC) liquid. Use the latter with caution.

Some practitioners use an ice block to freeze the lacerated site. The child is asked to hold the ice while a suture is rapidly inserted.

Removal of skin sutures
Suture marks are related to the time of retention of the suture, its tension and position. The objective is to remove the sutures as early as possible, as soon as their purpose is achieved. The timing of removal is based on common sense and individual cases. Nylon sutures are less reactive and can be left for longer periods. After suture removal it is advisable to support the wound with micropore skin tape (e.g. Steri-strips) for 1–2 weeks, especially in areas of skin tension.

Method

1. Use good light and have the patient lying comfortably.
2. Use fine, sharp scissors which cut to the point or the tip of a scalpel blade, and a pair of fine, non-toothed dissecting forceps that grip firmly.
3. Cut the suture close to the skin below the knot with scissors or a scalpel tip (Fig. 116.12a).
4. Gently pull the suture out towards the side on which it was divided—that is, *always towards the wound* (Fig. 116.12b).

When to remove non-absorbable sutures

For removal of sutures after non-complicated wound closure in adults, see Table 116.2.

Note: Decisions need to be individualised according to the nature of the wound and health of the patient and healing. In general, take sutures out as soon as possible. One way of achieving this is to remove alternate sutures a day or two earlier and remove the rest at the usual time. Steri-strips can then be used to maintain closure and healing.

Additional aspects

In children, tend to remove 1–2 days earlier. Allow additional time for backs and legs, especially the calf. Nylon sutures can be left longer

Fig. 116.12 *Removal of skin sutures:* **(a)** *cutting the suture;* **(b)** *removal by pulling towards wound*

Table 116.2 *Time after insertion for removal of sutures*

Area	Days later
Scalp	6
Face	3 (or alternate at 2, rest 3–4)
Ear	5
Neck	4 (or alternate at 3, rest 4)
Chest	8
Arm (including hand and fingers)	8–10
Abdomen	8–10 (tension 12–14)
Back	12
Inguinal and scrotal	7
Perineum	2
Legs	10
Knees and calf	12
Foot (including toes)	10–12

because they are less reactive. Alternate sutures may be removed earlier (e.g. face in women).

Foreign bodies
Penetrating gun injuries

Injuries to the body from various types of guns present decision dilemmas for the treating doctor. The following information represents guidelines, including special sources of danger to tissues from various foreign materials discharged by guns.

> Gunshot wounds

Airgun

The rule is to remove subcutaneous slugs but to leave deeper slugs unless they lie within and around vital structures (e.g. the wrist). A special common problem is that of slugs in the orbit. These often do little damage and can be left alone, but referral to an ophthalmologist would be appropriate.

0.22 rifle (the pea rifle)

The same principles of management apply but the bullet must be localised precisely by X-ray. Of particular interest are abdominal wounds, which should be observed carefully, as visceral perforations can occur with minimal initial symptoms and signs.

0.410 shotgun

The pellets from this shotgun are usually only dangerous when penetrating from a close range. Again, the rule is not to remove deep-lying pellets—perhaps only those superficial pellets that can be palpated.

Pressure gun injuries

Injection of grease, oil, paint and similar substances from pressure guns (Fig. 116.13) can cause very serious injuries, requiring decompression and removal of the substances.

Grease gun and paint gun

High-pressure injection of paint or grease into the hand requires urgent surgery if amputation is to be avoided. There is a deceptively minor wound to show for this injury, and after a while the hand feels comfortable. However, ischaemia,[1] chemical irritation and infection can follow, with gangrene of the digits, resulting in, at best, a claw hand due to sclerosis. Treatment is by immediate decompression and meticulous removal of all foreign material and necrotic tissue.

Oil injection

Accidental injection of an inoculum in an oily vehicle into the hand also creates a serious problem with local tissue necrosis. If injected into the digital pulp, this may necessitate amputation. Such injections are common on poultry farms, where many fowl-pest injections are administered.

Splinters under the skin

The splinter under the skin is a common and difficult procedural problem. Instead of using forceps or making a wider excision, use a disposable hypodermic needle to 'spear' the splinter (Fig. 116.14) and then use it as a lever to ease the splinter out through the skin.

Embedded fish hooks

Two methods of removing fish hooks are presented here, both requiring removal in the reverse direction, against the barb. Method 2 is recommended as first-line management.

Method 1

1. Inject 1–2 mL of LA around the fish hook.
2. Grasp the shank of the hook with strong artery forceps.
3. Slide a D11 scalpel blade in along the hook, sharp edge away from the hook, to cut the tissue and free the barb (Fig. 116.15)
4. Withdraw the hook with the forceps.

Method 2

This method, used by some fishermen, relies on a loop of cord or fishing line to forcibly disengage and extract the hook intact. It requires no anaesthesia and no instruments—only nerves of steel, especially for the first attempt.

1. Take a piece of string about 10–12 cm long and make a loop. One end slips around the hook, the other hooking around one finger of the operator.

Fig. 116.13 *Dangerous accidential injections into the hand*

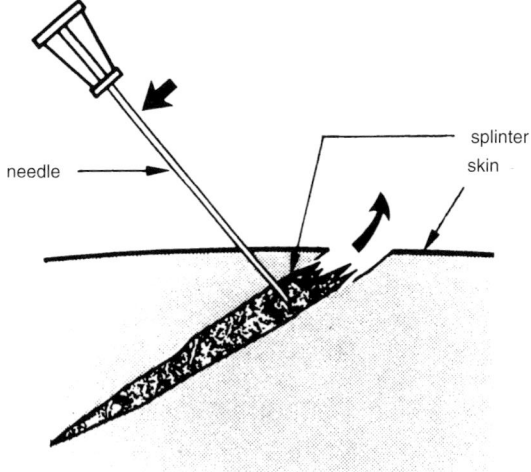

Fig. 116.14 *Removal of splinters in the skin*

Fig. 116.15 *Removal of fish hooks by cutting a path in the skin*

2. Depress the shank with the other hand in the direction that tends to disengage the barb.
3. At this point give a very swift, sharp tug along the cord.
4. The hook flies out painlessly in the direction of the tug (Fig. 116.16).

Note: You must be bold, decisive, confident and quick—half-hearted attempts do not work.

For difficult cases, some local anaesthetic infiltration may be appropriate. Instead of a short loop of cord, a long piece of fishing line double looped around the hook and tugged by the hand, or flicked with a thin ruler in the loop, will work.

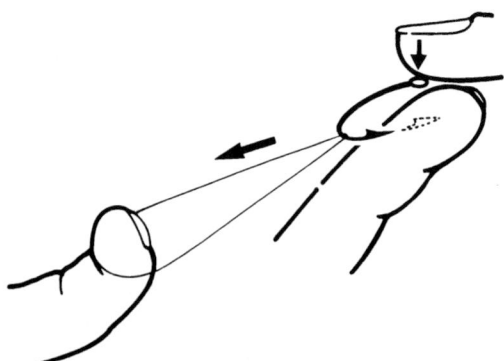

Fig. 116.16 *Fisherman's method of removing a fish hook intact*

Needlesticks and sharps injuries

Accidental skin puncture by contaminated 'sharps', including needles (with blood or blood-stained body fluids), is of great concern to all health care workers. Another problem that occurs occasionally is the deliberate inoculation of people such as police by angry sociopathic individuals. A needlestick accident is the commonest incident with the potential to transmit infections such as HIV and hepatitis B,C or D. The part of the venipuncture that is most likely to cause the accident is the recapping or re-sheathing of the needle. This practice should be discouraged.

Infections transmitted by needlestick accidents are summarised in Table 116.3. The risk from a contaminated patient is greatest with hepatitis (10–30%), while the risk of seroconversion or clinical infection after a needlestick with HIV-positive blood is very low (probably about 1 in 300).[4]

Prevention

- Avoid physically struggling with overdose victims or high-risk patients for lavage or venipuncture.
- Needles should not be recapped.
- Dispose of needles immediately and directly into a leak-proof, puncture-proof sharps container.
- Avoid contact with blood.
- Wear protective gloves (does not prevent sharps injury).

Management

- Squeeze out and wash under running tap water with soap and/or dilute sodium hypochlorite solution, e.g. Milton.
- Encourage bleeding.
- Obtain information about and blood from the sharps victim and the source person (source of body fluid). A known carrier of hepatitis B

Table 116.3 *Infections transmitted by needlestick accidents*

Viruses
Human immunodeficiency virus (HIV)
Hepatitis B,C,D
Herpes simplex
Herpes varicella-zoster
Bacteria
Streptococcal infections
Staphylococcal infections
Syphilis
Tuberculosis
Other
Malaria

surface antigen or an HIV-positive source person will facilitate early decision making.

Note: It takes three months to seroconvert with HIV so the patient may be infected but negative on initial tests.

Known hepatitis B carrier source person
- If injured person immune — no further action
- If non-vaccinated and non-immune
  - give hyperimmune hepatitis B gammaglobulin (within 48 hours)
  - commence course of hepatitis B vaccination

Known HIV-positive source person
Refer to consultant about relative merits of drug prophylaxis and serological monitoring.
Options
    zidovudine (AZT) + 3TC + indinavir prophylaxis within 8 hours,[5] for 6 weeks
        or
    serological monitoring 0,4,6,12,24 and 52 weeks[6]

Unknown risk source person
Take source person's blood (if consent is given) and sharps victim's blood for hepatitis B (HBsAg and anti-HBs) and (if high risk for HIV) HIV status tests. Commence hepatitis B vaccination if not vaccinated.

Note: Informed consent for testing and disclosure of test results for involved person should be obtained.

Tetanus prophylaxis

Tetanus is a very serious disease but completely preventable by active immunisation. Protection should be universal, especially if the childhood immunisation program is followed. However, all patients with wounds should be assessed for their tetanus status and managed on their merits. For severe wounds the possibility of gas gangrene should also be considered.

   Tetanus-prone wounds:
- compound fractures
- penetrating injuries
- foreign bodies
- extensive crushing
- delayed debridement
- severe burns
- pyogenic infection

For the primary immunisation of adults, tetanus toxoid (singly or combined with diphtheria if primary childhood course not given) is given as two doses 6 weeks apart with a third dose 6 months later. Booster doses of tetanus toxoid are given every 10 years or at the time of major injury occurring 5 years after previous dose.

Passive immunisation
Passive immunisation, in the form of tetanus immune globulin 250 units by IM injection, is reserved for non-immunised individuals or those of uncertain immunity wherever the wound is contaminated or has devitalised tissue. Wounds at risk include those contaminated with dirt, faeces/manure, soil, saliva or other foreign material; puncture wounds; wounds from missiles, crushes and burns.

The guide is outlined in Table 116.4.

Practice tips
- Have the patient lying down for suturing and parents of children sitting down.
- Avoid using antibiotic sprays and powders in

Table 116.4   *Guide to tetanus prophylaxis in wound management*

History of active tetanus immunisation	Clean, minor wounds		All other wounds	
	Tetanus toxoid	Tetanus immune globulin	Tetanus toxoid[1]	Tetanus immune globulin
Uncertain, or less than 3 doses	yes	no	yes	yes
3 doses or more	no[2]	no	no[3]	no[4]

1. Adult or child 8 years and over—use tetanus toxoid or ADT. Child 7 years or less, use tetanus toxoid or CDT or DTP (if due, on routine immunisation schedule).
2. Yes, if more than 10 years since last dose.
3. Yes, if more than 5 years since last dose.
4. Yes, if more than 10 years since last dose and tetanus-prone wound.

simple wounds—resistant organisms can develop.

- Consider tetanus and gas gangrene prophylaxis in contaminated and deep necrotic wounds.
- Give a tetanus booster if patient has not had one within 5 years for dirty wounds or within 10 years with clean wounds.
- Give tetanus immune globulin if patient is not immunised or if the wound is grossly contaminated.
- Never send patients home before thoroughly washing their hair and carefully examining for other lacerations.
- Any laceration in the cheek, mandible or lower eyelid may damage the facial nerve, parotid duct or lacrimal duct respectively.
- When a patient falls onto glass it takes bone to halt its cutting path. Assume all structures between skin and bone are severed.

References

1. Hansen G. *Practice tips.* Aust Fam Physician, 1982; 11:867.

2. Mashford L. *Antibiotic guidelines* (9th edn). Victorian Medical Postgraduate Foundation, 1996–97; 143–151.

3. Tierney LM et al. *Current medical diagnosis and treatment.* East Norwalk: Appleton and Lange, 1996, 1119–1120.

4. Spelman D. Transmission of infection by needlesticks, sharps and splashes. Aust Fam Physician, 1988; 17:681.

5. Gerberding JL. Drug therapy: management of occupational exposures to blood-borne viruses. N Engl J Med, 1995; 332:444.

6. Hammond L. AIDS and hepatitis B protection strategies. Aust Fam Physician, 1990; 19:657–661.

117

Common fractures and dislocations

—

The broken bone, once set together, is stronger than ever.

John Lyly (1554–1606)

Common fractures and dislocations usually apply to the limbs, the shoulder girdle and the pelvic girdle and their management requires an early diagnosis to ensure optimum treatment and to prevent complications. Early diagnosis depends on the physician being vigilant and on having knowledge of the less common conditions so that a careful search for the diagnosis can be made.

The diagnosis is dependent on a good history followed by a careful examination, good-quality X-rays appropriate to the injury (e.g. stress view) and, if necessary, special investigations. The golden rule is: if in doubt—X-ray. The family doctor should develop the habit of looking at a patient's X-rays. Such a back-up to the radiologist's report can help avoid missed diagnoses.

There are many pitfalls involved in managing fractures and dislocations. Many injuries, such as fractures of the arm and hand, seem trivial but they can lead to long-term disability. This chapter presents guidelines to help avoid these pitfalls.

General guidelines

- A fracture usually causes deformity but may cause nothing more than local tenderness over the bone, e.g. scaphoid fracture, impacted fractured neck of femur.
- The classic signs of fracture are:
  — pain
  — tenderness
  — loss of function
  — deformity
  — swelling/bruising
  — crepitus
- X-ray examination of the affected area of the upper limb should include views of joints proximal or distal to the site of the injury, and X-rays in both AP and lateral planes.
- If an X-ray is reported as normal but a fracture is strongly suspected, an option is to splint the affected limb for about 10 days and then repeat the X-ray.
- As a rule, displaced fractures must be reduced whereby bone ends should be placed in proper alignment and then immobilised until union occurs.
- Fractures should be monitored radiologically for loss of position, particularly in the first 1–2 weeks following reduction.
- Bone union is assessed clinically by reduced pain at the fracture site and reduced fracture mobility. It is assessed radiologically by X-ray features such as trabecular continuity across the fracture site and bridging callus.
- Non-union is caused by such factors as inadequate immobilisation, excessive distraction, loss of healing callus, infection or avascular necrosis.
- Stiffness of joints is a common problem with immobilisation in plaster casts and slings so the joints must be moved as early as possible. Early use is possible if the fracture is stable.
- A stress fracture is an incomplete fracture resulting from repeated small episodes of trauma, which individually would be insufficient to damage the bone. Stress fractures, especially in the foot, are most likely to result from sport, ballet, gymnastics and aerobics. Their incidence rises sharply at times of increased activity.[1]

- A dislocation is a complete disruption of one bone relative to another at a joint.
- A subluxation is a partial displacement such that the joint surfaces are still in partial contact.
- A sprain is a partial disruption of a ligament or capsule of a joint.
- Always consider associated soft-tissue injuries such as neuropraxia to adjacent nerves, vascular injuries and muscle compartment syndromes.

Testing for fractures[2]

This method describes the simple principle of applying axial compression for the clinical diagnosis of fractures of bones of the forearm and hand, but also applies to bones of the limbs.

Many fractures are obvious when applying the classic methods of diagnosis but it is sometimes more difficult if there is associated soft-tissue injury from a blow or if there is only a minor fracture such as a greenstick fracture of the distal radius.

If the bone suspected of fracture is compressed gently from end to end, the patient will feel pain. A soft-tissue injury of the forearm will show pain, tenderness, swelling and possibly loss of function. It will, however, not be painful if the bone is compressed axially—that is, in its long axis.

Walking is another method of applying axial compression, and this is very difficult (because of pain) in the presence of a fracture in the weight-bearing axis or pelvis.

Method

1. Grasp the affected area both distally and proximally with your hands.
2. Compress along the long axis of the bones by pushing in both directions, so that the forces focus on the affected area (fracture site; Fig. 117.1a). Alternatively, compression can be applied from the distal end with stabilising counterpressure applied proximally (Fig. 117.1b).
3. The patient will accurately localise the pain at the fracture site.

Principles of treatment of limb fractures

To reduce any fracture properly, the following steps must be taken (Fig. 117.2a).[3]

1. Disimpact the fragments, usually by increasing the deformity.

Fig. 117.1 *Testing for fractures:* **(a)** *axial compression to detect a fracture of the radius or ulna bones;* **(b)** *axial compression to detect a fracture of the metacarpal*

2. Re-establish the correct length of the bone.
3. Re-establish the correct alignment by proper reduction of the fracture.

The above steps will only be achieved with adequate anaesthesia, analgesia and relaxation. Maintenance of the reduction depends upon the moulding which utilises the intact periosteal bridge to hold the fracture fragments in a reduced position. Figure 117.2b illustrates the principle of moulding to maintain reduction.[3]

Fractures and dislocations of the face and skull

Skull fractures

Closed fractures without any neurological symptoms do not require active intervention. Depressed fractures may require elevation of the depressed fragment. Compound fractures of the

fracture (impacted)

Step 1. Disimpaction

Step 2. Establish length

Step 3. Establish alignment

Fig 117.2a *Principles of reduction of fractured bones*

Fig. 117.2b *Principles of moulding to maintain reduction: the arrows indicate the three point pressure areas required to maintain reduction*

vault require careful evaluation and referral. Special care is required over the midline as manipulation (usually by elevation) of any depressed fragment can tear the sagittal sinus, causing profuse and fatal bleeding.[4]

Base of skull fractures
These fractures are difficult to diagnose on radiography but their presence is indicated by bleeding from the nose, throat or ears. CSF may be observed escaping, especially through the nose, if the dura is also torn.

Treatment of basal fractures is based on prevention of intracranial infection and avoidance of excessive interference with the nose or ear, such as with packing and nasogastric tubes. An appropriate antibiotic is cotrimoxazole.[4]

'Malar' fracture
A fractured zygomaticomaxillary complex (malar) is a common body contact sports injury or injury resulting from a fight.

Clinical features:
- swelling of cheek
- circumocular haematoma
- subconjunctival haemorrhage
- palpable step in infraorbital margin
- flat malar eminence when viewed from above
- paraesthesia due to infraorbital nerve injury
- loss of function, i.e. difficulty opening mouth

Management
- head injury assessment
- exclude 'blowout' fracture of the orbit
- exclude ocular trauma
  — remove contact lenses if worn
  — check visual acuity
  — check for diplopia
  — check for hyphaema
  — check for retinal haemorrhage
- persuade patient not to blow nose (can cause surgical emphysema)
- if fracture displaced, refer for reduction under GA

Reduction methods
- elevation by temporal or intraoral approach— healing can be expected in 3–4 weeks
- some require interosseous wiring or plating or pinning

Fracture of mandible
A fracture of the mandible follows a blow to the jaw. The patient may have swelling (which can vary from virtually none to severe), pain, deformity, inability to chew, malalignment of the jaw and teeth and drooling of saliva. Intraoral examination is important as submucosal ecchymosis in the floor of the mouth is a pathognomonic sign.

A simple office test for a suspected fractured mandible is to ask patients to bite on a wooden tongue depressor (or similar firm object). Ask them to maintain the bite as you twist the spatula. If they have a fracture they cannot hang onto the spatula because of pain.[5]

X-rays: AP views and lateral obliques
an orthopantomogram provides a global view

First aid management

- check the patient's bite and airway
- remove any free-floating tooth fragments and retain them
- replace any avulsed or subluxed teeth in their sockets
  Note: Never discard teeth.
- first aid immobilisation with a four-tailed bandage (Fig. 117.3)

Treatment

Refer for possible internal fixation.
   A fracture of the body of the mandible will usually heal in 6–12 weeks (depending on the nature of the fracture and fitness of the patient).

Fig. 117.3 *Immobilisation of a fractured mandible in a four-tailed bandage*

Dislocated jaw

The patient may present with unilateral or bilateral dislocation. The jaw will be 'locked' and the patient unable to articulate or close the mouth.

Method of reduction

- Get the patient to sit upright with the head against the wall.

- Wrap a handkerchief around both thumbs and place the thumbs over the lower molar teeth, with the fingers firmly grasping the mandible on the outside.
- Firmly thrusting with the thumbs, push downwards towards the floor.

This action invariably reduces the dislocation, but the reduction can be reinforced by the fingers rotating the mandible upward as the thumbs thrust downwards.

Fractured vertebrae/spinal column

Cervical fractures, especially atlas (C1), axis (C2) and odontoid process, require early referral with the neck immobilised in a cervical collar, in a supine position. A hard collar is preferred but a soft collar with sandbags either side of the head to prevent movement will suffice.

Thoracolumbar fractures

Fractures or fracture dislocations of the thoracic and lumbar vertebrae, without neurological deficit, are classified as either stable or unstable.

Stable fractures

- compression fractures of vertebral body with < 50% loss of vertical height
- minor fractures
- laminar fractures

Treatment: rest on firm-to-hard bed for 10–28 days depending on symptoms, followed by a brace.
Special problems:

- retroperitoneal haematoma
- paralytic ileus
- associated kidney rupture with L_1 fractures
- underlying vertebral body pathology in the elderly, e.g. myeloma or metastases

Unstable fractures

Burst fractures and shearing fractures are usually unstable. They are often associated with partial or complete paraplegia and require urgent referral.

Fractures of sacrum and coccyx

No treatment apart from symptomatic treatment is required. Manual reduction per rectum can be attempted for significant forward displacement of the coccyx. Advise the use of a rubber ring or special cushion (such as a Sorbo cushion) when sitting. Excision of the coccyx may be considered for persistent discomfort.

Fractured rib

Features:

- pain over the fracture site especially with deep inspiration and coughing
- localised tenderness and swelling
- pain in the site upon whole chest compression
- X-ray confirms diagnosis and excludes underlying lung damage, e.g. pneumothorax. There is a high incidence of false negative fractures on X-ray, so caution is necessary
- suspect splenic, hepatic and renal trauma with lower rib fractures

Treatment

A simple rib fracture can be extremely painful. The first treatment strategy is to prescribe analgesics, such as paracetamol, and encourage breathing within the limits of pain. If pain persists in cases of single or double rib fracture with no complication, application of a rib support is most helpful.

The universal rib belt

A special elastic rib belt can provide thoracic support and mild compression for fractured ribs (Fig. 117.4). Despite its flexibility it gives excellent support and symptom relief while permitting adequate lung expansion. The elastic belt is 15 cm wide and has a Velcro grip fastening, so it can be applied to a variety of chest sizes.

Healing time

3–6 weeks; local discomfort may persist much longer.

Fractures of the clavicle

There is a history of a fall onto the outstretched hand or elbow although this fracture may also occur with a direct blow to the clavicle or the point of the shoulder. The patient has pain aggravated by shoulder movement and usually supports the arm at the elbow and clasped to the chest. The most common fracture site is at the junction of the outer and middle thirds, or in the middle third. Consider the possibility of neurovascular injury.

Treatment

- St John's elevated sling to support arm—for 3 weeks
- figure of eight bandage (used mainly for severe discomfort)
- early active exercises to elbow, wrist and fingers
- active shoulder movements as early as possible

Special problem

Fracture at the lateral end of the bone: this fracture is often subject to delayed or non union. Consider referral for open reduction.

Healing time

4–8 weeks.

The appropriate use of slings for fracture–dislocations is presented in Table 117.1.

Fig. 117.4 *Method of application of a universal rib belt*

Table 117.1 *Appropriate use of slings for fracture–dislocations*

Collar and cuff	Fractured shaft of humerus
Broad arm sling	Fractured forearm
	Fractured scapula
St John's high sling	Fractured clavicle
	Fractured neck of humerus
	Subluxed acromioclavicular joint
	Dislocated acromioclavicular joint
	Subluxed sternoclavicular joint

Fractures of the scapula

Fractures of the scapula may include:

- body of scapula: due to a crushing force, considerable blood loss, may be rib fractures
- neck of scapula (may involve joint)
- acromion process $\Big\}$ due to a blow or fall on
- coracoid process $\Big\}$ the shoulder

Treatment

- broad-based triangular sling for comfort
- early active exercises for shoulder, elbow and fingers as soon as tolerable
- a large glenoid fragment usually requires surgical reduction because of potential glenohumeral joint instability

Healing time
Several weeks to months.

Fractures of the sternum

These are treated symptomatically with analgesics but careful evaluation of thoracic injuries, including cardiac tamponade or myocardial contusion, is essential. A significantly depressed fracture should be referred. An ECG is advisable.

Acromioclavicular joint dislocation/ subluxation

A fall on the shoulder, elbow or outstretched arm can cause varying degrees of separation of the acromioclavicular joint, causing the lateral end of the clavicle to be displaced upwards.

Grades I & II	partial separation, involving tearing of the acromioclavicular capsule and ligaments
Grade III	complete tearing, also affecting the coracoclavicular ligaments

Treatment

- Analgesics
- St John arm sling (suitable for all injuries)
- Mobilisation exercises as soon as possible

and (for Grade III)

- a compression bandage (or long straps of adhesive low-stretch strapping) with padding at pressure points—elbows, clavicle and coracoid. The clavicle should be manipulated into its correct position and the forearm elevated: applying pressure from above (clavicle) and

below (elbow) to achieve compression, apply a bandage over the outer end of the clavicle and round the elbow joint which is flexed to 90°. The bandage or strapping is worn for 2–3 weeks.[6]

Many patients are unable to tolerate this method of treatment. Skin irritation or blisters are common. This occurs particularly with adhesive strapping and the deformity commonly requires correction after the removal of bandage or strapping. The same effect may be achieved with an orthotic device known as a Kenny-Howard sling or brace.

- The issue of internal fixation versus conservative treatment for a complete dislocation is controversial in that the bulk of patients treated conservatively have minimal residual symptoms. However, a significant proportion have residual symptoms in the form of AC joint pain and traction effects on the brachial plexus due to loss of scapular suspension. The patients most likely to have these symptoms are those with high grades of separation, involvement of the dominant shoulder and participation in employment or sports that place heavy physical demands on the shoulder girdle. If in doubt, referral within the first few weeks of injury for consideration of the pros and cons of conservative versus surgical treatment would be appropriate.

Sternoclavicular joint dislocation/ subluxation

This uncommon injury is caused by a fall or very heavy impact on the shoulder, causing the medial end of the clavicle to move forwards or anterior (making it prominent) or backwards. Plain X-rays are difficult to interpret but a CT scan is the ideal diagnostic method.

Special problem
Backward (inward) displacement of the clavicular end with danger to major blood vessels and trachea. This is one of the few potentially life-threatening orthopaedic injuries. Urgent referral for reduction is essential. Closed reduction can usually be achieved under anaesthesia. The reduction is nearly always stable.

Treatment
Forward subluxation or disclocation, unlike posterior dislocation, is nearly always unstable and

resists attempts at maintaining closed reduction. Despite the persistence of a medial clavicular swelling, most patients need a sling for only 1–2 weeks and the bulk of their pain settles over the following months. Surgery is generally only indicated for an unusually painful and chronic anterior sternoclavicular dislocation.

Dislocation of the shoulder

Dislocations of the shoulder joint can be caused by an impact on the arm by falling directly on the outer aspect of the shoulder, or by a direct violent impact, or by a forceful wrenching of the arm outwards and backwards.

Types of dislocation:

- anterior (forward and downward)—95% of dislocations
- posterior (backward)—diagnosis often overlooked
- recurrent anterior dislocation (recurrent posterior dislocation extremely rare)

Anterior dislocation of the shoulder

Management

AP and lateral X-rays should be undertaken to check the position and exclude an associated fracture. The arm should be assessed for the presence of neurological injury before reduction. Reduction can be achieved under general anaesthesia (easier and more comfortable) or with intravenous pethidine ± diazepam. The following methods can be used for anterior dislocation. Satisfactory analgesia and patient relaxation are vital to the success of any of the methods.

Kocher method

- elbow flexed to 90° and held close to the body
- slowly rotate arm laterally (externally)
- adduct humerus across the body by carrying point of elbow while simultaneously applying longitudinal traction along the line of the humerus
- rotate arm medially (internally)

Hippocratic method

Apply traction to the outstretched arm by a hold on the hand with countertraction from stockinged foot in the medial wall of the axilla. This levers the head of the humerus back. It is a good method if there is an associated avulsion fracture of the greater tuberosity.

Milch method (does not require anaesthesia or sedation)

- Patient reclines at 30° and with guidance slowly bends the elbow to 90°.
- Operator braces thumb against humeral head.
- The patient is asked to lift the arm (abduct) slowly with the elbow bent so that they can pat the back of their head (requires considerable reassurance and encouragement).
- At this position of external rotation, traction along the line of the humerus (with countertraction) achieves reduction.

Dependent arm in prone position method

- The patient is placed in prone position on bed or trolley with arm hanging limply over the edge and elbow fully extended.
- The shoulder may reduce spontaneously, especially with adequate analgesia.
- The technique may be enhanced by longitudinal traction applied to the arm.

Postreduction

- Reduction is complete if the hand can rest comfortably on the opposite shoulder.
- Confirm reduction by X-ray in two planes and again assess for unsuspected fractures, e.g. glenoid rim or greater tuberosity fractures.
- Keep the arm in a sling for 2 weeks.
- Apply a swathe bandage to the chest wall.
- After immobilisation, begin pendulum and circumduction exercises.
- Combined abduction and lateral rotation should be avoided for 3 weeks.

Posterior dislocation of the shoulder

This is the most commonly misdiagnosed major joint dislocation.[7] Posterior dislocation most often follows an epileptic seizure or electrical shock. The post-ictal patient with a painful shoulder has a posterior dislocation of the shoulder until proven otherwise. Less often this injury is caused by a fall onto the outstretched hand with the arm internally rotated or by a direct blow to the front of the shoulder. If any doubt persists about the diagnosis, a CT scan is appropriate.

The shoulder contour may look normal but the major clinical sign is painful restriction of external rotation which is usually completely blocked. Beware of the problem of pain in the shoulder after a convulsion. An 'axillary shoot through' X-ray view should be routinely ordered following shoulder trauma (Fig. 117.5).

Fig. 117.5 *X-ray (axillary view) illustrating posterior dislocation of the shoulder; the femoral head is pushed backwards with an impaction fracture anteriorly. If the patient prevents satisfactory positioning for X-ray, consider CT scan*

Reduction of posterior dislocation

Using appropriate analgesia or anaesthesia, apply traction to the shoulder in 90° of abduction (with the elbow at right angles) and laterally (externally) rotate the limb.

Recurrent anterior dislocation

Acute anterior shoulder dislocation may tear or stretch the anterior capsular ligaments from their bony origin. This may predispose to recurrent anterior dislocation or subluxation. (Recurrent posterior instability is rare.)

A simple procedure for reducing recurrent anterior dislocation:

- Get the patient to sit comfortably on a chair with legs crossed.
- The patient then interlocks hands and elevates the upper knee so that the hands grip the knee.
- The knee is gradually lowered until its full weight is taken by the hands. At the same time the patient has to concentrate on relaxing the muscles of the shoulder girdle. This method usually effects reduction without the use of force.

Recurrent dislocation often requires definitive surgery, depending on the frequency of dislocations and the degree of apprehension between episodes.

Pitfalls

- Nerve injury, especially axillary (circumflex) nerve.
- A fractured neck of the humerus, especially in the elderly, may mimic a dislocation.
- Associated fractures (greater tuberosity, head of radius, glenoid) may require internal fixation.
- Great difficulty with some reductions (this is often related to inadequate analgesia; the use of excessive force may result in fracture).
- Failing to X-ray all suspected dislocations before and after reduction; failing to obtain an axillary view to show posterior displacement or fractures of the humerus or glenoid.

Orthopaedic problems that cause difficulties in diagnosis and management are outlined in Table 117.2.

Fractured greater tuberosity of humerus

Treat with a combination of immediate mobilisation and rest in a sling unless grossly displaced, when surgical reduction is advisable. Shoulder stiffness can be a disabling problem, so early movement is encouraged with review in 7 days. This fracture should be monitored by X-ray within 2 weeks after injury. Undetected displacement may lead to mechanical impingement against the acromion. This fracture may also be an indication of the patient having had a transient glenohumeral dislocation.

Fractured surgical neck of humerus

This usually occurs in the elderly due to a fall onto the outstretched hand. The fragments may be impacted. The greater tuberosity may also be fractured. Watch out for associated dislocation.

Table 117.2 *Important orthopaedic problems that cause difficulties in diagnosis and management*

Shoulders
• Posterior dislocation of the shoulder
• Recurrent subluxations
• Unstable surgical neck fractures of humerus
• The avascular humeral head

Elbow
• Supracondylar fractures with forearm ischaemia
• Fracture of the lateral humeral condyle in children
• Fractured neck of radius in children
• The Monteggia fracture with dislocation of radial head

Wrist
• Scaphoid fractures
• Scapholunate dislocation
• The unstable Colles' fracture

Fingers
• Phalangeal fractures
• Intra-articular fractures
• Penetrating injuries of the metacarpophalangeal joint
• Gamekeeper's thumb (MCP joint)

The hip
• Developmental dysplasia of the hip
• Septic arthritis
• Slipped capital femoral epiphysis
• Subcapital fractures
• Stress fractures of the femoral neck in athletes
• Impacted subcapital femoral neck fracture in the elderly

Foot and ankle
• Stress fractures of the navicular
• Intra-articular fractures

In adolescents, fracture–separation of the upper humeral epiphysis occurs.

Treatment (no displacement or impaction)
• triangular sling
• when pain subsides (10–14 days) encourage pendulum exercises in the sling
• aim at full activity within 8–12 weeks post injury

Displaced fractures may require internal fixation. Severely comminuted fractures may predispose to post-traumatic osteoarthritis or humeral head avascular necrosis. Referral with a view to prosthetic hemiarthroplasty should be considered.

Healing
Union usually occurs in 4 weeks and consolidation at 6 weeks.

Pitfalls with fractures of the surgical neck
Minimally displaced fractures of the surgical neck of the humerus are usually managed conservatively, but overzealous early mobilisation

can lead to non-union.[7] If there is a communication of this fracture with joint fluid, movement washes away the fracture haematoma and leads to the development of true pseudoarthrosis. Judicious early immobilisation will avert this complication.

Always remember the cardinal fracture management rule: 'First ensure that stability of the fracture is sufficient to allow healing before prescribing rehabilitation exercises or early use of the extremity'.[7]

The management of various humeral fractures is summarised in Figure 117.6.

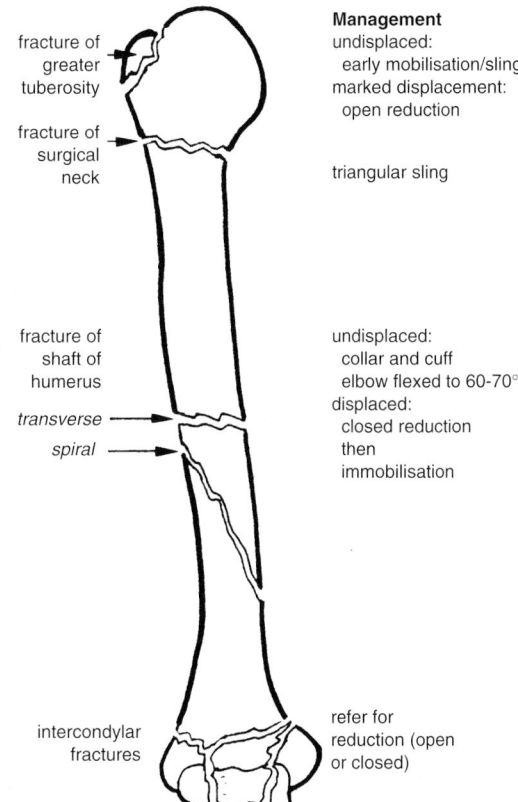

Fig. 117.6 *Various fractures of the humerus in adults*

Fracture of shaft of humerus
Humeral shaft fractures may be:

• spiral—due to a fall on the hand
• transverse or slightly oblique—fall on elbow with arm abducted
• comminuted—heavy blow

Caution: watch for radial nerve palsy.

Treatment

- Perfect bony opposition is not necessary; some overriding is acceptable but distraction of the fragments is not.
- Undisplaced fracture: collar and cuff with elbow flexed to 60–70°.
- Significantly displaced humeral shaft fractures may require manipulation under anaesthestic. However, the vast majority of shaft fractures realign to a satisfactory extent under gravitational effects in a sling once muscle spasm and oedema have subsided. A U-shaped hanging cast or slab enhances the gravitational effect and assists splintage.

Intercondylar fractures in adults

Intercondylar fractures, which may be T-shaped or Y-shaped, are usually caused by a fall on the point of the elbow which drives the olecranon process upwards, splitting the condyles apart. Fractures involving the joint can cause long-term problems of post-traumatic osteoarthritis and joint stiffness. Referral for reduction (closed or open) is appropriate.

Fractures and avulsion injuries around the elbow joint in children

Potentially severe deforming injuries include:

- supracondylar fractures
- fracture of the lateral humeral condyle
- fracture of medial humeral epicondyle (Fig. 117.7)
- fracture of neck of radius

Fractures around the elbow in children require referral to consultants experienced in radiology and fracture management.

Supracondylar fractures with forearm ischaemia

Supracondylar fractures represent about half of all elbow fractures in children; and most are extension fractures following falls onto the outstretched arm.

Pressure of the displaced bony fragments causing impingement on the brachial artery leads to impending forearm flexor compartment ischaemia and muscle death. Severe forearm pain is the most significant and important sign of ischaemia. Neuropraxia of the median, radial or ulnar nerves is common. These injuries almost invariably recover.

This diagnosis must always be assumed in displaced supracondylar fractures in children. Thus it is the general practitioner's responsibility to ensure treatment is expedited.

The fracture is reduced by hyperflexion of the elbow during traction (after lateral displacement has been corrected) and then immobilised in collar and cuff and stockinet vest. The fully flexed elbow with the usually intact posterior periosteal hinge provides fracture stability. Plaster casting is unnecessary and some would suggest contraindicated because of the significant risk of ischaemic contracture. Circulatory status requires monitoring in the first 24 hours following injury. The collar and cuff should be used for 6 weeks. The invariably stiff elbow quickly resolves without a need for formal therapy.

Fracture of the lateral humeral condyle

Fractures of the lateral humeral condyle also result from a fall onto the outstretched arm in children (Fig. 117.7). The fracture line passes vertically or obliquely through the lateral condyle and thus crosses the distal humeral growth plate. It occurs in an age group prior to the appearance of the epiphysis of the lateral epicondyle. Pain and swelling over the lateral elbow, but without the gross deformity of a supracondylar fracture

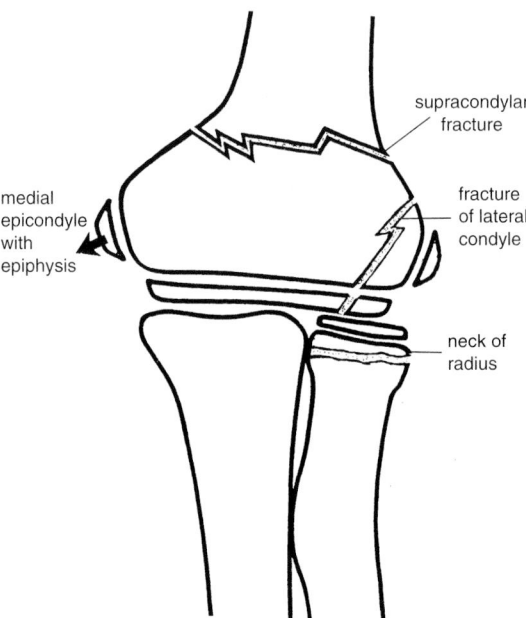

Fig. 117.7 *Fractures and avulsion injuries around the elbow joint in children*

of the humerus, could make one suspect this injury. The fracture is commonly overlooked on X-ray. Comparison views of the opposite elbow are particularly helpful in diagnosing this injury.

Recognition of the fracture and early open reduction and internal fixation with wires is vital to reduce the risk of premature plate closure. Such growth plate disturbance may result in a progressive valgus deformity of the elbow and the late development of an ulnar nerve palsy.

Fracture of the medial humeral epicondyle

This problem occurs typically in adolescents following a fall onto the outstretched hand. The medial epicondyle may be avulsed by massive flexor pronator muscle contraction together with abduction stresses on the forearm. Avulsion of the epicondyle occurs in the young patient before the epiphysis is united. If displaced this fracture is best treated by open reduction and internal fixation. Untreated injuries commonly result in non-union, elbow pain and restricted elbow extension.

Fractured neck of radius

This fracture is caused by a child falling on the outstretched hand. The fracture line is transverse and is situated immediately distal to the epiphysis.

The degree of tilt is critical. Up to 15° of tilt is acceptable but, beyond that, reduction (preferably closed) will be necessary. The head of the radius must never be excised in children.

Dislocated elbow

A dislocated elbow is caused by a fall on the outstretched hand, forcing the forearm backwards to result in posterior and lateral displacement (Fig. 117.8). The peripheral pulses and sensation in the hand must be assessed carefully. Check the function of the ulnar nerve before and after reduction.

Treatment

Attempt reduction with patient fully relaxed under anesthesia. It is important to apply traction to the flexed elbow but allowing it to extend approximately (20–30°) to enable correction of the lateral displacement and then the posterior displacement.

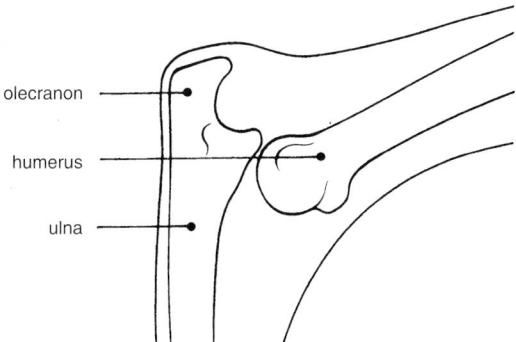

olecranon

humerus

ulna

Fig. 117.8 *Dislocated elbow: uncomplicated posterior dislocation*

Follow-up

Encourage early mobilisation with gentle exercises in between resting the elbow for 2–3 weeks in a collar and cuff with the elbow flexed above 90°, avoiding passive movements. A plaster cast should not be used because of the risk of ischaemic necrosis of muscle. This will minimise the possibility of myositis ossificans. Recurrent dislocation of the elbow is uncommon.

A simple method of reduction

This method reduces an uncomplicated posterior dislocation of the elbow without the need for anaesthesia or an assistant. The manipulation must be gentle and without sudden movement.

Method

1. The patient lies prone on a stretcher or couch, with the forearm dangling towards the floor.
2. Grasp the wrist and slowly apply traction in the direction of the long axis of the forearm (Fig. 117.9).
3. When the muscles feel relaxed (this might take several minutes), use the thumb and index finger of the other hand to grasp the olecranon and guide it to a reduced position, correcting any lateral shift.

Pitfalls

- incomplete reduction: ulna articulates with capitellum and not the trochlea
- injury to ulnar nerve (spontaneous recovery usually occurs after 6–8 weeks)
- associated fractures, e.g. coronoid process, which may cause instability

Fig. 117.9 *Dislocated elbow: method of reduction by traction on the dependent arm*

Fractured head of radius (adults)

If the fracture is very slight and undisplaced, treat conservatively with the elbow at right angles in a collar and cuff until pain subsides sufficiently to allow flexion/extension and pronation/supination exercises.

Elbow stiffness is a major problem even after apparently trivial radial head fractures. Early mobilisation is vital. Excision of the radial head should be considered for highly comminuted fractures which limit the ability to mobilise the elbow early or predispose to post-traumatic osteoarthritis. Associated distal radioulnar joint or wrist injuries are often overlooked.

Fractured olecranon

- Comminuted fracture (with little displacement): sling for three weeks and active movements.
- Transverse (gap) fracture: open reduction with screw or wire.

Monteggia fracture–dislocation of the radial head

Fractures of the proximal third of the ulna with dislocation of the radial head (Monteggia fracture–dislocation) (Fig. 117.10) has a history of mismanagement during treatment. The radial head dislocation is easily overlooked.

Redislocation or subluxation of the radial head is common.

Since surgical intervention is advisable, referral of displaced forearm fractures for early surgery is recommended. Surgical plating of the ulnar shaft maintains the radial head in a reduced position. Follow-up X-rays are mandatory to ensure that there has not been a late redislocation of the radial head.

Fig. 117.10 *Monteggia fracture–dislocation of the radial head; it is important not to miss a dislocated head of radius with a fracture of the proximal third of the ulna*

Fracture–dislocation in the lower forearm (Galeazzi injury)

This injury is usually caused by a fall on the hand and is a combination of a fractured radius (at the junction of its middle and distal thirds) and subluxation of the distal radioulnar joint. The patient should be referred, as open reduction is often required.

Fractures of the radius and ulna shafts

General features

It is more common to have both bones broken. Displaced fractures of both forearm bones in the adult require perfect reduction which can generally only be achieved by surgical reduction and plating. Less than satisfactory reduction interferes with normal pronation and supination. A fracture of one bone alone is uncommon and usually caused by a direct blow. For a fracture of one bone alone look for evidence of an associated dislocation of the other forearm bone. In children, greenstick fractures are common. Fractured radial shafts tend to slip and ulna fractures heal slowly. Dislocation of the head of the radius or inferior radioulnar joint can be missed if X-rays do not include the elbows and wrist joints.

Reduction

- A greenstick fracture is readily straightened by firm pressure.
- A complete fracture (spiral or transverse) is reduced by traction and rotation.
- A slight overlap and angulation is permissible in children but perfect reduction is essential in adults.
- A plaster cast should include both the elbow and the wrist joints.

Healing time: (adults) spiral fracture—6 weeks; transverse fracture—12 weeks

Colles' fracture of lower end of radius

A Colles' fracture, probably the most common of all fractures, is a supination fracture of the distal 3 cm of the radius, caused by a fall onto the outstretched hand.

Clinical features

- usually an elderly woman
- osteoporosis is common
- fall on dorsiflexed hand
- fracture features
  - impaction
  - posterior displacement and angulation
  - lateral displacement and angulation
  - supination
  - dinner fork deformity (Fig. 117.11)

Treatment

- if minimal displacement—below-elbow plaster for 4 weeks, then a crepe bandage
- if displaced: meticulous reduction under anaesthesia
  - set in flexion 10°, ulnar deviation 10° and pronation
  - below-elbow plaster 4–6 weeks (6 weeks maximum time)

Fig. 117.11 *Dinner fork deformity of Colles' fracture: a fracture of the distal head of the radius showing impaction and posterior displacement and angulation*

- unstable fractures may require an above-elbow cast initially with the forearm in pronation
- check X-ray at 10–14 days; position may be lost as swelling subsides and plaster becomes loose

Problems associated with Colles' fracture:

- watch for ruptured extensor pollicus longus tendon
- stiffness of the elbow, MCP joints and IP joints
- discomfort at inferior radioulnar joint due to disruption
- reflex sympathetic dystrophy

Pitfall: the unstable Colles' fracture[7]

With the advent of modern imaging techniques and power equipment it has become a simple procedure to pin unstable Colles' fractures percutaneously, even in the elderly. Thus severe deformities are now unacceptable. An early percutaneous pin is much simpler than a late osteotomy. Colles' fractures deserve more respect than they received in the past.

Remember the basic classification into intra-articular and extra-articular fractures. Restoring reasonable joint surface alignment is an important part of the treatment and fortunately is usually relieved with simple traction under local or general anaesthesia.

Smith's fracture of lower end of radius

This is often referred to as a 'reverse Colles''. It is caused by a fall on the back of the hand. The lower fragment is flexed and impacted on the upper fragment. It is reduced and immobilised for 6 weeks in a cast as for Colles' fracture but with the wrist extended. Unstable fractures may require an above-elbow cast initially with the forearm in supination.

Ulna styloid fracture

Treat symptomatically. Delayed or non union is common, but rarely symptomatic.

Radial styloid fracture

Undisplaced: plaster slab for 3 weeks
Displaced: closed reduction and plaster slab for 6 weeks
if this fails—open reduction

Scaphoid fractures

Scaphoid fractures account for almost 75% of all carpal injuries, but are rare in children and the elderly.[8] If a scaphoid fracture is suspected in the presence of a normal X-ray of wrist, a follow-up X-ray should be arranged in 2 weeks. Isotopic bone scan may be indicated in cases where suspicion of fracture is high despite normal X-rays. For undisplaced fractures, 8 weeks in a below-elbow scaphoid cast usually suffices. Displaced fractures of the scaphoid require reduction (either open or closed) and, if unstable, internal fixation.

All scaphoid fractures require late X-ray evaluation of treatment to diagnose non-union before they become symptomatic from late degenerative changes. Early bone grafting of a non-union can prevent fragment collapse and radioscaphoid degenerative changes.

Pitfall

The fracture may not be apparent on routine wrist X-rays. Specific scaphoid views should be requested.

Scapholunate dissociation

This not uncommon carpal injury results from disruption of the scapholunate interosseous ligament and palmar radiocarpal ligaments. It results in a gap appearing between the scaphoid and lunate bones (the so-called 'Terry-Thomas' sign on plain anterior-posterior X-rays of the wrist) and the scaphoid rotating into a vertical position on lateral X-rays. It is associated with pain in the wrist on dorsiflexion.

Early diagnosis with referral simplifies treatment. This injury has only been recognised in recent times.

Fractures of the hands and fingers
Thumb fractures

The thumb's special function renders injuries more difficult than other digits. Fractures well clear of the joints in the proximal and distal phalanges are treated in a similar way to other digits. However, intra-articular injuries are more common and internal fixation is more likely on the thumb than other digits.[9]

Bennett's fracture

This is a fracture–dislocation of the first carpometacarpal joint. The larger fragment of the first metacarpal dislocates proximally and laterally (Fig. 117.12).

Treatment

Under anaesthesia the thumb is reduced using the forces indicated (Fig. 117.12). A scaphoid plaster is applied with the thumb in the open grasp position. If anatomical reduction cannot be achieved by closed means then open reduction and internal fixation is indicated. Percutaneous pinning with wires under X-ray control is also commonly used to hold an anatomical reduction.

Gamekeeper's thumb

This problematic injury of the metacarpophalangeal joint is presented in more detail on page 1186.

Metacarpal fractures

Metacarpal fractures can be stable or unstable, intra-articular or extra-articular, and closed or

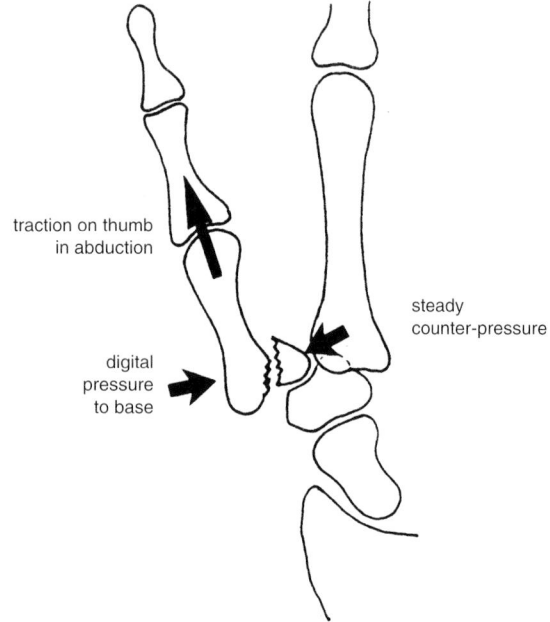

Fig. 117.12 *Method of reduction of a Bennett's fracture—dislocation of the first carpometacarpal joint*

open. They include the 'knuckle' injuries resulting from a punch which is prone to cause a fracture of the neck of the fifth metacarpal. As a
general rule, most metacarpal (shaft and neck)
fractures are treated by correcting marked dis-
placements with manipulation (under anaesthesia) and splinting with a below-elbow, padded
posterior plaster slab that extends up to the
dorsum of the proximal phalanx and holds the
metacarpophalangeal joints in a position of function (Fig. 117.13).[4]

Fig. 117.13 *Fracture of the metacarpal: showing position
of function with posterior plaster slab and
the hand gripping a roll of felt padding*

There is often a tendency for metacarpal fractures to rotate and this must be prevented. This
is best achieved by splinting the MCP joints at
90° which corrects any tendency to malrotation.
If there is gross displacement, shortening or rotation then surgical intervention is indicated. A felt
pad acts as a suitable grip. The patient should
exercise free fingers vigorously. Remove the
splint after 3 weeks and start active mobilisation.

Phalangeal fractures

These fractures result from either direct trauma
causing a transverse or a comminuted fracture
or a torsional force causing an oblique fracture.
The tendency to regard fractures of phalanges
(especially middle and proximal phalanges) as
minor injuries (with scant attention paid to
management and particularly to follow-up care)
is worth highlighting. These fractures require as
near perfect reduction as possible, careful splintage and, above all, early mobilisation once the
fracture is stable—usually in 2–3 weeks.

Nevertheless, overzealous mobilisation can be
as dangerous as prolonged immobilisation. Early
operative intervention should be considered if
the fracture is unstable.

Angulation is usually obvious but it is most
important to check for rotational malalignment,
especially with torsional fracture. A simple
method is to get the patient to make a fist of the
hand and check the direction in which the nails
are facing. Furthermore each finger can be

flexed in turn and checked to see if the fingertips
point towards the tubercule of the scaphoid
(palpable halfway along the base of the thenar
eminence and 1.5 cm distal to the distal wrist
crease).

The phalanges

- *Distal phalanges:* usually crush fractures; generally heal simply unless intra-articular. Disturbance of nail growth is common.
- *Middle phalanges:* tend to be displaced and
unstable—beware of rotation.
- *Proximal phalanges:* of the greatest concern,
especially of the little finger; intra-articular fractures usually need internal fixation.

Treatment

*Non-displaced phalanges with no rotational mal-
alignment.* Strap the injured finger to the adjacent normal finger with an elastic garter or
adhesive tape for 2–3 weeks, i.e. 'buddy strapping' (Fig. 117.14). Start the patient on active
exercises.

or

If pain and swelling is a problem, splint the
finger with a narrow dorsal or anterior slab (a
felt-lined strip of malleable aluminium can be
used) (Fig. 117.15). An alternative is to bandage
the hand while the patient holds a tennis ball or
appropriate roll of bandage in order to maintain
appropriate flexion of all interphalangeal joints.

*Displaced phalangeal fractures (usually proximal
and middle).* With suitable anaesthesia correct
the deformity by traction and direct digital pressure. Maintain correction by splintage for 2–3
weeks. Ensure flexion at the interphalangeal

Fig. 117.14 *Treatment of non-displaced phalanges by
'buddy strapping': the fractured finger is
strapped to an adjacent healthy finger*[4]

Fig. 117.15 *Method of splinting a phalangeal fracture of the index finger by a posterior plaster slab* [4]

joints with a dorsal padded plaster slab from above the wrist to the base of the fingernail (Fig. 117.15).

Intra-articular phalangeal fractures

Intra-articular phalangeal fractures are a great problem in management as subsequent stiffness of even a single interphalangeal joint can be a significant disability. Subsequent degenerative changes are common.

These fractures often occur in association with subluxation or dislocation of the joint. Reduction and fixation of the fracture may be an integral part of restoring joint stability. Displaced intra-articular phalangeal fractures, especially with joint instability, require referral.

Mallet finger

Refer to page 1184.

Penetrating injuries to the hand

Assessing these injuries requires a careful history and examination. The pugilist who sustains a seemingly minor cut over a 'knuckle' may have a tooth-penetrating injury to the metacarpophalangeal joint. In the flexed position the dorsal hood is drawn over the joint. The point of penetration of the hood retracts as the finger extends and 'locks' saliva into the joint. This injury invariably results in a severe septic arthritis unless aggressively treated with surgical debridement and high-dose antibiotics. Given the common occurrence of oral pathogens, antibiotic cover should include anaerobic organisms.

Dislocated fingers

For dislocated fingers immediate reduction is advisable. Test for an associated fracture and X-ray if appropriate. General anaesthesia may be necessary for reduction of a dislocated thumb.

Simple reduction of a dislocated interphalangeal joint

This method employs the principles of using the patient's body weight as the distracting force to achieve reduction of the dislocation. It is relatively painless and very effective.

> ### Method

1. Face the patient, both in standing positions.
2. Firmly grasp the distal part of the dislocated finger. A better grip is achieved by wrapping simple adhesive tape around the end of the finger.
3. Request the patient to lean backward, while maintaining the finger in the fixed position (Fig. 117.16).
4. As the patient leans back, sudden, painless reduction should spontaneously occur.

Splint the joint for 3 weeks to allow soft tissue healing.

> ### Pitfalls

- instability—torn collateral ligaments: unstable in lateral direction
- interposed volar plate—postreduction full flexion absent
- fractures of base of phalanx

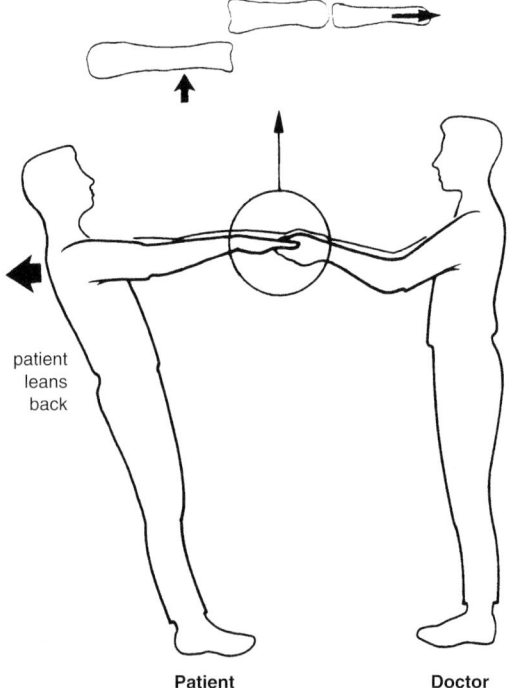

Fig. 117.16 *Reduction of a dislocated finger*

• extensor mechanism rupture, e.g. buttonhole deformity at PIP joint or mallet finger deformity at DIP joint

These problems may need surgical reduction.

Fractures of the pelvis

Fractures of the pelvic ring are either:

1. stable: a single fracture
2. unstable: a break at two sites or association with disruption of the symphysis pubis or sacroiliac articulation

Treatment

Stable pelvic fracture:

• symptomatic, especially analgesics
• bed rest as pain symptoms dictate
• attempt walking with an aid as soon as comfortable

Unstable fractures: these are usually serious with possible associated visceral damage or blood loss. Patients should be referred for expert help.

Femoral fractures

Femoral neck fractures include:

• subcapital fractures
• intertrochanteric fractures
• stress fractures in the young

Subcapital fractures are usually treated by pinning. Greatly displaced subcapital fractures in the elderly have a high risk of femoral head vascular necrosis. Thus prosthetic replacement of the femoral head may be considered as a primary option.

A trap can be the impacted subcapital fracture that may allow partial weight bearing, thus making radiological investigation essential in elderly patients complaining of hip pain. The fracture may not be evident on plain X-rays. If suspicion of fracture is still high, a bone scan should be performed.

Beware of the teenage athlete who complains of hip pain after running. Exclude a slipped upper femoral epiphysis and then a stress fracture. A technetium bone scan will detect the fracture. A stress fracture may displace without warning, posing a serious risk of femoral head avascular necrosis. Thus, stress fractures must be considered for prophylactic pinning.

A summary of the management of other femoral fractures is presented with Figure 117.17.

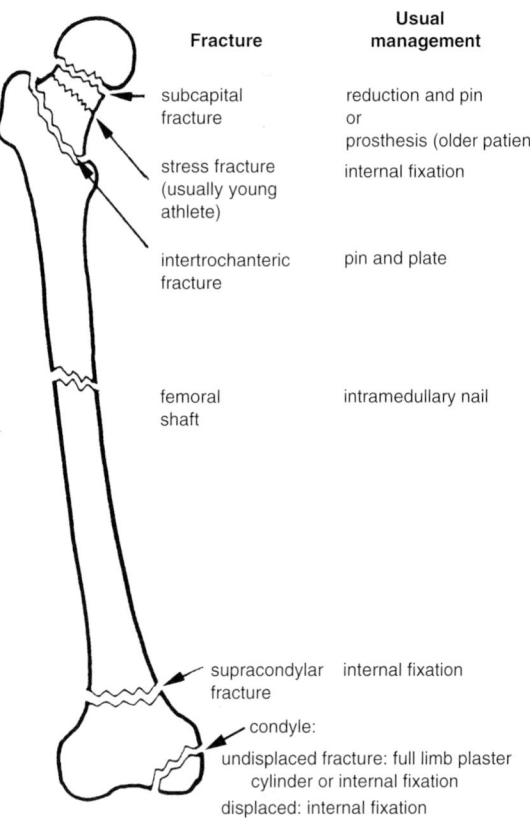

Fracture	Usual management
subcapital fracture	reduction and pin or prosthesis (older patient)
stress fracture (usually young athlete)	internal fixation
intertrochanteric fracture	pin and plate
femoral shaft	intramedullary nail
supracondylar fracture	internal fixation
condyle:	undisplaced fracture: full limb plaster cylinder or internal fixation displaced: internal fixation

Fig. 117.17 *Management of basic fractures of the femur*

Dislocations of the lower limbs
Posterior dislocation of the hip

This causes a very painful shortened leg which is held adducted, medially rotated and slightly flexed.

Management

• adequate analgesia, e.g. IM pethidine
• X-rays to confirm diagnosis and exclude associated fracture
• reduction of the dislocated hip under relaxant anaesthesia
• follow-up X-ray to confirm reduction and exclude any fracture not visible on the first X-ray
• Intra-articular bone fragments need to be excluded by CT scanning

Dislocated patella

The dislocated patella, which occurs mainly in children and young adults, especially girls, is always displaced laterally. Immediate reduction can be attempted by placing the thumb under the lateral edge of the patella and pushing it medially as the knee is extended. This may be attempted without anaesthesia or by using pethidine and intravenous diazepam as a relaxant.

X-rays with anteroposterior, lateral, skyline and intracondylar views should be taken to exclude an associated osteochondral fracture.

The usual RICE treatment should be given initially and crutches provided. Rest of the injured knee is achieved using a knee splint with the knee held in extension and crutches for 4–6 weeks.

Weight bearing is permitted when the swelling has subsided and the patient is gradually taken off the crutches. Introduce quadriceps exercises with the knee in extension.

Recurrent dislocation/subluxations in young females (14–18 years) requires surgery—combined tibial tubercle transfer with lateral release of the capsule. Immediate surgery in the acute phase is undertaken only in the presence of haemarthrosis with an osteochondral fracture.

Fractures of the patella

- Fractures without displacement: walking plaster cylinder 4 weeks.
- Displaced single transverse fracture: surgical reduction with Kirschner wires.
- Displaced and comminuted fracture: refer for patellectomy.

Fractures of both tibia and fibula

The nature and management of these fractures vary considerably. Some fractures are caused by blunt injuries, such as a blow from a motor car bumper, while twisting forces cause a spiral fracture of both bones at different levels. As a general rule, referral of patients to a specialist is necessary, especially where soft-tissue damage is significant. Management of fractures with minimal soft-tissue damage can be summarised thus:

- No or minimal displacement: full-length cast as for isolated fracture of tibia.
- Displacement: reduction under general anaesthesia, then application of cast as above (meticulous alignment essential).
- Period of immobilisation: adults 16 weeks, children 8 weeks.

Fracture of fibula[8]

An isolated fracture of the fibula is usually due to stress or to a direct blow. The patient is generally able to stand and move the knee and ankle joints. However, most spiral fractures are associated with injuries of the ankle or knee. The ankle in particular should be examined and X-rayed.

Treatment is usually with analgesics to control the pain and no more than a crepe bandage or a walking stick is necessary. A below-knee walking plaster for about three weeks will help those with severe discomfort.

Fracture of the tibial shaft

A fracture of the tibia alone is uncommon in adults but more common in children, due to a twisting injury. Reduction may not be necessary in some patients. Many can be reduced to a satisfactory position in the anaesthetised patient by letting the fractured leg hang over the edge of the table with the knee at a right angle.

A padded cast from the groin to the metatarsal necks is applied with the knee joint at 10° of flexion, and the ankle at a right angle. This should be maintained for 3–4 months.

Fracture around the ankle

The ankle is one of the areas liable to fractures. The commonest mechanism is forceful inversion of the foot, which can cause fracture of the fibula on a level with the joint line and tearing of the lateral collateral ligament. Other injuries can also occur such as fracture of the medial malleolus and tearing of the tibiofibular syndesmosis. At least three views on X-ray are needed: anteroposterior, lateral and a half oblique 'mortise' view.

Undisplaced, uncomplicated fractures are treated with a plaster cast from just below the knee to the toes for 6–8 weeks. The foot must be plantigrade, i.e. with the foot at 90° to the leg and neither in varus nor in valgus.[8] Fractures treated in plaster need X-ray monitoring. Unsuspected displacement may occur as swelling subsides and the plaster loosens. Occult displacement of the fracture leading to mal-union will predispose to ankle osteoarthritis. Fractures that are displaced or cause instability of the ankle joint require surgery to achieve stability followed by a longer period of immobilisation.

Stress fractures of the foot

Stress fractures of the navicular, calcaneus and metatarsal bones can be found in otherwise healthy people from the age of seven onwards. Long-distance runners and high-performance athletes are also susceptible.

Clinical features

- localised pain during weight-bearing activity
- localised tenderness and swelling (not inevitable)
- plain X-rays are necessary but show no fracture in about 50% of cases[6]; X-rays can be repeated in 2–3 weeks if a fracture is suspected
- a nuclear bone scan may confirm the diagnosis

Navicular

This hitherto unrecognised stress fracture has become apparent with the advent of CT scanning, which shows up the fracture better than nuclear scanning. It is seen in athletes involved with running sports and presents as poorly localised mid-foot pain. Plain X-ray is usually normal. The fracture, like the scaphoid fracture, is difficult to manage since delayed union and non-union are common. Cast immobilisation for 8 weeks may avoid the need for an operation.

Metatarsal bones

The second metatarsal is probably the most common site of all for stress fracture because it is invariably the largest metatarsal and absorbs a greater load than the others.[1]

Treatment

- rest is the basis of treatment
- resting the foot with crutches for 6 weeks provides optimal healing
- healing usually takes 6–8 weeks
- gradual slow resumption of activity

Fractures of the toes

Most toe injuries are easy to treat but, like the fingers, the great and little toes demand special attention. Intra-articular injuries of the great toe (unless undisplaced) should be treated by internal fixation.

Buddy strapping can be used for many uncomplicated fractured phalanges of the toes, which tend to angulate and rotate more readily and are often harder to control than finger fractures. Strapping them to their adjacent toes on both sides simultaneously tends to counteract this problem.

Like the little finger, the little toe is injured by forceful abduction and if allowed to heal in that position may leave difficulties in wearing shoes.[9]

Approximate average immobilisation times for various fractures are given in Table 117.3.

Dislocation of toes

Dislocations occur mainly at the metatarsophalangeal joint and are rare; they require special care because of the strong tendons crossing the joint. Perfect reduction of the dislocated great toe is essential and it should be supported by a below-knee plaster cast extending beyond the toes. Temporary internal fixation with a Kirschner wire or open ligamentous repair may be required.[9]

Analgesia and relaxation

For the reduction of dislocations, analgesia and relaxation is appropriate. Resuscitation facilities and an experienced practitioner are required to handle this procedure. All drugs should be given intravenously and titrated to achieve the desired effect. Adverse effects include respiratory depression and hypotension.[10] The choice of agents is presented in Table 117.4.

Plastering tips
Plaster of Paris

The bucket of water

- Line the bucket with a plastic bag for easy cleaning.
- The water should be deep enough to allow complete vertical immersion.
- Use cold water for slow setting.
- Use tepid water for faster setting.
- Do not use hot water: it produces rapid setting and brittle plaster.

The plaster rolls

- Do not use plaster rolls if water has been splashed on them.
- Hold the roll loosely but with the free end firm and secure (Fig. 117.18).
- Ensure that the centre of the plaster is fully wet.

Table 117.3 *Healing of uncomplicated fractures (adults)*

Fracture	(Approximate) average immobilisation time (weeks)
Rib	3–6 (healing time)
Clavicle	4–8 (2 weeks in sling)
Scapula	weeks to months
Humerus	
• neck	3–6
• shaft	8
• condyles	3–4
Radius	
• head of radius	3
• shaft	6
• Colles'	4–6
Radius and ulna (shafts)	6–12
Ulna—shaft	8
Scaphoid	8–12
Metacarpals	
• Bennett's #	6–8
• Other MCs	3–4
Phalanges (hand)	
• proximal	3
• middle	2–3
• distal	2–3
Pelvis	rest in bed 2–6
Femur	
• femoral neck	according to surgery
• shaft	12–16
• distal	8–12
Patella	3–4
Tibia	12–16
Fibula	0–6
Both T and F	16
Pott's fracture	6–8
Lateral malleolus avulsion	3
Calcaneus	
• minor	4–6
• compression	14–16
Talus	12
Tarsal bones (stress #)	8
Metatarsals	4
Phalanges (toes)	0–3

Important principles
• Children under 8 years usually take half the time to heal.
• Have a check X-ray in 1 week (for most fractures).
• Radiological union lags behind clinical union.
Note: There can be considerable variation in immobilisation times depending on factors such as trauma degree and soft tissue injuries.

• Drain surface water after removal from the bucket.
• Gently squeeze the roll in the middle: do not indent.

Table 117.4 *Analgesic and relaxant/sedative agents*

	IV dose	Antidote
Relaxant/ sedative agent		
Diazepam	0.1–0.2 mg/kg (5–10 mg)	Flumazenil
Midazolam	0.05–0.1 mg/kg (2–5 mg)	Flumazenil
Analgesic agent		
Fentanyl	1–2 μg/kg (50–100 μg)	Naloxone
Morphine	0.1–0.2 mg/kg (5–15 mg)	Naloxone
Pethidine	1–2 mg/kg (50–100 mg)	Naloxone

Padding
• Use Velband or stockinet under the plaster.
• With Velband, moisten the end of the roll in water to allow it to adhere to the limb.
• For legs, make extra padding around the ankle and heel.
• Avoid multiple layers of padding.

Method
• Use an assistant to support the limb where possible (e.g. hold the arm up with fingers of stockinet).
• Lay the bandage on firmly but do not pull tight.
• Lay it on quickly.
• Overlap the bandage by about 25% of its width.

Fig. 117.18 *Holding the plaster roll*

References

1. Quirk R. Stress fractures. Aust Fam Physician, 1993; 22:300–307.

2. Brentnall E. Diagnosing a fracture. Aust Fam Physician, 1990; 19:948.

3. McMenimen PJ. Management of common fractures of the upper limb. Aust Fam Physician, 1987; 16:783–791.

4. Cook J, Sankaran B, Wasunna A. *Surgery at the district hospital: obstetrics, gynaecology, orthopaedics and traumatology.* Geneva: World Health Organisation, 1991, 75–162.

5. Brentnall E. Spatula test for fracture of mandible. Aust Fam Physician, 1992; 21:1007.

6. Peterson L, Renström P. *Sports injuries: their prevention and treatment.* Sydney: Methuen, 1986, 179–181.

7. Young D, Murtagh J. Pitfalls in orthopaedics. Aust Fam Physician, 1989; 18:645–660.

8. Apley AG, Solomon L. *Apley's system of orthopaedics and fractures.* Oxford: Butterworth-Heinemann, 1993, 601–604.

9. Carter G. Fractures and dislocations of fingers and toes. Aust Fam Physician, 1993; 22:310–317.

10. Mohammed KD, Sonnabend DH. A GP's guide to the reduction of dislocations. Mod Med Aust, 1996; 39(2):100–108.

Further reading

Apley AG, Solomon L. Apley's system of orthopaedics and fractures (9th edn), Oxford: Butterworth-Heinemann, 1993.

118

Major trauma

—

*Until homo sapiens becomes more sapient I can see
no prospect of his ever avoiding the foolishness of
war or of his learning that two automobiles cannot
occupy the same spot at the same time, especially
when they come from opposite directions. Broken
bones and lacerated wounds are therefore likely to
require surgical attention for as long as this would-be
clairvoyant can see into the future.*

Evarts A. Graham 1950
Postgraduate Medicine

Major trauma, which is the third leading cause
of death in Australia, is where one or more areas
of the body (head and neck, chest, spine,
abdomen and pelvis, limbs) is damaged by
severe external trauma.

Critical injury is the situation where damage
leads to failure of one or more of the vital
systems (nervous, cardiovascular, respiratory,
urinary, gastrointestinal).

About 50% of deaths from major trauma occur
within seconds to minutes and 35% occur in
1–2 hours. These are the so-called golden hours
where early intervention can be lifesaving.

Death is usually caused by:

- airway obstruction
- hypotension due to blood loss
- head injury

The early management of severe trauma is now
a specialised part of emergency medicine
training.

Important guidelines

- For each death in a motor vehicle accident 30
  people sustain injuries.[1]

- Almost two-thirds of road accident deaths
  occur before arrival at a hospital.
- All patients with multiple injuries should
  receive high-flow oxygen.
- Another simple and important measure is to
  elevate the legs of a patient with signs and
  symptoms of significant blood loss.
- Having cleared the airway in a trauma victim,
  the restoration of effective breathing takes the
  highest priority.
- Do not forget to consider severe neck injury
  and thus spinal cord injury in patients with
  head trauma.
- Deterioration in conscious level may be due to
  hypoxia or hypoperfusion rather than primary
  brain injury.
- Consider the possibility of a reversible cause of
  altered conscious state that may have precipitated the head injury.
- Remember the possibility of myocardial infarction in a middle-aged or elderly patient presenting with major trauma and shock.
- The normal circulatory blood volume is
  5 litres. Young adults can usually compensate
  for a loss of up to 1500–2000 mL but others
  develop hypotension.
- Bleeding from superficial lacerations such as
  the scalp must not be ignored: the blood loss
  may be sufficient to tip the patient with multiple trauma into 'shock'.

The information in this chapter is a guide to help
practitioners cope with major trauma when
working in circumstances relatively remote from
a major trauma centre. Emergency lifesaving
measures may have to be taken before stabilising the victim or victims for evacuation to an
appropriate management facility.

Assessment and management priorities[2]

The following stepwise approach is recommended. It is very important to wear gloves, an apron and eye protection during this process.

1. Rapid primary survey and resuscitation of vital functions
   A Airway maintenance with protection of the cervical spine
   B Breathing and ventilation
   C Circulation and haemorrhage control
   D Dysfunction of the central nervous system
   E Exposure: completely undress the patient (if appropriate)

   Resuscitation of vital functions involves simultaneous attention to the airway with high-flow oxygenation and insertion of an intravenous line.
2. Detailed secondary survey.
3. Definitive care, including evacuation (if necessary).

The three basic X-rays for blunt trauma are presented in Table 118.1.

Airway management

During the process of airway management it is vital to protect the cervical spine which should be stabilised with the hands and kept in a neutral position. Ideally, a conforming hard cervical collar should be used.

If the patient cannot reply to commands or questions, open the mouth and check the upper airway.

- Clear debris and remove liquid vomit with a rigid sucker.
- Remove dentures or solid foreign objects with Magill forceps.
- Lift the chin and ventilate with bag and mask using high-flow oxygen.
- A Guedel airway may be needed to maintain the airway.
- Intubation may be necessary if the gag reflex is absent and if there is a flail segment of the chest—a cuffed endotracheal tube is the safest method. An orotracheal tube is preferred to nasotracheal intubation.
- If endotracheal intubation is not possible, perform a cricothyroidotomy.

Cricothyroidotomy

Emergency surgical access to the upper airway is a rare necessity but it can be a simple life-saving procedure.

Adults

- patient supine and neck extended
- palpate the groove between the cricoid and thyroid cartilage
- make a short (2–3 cm) transverse incision through the skin and cricothyroid membrane (Fig. 118.1)
  — ensure the incision is *not* made above the thyroid cartilage
- insert an endotracheal or tracheostomy tube. If unavailable, any piece of plastic tubing will do or even the shell of a ballpoint pen.

Children

- do not perform a stab wound in children because of poor healing
- use a 14–15 g intravenous cannula
- pierce the cricothyroid membrane at an angle of 45°
- free aspiration of air confirms correct placement

Fig. 118.1 *Cricothyroidotomy (in adult)*

Table 118.1 *Three basic X-rays for blunt trauma*

Chest

Cervical spine (lateral view)

Pelvis

- a 3.0 mm endotracheal tube connector fits into the end of the cannula or a 7.0 mm connector into a 2 mL or 5 mL syringe barrel connected to the cannula
- the connector is attached to the oxygen circuit; this system will allow oxygenation for about 30 minutes but carbon dioxide retention will occur

Breathing

Ensure the endotracheal tube is placed in the trachea. Auscultate in three areas: epigastrium, left lateral chest, right lateral chest. Check movement on both sides of chest. The respiratory rate should be noted.

If the upper airway has been cleared but respiratory distress is still present, possible causes include pneumothorax and/or haemothorax. If respiration is not markedly embarrassed, a chest X-ray should be taken with a view to insertion of a thoracostomy tube.

Tension pneumothorax

If respiratory distress is developing rapidly a tension pneumothorax could be responsible. Symptoms include dyspnoea, cyanosis and a tympanitic expanded hemithorax. A lifesaving procedure is the insertion of an intercostal catheter or needle attached to a 20 mL syringe in the second intercostal space in the mid-clavicular line and connecting it to an underwater seal. The site is at least two finger-breadths from the edge of the sternum, so that damage to the internal mammary artery is avoided.

Ruptured diaphragm

The possibility of rupture of the diaphragm should be kept in mind, especially if there is chest and abdominal trauma, although it is often very difficult to diagnose at first presentation. This condition can manifest itself at a variable time after injury, whether it be by persistent symptoms such as vomiting and respiratory distress or by signs of the presence of the stomach in the left hemithorax.

Chest drain insertion[3]

Thoracostomy tubes are usually inserted for combined haemopneumo-thoraces, that is, to clear blood and/or air from the pleural cavity. A preliminary X-ray should be taken to ensure that either blood or air is interposed between the chest wall and the lung.

Position: 4th or 5th intercostal space
        mid-axillary line

Note: The diaphragm is often raised to a surprising degree so assume it is at the level of the nipple and make the site of insertion at or above this level.

Method

With a scalpel a 2 cm incision is made through the skin and the underlying muscle in an intercostal space, sufficiently deep to be somewhere near the pleura. A skin incision alone is not suitable, as excessive force will then be required to introduce the tube. The tube can be inserted in the usual manner mounted on a trocar, but a less traumatic method is to incise through the pleura and insert the index finger to ensure entry into the pleural cavity. The end of the tube is then grasped with a large artery forceps and placed in the pleural cavity, fed in several inches and secured (see Figs 118.2 and 118.3).

Some air may enter the pleural cavity using this method, but it is expelled once the tube is connected to underwater seal drainage. If underwater seal drainage is not available, a flap valve can be fashioned by tying a cylinder of surgical rubber glove onto the open end of the tube. Similar devices are available commercially and are present in most emergency departments; however, they can easily get blocked with blood if a haemothorax is present.

Fig. 118.2 *Thoracostomy: a finger is introduced into the pleural cavity*

Circulation and haemorrhage control

A rapid assessment is made of the circulation and possible blood loss. Haemostasis should be achieved with direct pressure rather than the use

Fig. 118.3 *Thoracostomy: the drainage tube is introduced into the pleural cavity with a large artery forceps*

of tourniquets. Multiple packs into wounds should be avoided. Two important monitors are a cardiac monitor and a central venous line.

To replace blood loss two peripheral lines should be inserted into the cubital fossa, if possible. The larger the needle gauge the better; for example, the rate of flow in mL per minute for a 14 g cannula is 175–220 and for a 16 g cannula is 100–150. Flow rates are improved by using pressure bags to 300 mmHg.

Cutdown can be used and if problems occur an interosseous infusion is a suitable alternative (refer p. 792). A colloid solution (e.g. Haemaccel) should be used initially with one litre infused rapidly. If there are two lines a crystalloid solution such as normal saline or Hartman's solution can be used on one side and Haemaccel on the other line.

Blood is required after a major injury or where there has been a limited response to two litres of colloid.[2] Blood should be warmed before use. The pneumatic antishock suit has only been shown to be useful in 'shocked' patients, especially those suspected of having fractures of the pelvis and legs. Massive amounts of blood loss can be associated with these fractures (Table 118.2). It must be remembered that young patients can compensate well for surprising degrees of blood loss and maintain normal vital signs simply by increasing the cardiac stroke volume. Such patients can collapse dramatically.

Peripheral circulatory failure (shock) signifies an acute reduction of tissue perfusion and seriously affects vital organs such as the kidneys. It can be minimised or prevented by early aggressive resuscitation. Apart from blood and fluid loss other causes include respiratory failure (adult respiratory distress syndrome or shock lung), myocardial infarction and pancreatitis.

Cardiac tamponade

This serious problem should be diagnosed in the presence of an elevated JVP and a narrow pulse pressure, especially if a penetrating wound is present (Table 118.3). Diagnostic percutaneous needle paracentesis is made by inserting a long wide-bore needle and syringe (which can be connected to a three-way tap) into the epigastrium just between the xiphisternum and the left costal margin. It is advanced slowly towards the heart by aiming it towards the tip of the left scapula. The pericardium is reached after advancing 3–4 cm. If the ventricular wall is

Table 118.2 *General rules for acute blood loss with trauma (after Rogers)*[4]

Normal circulating volume	*5000 mL*
< 10% (500 mL) loss	no significant change
10–20% (500–1000 mL) loss	tachycardia, postural hypotension
20–40% (1000–2000 mL) loss	progressive hypotension, anxious, confused, pale
> 40% (2000 mL) loss	circulatory failure, ashen, confused, lethargic
Potential concealed loss with fractures	
Tibia and fibula	750 mL
Neck of femur	1000–1500 mL
Shaft of femur	1500–2000 mL
Pelvis	up to 5000 mL

Table 118.3 *Signs of pericardial tamponade*

Beck's triad
1. JVP elevated
2. muffled heart sounds
3. hypotension

Narrowed pulse pressure

Tachycardia

Pulsus paradoxicus

Treatment
1. oxygen
2. relieving paracentesis
3. thoracotomy

struck there is a scraping, moving sensation transmitted to the hand.

Head injury

Head injury is the main cause of death in major trauma. A Glasgow coma scale (p. 698) can be used to assess cerebral status. A useful simplified method of recording the conscious state is to use a five-level system rating.

1. awake
2. confused
3. responds to shake and shout
4. responds to pain
5. unresponsive coma

Unequal pupils

It is worth noting that relatively minor blunt trauma to the eye region will cause a traumatic mydriasis.[3] Unequal pupils in a conscious patient whose conscious level is not deteriorating is usually not significant in patients with head injury.

The single physical sign that outweighs all others in head injury assessment is the level of consciousness. If this is satisfactory, there is little cause for concern.

Emergency exploratory burr hole[3]

After a head injury, a rapidly developing mass lesion is heralded by a deteriorating conscious level (e.g. Glasgow coma scale 15 to 3); a rising blood pressure (e.g. $^{140}/_{70}$ to $^{160}/_{100}$); slowing respirations (16 to 10); a slowing pulse (70 to 55) and a dilating pupil. In such conditions an urgent burr hole is indicated even in the absence of a plain X-ray and a CT scan of the head. Even elevating a depressed fracture may be sufficient to alleviate the pressure.

Method (in absence of neurosurgical facilities)

- Ideally performed in an operating theatre.
- The patient is induced, paralysed, intubated and ventilated (100% oxygen).
- Dehydrating dose of 20% mannitol (1 g/kg IV in one hour) administered.
- After shaving the scalp, a mark is made over the site of external bruising, especially if a clinical fracture is obvious. A 5 cm long incision is made over the site of external bruising or swelling. Otherwise the burr hole is made in the low temporal area. A vertical incision is made above the zygoma, and the skull is trephined 2–3 cm above it (Fig. 118.4). This is the site of the classical middle meningeal haemorrhage.
- The clot is gently aspirated and the skin is loosely sutured around the drain.
- If there are difficulties controlling the bleeding, the intracranial area is packed with wet balls of Gelfoam or similar material.
- Other areas that can be explored in the presence of subdural haematoma include:
  — frontal region: a suspicion of an anterior fossa haematoma, e.g. a black eye
  — parietal region: haematoma from the posterior branch of the middle meningeal artery (Fig. 118.4).

Fig. 118.4 *Three sites suggested for burr holes:* **(1)** *low in the temporal region will disclose a classical middle meningeal artery bleed; on division of the muscle, haematoma should be found between the muscle and the fracture line;* **(2)** *frontal region;* **(3)** *parietal region*

Spinal injuries

Severe injuries of the upper cervical spine are immediately fatal. Patients with quadriplegia from cervical spine injury or paraplegia from thoracic or lumbar spine injuries require transfer to a spinal injury unit.

Remarkable recovery from quadriplegia due to cervical spine injury may follow prompt reduction of flexion-rotation injuries with bilateral facet dislocation in a spinal unit. Open reduction may be required.[5]

If these problems are present, insert an indwelling catheter and aim to avoid pressure sores by frequent (2 hourly) turning.

Signs of spinal injury include:[3]

- priapism in the male patient
- hypotension with bradycardia
- decreased motor power and sensation below the lesion
- decreased anal sphincter tone

Urinary catheterisation

A catheter should be inserted to measure the patient's rate of urine output. A perurethral approach is used if there is no contraindication, such as evidence of urethral injury. Contraindications include: blood at the meatus; perineal bruising; impalpable or high-riding prostate; inability to pass urine; inability to pass a catheter; or simply clinical suspicion of major clinical pathology.

If a patient has a ruptured urethra, attempted insertion of a catheter can convert a partial tear into a complete tear, or may introduce infection.

Nasogastric intubation

Nasogastric intubation can be both therapeutic (especially with pronounced gastric distension) and diagnostic.

Special caution is required in the presence of a maxillary fracture or a fracture of the cribriform plate.

Diagnostic peritoneal lavage

Intra-abdominal bleeding has to be considered according to the nature of the trauma and stability of the circulation. The ideal investigation is a CT scan to detect injuries. Peritoneal lavage is a reliable bedside test to demonstrate haemoperitoneum. It requires minimal equipment. The only relative contraindications are previous intra-abdominal surgery (except uncomplicated appendicectomy or cholecystectomy) and pregnancy.

Method[3]

- Empty bladder, by catheterisation if necessary.
- Inject local anaesthetic with a 23 g, 32 mm needle just below the umbilicus at an angle of 45° towards the pelvis.
- A stab incision is made at this site at the same angle so that it extends through the linea alba.
- Insert the trocar of the peritoneal dialysis kit.
- Pass the catheter into the peritoneal cavity and withdraw the trocar.
- Attach a syringe and aspirate for blood.
- If negative: infuse 1L of normal saline.
- Cut the drip tubing and place the end in a transparent container below the bed to allow the lavage fluid to drain by gravity.
- If the fluid is clear or lightly bloodstained, the test is negative.
- If the fluid is heavily bloodstained, the test is positive.
- Bile-stained fluid is an absolute indication for urgent laparotomy.

Think of associations

When certain injuries, especially bony fractures, are found it is important to consider associated soft-tissue injuries. Table 118.4 presents possible associated injuries with various fractures, while Table 118.5 outlines possible associated injuries with various physical signs or symptoms.

Roadside emergencies

The first 2 hours after injury can be vital: proper care can be lifesaving, inappropriate care can be damaging. Proper acquaintance with resuscitation procedures is important. The first step is for someone to notify the police and ambulance or appropriate emergency service. The site of an accident should be rendered safe by eliminating as many hazards as possible, e.g. turning off the ignition of a vehicle, warning people not to smoke, moving victims and workers out of danger of other traffic.

Attention should be given to:

- the airway and breathing
- the cervical spine: protect the spine
- circulation: arrest bleeding
- fractured limbs (gentle manipulation and splintage)
- open wounds, especially open chest wounds, should be covered by a firm dressing

Table 118.4 *Associated injuries related to specific fractures*

Fracture	Associated injuries to consider
Ribs	Pneumothorax Haemothorax Ruptured spleen (lower left 10–11) Ruptured diaphragm (lower left 10–11)
Sternum	Ruptured base of heart with tamponade Ruptured aorta
Lumbar vertebra	Ruptured kidney (L_1, L_2) and other viscera, e.g. pancreas (L_2)
Pelvis	Heavy blood loss Ruptured bladder Ruptured urethra Fractured femur
Temporal bone of skull	Cerebral contusion Extradural haematoma Subdural haematoma
Femur	Blood loss, possible > 1 L

Table 118.5 *Associated serious injuries and typical clinical features*

Physical sign or symptom	Associated serious injury
Subconjunctival haematoma with no posterior limit	Fractured base of skull
Sublingual haematoma	Fracture of mandible
Surgical emphysema	Pneumothorax with pleural tear Ruptured trachea
Unequal pupils	Cerebral compression, e.g. extradural haematoma Trauma to II and III cranial nerves Eye injuries, including traumatic mydriasis Brainstem injuries
Shoulder tip pain without local injury	Intra-abdominal bleeding, e.g. ruptured spleen Intra-abdominal perforation or rupture, e.g. perforated bowel
Bluish-coloured umbilicus	Intra-abdominal bleeding, e.g. ruptured ectopic pregnancy

Major haemorrhage is a common cause of death in the first few hours. Lacerated organs and multiple fractures can lose 250mL of blood a minute; pressure should be applied to control haemorrhage where possible. Colloids that can be administered intravenously for blood loss include Haemaccel.[6]

Most convulsions after trauma are due to hypoxia and will subside when it is corrected by adequate care of the airway; if not, IV anticonvulsant medication may be given.

Intramuscular narcotic injections (morphine, pethidine) and alcohol 'to settle the victim's nerves' must be avoided. The use of inhalational analgesia such as nitrous oxide (usually carried in ambulances) may provide some pain control. When the patient is under control, he or she should be shifted into the coma position (Fig. 118.5).

Administration of first aid to the injured at the roadside

A simple guide is as follows:

1. Check airway and breathing (being mindful of cervical spine)
   a. Check oral cavity

Fig. 118.5 *The coma position*

? tongue fallen back
? dentures or other foreign matter in mouth
Clear with finger and place in oral airway if available, or hold chin forward.

b. Check breathing
   if absent, commence artificial respiration if feasible.

2. Check circulation
   If pulse absent, commence external cardiac massage if possible.

3. Check for haemorrhage, especially bleeding from superficial wounds. Apply a pressure bandage directly to the site.

4. Check for fractures, especially those of the cervical spine.

Rules to remember

- Immobilise all serious fractures and large wounds before shifting.
- Always apply traction to the suspected fracture site.
- Splint any fractured limbs with an air splint, wooden splint or to body, e.g. arm to chest, leg to leg.
- For a suspected or actual fractured neck, apply a cervical collar, even if made out of newspaper, but have a hard collar (not soft) available. Keep the head held firmly in a neutral position with gentle traction (avoid flexion and torsion).
- Lay patients on their back with head supported on either side.

5. Shifting the patient
   - Immobilise all fractures.
   - Lift the casualty without any movement taking place at the fracture site, using as much help as possible.
   - Always support the natural curves of the spine.

- Protect all numb areas of skin (e.g. remove objects such as keys from the pockets).

6. The unconscious patient
   - Transport the casualty lying on the back if a clear airway can be maintained.
   - If not, gently move into the coma position.

7. Reassure the patient (if possible)
   - Reassurance of the casualty is most important.
   - Conduct yourself with calmness and efficiency.

8. Help the medical team
   Take notes of your observations at the accident, e.g. record times, colour of casualty, conscious level, respiration, pulse, blood pressure.

References

1. Trinca G, Murtagh JE. Road accident trauma—facts and trends. Aust Fam Physician, 1984; 13:239.

2. Skinner D, Driscoll P, Earlam R. *ABC of major trauma*. London: BMJ, 1991, 1–13.

3. Webster V. *Trauma*. Melbourne: RACGP, CHECK Programme, 1996, Unit 293, 3–14.

4. Rogers I. *Guidelines for the management of common emergencies in the emergency department* (2nd edn). Auckland Hospital Dept of Emergency Medicine, 1996, 14.

5. Ryan P. *A very short textbook of surgery* (2nd edn). Canberra: Dennis and Ryan, 1990, 75–77.

6. Walpole BG. Roadside emergencies. Aust Fam Physician, 1984; 13:249–253.

119

The doctor's bag and other emergency equipment

—

Almost everyone who goes to bed counts upon a full night's rest: like a picket at the outposts, the doctor must be ever on call.

Karl F. Marx (1796–1877)

General practitioners who perform home visits and nursing home visits require the traditional doctor's bag that includes the basic tools of trade, drugs (including those for emergency use), stationery and various miscellaneous items. Country doctors will by necessity use their bag for more emergency home and roadside calls.[1] These recommended contents are simply a guide for cross-checking.

Essential requirements for the bag

- sturdiness
- lockable, e.g. combination lock
- ready interior access
- uncluttered
- disposable single-use items
- light, portable equipment
- regular checks to ensure non-expired drugs
- storage in a cool place (not boot of car)

Stationery (checklist)

- Practice letterhead and envelopes
- Prescription pads
- Hospital admission forms
- Sickness/off-work certificates
- X-ray, pathology referral forms
- Accounting forms

- Dangerous drugs record books
- Continuation notes
- Large adhesive labels to record visit (attach later to patient's history)
- Tie-on labels for emergencies
- Recommendation forms (to psychiatric/mental hospitals)
- Pens

Miscellaneous items

Quick reference cards
- the Doctor's Bag checklist[1,2,3]
- dosage details of drugs, all age groups
- important telephone numbers

Local map
Phonecard or coins for public telephone use
Handbook of emergency medicine

Equipment

- Sphygmomanometer (aneroid)
- Stethoscope
- Diagnostic set (auriscope + ophthalmoscope)
- Tongue depressors
- Tourniquet
- Small needle disposal bottle
- Scissors
- Syringes 2, 5, 10 mL
- Needles 19, 21, 23, 25 g
- Scalp veins (butterfly) needles
- IV cannulae 16 g, 18 g, 20 g
- Alcohol swabs
- Micropore tape
- Thermometer

- Artery forceps
- Urine testing sticks
- Pathology specimen bottles
- Skin swabs, throat swabs
- Torch
- Patellar hammer
- Oral airway, e.g. Revivatube, Resuscitube (Fig. 119.1), Guedel
- Scalpel (disposable)
- File (for glass ampoules)
- Examination glove

Fig. 119.1 *The two-way Resuscitube*

Drugs

Drugs (oral)
Samples of commonly used:

- analgesics
- antibiotics
- antidiarrhoeal agents
- antiemetics
- antihistamines
- sedatives

Glyceryl trinitrate (nitroglycerin)
Soluble aspirin (for myocardial infarction)
Sumatriptan (Imigran)

Drugs (sprays)
Glyceryl trinitrate
Salbutamol aerosol

Drugs (topical)
Anaesthetic eyedrops

Drugs (injectable)
Refer to Tables 119.1 and 119.2.

Drugs (suppositories)
Indomethacin

The country doctor's bag

Country doctors, especially in isolated areas, usually carry additional equipment in their motor vehicles when called to the scene of an accident or other emergency. The equipment will vary according to geographic factors, the ambulance service and the special interests and enthusiasm of the practitioner.

Accident kit
The following list represents the contents of an isolated country doctor's kit; it will occupy a standard briefcase only.

- Flashlight and spare batteries
- Sterile compression bandages
- Steri-strips (large and small)
- Plastic container of antiseptic
- Wide-bore needle
- Sterile suture set
- Suture material
- Gillies' forceps
- Small scissors
- Large scissors (for cutting clothing)
- Artery forceps × 2
- Laerdal pocket mask (Fig. 119.2)
- Medium-sized torch
- Rigid cervical collar
- Triangular bandages × 2
- Crepe bandages × 2
- Air splints × 2

Fig. 119.2 *The Laerdal pocket mask*

Table 119.1 *Injectable drugs (ideal kit)*

Drug	Presentation	Indications
Adrenaline†	1 mg/mL	hypersensitivity reactions and anaphylactic shock; * bronchial asthma; ventricular asystole; croup; ventricular fibrillation (to assist CPR)
Atropine sulphate	0.6 mg/1 mL	bradycardia (after myocardial infarction); * ureteric colic; organophosphate poisoning (Malathion)
Benztropine mesylate†	Cogentin 2 mg/2 mL	acute dystonia
Benzylpenicillin†	600 mg with 2 mL water	meningococcaemia, pneumonia (adults)
Dexamethasone	4 mg/1 mL	status asthmaticus (esp. elderly); croup
Diazepam†	10 mg/2 mL	status epilepticus and other convulsions such as eclampsia; sedation in acute anxiety and severe tension headache; psychiatric emergencies
Dihydroergotamine	1 mg/mL	severe migraine
Ergometrine maleate	0.25 mg/1 mL	uterine bleeding; abortion or postpartum haemorrhage
Frusemide†	Lasix 20 mg/2 mL	left ventricular failure, acute pulmonary oedema
Glucagon†	1 mg + 1 mL solvent	hypoglycaemia
Glucose 50%	5 g/10 mL	hypoglycaemic coma
Haloperidol†	Serenace 5 mg/1 mL	psychiatric emergencies such as severe agitation, psychoses
Hydrocortisone† sodium succinate	Solu-cortef 100 mg/2 mL 250 mg/2 L	anaphylactic shock; status asthmaticus; Addisonian crisis; thyrotoxic crisis; acute allergies
Hyoscine butylbromide	Buscopan 20 mg/1 mL	* ureteric and biliary colic; acute pancreatitis
Lignocaine	Xylocard 100 mg/5 mL (IV)	ventricular arrhythmias, especially ventricular tachycardia and fibrillation; migraine; severe tinnitus
Metoclopramide† or Prochlorperazine	Maxolon 10 mg/2 mL Stemetil 12.5 mg/ mL	severe vomiting (e.g. Ménière's disease, gastritis); acute labyrinthitis; migraine
Morphine sulphate†	15 mg/1 mL	acute pulmonary oedema; relief of severe pain (not due to muscular spasm) such as myocardial infarction
Naloxone (more than one ampoule)†	Narcan 0.4 mg/ mL	opiate respiratory depression
Pethidine	100 mg/2 mL	severe pain such as ureteric and biliary colic
Phytomenadione (vitamin K)	Konakion 10 mg/mL	anticoagulant overdose with haemorrhage
Promethazine†	Phenergan 50 mg/2 mL	acute allergic conditions, * antiemetic
Salbutamol	Ventolin 0.5 mg/mL	bronchial asthma, other bronchospasm
Sumatriptan	Imigran 6 mg/0.5 mL	severe migraine, cluster headache
Water	5 mL	diluent

* May be useful as an alternative drug   † essential drugs

- Disposable scalpel with blade
- Safety pins
- Sterile gauze
- Urinary catheter
- Makeshift hook to suspend IV fluid pack
- IV infusion tubing
- Bottle of Haemaccel × 2
- Fluid pack

- 1 litre IV fluid (N saline)

The contents of this bag provide the equipment to cope with common accidents, including:

- bleeding wounds, e.g. arterial bleeders
- tension pneumothorax
- fractured cervical spine

Table 119.2 *Additional cardiopulmonary drugs (optional)*

Injectable drugs	Presentation	Indications
Adenosine	Adenocor 6 mg/2 mL	supraventricular tachycardia
Isoprenaline	Isuprel 1 mg/mL	bradycardia unresponsive to atropine
Metaraminol bitartrate	Aramine 10 mg/mL	non-hypovolaemic shock; anaphylaxis drug-induced, associated with spinal anaesthesia, ? cardiogenic
Terbutaline	Bricanyl 0.5 mg/mL	bronchospasm; asthma; bronchitis; smoke inhalation
Verapamil	Isoptin 5 mg/2 mL	supraventricular tachycardia (with adequate blood pressure)
Heparin	5000 U/mL	thromboembolism, myocardial infarction

Note: The author recommends the MIN-I-JET syringe packs for ideal emergency use. The range includes Naloxone 5 mL, aminophylline, atropine, adrenaline, dextrose, lignocaine, isoprenaline, sodium bicarbonate.

- fractured limbs
- fractures of the shoulder girdle
- snake bites

In addition, some country doctors carry a trephine to cope with the extradural haematoma.

Resuscitation kit

The country doctor can carry an oxyresuscitator unit with the following standard items:

- Oxygen
- Suction
- Laryngoscopes
- Endotracheal tubes
- Oropharyngeal airways, e.g. Guedel
- Endotracheal adaptor
- Face mask, e.g. Laerdal pocket mask (with one-way valve), or Concorde mask

The base of the unit contains:

- Paediatric tracheostomy tube
- Self-retaining tourniquet
- Intravenous infusion needle
- Intravenous infusion tubing
- Haemaccel 500 mL
- Disposable scalpel ⎫
- Chromic catgut ⎬ for intravenous cutdown
- Mosquito forceps ⎭
- Magill's forceps

Other equipment that could be carried:

- A balloon resuscitator and sucker + oxygen cylinder (instead of the oxyresuscitator)
- Normal saline or Hartman's solution
- Sodium bicarbonate (100 mL)
- Portable ECG and defibrillator, e.g. Heartstart

Precautions at the scene of the accident[4,5]

- Don't become a casualty yourself.
- Do not speed to the accident.
- Be alert for other traffic, hazardous material, HIV contamination, power lines, petrol and other inflammable material, jagged edges.
- Turn ignition off as first measure.
- Ensure proper triage: check airways of all victims first, attend to cervical spine injuries and arrest bleeding.
- Recruit bystanders for simple tasks.
- Control the accident scene: stop traffic with proper lights and signs.

Practice tips

- Check your doctor's bag every month for drugs that may be expired, damaged or in short supply (your practice nurse can do this).
- Replace any used drugs or materials the day after use.
- Always have your bag handy but don't carry it in the car in hot weather. It is best to be able to grab it from a safe accessible spot when you leave for an emergency.
- Drugs of addiction (pethidine and morphine) may be kept separate and then taken from their secure place when their use is anticipated, e.g. myocardial infarction, severe biliary or renal colic.
- Keep a spare kit in your surgery if you or your assistants or locums perform a lot of emergency work.

- Familiarise yourself with the layout of your bag (including ampoule files) so that using it in urgent circumstances is efficient.
- Use a large intravenous cannula wherever possible if rapid infusion is required.

References

1. Murtagh J. Drugs for the doctor's bag. Australian Prescriber, 1996; 19(4):89–92.

2. Hogan C. The management of emergencies in general practice. Aust Fam Physician, 1989; 18:1211–1219.

3. Troller J. The doctor's bag. Essential requirements. Current Therapeutics, August 1990; 64–65.

4. Walpole BG. Roadside emergencies. Aust Fam Physician, 1984; 13(4):249–253.

5. Murtagh J. *Medical emergencies*. Melbourne, RACGP CHECK Programme, 1987; 189:19–22.

120

The treatment room and equipment

—

Planning

A treatment room is best planned by those who will run and use it, including the nursing sister of the practice. It is wrong to assume that an architect knows best. The function of the room has to be considered: is it to be used exclusively for minor surgery and accidents and emergencies; or is it a general purpose room that can act as the sister's room or as a second consulting room?

Some practitioners may choose to install expensive equipment such as X-ray units, special sterilisers, microscopes, ECG units, electrotherapeutic units such as ultrasonography or interferential machines, and portable defibrillators; others can cope with the simplest equipment.

The room

The function of the room will determine some of the requirements. Access is important if the room is used as an emergency room: can a patient in a wheelchair, or on crutches or on a stretcher be moved comfortably in and out of the treatment room? How close is the room to the ambulance access for transfer of the critically ill?

Some doctors prefer a mobile couch; others prefer a couch placed in the centre of the room.

The room does not need a desk: one option is to use a mobile tray that can hold records and other writing material and can also be used as a dressing table.

Floor space is important, hence most equipment should be stored on accessible shelves or bench tops. The floors should be washable and non-slip (not carpeted) and the walls should be washable.

A mobile overhead light is ideal. A central theatre light, however, is too expensive and an alternative is to use angle-poise lamps at each end of the couch.

An intravenous drip stand and bottle doubles for intravenous fluids and eye irrigation, but it is preferable to have a hook from the ceiling or wall to support an intravenous drip.

Other important practical questions include:

- Are there enough lights, power sockets and taps?
- Can taps be turned off by the elbow after scrubbing?
- Is there adequate ventilation for a steriliser?
- Is there ready access from the main consulting room to the treatment room?
- Is a push button 'intercom' practical?

Resuscitation equipment

Sick people attend surgeries and unfortunately they sometimes have an unpredictable habit of 'collapsing', occasionally with a cardiopulmonary arrest. Any injection of local anaesthetic has the potential to produce a convulsion. Thus it is imperative to have resuscitation equipment available to cope with emergencies such as:

- bronchial asthma
- cardiac arrest
- acute blood loss and continuing haemorrhage
- convulsions, including febrile convulsions

Resuscitation equipment ideally should include:

- an oxygen unit
- suction
- a compressed air pump, nebuliser, solutions and masks
- intravenous equipment and fluids
- an oral airway (Resuscitube or Guedel airway)
- a doctor's bag with standard drugs
- a defibrillator
- Ambubag or Air-viva

Commercially available resuscitation (air or oxygen and suction) units include the oxy-viva (CIG), Modulaide oxygen (Laerdal) and Dr Blue Bag (CIG).

Basic equipment

When equipping the practice do not purchase more than you need. It should be remembered that many hospitals replace instruments at a stage when they are still useful, and these, as well as adequate trolleys, couches and instrument or suture trays, tables and microscopes can be purchased inexpensively.

Standard surgical instruments include scalpels and blades (disposable items available), artery forceps, Gillies' forceps, Allis' forceps, dissecting forceps, splinter forceps, scissors, Magill's forceps, bone forceps, probes and sponge-holding forceps. Important accessories include syringes, needles, suture material, local anaesthesia, float bowls, gauze and swabs.[1]

Dressing and suture materials are important considerations. Dressing kits, already prepacked and sterilised, are available commercially or can be obtained through the local hospital, especially for country practitioners.

Sharps disposable containers are essential to eliminate as far as possible the risk of accidental puncture from used needles.

The microscope is an invaluable item of equipment in the practice.

Special equipment

Practitioners exhibit varying skills and interest in the different surgical disciplines. Recommended equipment to manage basic problems includes:

Ear, nose and throat—auriscope, head mirror, aural specula, laryngeal mirror, nasal specula, nasal packing, nasal packing forceps, BIP (bismuth iodoform paraffin) paste, spirit burner, topical anaesthesia, ear syringe, wax curette, Waxsol drops, dental broach, small Foley catheter, cupped alligator forceps, foreign body remover, eustachian catheter, Epistat nasal catheter, Merocel ear wick and nasal pack.

Eyes—binocular loupe, dental burr, meibomian clamp, eye stream, Minims (e.g. fluorescein and amethocaine), eye testing charts (46 cm and 305 cm), multiple pinholes, sterile cotton buds, non-allergenic tape, eye pads, eyebrow tweezers.

Skin—liquid nitrogen, electrodiathermy unit, small dermatome, punch biopsy punches (disposable), Wood's light, e.g. 'the black light', 20% potassium hydroxide (for dermatophyte diagnosis).

The cryosurgical unit, complete with cylinder of gas and cryoprobe, is an excellent though expensive unit.

A wide-bore trocar and cannula (with expellor) is needed for subcutaneous insertion of hormone implants.

Musculoskeletal—plaster, open toe cast shoe (to allow walking on leg plaster), plaster cutters, air splints, aluminium-backed foam splints. Soft cervical collars, lumbar supports (e.g. McKenzie roll), crutches. Special electrotherapy equipment, e.g. ultrasound.

Genitourinary—specula, uterine sound, intrauterine contraceptive devices, tenaculum, urinary catheter.

Anorectal—proctoscope, gloves, haemorrhoid ligatures, suppositories, enemas (e.g. Microlax). Haemorrhoid (Gabriel) injection syringe and needle with ampoules of 5% phenol in almond oil.

Respiratory—vitalograph, peak flow meter, air pump, nebuliser and accessories. Hand-held nebulisers and spacers for inhaler technique demonstration.

Pharmaceutical preparations

The emergency injectable drugs such as adrenaline, morphine and diazepam can be located in locked cupboards or in the doctor's bag.

Many topical preparations have a multiplicity of uses. These include various antiseptics, topical freezing preparations such as ethyl chloride, ether, trichloracetic acid, podophyllin paint, silver nitrate, phenol of various strengths, salicylic acid paste, ethanolamine 5%, and Stingose.

Office sterilisation

Sterilisation of office equipment is a very important issue, especially with items and instruments that breach the body surface. These must be sterile, that is, free from all infections and potentially infectious matter[2,3] including bacteria, viruses, chlamydia, rickettsia, mycoplasma, protozoa and spores. The blood and body fluids of all patients must be treated as potentially infectious for blood-borne diseases such as AIDS, hepatitis B and hepatitis C. Endoscopy equipment in particular requires special attention. The practitioner is responsible for preventing cross-infection in the practice and hence careful attention to correct decontamination of medical instruments is essential.

Distinctions between main techniques

- *Decontamination*—a general term to cover methods of cleaning, disinfection and sterilisation for removal of microbial contamination from medical equipment such as to render it safe.[2]
- *Cleaning*—a process by which micro-organisms and biohazardous materials are removed from the surface of an object.
- *Disinfection*—inactivation of vegetative bacteria, viruses and fungi, but not necessarily of bacterial spores.
- *Sterilisation*—complete destruction or removal of micro-organisms and their spores from materials.

Many doctors still use the misnomer 'steriliser' when referring to a hot water disinfector, which does not kill all bacterial spores. The principal methods of decontamination are steam under pressure (autoclaves), dry heat (hot air ovens), boiling water and chemical disinfectants. The use of sterile single-use instruments and other equipment removes the need for any procedures to decontaminate instruments.

As soon as possible after use, instruments *must* undergo preliminary cleaning.

Sterilisation techniques[2]
Heat disinfectants
1. Steam under pressure (autoclave)
This is the most reliable method of sterilising instruments. However, if the instruments were not cleaned properly beforehand they would not necessarily be rendered sterile. The steam steriliser should have a drying cycle.

Recommended sterilisation times and temperatures for autoclaves are:

Temperature (°C)	Time (minutes)
121	15
126	10
134	3.5

2. Hot air ovens
Recommended times and temperatures for dry heat are:

Temperature (°C)	Time (minutes)
160	60
170	40
180	20

3. Hot water disinfectors
To ensure destruction of the HIV virus it is important to boil the instruments for 10–30 minutes. The recommended time is 30 minutes. If another instrument is added to the load, timing must start anew.

Cold or chemical disinfectors
Chemical disinfection is an uncertain process and should only be used when more effective heat treatment is inappropriate. It is suitable for medium-risk items such as thermometers or flexible endoscopes which can be damaged by heat or steam.
1. *Alcohol.* e.g. ethyl or isopropyl alcohol as 70% v/v in water. Alcohol does not kill spores.
Note: Surgical spirit should be avoided for routine disinfection purposes.
2. *Glutaraldehyde.* A 2% solution of alkaline glutaraldehyde is suitable for disinfection of fibreoptic equipment, which should be thoroughly washed in water and detergent immediately after use.
3. *Hypochlorite.* Hypochlorites as a solution of sodium hypochlorite, e.g. 'Milton' bleach, or as sodium dichloroisocyanurate (NaDCC)

Table 120.1 *Risk categories and types of instrument decontamination*[2]

Risk instruments		
High risk	**Medium risk**	**Low risk**
Surgical scissors	Vaginal specula for vaginal	Ear syringe nozzles
Metal/plastic forceps	examination	Skin thermometer
Stitch cutters	Ring pessaries	
Intrauterine device sets	Ring diaphragms	
Uterine sounds	Proctoscopes	
Tenacula	Nasal specula	
Hypodermic needles	Tongue depressors	
Vaginal specula used for inserting	Laryngeal mirrors	
IUDs	Thermometers	
Recommended method of decontamination		
Sterilise or single-use (presterile)	Sterilise by autoclaving or dry heat or single-use (non-presterile)	Sterilise or boil (nozzles) especially if skin breaks or infection suspected
Alternatives		
None	Boil if suitable or none	Chemical disinfection or wash

Note: All scrubbing brushes and bottle brushes used for cleaning purposes must themselves be autoclaved or disinfected regularly. Reprinted with permission from *A code of practice for sterilisation of instruments and control of cross-infection*, published by the BMA.

tablets or granules have a wide microbicidal activity.

Table 120.1 summarises categories of risk and types of instruments decontaminated in general practice.[2]

Summary

The recommendations about the contents of the treatment room are not intended to be complete or a mandatory survival package. Some practitioners manage comfortably with basic equipment such as an Air-viva, a standard doctor's bag and a handful of instruments. Others have very advanced rooms with equipment compatible with their special interests and geographical location. The medical equipment can be obtained from suppliers, and some equipment has been designed by doctors who market their own concepts.

An autoclave is undoubtedly the most efficient method of sterilising reusable medical instruments,[3] although great diligence must be exercised in the cleaning of the equipment beforehand and in the care of the autoclave. General practitioners should consider using single-use presterilised material wherever possible and employing the services of nearby hospital sterilising departments for sterilisation of instruments. The most effective way to avoid cross-infection via injection is through the use of single-dose vials.

The efficiently managed treatment room should have an accurate record of procedures and list of current stock (including expiry dates, service dates and faulty equipment). There is no doubt patients and therapists benefit from an efficient treatment room.

References

1. Murtagh J, Troller J. Establishing a treatment room. Aust Fam Physician, 1989; 18:22–24.

2. Dawson J. *A code of practice for sterilisation of instruments and control of cross-infection*. London: British Medical Association, 1989, 31–52.

3. Hammond L. Office sterilisation. Aust Fam Physician, 1990; 19:693.

121

Common sporting injuries

—

Although there is considerable overlap between injuries occurring during everyday activities and those of sporting and recreational activities, there are many injuries that are characteristic to sports people. Many of these injuries are the result of trauma of various degree and include the many varieties of fractures, dislocations and soft tissue injuries.

Injuries to the eye

Blunt injuries to the eye are common in sport. Examples include tennis and squash balls, cricket balls and baseballs, and fists and fingers associated with body contact sports. Haemorrhage is the most common problem and occurs throughout the eye: subconjunctivally; in the anterior chamber (hyphaema); into the vitreous; and underneath the retina or choroid.

Another common problem is a corneal abrasion where a small wound can be caused by a foreign body, a fingernail or a contact lens. It needs to be treated with great respect.

Hyphaema

With hyphaema, bleeding from the iris collects in the anterior chamber of the eye. The danger is that, with exertion, a secondary bleed from the ruptured vessel could fill the anterior chamber with blood, blocking the escape of aqueous humour and causing a severe secondary glaucoma. Loss of the eye can occur with a severe haemorrhage. It is likely to happen between the second and fourth day after the injury.

Management

- First, exclude a penetrating injury.
- Avoid unnecessary movement: vibration will aggravate bleeding. (For this reason, do not use a helicopter if evacuation is necessary.)
- Avoid smoking and alcohol.
- Do not give aspirin (can induce bleeding).
- Prescribe complete bed rest for 5 days and review the patient daily.
- Apply padding over the injured eye for 4 days.
- Administer sedatives as required.
- Beware of 'floaters', 'flashes' and field defects.

Arrange ophthalmic consultation after one month to exclude glaucoma and retinal detachment. No sport before this time.

Generally, recovery runs an uneventful course. If secondary bleeding occurs (usually the second, third or fourth day) the patient should be transported immediately to the nearest eye hospital. Evacuate by air (not by helicopter) only if the cabin altitude can be kept below 1300 metres (4000 feet). It is important to prevent vomiting and expansion of air within the eye.

Protective spectacles should always be worn when playing squash. People with monocular vision should be advised not to participate in this sport.

Knocked out or broken teeth

If a permanent (second) tooth is knocked out it can be saved by immediate proper care. Likewise, a broken tooth should be saved and urgent dental attention sought.

The knocked-out tooth

- Place the tooth in its original position, preferably immediately (Fig. 121.1): if dirty, put it in milk before replacement or, better still, place it under the tongue and 'wash it' in saliva. Do not use water, and do not wipe or touch the root.
- Fix the tooth by moulding strong silver foil (e.g. a milk bottle top or cooking foil) over it and the adjacent teeth.
- Refer the patient to his or her dentist or dental hospital as soon as possible.

Note: Teeth replaced within half an hour have a 90% chance of successful reimplantation.

Fig. 121.1 *Replacement of a knocked-out tooth*

Injuries to the nose

Common injuries to the nose include epistaxis and fractures of the nasal bones.

Epistaxis

First aid is simple tamponade, which is invariably effective. The soft cartilaginous part of the nose should be pinched between the finger and thumb for 5–10 minutes. The head should be kept bent slightly forward. Packing of the nose may be required.

Fracture of the nose

If deformity is present the patient should be referred for reduction within 7 days.

Septal haematoma

Special care has to be taken of a septal haematoma, which has a tendency to become infected (p. 1133).

Shoulder injuries

Common shoulder injuries acquired in sporting activities include:

- dislocated or subluxed acromioclavicular joint (p. 1150)

- fractured clavicle (p. 1149)
- dislocated shoulder (p. 1151)
- supraspinatus tendinitis (p. 574)

Swimmer's shoulder

Painful shoulders occur in about 60% of elite level swimmers during their career. The basic disorder is rotator cuff tendinitis, particularly supraspinatus tendinitis, which is considered to be associated with abnormal scapular positioning and cervicothoracic dysfunction. The best treatment is prevention, which aims at rotator cuff strengthening exercises, better scapulothoracic control, including correction of thoracic extension if it is decreased, and scapular stabilisation exercises.[1]

Elbow injuries

Soft-tissue disorders of the elbow are extremely common. Two types of tennis elbow are identifiable. 'Backhand' tennis elbow or lateral epicondylitis (p. 585) and 'forehand' tennis elbow or medial epicondylitis, which is also known as golfer's elbow or baseball pitcher's elbow. These common problems, often unrelated to sporting activity, are presented in more detail in Chapter 58.

Hand injuries

Hand and finger injuries are very important in sporting activities and include fractures and dislocations of phalanges and metacarpals. A mallet finger is a common injury and can result from overuse.

Ligamentous disruption of finger joints can cause instability and require early referral. An example is gamekeeper's thumb, often encountered in skiers, where there is complete tearing of the medial ligament of the metacarpophalangeal joint.

Mallet finger

A mallet finger is a common sports injury caused by the ball (football, cricket ball or baseball) unexpectedly hitting the finger tip and forcing the finger to flex. Such a forced hyperflexion injury to the distal phalanx can rupture or avulse the extensor insertion into its dorsal base. The characteristic swan neck deformity is due to retraction of the lateral bands and hyperextension of the proximal interphalangeal joint.

The 45° guideline

Without treatment, the eventual disability will be minimal if the extensor lag at the distal joint is less than 45°; a greater lag will result in functional difficulty and cosmetic deformity.

Treatment

Maintain hyperextension of the distal interphalangeal joint for 6 weeks, leaving the proximal interphalangeal joint free to flex.

Equipment

- Friar's balsam (will permit greater adhesion of tape)
- Non-stretch adhesive tape, 1 cm wide: two strips approximately 10 cm in length

Method

1. Paint finger with Friar's balsam (compound benzoin tincture).
2. Apply the first strip of tape in a figure of eight configuration. The centre of the tape must engage and support the pulp of the finger. The tapes must cross dorsally at the level of the distal interphalangeal joint and extend to the volar aspect of the proximal interphalangeal joint without inhibiting its movement (Fig. 121.2a).

3. Apply the second piece of tape as a 'stay' around the midshaft of the middle phalanx (Fig. 121.2b).

Reapply the tape wherever extension of the distal interphalangeal joint drops below the neutral position (usually daily, depending on the patient's occupation). Maintain extension for 6 weeks.

Surgery

Open reduction and internal fixation are reserved for those cases where the avulsed bony fragment is large enough to cause instability, leading to volar subluxation of the distal interphalangeal joint.

Tenpin bowler's thumb

Tenpin bowler's thumb is a common stress syndrome in players. It usually presents as a soft-tissue swelling at the base of the thumb web, with associated pain and stiffness of the digits used for bowling. It may cause a traumatic neuroma of the digital nerve at this site with associated hyperaesthesia.

Management

- rest
- massage
- bevel the bowling ball holes to reduce friction
- an intralesional injection (Fig. 121.3) of 0.25 mL of long-acting corticosteroid mixed with local anaesthetic (resistant cases)

Fig. 121.2 *Mallet finger:* **(a)** *application of first tape;* **(b)** *application of 'stay' tape*

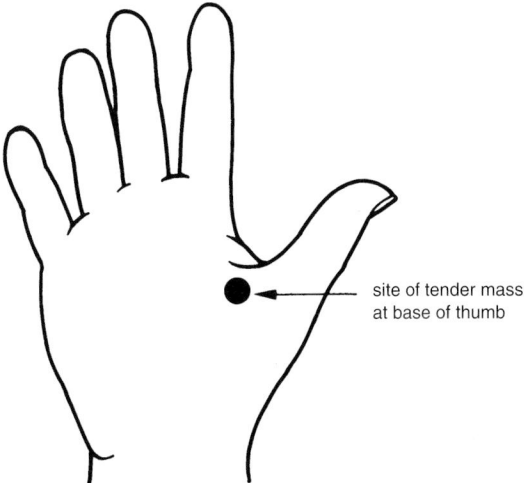

site of tender mass at base of thumb

Fig. 121.3 *Tenpin bowler's thumb*

Snow skiing injuries

The most common injuries encountered in snow skiing are soft-tissue injuries and fractures and dislocations.

A study by Robinson showed that the six most common skiing injuries were: strains to the medial collateral ligament of the knee 24.3%; contusions of soft tissue (excluding head and neck) 17.6%; lacerations 15.5%; neck and back injuries 7.8%; fractures 7.6%; and dislocations.[2]

There has been a large decrease in injuries relative to participation in the past decade because of improved equipment and attention to safety. The most common fractures in skiers are those involving the tibia and fibula, especially spiral fractures. Other common fractures are of the clavicle, wrist and humerus. Dislocation of the shoulder region (glenohumeral joint and acromioclavicular joint) are due to falls on hard impacted snow.

Skier's thumb[3]

A special injury is skier's thumb (also known as gamekeeper's thumb) in which there is ligamentous disruption of the metacarpophalangeal joint with or without an avulsion fracture of the base of the proximal phalanx at the point of ligamentous attachment. This injury is caused by the thumb being forced into abduction and hyperextension by the ski pole as the skier pitches into the snow.

Diagnosis is made by X-ray with stress views of the thumb. Incomplete tears are immobilised in a scaphoid type of plaster for 3 weeks, while complete tears and avulsion fractures should be referred for surgical repair.

Spinal problems

Spinal dysfunction, particularly of the neck and low back, are very common problems in sport, as for the general population.

Serious problems include pars interarticularis fractures, spondylolisthesis, disc disruptions with prolapse and, rarely, vertebral body fracture. The common problems are the various facet joint syndromes and musculoskeletal strains, which are managed conservatively as outlined in Chapters 33 and 56. The key to management is a conservative approach with a back education and exercise program.

Injuries to the lower limbs

Injuries due to trauma and overuse of the lower limbs comprise the most frequent group of sports-related disorders requiring medical attention.

The three main causes of overuse trauma are:

- friction, e.g. peritendinitis
- stress or overload, e.g. hamstring tear, tibial stress fracture
- ischaemia, e.g. anterior compartment syndrome

Overuse leg syndromes

Increased community participation in physical activity, including running and jogging, has resulted in a concomitant increase in overuse leg injuries, especially in the lower leg with its weight-bearing load. The common cause is repetitive trauma where the forces involved overwhelm the tissue's ability to repair adequately. Common causes of chronic leg pain include hamstring injuries and injuries to the lower leg.

Principles of management
Prevention:

- maintain ideal weight
- good nutrition
- adequate preparation
- warm-up exercises for the legs
- proper footwear
- proper activity planning

Treatment of injury
- Rest, or relative rest: the patient is allowed to perform activities that do not aggravate the injury.
- Ice: apply an ice pack for 20–30 minutes every 2 hours while awake during the first 48–72 hours post injury.
- Compression: keep the injured muscle or tissue firmly bandaged for at least 48 hours.
- Elevation: rest the leg on a stool or chair until the swelling subsides.
- Correction of predisposing factors (intrinsic or extrinsic), e.g. orthotics for malalignment, correction of training errors.
- NSAIDs for painful inflammatory response.
- Physical therapy, e.g. stretching, mobilisation when acute phase settled.

Groin pain

Groin pain is a particularly common condition among athletes.

Acute groin pain

Acute conditions such as muscle and musculotendinous strains,[4] and overuse injuries such as tendinitis and tendoperiostitis, are generally readily diagnosed and treated. Diagnostic difficulties can arise because of referred pain from the lumbosacral spine, hip and pelvis. More common acute groin injuries include injuries to the following muscles and their tendons (Fig. 121.4).

- adductor longus, e.g. musculotendinous strains
- rectus femoris
- sartorius
- iliopsoas

Other injuries include:

- SUFE in adolescents
- avulsion fractures in adolescents, e.g. rectus femoris and sartorius on the iliac spines

Chronic groin pain

There are many causes of chronic groin pain, with bone and joint abnormalities being more likely causes. Important causes include:

- muscle and musculotendinous lesions, e.g. adductor longus tendoperiostitis
- bursitis, e.g. iliopsoas bursitis

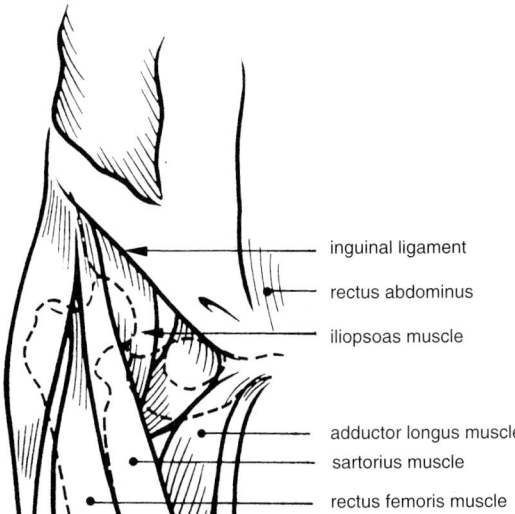

- osteitis pubis (pubic symphysis)
- stress fractures, e.g. femoral neck and pubic rami
- sacroiliac and hip joint disorders, e.g. osteoarthritis hip/tumour
- lumbar spine: L1/L2 or L2/L3 disc
- 'occult' inguinal or femoral hernia

Investigations

- X-ray of pelvis (AP, lateral, oblique)
- tomography of pubic symphysis (to detect osteitis pubis and pubic instability)
- bone scan to detect stress fractures or osteitis pubis
- herniography
- CT scan or MRI or ultrasound (increasing potential)

Jock itch

Jock itch, or tinea cruris, is a common infection in the groin area of young men, especially athletes, who are subjected to chaffing in the groins from tight shorts and nylon 'jock straps'. The feet should be inspected for evidence of tinea pedis. The dermatophyte is transmitted by towels and other objects, particularly in change rooms and communal showers (p. 969).

Hamstring injuries

Hamstring strains are common in athletes. The short head of biceps femoris is the most commonly strained component of the hamstring group.

Clinical features:

- a history of a 'pull', 'twinge', 'tear' or 'twang' in the back of the thigh
- a soreness and lump develops (with a severe tear a person can collapse)
- localised tenderness
- limitation of straight leg raising
- pain on resisted or active knee flexion or hip extension
- bruising (usually in popliteal fossa) may be present

Management

The immediate goals of treatment of the acute injury are to relieve pain and minimise swelling.

- RICE for 72 hours
- NSAIDs, e.g. aspirin or indomethacin
- stretching exercises
  — passive stretching after ice treatment

inguinal ligament

rectus abdominus

iliopsoas muscle

adductor longus muscle

sartorius muscle

rectus femoris muscle

Fig. 121.4 *Muscles in the groin region subject to musculotendinous injuries in the athlete*

— then active stretching
— then isometric contraction exercises

Haematomas in muscle ('corked thigh')

Haematomas can be intramuscular, intermuscular or interstitial. They usually result from a sharp blow, e.g. knee to the thigh or kick in the anterior compartment of the leg.

An intramuscular haematoma can cause an acute compartment syndrome which may require urgent decompression. One objective of treatment is to prevent excessive scarring. Other complications include infection, cyst formation, thrombophlebitis and myositis ossificans.

Management
• RICE treatment with emphasis on cooling
• non-weight-bearing, using crutches initially
• consider admission to hospital or a day surgical unit to check progress
• referral for expert advice may be appropriate because of the potentially serious nature of the injury

Injuries to the knee

Knee injuries are common, have multiple clinical disorders and are potentially disastrous to the athlete. The various injuries and overuse syndromes are presented in considerable detail in Chapter 61, on the painful knee.

Acute injuries
Acute injuries (pp. 635–638) include:

• meniscal tears
• ligamentous tears and strains (of varying degrees)
   — anterior cruciate ligament
   — posterior cruciate ligament
   — medial collateral ligament
   — lateral collateral ligament

Overuse syndromes
The knee is very prone to overuse disorders (pp. 638–641). The pain develops gradually without swelling, is aggravated by activity and relieved with rest. It can usually be traced back to a change in the sportsperson's training schedule, footwear, technique or related factors. It

may also be related to biomechanical abnormalities, ranging from hip disorders to disorders of the feet.
   Overuse injuries include:

• patellofemoral pain syndrome (jogger's knee/runner's knee)
• patellar tendinitis (jumper's knee)
• synovial plica syndrome
• infrapatellar fat-pad inflammation
• anserinus bursitis/tendinitis
• biceps femoris tendinitis
• semimembranous bursitis/tendinitis
• quadriceps tendinitis/rupture
• popliteus tendinitis
• iliotibial band friction syndrome (runner's knee)
• the hamstrung knee

A careful history followed by systematic anatomical palpation around the knee joint will pinpoint the specific overuse syndrome.

Overuse injuries to lower leg

A summary of the clinical and management aspects of various injuries is presented in Table 121.1 and in Figure 121.5.

Common causes of chronic lower leg pain in sportspeople include:[5]

• medial tibial stress syndrome (previously called shin splints)
• stress fractures (Fig. 121.6)
• exertional compartment syndrome, especially anterior compartment
• tibialis anterior tenosynovitis (Fig. 121.7)
• chronic muscle strains

These problems are invariably due to excessive physical demands in athletes striving for the ultimate performance or in the occasional athletes who have made inadequate preparation for their activity. Training errors contribute to a large proportion (60%) of overuse injuries.[5]

Principles of treatment
1. rest or relative rest
2. exercise program (where appropriate)
3. correction of predisposing factors, e.g.
   — training errors
   — unsuitable footwear
   — inadequate warm-up
   — malalignment
4. analgesics: use NSAIDs only if it is true inflammatory pain (pain at rest)

Table 121.1 *Clinical comparisons of overuse syndromes in lower leg*

Syndrome	Symptoms	Cause	Treatment
Anterior compartment syndrome	Pain in the anterolateral muscular compartment of the leg, increasing with activity. Difficult dorsiflexion of foot, which may feel floppy.	Persistent fast running (e.g. squash, football, middle-distance running).	Modify activities. Surgical fasciotomy is the only effective treatment.
Iliotibial band tendinitis	Deep aching along lateral aspect of knee or lateral thigh. Worse running downhill, eased by rest. Pain appears after 3–4 km running.	Running up hills by long-distance runners and increasing distance too quickly.	Rest from running for 6 weeks. Special stretching exercises. Correct training faults and footwear. ? injection of LA and corticosteroids deep into tender areas.
Tibial stress syndrome or shin splints	Pain and localised tenderness over the distal posteromedial border of the tibia. Bone scan for diagnosis.	Running or jumping on hard surfaces.	Relative rest for 6 weeks. Ice massage. Calf (soleus stretching). NSAIDs. Correct training faults and footwear.
Tibial stress fracture	Pain, in a similar site to shin splints, noted after running. Usually relieved by rest. Bone scan for diagnosis.	Overtraining on hard (often bitumen) surfaces. Faulty footwear.	Rest for 6–10 weeks. Casting not recommended. Graduated training after healing.
Tibialis anterior tenosynovitis	Pain, over anterior distal third of leg and ankle. Pain at beginning and after exercise ± swelling, crepitus. Pain on active or resisted ankle dorsiflexion.	Overuse—excessive downhill running.	Rest, even from walking. Injection of LA and corticosteroid within tendon sheath.
Achilles tendinitis	Pain in the Achilles tendon aggravated by walking on the toes. Stiff and sore in the morning after rising but improving after activity.	Repeated toe running in sprinters or running uphill in distance runners.	Relative rest. Ice at first and then heat. 10 mm heel wedge. Correct training faults and footwear. NSAIDs.

Fig. 121.5 *Common sites of overuse injuries in the lower leg*

Stress fractures

Stress fractures are an important cause of lower leg pain and foot pain in sport, accounting for 5–15% of injuries.[5] Stress fractures occur in the tibia and fibula and in the foot (navicular, calcaneus and metatarsals). The important clinical factor is to keep stress fractures in mind and X-ray the tender area. If the X-ray is negative and there is a high index of suspicion, a radionuclide scan should be ordered.

In the tibia, stress fractures occur mainly in the proximal metaphysis and the junction of the middle and distal thirds of the shaft. In the fibula they usually occur 5–7 cm above the tip of the lateral malleolus (Fig. 121.6).

Fig. 121.6 *Typical sites of stress fractures in athletes in the tibia and fibula*

These stress fractures usually occur after prolonged and repeated heavy loading such as long-distance running or repeated jumping.

Torn 'monkey muscle'

The so-called torn 'monkey muscle', or 'tennis leg', is actually a rupture of the medial head of gastrocnemius at the musculoskeletal junction where the Achilles tendon merges with the muscle (Fig. 121.8). It is not a torn plantaris muscle as commonly believed. This painful injury is common in middle-aged tennis and squash players who play infrequently and are unfit.

Clinical features:
- a sudden sharp pain in the calf (the person thinks he/she has been struck from behind, e.g. a thrown stone)
- unable to put heel to ground
- walks on tip toes
- localised tenderness and hardness
- dorsiflexion of ankle painful
- bruising over site of rupture

Management
- RICE treatment for 48 hours
- ice packs immediately for 20 minutes and then

Fig. 121.7 *Site of tibialis anterior tenosynovitis*

Fig. 121.8 *'Tennis leg' or 'monkey muscle'—illustrating typical site of rupture of the medial head of gastrocnemius at the junction of muscle and tendon (left leg)*

every 2 hours when awake (can be placed over the bandage)
- a firm elastic bandage from toes to below the knee
- crutches can be used if severe
- a raised heel on the shoe aids mobility
- commence mobilisation after 48 hours rest, with active exercises
- phyiotherapist supervision for gentle stretching massage and then restricted exercise

Sprained ankle

There are two main ligaments that are subject to heavy inversion or eversion stresses, namely the lateral ligaments and the medial ligaments respectively. Most of the ankle 'sprains' or tears involve the lateral ligaments (up to 90%) while the stronger tauter (deltoid) ligament is less prone to injury.

The lateral ligament complex involves three main bands: the anterior talofibular (ATFL), the calcaneofibular (CFL) and the posterior talofibular ligament (PTFL) (Fig. 121.9).

Mechanism of injury to lateral ligaments[6]

Forced inversion causes about 90% of all ankle injuries.

Most sprains occur when the ankle is plantarflexed and inverted such as when landing awkwardly after jumping or stepping on uneven ground.

Inversion

Foot in plantar flexion: ATFL injury likely (50–60%)
Foot in neutral: CFL injury likely (10%)

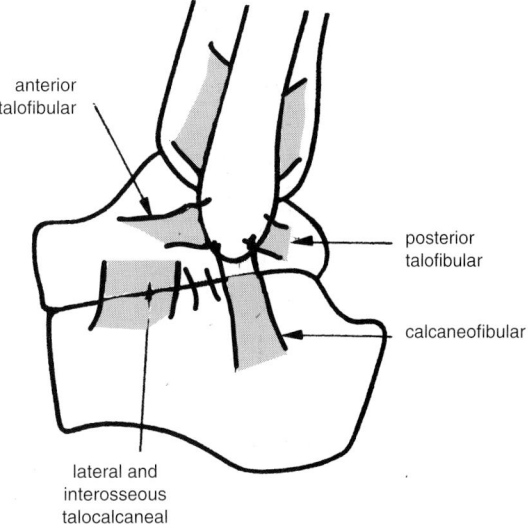

Fig. **121.9** *Lateral ligaments of the ankle*

Foot in dorsiflexion: PTFL injury likely (5%)

Note: Combined ATFL and CFL injury (15–25%).

Eversion

Foot in plantar flexion or neutral: medial ligament (mainly anterior part)

The classification of ankle injuries is presented in Table 121.2.

Clinical features of sprained lateral ligaments

Common features
- ankle 'gives way'
- difficulty in weight bearing
- discomfort varies from mild to severe

Table 121.2 *Classification of injuries to ankle ligaments (adapted from Litt)*[6]

Grade	Functional/clinical	Ligamentous stability	Stress X-rays
I (mild)	minimal pain and swelling minimal bleeding full range of motion heel and toe walking	minor ligamentous injury with only a partial tear of the ligament stable ankle joint	normal
II (moderate)	moderate to severe pain and swelling considerable bleeding decreased range of motion difficulty in weight bearing and ambulation	similar to Grade I only more severe partially unstable joint	anterior draw 4–14 mm Talar tilt 5–10°
III (severe)	minimal to severe pain and swelling pronounced bleeding minimal range of motion unable to weight bear	complete ligamentous rupture with unstable joint	anterior draw > 15 mm Talar tilt > 20°

- bruising (may take 12–24 hours) indicates more severe injury
- may have functional instability: ankle gives way on uneven ground

Physical examination (perform as soon as possible)

- note swelling and bruising
- palpate over bony landmarks and three lateral ligaments
- test general joint laxity and range of motion
- a common finding is rounded swelling in front of lateral malleolus (the 'signe de la coquille d'oeuf')
- test stability in AP plane (anterior draw sign)
- talar tilt test (inversion stress test)

Is there an underlying fracture?[7]

For a severe injury the possibility of a fracture—usually of the lateral malleolus or base of fifth metatarsal—must be considered. If the patient is able to walk without much discomfort straight after the injury, a fracture is unlikely.

Indications for X-ray include:[7]

- inability to weight bear immediately after injury
- marked swelling and bruising soon after injury
- marked tenderness over the bony landmarks
- marked pain on movement of the ankle
- crepitus on palpation or movement
- point tenderness over the base of the fifth metatarsal
- special circumstances, e.g. litigation potential

Management

The treatment of ankle ligament sprains depends on the severity of the sprain. Most grade I and II sprains respond well to standard conservative measures and regain full, pain-free movement in 1–6 weeks, but controversy surrounds the most appropriate management of grade III sprains.

Grade I sprain

R   rest the injured part for 48 hours, depending on disability
I   ice pack for 20 minutes every 3–4 hours when awake for the first 48 hours
C   compression bandage, e.g. crepe bandage
E   elevate to hip level to minimise swelling
A   analgesics, e.g. paracetamol ± codeine
R   review in 48 hours, then 7 days
S   special strapping

Use partial weight bearing with crutches for the first 48 hours or until standing is no longer painful, then encourage early full weight bearing and a full range of movement with isometric exercises.[7] Use warm soaks, dispense with ice packs after 48 hours. Walking in sand, e.g. along the beach, is excellent rehabilitation. Aim towards full activity by 2 weeks.

Special strapping

A firm support for partial tears in the absence of gross swelling provides excellent symptomatic relief and early mobilisation.

Method

- Maintain the foot in a neutral position (right angles to leg) by getting patient to hold the foot in that position by a long strap or sling.
- Apply small protective pads over pressure points.
- Apply one or two stirrups of adhesive low-stretch 6–8 cm strapping from halfway up medial side, around the heel and then halfway up the lateral side to hold foot in slight eversion (Figs 121.10 a,b).
- Apply an adhesive bandage, e.g. Acrylastic (6–8 cm) which can be rerolled and reused.
- Reapply in 3–4 days.
- After 7 days, remove the bandage and use a non-adhesive tubular elasticised support until full pain-free movement is achieved.

Grade II sprain

RICE treatment (as above) for 48 hours but ice, e.g. ACE wrap, should be every 2–3 hours and no weight bearing (use crutches) for 48 hours. Then permit partial weight bearing with crutches and begin the active exercise program. Follow-up and supportive strapping as for Grade I. Note that the ice packs can be placed over the strapping.

Grade III sprain

It would be appropriate to refer this patient with a complete tear. Initial management includes RICE and analgesics and an X-ray to exclude an associated fracture. The three main treatment approaches appear to be equally satisfactory.

Surgical repair

Some specialists prefer this treatment but it is usually reserved for the competitive athlete who demands absolute stability of the ankle.

angle and those who need to be mobile and protected in order to work. The plaster is maintained until the ligament repairs, usually 4–6 weeks. The patient can walk normally when comfortable with a rockered sole or open cast walking shoe.

Strapping and physiotherapy

This approach is generally recommended. After the usual treatment for a Grade II repair, including the strapping as described, a heel lock (Fig. 121.10c) should be used. The patient continues on crutches and appropriate physiotherapy is given with care so that the torn ends are not distracted. Strengthened balance is achieved by the use of elastic bands, swimming and cycling.

Non-response to treatment

There are some patients who, despite an apparently straightforward ankle sprain, do not respond to therapy and do not regain a full range of movement. In such patients alternative diagnoses in addition to ligament tearing must be considered (Table 121.3). These require careful clinical assessment and further investigation such as bone scans.

stirrups
of adhesive
tape

Fig. 121.10a,b *Supportive strapping for a sprained ankle:* **Step 1** *apply protective pads and stay tape;* **Step 2** *apply stirrups to hold foot in slight eversion*

Plaster immobilisation

This is usually reserved for patients who are unable actively to dorsiflex their foot to a right

Fig. 121.10c *Supportive strapping for a sprained ankle:* **Step 3** *apply an ankle lock tape*

Table 121.3 *Unstable ankle injuries to be considered in delayed healing (after Brukner)*[7]

Osteochondral fracture of the talar dome
Dislocation of the peroneal tendons
Sinus tarsi syndrome
Anteroinferior tibiofibular ligament injury
Post-traumatic synovitis
Anterior impingement syndrome
Posterior impingement syndrome
Anterior lateral impingement
Rupture of posterior tibial tendon
Reflex sympathetic dystrophy
Other fractures
• base 5th metatarsal (avulsion)
• lateral process of talus
• anterior process of the calcaneus
• tibial plafond
• stress fracture navicular

Heel disorders

Important causes of heel pain and other disorders resulting from overuse sporting activities include:

• Achilles tendon disorders
  — tendinitis/peritendinitis
  — tear: partial or complete
• bruised heel
• 'pump bumps'/bursitis
• calcaneal apophysitis
• plantar fasciitis (p. 650)
• talon noir
• blisters

Achilles tendinitis/peritendinitis[9]

The inflammation that occurs as a combination of degenerative and inflammatory changes due to overuse may appear either in the tendon itself or in the surrounding paratendon. The latter is called peritendinitis rather than tenosynovitis because there is no synovial sheath.

Clinical features:

• history of unaccustomed running or long walk
• common in runners who change routine
• usually young to middle-aged males
• aching pain on using tendon
• tendon feels stiff, especially on rising
• tender thickened tendon
• palpable crepitus on movement of tendon

Ultrasound examination
This is very useful in differentiating between tendinitis, peritendinitis, focal degeneration and a partial tear.

Preventive measures
• warm-up and stretching exercises in athletes
• good quality shoes
• 1 cm heel raise

Treatment
• Rest: ? crutches in acute phase, plaster cast if severe
• Cool with ice in acute stage, then heat
• NSAIDs
• 1–2 cm heel raise under the shoe
• ultrasound and deep friction massage
• mobilisation, then graduated stretching exercises

Note: Ensure adequate rest and early resolution because chronic tendinitis is persistent and very difficult to treat.

Avoid corticosteroid injection in acute stages and never give into tendon. Can be injected *around* the tendon if localised and tender.

Partial rupture of Achilles tendon

Clinical features:

• a sudden sharp pain at the time of injury
• sharp pain when stepping off affected leg
• usually males >30 sporadically engaged in sport
• history of running, jumping or hurrying up stairs
• a tender swelling palpable about 2.5 cm above the insertion
• may be a very tender defect about size of tip of little finger

Treatment
If palpable gap—early surgical exploration with repair.

If no gap, use conservative treatment:

• initial rest (with ice) and crutches
• 1–2 cm heel raise inside shoe
• ultrasound and deep friction massage
• graduated stretching exercises

Convalescence is usually 10–12 weeks.[8] A poor response to healing manifests as recurrent pain and disability, indicates surgical exploration and possible repair.

Complete rupture of Achilles tendon

This common problem in athletes occurs in a possibly degenerated tendon subjected to a sudden increased load, e.g. a skier with foot anchored and ankle dorsiflexed.

Clinical features:

- sudden onset of intense pain
- patient usually falls over
- feels more comfortable when acute phase passes
- development of swelling and bruising
- some difficulty walking, especially on tip toe

Diagnosis

- palpation of gap (best to test in first 2–3 hours as haematoma can fill gap)
- positive Thompson's test (Figs 121.11 a,b)

Note: The injury may be missed because the patient is able to plantar flex the foot actively by means of the deep long flexors to the foot.

Treatment

Early surgical repair (within 3 weeks).

(a)

(b)

Fig. 121.11 *Thompson's calf squeeze test for ruptured Achilles tendon:* **(a)** *intact tendon, normal plantar flexion;* **(b)** *ruptured tendon, foot remains stationary*

'Pump bumps'

A 'pump bump' is a tender bursa over a bony prominence lateral to the attachment of the Achilles tendon. This is caused by inflammation related to poorly fitting footwear irritating a pre-existing enlargement of the calcaneus. Treatment is symptomatic and attention to footwear.

Talon noir

Talon noir or 'black heel', which has a black spotted appearance on the posterior end of the heel, is common in sportsmen and women, especially squash players. It tends to be bilateral and is caused by the shearing stresses of the sharp turns required in sport. The diagnosis is confirmed by gentle paring away of the hard skin containing old blood.

Disorders of the feet and toes

Common problems include:

- fractures of toes
- foot strain
- ingrowing toenails
- 'black' nails
- bony outgrowth under the nail (subungual exostosis)
- calluses
- athlete's foot (tinea pedis)
- plantar warts

Black nails ('soccer toe')

Black or 'bruised' nails are due to subungual haematoma caused by trauma. The problem can be acute or chronic and is seen in the great toes. Acute cases are usually the result of the toe being trodden on, while chronic cases are the result of wearing ill-fitting shoes (too narrow or loose) or the toenails being left too long.

The problem is encountered commonly in sports that involve deceleration forces and include running (especially cross-country with downhill running), netball, basketball, tennis, football and skiing.

Treatment

An acute subungual haematoma should be decompressed with a hot needle or other procedure through the nail. A chronic non-painful problem should be left to heal. The toenails will become dystrophic and be replaced by 'new' nails.

Attention should be paid to the footwear either by changing it or by placing protective padding in the toes of the running shoes or boots.

Injuries in adolescents

If an adolescent engaged in sport presents with pain in the leg it is important to consider the following problems.

- slipped capital femoral epiphysis (p. 603)
- avulsion of epiphyses, e.g. ischial tuberosity (hamstring)
- stress fracture
- Osgood-Schlatter's disorder
- Scheuermann's disorder
- idiopathic scoliosis

References

1. Fitzpatrick J. Shoulder pain a real wet blanket. Australian Dr Weekly, 5 February 1993; 56.

2. Robinson M. Hazards of alpine sport. Aust Fam Physician, 1991; 20:961–970.

3. Elliott B, Sherry E. Common snow skiing injuries. Aust Fam Physician, 1984; 13:570–574.

4. Zimmermann G. Groin pain in athletes. Aust Fam Physician, 1988; 17:1046–1052.

5. James T. Chronic lower leg pain in sport. Aust Fam Physician, 1988; 17:1041–1045.

6. Litt J. The sprained ankle. Aust Fam Physician, 1992; 21:447–456.

7. Brukner P. The difficult ankle. Aust Fam Physician, 1991; 20:919–930.

8. Sloane PD, Slatt LM, Baker RM. *Essentials of family medicine*. Baltimore: Williams and Wilkins, 1988, 253–259.

9. Bruckner P, Khan K. *Clinical sports medicine*. Sydney: McGraw-Hill, 1995, 426–435.

PART 11

ABORIGINAL HEALTH

———

122

The health of Aboriginal and Torres Strait Islander peoples

—

Health does not just mean the physical well being of the individual but refers to the social, emotional and cultural well being of the whole community. This is a whole of life view and includes the cyclical concept of life-death-life. Health services should strive to achieve the state where every individual can achieve their full potential as human beings (Aborigines) and thus bring about the total well being of their communities. This is an evolving definition (process).

National Aboriginal Community Controlled
Health Organisation, September 1993

The major health challenge in Australia (and several other developed countries) is the health status of Aboriginal people which continues to be dramatically worse than that of other Australians. In some cases, it appears that the gap may be widening, especially for women.[1]

Life expectancies in 1992–94 for Aboriginal and Torres Strait Islander men and women were 15–20 years below those of other Australians. The contrast with other Australians is most marked at 25–54 years. Diseases of the circulatory system, injury and poisoning, respiratory illness and neoplasms continue to be important causes of death. Deaths from infectious diseases and genitourinary disorders continue to occur at much higher rates than among other Australians.

The increasing incidence of diabetes is of great concern, especially in those changing from a traditional diet to inappropriate westernised diets. Death rates from diabetes in 1992–94 were 12 times higher for men and nearly 17 times higher for women than the rates for other Australians.[1]

The level of infant and maternal mortality continues to be a concern. After great reductions in infant mortality rates in the 1970s there has been a levelling off, with rates remaining 3–5 times higher than those of other Australians. About 30% of maternal deaths occur in Aboriginal and Torres Strait Islander women, who contribute only about 3% of confinements.[1]

Other key facts and checkpoints

- Consider the importance of cultural issues in a consultation with an Aboriginal Australian or Torres Strait Islander.
- If assistance is required with a cultural issue, consider involving an Aboriginal and Torres Strait Islander health worker in the consultation.
- Always consider multiple medical conditions in the sick person.
- Remember the importance of opportunistic screening in Aboriginal and Torres Strait Islander patients for relatively common conditions, e.g.
  - NIDDM (20–50% incidence)
  - hypertension
  - hepatitis B
  - STD screening with Pap smears
  - anaemia in children
  - hearing in children
- Cervical cancer is 6–8 times more common in Aboriginal and Torres Strait Islander women.
- Approximately 50% of Aboriginal and Torres Strait Islander children have chronic tympanic membrane perforations, with very significant consequences for language development and school achievement.

- BCG and hepatitis B vaccination are recommended for newborn Aboriginal and Torres Strait Islander children.
- Influenza and pneumococcal vaccines are recommended for adult Aboriginal Australians and Torres Strait Islanders over 50 years.

National survey

The first national survey of the health of Aboriginal Australians and Torres Strait Islanders, completed in 1994, highlighted considerable differences in reported health status according to place of residence.[1] Interestingly, most survey participants (88%) considered themselves to be in good to excellent health.

The survey highlighted the following disorders.

- asthma
- ear and hearing problems
- diabetes
- hypertension
- kidney disorders
- heart disease
- skin disorders
- eye problems, including trachoma
- nutritional status (esp. obesity)
- substance abuse, e.g. alcohol, marijuana, petrol sniffing
- dental problems (a reversed trend of dental caries)

The many reasons for the lower health status of Aboriginal Australians and Torres Strait Islanders include poverty, dispossession, geographical isolation, high population mobility, temperature extremes in central Australia, increased exposure to infectious diseases, especially in subtropical areas, and lack of appropriate service deliveries.

Poor living conditions contribute to poor health outcomes such as substance abuse, domestic violence, other social dysfunction and child malnutrition. Other environmental health issues such as lack of adequate shelter, lack of basic amenities such as clean running water and adequate sewage disposal facilities, and often lack of refrigeration in hot climates all impact on Aboriginal health. Diseased dogs have been shown to be an important reservoir of infections for humans, and Aboriginal people are at special risk of cross-infection.[2] Thus, controlling parasitic infections in their dogs will improve the health of the people.

Aboriginal culture and the doctor–patient relationship

An understanding of Aboriginal cultural issues is fundamental to successful management outcomes. Doctors should realise that, while examining Aboriginal patients, they are themselves being examined. When Aboriginal Australians visit the doctor they bring their own cultural expectations with them. 'A poster or coffee table book on Aboriginal culture in the waiting room may form a simple bridge to acceptance.'[3] Aboriginal people are often rather shy and communicate more indirectly than Europeans on important sensitive issues. They may use silence while waiting for answers and this could be a cue for the doctor to use a new line of approach.[4] It is important for doctors working in Aboriginal communities to have an appreciation of and respect for Aboriginal culture and be aware of its significance in health and behaviour.

An Aboriginal patient may feel more relaxed if accompanied by a relative, who can witness what the doctor said and reinforce it later.

It is important to understand that Aboriginal people and culture must not be seen as homogeneous but rather as diverse, with each group needing a special understanding of its cultural issues.

Women's business

The Aboriginal concept of 'women's business' can be defined as the range of experience and knowledge that is the exclusive preserve and domain of Aboriginal women. It encompasses issues about menstruation, pregnancy, childbirth and contraception.[5] Such matters are traditionally not discussed directly but are conveyed indirectly through stories, ceremonies and songs. For more traditional women it is taboo to talk about women's health issues to male doctors or male health workers, or to be physically examined by them. Apart from the sense of shame and embarrassment, it represents a transgression of their natural law.[6]

Men's business

Similarly, the cultural issue of men's business needs to be understood and respected. This applies to manhood initiation rites, circumcision, sexuality and sexually transmitted diseases.

Sorry business

Sorry business is the process of grieving, and this needs to be clearly understood. There is a cultural obligation for mourners to grieve the death of a relative in a special way. This involves changing their appearance and a deliberate avoidance of any mention of the deceased person's name or any portrayal of his or her likeness.[5] The place where the person died is deserted for a certain time and then smoked out.

Common problems in children[7]

Aboriginal children suffer the same spectrum of health problems as children in developing countries and communities throughout the world, and the infant mortality rate remains high. The major problems are malnutrition, diarrhoeal disease, skin infections and respiratory tract infection. Common problems are presented in Table 122.1

Acute respiratory tract infections are a common reason for admission to hospital. Bacterial pneumonias occur more commonly than in non-Aboriginal children and usually present late. Chronic upper respiratory tract disease is typical in younger children and mucopurulent nasal discharge is present in most preschool children.[7] Inappropriate treatment of respiratory tract infection will predispose to a high incidence of low-grade lower respiratory tract

Table 122.1 *Common clinical problems in children*

Perinatal
Low birth weight
Asphyxia
Infections

Preschool
Malnutrition
Anaemia
Respiratory infection
Diarrhoeal disease
Hepatitis B
Skin infection/infestation
Urinary tract infection
Meningitis
Joint and bone infection

Later childhood and adolescence
Bacterial and viral infections
Parasitic infestation
Streptococcal infection
• rheumatic fever
• glomerulonephritis
Trauma
Substance abuse

disease in later childhood and classic bronchiectasis.

Chronic suppurative otitis media, which is almost universal in preschool children, is often refractory to treatment and can lead to significant hearing impairment in many children. It can develop without apparent preceding acute otitis media and may be related to poor nutrition and anaemia. The basic treatment is ear toilet with povidone-iodine solution, followed by dry mopping with rolled toilet paper/tissue 'spears', or initial use of the 'spears' followed by acetic acid drops.

Skin infection and infestation are almost as prevalent as respiratory tract disease. Scabies is endemic and occasionally reaches epidemic proportions. It can be a very debilitating problem and can present in very young infants, in the first few weeks of life.[7]

Anaemia, usually iron deficiency, is found in at least 25% of children. Apart from reduced intake, intestinal loss from hookworm and other parasitic infection is an important factor. Treatment includes deworming in addition to iron supplements.

Diarrhoeal disease is a very common reason for hospital admission. Causes of infective gastroenteritis include rotavirus, bacteria including shigella, salmonella and campylobacter, and parasites such as *Giardia lamblia*, Strongyloides and Cryptosporidium.

Other important and serious problems encountered more frequently in Aboriginal children include bacterial meningitis (especially due to *Haemophilus influenzae*), septic arthritis and osteomyelitis, pyomyositis, *Streptococcus pyogenes* infections with associated glomerulonephritis and rheumatic fever, urinary tract calculi, urinary tract infection, hepatitis B and petrol sniffing.

The ability to achieve appropriate levels of immunisation in these communities will have enormous health benefits. Poliomyelitis, diphtheria, pertussis and tuberculosis are now rare and it is hoped that hepatitis B and *Haemophilus influenzae* infections will be drastically reduced.

Specific disorders requiring attention

The general practitioner attending Aboriginal and Torres Strait Islander patients has to develop special skills in the diagnosis and management of the following health concerns:

- diabetes mellitus
- trauma
- substance abuse, including alcohol and smoking
- ear and eye infections
- respiratory disorders: upper and lower RTIs, asthma
- skin disorders, e.g. fungal infections, impetigo, leg ulcers, cellulitis, boils
- parasitic infestations, e.g. scabies, lice
- gastrointestinal infections, e.g. Campylobacter enteritis, giardiasis, Shigella
- sexually transmitted disease
- psychosocial dysfunction
- bites and stings
- severe infections, e.g. meningitis, rheumatic fever, septicaemia
- hepatitis B
- tropical diseases (where applicable)
- worm infestation

However, the general management of medical disorders follows the principles and treatment guidelines outlined in this book. Antibiotic guidelines for use by Aboriginal health workers in rural Aboriginal communities are available.[8]

Ear infections[8,9]

Otitis externa and otitis media with its acute and chronic complications are major health problems in rural Aboriginal and Torres Strait Islander children. Acute otitis media should be treated early and aggressively with antibiotics to prevent chronic suppurative otitis media which is very difficult to cure once established.

Treatment guidelines

- acute otitis media — amoxycillin (o) or co-trimazole (o) or procaine penicillin (IM) for 5 days; if no response, consider amoxycillin/clavulanate or cefaclor
- acute suppurative otitis media — antibiotics (as above) + dry mop ear
- chronic suppurative otitis media — wash with acetic acid 0.25% or water or povidone-iodine 5% solution (preferred) using a 20mL syringe with plastic tubing 1, 2 or 3 times daily, then dry mop with rolled toilet paper 'spears', or dry mop first then instil 2 drops of acetic acid 1% until dry. Teach this method to family members. If available, suction kits are useful
- otitis externa — gently clean out debris with toilet paper 'spears' followed by acetic acid 0.25%; insert Kenacomb or Sofradex drops or ointment 12 hourly on a gauze wick
- acute mastoiditis — parenteral flucloxacillin/dicloxacillin and hospitalisation

Eye infections[8]

Treatment guidelines

- *Periorbital cellulitis and penetrating eye trauma.* Arrange evacuation to hospital; if critically ill or delay in transfer give empirical treatment with ceftriaxone IM or IV once daily. Add gentamicin IM or IV as single dose for a child < 3 months or patients with other risk factors such as diabetes.
- *Conjunctivitis.* Take two swabs (one for microculture and one for chlamydia). Apply topical chloramphenicol eyedrops plus ointment.
- *Neonatal gonococcal ophthalmia and chlamydia infection*: refer page 477.
- *Gonococcal conjunctivitis.* Procaine penicillin (IM) statim or single dose oral therapy with amoxycillin plus probenecid, e.g. 3g + 1g in adult. Use ceftriaxone IM if penicillin-resistant.
- *Trachoma.* These patients have 'scratchy' eyes and watery discharge ± red eye.
  — if over 6 kg and not pregnant: azithromycin (o) as single dose
  — if under 6kg or pregnant: erythromycin or roxithromycin (o) for 14 days or oily tetracycline eyedrops 1 bd for 3–6 weeks
  — check and treat household contacts
  — check routinely for 'follicles' of trachoma

Skin and soft-tissue infections

Skin infections are the commonest presenting problem in many clinics.[10] These include a high incidence of scabies and tinea corporis (ringworm), boils and carbuncles, infected wounds, impetigo and cellulitis. The most serious complication of skin infections is post-streptococcal glomerulonephritis secondary to *Streptococcus pyogenes* infection. Scabies is the most common skin infestation and commonly starts as an itchy rash with pinhead papules in the web spaces of the fingers.

Recommended treatment (in summary)[8,9]

Impetigo and other skin sores
- soak and remove crusts with povidone-iodine or cetrimide/chlorhexadine
- antibiotic treatment (if required)

    Bicillin All-Purpose IM, statim dose

    or

    erythromycin (o) 12 hourly or roxithromycin (o) daily for 10 days

Cellulitis (mild–moderate) and erysipelas
    Bicillin All-Purpose IM on days 1 and 3 or daily for 3–5 days

    or

    procaine penicillin IM daily for 5 days
    If no improvement: flucloxacillin/dicloxacillin plus probenecid (as below)

Boils, carbuncles, abscesses, bullous impetigo
    flucloxacillin/dicloxacillin (o) + probenecid (o) 12 hourly for 5–10 days

Suppurative wound infections
- use local measures such as aseptic dressings and topical antiseptics
- if necessary, add flucloxacillin/dicloxacillin (as above); consider clindamycin

Tinea corporis (ringworm)
- use benzoic acid ointment, Whitfield's ointment or one of the imidazole preparations: apply 1–3 times daily for 4–6 weeks
- continue topical therapy for 2 weeks after resolution
- systemic agents may be necessary

Scabies
- apply permethrin 5% cream or benzyl benzoate 25% emulsion (pp. 967–968)
- for children less than 2 months use sulphur 5% cream for 2–3 days

    or

    crotamiton 10% cream daily for 3–5 days
- for infected scabies use flucloxacillin/dicloxacillin or erythromycin

Pityriasis versicolor (white spot)
Refer to page 987.

Worm infestations

Intestinal helminths are common in tropical northern Australia. Symptoms may include diarrhoea and abdominal pain with or without distension. Anaemia is common with hookworm infestation. Refer to page 102 for more information.

> ### Treatment[8]
- *Hookworm, roundworm, threadworm*—pyrantel embonate or imbendazole or albendazole
- *Whipworm*—mebendazole or albendazole
- *Strongyloidiasis*—albendazole or thiabendazole
- *Cutaneous larva migrans*—albendazole or thiabendazole

Community worm program. In selected communities a worm eradication program is recommended for children between the ages of 6 months and 12 years with either pyrantel embonate or albendazole.

Sexually transmitted diseases

In the management of STDs it is important to be aware of the significance of men's and women's 'business'; that is, the cultural sensitivities regarding men's and women's special gender feelings and issues which need to be observed when discussing STDs with Aboriginal and Torres Strait Islander patients. For some women it is inappropriate for a male doctor to discuss such issues with them but appropriate for a female doctor, nurse or health worker to do so. Similarly, it may be inappropriate for a female health worker to discuss STDs with a male patient.

Always undertake a full STD screen in patients presenting with an STD. Screening consists of counselling, taking blood for RPR, hepatitis B and HIV, urethral and cervical swabs for gonococcus and chlamydia, ulcer swabs, viral media swab for possible herpes, 'snip' biopsy (where appropriate) for Donovanosis or malignancy, and urine for MCU.[8] First voided urine for polymerase chain reaction (PCR) for gonococcus and chlamydia is an important investigation, especially for those who refuse swabs. Follow-up after therapy and contact tracing, screening, treatment and notification are all necessary.

Specific treatment
(Refer also to Chap. 98)

Urethritis and cervicitis
amoxycillin 3 g (o) + probenecid 1 g (o)—single dose
plus azithromycin 1 g(o) as single dose

Genital sores
Herpes simplex, syphilis and Donovanosis are much more common than chancroid and lymphogranuloma venereum. Serology for syphilis is essential. Advise to avoid sex and for males to use condoms until treatment is completed and lesions well healed.

Syphilis
benzathine penicillin 1.8 g IM as single dose

Donovanosis (granuloma inguinale)
azithromycin 0.5–1 g (o) once daily for 7 days[8]
or
1 g (o) once weekly for 4 weeks
(if not pregnant or breast-feeding); if so, give erythromycin or roxithromycin[8]

Herpes simplex
See pages 946–947.

Genital warts
See page 949.

Pelvic inflammatory disease
If sexually acquired, it is usually due to *Neisseria gonorrhoeae* or *Chlamydia trachomatis* (less likely). For treatment, see page 946.

Vaginal infections
(Refer Chap. 98 for treatment.) *Trichomonas vaginalis* is usually sexually transmitted, while *Candida albicans* and bacterial vaginosis is not.

Practice tips
- Anaemia is common in Aboriginal and Torres Strait Islander children—be on the lookout for it. Consider giving pyrantel embonate or mebendazole in a hookworm endemic area.
- Asthma is common—consider it in coughing children.
- In children with failure to thrive consider insufficient food, urinary tract infection, GIT infection or parasites and recurrent illness.

- Beware of diarrhoea in children—attend to fluid and electrolyte replacement.
- Think pelvic inflammatory disease in the woman of child-bearing age presenting with abdominal pain. Be watchful for penicillinase producing *Neisseria gonorrhoeae* (although it remains uncommon in Aboriginal and Torres Strait Islander communities).
- Consider the possibility of rheumatic fever or glomerulonephritis with *Streptococcus pyogenes* throat infection and treat with an optimal course of antibiotics, e.g. single injection of benzathine penicillin.
- In tropical areas consider diseases such as melioidosis, dengue and Ross River infection.
- Promote immunisation programs.
- Measles can be a very serious disease in Aboriginal children and is highly contagious.
- In the fitting or aggressive patient alcohol withdrawal is the commonest cause but the possibility of petrol sniffing should also be considered.
- Renal failure is more common in Aboriginal and Torres Strait Islander people: look for it if proteinuria, diabetes, hypertension, general debility, recurrent infections.
- Donovanosis (granuloma inguinale), which can be chronic and progressive, presents initially as raised beefy nodules or sores. Microscopy of scrapings or snip or pinch biopsy will confirm diagnosis.[8]
- If routine swabs for gonococcus and chlamydia infection are unobtainable for cultural reasons, use urine polymerase chain reaction (PCR) testing.
- Medroxyprogesterone acetale (Depo-Provera) is a very useful contraceptive agent but always adhere to guidelines for informed consent.
- Because compliance with medication may be a problem with some patients, once-a-day therapy is recommended where possible.

References
1. Reid J (Chair). *Australia's health 1996.* Canberra: Australian Institute of Health and Welfare, 1996, 21–30.
2. Palmer A, Presson B. *Aboriginal community canine parasitic disease and population control coupled with field test programs.* Darwin: DAA, 1990.

3. Hill P. Aboriginal culture and the doctor–patient relationship. Aust Fam Physician, 1994; 23:29–32.

4. Eades D. They don't speak an Aboriginal language, or do they? In: Keen I ed. *Being black: Aboriginal cultures in 'settled' Australia*. Canberra: Aboriginal Studies Press, 1991, 97–115.

5. O'Connor M. Women's business. Aust Fam Physician, 1994; 23:40–44.

6. National Aboriginal Health Strategy Working Party. *A National Aboriginal Health Strategy*. Canberra: Department of Aboriginal Affairs, 1989, 193.

7. Walker A. Common health problems in Northern Territory Aboriginal children. Aust Fam Physician, 1994; 23:55–62.

8. Mashford ML (Chairman). Antibiotic Guidelines for Central and Northern Australia and other remote areas. In: *Antibiotic guidelines* (9th edn). Melbourne: Therapeutic Guidelines, 1997, 175–202.

9. Central Australian Rural Practitioners Association (CARPA). *Standard treatment manual*. Alice Springs, 1992.

10. Crowe C. Common illnesses (Aboriginal health). Aust Fam Physician, 1995; 24:1469–1474.

PART 12

EVERYDAY PRACTICE TIPS

———

123

Nitty-gritty problems A–Z (a summary)

—

Mind like parachute, useless if not open.

Chinese saying

Acne (mild to moderate)

(refer page 983)

Topical

1. Use isotretinoin 0.05% gel or tretinoin 0.05% cream, apply each night (especially if comedones).
2. After 2 weeks, add benzoyl peroxide 2.5% or 5% gel. That is, after 2 weeks, maintenance treatment is:
   - isotretinoin 0.5% gel at night
   - benzoyl peroxide 2.5% or 5% mane
   Maintain for 3 months and review.
3. Alternative treatments:
   clindamycin topical
        or
   erythromycin 2% gel
        or
   azelaic acid, apply bd

Clindamycin regimen

Use clindamycin HCl in alcohol. Apply to each comedone with fingertips twice daily.
- A ready clindamycin preparation is Clindatech.
- Clindamycin is particularly useful for pregnant women and those who cannot tolerate antibiotics or exfoliants.

Oral antibiotics

Use if acne is resistant to topical agents or for inflammatory acne:

   tetracycline 1 g per day or doxycycline 100 mg per day or minocycline 50 mg bd for 4 weeks (or up to 10 weeks if slow response) then reduce according to response, e.g. doxycycline 50 mg for 8 weeks. Give a 12 week minimum trial.

Other therapies

Severe cystic or recalcitrant acne (specialist care)
- isotretinoin, oral
- dapsone

Alopecia androgenetica (male pattern baldness): also for women with hair thinning

Possible drug therapy (limited value):
   Minoxidil 2% or 5%
   1 mL bd to *dry* scalp
   Oral finasteride for men
   Spironolactone or cyproterone for women

Alopecia areata (patchy hair loss)

Potent topical corticosteroids (class III or IV).
Intradermal injections of triamcinolone
      (Kenacort A10)
           or
Minoxidil 2% or 5%
      1 mL bd applied to scalp (for 4 + months)

Anal fissure

- Apply glyceryl trinitrate 0.2% ointment (e.g. Rectogesic) bd to lower anal canal (refer p. 288)
- Avoid constipation—high-residue diet
- Hot baths to relax sphincter

If persistent/severe:
   external sphincterotomy
      or
   digital anal dilatation with four fingers for 4 minutes under anaesthesia
      or
   injection botulinum toxin into sphincter

Angina

(refer p. 347)

- Modification of risk factors
- Regular exercise (e.g. walking 20 minutes a day) to threshold of angina
- Relaxation program

Mild and stable

- aspirin 100 mg (o) daily
- glyceryl trinitrate (sublingual prn)

Moderate and stable

- as above
   +
- beta-blocker, e.g. atenolol 50–100 mg (o) daily
- glyceryl trinitrate (ointment and patches) daily

(12–16 hours only)
   or
isosorbide mononitrate 60 mg (o) SR tablets mane (16 hour span)

Add if necessary

- a dihydropyridine calcium channel blocker, e.g. nifedipine or amlodipine
   or
- a potassium channel opener e.g. nicorandil

Anorexia (simple) in children/infants

Acid or alkaline gentian mixture (preferably alkaline)
   5–10 mL 30–60 minutes before meals, tds
Acid or alkaline gentian mixture (for infants)
   4 mL 30–60 minutes before feeds
      or
Incremin mixture
   < 2 years: 2.5 mL daily
   > 2 years: 5 mL daily

Antibiotics (when to take)

(refer Table 123.1)

Anxiety

(refer Chap. 108)

Aphthous ulcers (canker sores)

Precautions: consider blood dyscrasia, denture pressure, Crohn's disease, pernicious anaemia

Table 123.1   *Ingestion of oral antibiotics in relation to food*

Antibiotic	Advice with respect to food
Amoxycillin	May be taken with food but not essential
Amoxycillin/clavulanic acid	Take with food
Ampicillin	As above
Cefaclor	As above
Cephalexin	As above
Ciprofloxacin	As above
Clindamycin	As above
Cloxacillin	Take on an empty stomach
Cotrimoxazole	Take with food
Doxycycline	Take with food or milk
Erythromycin base	Take on an empty stomach
Erythromycin estolate and ethylsuccinate	Take with food but not essential
Erythromycin stearate	Take on an empty stomach
Flucloxacillin	Take on an empty stomach
Griseofulvin	Take with food
Ketaconazole	Take with food
Metronidazole	Take after food
Minocycline	Take with food or milk
Penicillins	Take on an empty stomach
Tetracycline	Take on an empty stomach
Tinidazole	Take with food
Trimethoprim	Take with food

Note: 'Take on an empty stomach' means about 1 hour before food.

Minor ulcer: < 1 cm in diameter—lasts 10–14 days
Major ulcer: > 1 cm in diameter—lasts weeks

Treatment methods (use early when ulcer worse)
Consider applying a wet, squeezed-out, black teabag directly to the ulcer regularly (the tannic acid promotes healing).

Symptomatic relief
Apply topical lignocaine, e.g. 2% jelly or 5% ointment with cotton bud: after 2 minutes apply lignocaine gel or paint, e.g. SM-33 adult paint formula or SM-33 gel (children) every 3 hours.

Healing
Tetracycline suspension rinse
• empty contents of 250 mg capsule into 20–30 mL of warm water and shake it
• swirl this solution in the mouth for 5–10 minutes every 3 hours or apply the solution soaked in cotton wool wads to the ulcers (has a terrible taste)
or
Triamcinolone 0.1% (Kenalog in orabase) paste apply 8 hourly and nocte (preferred method)
or
10% chloramphenicol in propylene glycol apply with cotton bud for 1 minute (after drying the ulcer) 6 hourly for 3–4 days
or
Beclomethasone spray onto ulcer tds
or
Sucralfate 1 g in 20–30 mL of warm water. Use this as a mouthwash.

Asthma
(refer pp. 1051–1062)

Athlete's foot (tinea pedis)
(refer p. 985)
• Use antifungal powder between toes after drying.
• Wear open sandals or shoes with porous soles and uppers (if possible).
• Keep feet clean and dry at all times.
• Wear cotton or woollen sockettes (avoid synthetics).
• Charcoal inner soles (in every shoe).
• Clotrimazole 1% or miconazole 2% cream or lotion (after drying) bd or tds for 2–3 weeks

(an alternative to the imidazoles is topical ketoconazole or terbinafine).
If widespread and smelly vesiculobullae (take scrapings) use terbinafine (o) for 2–6 weeks.

Back pain
Acute low back pain
(refer Chap. 33)

Non-specific 'mechanical' disorder (no radicular pain)

Investigations
• nil needed (review in 4–6 weeks)

Management
• no bed rest (unless severe spasm → 2 days rest: consider antispasmodic, e.g. diazepam and topical ice packs)
• back education
• normal daily activities: keep active, return to work (if possible)
• non-opioid analgesics, e.g. paracetamol 4–6 hourly
• NSAIDs: 10–14 days (only if evidence of inflammation)
• physical therapy—for localised segment e.g. stretching, muscle energy therapy, mobilisation

Follow-up
• 3–7 days, then at 2 weeks
If symptoms persist:
• referral for spinal mobilisation/manipulation
• exercise program

Pain with radicular symptoms
If abnormal neurological signs, e.g. foot drop, investigate with plain X-ray, CT scan ± MRI. Consider urgent surgical referral—for guidelines see page 316.

If no abnormal signs
• bed rest 2–3 days
• back education
• analgesics (non-opioid) 4–6 hourly
• NSAIDs: 10–14 days (if inflammation)
• resume activity ASAP
• maintain fitness/exercises

Consider other modalities
- physiotherapy ? traction with care
- hydrotherapy

Regular follow-up—can resolve within 3 months

Chronic low back pain (pain > 3 months)

Investigations
Plain X-ray, ESR, urine analysis, PSA (male> 50)

Management
- back education
- normal activities
- analgesics, e.g. paracetamol
- NSAIDs: 10–14 days (if inflammation)
- exercise program
- trial of manipulation (if untried) × 3, if no contraindications
- referral for physiotherapy

Acute thoracic back pain

Investigations
- usually nil if < 50 years
- older or chronic pain: plain X-ray
  - CT scan (if suspect tumour)

Management
- continued activity
- analgesia (if required), e.g. paracetamol (around clock)
- back education program
- spinal manipulation (very effective)
- spinal mobilisation (if manipulation contra-indicated)
- exercise program, especially extension exercises
- posture education

Bed sores (pressure sores)

(refer page 1003)
The decubitus ulcer is typically undermined at the edges.

Prevention
- Good nursing care including turning patient every 2 hours
- Special care of pressure areas, including gentle handling

- Special beds, mattresses (e.g. air-filled ripple) and sheepskin to relieve pressure areas
- Good nutrition and hygiene
- Control of urinary and faecal incontinence
- Avoid the donut cushion

Treatment of ulcer
Use above measures, plus:
- Clean base with saline solution (applied gently via a syringe) or Intra Site Gel.
- General guidelines for dressings:
  - deep ulcers: alginates, e.g. Tegagel
  - shallow ulcers: hydrocolloids, e.g. Duo-derm, Cutinova Hydro
  - dry or necrotic ulcers: hydrogels, e.g. IntraSite
  - heavy exudative ulcers: foams, e.g. Lyofoam
- Give vitamin C, 500 mg bd.
- Give antibiotics for spreading cellulitis (other-wise of little use).
- Healing is usually satisfactory but, if not, surgical intervention with debridement of necrotic tissue and skin grafting may be necessary.

Bee stings

- scrape off stinger (if still present)—don't squeeze it
- apply cold packs
- apply vinegar, Stingose or methylated spirits
- oral antihistamines (if necessary)

Belching (aerophagia)

(patient swallows air without admitting it)

- make patient aware of excessive swallowing
- avoid fizzy (carbonated) soft drinks
- avoid chewing gum
- don't drink with meals
- don't mix proteins and starches
- eat slowly and chew food thoroughly before swallowing
- eat and chew with the mouth closed

If persistent
  Simethicone preparation, e.g. Mylanta II, Phazyme

If desperate
  Place one small cork between the back teeth after meals for 30 minutes.

Bell's palsy

Prednisolone 60 mg daily for 3 days then taper to zero over next 7 days (start within 3 days of onset)

- adhesive tape or patch at night over eye if corneal exposure
- consider artificial tears if eye dry
- massage and facial exercises during recovery
- about 90% spontaneous recovery

Bladder dysfunction (in women during night)

Women with urethral syndrome constantly wake at night with urge to micturate but produce only a small dribble of urine.

- instruct patient to perform a pelvic lift exercise by balancing on upper back, lifting her pelvis with knees flexed and holding position for 30 seconds
- squeeze pelvic floor inwards (as though holding back urine or faeces)
- repeat a few times

Blepharitis

Precautions: corneal ulceration, recurrent staphylococcal infections

Treatment
- eyelid hygiene—clean with a cotton bud dipped in 1:10 dilution of baby shampoo, once or twice daily
- artificial tears, e.g. hypromellose 1%
- tetracycline 1% or bacitracin ointment to lid margins 3–6 hourly
- control scalp seborrhoea with medicated shampoos, e.g. ketoconazole
- if chronic: short-term use of hydrocortisone ointment

Body odour

Cause: poor hygiene, excessive perspiration and active skin bacteria
Main focus: axilla and groin
Precautions: consider uraemia, vaginitis

Treatment method
- scrub body, especially groins and axillae, with deodorant soap at least morning and night
- try an antibacterial surgical scrub

- keep clothes clean, launder regularly
- choose suitable clothes—natural fibres, e.g. cotton, not synthetics
- use an antiperspirant deodorant
- alternative soap—pine soap
- diet: avoid garlic, fish, asparagus, onions, curry
- reduce caffeine (coffee, tea and coca cola drinks), which stimulates sweat activity
- shave axillary hair
- axillary wedge resection for excessive perspiration

Boils (recurrent)
- obtain swabs
- 3% hexachlorophane body wash daily
- mupirocin to the lesions and nares
- antibiotics (according to swabs), e.g. erythromycin 500 mg bd for 10 days (may require up to 3 months)

Breath-holding attacks
(refer p. 770)
- reassure parents
- advise firm discipline
- try to avoid precipitating incidents

Bronchiolitis
(refer p. 790)
Usually children 2 weeks to 9 months
Auscultation
- widespread fine crackles
- expiratory wheezes

Admit to hospital
- minimal handling/good nursing care
- observations with pulse oximeter
- oxygen: maintain $P_aO_2 > 90\%$
- maintain hydration

Bruxism (teeth grinding)
- Practise keeping teeth apart.
- Slowly munch an apple before retiring.
- Practise relaxation techniques, including meditation, before retiring (bruxism is related to stress).
- Place a hot face towel against the sides of the face before retiring to achieve relaxation.
- If this fails and bruxism is socially unacceptable during the night, use a mouthguard.

Burning feet syndrome

Anterior burning pain in forefoot—consider tarsal tunnel syndrome (refer p. 617) or peripheral neuropathy, e.g. from diabetes or vascular insufficiency.

Burns

Management depends on extent and depth (burns are classified as superficial or deep).

Small burns should be immersed in cold water immediately, e.g. tap water for 20 minutes.

Chemical burns should be liberally irrigated with water.

Refer the following burns to hospital:
- > 10% surface area, especially in a child (see rule of 9s, p. 964)
- all deep burns
- burns of difficult or vital areas, e.g. face, hands, perineum/genitalia, feet
- burns with potential problems, e.g. electrical, chemical, circumferential.

Always give adequate pain relief.

Treatment of superficial burns

Most scalds cause partial thickness (superficial) burns. Smear the clean burnt or scalded area with silver sulfadiazine with chlorhexadine (Silvazine) cream with a sterile gloved hand or spatula (3 mm thick layer).

Exposure (open method)

- keep open without dressings (good for face, perineum or single surface burns)
- renew coating of cream every 24 hours

Dressings (closed method)

- suitable for circumferential wounds
- cover creamed area with non-adherent tulle, e.g. paraffin gauze
- dress with an absorbent bulky layer of gauze and wool
- use a plaster splint if necessary

Burns to hands

A first aid method for partial thickness burns to hands is to place the hand in a suitable plastic bag containing a liberal quantity of Silvazine. If a sterile plastic bag is unavailable a standard household bag will suffice.

Then apply a crepe bandage around the hand, leaving the fingers and thumb free so that the fingers can move freely in the bag. Consider placing the arm in a sling. Change the bag every day or second day to review the wound. Leave blisters intact.

Calluses

- Remove the cause.
- Proper footwear is essential, with cushion pads over callosities.
- Pare with a sterile sharp scalpel blade.

'Cellulite'

The best way to overcome 'cellulite' is to keep to ideal weight. If overweight, lose it slowly and exercise to improve the muscle tone in the buttocks and thighs.

Chickenpox

(refer p. 759)
- rest in bed until feeling well
- give paracetamol for fever
- drink ample fluids
- calamine lotion to relieve itching
- daily bathing with sodium bicarbonate (half a cup added) or Pinetarsol (preferable) in bath water
- antihistamines for itching
- aciclovir, famciclovir or valaciclovir in immunocompromised and those over 15 years

Chilblains

Precautions: think Raynaud's
protect from trauma and secondary infection
do not rub or massage injured tissues
do not apply heat or ice

Physical Rx: elevate affected part
warm gradually to room temperature

Drug Rx: apply glyceryl trinitrate vasodilator spray or ointment or patch (use plastic gloves and wash hands for ointment)

Other Rx: rum at night
nifedipine

Chloasma

see Melasma

Cold sores

At the first sensation of development

- apply an ice cube to site for 5 minutes every 60 minutes (first 12 hours)
- apply idoxuridine 0.5% preparation hourly at onset

or

saturated solution of menthol in SVR

or

povidone-iodine 10% cold sore paint on swab stick 4 times a day until disappearance

or

aciclovir cold sore cream, 5 times a day for 5 days

Common cold

- rest 24–48 hours if feeling weak
- aspirin or paracetamol (up to 8 tablets a day for adults)
- steam inhalations using menthol or Friar's balsam
- gargle aspirin in lemon juice for a sore throat
- vitamin C—2 g a day for 5–7 days
- increase fluid intake
- stop smoking (if applicable)
- use cough drops or syrup for a dry troublesome cough

Conjunctivitis

(refer p. 478)

Bacterial conjunctivitis

Limit spread: use of separate towels and good ocular hygiene.

Mild: saline irrigation or propamidine isethionate 0.1% (Brolene)

More severe: polymyxin B sulphate compound drops (Neosporin) 1–2 drops 4–5 times daily for up to 7 days (depending on response). An ointment of similar composition can be used at night.

If pseudomonas and other coliform: topical gentamicin and tobramycin.

Viral conjunctivitis

Symptomatic care only; limit cross-infection.

Herpes simplex

aciclovir 3% eye ointment 5 times daily for 14 days, or for at least 3 days after healing
atropine 1% eyedrops 1 drop 12 hourly (best under specialist supervision)

Constipation (idiopathic)

- patient education, including 'good habit'
- adequate exercise
- plenty of fluids, e.g. water, fruit juice
- avoid laxatives and codeine compounds
- optimal bulk diet

If unsuccessful

- ispaghula (or psyllium granules), e.g. adults: 1 sachet in water bd

Corns on feet

- Remove cause of friction and use wide shoes.
- Use corn pads.
- Soften corn with a few daily applications of 15% salicylic acid in collodion or commercial 'corn removers' (salicylic acid), then pare.

'Cracked' and dry lips

- Use a lip balm with sunscreen, e.g. Sunsense 15 lip balm.
- Women can use a creamy lipstick.
- Vaseline helps.

'Cracked' hands and fingers

- Wear protective work gloves: cotton-lined PVC gloves.
- Use soap substitutes, e.g. Cetaphil lotion, Dove.
- Apply 2–5% salicylic acid and 10% liq picis carb in white soft paraffin ointment.

or

- Corticosteroid ointment: class II–III.

'Cracked' heels

- Soak feet for 30 minutes in warm water containing an oil such as Alpha-Keri or Derma Oil.
- Pat dry, then apply a cream such as Nutraplus (10% urea) or Eulactol heel balm. Hydrocortisone 0.5% cream for resistant cases.
- For severe cases use sorbolene cream with 20% glycerol and 30% urea (test skin sensitivity first).

Cramps (nocturnal cramps in legs)

Precautions: treat cause (if known), e.g. tetanus, drugs, sodium depletion, hypothyroidism.

Physical
- muscle stretching and relaxation exercises: stretch calf for 3 minutes before retiring (Fig. 123.1) then rest in chair with the feet out horizontally to the floor with cushion under tendoachilles (10 minutes)
- massage and heat to affected muscles
- try to keep bedclothes off feet and lower part of legs—use a doubled-up pillow at the foot of the bed

Drugs
- quinine sulphate 300 mg nocte
  or
- biperiden 2–4 mg nocte

Note: Tonic water before retiring may help.

Croup

(refer p. 789)
- get child to inhale humidified steaming air, e.g.

Fig. 123.1 *Leg-stretching exercise for cramp*

in bathroom with hot water taps running (minor obstruction usually resolves after 30–60 minutes)
- paracetamol mixture 4–6 hourly
- no place for cough medicine or antibiotics
- support child on pillows
- keep child calm
- consider nebulised budesonide or oral steroids

If significant laryngeal obstruction:
- hospitalisation—nurse in intensive care
- nebulised adrenaline 1:1000 solution (0.5 mL/kg/dose) run with oxygen 8L/min
  ↓
- dexamethasone IV 0.2 mg/kg, followed by oral steroids
  ↓
- artificial airway (nasotracheal intubation or tracheostomy) if irreversible obstruction

Crying baby

Checklist: hunger; wet or soiled nappy; teething; colic; infection; loneliness; or seeking attention.

Dandruff

Dandruff (pityriasis capitis) is mainly a physiological process, the result of normal desquamation of scale from the scalp. It is most prevalent in adolescence and worse around the age of 20.

Treatment
Shampoos:
  zinc pyrithione, e.g. Dan-Gard
    or
  selenium sulphide, e.g. Selsun
Method: massage into scalp,leave for 5 minutes, rinse thoroughly—twice weekly

Persistent dandruff with severe flaking and itching indicates seborrhoeic dermatitis or psoriasis.

Treatment
  coal tar + salicylic acid compound (Sebitar) shampoo
    or
  Ionil T plus shampoo
Method: as above, followed by Sebi Rinse or ketoconazole (Nizoral) shampoo

If persistent, especially itching, and Nizoral shampoo ineffective use a corticosteroid, e.g. betamethasone scalp lotion.

Dizzy turns in elderly women

If no cause such as hypertension is found, advise them to get up slowly from sitting or lying and to wear firm elastic stockings.

Dizzy turns in girls in late teens

- common due to blood pressure fluctuations
- give advice related to stress, lack of sleep, or excessive activity
- reassure that it settles with age (rare after 25 years)

Dry hair

- Don't shampoo every day.
- Use a mild shampoo (labelled for 'dry or damaged hair').
- Use a conditioner.
- Snip off the split or frayed ends.
- Avoid heat, e.g. electric curlers, hair dryers.
- Wear head protection in hot wind.
- Wear a rubber cap when swimming.

Dry skin

- Reduce bathing and frequency and duration of showering.
- Bathe and shower in tepid water.
- Use a soap substitute, e.g. Dove, Neutrogena, Cetaphil lotion or aqueous cream.
- Rub in baby oil after patting dry.
- Avoid wool next to skin (e.g. wear cotton).
- Use emollients, e.g. Alpha-Keri lotion, Nutra D cream.
- Use moisturisers with 10% urea, e.g. Calmurid, Nutraplus.
- Use dilute corticosteroid ointment if resistant local patches.
- Advise a good diet and plenty of water to drink.

Dysmenorrhoea (primary)

Mild: explanation
    healthy lifestyle
    practise relaxation, e.g. yoga
    pelvic floor exercises
    apply warmth to area (hot water bottle)

Medication for moderate to severe pain: simple analgesics, e.g. paracetamol
    prostaglandin inhibitors (from first sign of menses)
    e.g. mefenamic acid 500 mg tds

    naproxen 500 mg statim then 250 mg tds
combined oral contraceptive pill
    e.g. low oestrogen triphasic pill

Ear exostoses ('surfer's ear')

These bony overgrowths are caused by water retention in the ear.

Prevention
- Use plugs to waterproof ear.
- Dry thoroughly with hair dryer after swimming.

Ectropion

- requires surgical repair (local anaesthetic)
- use a mild ointment prior to surgery

Entropion

If unsuitable for surgery, use a strip of hypo-allergenic, non-woven surgical tape (1 cm × 3 cm) to evert lid and secure to cheek (Fig. 123.2).

adhesive tape —   3 cm

1 cm

Fig. 123.2 *Treatment of entropion*

Enuresis (bedwetting)

(refer p.749)

The bed-wetting alarm, particularly a body-worn alarm, such as the Malem night trainer, is generally regarded as the most effective method. If the child has an emotional problem, counselling or hypnotherapy may be desirable. Tricyclic anti-depressants may be effective in some children. Best pharmaceutical option is desmopressin acetate, 1 spray in lower part of nostril per night.

Epistaxis

Simple tamponade

- pinch 'soft' part of nose between thumb and finger for 5 minutes
- apply ice packs to bridge of nose (Fig. 123.3)

Simple cautery of Little's area (under local anaesthetic e.g. Cophenylcaine forte nasal spray ±5% cocaine solution)

use one of 3 methods: electrocautery trichloracetic acid or silver nitrate stick (preferred)

Persistent anterior bleed

Merocel (surgical sponge) nasal tampon or Kaltostat pack

'Trick of the trade' for recurrent anterior epistaxis:

- apply topical antibiotic, e.g. Aureomycin ointment, bd or tds for 10 days
  or (better option) Nasalate nasal cream tds for 7–10 days
  or Rectinol ointment

Severe posterior epistaxis

Use a Foley's catheter or an Epistat catheter.

Eye: dry

Usually elderly patient complaining of a chronic gritty sensation—due to reduced tear secretion.

- artificial tear drops, e.g. polyvinyl alcohol solution or hypromellose 0.5%

ice pack

Fig. 123.3 *First-line treatment for epistaxis*

Eyelashes: ingrowing (trichiasis)

Perform epilation using eyebrow tweezers (available from chemists).
Regular epilation may be necessary.
Severe cases: electrolysis of hair roots

Eyelid 'twitching' or 'jumping'

Advise that cause is usually stress or fatigue.
Reassure and counsel.
Consider prescribing clonazepam if severe.

Blepharospasm (which may cause uncontrolled blinking) can be treated with botulinum toxin injected into the orbicularis oculi muscle.

Fever in children

(refer p. 500)

- undress to singlet and nappy or underpants (avoid shivering)
- paracetamol 20 mg/kg statim then 15 mg/kg every 4 hours
- copious fluids, especially water

Note: Sponging with lukewarm water and using fans is unnecessary.

Fibromyalgia

Consider: clonazepam (Rivotril) 0.5 mg nocte
or
antidepressant, e.g. amitriptyline, SSRI group

Flashburns to eyes

Cause: intense ultraviolet light burns to corneas (keratitis), e.g. arc welding, UV lamps, snow reflection
Precautions: foreign bodies
continued use of topical anaesthetics (once only)

Treatment

- topical long-acting LA drops, e.g. amethocaine, statim
- homotropine 2% eyedrops, 1–2 drops statim
- broad spectrum antibiotic eye ointment, bd in lower fornix (48 hours)
- analgesics, e.g. codeine + paracetamol
- eye padding for 24 hours, then review

Folliculitis: of groin

Folliculitis of the groin area is common in women who shave. It tends to recur.

- Use tea tree lotion daily for folliculitis.
- Prior to shaving apply 'tea tree wash'.
- If persistent, use povidone-iodine or chlorhexidine (Hibiclens) solution.
- If severe, use mupirocin 2% (Bactroban) ointment.

Folliculitis: of trunk from spa baths

Due to pseudomonas or *Staphylcoccus aureus*

- Rx—ciprofloxacin 500 mg (o) bd for 7 days

Foot ache

- Avoid wearing high heels.
- Wear insoles to support the foot arch.
- Perform foot exercises.
- Soak the feet in a basin of warm water containing therapeutic salts (Epsom salts is suitable).
- Massage feet with baby oil followed by a special ribbed wooden foot massager.

Foot odour (smelly and sweaty feet)

Includes pitted keratolysis secondary to hyperhidrosis (common in teenagers)

Treatment
- education and reassurance
- wear cotton or woollen socks
- aluminium chloride 20% in alcohol solution (Driclor, Hidrosol) or Neat Feet—apply nocte for one week, then 1–2 times weekly as necessary
- shoe liners, e.g. 'Odor eaters'; charcoal inner soles
- apply undiluted Burow's solution after a shower or bath
- the teabag treatment (if desperate)
  — prepare 600 mL of strong hot tea (from two teabags left in water for 15 minutes)
  — pour the hot tea into a basin with 2 litres of cool water
  — soak the feet in this for 20–30 minutes daily for 10 days, then as often as required

Freckles and lentigines (sun spots)

- Reassure the patient.
- Use a sunscreen.
- Otherwise, rather than use 'fade cream', use fresh lemon juice. Squeeze lemon juice (½ lemon) into a small bowl and apply the juice with a cotton ball to the spots daily. Continue for 8 weeks.
- Apply tretinoin 0.05% cream daily at night, if necessary.

Frostbite

Treatment depends on severity.

Precautions: watch for secondary infection, tetanus, gangrene

Physical Rx: • elevate affected limb
- rewarm in water just above body temperature 40°C (104°F) or use body heat, e.g. in axillae
- avoid thawing or refreezing
- surgical debridement
- don't debride early (wait until dead tissue dried)
- don't drink alcohol or smoke
- for blistering, apply warm water compresses for 15 minutes every 2 hours

Drug Rx: • analgesics

Gastroenteritis

(refer pp. 401–403)

Genital herpes

(refer p. 946)

Topical
- aciclovir cream, apply 5 times daily for 5 days
or
- 10% povidone-iodine paint for several days

Oral
- aciclovir 200 mg 5 times a day for 7–10 days (or famciclovir or valaciclovir)

Genital warts

(refer p. 949)

Use podophyllin 25% solution in tinct. benz. co.
or
podophyllotoxin 0.5% paint

Geographical tongue

- explanation and reassurance
- no treatment if asymptomatic
- Cepacaine gargles, 10 mL tds, if tender

Gingivitis

- use dental floss regularly (twice a day)
- brush carefully at gumline with Sensodyne (pink) toothpaste
- perform gum massage between thumb and index finger
- use Listerine mouthwash or dilute hydrogen peroxide
- take Vitamin C—2 g daily

Gout (acute attack)

- bed rest
- keep weight of the bedclothes off the foot with a bed cradle or pillow under bedclothes
- avoid aspirin (it may exacerbate gout)
- indomethacin 100 mg (o) statim, 75 mg 2 hours later, then 50 mg (o) 8 hourly; relief can be expected in 24–48 hours
- add an antiemetic, e.g. Maxolon 10 mg (o)
- consider an intra-articular injection of corticosteroid, e.g. 10 mg/mL triamcinolone under a digital nerve block

or

prednisolone 40 mg/day for 3–5 days, then taper by 5 mg over 10 days

or

corticotrophin (ACTH) IM in difficult cases
- consider colchicine (only if NSAIDs not tolerated) 0.5–1 mg statim then 0.5 mg every 2 hours

Haemorrhoids

(refer p.289)

Halitosis

- Exclude dental disease, malignancy, pulmonary TB, nasal and sinus infection.
- Consider drugs as a cause.
- Avoid onions, garlic, peppers, spicy salami and similar meats.
- Avoid strong cheeses.
- Avoid smoking and excessive nips of alcohol.
- Brush teeth regularly during day—immediately after a meal.
- Rinse mouth out with water after meals.
- Avoid fasting for long periods during the day.
- Gargle with mouthwash, e.g. Listerine.
- Use dental floss regularly to clean the teeth.

Tip: use an oil/water wash, e.g. equal volumes of aqueous Cepacol and olive oil, gargle a well-shaken mixture and spit out, qid.

Hangover

Preventive advice:

- Drink alcohol on a full stomach.
- Select alcoholic drinks that suit you: avoid champagne.
- Avoid fast drinking—keep it slow.
- Restrict the quantity of alcohol.
- Take two soluble aspirin before retiring.
- Drink three large glasses of water before retiring.

Treatment
- Drink ample fluids because of relative dehydration effect of alcohol.
- Take soluble aspirin, e.g. Aspro Clear (600 mg), Alka-Seltzer.
- Drink orange juice or tomato juice, with added sugar.
- A drink of honey in lemon juice helps.
- Coffee and tea are suitable beverages.
- Have a substantial meal but avoid fats.

Hay fever (allergic rhinitis)

(refer p. 1038)

- patient education
- allergen avoidance (if possible)
- non-sedating antihistamines
    — astemizole 10 mg daily, or
    — loratadine 10 mg daily, or
    — terfenadine 60 mg bd, or
    — cetirizine 10 mg daily or bd, or
    — fexfenadine 60 mg bd
- consider levocabastine nasal spray bd → qid

Alternative treatments

- inhaled sodium cromoglycate

or

- inhaled corticosteroids (beclomethasone or budesonide) preferable
- use sodium cromoglycate (Opticrom) drops for eye irritation

Head banging or rocking in toddlers

This is common < 4 years when going to sleep, especially in 3 year olds. Reassure parents that problem settles by 4–5 years.

Heartburn (dyspepsia)

(refer pp. 439–40)

- patient education
- lifestyle changes
  — maintain ideal weight (very important)
  — stress management
  — reduce or cease smoking
  — reduce or cease alcohol intake
  — reduce or cease coffee and chocolate
  — avoid fatty foods, e.g. pastries
- antacids (alginate/antacid mixture)
  — Gaviscon liquid or Mylanta plus liquid 10–20 mL, on demand or 2 hours after meals
    20–30 mL at bedtime
- consider H$_2$ receptor antagonists, proton pump blocker or prokinetic agent

Hiccoughs (hiccups)

Simple brief episodes:

- rebreathing air in a paper bag (as for hyperventilation)
- breath holding
- sucking ice/swallowing iced water
- catheter inserted quickly in and out of nose
- pressure on the eyeballs

Persistent (assuming exclusion of organic diseases):

- chlorpromazine orally or IV
        or
- sodium valproate

Consider acupuncture, hypnosis or phrenic nerve block.

Hirsutism

- Exclude adrenal or ovarian pathology.
- Initial investigation: s. testosterone and DHEAs
- Use bleaching, waxing or depilatory creams, or shave.
- Do not pluck hairs, especially around the lips and chin.
- Plucking stimulates hair growth but shaving appears to have no effect.
- Electrolysis or laser epilation may help.

- Drug treatment: spironolactone 100–200 mg daily; takes 6–12 months to respond.
- Alternatives: cyproterone acetate

Hoarseness

Common causes: viral URTI (acute laryngitis), non-specific irritative laryngitis, vocal abuse, nodules and polyps, intubation, oesophageal reflux.
- chronic: children—'screamer's nodules'
          adults—non-specific laryngitis, e.g. smoking

Exclude: imminent airway obstruction, e.g. croup, epiglottitis, malignancy, hypothyroidism; other severe infections, e.g. diphtheria, TB, foreign body, allergy, goitre.

Diagnosis: larynx must be visualised.

Management
- acute: treat according to cause
           vocal rest or minimal usage at normal conversation
           avoid irritants, e.g. dust, tobacco, alcohol
           consider inhalations (p. 1226) and cough suppressants
- chronic: establish diagnosis
           consider specialist ENT referral

Hyperventilation

- Get patient to breathe in and out of a paper bag.
- If a paper bag is unavailable, rebreathe air from cupped hands over nose and mouth.
- Encourage patient to learn to slow down breathing.
- Investigate the possibility of phobias.
- Advise cutting out caffeine and nicotine.

Impetigo

(refer p. 767)
- If mild and limited: antiseptic cleansing and removal of crusts with gentle washing and an antibacterial soap or chlorhexidine or povidone-iodine. Apply mupirocin (Bactroban) tds for 7–10 days.
- If extensive: flucloxacillin/dicloxacillin, cephalexin or erythromycin (o) for 7 days.

Impotence

(refer p. 937)

Incontinence of urine

(refer p. 709)

- Search for a cause: refer to a consultant.
- Avoid various drugs, e.g. diuretics, psychotropics, alcohol.

In women:

- bladder retraining and pelvic floor exercises (mainstay of treatment)
- physiotherapist referral

Consider incontinence aids:

- absorbent pads and special pants
- condoms and catheters; urinary drainage bags
- absorbent sheeting

Infantile colic

Usually an infant 2–16 weeks old
(refer p. 254)
Avoid medications if possible but consider:
simethicone preparations, e.g. Infacol wind drops
or
dicyclomine, e.g. Merbentyl syrup
or
Donnalix infant drops

Influenza

- Rest in bed until fever subsides and patient feels better.
- Analgesics: codeine compound tablets (helps cough and discomfort) or aspirin.
- Drink as much water and fruit juice as possible; freshly squeezed lemon juice and honey preparations help.
- Consider vitamin C, 2 g daily.

Ingrowing toenails

- Cut nails properly: cut across so that the cut slopes towards the centre of the nail and do not cut towards the edges (Fig. 123.4).
- Fashion the toenails so that the corners project beyond the skin.
- Wear good-fitting shoes (avoid tight shoes).
- Keep toe area clean and dry.

Insect stings

- Wash site with large quantities of cool water.
- Apply vinegar (liberal amount) or aluminium

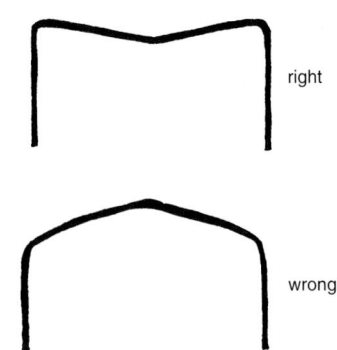

Fig. 123.4 *Correct method of cutting toenails*

sulfate 20% solution (Stingose) for about 30 seconds.

- Apply ice for several seconds.
- Use soothing anti-itch cream or 3–5% lignocaine, e.g. Dermocaine gel ointment, if very painful.

Insomnia

Exclude and treat

- drugs, e.g. caffeine, alcohol, beta-blockers
- anxiety, stress
- depression
- restless legs syndrome
- sleep apnoea
- nightmares
- physical disorders, e.g. CCF, arthritis
- bed-wetting
- reflux disease

Management

- Give explanation and reassurance (treat cause if known, e.g. depression).
- Try to recognise what helps patient to settle best, e.g. warm bath, listening to music.
- Establish a routine before going to bed.
- Avoid alcohol and drinks containing caffeine in evening.
- Avoid a heavy evening meal.
- Try a drink of warm milk before retiring.
- Organise a comfortable quiet sleep setting.
- Sex last thing at night where appropriate is usually helpful.
- Try relaxation therapy, meditation, stress management.
- Consider hypnosis.
- If all conservative means fail, try zopiclone (Imovane) 7.5 mg (o) at night (limit to 2 weeks) or temazepam 10–20 mg (o) or zolpidem 5–10 mg (o).

Intertrigo (due to *Candida albicans*)

- Treat underlying problem, e.g. obesity, diabetes.
- Apply clotrimazole or miconazole or nystatin preparation (use ketoconazole if resistant).
- Apply Burow's solution compresses if weeping.
- Keep area dry and skin folds apart (if possible).
- Apply zinc oxide powder, e.g. Curash.

Irritable bowel

- reassurance and patient education
- stress management/relaxation
- avoid foods that 'irritate', smoking, alcohol, laxatives, codeine
- high-fibre diet (for constipation without flatulence)
- medications to consider:
  constipation dominant
  — metamucil 1 teaspoon bd
  pain/distension dominant
  — mebeverine HCl (Colofac) 135 mg tds
  or
  peppermint oil capsules 1–2 (o) tds
  diarrhoea dominant
  — loperamide 2 mg (o) after each loose bowel motion

Jet lag

(refer p. 104)

Jitters

(pre-occasion jitters/performance anxiety)
Propranolol 10–40 mg (o) 30–60 minutes before the event or performance.

Jock itch

see Tinea cruris

Keloid or hypertrophic scar

Various methods (refer p. 1009)
Multiple pressure injections:
- Spread film of corticosteroid solution over scar.
- Apply multiple pressure through solution with a 21 g needle held tangentially (about 20 superficial stabs per cm^2).
- Avoid bleeding.

- Repeat in 6 weeks.
  or
intralesional injection of triamcinolone
  or
topical class III–IV corticosteroid ointment with occlusion

Keratoacanthoma

Surgical excision and histology (refer p. 1012)
Note: Can be misdiagnosed as SCC.

Keratoses (seborrhoeic and solar)
Seborrhoeic keratoses
Management
- usually nil apart from reassurance
- does not undergo malignant change
- can be removed for cosmetic reasons
- light cautery to small facial lesions
- may drop off spontaneously
- if diagnosis uncertain, remove for histopathology

Decolourisation or removal:
- liquid nitrogen (regular applications, e.g. every 3 weeks)
  or
- concentrated phenol solution (with care) repeat in 3 weeks
  or
- trichloroacetic acid: apply to surface and instil with multiple small needle pricks (25 g) repeat twice weekly for 2 weeks

Solar keratoses
Management
- reduce exposure to sunlight
- can disappear spontaneously
- liquid nitrogen if superficial
  or
- 5-fluorouracil 5% cream daily for 3–4 weeks
- surgical excision for suspicious and ulcerating lesions
- biopsy if doubtful

Lactation suppression

- avoid nipple stimulation
- refrain from expressing milk
- use well-fitting brassiere
- bromocriptine (Parlodel) 2.5 mg (o) bd for 10–14 days—nausea is a problem
- avoid oestrogens

Laryngitis

- avoid talking
- drink ample fluids
- avoid cigarettes
- use steam inhalations (5 minutes bd)

Leg ulcer

(refer p. 1001)

Lice

(refer p. 767)

Head lice

pyrethrins/piperonyl butoxide foam or shampoo, e.g. Lyban 5% foam (alternatives: permethrin 1%, Maldison 1%)
apply to wet hair, leave at least 10 minutes and wash off
repeat in one week
use Vaseline for eyelids

Pubic lice

permethrin 1% lotion
or
pyrethrins 0.165% with piperonyl butoxide 2% in foam base
apply to affected area, leave for 10 minutes then wash off
repeat after 7 days (may be third treatment)
shaving pubic hair is recommended

Lichen planus

(troublesome, e.g. itching)

- topical fluorinated steroids under plastic occlusion
- consider intralesional injections of triamcinolone for hypertrophic areas

Mastalgia (cyclical)

- vitamin B complex with B_6 (100 mg) daily
- evening primrose oil 4–6 g (o) daily
- mefenamic acid 500 mg tds

(try first)

Consider:
bromocriptine 2.5 mg bd
danazol 200 mg daily

Melasma (chloasma)

2% hydroquinone in sorbolene cream

Ménière's syndrome

Long-term management

- explanation and advice
- avoid excessive intake of salt, coffee and tobacco
- sodium depleting diuretic
- consider: betahistine (Serc) or diazepam
- oral urea 20–30 g in orange juice and prochlorperazine 25 mg suppository (with warning of attack)

Acute attack

- diazepam 5 mg IV ± prochlorperazine 12.5 mg IM

Menopause syndrome

(refer pp. 857–863)

Migraine attack

(refer pp. 522–524)
First signs of attack:

1st line:	soluble aspirin 2–3 tablets (o)
	+
	metoclopramide 10 mg (o)
2nd line:	ergotamine (tablets, suppository or medihaler)
	or
	sumatriptan 100 mg (o) or 6 mg (SC) injection
	repeat in 2 hours if necessary

Severe attack: metoclopramide 10 mg (2 ml) IM or IV plus dihydroergotamine 1 mg IM or 0.5 mg IV slowly
(rule: IM in the home, IV in hospital)

Migraine prophylaxis

(for > 2 attacks per month)

- propranolol 40 mg (o) bd increasing up to 320 mg daily if necessary
or
- pizotifen 0.5 mg (o) nocte increasing to 3 mg if necessary

Milker's nodules

- self-limiting and remits in 5–6 weeks
- can give intralesional injection of corticosteroid

Molluscum contagiosum

Refer pages 753 and 949 for various treatments.

In the surgery the best treatment is application of liquid nitrogen or lifting the lesion open with a needle or fine pointed stick and instilling 10% povidone-iodine or 2.5% phenol.

Note: Be careful not to overtreat or run the risk of scarring.

Monkey muscle tear

(refer p. 1190)

- RICE treatment for 72 hours
- compress with firm elastic bandage (toes to below knee)
- crutches if necessary
- raised heel on shoe
- physiotherapist referral
- active exercises after 48 hours

Morning-after pill

(must be used within 72 hours)

- use high-oestrogen pill (Yuzpe method)
    50 μg EO + 250 μg LNG (Nordiol) $\times$ 2 pills (or equivalent dose in other pills)
    repeat in 12 hours
- add an antiemetic, e.g. metoclopramide 10 mg (o)

Morning sickness

- invariably disappears by end of first trimester
- explanation and reassurance
- simple measures
    — small frequent meals
    — fizzy soft drinks
    — avoid stimuli such as cooking smells
    — avoid oral iron
    — be careful cleaning teeth

Medication (for severe cases):

- pyridoxine 50–100 mg (o) bd
- add metoclopramide 10 mg (o) 2–3 times a day if still present

Mouth: angular fissures

- check dentures and hygiene
- apply dimethicone cream for protection
- if persistent and/or for suspected candida, use antifungal cream

Mouth: bad taste

- look for cause, e.g. teeth, gums, depression
- consider Ascoxal tablets, 1–2 tabs dissolved in 25 mL warm water as mouthwash for 2 rinses up to 5 times daily

Mouth ulcers

(as for aphthous ulcers)

Nappy rash

The main factor is dampness due to urine and faeces.

Irritant dermatitis

- Keep the area dry.
- Change wet or soiled napkins often—disposable ones are good.
- Wash gently and pat dry (do not rub).
- Avoid excessive bathing and soap.
- Avoid powders and plastic pants.
- Use emollients to keep skin lubricated e.g. zinc oxide and castor oil cream
                        or
            nappy rash cream formula
                sol. al. acetate   16%
                wool fat   33%
                camphor   1%
                zinc cream   add to 100
                sig: apply each change

If: atopic dermatitis: 1% hydrocortisone
    seborrhoeic dermatitis: 1% hydrocortisone and ketoconazole ointment
    Candida albicans: topical nystatin at each nappy change
    widespread nappy rash: 1% hydrocortisone and nystatin ointment or clotrimazole cream (qid after changes)

Neck pain

(refer Chap. 56)

Nightmares
Adults

- check whether due to medication
- 4 week trial of phenytoin
- diazepam at night can be used

Children
- no active treatment is usually needed for parainsomnias (nightmares, sleep talking or sleep walking) in children
- usually self-limiting
- if persistent or severe: 6 week trial phenytoin or imipramine

Nipples: cracked

(refer p. 894)
- Get baby to latch onto breast fully and properly.
- Do not feed from the affected breast—rest the nipple for 1–2 feeds.
- Express the milk from that breast by hand.
- Start feeding gradually with short feeds.
- Take paracetamol 1 g just before feeding to relieve the pain.
- Avoid drying agents such as spirits, creams and ointments.

Nipples: sore

- Use a relaxed feeding technique.
- Try to use the 'chest to chest, chin on breast' feeding position.
- Start feeding from the less painful side first if one nipple is very sore.
- Express some milk first to soften and 'lubricate' the nipple.
- Never pull the baby off the nipple: gently break the suction with your finger.
- Apply covered ice to the nipple to relieve pain.
- Keep the nipples dry (exposure to air or to hair dryer).
- Do not wear a bra at night.
- If wearing a bra by day, try Cannon breast shields.

Nose: offensive smell from

Ensure no foreign body present.
- mupirocin 2% nasal ointment
    instil 2 or 3 times a day
        or
- Kenacomb ointment
    instil 2 or 3 times a day

Nose: stuffy, running

- blow nose hard into disposable paper tissue or handkerchief until clear
- nasal decongestant for 2–3 days only
- steam inhalations with Friar's balsam or menthol

Fig. 123.5 *Steam inhalation*

preparations—use 1 teaspoon to 500 mL boiled water in old container (Fig. 123.5)

Obesity

(refer pp. 727–730)

Obsessive compulsive disorder

- refer for group therapy
- clomipramine (Anafranil)
    50–75 mg (o) nocte, increasing every 2 to 3 days to 150–250 mg orally (o) nocte
        or
    SSRI antidepressant, e.g. fluoxetine

Oily hair

- Shampoo daily with a 'shampoo for oily hair'.
- Massage the scalp during the shampoo process.
- Leave the shampoo on for at least 5 minutes.
- Avoid hair conditioners.
- Avoid overbrushing.
- Attend to lifestyle factors: relaxation and balanced diet are important.

Otitis externa

- aural toilet—dry mopping
- dressing with insertion of 4 mm Nufold gauze impregnated with ointment (as below)
- topical combined ointment or drops, e.g. Kenacomb or Sofradex or Locacorten-Vioform

- consider wick insertion

See also Tropical ear.

Otitis media

(refer pp. 467–469)

Children
- rest patient in warm room with adequate humidity
- paracetamol suspension of pain (high dosage)
- decongestants only if nasal congestion
- amoxycillin (1st choice) 40–50 mg/kg/day in three divided doses for 10 days; cephalosporin, e.g. cefaclor (2nd choice)
- follow-up: evaluate hearing at 10 days

Adults
- analgesics
- nasal decongestants only for nasal congestion
- antibiotics 5 day course:

1st choice: amoxycillin 750 mg (o) 12 hourly
or 500 mg (o) 5 hourly
or
amoxycillin/clavulanate 500mg/
125 mg (o) tds

2nd choice: doxycycline or cefaclor
or roxithromycin

Panic attack

(refer p. 1047)

- general support, explanation and reassurance
- stress management
- rebreathe into a paper bag if hyperventilating
- initial treatment
oxazepam 15–30 mg (o)
or
alprazolam 0.25–0.5 mg (o)
or
diazepam 5 mg(o)

Prophylaxis
Consider:
- alprazolam 0.25–6 mg (o) in 2–4 divided doses
or
- tricyclic antidepressants

Paronychia: acute

Uncomplicated with localised pus:
- simple elevation of nail fold (Fig. 123.6) or puncture the fold close to the nail to drain pus

Fig. 123.6 *Treatment of paronychia by elevating the nail fold*

- advice on hygiene
- antibiotics rarely necessary
- exclude diabetes

Complicated with subungual extension:
- small vertical incision alongside the nail
or
- removal of nail in part or totally
- exclude diabetes

Paronychia: chronic

- usually due to a secondary invading organism
- culture organisms
- exclude diabetes

Attend to causation
- Minimise contact with water, soap, detergents, lipid solvents and other irritants.
- Keep hands dry (avoid wet work if possible).
- Wear cotton lined gloves for maximum of 15 minutes.

Topical medications to nail folds
2% thymol in alcohol qid
or
10% sulphacetamide in alcohol

For Candida (if cultured)
tincture miconazole bd
or
clotrimazole topical preparations

Perianal haematoma

Within 24 hours of onset:
- simple aspiration of blood
or
- surgical drainage under LA

Within 24 hours to 5 days of onset:
- express thrombus through small incision under LA

Day 6 onwards:
• leave alone unless very painful or infected

Periodic limb movement disorder (nocturnal myoclonus)

clonazepam 1mg (o) nocte increasing to 3 mg (o) nocte

or

sodium valproate 100 mg (o) nocte

Perioral dermatitis

• tetracycline 250 mg bd for 8 weeks
• consider topical 2–4% sulphur and 2% salicylic acid in aqueous or sorbolene cream
• consider ketoconazole 2% cream
• avoid corticosteroids

Perspiration: excessive

• use an antiperspirant deodorant
• reduce caffeine intake
• avoid known aggravating factors
• refer for axillary wedge resection

Photoageing/wrinkles

Prevention
• Avoid exposure to the sun.
• Use an SPF 15⁺ sunscreen during the day.
• Wash with a 'neutral' mild soap, e.g. Neutrogena (max. twice daily) and pat dry.

Treatment
• tretinoin (Retin-A) cream
  apply once daily at bedtime (on dry skin) test for skin irritation by gradual exposure, e.g. 5 minutes at first (wash off), then 15 minutes until it can be left overnight
• Lac-Hydrin (USA)
  12% solution may be effective alternative; other lactic acid preparations may be useful

Pityriasis rosea

• explanation and reassurance
• bathe and shower as usual—use a neutral soap, e.g. Neutrogena, Dove
• use a soothing bath oil, e.g. QV bath oil, Hamilton bath oil

• for itching: urea cream or calamine lotion with 1% phenol
• expose rash to sunlight (avoid sunburn)

Pityriasis versicolor (tinea versicolor)

(refer p. 987)
selenium sulfide (Selsun shampoo) (see p. 987 for instructions)

or

econazole 1% (Pevaryl) foaming solution
• apply to wet body (after shower)
• rub in from head to toe
• do not rinse, allow to dry
• shower off next morning
• apply for 3 consecutive days once weekly for 3 weeks

or

clotrimazole, miconazole or econazole cream/lotion applied nocte for 2–4 weeks

or

terbinafine 1% cream bd for 2 weeks
ketoconazole cream bd for 10 days in severe or resistant cases.

Plantar warts

(refer pp. 655–656)
• pare wart with a 21 g scalpel blade
• apply Upton's paste to wart each night and cover (after paring)

or

• apply paste of 70% salicylic acid in raw linseed oil after paring; occlude for one week; review; pare; apply liqud nitrogen; review

or

• apply liquid nitrogen
  repeat in one week, then as necessary

or

  (at home) 16% salicyclic acid and 16% lactic acid paint, apply daily

Premenstrual tension

• explanation and reassurance
• advise recording a daily symptom diary for 2–3 months
• attend to lifestyle factors
  — diet
  — exercise
  — relaxation
• medication (refer pp. 853–856)
  moderate dose COC with 50μg ethinyl oestradiol

otherwise
pyridoxine 100 mg/day
or
evening primrose oil capsules 1 g bd
(day 12 to day 1 of next cycle)
- severe PMT
  — fluoxetine 20 mg daily 10 days before menstruation

Prickly heat (miliaria/heat rash)
- Keep the skin dry and cool, e.g. fan, air-conditioner.
- Dress in loose-fitting cotton clothing.
- Reduce activity.
- Avoid frequent bathing and overuse of soap.

Rx: Lotion: salicylic acid 2%, menthol 1%, chlorhexidine 0.5% in alcohol
or
Egozite (infants), Isophyl (adults)
If severe: hydrocortison + clotrimazole cream
Prevention: Ego Prickly Heat powder

Proctalgia fugax
- Use salbutamol inhaler, two puffs, when awakened by pain.
- Consider glyceryl trinitrate spray for the pain or prophylactic quinine bisulphate before retiring.

Prostate: benign prostatic hypertrophy
Initial trial:
- avoid caffeine
- avoid wheat, dairy and yeast products
- zinc and vitamin C tablets, e.g. Zinvit-C 250 tds

Consider:
- terazosin (as directed) or prazosin 0.5 mg (o) nocte for 3–7 days then 0.5 mg bd
    adjust to maintenance dose 1–2 mg (o) bd, then to maximum 2 mg bd
- finasteride 5 mg (o) daily for at least 6–12 months

Pruritis ani
(refer pp. 291–293)
Treat cause, e.g. dermatitis.

General measures
- Stop scratching.
- Bathe carefully: avoid hot water, excessive scrubbing and soaps.
- Use bland aqueous cream, Cetaphil lotion or Neutrogena soap.
- Keep area dry and cool.
- Keep bowels regular and wipe with cotton wool soaked in warm water.
- Wear loose-fitting clothing and underwear.
- Avoid local anaesthetics and antiseptics.

If still problematic and a dermatosis probably involved use:
hydrocortisone 1% cream
or
hydrocortisone 1% cream with clioquinol 0.5–3% or with clotrimazole 1%

If isolated area and resistant:
infiltrate 0.5 mL triamcinolone intradermally

If desperate:
fractionated X-ray therapy

Pruritus vulvae
(refer p. 968)
Management depends on cause, e.g. candidiasis

General measures
- Attend to hygiene and excessive sweating.
- Keep genital area dry and wash thoroughly at least once a day.
- Avoid overzealous washing.
- Do not wear pantyhose, tight jeans or tight underwear, or use tampons.
- Do not use vaginal douches, powders or deodorants.
- Use aqueous cream or Cetaphil lotion rather than toilet soap.

Psoriasis
(refer to pp. 979–981)
General:
- tar baths, e.g. Pinetarsol or Polytar
- tar shampoo, e.g. Polytar, Ionil-T
- sunlight (in moderation)

For stable plaques on limbs or trunk:
- apply dithranol 0.1% cream to affected area at night, leave 20–30 minutes, wash off under shower and increase strength every 5 days to 1% (up to maximum 2 hours)

- then apply topical fluorinated corticosteroid in the morning

An alternative method
- dithranol 0.1%, salicylic acid 3%, LPC 10% in white soft paraffin
- leave overnight (warn that dithranol stains— use old pyjamas and sheets)
- review in 3 weeks then gradually increase strength of dithranol to 0.25%, then 0.5%, then 1%; cut down frequency to 2–3 times per week
- shower in the morning and then apply topical fluorinated corticosteroid

For milder stabilised plaques:
- salicylic acid 3%, LPC 8% in sorbolene
apply bd or tds
          or
topical fluorinated corticosteroids
          or
calcipotriol, apply tds

For resistant plaque:
- topical fluorinated corticosteroids (II–III class) with occlusion
- intralesional injection of triamcinolone mixed (50:50) with LA or normal saline (Fig. 123.7)

Fig. 123.7 *Intralesional injection for psoriasis*

Renal (or ureteric) colic
- pethidine and metoclopramide (10 mg) injection statim:
     give IM or by IV titration
- indomethacin suppositories (take home for any further pain)
     limited to two a day

Restless legs (Ekbom's syndrome)
Exclude diabetes, various drugs e.g. antidepressants, neuroleptics, β blockers, uraemia, hypothyroidism and anaemia. It is mainly a functional disorder affecting the elderly.

- diet: eliminate caffeine and follow a healthy diet
- exercises: gentle stretching of legs, particularly of hamstrings and calf muscles, for at least 5 minutes before retiring (Fig. 123.8)

Fig. 123.8 *Stretching exercise for restless legs*

Medication
1st choice: clonazepam 1 mg, one hour before retiring
2nd choice: diazepam
May help: codeine, levodopa, baclofen, propranolol
Generally unhelpful: carbamazepine, quinine, antipsychotics and antidepressants

Ringworm (tinea corporis)
- clotrimazole 1%, miconazole 2% or ketoconazole 2% cream; apply bd for 5–6 weeks (ensure 4 weeks past apparent cure)
- may require griseofulvin or terbinafine if no response

Rosacea
- tetracycline 250 mg bd or qid
     (doxycycline 100 mg daily)

until improved, then
- tetracycline 250 mg daily
     (doxycycline 50 mg)
for at least 8–10 weeks

Second line: erythromycin (in similar dose)
Resistant cases: metronidazole 200 mg bd for 10 days

Topical agents
- 2% sulphur in aqueous cream (milder cases)
          or
- metronidazole gel bd (more severe cases)

Rough stippled skin (keratosis pilaris)

Rough skin in children and adolescents on outer aspects of thighs and upper arms
• reassurance and education

If needed for temporary treatment select from:
• moisturisers with urea, e.g. Calmurid
• 3% salicylic acid ointment
• topical retinoid creams

Roundworms (acariasis)

• pyrantel (various preparations)
    20 mg/kg (to max. of 750 mg) as single dose

Scabies (all types)

• permethrin 5% cream (if > 2 months of age) apply to whole body from jawline down leave overnight and wash off—single application
        or
benzyl benzoate 25%

Seborrhoeic warts/keratoses

• *see* Keratoses (p. 1223)

Shingles (herpes zoster)

(refer pp. 995–996)
• use menthol in flexible collodion for the rash
• for severe cases (within 72 hours of development of rash) aciclovir 800 mg 5 times daily or famciclovir 250 mg tds or valaciclovir 1000 mg tds for 7 days

Postherpetic neuralgia
• consider topical capsaicin cream (Capsig); apply 3–4 times a day; antidepressants or carbamazepine (especially for lancinating pain)

Sinusitis: acute

(refer pp. 490–491)
• look for nasal pathology such as polyposis and dental problems
• analgesics
• steam inhalations (Fig. 123.5)
• pseudoephedrine tablets
• antibiotics (1st choice)—for 7–10 day course
        amoxycillin
                or

        amoxycillin/potassium clavulanate (if amoxycillin-resistant)
                or
        doxycycline

Sinusitis: chronic

Sinusitis persisting longer than 2 weeks, despite repeated antibiotic and decongestant therapy, is common in general practice. Postnasal drip with cough, especially at night, is a feature.
• steam inhalations with Friar's balsam or menthol (best is menthol Co APF inhalation)
• vitamin C (sodium ascorbate) 2–4 g daily (a powder can be obtained and mixed with orange juice)

Smoking

Quitting tips (refer pp. 149–150)

Snoring

If abnormal, refer to a sleep laboratory for assessment and management of obstructive sleep apnoea syndrome and other abnormalities.
  If functional, give the following advice to consider:
• Obtain and maintain ideal weight.
• Avoid drugs, e.g. sedatives, hypnotics.
• Avoid sleeping on the back—consider sewing tennis balls on back of nightwear or wear bra (with tennis balls) back to front.
• Keep neck extended with a soft collar at night.
• Provide partner with appropriate ear plugs!

Stinging fish

Injury due mainly to sharp spines, e.g. stonefish.
• bathe or immerse part in very warm to hot water
• consider infiltration with local anaesthetic

Stitch in side

A stitch in the epigastric or hypochondrium is sharp pain due to cramping in the diaphragm.
• Stop and rest when the pain strikes during activity. Then walk—don't run.
• Apply deep massage to the area with the pulps of the middle three fingers.
• Perform slow deep breathing.

Prophylaxis

- undertake a program of abdominal breathing prior to activity.

Stuttering

Recommend medical hypnotherapy if there are no contraindications.

Stye in eye

- Apply heat with direct steam from a thermos (Fig. 123.9) onto the closed eye or by a hot compress (helps spontaneous discharge).
- Perform lash epilation to allow drainage (incise with a D_{11} blade if epilation doesn't work).
- Only use topical antibiotic ointment, e.g. chloramphenicol, if infection spreading locally, and systemic antibiotics if distal spread noted by preauricular adenitis.

Fig. 123.9 *Steaming a painful eye*

Subconjunctival haemorrhage

- Patient explanation and reassurance is necessary.
- It absorbs over two weeks.
- Although no local therapy is necessary, bathing with a weak salt solution twice daily helps.

Sunburn

(refer p. 988)

- aspirin (for pain)

- promethazine (for sedation/itching) only if necessary

Topical:

- hydrocortisone 1% ointment or cream for unblistered severe cases (early)
    repeat in 2–3 hours, then next day (not after 24 hours)
        or
- bicarbonate of soda paste, applied 2 hourly
        or
- oily calamine lotion

Sweating (excessive)

General hyperhidrosis

- explanation and reassurance
- trial of probanthine aluminium chloride 20% in alcohol solution if localised area

Axillary hyperhidrosis

Treatment:

- explanation and reassurance
- *see* treatment of body odour
- aluminium chloride 20% in alcohol solution (Driclor); apply nocte for one week, then 1–2 times weekly or as necessary

Surgery

Wedge resection of a small block of skin and subcutaneous tissue from axillary vault. Define sweat glands with codeine starch powder. The area excised is usually about 4 cm × 2.5 cm.

Tear duct (nasolacrimal duct) blockage in child

- if conjunctivitis present
    chloramphenicol eyedrops
- perform regular massage from inner canthus to base of nose (teach mother) at least twice daily
- if persistent in infant: requires nasolacrimal probing at 4 months—otherwise leave to 6 months or so as it may resolve

Teething

Precautions: exclude other possible causes of irritability in a teething child, e.g. UTI, meningitis, otitis media. Teething doesn't cause fever.

Treatment:

- paracetamol
- trimeprazine or other antihistamine (o) nocte

Chewing
- teething ring (kept cold in the refrigerator)

  or
- baby can chew on a clean, cold, lightly moistened facewasher (a piece of apple can be placed in the facewasher)

  or
- parent can massage gum with forefinger wrapped in a soft cloth or gauze pad (Ora-sed gel can be massaged into gums every 3 hours if extremely troublesome)

Temporomandibular joint dysfunction

Refer to the various exercise techniques on pages 492–493. Most effective and simplest method is placing a piece of soft wood, e.g. carpenter's pencil, firmly against back molars and biting rhythmically on the object with a grinding movement for 2–3 minutes at least 3 times a day.

Tennis elbow
(refer p. 585)

Tension headache
- explanation and reassurance
- remove source of anxiety (if possible)
- counselling
- relaxation techniques/meditation
- consider cervical spine as factor and treat any dysfunction with mobilisation, massage and exercises
- aspirin or paracetamol for pain

Threadworms
- explanation and reassurance
- pyrantel (various oral preparations)
  20 mg/kg (up to max. of 750 mg) as a single dose
  repeat after 1 week if a heavy infection

Thrush (moniliasis)
In infants: nystatin oral drops or miconazole oral gel 1 mL held in mouth as long as possible 4 times daily
In adults: amphotericin, 1 lozenge (10 mg) dissolved slowly in mouth 6 hourly for 10 days

  or

miconazole oral gel 50 mg 6 hourly dropped on tongue and held in mouth as long as possible

Vaginal thrush
(refer pp. 870–871 and 1235)

Thumb sucking
- not a concern before 6–7 years
- usually ceases spontaneously
- no specific treatment/medication
- avoid drawing attention
- distract child with other activities
- refer if prolonged and excessive

Tick bites
(refer p. 1119)

Tinea capitis
Griseofulvin 500 mg (o) for 6–8 weeks
- Children: 10 mg/kg day (max. 250 mg)
Also — take hair plucking and scale for culture
— Selsun shampoo twice weekly
— topical clotrimazole or miconazole

Tinea cruris (jock itch)
- Soak the area in a warm bath and dry thoroughly.
- Apply clotrimazole 1% or miconazole 2% or ketoconazole 2% cream; rub in a thin layer bd for 3–4 weeks.
- When almost healed, apply tolnaftate dusting powder bd for 3–4 weeks.
- If itch severe: add 1% hydrocortisone cream.
- If weeping: apply Burow's solution compresses.

Tinea pedis (athlete's foot)
(refer p. 985)
- patient education
- keep feet clean and dry
- use antifungal powder between toes after drying
- wear socks of natural absorbent fibres (avoid synthetics)
- wear open sandals or shoes with porous soles and uppers (if possible)
- use thongs in public showers
- keep toe spaces separated if interdigital

Rx: clotrimazole 1% or miconazole 2% cream or
lotion; apply bd or tds for 2–3 weeks
or
ketoconazole 2% cream bd
if widespread or smelly vesiculobullae (take
scrapings), use griseofulvin (Griseostatin)
330 mg (o) daily for 6 weeks
or
terbinafine 250 mg (o) daily for 2–6 weeks

Tinea of toenails and fingernails (tinea unguium)

- usually associated with tinea pedis
- nails show white spots; may be yellow and crumbling
- starts at the edge of periphery and spreads towards base

Treatment:
- cut affected nail well back, elevate the nail slightly at the edges and apply tincture of miconazole (Daktarin) to and under the nail bd for several weeks
or
apply terbinafine
or
apply amorolfine nail lacquer
- terbinafine (Lamisil) 250 mg (o) daily
  — fingernails 4 weeks
  — toenails 12 weeks

Tinnitus

Precautions:
- exclude wax, drugs including marijuana, vascular disease, depression, aneurysm, vascular tumours, venous hum (jugular vein)
- beware of lonely elderly people living alone (suicide risk)

Management includes:
- educate and reassure the patient
- relaxation techniques
- background 'noise', e.g. music playing during night for masking
- tinnitus maskers
- hearing aids

Consider psychological counselling or hypnotherapy.

Drug trials to consider (limited efficacy)
- betahistine (Serc) 8–16 mg daily (max. 32 mg)
- carbamazepine

- antidepessants
- sodium valproate

Acute severe tinnitus
- lignocaine 1% IV slowly (up to 5 mL)

Tongue problems
- geographical tongue: reassurance and Cepacaine gargles 10 mL tds if tender
- black or hairy tongue: this is basically a harmless condition related to smoking and antibiotic treatment
Rx (if patient pressure):
  — brush with toothbrush using sodium bicarbonate paste
or
  — suck fresh pineapple pieces

Torticollis (acute wry neck)
Muscle energy therapy, which is simple to use and highly effective, is described on page 563.

Travel sickness
Oral preparations:
- dimenhydrinate (Andrumin, Dramamine, Travacalm)
or
- promethazine theoclate (Avomine)
or
- hyoscine (Kwells)

Take 30–60 minutes before the trip
repeat 4–6 hourly during trip
(maximum 4 doses in 24 hours)

Dermal:
- hyoscine dermal disc (Scop)
  apply to dry hairless skin behind ear 5–6 hours before travel, leave on for 3 days

Tremor: essential
Usually no specific treatment, apart from explation and reassurance. Can use propranolol (first choice) 40 mg bd (or more) or primidone.

Tropical ear
For severe painful otitis externa in tropics:
- prednisolone (orally) 15 mg statim, then 10 mg 8 hourly for 6 doses followed by
- Merocel ear wick

- topical Kenacomb or Sofradex drops for 10 days

Umbilical discharge

Usually infected (fungal or bacterial) dermatitis, often with offensive discharge.

  Precautions: consider umbilical fistula, carcinoma, umbilical calculus.

Management:
- swab for micro and culture
- toilet—remove all debris and clean
- keep dry and clean—daily dressings
- consider Kenacomb ointment

Umbilical granuloma in infants

Apply a caustic pencil gently daily for about 5 days.

Urticaria (hives)

(refer p. 971)
- search for cause, e.g. drugs, food, infestation
- food check: nuts, chocolate, cheese, fish, eggs

Rx: antihistamines: e.g. cetirizine 10–20 mg daily,
          loratadine, astemizole or fexofenadine
- lukewarm baths with Pinetarsol or similar soothing bath oil
- topical 0.5% hydrocortisone—apply every 4 hours for itching

If severe: prednisolone 50 mg once daily for 10–14 days

Vaginal thrush (monilial vaginitis)

- Bathe genital area bd or tds with sodium bicarbonate (especially before using treatment).
- Dry area thoroughly.
- Wear loose-fitting cotton underwear.
- Avoid wearing tight clothing or using tampons.
- Avoid vaginal douches, powders and deodorants.

Rx: can use amphotericin, clotrimazole, econazole, isoconazole, miconazole or nystatin. Examples:
- clotrimazole 500 mg vaginal tablet statim, and clotrimazole 2% cream applied to vagina and vulva (for symptomatic relief)
    or (especially if recurrent or recalcitrant)
- nystatin pessaries, once daily for 7 days

and/or nystatin vaginal cream 4 g once daily for 7 days
            or (if recalcitrant)
- fluconazole 150 mg (o) as a single dose or 100 mg (o) daily for 14 days

Varicose ulcers

(refer pp. 1002–1003)

Vitiligo

Consider a trial of topical corticosteroids e.g. hydrocortisone 1% for 6 months then methylprednisolone aceponale 0.1% for 6 months

Warts: common

- soak the wart/s in warm soapy water
- rub back the wart surface with a pumice stone
- apply the paint (protect the surrounding skin with vaseline), e.g. formalin 5%, salicylic acid 12%, acetone 25%, collodion to 100%, apply once daily
            or
(adult) 16% salicylic acid, 16% lactic acid in collodion paint, apply once daily
(children) 8% salicylic acid, 8% lactic acid in collodion

Whiplash

(refer p. 564)

Wrinkles

(refer p. 1228)

Writer's cramp

- education and reassurance
- avoid holding pen too tight
- clonazepam 0.5 mg bd (if persisting)

          *   *   *

Ionising radiation illness

Although this is fortunately not an everyday problem and hopefully never will be to readers, it is worthwhile to conclude with an overview of the clinical consequences of radioactive fallout. The nuclear disasters in Eastern Europe highlighted the paucity of knowledge available to the general practitioner about the known clinical effects of the radioactive elements (mainly iodine and caesium) that are discharged into the atmosphere.

  Apart from nuclear accidents, the effects of

excessive ionising radiation can follow accidental exposure in hospitals and industry, and in the use of atomic weaponry. Ionising radiation can be either penetrating (X-rays, gamma rays, neutrons) or non-penetrating (alpha or beta particles).

The revised *Système International* (SI) nomenclature uses the sievert (SV) as the unit of radiation dose to body tissue. It is the absorbed dose weighted for the damaging effect of the radiation. As a guideline the annual background radiation is approximately 2.5 millisievert and a typical X-ray is 0.5 millisievert.

The general principles of radiation exposure are:

- The closer to the focus of radiation, the more devastating the injury.
- Radiation illness can vary from mild vomiting to acute leukaemia.
- The most sensitive tissues are the brain, the gastrointestinal mucosa and bone marrow.
- The dividing (mitotic) cells of blood, the gastrointestinal tract, skin, lenses and gonads are especially vulnerable.

Severe acute radiation sickness

The extent of the radiation damage depends on the dose of radiation. The typical clinical effects are presented in Table 123.2. The acute effects include the cerebral or CNS syndrome, haemopoietic syndrome, gastrointestinal syndrome and the skin and mucous membrane syndrome (radiation dermatitis).

Acute lethal injury

The lethal problems that can result from acute exposure to radiation are due to haemopoietic failure, gastrointestinal mucosa damage, central nervous system damage and widespread vascular injury (Fig. 123.10).

Death is usually due to haemorrhage, anaemia or infection secondary to haemopoietic failure (mainly leukaemia). Lymphocytes are the most sensitive cells, then leucocytes, erythrocytes and platelets. Where death doesn't occur, recovery of cells can take months.

High doses of radiation produce irradiation of the brain, leading to the cerebral syndrome. This is characterised by nausea, vomiting, listlessness and drowsiness followed by convulsions, ataxia and, usually quickly, death.

The gastrointestinal syndrome, which is maximal 3–5 days after exposure, is caused by destruction of the crypt cells in the mucosa. It is characterised by intractable nausea and vomiting (which responds poorly to antiemetic drugs) and diarrhoea with subsequent severe fluid and electrolyte imbalance.

Table 123.2 *Clinical effects of radioactive fallout from a nuclear accident (using Chernobyl as a reference)*

Radiation dose expressed in sieverts*	Distance from focus (approximate)	Typical clinical effects (variable time of onset)	Mortality risk
10–50	1 km	Nausea, vomiting, diarrhoea, Cerebral syndrome Fever Fluid and electrolyte imbalance Acute leukaemia	100% Rapidly fatal
6–10	2–3 km	Nausea, vomiting, diarrhoea Rash Acute leukaemia/agranulocytosis	80–100%
2–6	4–6 km	Nausea, vomiting Rash Leukaemia/agranulocytosis Alopecia Cataracts	50%
1–2	7–8 km	Nausea, vomiting Agranulocytosis (mild)	Not immediate Long-term cancer risk
0–1	9 km and over	Nausea, vomiting	Not fatal

* 1 sievert = 10 REM (older unit)
  typical X-ray = 0.5 millisievert

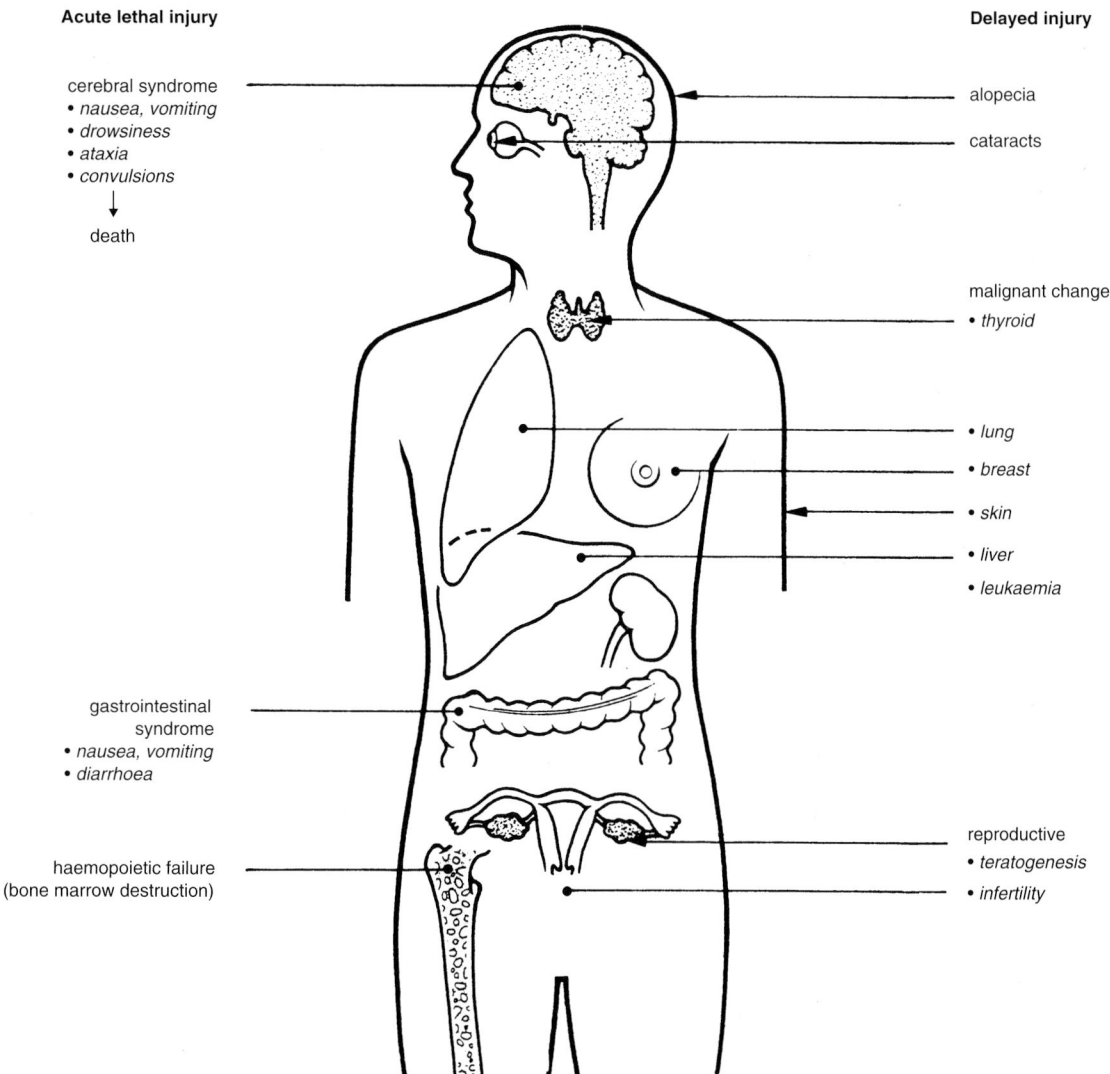

Acute lethal injury

cerebral syndrome
• *nausea, vomiting*
• *drowsiness*
• *ataxia*
• *convulsions*

↓

death

gastrointestinal
syndrome
• *nausea, vomiting*
• *diarrhoea*

haemopoietic failure
(bone marrow destruction)

Delayed injury

alopecia

cataracts

malignant change
• *thyroid*

• *lung*
• *breast*
• *skin*
• *liver*
• *leukaemia*

reproductive
• *teratogenesis*
• *infertility*

Fig. 123.10 *Clinical effects of radiation illness*

The acute effects on the skin and mucous membrane include erythema, epilation, blistering, purpura, destruction of fingers and secondary infection. Total loss of body hair, particularly alopecia, is a serious prognostic sign.

Mild acute radiation sickness

The main symptoms are malaise, weakness, anorexia, nausea and vomiting. The blood film is affected with diminished production of the blood cells. Lymphocytes are the most sensitive and lymphopenia develops within several days with a fall in all white cells and platelets within another three weeks.

Delayed effects

Other organs with a tendency to absorb radiation do not show immediate effects but will undergo malignant change. The thyroid gland is the most vulnerable. Others include the lungs, kidney, liver and breast, skin and salivary glands.

Acute myeloid leukaemia is a common sequela. Other late sequelae include infertility, teratogenesis, skin changes and cataracts.

Management

Acute radiation sickness is a medical emergency and arrangements must be made for immediate referral to hospital. Contaminated clothing should be removed and substituted with protective clothing.

Response to treatment obviously depends on the extent, degree and localisation of tissue damage.

For distressing nausea and vomiting use:
metoclopramide 10 mg IM or IV (slowly) injections

or
chlorpromazine 25–50 mg IM 4–6 hourly

Treatment might include:
• fluid and electrolyte replacement
• ultra isolation techniques to prevent infection
• antibiotics are necessary
• bone marrow transplantation
• platelet or granulocyte transfusion

APPENDICES

———

INFANT GIRLS

NAME   BIRTH DATE   NO.

WEIGHT

The child is weighed without
clothing except light under
garments.

LENGTH

The child lies relaxed on a
firm surface. The soles of
the feet are held against
a firm upright at the
zero mark on a
parallel rule & a
movable square
is brought
against the
vertex. The
head is held
so the eyes
face the
ceiling.

MONTHS

MONTHS

HEAD CIRCUMFERENCE

WEEKS

INFANT BOYS

NAME   BIRTH DATE   NO.

WEIGHT

The child is weighed without clothing except light under garments.

LENGTH

The child lies relaxed on a firm surface. The soles of the feet are held against a firm upright at the zero mark on a parallel rule & a movable square is brought against the vertex. The head is held so the eyes face the ceiling.

HEAD CIRCUMFERENCE

GIRLS

NAME   BIRTH DATE   NO.

LENGTH
The child lies relaxed
on a firm surface. the
soles of the feet are held
against a firm upright
at the zero mark on a
parallel rule & a
movable square is
brought against the
vertex. The head is
held so the eyes face
the ceiling.

HEIGHT
The child's heels should
be near together. Heels
buttocks & occiput
should be against
a vertical upright.

WEIGHT
The child is weighed without
clothing except light undergarments.

AGE IN YEARS

3 4 5 6 7 8 9 10 11 12

97 90 75 50 25 10 3

BOYS

NAME

BIRTH DATE

NO.

LENGTH

The child lies relaxed
on a firm surface. the
soles of the feet are held
against a firm upright
at the zero mark on a
parallel rule & a
movable square is
brought against the
vertex. The head is
held so the eyes face
the ceiling.

HEIGHT

The child's heels should
be near together. Heels
buttocks & occiput
should be against
a vertical upright.

WEIGHT

The child is weighed without
clothing except light undergarments.

AGE
IN YEARS

AGE
IN YEARS

NORMAL PEAK EXPIRATORY FLOW RATES

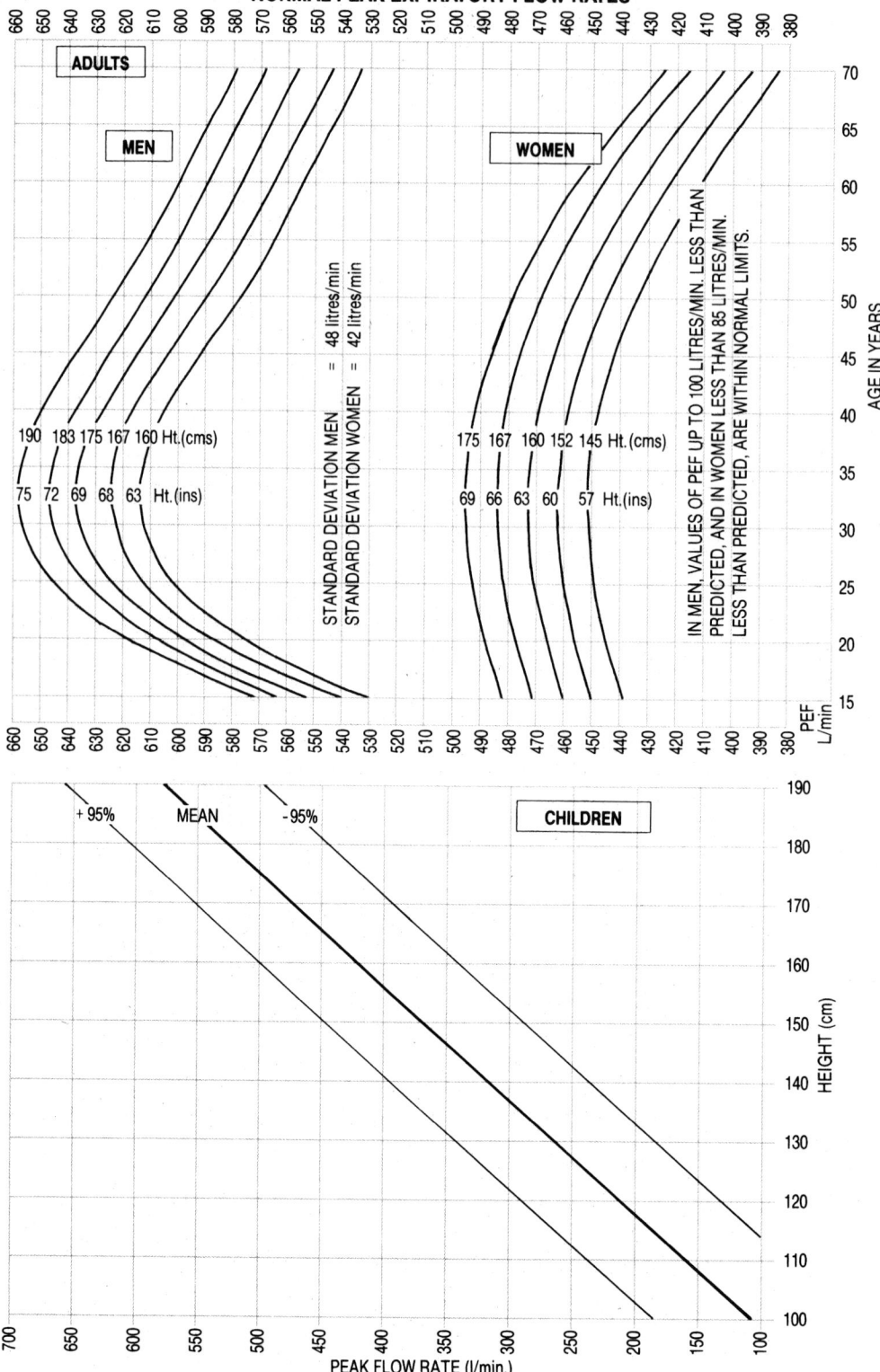

THE AUSTRALIAN NUTRITION FOUNDATION
Weight For Height Chart
(For Men and Women from 18 years onward)

Based on Body Mass Index (BMI) in Range of 18, 20, 25, 30.

HEIGHT IN CENTIMETRES (FEET & INCHES) — WITHOUT SHOES

Index

abdomen, acute, 247–8
abdominal aortic aneurysm, 257–8
abdominal distension, 248
abdominal examination, 251
abdominal pain
    acute abdomen, 247–8
    in children, 253–7
    chronic pain, 248–9, 265
    in elderly, 257–60
    recurrent, 256–7, 265–6
    in women, 840–51
abnormal uterine bleeding, 835–9
Aboriginal health, 78, 1199–1205
abortion, 894
abrasions, 1134
abscess
    amoebic liver, 99, 203
    breast, 822
    cerebral, 697
    pelvic, 259
    perianal, 289
absence seizures, 510, 1064
abuse
    children, 776–81
    sexual, 778, 876–8
    women, 874–7
ACE inhibitors
    cough, 372
    heart failure, 456–7
    hypertension, 1082–3
acetazolamide
    in altitude sickness, 107
    in glaucoma, 718
achalasia, 446–7
Achilles tendon, 650, 1194
    bursitis, 650, 1195
    rupture, 1194–5
    tendinitis, 650, 1194
aciclovir
    for genital herpes, 946–8
    for herpes simplex, 996–7
    for herpes zoster, 995–6
    for keratitis, 480
acne, 983–4, 1209
acoustic neuroma, 429
acral lentiginous melanoma, 1023
acromegaly, 170
acromioclavicular
    dislocation, 1150
    osteoarthritis, 578
    subluxation, 1150
actinomycosis
    lumpy jaw, 553
    pelvis, 849
acute abdomen, 247–8
acute anaphylaxis, 1037, 1113
acute appendicitis, 255, 259–60

acute calcific periarthritis, 280–1
acute cholangitis, 543
acute cholecystitis, 263–4
acute disturbed patient, 413–14
acute diverticulitis, 264–5
acute epiglottitis, 788–90
acute gastroenteritis, 401–5
acute idiopathic demyelinating
    polyneuropathy, 240–1
acute leukaemia, 183–4
acute mountain sickness, 97
acute myocardial infarction, 342–3,
    351–4
acute pancreatitis, 264
acute pericarditis, 344
acute pulmonary oedema, 1113
acute pyelonephritis, 175–8
acute retention of urine, 259
acute skin eruptions, 989–98
acute torticollis, 563–4
Addison's disease, 171
adenovirus infection
    of eye, 478
    of throat, 680
adhesive capsulitis, shoulder, 576–7
adhesive skin tape, for mallet finger,
    1184–5
adjustment disorder with anxious mood,
    1049
adolescent
    eating disorders, 796
    general health, 795–9
    psychiatric disorders, 421
    scoliosis, 325–6
adrenal cortex disorders, 169–70
adverse drug reactions, 63, 126, 147–8
aerophagy, 435, 1212
ageing and disease, 55–6
agoraphobia, 1047
AIDS, see human immunodeficiency
    virus infection
air travel, 104
alcohol, abuse of, 150–1, 1029–35
alcoholic liver disease, 544
Alcoholics Anonymous, 1034
alkaline phosphatase, 537
allergic alveolitis, 460
allergic conjunctivitis, 480, 1038–9
allergic contact dermatitis, 976
allergic disorders, 1036–41
allergic rhinitis, 1038–41
allopurinol, 282
alopecia androgenetica, 1209
alopecia areata, 1209
alpha fetoprotein, 880
ALTE, 794
altitude sickness, 107

Alzheimer's disease, 59–62, 415–16
amaurosis fugax, 718–19, 1128–30
amblyopia, 715
ambulatory monitoring, 342, 1075
amenorrhoea, 838
amiodarone, 672, 677
amitriptyline, 134
amnesic episodes, 511
amniocentesis, 880
amoebiasis, 92–3, 203
amoebic liver abscess, 99
amphetamines, 152
amputated finger, 1138
Amsler grid, 714
amyloidosis, 123
anabolic steroids, 153–4
anaemia, 127, 131–2, 156–61
    childhood, 161
    iron deficiency, 157–9
    macrocytic, 159–60
    microcytic, 157
    normocytic, 160–1
anal discharge, 290–1
anal fissure, 288, 1210
anaphylaxis, 792, 1037, 1113
aneurysm
    of abdominal aorta, 257–8
    dissecting, 343, 354
angina pectoris, 342–3, 347–50, 1210
angiodysplasia, 291
angioedema, 1113
angiography, 342, 620
angry patient, 45
ankle examination, 647–8
ankle pain, 644–58
ankle sprain, 649, 1191–4
ankylosing spondylitis, 282–3, 309–10
anorectal disorders, 287–93
anorexia, in children and infants, 1210
anorexia nervosa, 736–7
anovulation, 837–9
anserinus tendinitis, 640
antacids, 439–40
antenatal care, 878–85
antepartum haemorrhage, 889
anterior compartment
    syndrome, 1189
anterior cord syndrome, 566
antibiotics, 1096–9, 1210
anticipatory guidance, 5, 89
anticoagulants, 355–7
anticonvulsants, see antiepileptics
antidepressants, 133–5
antiemetics, 105, 549–50
antiepileptics, 1065–7
antihistamines, 106, 1040
antinuclear antibodies, 224, 280

antioxidants, 69–70
antiparkinsonian drugs, 235–7
anxiety, 1043–50
aortic stenosis, 505–6
aphthous ulcers, 1211
Apley grind/distraction test, 632
apnoea, sleep, 691–2
appendicitis, 255, 259
arcobase, 141
arm pain, 580–5
   arthritis conditions, 593–4
   carpal tunnel syndrome, 588–90
   in children, 583–4
   in elderly, 585
   neurovascular disorders, 592–3
   olecranon bursitis, 588
   de Quervain's tenosynovitis,
     591–2
   tennis elbow, 585–8
   trigger finger/thumb, 590–1
arrhythmias, 671–7
arterial ischaemic ulcer, 1001–2
arthralgia, *see* arthritis
arthritis, 267–85
   in children, 272–4
   in foot, 651–2
   in hand, 593–4
   in hip, 604
   in knee, 641
arthroscopy, 482
asbestos, and mesothelioma, 461
ascorbic acid, *see* vitamin c
aspirated foreign body, 791–2
aspiration
   of breast lump, 827–8
   of hydrocele, 907
   for pneumothorax, 354–5
aspirin, 1102–3
   in angina, 349,1210
   in arthritis, 276, 279
   in gastrointestinal bleeding, 512,
     1101
   in migraine, 523
   in myocardial infarction, 352
   in tension headache, 521
   in TIAs, 1130
   in URTIs, 378
asteatotic eczema, 970, 975
asterixis, 536
asthma
   bronchial, 70, 449, 1051–62
   cardiac, 449
   childhood, 790–1, 1061
asthma action plan, 1060
asthma management plan, 1054–6
astigmatism, 716
astringents, 961
asymptomatic bacteriuria, 175
ataxia, 238–9, 659–60
atenolol
   in angina, 349, 1210
   in arrhythmias, 677
   in hypertension, 1082
   in migraine, 524
   in myocardial infarction, 353
athletes
   little athletes, 603, 633
   overuse of legs, 1188–9
athlete's foot, *see* tinea pedis
atlanto-axial subluxation, 567
atopic dermatitis, 751, 972–5
atrial fibrillation, 675–6, 1131
atrial flutter, 675–6
atrial premature beats, 672

atrophic vaginitis, 870
atropine, 1125, 1176
attention deficit hyperactivity disorder,
   772
atypical facial pain, 495
atypical pneumonia, 216, 379
audiometry, 388
aura, in migraine, 522–3
autism, 773–4
autonomic neuropathy, 143, 505–6
avascular necrosis
   femoral head, 1161
   humeral head, 1153
axial loading test, 313
azoospermia, 928–9

back
   manipulation of, 314–15, 1221
   mobilisation of, 314–15, 1221
   trigger points on, 314
back pain
   low/lumbar, 295–317, 1211–12
   thoracic, 318–330, 357–8, 1212
backache, *see* back pain
bacteraemia, 503
bacterial endocarditis,
     see infective endocarditis
bacterial infections, puzzling, 206–17
bacterial vaginosis, 872
bacteriuria, 175
bad news, breaking of, 40–1
Baker's cyst, 632
balanitis, 913
baldness, 1209
balloon tamponade, 350
banned drugs in sport 154–5
barbiturate dependence, 420
barotrauma, 472–3
Barrett's oesophagus, 439
basal cell carcinoma, 1013
BATHE technique, 13
BCG vaccinations, 208
Becker's naevus, 1020
Beckwith-Wiedemann
     syndrome 727
beclomethasone, in asthma, 1056–7
bed sores, 1003, 1212
bee stings, 1117, 1212
behaviour disorders of children, 769–75
behaviour modification, 68, 1032
belching, 1212
Bell's palsy, 1213
benign intracranial hypertension, 530
benign positional vertigo, 432–3
benign prostatic hyperplasia, 919–21
benign tumours, 181
benzodiazepines, 420, 1049–50, 1099
benzylpenicillin, 788, 1176
bereavement, 39, 691
beta 2 agonists, in asthma, 1057–8
bicipital tendinitis, 577
beta-blockers
   in angina, 349, 1210
   in anxiety, 1046
   in arrhythmias, 672, 677
   in hypertension, 1082–3
   in migraine, 524
   in myocardial infarction, 353
biceps femoris tendinitis, 640
bicipital tendinitis, 577
biguanides, for diabetes, 142
bilharzia, 101
biliary pain, 263
bilirubin, 532–3, 537
Billing's ovulation method, 811

biopsy
   breast, 827–8
   punch, 1016–17
   shave, 1016–17
bipolar disorder, 418–19, 421
bird fancier's lung, 460
bites, 1115–16, 1138–9
   cats, 1139
   dogs, 1138–9
   human, 1138
   snakes, 1115–16
   spiders, 1115–17
   ticks, 1119
'black' nails, 1195
blackout, 509, 699
blackwater fever, 100, 706
bladder
   dysfunction, 1213
   outflow obstruction, 919–20
   tumours, 705
bleeding disorder, 333–6
blepharitis, 482–3, 1213
blepharospasm, 242
blindness, 712, 718
blood groups, in pregnancy, 880
blood loss, 513–14, 1124
blood pressure
   diastolic, 1071
   levels, 1071–2
   measurement, 1073–6
   systolic, 1071
blood transfusion, 513–14, 1124
blue fingers syndrome, 592
blue naevus, 1022
body language, 31
body mass index, 726
body odour, 1213
boil (furuncle), 956, 1213
bone forceps, for skin tag, 1007
bone, fractures of, *see* fractures
Bordetella pertussis, 766
Bornholm disease, 319
Borrelia burgdorferi,
     see Lyme disease
botulinum A toxin, 242
botulism, 216
Bouchard's nodes, 270
bowed legs, *see* genu varum
bowel disorders
   inflammatory bowel disease,
     405–6
   irritable bowel syndrome, 406–7
   large bowel obstruction, 261–2
   small bowel obstruction, 261
Bowen's disease, 1013
brachial plexus lesions, 573
bradycardia, 671, 677
brain stem lesions: 'locked-in' syndrome,
   1130
brain syndrome
   acute, 414–16
   chronic, 61, 415
breast
   abscess, 822
   aspiration of, 827–8
   cancer, 829
   clinical examination, 825–6
   cyst, 830
   engorged, 892–3
   lumps, 824–33
   pain, 818–23
   self-examination, 825–6
breast-feeding, 770, 791, 892, 1213
breath-holding attacks, 770, 1213

breathlessness, 448
bromocriptine, 237, 821, 855, 893,
bronchial carcinoma, 182, 381, 461
bronchiectasis, 382–3
bronchiolitis, 790, 1213
bronchitis
    acute, 379
    chronic, 379, 457–8
bronchodilators, 458, 1056–8
bronchoscopy, 374
brucellosis, 212–13
bruising and bleeding, 331–6
bruxism, 1213
Buerger's test, 619
bulimia, 737
bunions
    lateral (Tailor's), 654
    medial (hallux valgus), 654
burning feet syndrome, 1214
burnout, 693
burns, 1214
bursitis
    infrapatellar, 640
    olecranon, 588
    prepatellar, 640
    subacromial, 576
    trochanteric, 605
butterfly rash, 123
buttock pain, 597–607

C-reactive protein
    in arthritis, 273–5
    in infective endocarditis, 210
    in giant cell arteritis, 230
    in rheumatic fever, 274
    in sick children, 783
caffeine, 1077
CAGE questionnaire, 1031
calcium antagonists, 349, 1081–3, 1210
calcium channel blockers, see calcium
    antagonists
calcium pyrophosphate, 281, 634
callus on foot, 655, 1215
Campylobacter jejuni, 98, 396, 403–6
cancer, 73, 181–6
    breast, 73, 825–30
    caecum, 183
    cerebral, 528–9
    cervix, 73, 804–9
    childhood, 181
    colorectal, 73, 367–8
    kidney, 183
    leukaemia, 183–4
    liver, 533, 537
    lung, 79, 182, 381, 461
    lymphoma, 184–5
    as a masquerade, 127
    melanoma, 1023–6
    metastatic, 185
    myeloma, 185
    oesophagus, 446
    ovary, 183, 847
    pain control, 47–52
    pancreas, 543–4
    penis, 915
    prevention, 69
    prognosis, 69
    prostate, 921–2
    skin, 1006, 1013
    spine, 309–10, 320
    stomach, 442–3
    symptom control, 52–3
    testes, 908–9

thyroid, 169
candida infection
    intertrigo, 969
    oral, 685
    pruritus vulvae, 968–9
    sexually transmitted, 943, 1201–2
    vaginitis, 870–2, 1235
cannabis dependence, 153
captopril, 456, 1082–3
carbamazepine
    bipolar disorder, 419
    epilepsy, 509–10, 1065
    neuralgias, 494
carcinoid syndrome, 185
carcinoid tumours, 185
carcinoma, see cancer
cardiac arrest, 1121–5
cardiac arrhythmias, 671–7
cardiac enzymes, 352
cardiac failure, see heart failure
cardiac resuscitation, 1121–5
cardiac tamponade, 1169–70
cardiogenic shock, 353
cardiomyopathy, 449
cardiopulmonary arrest, 784, 1121–5
cardiopulmonary resuscitation
    children, 784
    adults, 1121–5
carotid sinus massage, 675
carpal tunnel syndrome, 588–90
    injection for, 590
    tests for, 589
carvediol, 456
cat bites, 1139
cat-scratch disease, 1140
cataracts, 123, 716–17
cauliflower ear, 1133
cavernous sinus a-v fistula, 485
CD4 (T helper cell), 189
CD8 (T suppressor cell), 189
cefotaxime, 789–90, 1096
cellulite, 1214
cellulitis, 624
centipede bite, 1118
central cord syndrome, 566
central retinal artery occlusion, 720–1
central retinal vein thrombosis, 721
cephalosporins, 789–90, 1096
cerebellar ataxia, 233
cerebellar tumours, 232–3
cerebral haemorrhage, 576, 697, 1127–8
cerebral metastases, 185, 516
cerebral palsy, 755
cerebral tumours, 528–9
cerebrospinal fluid, 529–30, 755, 788
cerebrovascular disease, 1127–31
cervical cancer, 73, 803–9
cervical disc disruption, 565
cervical dystonia, 242
cervical intraepithelial neoplasia, 804
cervical lymphadenopathy, 552–3
cervical myelopathy, 566
cervical rib, 582
cervical spine
    clinical disorders, 561–7
    dysfunction, 172–3, 561–2
    examination, 558–60
    headache, 525–6
cervical spondylosis, 562–3
cervicitis, 946
cervix
    cancer, 73, 803–9
    intraepithelial neoplasia, 805
    smear, 805–8

chalazion, 482
chancroid, 943
charcoal, in treatment of poisoning,
    785–6
chemotherapy, 185
chest
    auscultation, 451–2
    examination, 373–4
    pain, 337–59
chest wall, 357
Cheyne Stokes breathing, 698
chickenpox, 759, 1214
chilblains, 1214
child abuse, 776–81
childhood absence seizures, 508–10
children
    Aboriginal problems, 1201–2
    abuse of, 776–81
    behaviour disorders, 769–75
    developmental problems, 743
    general approach to, 741–6
    infectious diseases, 758–67
    neglect, 777–8
    serious diseases of, 743, 782–3
    sexual abuse of, 779–80
    specific problems, 747–57
    and travel, 103–4
chills, 496–7
Chlamydia
    C. pneumoniae, 379
    C. psittaci, 212, 216
    C. trachomatis, 216, 945
Chlamydial infection
    ornithosis, 212, 216
    psittacosis, 216
    sexually transmitted disease, 943–5
    trachoma, 477, 480
chloasma, see melasma
choking, 700
chloroquine, 94–6, 100
cholangitis, ascending, 533, 543
cholecystectomy, 264
cholecystitis, 263–4
cholera, 97, 405
cholestatic jaundice, 537, 543
cholesterol, 79, 1090–3
chondrocalcinosis, 634
chorionic villus sampling, 880
chronic bronchitis, 457
chronic cough, 375, 376, 379, 380–1
chronic fatigue syndrome, 693–5
chronic lymphocytic leukaemia, 184
chronic myeloid leukaemia, 184
chronic obstructive airways disease,
    457–9
chronic pain, 48–50
chronic renal failure, 218–22
cigarette smoking, 80, 68–71, 148–50
ciguatera, 103
ciprofloxacin, 92–3, 100, 998, 1098
circumcision, 914
cirrhosis, 544
citalopram, 134
claudication
    arm, 582
    intermittent, 613, 620–1
    jaw, 527
    neurogenic, 613
    vascular, 613
clavicle
    dislocation, 1150–1
    fracture, 1149
clergyman's knee, 640
clonazepam, 1065–6, 1069

clonidine, 1083
clostridial infections, 216
Clostridium botulinum, 216
Clostridium difficile, 396
Clostridium tetani, 216
Clostridium welchii: gas gangrene, 216
club foot, 753
clubbing, 124, 383, 451
cluster headache, 524–5
coagulation disorders, 335
coarctation of the aorta, 1072–3
cocaine dependence, 151–2
coccydynia, 296
coeliac disease, 400, 403
cognitive state, 59–61, 410
Colagiuri and Craig model, of emotional
        responses to infertility, 929–30
colchicine, 282
cold, common, 377, 1215
cold sores (herpes labialis), 996–7, 1215
colic
        biliary, 263
        general patterns, 252–3
        infantile, 254, 747, 1222
        renal, 263
        ureteric, 263, 1230
colitis, 405–6
collapse, 506–7, 699, 783
colorectal cancer, 73, 367–8
coma
        causes, 696–8
        cocktail for, 701
        Glasgow scale, 698
common cold, 377, 1215
common presenting problems, 5–7
communicable diseases, 79
communication skills, 25–33
complex partial seizures, 509–10, 770
conduct disorders in children, 769–75
confrontation, 19
confusion, 57–60
congenital dislocation of hip, 72, 601–2,
        753
conjunctivitis, 478–80, 1215
connective tissue disorders, 223–30, 280
Conn's syndrome, 1073
constipation, 360–9, 1215
consultation models, 17–24
consulting skills, 17–24
contact dermatitis, 976
contact lens, 484
continuity, of patient care, 4–5
contraception, 810–17
contraceptive pill, 811–14
contusion, 1132–4
conversion reaction, 688, 1120
convulsions, *see* seizures
coral cuts, 1139
corked thigh, 1188
corns, on feet, 655, 1215
coronary angioplasty, 350
coronary heart disease, 342–3, 347–52
corticosteroids
        in asthma, 1056–7, 1061, 1114
        in atopic dermatitis, 974–5
        in carpal tunnel, 590
        intra-articular injection, 277, 279
        intradermal injection, 981, 1017
        intralesional injection, 586–93, 981
        parenteral, 279, 936, 1056–7, 1113–14
        in psoriasis, 980–1
        in sunburn, 988
        topical, 962–3, 974–5, 980–1
costochondritis, 346, 821

costovertebral joint dysfunction, 321
cough, 371–84
cough mixtures, 383–4
counselling, 35–42
        adolescent, 797
        in breast cancer, 831
        family, 13–14
        in HIV infection, 193–5
        sexual, 935–6
        skills, 35–42
        subfertile couple, 929–30
country doctor's bag, 1175–6
Coxiella burnetti, 212–13
cracked hands, 975, 1215
cracked heels, 975, 1215
cracked lips, 1215
crackles, in chest, 382–3, 449–51
cramps
        nocturnal, 625–6, 1216
        in pregnancy, 884
creams, rules for use, 963–4
creatinine, serum levels, 219–21
CREST syndrome, 122
Creutzfeld-Jakob disease, 205, 410
cricothyroidotomy, 1167
crisis management, 38–9
critical appraisal, of published research,
        117
Crohn's disease, 406
croup, 377, 789–90, 1216
cruciate ligament injury, 636–8
crying baby, 747, 1216
cryotherapy, 1015–16
crystal deposition disease, 280–2
Cushing's disease, 170, 727
Cushing's syndrome, 170, 727
cutaneous larva migrans, 102
cutaneous leishmaniasis, 101
cutaneous myiasis, 102
cutdown, intravenous, 1124
cyanosis, 124
cyproterone acetate, 922
cyst
        implantation, 1008
        meibomian, 482
        ovarian, 845–6
        sebaceous, 1008
cystic fibrosis, 404
cystitis, 175–8
cytomegalovirus, 199, 201–2

dacryocystitis, 483
dandruff, 1216
dangerous behaviour, 421–2
de Quervain's tenosynovitis, 591–2
deadly infections of world, 204–5
deafness, 385
death rattles, 52
death, sudden, 1121
decubitus ulcers, 1003
deep venous thrombosis, 624
defibrillation, 1123–5
delirium, 60, 414–15
delirium tremens, 1034
delusions, 410
demanding patients, 43–4
dementia, 60–2, 415–16
dementia vs depression, 60–1
dendritic ulcer, 479–80
dengue fever, 100–1, 203
dental caries, 490
dental disorders, 490
depression, 60–1, 126–7, 130–6, 419–20
        in children, 132

        in elderly,132
        major, 130–1
        masked, 126–7, 131–2
        minor, 131
        postnatal, 896
dermatitis, 972
        atopic, 972–6
        contact, 976
        dyshydrotic, 975
        lichen simplex, 976
        nummular (discoid), 976
        pityriasis alba, 976
        seborrhoeic, 752, 977–9
dermatitis artefacta, 1004
dermatitis herpetiformis, 968–9
dermatofibroma, 1012
dermatomes
        cervical, 560
        lumbar, 612
        thoracic, 323
dermatomyositis, 227–8
dermatoscope, 959, 1024
desmopressin, 750
developmental disability and delay,
        754–7
developmental dysplasia of hip, 72,
        601–2, 753
developmental milestones, in child, 742
diabetes insipidus, 171
diabetes mellitus, 137–45
diabetic ketoacidosis, 145
diagnosis
        disease-centred, 85
        a model of, 125–9
        patient-centred, 85
        strategy for, 125
diagnostic facies, 122–3
diaphragm, rupture of, 1168
diarrhoea, 92–4, 393–408
diazepam
        in anxiety, 1046–50
        in disturbed patient, 413–15
        in febrile convulsions, 787
        in status epilepticus, 1069
diet, 53, 68, 1069
difficult problems, 43
        management strategies, 43–6
digital rectal examination, 921–2
digoxin, 456–7, 675–7
dihydroergotamine, 523–4
diphtheria, 685
diplopia, 231–2, 1128–9
disc disruption
        acute, 295, 305–6, 565–6
        chronic, 305–6, 565–6
discitis, 304
dislocations
        acromioclavicular joint, 1150
        elbow, 1155–6
        fingers, 1161
        hip, 1162
        jaw, 1149
        patella, 1162
        scapholunate, 1158
        shoulder, 1151–2
        sternoclavicular joint, 1151
        toes, 1164
disodium cromoglycate
        for allergic rhinitis, 1040–1
        in asthma, 1057–8
dissecting aneurysm, 343, 354
distracting children, 743
disturbed patient, 409–25
disulfiram (Antabuse), 1034

dithranol, for psoriasis, 980
diuretics
    adverse effects, 148, 281, 1082–4
    in heart failure, 456, 1113–14
    in hypertension, 1081–4
diverticular disease, 264–5, 407
diverticulitis, 264–5
dizziness, 426–34
dizzy turns
    in elderly women, 431, 1217
    in girls, 431, 1217
doctor's bag, emergency use, 1175–8
doctors, characteristics of, 28–30
dog bites, 1139–40
domestic violence, 874–7
Donovanosis, 943
dothiepin, 134
Down syndrome, 755
doxepin, 134
doxycycline
    in acne, 983, 1209
    in malaria, 95–6, 100
    in perioral dermatitis, 985
    in rosacea, 984, 1230
    in STDs, 943–6
dream drawing in children, 774–5
drop attacks, 700
drowning, 792
drug abuse, 147–55, 1049
drug dependence, 147–55, 1049
drug eruptions, 992–3
drug history, 126
drug reactions, 63, 147–8, 992–3
drugs
    adverse reactions, 63, 126, 147–8,
      992–3
    as a masquerade, 126, 992
    monitoring, 1104
    rational prescribing, 1094
    in sport, 154–5
    in travellers,108
dry hair, 1217
dry skin, 987–8, 1217
duodenal ulcer, 441–2
dying patients, communicating with,
    53–6
dysentery, 92, 99, 404–5
dysfunctional uterine bleeding, 836–8
dyskinesia, 235–6
dyslexia, 756–7
dyslipidaemia, 1090–3
dysmenorrhoea, 847–8, 1217
dyspepsia, 435–43
dysphagia, 445–7
dysplastic naevi, 1022
dyspnoea, 448–62
dysrhythmias, *see* arrhythmias
dystonia, 242, 418
dysuria, 703–5

ear infections, 467–72
    in Aborigines, 1202
ear pain, 463–73
easy bruising syndrome, 335
eating disorders, 736–7
Ebola virus, 205
ᴱBV, *see* Epstein-Barr virus
ecchymoses, 331
ECG, *see* electrocardiogram
echocardiography, 342
eclampsia, 888
ectopic heartbeats, 672–3
ectopic pregnancy, 843–4

ectopic testis, 910
ectropion, 1217
eczema, *see* dermatitis
elbows
    dislocation of, 1155–6
    examination of, 582–3
    fractures of, 1154–5
    pain in, 583–8
    pulled, 583–4
    tennis elbow, 585–8
elderly patient, 55–64, 1095–6
electric shock, 1119–20
electrocardiogram, 341
electroconvulsive therapy, 135
electroencephalography, 508, 1063
ELISA test, 191
embolus
    cerebral, 1127–9
    lower limb, 619
    pulmonary, 343, 355
emergencies in children, 782–94
emergency care, 1111–26
emergency drugs, 1175–7
emesis, induced after poisoning, 785–6
emollients, 961
emphysema, 457
emporiatics, 91
empyema, 498–500
emulsions, 961
encephalitis, 787–8
encopresis, 750–1
endocarditis, infective, 209–212
endocrine disorders, 163–71
endometriosis, 848–9
endoscopy, 438, 441, 512
endotracheal intubation, 1167
engorged breasts, 892–3
Entamoeba histolytica, 923
enterobacteria, 92, 393, 397
enterovirus, 92, 393
entrapment neuropathies, *see* nerve
    entrapment
entropion, 1217
enuresis, 749–50, 1217
eosinophilia, 1038
epicondylitis
    lateral, 585–7
    medial, 587–8
epidermis, 958
epididymal cysts, 908
epididymo-orchitis, 900–1
epidural injection, 314
epiglottitis, acute, 684, 788–90
epilepsy, 508–10, 699–700, 1062–9
    benign rolandic, 508
    children, 508
    juvenile myoclonic, 508
    temporal lobe, 509
episcleritis, 481
epispadius, 915
epistaxis, 1184, 1218
Epstein-Barr mononucleosis, 199–201,
    682–9, 765, 992
Epstein-Barr virus, 198–9
ERCP, 536
erectile dysfunction, 937–8
ergotamine, 523–4
erysipelas, 624
erysipeloid, 594
erythema, 992–3
    in newborn, 751
erythema infectiosum, 763
erythema multiforme, 994
erythema nodosum, 994

erythermalgia, 593
erythrasma, 970
erythrocyte sedimentation rate, *see* ESR
erythromycin
    in acne, 983, 1204
    in atypical pneumonia, 216
    in penicillin resistance, 1100
    in sore throat, 683
Escherichia coli, 92, 393, 404
ESR, 156
    arthritis, 273, 283
    back pain, 302, 325
    bacterial infections, 211
    connective tissue disorders, 224–5
    giant cell/temporal arteritis, 230, 527,
      721
    myeloma, 185
euthanasia, 54
Ewing's sign 519, 528
exercise tolerance test, 341
exercises
    back, 83, 313
    knee, 642
    neck, 562–5
expired air resuscitation, 1121
extradural haematoma, 1170
extrinsic allergic alveolitis, 460
eye
    dry, 1218
    infections, 477–84
    injuries, 485, 1183
    red and tender, 475–85
eyelashes, ingrowing, 1218
eyelid laceration, 1137
eyelid 'twitching', 1218

Fabere test, 605
face, as a mirror of disease, 121–2
facial migraine, 494
facial neuralgias, 493–5
facial pain, 487–95
facial rash, 983–5
facial (seventh) cranial nerve, 122
facilitation, 19
factitious fever, 497
faecal impaction, 259, 365–6
failure to thrive, 734–6
faints, 505
falciparum malaria, 94–5, 99–100
falls in elderly, 63
family, 9–15
family counselling, 13–14
family dynamics, 10–11
family dysfunction, 10
family history, 71
family life cycle, 11–13
family planning, 810–17
family practice, definition, 32
farmer's lung, 460
fat necrosis, of breast, 830
fat pad disorders, 650
fatigue, 687–95
    chronic fatigue syndrome, 693–5
fatty liver, 533, 545
favism, 535
febrile convulsion, 787
female infertility, 926–7
femoral cutaneous nerve entrapment,
    613, 616
ferritin, serum, 156–9
fertility, 925–31
fertility control, 800
fetor hepaticus, 537

FEV, *see* forced expiratory volume
fever, 497–503
  in children, 500, 1218
  in elderly, 500
  patterns, 498–500
  in returned travellers, 99–100
  of unknown origin, 501–3
fibre, 68, 366
fibroadenoma, 830
fibrocystic disease, *see* cystic fibrosis
fibroepithelial polyps, *see* skin tags
fibromyalgia, 328–9, 695, 1218
fibrosing alveolitis, 460
fifth disease, 763
filoviruses, 205
finger, amputation, 1138
finger clubbing, 124, 383, 451
Finklestein's test, 591–2
fish hook removal, 1141
fish stings, 1118, 1231
fissure in ano, 287, 1210
fits, 505–11
fixed drug eruption, 993
flashburns to eyes, 484, 1218
flat feet, 753
flatulence, 435
floaters, visual 713, 722
fluid depletion, 401–3
fluid replacement, 401–3
flumazenil, 701
fluorescein angiography, 714, 721
fluorescein, for eyes, 476, 480
fluoxetine, 134–5, 855
flutamide, 922
flying, fitness for, 105
foetus
  abnormalities, 879–82
  position, 879–82
folate deficiency, 158–60
folic acid, 160
follicle stimulating hormone, 925–9
folliculitis, 997–8, 1219
food, *see* nutrition
food poisoning, 92–4, 396–7
foot
  aching, 652, 1219
  diabetic, 144
  examination, 647–8
  odour, 1219
  pain, 644–58
  strain, 652
forced expiratory volume, 452–3
forced vital capacity, 452–3
foreign bodies
  ear, 466–7
  eye, 718
  gunshot, 1140–1
  inhaled, 376, 449, 792
  pressure gun, 1141
  splinters, 1141
  stomach, 787
foreskin hygiene, 913–14
Fournier's gangrene, 902
fourth disease, 763
fractures, 1145–64, 1171–3
  ankle, 1163
  Bennett's, 1159
  clavicle, 1149
  coccyx, 1145
  Colles', 1157
  elbow, 1154–5
  femur, 1161–2
  fingers, 1159–60
  foot, 1163–4

humerus
  greater tuberosity, 1152
  shaft, 1154
  surgical neck, 1153
intercondylar, 1154
malar, 1147
mandible, 1147
metacarpals, 1159
metatarsals, 1163–4
Monteggia, 1157
navicular, 1163
nose, 1184
patella, 1162
pelvis, 1161
phalanges, 1159–60
radius, 1156–7
radius and ulna, 1157–8
rib, 1149
sacrum, 1148
scaphoid, 1159
scapula, 1150
skull, 1147, 1172
sternum, 1150, 1172
thumb, 1159
tibia and fibula, 1162–3
ulna, 1157
vertebrae, 1148
fragile X syndrome, 755–6
freckles, 1020, 1219
Freiberg's disease, 648
frenuloplasty, 914
frontal sinusitis, 527–8
frostbite, 1219
frozen shoulder, 576
frusemide, 456–7, 1113
FSH, *see* follicle stimulating hormone
functional dyspepsia, 440–1
funnel-web spider bite, 1115–16
'funny turns', 505–11
furuncle (boil), 956, 1213
furunculosis of ear, 471–2
fussing in infants, 747

gait disorders, 659–61
gall bladder
  acute cholecystitis, 263–4, 543
  ascending cholangitis, 543
gallstones, 543
gamekeeper's thumb, 1159, 1186
gamma-benzene hexachloride, 867–8, 1231
gamma-glutamyl transferase
  in alcohol abuse, 1031
  liver function tests, 537
ganglion, 1015
gangrene
  Fournier's, 902
  gas, 216
gas transfer factor, 453
gastric cancer, 442–3
gastric lavage, 787
gastritis, 435
gastrocnemius muscle tear, 1190–1
gastroenteritis, 401–3, 404–5
gastrointestinal bleeding, 512–14
gastro-oesophageal reflux, 381, 439–40
gastro-oesophageal varices, 513
gatekeeper role, 23
gay bowel syndrome, 395
general practice, 3
  common disorders in, 5–7
  definition, 3
  skills of, 17

genital herpes, 946–8, 1219
genital infections, 942–52
genital warts, 949
genogram, 11–12
genu recurvatum, 630
genu valgum, 630, 753
genu varum, 630, 753
geographical tongue, 1220
German measles, *see* rubella
giant cell arteritis, 228–9
Giardia lamblia, 92–3, 405
giardiasis, 92–3, 405
giddiness, 426–8
Gilbert's syndrome, 534, 537
gingivitis, 1220
glandular fever, *see*
          Epstein-Barr mononucleosis
Glasgow coma scale, 698
glaucoma, 481–2, 717–18
glibenclamide, for diabetes mellitus, 142
global amnesia, 511
globus hystericus, 447
glomerulonephritis, 218, 706
glossopharyngeal neuralgia, 495
glucagon, 144, 1114, 1176
glucose tolerance test, 138
gluten-free diet, 400
gluteus medius tendinitis, 605–6
glyceryl trinitrate
  for acute heart failure, 1113
  for acute myocardial
          infarction, 352, 1114
  for angina, 347
glycosylated haemoglobin, 140
GnRH, *see* gonadotrophin
          releasing hormone
goitre, 164–9
gold salts, 279
golfer's elbow, 587–8
gonadotrophin releasing
          hormone, 925–8
gonococcal arthritis, 268
gonorrhoea, 945
goserelin, 922
gout, 280–2, 652, 1220
granuloma, *see* pyogenic granuloma
granuloma annulare, 1011
granuloma inguinale, 943
granuloma of umbilicus, 751, 1235
Grave's disease, 168
grieving, 53
groin lumps, 903
groin pain, 596, 1187
Grover's disease, 971
Guillain-Barré syndrome, 240–1
gun injuries, 1140–1
guttate psoriasis, 991–2
gynaecomastia, 831

H_2-receptor antagonists, 440–3
Haemaccel, 1113, 1169, 1177
haemarthrosis of knee, 626, 636
haematemesis, 512–14
haematocele, 908
haematoma
  intracerebral, 1170
  muscle, 1188
  nasal septum, 1133
  perianal, 288
  pinna, 1133
  pretibial, 1134
  subdural, 1170
haematospermia, 916

haematuria, 705–8
haemochromatosis, 124, 138, 162, 534
haemoglobin E, 159
haemolytic anaemia, 160
haemophilia, 334–6
Haemophilus influenzae, 75
haemoptysis, 376
haemorrhoids, 289–90
halitosis, 129, 1220
hallucinations, 410, 416–17
hallux rigidus, 651
hallux valgus, 654
halo naevus, 1021–2
haloperidol, 414–19
hamstring injuries, 1187–8
hand
    arthritis in, 594
    common disorders, 589–4
    infections, 594
    injuries, 1184–6
hand, foot and mouth disease, 997
hangover, 1220
Hashimoto's disease, 165
HAV, *see* hepatitis A
hay fever, 1038–41, 1220
HBV, *see* hepatitis B
HCV, *see* hepatitis C
HDV, *see* hepatitis D
head banging/rocking 770, 1221
head injury, 696–8, 1170
headache, 515–31
    in children, 519–20
    cluster, 524–5
    combination, 526
    cough, 530
    drug causes, 517
    in elderly, 520
    'ice-cream', 530
    migraine, 521–4
    occipital, 525
    sex, 530
    tension, 520–1
health education, 76–83
health goals and targets, 78–81
health promotion, 76–83
hearing problems, 385–92
heart failure, 452–7
heartburn, 439–40, 1221
heartsink patient, 44
heat rash, 1229
Heberden's nodes, 270
heel pain, 649–51, 1194–6
Helicobacter pylori infection, 442
hemianopia, 714
hemicrania, chronic paroxysmal, 495, 529
hemifacial spasms, 242
hemiparesis, 238, 1129
Henoch-Schönlein purpura, 227–8, 335
heparin, 333, 353
hepatitis
    A (HAV), 97, 539–40
    acute alcoholic, 545
    autoimmune, 544
    B (HBV), 97, 541–2
    C (HCV), 541
    cholestatic, 543
    chronic active, 542
    chronic viral, 544
    D (HDV), 542
    E (HEV), 542
hepatocellular carcinoma, 533, 537
hepatomegaly, 536
hernia
    femoral, 903–4

inguinal, 903–5
herpangina, 684
herpes labialis (cold sores), 997, 1215
herpes simplex, 996–7
    genital, 946–7
    keratitis, 480
    primary, 766–7
herpes zoster, 767, 995–6
herpes zoster ophthalmicus, 484
hiatus hernia, 435–40
hiccoughs, 53, 128–9, 1221
hiccups, *see* hiccoughs
hidden agenda, 128
high-risk obstetric care, 886–9
hilar lymphadenopathy, 459
hip
    clicking, 606
    developmental dysplasia, 72, 601–2, 753
    examination, 599–601
    fracture, 1161–2
    osteoarthritis, 604
    pain, 596–607
    pain in children, 601–3
    septic arthritis, 603
hip pocket nerve syndrome, 598–9
Hirschsprung's disease, 365
hirsutism, 1221
HIS, bundle of, 676
histiocytosis X, 982
history taking, 18–19, 71–2
HIV, *see* human
                immunodeficiency virus
                infection
HLAB$_{27}$ antigen, 273, 283
hoarseness, 1221
Hodgkin's disease, 184
holistic health, *see* whole person approach
hookworm, 102
hormone replacement therapy, 859–63
Horner's syndrome, 382
house-dust mites, 1038
housemaid's knee, 640
HSV, *see* herpes simplex
human bite wounds, 1138
human immunodeficiency
                virus infection, 187–97, 198–9, 951, 991
hydralazine, 456–7, 1084
hydrocele, 907
hydroxychloroquine, 224, 279
hyoscine, 53, 106
hyperaldosteronism, 1072–3
hyperbilirubinaemia, 532–4
hypercalcaemia, 171
hypercholesterolaemia, 79, 1090–3
hyperglycaemia, 138–9, 145
hyperkalaemia, 688, 1082
hyperlipidaemia, 1090–3
hypermetropia, 716
hyperparathyroidism, 170–1
hypertension, 1071–89
    diastolic, 1071
    and headache, 530
    malignant, 1084
    in pregnancy, 888, 1087
    refractory, 1086
    secondary, 1072–3
    systolic, 1085
hyperthermia, 497
hyperthyroidism, 166–9
hypertrophic scar, 1009
hyperuricaemia, 280

hyperventilation, 1049, 1114
hyphaema, 1183
hypoglycaemia, 145, 701, 1114
hypokalaemia, 688, 1073
hypomania, 418–19
hypoparathyroidism, 171
hypopituitarism, 170
hypospadius, 914
hypotension, 164, 505, 1082
hypothyroidism, 164–6
hypsarrhythmia, 508
hysteria, 688, 1120

'ice-cream' headache, 551
idiopathic adolescent scoliosis, 326
idiopathic oedema, 731
idiopathic thrombocytopenic purpura, 335
idoxuridine, antiviral uses, 997, 1215
IHD, *see* ischaemic heart disease
iliofemoral thrombophlebitis, 624
iliotibial band friction syndrome, 640, 1188–9
illicit drugs, 126–7, 151–5
illness education, 76
illusions, 410
imipramine, 134, 750
immunisation program, 74–5, 745
immunity, 69–70
impetigo, 752, 767, 1221
implantation cyst, 1008
impotence, 937–8, 1221
in-toeing, 753
in-vitro fertilisation, 930
incontinence, urinary, 709–10, 1222
indigestion, *see* dyspepsia
indomethacin, in
    arthritis, 279
    gout, 282, 1220
    spondyloarthropathy, 284
    ureteric colic, 263, 1230
infantile colic, 254, 747, 1222
infantile spasms, 508
infectious diseases, 758–9
infectious mononucleosis, *see*
                Epstein-Barr mononucleosis
infective endocarditis, 209–12
infertility, 925–30
inflammatory bowel disease, 405–6
influenza, 74, 378, 1222
infrapatellar bursitis, 640
ingrowing toe-nails, 656–7, 1222
inguinoscrotal lumps, 903–11
inhaled foreign body, 376, 453, 791–2
injuries
    fractures, 1145–64
    major, 1166–73
    sporting, 1183–96
insect bites and stings, 1117–18
insomnia, 771, 1222
inspection, as a clinical skill, 121
insulin, 140–1
intellectual disability, 755
intermenstrual bleeding, 838
intermittent claudication, 610–11
international normalised ratio (INR), 355–6, 1131
interstitial lung diseases, 459–60
intertrigo, 1223
intervertebral disc, *see*
                disc disruption
interviewing techniques, 19–20
intestinal infections, 92–4, 393–7, 401–5

intestinal ischaemia, 258, 395
intestinal obstruction, 260–1
Intra Site Gel, 1003–4
intracerebral haemorrhage, 1127–8
intracerebral tumours, 529–30
intracranial pressure, 529–30
intraosseous infusion, 792–3
intrauterine contraceptive device, 815–16
intravenous cutdown, 1125
intravenous pyelography/urography, 262, 708
intussusception, 255, 793
ionising radiation illness, 1235–7
ipecacuanha, 785–6
iridocyclitis, 283, 481
iritis, *see* uveitis
iron
    deficiency, 157–9, 160–1
    poisoning, 785–7
    therapy, 158–9, 161
iron deficiency anaemia, 157–9, 161
irritable bowel syndrome, 265, 406–7, 1223
irritable colon, *see* irritable bowel
irritant contact dermatitis, 976
ischaemia of lower limb, 618–21
ischaemic colitis, 400–1
ischaemic heart disease, 342–3, 347–50
isoniazid, 209, 383
isosorbide dinitrate, 349
itch, of genitals, 949–50
itching, *see* pruritus
IVU, *see* intravenous pyelography/
    urography

Jacksonian epilepsy, 510
Japanese encephalitis, 97, 203
jaundice, 533–46
    in children, 538
    in pregnancy, 544–5
jealousy, morbid, 421
jellyfish stings, 1118
jetlag, 104
jitters, 1046–8, 1223
jock itch, *see* tinea cruris
jogger's knee, 638
jugular venous pressure, 454
jumper's knee, 639
juvenile ankylosing spondylitis, 274
juvenile chronic arthritis, 272–3
juvenile myoclonic epilepsy, 508
juvenile plantar dermatosis, 648

Kaposi's sarcoma, 189–91, 1014
Kawasaki's disease, 764
keloid, 1009, 1222
keratitis, 480
keratoacanthoma, 1012, 1223
keratoconjunctivitis, 482
keratolysis, pitted, 648–9
keratolytics, 961
keratoses
    seborrhoeic, 1011, 1223
    solar, 1012, 1223
keratosis pilaris, 1231
kerion, 986
ketoacidosis, 145
ketoconazole, 871, 895–7
kidney
    carcinoma, 183
    failure, 218–22
    and hypertension, 1072–3
Kienböck's disorder, 593–4

Klinefelter's syndrome, 927
knee
    examination, 630–2
    jumper's, 639
    ligament injuries, 635–8
    locking, 630–1
    meniscus injuries, 635
    overuse syndromes, 638–40
    pain in, 627–34
        children, 633–4
        elderly, 634–5
knock knees, *see* genu valgum
knocked out tooth, 1183–4
Kohler's disease, 648
Korsakoff's encephalopathy, 1030

labyrinthitis, 432
lacerations, 1134–8
Lachman test, 637
lactate dehydrogenase, 352
lactation, 892–4
lactation cysts, 830
lactation suppression, 893, 1223
lactose intolerance, 403
large bowel obstruction, 260–1
laryngeal dystonia, 242
laryngitis, 1224
laryngotracheobronchitis, *see* croup
laser treatment
    eyes, 721
    prostate, 920
latex allergy, 1037
Laurence-Moon-Biedl syndrome, 727
laxatives, 366–7
lead poisoning, 757
Leber's hereditary optic atrophy, 719
left heart failure, 454
leg
    compartment syndrome, 1188–9
    ischaemia, 618–21
    occlusive vascular disease, 618
    pain, 609–25
    swelling, 663–5
    ulceration, 1001–2
Legionella pneumonia, 216
Leishmaniasis, 101
Lennox-Gastaut syndrome, 508
lentigines, 1020
lentigo maligna, 1023
leptospirosis, 212–14
leucoplakia, 1013
leucotriene antagonists, 1056–61
leukaemia
    acute lymphocytic, 183–4
    acute myeloid, 183–4
    chronic lymphocytic, 184
    chronic myeloid, 184
leuprorelin acetate, 922
levator ani spasm, *see* proctalgia fugax
levodopa, 235–7
LHRH agonists, 922
lice
    head, 752, 767–8, 1224
    pubic, 950, 1224
lichen planus, 968, 1224
lichen simplex chronicus, 975
life-threatening disorders, 126
lifestyle, 68–70, 89
lightning strike, 1120
lignocaine, 524, 677, 1120, 1125
limp, 661–3
lip laceration, 1136–7
lipoedema, 665

lipoma, 1014–15
liquid nitrogen therapy, 1015–16
listerosis, 214–15
literature search, 115
lithium 419
lithotripsy, 263
liver
    abscess, 89
    cirrhosis, 544
    failure, 544–5
    function tests, 537
    hepatoma, 533
    investigations, 536–7
'locked-in' syndrome, 1130
Lomotil, 92
loperamide, 92
lotions, 961
lower motor neurone signs, 232, 660
lower respiratory tract infection, 377–80
lumbago, *see* back pain
lumbar puncture, 699, 787–8
lumbar spine dysfunction, 173, 294–305
lumbar spine examination, 299–302
lumbar spondylosis, 307–8
lung
    abscess, 371, 376
    biopsy, 374
    carcinoma, 381, 461
    collapse, 452
    crackles, 382, 449, 451–2
    function tests, 452–3
    radioisotope scanning, 374
luteinising hormone, 925–9
LUTS, 918–19
Lyme disease, 214, 284
lymphadenitis, 553
lymphangitis, 594
lymphogranuloma venerum, 943
lymphoma, 184–5

macrocytic anaemia, 159–60
macrocytosis, 159–60
macular abnormality, 721
macular degeneration, 721
Maggylamp, 851, 913
magnetic resonance imaging
    acoustic neuroma, 431
    aortic aneurysm, 259
    back pain, 303
    CVAs, 1127
    epilepsy, 1063
    funny turns, 507
    headache, 529
    multiple sclerosis, 239
    sciatica, 567
major trauma, 1166–73
malabsorption, 400
malaise, 687
malar flush, 123
malaria, 94–6, 99–100, 202–3
male infertility, 927–9
male pattern baldness, 1209
Malgaigne's bulgings, 903
malignant disease, 181–6
    prevention, 69–70
malignant melanoma, 1022–6
mallet finger, 1184–5
Mallory-Weiss syndrome, 513
malnutrition, 78, 735–6
maltoma, 442
mammary duct ectasia, 831
mammary dysplasia, 829–30
management phase, of consultation,

21–2
mania, 418–19, 421
manic-depressive disorders, *see* bipolar
    disorder
manipulation, spinal, 314–15, 327, 562
Mantoux test, 208–9
MAOI, *see* monoamine
    oxidase inhibitors
Marfan's syndrome, 122
marijuana, *see* cannabis dependence
marine animals, bites and stings, 987
marital disharmony, 14–18
masquerades, 71, 126–8
mastalgia, 818–23, 1224
mastitis, 821–2, 894–5
masturbation, 508
maxillary sinusitis, 490–1
McMurray's test, 632
mean corpuscular volume, 157, 1031
measles, 760–1
meatal stenosis, 914
medicines in pregnancy, 889–90
medulloblastoma, 429, 528
mefloquine, 95–6, 100
megacolon, 361, 368–9
megaloblastic anaemia, 159–60, 889
meibomian cyst, 482
Meige's syndrome, 242
melaena, 291, 512–13
melanocytic naevi, 1020
melanoma, malignant, 1023–6
melasma, 123, 1224
melioidosis, 103
Ménière's syndrome, 433, 1224
meningitis, 529, 787–8
meningococcaemia, 788
meningococcal infection
    in children, 788
    in travellers, 96
meniscus injuries, 635
menopause, 857–63
menorrhagia, 835–8
men's business (Aboriginal health), 1200
menstrual cycle, 842, 926
menstruation, 926
mental state examination, 59, 412
meralgia paraesthetica, 616–17
mesenteric adenitis, 256
mesenteric artery occlusion, 258
mesenteric ischaemia, 258
mesothelioma, 461
metastatic cancer, 185–6
metatarsalgia, 653
metformin, for diabetes mellitus, 141–2
methadone, 154, 420, 1103
methyldopa, 349
methysergide, 524–5
metoclopramide
    in migraine, 523–4
    with morphine, 353, 1113–14
    in pregnancy sickness, 884
metoprolol, *see* atenolol
microalbuminuria, 709
microcytic anaemia, 132
Microsporum canis, 875
micturition
    disorders, 703–10
    frequency, 703
migraine, 521–4, 722, 1224
migrainous neuralgia, *see*
    cluster headache
milia, 751
miliaria, 751
milker's nodules, 1011, 1224

mini-mental status examination, 59
minocycline, 984
mittelschmerz, 845
mixed connective tissue disease, 223
mobilisation, spinal, *see*
    manipulation
moclobemide, 134
mollusc bite, 1118
molluscum contagiosum, 949, 1010–11,
    1224
'monkey muscle' tear, 1190, 1225
monoamine oxidase inhibitors, 134
morbidity patterns, 67–8
morning after pill, 815, 1225
morning sickness, 884, 1225
morphine
    in analgesia, 1103
    in doctor's bag, 1176
    in heart failure, 1113–14
    in myocardial infarction, 352, 1114
    in palliative care, 49–52
morphoea, 227
mortality patterns, 49–52, 67–8
Morton's metatarsalgia, *see*
    Morton's neuroma
Morton's neuroma, 654
mosquitoes and infections, 94, 108
motion sickness, 105–6
motor neurone disease, 232, 687
motor weakness, 232, 661
mountain sickness, 407
mouth, angular fissures of, 1225
mouth, bad taste, 1225
mouth-to-mouth resuscitation, 1122–3
mouth ulcers, *see* aphthous ulcers
movement disorders, 659–61
    iatrogenic, 418
MRI, *see* magnetic
    resonance imaging
mucocele, 1009
multiple myeloma, 185
multiple sclerosis, 238–9
mumps, 764–5
Murphy's sign, 263
mushroom poisoning, 397
myasthenia gravis, 241
Mycobacterium ulcerans, 1001
mycoplasma infections, 216
mycoplasma pneumonia, 216
myelodysplastic syndromes, 160
myelopathy, 566
myiasis, 102
myocardial infarction, 342–3, 351–4, 1114
myocardial ischaemia, 342–3
myofascial trigger points, 328
myopia, 716
myxoedema, 164–6
myxoedema madness, 167

naevus
    blue, 1022
    common acquired, 1020
    compound, 1020
    dysplastic, 1022
    flammeus, 751
    halo, 1021
    intradermal, 1021
    junctional, 1021
    melanocytic, 1020–2
    Spitz, 1022
naloxone, 1165, 1176
naltrexone, 420
nappy rash, 752, 981–2, 1225

narcolepsy, 510, 693
narcotics, dependence, 151–3, 420
nasal polyps, 1039
nasogastric intubation, 1171
nasolacrimal duct blockage, 477, 1232
natural contraceptive methods, 811, 816
nausea, 547–50
near drowning, 792
neck
    examination, 558–60
    lumps, 551–3
    pain in, 555–67
needlestick injuries, 1142–3
neglect
    of children, 778
    of elderly, 60
Neisseria gonorrhoea, 945–6
neonatal conjunctivitis, 477
neonatal hypothyroidism, 165–6
neonatal pustular dermatosis, 751
nephroblastoma, 183
nerve entrapment
    common peroneal, 617
    lateral cutaneous nerve of thigh, 616
    median 588–90
    obturator, 615
    posterior tibial, 617
    sciatic, 614–16
neuralgias, 493–5
neurofibroma, 1015
neuroleptic malignant syndrome, 418,
    497
neurological dilemmas, 231–42
neuropathy, 143, 565, 999
neurotic excoriations, 1004
neurosyphilis, 207
nicotine, 148–50
nifedipine, 349, 1082–4, 1200
nightmares, 1225
nipples
    cracked, 894, 1226
    discharge from, 825
    inverted, 894
    sore, 893, 1226
nocturnal cramps, 625–6, 1216
nocturnal enuresis, 749–50
nocturnal myoclonus, 1228
noise-induced hearing loss, 391–2
non-Hodgkin's lymphoma, 184–5
non-insulin dependent diabetes, 141–2
non-specific urethritis, 945
non-verbal communication, 31
normocytic anaemia, 160–1
nose
    bleeding, 1217–18
    injuries, 1184
    offensive smell, 1226
    stuffy, running, 1226
NSAIDs, 276–82, 443, 512, 1100–2
nummular eczema, 975
nutrition
    advice, 68–9
    in pregnancy, 882–3
nystagmus, 430–1

obesity, 727–30
obsessional compulsive disorder, 1048,
    1226
obstetric care, 879–85
obstructive jaundice, 537, 543
obstructive lung disease, 457–9
obstructive sleep apnoea, 691–2
occipital neuralgia, 525–6, 561

occupational causes of cancer, 183
occupational health, 71
occupational pulmonary disease, 460–1
ocular pain, relief by heat, 482
oedema, 730–1
oesophageal achlasia, 446–7
oesophageal atresia, 549
oesophageal carcinoma, 446
oesophageal dysmotility, 445–6
oesophageal pain, 344
oesophageal reflux, 355, 446–7
oesophageal rupture, 354
oesophageal stricture, 446
oesophageal ulceration, 447
oesophagitis, 344, 446
oestrogen
    deficiency, 857–9
    replacement, 879–81
oily hair, 1226
ointments, rules for, 963–4
olecranon bursitis, 588
oligomenorrhoea, 838
ophthalmic zoster, 484
ophthalmoscope, 146, 519, 717, 1079
opioid dependence, 151–2, 420
opioid overdosage, 702
opportunistic health promotion, 77
oppositional behaviour, 770
optic chiasma tumours, 714
optic fundi, 146, 714, 1079
optic neuritis, 722–3
oral anticoagulants, 355–7
oral contraceptives, 811–14
orbital cellulitis, 483
orchidectomy, 922
orchitis, 901
orf, 1011
oromandibular dystonia, 242
orthopnoea, 448
orthostatic hypotension, 505
Osgood-Schlatter disorder, 634
osteoarthritis, 275–7
    acromioclavicular, 578
    of foot, 651–2
    of hand, 593–4
    of hip, 604
    of knee, 640–1
    lumbar spine, 307–8
    of neck, 562–3
osteochondritis dissecans, 634
osteoid osteoma, 320, 609, 646
osteomyelitis, 295, 662
osteonecrosis, 635
osteoporosis, 71, 863–4
otalgia, see ear pain
otic barotrauma, 472–3
otitis externa, 470–1, 1226
otitis media, 467–9, 1227
otosclerosis, 391
out-toeing, 753
ovaries
    cancer, 183, 847
    cyst, 845–6
    polycystic disease, 929
    torsion, 846
    tumours, 845–7
overlap syndrome, 223
overseas travel, see travel medicine
overuse syndromes
    of knee, 638–41
    of leg, 1189–90
ovulation, 926–8
oxygen, administration of, 1112

pacemaker, 677
Paget's disease of bone, 663
Paget's disease of nipple, 825
pain
    abdominal, 247–66
    ankle, 644–58
    anorectal, 287–9
    arm, 580–95
    back
        low back, 295–317
        thoracic, 318–30
    cancer, 48–51
    chest, 337–59
    ear, 463–73
    eye, 475–85
    facial, 487–95
    foot, 644–58
    hand, 580–94
    head, 515–31
    heel, 649–51
    hip and buttock, 596–607
    joint, 267–85
    knee, 627–34
    leg, 609–25
    neck, 555–67
    oesophageal, 344
    pelvic, 849–51
    scrotal, 899–902
    shoulder, 568–79
    thoracic spine, 318–330
palliative care, 36–42, 47–54
palpitations, 666–77
PAN, see polyarteritis nodosa
Pancoast's syndrome, 570
pancreatic disease
    acute pancreatitis, 264
    carcinoma, 543–4
    chronic pancreatitis, 264
    cystic fibrosis, 372, 400–1
    ERCP, 536
panic attack, 1047, 1227
panic disorder, 1046–7
Papanicolaou smear, 803–8
papilloedema, 519, 1079
papillomas, see warts
papular urticaria, 752
parainsomnia, 771
paraneoplastic effects, 181–2
paranoia, 63, 424
paraphimosis, 912–13
paraphrenia, 63
paraplegia, 53
parasuicide, 422–3, 798
parathyroid disorders
    hyperparathyroidism, 170–1
    hypoparathyroidism, 171
parent-child interaction, 742
Parkinson's disease, 235–8
paronychia
    acute, 658, 1227
    chronic, 658, 1227
parvovirus infection ('fifth disease'), 763
patch testing, 976, 1037
patellar tendinitis, 628, 639, 1189
patellofemoral syndrome, 638–9
patient-centred care, 85–90
patient education, 5, 82–3
Paul Bunnell test, 200–1, 765
peak expiratory flow rate
    measurement, 1053
peanut allergy, 1037
pediculosis capitis, 767
pediculosis pubis, 950, 1224

Pellegrini-Steida disease, 638
pelvic inflammatory disease, 849–51, 946
pelvic pain, 840–51
penicillin
    allergy, 922–3, 1097
    benzyl penicillin, 788, 1096
    phenoxymethyl penicillins, 683, 1096
    sensitivity and toxicity, 992–3, 1097
    skin eruptions, 992–3
penis
    cancer, 915
    disorders of, 912–16
    small penis anxiety, 940
    ulcers, 915
    warts, 915
peptic stricture, 446
peptic ulcer
    acute bleeding, 512–13
    clinical features, 441, 1102
    complications, 441
    duodenal, 441
    gastric, 441–2, 512, 1102
    perforated, 261
    treatment, 441–2
perennial rhinitis, 1038–9
perianal abscess, 289
perianal haematoma, 288–9, 1227
perianal skin tag, 289
perianal warts, 290
periapical dental abscess, 491
pericarditis, 344
perichondritis, 472
pericoronitis, 490
perimetry, 430
periodic health examination, 70–1
periodic limb movement disorder, 1228
perioral dermatitis, 985, 1228
peripheral neuropathy, 143, 660, 999
peripheral vascular disease
    arteriosclerosis, 618–20
    diabetic foot, 143
    intermittent claudication, 620
pernicious anaemia, 160
peroneal nerve entrapment, 617
personal health records, 5, 744–5
personality disorders, 423–5
perspiration, excessive, 1228
Perthe's disorder, 602–3
pertussis, 766
petechiae, 331, 956
pethidine, 262, 525, 1103, 1176
petit mal epilepsy, see
    absence seizures
petrol sniffing, 1120, 1204
Peyronie's disease, 916
phaeochromocytoma, 1073
Phalen's test, 589
pharyngitis, 679–85
phenol treatment
    for hydroceles, 907
    for ingrowing toenails, 657
phenolphthalein, 367, 993
phenothiazines, 148, 414–18
phenoxymethyl penicillin, 683
phimosis, 912
phlegmasia dolens, 624
phobic disorder, 1047–8
photoageing, 1228
photosensitivity, 993
phototherapy, 980
physiognomy, 121
phytoestrogens, 862–3
pigmentation disorders, 124
pigmented skin lesions, 1019–26

pill, *see* oral contraceptives
pill failure, 815
pinguecula, 484
pinhole test for blurred vision, 716
pitfalls in diagnosis, 126–7
pitted keratolysis, 648
pituitary disorders, 170–1
pityriasis alba, 751, 975
pityriasis rosea, 990, 1228
pityriasis versicolor, 987, 1228
pivot shift test, 637
pizotifen, 524–5
plague, 98
plantar dermatosis, juvenile, 649
plantar fasciitis, 650–1
plantar response, 232, 238, 698
plantar warts, 655–6, 1229
plasmapheresis, 241
Plasmodium falciparum, 94, 99
plastering tips, 1164–5
platelet disorders, 335
pleural chest pain, 344
pleural effusion, 452, 461
pleurisy, 344, 357
PLISSIT model, 35, 936
pneumoconiosis, 461
pneumocystitis carinii, in AIDS, 189–90,
    372
pneumocystitis pneumonia, 189, 372
pneumonia, 216, 379–80, 450
pneumothorax, 344–5, 354–5, 452
podalgia, *see* foot pain
podophyllin/podophyllotoxin, 949, 1009
poisoning, 785–7
poliomyelitis, 74–5
polyarteritis nodosa, 228–9
polycystic ovarian syndrome, 929
polymyalgia rheumatica, 229–30, 578
polymyositis, 226–7
pompholyx, 975
popliteal cyst, 630
population groups, for health
    promotion, 78
porphyria, 248–9, 708
post-traumatic stress disorder, 1048–9
postcoital contraception, 815, 1225
posterior inferior cerebellar artery, 427
postherpetic neuralgia, 996
postmenopausal bleeding, 839
postnatal blues, 895
postnatal care, 891–6
postnatal depression, 896
postpartum haemorrhage, 895
postpartum hypothyroidism, 896
postural hypotension, 164, 505, 1082
postviral syndrome, 688
pox virus lumps, 1010–1
Prader-Willi syndrome, 726–7, 756
prazosin
    in hypertension, 1082–4
    in prostatism, 920
pre-eclampsia, 888
precordial catch, 347
pregnancy
    antenatal care, 878–85
    epilepsy, 1067
    high-risk, 886–9
    sickness, 884
    travel, 103
premature beats
    atrial, 672
    ventricular, 672
premature ejaculation, 939–40
premenstrual syndrome, 853–6, 1229

prepatellar bursitis, 628, 640
presbyacusis, 391
presbyopia, 716
prescribing
    analgesics, 1102–4
    antibiotics, 1096–9
    anticoagulants, 355–7
    elderly, 63–4, 1095
    NSAIDs, 1101–2
    psychotropics, 1099–1100
prescription writing, 1104–5
pressure gun injuries, 1141
pressure sores, 1003–4
prevention, 65–75
priapism, 915–16
prickly heat, 1229
Prinzmetal's syndrome, 348
proactive behaviour, 75–8
probability diagnosis, 125
procaine penicillin, 683–4, 949, 1139
Prochaska & Di Clemente model of
    change, 1032–3
proctalgia fugax, 288, 1229
progestogens, in
    contraceptive pill, 814–15
    HRT, 859–62
    menorrhagia, 837–8
prolactin, 926–9
prolapsed intervertebral disc, 295, 305–6,
    565–6
propranolol
    in anxiety, 1048
    in hypertension, 1082
    in migraine, 524
    in performance jitters, 1223
prostate
    carcinoma, 921–2
    hyperplasia, 919–21, 1229
prostatectomy, 920–1
prostatic specific antigen, 921–2
prostatism, *see* LUTS
prostatitis
    acute, 917–18
    chronic, 917–18
prostatodynia, 917–18
proteinuria, 708–9
proton pump blockers, 440, 441–2
protozoal infections, 198–204
pruritus
    ani, 291–3, 1229
    generalised, 965–71
    vulval, 968–9, 1229
pseudogout, 280–1, 634
pseudohaematuria, 708
pseudomembranous colitis, 396
psittacosis, 214
psoriasis, 283, 979–81, 1229–30
psychosexual disorders, 937–41
psychosocial factors, 128
psychotherapy, *see* counselling
psychotropic drugs, 1099–1100
pterygium, 484
ptosis, 241
pubic lice, 950, 1224
puerperal fever, 895
pulled elbow, 583–4
pulmonary embolism, 343, 355
pulmonary fibrosis, 460
pulmonary oedema, 454–7
pulse forms, 669
punch biopsy, 1016–17
purpura, 331–6, 956
PUVA, for psoriasis, 980
pyelonephritis, acute, 175, 178–9

pyloric stenosis, 549, 793
pyogenic arthritis, 268, 641
pyogenic granuloma, 1020
pyrexia of unknown origin, *see* fever of
    unknown origin
pyridoxine, 820–1, 855, 884
pyrophosphate arthropathy, 280–1, 634

Q fever, 212–13
quadriceps exercises, 642
quadriceps injuries, 638
Queensland tick typhus, 103
de Quervain's tenosynovitis, 591–2
quinidine, 672
quinine sulphate, 624–5, 1216
quinsy, 684
quitting smoking, 149–50

rabies, 97
radiation injury, 1235–8
radiculopathy, 305–6, 565–6
Ramsey-Hunt syndrome, 464, 995
rapport-building techniques, 18, 31
rash
    diagnostic approach, 956–8
    eruptions, 989–98
rational prescribing, 1094–1107
Raynaud's phenomenon, 592–3
reactive arthritis, 283
rebelliousness, 771, 796
rectal bleeding, 291
rectal examination, 364–5, 921–2
rectal ulcer syndrome, 288
red-back spider bites, 1115–16
red eye, 475–85
red reflex, 717
referred pain, *see* pain: thoracic spine
reflex sympathetic dystrophy, 593,
    609–11
reflexes
    spinal, 302–3, 559–60
    UMN lesions, 232
reflux oesophagitis, 439
refractive errors, 715–16
refractory hypertension, 1086
Reiter's syndrome, 283
reliability, 112
renal artery stenosis, 1072–3
renal colic, 262–3, 1230
renal failure, 218–22
renal function, 219–20
renal hypertension, 1072–3
renal tumours, 183
Rendu-Osler-Weber syndrome, 512
repairs, 1134–8
    eyelid, 1137
    lip, 1136–7
    tongue, 1137–8
research, 110–17
resorcinol, 962
respiration
    artificial, 1121–3
    Cheyne-Stokes, 698
    Kussmaul's, 698
respiratory failure, 1121, 1167
respiratory function tests, 452–3
respiratory symptoms, 374–6, 448–9
restless legs, 1230
resuscitation
    cardiopulmonary, 784, 1121–5
    equipment, 1179–81
retention of urine, 259

retina, abnormalities, 1079
retinal detachment, 619
retinitis pigmentosa, 718
retinoblastoma, 715
retinoic acid, for acne, 983
retractable testis, 909
retrobulbar neuritis, 722
Reye syndrome, 758
rhesus status, 879–80
rheumatic fever, 274–5
rheumatoid arthritis, 277–80, 567
rhinitis, allergic, 1038–40
rhinophyma, 984, 1030
rhinorrhoea, 377–8
ringworm, 986, 1230
risk factors, in health promotion, 80–1
risus sardonicus, 216
roadside emergencies, 1171–3
rodent ulcer, *see* basal
      cell carcinoma
roller injuries to legs, 625
Romberg's test, 659
rosacea, 984, 1230
roseola infantum, 763–4
Ross River fever, 203–4
rotator cuff injuries, 572–6
rotavirus, 393, 401
rough skin, 1231
roundworms, 1231
rubella, 761–2, 883
rubeola, *see* measles
runner's knee, 639–40, 1188–9

sacroiliac strain, 604–5
sacroiliitis, 282–3, 308–9, 604
salbutamol, in asthma, 1056–8
salicylic acid, topical use, 962
salmonella infections, 98–100, 405
salpingitis, 849–50, 946
sarcoidosis, 459–60
Sarcoptes scabiei, 967–8
scabies, 967–8, 1231
scalp lacerations, in children, 1139
scarlet fever, 765
scars, 956, 1009
Scheuermann's disorder, 325–6
schistosomiasis, 101
schizophrenia, 416–18
Schober's test, 308–9
school exclusions, 760
sciatica, 305–6, 315–16, 614–16, 1211
scleritis, 481
scleroderma, *see* systemic sclerosis
scoliosis, 72, 326
scorpion sting, 1118
scotomas, 713, 721
screening, 73–5
scrotal lumps, 905–8
scrotal pain, 899–902
scrotal skin, 902
scrub tyhpus, 102–3
scurvy, 332
sea stingers, 118
sea travel, 107
seafood toxicity, 397
sebaceous cysts, 1008
sebaceous hyperplasia, 751
seborrhoeic dermatitis, 752, 977–9
seborrhoeic keratoses, 1011, 1231
secondary syphilis, 991
seizures
    absence, 510
    convulsive, 509, 1062

    generalised, 509, 1063–4
    non-convulsive, 509, 1062
    partial
        complex, 509, 1062
        simple, 509–10, 1062
selective serotonin reuptake inhibitors,
    134
selegiline, 237
selenium sulfide, 987
semen analysis, 928
seminoma, 908–9
senile dementia, 60–2, 415–16
septic arthritis, 268, 603
septicaemia, 503
serotonin noradrenaline reuptake
    inhibitors, 135
serotonin syndrome, 135
sesamoiditis, 653
Sever's disease, 648
sex headache, 530
sex in pregnancy, 883
sexual assault, 876–7
sexual counselling, 935–6
sexual dysfunction, 932–41
sexual history, 934
sexual myths, 935
sexuality in the elderly, 940–1
sexually transmitted diseases, 942–52
    in Aboriginals, 1203
    in travellers, 98
shared care, 145, 878
shave biopsy, 1016–17
Shigella, dysentery, 405
shin splints, 1189
shingles (herpes zoster), 995–6, 1231
shoulder
    dislocation, 578, 1151–2
    examination, 571–3
    frozen, 576
    pain, 568–79
Shy-Drager syndrome, 428
sibling rivalry, 772
sick sinus syndrome, 671
sigmoid volvulus, 252
sigmoidoscopy, 73, 364–5
sildenafil (Viagra), 938
silver sulphadiazine
    (Silvazine), 1214
simple partial seizures, 510
simple purpura, 335
sinus arrhythmia, 670–3
sinusitis
    acute, 491–2, 527, 1231
    chronic, 1231
skier's thumb, 1186
skiing injuries, 1186
skills
    communication, 25–33
    of general practice, 17
skin
    cancer, 1013–14
    common problems, 973–88
    diagnostic approach, 955–64
    eruptions, 989–98
    pigmented lesions, 1019–26
    repair, 1134–6
    scrapings, 960–1
    terminology of lesions, 955–6
    terminology of topical agents, 961–2
    ulcers, 999–1005
    wounds, 1132–43
skin splinters, 1141
skin tags, 289, 1007
SLE, *see* systemic lupus

    erythematosus
sleep apnoea, 691–2
sleep disturbances, 691–2, 771
sleeping sickness,
    see trypanosomiasis
slipped capital femoral epiphysis, 603,
    662
slump test, 301–2
small bowel obstruction, 261
smoking, 80, 148–50
snake bite, 1115
snake envenomation, 1115
snapping hip, 606
snoring, 692, 1231
snuffling infant, 749
sodium valproate
    in bipolar disorder, 419
    in epilepsy, 509–10, 1065–7
solar keratosis, 1012, 1223
sore throat, 679–86
spasmodic torticollis, 242
spastic gait, 660
specific learning disabilities, 756–7
speculum examination, 806
speech and language, 742
sperm counts, 928
spermatocele, 906–7
spermicides, 816
sphygmomanometer use, 1073–6
spider bites, 1115–17
spider naevi, 123
spinal canal stenosis, 307–8, 610–14
spinal cord disorders, 1171
spinal dysfunction, 172–3, 294–306,
    318–29
spinal injuries, 1171
spine
    cervical, 172
    lumbar, 173, 295–316
    manipulation, 314–15, 327, 562
    mobilisation, 314–15, 327, 562
    thoracic, 172–3, 318–29
spirometry, 452
Spitz naevus, 1022
spleen, rupture of, 1172
spondyloarthropathies, 282–4, 308–9
spondylolisthesis, 306–7
sporotrichosis, 594
sporting injuries, 1183–95
sprained ankle, 649, 1191–4
sputum, 374–6
squamous cell carcinoma, 1013
Staphylococcus aureus
    in diarrhoea, 393
    in mastitis, 821
    in skin infection, 752, 767, 956, 997
status asthmaticus, 1114
status epilepticus, 1069, 1114
stealing, 771
steatorrhoea, 398
Steele-Richardson syndrome, 235
sterilisation
    of instruments, 1181–2
    of men, 817
    of women, 817
steroid injections
    for ganglion, 1015
    for skin lesions, 1017
Steven-Johnson syndrome, 994
stinging fish, 1118, 1231
stitch, in side, 347, 1231
Stoke-Adams attack, 429, 701
Stott and Davis model, 18
strabismus, 715

strangulated hernia, 905
street drugs, 151–3
Streptococcus pyogenes
    in genital tract, 851, 895
        in skin infection, 752, 767
        in tonsillopharyngitis, 683
streptokinase, in AMI, 352–3
stress fractures, 653–4, 1189
stroke, 1127–8
strongyloidiasis, 102
stupor, 696
stuttering, 772, 1232
styes, of eyes, 482, 1232
subacromial bursitis, 576
subacute thyroiditis, 169
subarachnoid haemorrhage, 529, 1128
subconjunctival haemorrhage, 481, 1232
subdural haematoma, 1170–1
subscapularis injuries, 571–3
sucking blisters, 751
sudden infant death syndrome, 793–4
sudden visual loss, 718–21
sugar intolerance, 403
suicide, 71, 135–6, 422–3, 798
suicide risk, 135–6
sulphonylureas, 142
sulphur, topical use, 962
sumatriptan, 523–5
sunburn, 988, 1232
superficial thrombophlebitis, 623
supraspinatus tendinitis, 575–6
supraventricular tachycardia, 672–5
surfer's ear, 1217
suture methods, 1134–7
suture removal, 1139–40
swallowed foreign objects, 787
sweating, excessive, 1232
swimmer's shoulder, 574, 1184
syncope, 700
synovial plica syndrome, 641
syphilis, 206–7, 948–9, 991
syringing of ears, 467
systemic lupus erythematosus, 223–5, 280
systemic sclerosis, 225–6, 280

T cells, 188
tachycardia
    sinus, 673
    supraventricular, 669, 673–5
    ventricular, 677
talon noir, 1020
tampon removal, 872
tampon toxic shock syndrome, 872–3
tardive dyskinesia, 418
tarsal cyst, *see* meibomian cyst
tarsal tunnel syndrome, 617
teardruct blockage, 1232
teeth
    dry socket, 490
    infected, 490
    knocked out, 1183–4
    pitted, 748
teething, 748, 1232
telangiectasia, 123
temper tantrums, 769–70
temperature measurement, 497–8
temporal arteritis, 228, 526–7, 721
temporal lobe epilepsy, *see* complex
        partial seizures
temporomandibular joint dysfunction,
        492–3, 1233
tendinitis
    Achilles, 650, 1189

bicipital, 577
gluteus medius, 605–6
patellar, 628, 639
de Quervain's, 591–2
supraspinatus, 674–6
tendon sheath, injection of, 592
tennis elbow, 585–8
tenpin bowler's thumb, 1185
tension headache, 520–1, 1233
tension pneumothorax, 1168
terbutaline, in asthma, 1056–8
terminal care, *see* palliative care
testes
    cancer of, 908–9
    dysfunction of, 927–9
    ectopic, 910
    pain in, 899–902
    retractile, 909–10
    small, 906, 927
    torsion of, 900–1
    tumours of, 908–9
    undescended, 909–10
testicular self-examination, 909
testicular trauma, 902
tetanus
    features, 216
    immunisation, 745, 1143
tetracyclic antidepressants, 134
Texidor's twinge, 347
thalassaemia
    major, 159
    minor, 159
theophylline, 1056–8
thermometer, use of, 497–8
thiamine (vitamin B$_1$), 821–3, 1034
thiazides
    adverse effects, 148, 993, 1082–3
    gout, cause of, 281
    in heart failure, 456
    in hypertension, 1081–4
Thompson's calf squeeze test, 1195
thoracic back pain, 319–30
thoracic outlet syndrome, 581–2
thoracic spine
    deformity, 324–6
    pain, 172–3, 319–30
threadworms, 1233
threatened miscarriage, 894
throat, painful, 679–86
thrombocytopenia, 331–5
thrombophlebitis, 623–4
thrush (moniliasis), 1233
thrush, vaginal, 870–1, 1235
thumb
    fracture, 1159
    gamekeeper's 1186
    sucking of, 748–9
    tenpin bowler's, 1185
    trigger, 590–1
thymoma, 241
thyroid crisis, 169
thyroid disease
    hyperthyroidism, 166–9
    hypothyroidism, 164–7
    investigations, 163–4
thyroid function tests, 163–4
thyroid stimulating hormone (TSH), 163
thyroiditis
    acute, 680
    cancer, 169
    chronic (autoimmune), 165
    postpartum, 896
    subacute, 167
thyrotoxicosis, *see* hyperthyroidism

thyroxine, 165
TIA, *see* transient ischaemic attack
tibial nerve block, 651
tibial stress fracture, 1189
tibialis anterior tenosynovitis, 1189–90
tibialis posterior tendon rupture, 653
tick bites, 1119
'ticket of entry', 128
tics, 242
Tietze's syndrome, 821
timolol eyedrops, 718
tinea
    tinea capitis, 986, 1233
    tinea corporis, 986, 1230
    tinea cruris, 969, 1233
    tinea incognito, 986
    tinea manum, 986
    tinea nigra, 1020
    tinea pedis, 985, 1121, 1233
    tinea unguium, 986, 1234
Tinel sign, 589
tinnitus, 1234
tiredness, 687–95
titubation, 234
toenails
    ingrowing, 656–7
    paronychia, 658
togavirus (rubella), 761–2
tongue
    disease, 1234
    enlarged, 123
    geographic, 1219, 1234
    wound, 1137–8
tonic-clonic seizures, 509, 699, 1064–9
tonometry, 717
tonsillitis, 683–4
tonsils, 681–5
tooth, knocked out, 1183–4
TORCH organisms, 198
Torres Strait Islander health,
        see Aboriginal health
torsade de pointes, 667, 671
torsion of ovarian cyst, 846
torsion of testis, 899–900
torticollis, 563–4, 1234
total lung capacity, 453
Tourette's disorder, 421, 773
toxic erythema, 992–3
toxic shock syndrome, 872–3
toxoplasmosis
    in AIDS, 189
    primary infection, 199, 202
tracheostomy, 1167
trachoma, 477, 480
traction
    to lumbar spine, 315, 1212
    to neck, 566
transcutaneous electrical nerve
        stimulation (TENS), 89, 315
transferrin, 158
transient ischaemic attack, 1128–30
tranylcypromine, 134
travel medicine, 91–109
travel sickness, 105–6, 1234
traveller's diarrhoea, 92–4, 405
traveller's medical kit, 107
treatment room, 1179–82
tremor, 232
    benign essential, 233–4, 1234
    intention, 233
    Parkinson's, 233
    postural, 233
Trendelenburg's test
    of hip, 600

of veins, 622–3
Treponema pallidum, 206–7, 948
triangular flap wound, 1136
trichiasis, *see* eyelashes, ingrowing
Trichomonas vaginalis, 871–2
Trichophyton infections, 985–6
trichuriasis, 102
tricyclic antidepressants, 134
trigeminal neuralgia, 493–4, 530
trigger finger, 590–1
trigger points, 314, 328
trigger thumb, 590–1
triglycerides, 1090–4
trochanteric bursitis, 605–6
trophic ulcers, 1004
tropical ear, 471, 1234
tropical medicine, 99–103
trypanosomiasis, 101
tsetse fly, 101
tubal ligation, 817
tuberculin test, *see* Mantoux test
tuberculosis
    extrapulmonary, 208
    genitourinary, 179–80
    as masquerade, 127
    pulmonary, 208–9, 383
tumour markers, 183
tumours
    benign *vs* malignant, 181
    elliptical excision for, 1017–18
    as masquerade, 127
    skin, 1013
tuning fork tests, 387–8
Turner's syndrome, 123
typhoid, 97, 100–1, 405
typhus, 97

ulcerative colitis, 405–6
ulcers
    aphthous, 1211
    arterial, 1002–3
    basal cell carcinoma, 1013
    decubitus, 1003–4
    genital, 946–7
    leg, 1001–2
    Marjolin's, 999
    peptic, 441–2
    pressure, 1003
    stasis, 1002
    trophic, 1004
    venous, 1002–3
ultrasound, use in
    AAA, 258
    abdominal pain, 252
    Achilles tendon injuries, 648, 650, 1194
    appendicitis, 260
    breast disease, 827–32
    gallstone disease, 264–5, 536
    groin pain, 1187
    hip pain, 601
    knee pain, 632
    pelvic pain, 842–6
    pregnancy, 880–1
    shoulder pain, 573
    urinary tract, 221, 708
    vascular disease, 613, 620, 624, 1130
ultraviolet radiation
    photosensitivity, 993
    for psoriasis, 980
    sunburn, 988
umbilical discharge, 1234
umbilical granuloma, 1235
umbilical hernia, 911

unconsciousness, 696–702
undescended testes, 909–10
undifferentiated illness, 125
undulant fever, 499
Unna's boots, 1003
'unsafe' ear, 464
upper motor neurone signs, 232, 566, 659–60
upper respiratory tract infection, 371–2, 377–8
Upton's paste, 656
uraemia, 219, 697, 1003
ureteric colic, 262–3, 1230
urethral meatus disorders, 914
urethral syndrome, 175
urethritis, 944–5
uric acid, 280
urinary incontinence, 709, 1221
urinary retention, 259
urinary tract infection, 175–80, 704, 886–8
urine, 175–7, 703–8
URTI, *see* upper respiratory tract infection
urticaria, 971, 1235
uterine bleeding
    abnormal, 834–9
    dysfunctional, 836–8
uveitis, 481, 718

vaginal discharge, 866–73
vaginal tampon, removal of, 872
vaginal thrush, 870–1, 1235
vaginitis, 870–2, 944
validity, in research, 112
valproate, sodium, *see*
    sodium valproate
varicella (chickenpox), 759–60, 1241
varicocele, 906–8, 928
varicose veins, 621–3
vascular disease, 68
vasculitides, 226–30, 284
vasculitis, 227
vasectomy, 817
vasodilators
    for chilblains, 1214
    for heart failure, 456–7
    for hypertension, 1081–3
    for ischaemic heart disease, 349, 352–3
venereal warts, 949
venous thrombosis, 624
venous ulcers, 1002–3
ventricular aneurysm, 354
ventricular extrasystoles, 672
ventricular fibrillation, 676–7, 1123–5
ventricular premature beats, 672
ventricular tachycardia, 671, 677
verapamil
    for angina, 350
    for arrhythmias, 672–7
    for hypertension, 1081–3
vertebrae dysfunction, *see*
    spinal dysfunction
vertigo, 426–7
vestibular lesions, 432–3
vestibular migraine, 433
vestibular neuronitis, 432
vestibulo-ocular reflexes, 431
violent behaviour, 421–2
viral conjunctivitis, 478–80
viral exanthem, 763
viral infections, baffling, 198–205

visual acuity, 72
visual-evoked responses, 239, 431
visual failure, 713–23
visual fields, 713–14
vital capacity, 453
vitamin A, 69
vitamin B$_1$ (thiamine), 821–3, 1034
vitamin B$_2$ (riboflavin), 1034
vitamin B$_6$ (pyridoxine), 821–3, 855
vitamin C (ascorbic acid), 70, 335, 378, 1004, 1215, 1222
vitamin D, 864
vitamin E, 69–70
vitamin K, 334
vitreous detachment, 722
vitreous haemorrhage, 720
vomiting, 248–50, 401–5, 547–50, 737
von Willebrand's disease, 332–4

walking difficulty, 659–65
warfarin, 355–7
warts
    common, 1009, 1235
    filiform, 1010
    genital, 949, 1010
    perianal, 291
    plane, 1009
    plantar, 655–6, 1228
    seborrhoeic, *see* keratoses
wasp stings, 1118
wax in ears, 464
wedge resection
    of ear, 1013
    of lip, 1013
Wegener's granulomatosis, 230
weight and height charts,
    see Appendices I-IV
weight gain, 724–31
weight loss, 732–8
Weil's disease, 212–14
Wernicke's encephalopathy, 1030
wet film, 868–9
wheeze, 449
whiplash syndrome, 564–5
whole person approach, 85–90
whooping cough, 766
Williams syndrome, 756
Wilm's tumour, 185
Wilson's disease, 233, 533–4
Wolff-Parkinson-White syndrome, 672, 677
'women's business', 1200
Wood's light, 959–60
wound suturing, *see* wounds, repair of
wounds, repair of, 1134–9
wringing exercises, for tennis elbow, 586
wrinkles, 1228
writer's cramp, 1235
writing a paper, 115–16
wry neck, 563–4

xylocaine, *see* lignocaine

yellow fever, 96, 203
Yersinia colitis, 92

zidovudine, in HIV, 192–3
zolmitriptan, 524
zoonoses, 212–15